UNIVERSITY OF ROCHESTER LIBRARIES
3 9087 01866159 7
AF779728

CHRONIC LUNG DISEASE IN EARLY INFANCY

LUNG BIOLOGY IN HEALTH AND DISEASE

Executive Editor

Claude Lenfant
Director, National Heart, Lung and Blood Institute
National Institutes of Health
Bethesda, Maryland

1. Immunologic and Infectious Reactions in the Lung, *edited by C. H. Kirkpatrick and H. Y. Reynolds*
2. The Biochemical Basis of Pulmonary Function, *edited by R. G. Crystal*
3. Bioengineering Aspects of the Lung, *edited by J. B. West*
4. Metabolic Functions of the Lung, *edited by Y. S. Bakhle and J. R. Vane*
5. Respiratory Defense Mechanisms (in two parts), *edited by J. D. Brain, D. F. Proctor, and L. M. Reid*
6. Development of the Lung, *edited by W. A. Hodson*
7. Lung Water and Solute Exchange, *edited by N. C. Staub*
8. Extrapulmonary Manifestations of Respiratory Disease, *edited by E. D. Robin*
9. Chronic Obstructive Pulmonary Disease, *edited by T. L. Petty*
10. Pathogenesis and Therapy of Lung Cancer, *edited by C. C. Harris*
11. Genetic Determinants of Pulmonary Disease, *edited by S. D. Litwin*
12. The Lung in the Transition Between Health and Disease, *edited by P. T. Macklem and S. Permutt*
13. Evolution of Respiratory Processes: A Comparative Approach, *edited by S. C. Wood and C. Lenfant*
14. Pulmonary Vascular Diseases, *edited by K. M. Moser*
15. Physiology and Pharmacology of the Airways, *edited by J. A. Nadel*
16. Diagnostic Techniques in Pulmonary Disease (in two parts), *edited by M. A. Sackner*
17. Regulation of Breathing (in two parts), *edited by T. F. Hornbein*
18. Occupational Lung Diseases: Research Approaches and Methods, *edited by H. Weill and M. Turner-Warwick*
19. Immunopharmacology of the Lung, *edited by H. H. Newball*
20. Sarcoidosis and Other Granulomatous Diseases of the Lung, *edited by B. L. Fanburg*
21. Sleep and Breathing, *edited by N. A. Saunders and C. E. Sullivan*
22. *Pneumocystis carinii* Pneumonia: Pathogenesis, Diagnosis, and Treatment, *edited by L. S. Young*
23. Pulmonary Nuclear Medicine: Techniques in Diagnosis of Lung Disease, *edited by H. L. Atkins*
24. Acute Respiratory Failure, *edited by W. M. Zapol and K. J. Falke*
25. Gas Mixing and Distribution in the Lung, *edited by L. A. Engel and M. Paiva*

26. High-Frequency Ventilation in Intensive Care and During Surgery, *edited by G. Carlon and W. S. Howland*
27. Pulmonary Development: Transition from Intrauterine to Extrauterine Life, *edited by G. H. Nelson*
28. Chronic Obstructive Pulmonary Disease: Second Edition, *edited by T. L. Petty*
29. The Thorax (in two parts), *edited by C. Roussos and P. T. Macklem*
30. The Pleura in Health and Disease, *edited by J. Chrétien, J. Bignon, and A. Hirsch*
31. Drug Therapy for Asthma: Research and Clinical Practice, *edited by J. W. Jenne and S. Murphy*
32. Pulmonary Endothelium in Health and Disease, *edited by U. S. Ryan*
33. The Airways: Neural Control in Health and Disease, *edited by M. A. Kaliner and P. J. Barnes*
34. Pathophysiology and Treatment of Inhalation Injuries, *edited by J. Loke*
35. Respiratory Function of the Upper Airway, *edited by O. P. Mathew and G. Sant'Ambrogio*
36. Chronic Obstructive Pulmonary Disease: A Behavioral Perspective, *edited by A. J. McSweeny and I. Grant*
37. Biology of Lung Cancer: Diagnosis and Treatment, *edited by S. T. Rosen, J. L. Mulshine, F. Cuttitta, and P. G. Abrams*
38. Pulmonary Vascular Physiology and Pathophysiology, *edited by E. K. Weir and J. T. Reeves*
39. Comparative Pulmonary Physiology: Current Concepts, *edited by S. C. Wood*
40. Respiratory Physiology: An Analytical Approach, *edited by H. K. Chang and M. Paiva*
41. Lung Cell Biology, *edited by D. Massaro*
42. Heart–Lung Interactions in Health and Disease, *edited by S. M. Scharf and S. S. Cassidy*
43. Clinical Epidemiology of Chronic Obstructive Pulmonary Disease, *edited by M. J. Hensley and N. A. Saunders*
44. Surgical Pathology of Lung Neoplasms, *edited by A. M. Marchevsky*
45. The Lung in Rheumatic Diseases, *edited by G. W. Cannon and G. A. Zimmerman*
46. Diagnostic Imaging of the Lung, *edited by C. E. Putman*
47. Models of Lung Disease: Microscopy and Structural Methods, *edited by J. Gil*
48. Electron Microscopy of the Lung, *edited by D. E. Schraufnagel*
49. Asthma: Its Pathology and Treatment, *edited by M. A. Kaliner, P. J. Barnes, and C. G. A. Persson*
50. Acute Respiratory Failure: Second Edition, *edited by W. M. Zapol and F. Lemaire*
51. Lung Disease in the Tropics, *edited by O. P. Sharma*
52. Exercise: Pulmonary Physiology and Pathophysiology, *edited by B. J. Whipp and K. Wasserman*
53. Developmental Neurobiology of Breathing, *edited by G. G. Haddad and J. P. Farber*
54. Mediators of Pulmonary Inflammation, *edited by M. A. Bray and W. H. Anderson*

55. The Airway Epithelium, *edited by S. G. Farmer and D. Hay*
56. Physiological Adaptations in Vertebrates: Respiration, Circulation, and Metabolism, *edited by S. C. Wood, R. E. Weber, A. R. Hargens, and R. W. Millard*
57. The Bronchial Circulation, *edited by J. Butler*
58. Lung Cancer Differentiation: Implications for Diagnosis and Treatment, *edited by S. D. Bernal and P. J. Hesketh*
59. Pulmonary Complications of Systemic Disease, *edited by J. F. Murray*
60. Lung Vascular Injury: Molecular and Cellular Response, *edited by A. Johnson and T. J. Ferro*
61. Cytokines of the Lung, *edited by J. Kelley*
62. The Mast Cell in Health and Disease, *edited by M. A. Kaliner and D. D. Metcalfe*
63. Pulmonary Disease in the Elderly Patient, *edited by D. A. Mahler*
64. Cystic Fibrosis, *edited by P. B. Davis*
65. Signal Transduction in Lung Cells, *edited by J. S. Brody, D. M. Center, and V. A. Tkachuk*
66. Tuberculosis: A Comprehensive International Approach, *edited by L. B. Reichman and E. S. Hershfield*
67. Pharmacology of the Respiratory Tract: Experimental and Clinical Research, *edited by K. F. Chung and P. J. Barnes*
68. Prevention of Respiratory Diseases, *edited by A. Hirsch, M. Goldberg, J.-P. Martin, and R. Masse*
69. *Pneumocystis carinii* Pneumonia: Second Edition, *edited by P. D. Walzer*
70. Fluid and Solute Transport in the Airspaces of the Lungs, *edited by R. M. Effros and H. K. Chang*
71. Sleep and Breathing: Second Edition, *edited by N. A. Saunders and C. E. Sullivan*
72. Airway Secretion: Physiological Bases for the Control of Mucous Hypersecretion, *edited by T. Takishima and S. Shimura*
73. Sarcoidosis and Other Granulomatous Disorders, *edited by D. G. James*
74. Epidemiology of Lung Cancer, *edited by J. M. Samet*
75. Pulmonary Embolism, *edited by M. Morpurgo*
76. Sports and Exercise Medicine, *edited by S. C. Wood and R. C. Roach*
77. Endotoxin and the Lungs, *edited by K. L. Brigham*
78. The Mesothelial Cell and Mesothelioma, *edited by M.-C. Jaurand and J. Bignon*
79. Regulation of Breathing: Second Edition, *edited by J. A. Dempsey and A. I. Pack*
80. Pulmonary Fibrosis, *edited by S. Hin. Phan and R. S. Thrall*
81. Long-Term Oxygen Therapy: Scientific Basis and Clinical Application, *edited by W. J. O'Donohue, Jr.*
82. Ventral Brainstem Mechanisms and Control of Respiration and Blood Pressure, *edited by C. O. Trouth, R. M. Millis, H. F. Kiwull-Schöne, and M. E. Schläfke*
83. A History of Breathing Physiology, *edited by D. F. Proctor*
84. Surfactant Therapy for Lung Disease, *edited by B. Robertson and H. W. Taeusch*

85. The Thorax: Second Edition, Revised and Expanded (in three parts), *edited by C. Roussos*
86. Severe Asthma: Pathogenesis and Clinical Management, *edited by S. J. Szefler and D. Y. M. Leung*
87. *Mycobacterium avium*–Complex Infection: Progress in Research and Treatment, *edited by J. A. Korvick and C. A. Benson*
88. Alpha 1–Antitrypsin Deficiency: Biology • Pathogenesis • Clinical Manifestations • Therapy, *edited by R. G. Crystal*
89. Adhesion Molecules and the Lung, *edited by P. A. Ward and J. C. Fantone*
90. Respiratory Sensation, *edited by L. Adams and A. Guz*
91. Pulmonary Rehabilitation, *edited by A. P. Fishman*
92. Acute Respiratory Failure in Chronic Obstructive Pulmonary Disease, *edited by J.-P. Derenne, W. A. Whitelaw, and T. Similowski*
93. Environmental Impact on the Airways: From Injury to Repair, *edited by J. Chrétien and D. Dusser*
94. Inhalation Aerosols: Physical and Biological Basis for Therapy, *edited by A. J. Hickey*
95. Tissue Oxygen Deprivation: From Molecular to Integrated Function, *edited by G. G. Haddad and G. Lister*
96. The Genetics of Asthma, *edited by S. B. Liggett and D. A. Meyers*
97. Inhaled Glucocorticoids in Asthma: Mechanisms and Clinical Actions, *edited by R. P. Schleimer, W. W. Busse, and P. M. O'Byrne*
98. Nitric Oxide and the Lung, *edited by W. M. Zapol and K. D. Bloch*
99. Primary Pulmonary Hypertension, *edited by L. J. Rubin and S. Rich*
100. Lung Growth and Development, *edited by J. A. McDonald*
101. Parasitic Lung Diseases, *edited by A. A. F. Mahmoud*
102. Lung Macrophages and Dendritic Cells in Health and Disease, *edited by M. F. Lipscomb and S. W. Russell*
103. Pulmonary and Cardiac Imaging, *edited by C. Chiles and C. E. Putman*
104. Gene Therapy for Diseases of the Lung, *edited by K. L. Brigham*
105. Oxygen, Gene Expression, and Cellular Function, *edited by L. Biadasz Clerch and D. J. Massaro*
106. $Beta_2$-Agonists in Asthma Treatment, *edited by R. Pauwels and P. M. O'Byrne*
107. Inhalation Delivery of Therapeutic Peptides and Proteins, *edited by A. L. Adjei and P. K. Gupta*
108. Asthma in the Elderly, *edited by R. A. Barbee and J. W. Bloom*
109. Treatment of the Hospitalized Cystic Fibrosis Patient, *edited by D. M. Orenstein and R. C. Stern*
110. Asthma and Immunological Diseases in Pregnancy and Early Infancy, *edited by M. Schatz, R. S. Zeiger, and H. N. Claman*
111. Dyspnea, *edited by D. A. Mahler*
112. Proinflammatory and Antiinflammatory Peptides, *edited by S. I. Said*
113. Self-Management of Asthma, *edited by H. Kotses and A. Harver*
114. Eicosanoids, Aspirin, and Asthma, *edited by A. Szczeklik, R. J. Gryglewski, and J. R. Vane*
115. Fatal Asthma, *edited by A. L. Sheffer*
116. Pulmonary Edema, *edited by M. A. Matthay and D. H. Ingbar*

117. Inflammatory Mechanisms in Asthma, *edited by S. T. Holgate and W. W. Busse*
118. Physiological Basis of Ventilatory Support, *edited by J. J. Marini and A. S. Slutsky*
119. Human Immunodeficiency Virus and the Lung, *edited by M. J. Rosen and J. M. Beck*
120. Five-Lipoxygenase Products in Asthma, *edited by J. M. Drazen, S.-E. Dahlén, and T. H. Lee*
121. Complexity in Structure and Function of the Lung, *edited by M. P. Hlastala and H. T. Robertson*
122. Biology of Lung Cancer, *edited by M. A. Kane and P. A. Bunn, Jr.*
123. Rhinitis: Mechanisms and Management, *edited by R. M. Naclerio, S. R. Durham, and N. Mygind*
124. Lung Tumors: Fundamental Biology and Clinical Management, *edited by C. Brambilla and E. Brambilla*
125. Interleukin-5: From Molecule to Drug Target for Asthma, *edited by C. J. Sanderson*
126. Pediatric Asthma, *edited by S. Murphy and H. W. Kelly*
127. Viral Infections of the Respiratory Tract, *edited by R. Dolin and P. F. Wright*
128. Air Pollutants and the Respiratory Tract, *edited by D. L. Swift and W. M. Foster*
129. Gastroesophageal Reflux Disease and Airway Disease, *edited by M. R. Stein*
130. Exercise-Induced Asthma, *edited by E. R. McFadden, Jr.*
131. LAM and Other Diseases Characterized by Smooth Muscle Proliferation, *edited by J. Moss*
132. The Lung at Depth, *edited by C. E. G. Lundgren and J. N. Miller*
133. Regulation of Sleep and Circadian Rhythms, *edited by F. W. Turek and P. C. Zee*
134. Anticholinergic Agents in the Upper and Lower Airways, *edited by S. L. Spector*
135. Control of Breathing in Health and Disease, *edited by M. D. Altose and Y. Kawakami*
136. Immunotherapy in Asthma, *edited by J. Bousquet and H. Yssel*
137. Chronic Lung Disease in Early Infancy, *edited by R. D. Bland and J. J. Coalson*

ADDITIONAL VOLUMES IN PREPARATION

Diagnostic Pulmonary Pathology, *edited by P. T. Cagle*

Multimodality Treatment of Lung Cancer, *edited by A. T. Skarin*

Cytokines in Pulmonary Infectious Disease, *edited by S. Nelson and T. Martin*

Asthma's Impact on Society: The Social and Economic Burden, *edited by K. B. Weiss, A. S. Buist, and S. D. Sullivan*

Asthma and Respiratory Infections, *edited by D. P. Skoner*

New and Exploratory Therapeutic Agents for Asthma, *edited by M. Yeadon and Z. Diamant*

Particle–Lung Interactions, *edited by P. Gehr and J. Heyder*

Pulmonary and Peripheral Gas Exchange in Health and Disease, *edited by J. Roca, R. Rodriguez-Roisen, and P. Wagner*

Environmental Asthma, *edited by R. K. Bush*

Tuberculosis: A Comprehensive International Approach, Second Edition, *edited by L. B. Reichman and E. S. Hershfield*

Sleep and Breathing in Children: A Developmental Approach, *edited by G. M. Loughlin, J. L. Carroll, and C. L. Marcus*

The opinions expressed in these volumes do not necessarily represent the views of the National Institutes of Health.

CHRONIC LUNG DISEASE IN EARLY INFANCY

Edited by

Richard D. Bland

University of Utah School of Medicine
Salt Lake City, Utah

Jacqueline J. Coalson

University of Texas Health Science Center
San Antonio, Texas

MARCEL DEKKER, INC. NEW YORK • BASEL

ISBN: 0-8247-9871-6

This book is printed on acid-free paper.

Headquarters
Marcel Dekker, Inc.
270 Madison Avenue, New York, NY 10016
tel: 212-696-9000; fax: 212-685-4540

Eastern Hemisphere Distribution
Marcel Dekker AG
Hutgasse 4, Postfach 812, CH-4001 Basel, Switzerland
tel: 41-61-261-8482; fax: 41-61-261-8896

World Wide Web
http://www.dekker.com

The publisher offers discounts on this book when ordered in bulk quantities. For more information, write to Special Sales/Professional Marketing at the headquarters address above.

Copyright © 2000 by Marcel Dekker, Inc. All Rights Reserved.

Neither this book nor any part may be reproduced or transmitted in any form or by any means, electronic or mechanical, including photocopying, microfilming, and recording, or by any information storage and retrieval system, without permission in writing from the publisher.

Current printing (last digit):
10 9 8 7 6 5 4 3 2 1

PRINTED IN THE UNITED STATES OF AMERICA

WF
600
L963
1999
V.137

INTRODUCTION

I believe there is general acceptance that chronic lung disease in early infancy has its origin in abnormal lung development. One of the most common expressions of abnormal lung development is bronchopulmonary dysplasia (BPD). Our appreciation of this condition is relatively recent: it developed just over 30 years ago following the seminal observations of Northway et al. in 1967 (1). Since then, considerable research has been done to clarify the cause of BPD, to treat it, and to understand its relationship to chronic lung disease in early infancy and later.

In 1979, the report of a workshop on BPD (2) provided a blueprint for research that, if followed, should have improved the condition of newborns with BPD. In the Foreword of this report, I wrote: ''We hope that the interested scientific communities will respond to the challenge that these recommendations offer.''

About 10 years later, in 1988, Northway wrote: ''The short history of BPD has coincided with a remarkable increase in the 'intensity' of care provided not only to premature infants with respiratory failure, but also to children and adults with respiratory failure.'' And, he concluded later: ''History has focused on the occurrence of BPD in the premature infant. In the future, that focus may very well have to be broadened'' (3).

Since then, research has continued and its translation into better care has accelerated considerably. However, BPD has become a bigger public health problem, largely because of the immense success of neonatologists in saving the lives of babies born more and more prematurely. Thus, the incidence and severity of BPD have increased. Further, as noted by the editors of this volume in their Preface, the features and patterns of the disease have changed greatly.

In a way, this book commemorates the 30th anniversary of Dr. Northway's work, which brought to the attention of the research and medical communities a public health problem that has become more serious since that time. But, at the same time, it is a celebration of the tremendous research accomplishments of the last 30 years. As mentioned previously, the field has become much more complex, but the prospects for solutions have also become greater. For example, we can watch with positive expectations our evolving knowledge about the role of retinoic acid in the formation of alveoli!

I know for a fact that Drs. Richard Bland and Jacqueline Coalson committed themselves wholeheartedly to the development and realization of this volume. The personal time they devoted to it has been considerable and, as we look at the end product, we can only express admiration and gratitude. Indeed, the field is well served by this volume, which brought together experts in their fields. There is no doubt that this volume will be an inspiration to both researchers and clinicians. For the Lung Biology in Health and Disease series of monographs, this is another landmark for which I am most appreciative.

Claude Lenfant, M.D.
Bethesda, Maryland

References

1. Northway WH Jr, Rosan RC, Porter DY. Pulmonary disease following respiratory therapy of hyaline-membrane disease: Bronchopulmonary dysplasia. N Engl J Med 1967; 276: 357.
2. Workshop on Bronchopulmonary Dysplasia. J Ped 1979; 85(5).
3. Northway WH. Historical perspectives in bronchopulmonary dysplasia. In: Merritt TA, Northway WH, Boynston BP, eds. *Bronchopulmonary Dysplasia.* Oxford: Blackwell Scientific, 1988.

PREFACE

This book is about pulmonary pathology produced by progress in the practice of perinatal pediatrics. Chronic lung disease in early infancy was an unknown entity little more than three decades ago. Its appearance coincided with the initial efforts at positive pressure mechanical ventilation to rescue infants who suffered life-threatening respiratory distress, usually from underdeveloped lungs. When Northway and associates first described the clinical, radiographic, and pathological features of this disease, which they called bronchopulmonary dysplasia, few infants with respiratory failure survived, and most of those who did survive weighed at least 2 kg at birth. In the intervening years, there has been remarkable progress in our understanding, treatment, and prevention of acute respiratory distress after premature birth. Important discoveries in both basic and applied biomedical research paved the way for extraordinary success in the clinical care of infants who were born too soon. Widespread use of prenatal glucocorticoid and postnatal surfactant treatment, acceptance of modest hypercapnia with less aggressive application of positive pressure breathing, improved nutritional support, and meticulous attention to detail in the delivery of intensive care have spawned survival of extremely tiny, premature infants who are most vulnerable to experience the persistent need for assisted ventilation. Thus, the incidence of this type of chronic lung disease remains high, although the pattern of clinical signs and symptoms, radiographic images, and pathological features of the disease have changed considerably, probably reflecting the degree of lung immaturity of these tiny infants, as well as the many modifications in their management that have occurred over the past several years.

This book is divided into five parts. Part I focuses on major clinical aspects of the disease, with particular attention to its evolution over the past decade, during which time rapid technological developments and widespread applications of new therapies, notably prenatal glucocorticoids and postnatal surfactants, have had their greatest impact. Part II examines normal and abnormal alveolar and airway development. Part III focuses on both normal and abnormal development of lung circulation and interstitium. Part IV centers on mechanisms of injury and repair, and, finally, Part V discusses relevant animal models for studying the disease process during its evolution and during recovery.

Our goals in planning this book were to (1) present the important clinical and pathological features of a disease that represents a major cause of long-term hospitalization, slow growth, and recurrent respiratory ailments in early childhood; (2) provide a timely, comprehensive review of what is known about lung development, injury, and repair as they might relate to the pathogenesis of chronic lung disease of early infancy; (3) define what relevant information needs to be learned and how we might learn it; and (4) relate this information to potential therapeutic and preventive strategies. To accomplish these goals, we invited world-renowned experts from many scientific disciplines and medical fields to contribute their knowledge and ideas on this important subject. We are extremely grateful to the authors for their efforts, which we hope will facilitate better understanding of how the lungs develop both structurally and functionally, how this development may be altered as a result of injury and subsequent repair, and how these processes may be modified by effective therapy or, better yet, prevention.

We are especially grateful to Sharon Marron for her outstanding administrative efforts in organizing the submission of chapters and ensuring successful completion of this work.

Richard D. Bland
Jacqueline J. Coalson

CONTRIBUTORS

Steven H. Abman, M.D. Professor and Director, Pediatric Heart and Lung Center, University of Colorado School of Medicine, Denver, Colorado

Kurt Albertine, Ph.D. Professor, Departments of Pediatrics, Medicine, and Neurobiology/Anatomy, University of Utah Health Sciences Center, Salt Lake City, Utah

Solomon Alkrinawi, M.D. Fellow, Pediatric Pulmonology, University of Manitoba, Winnipeg, Manitoba, Canada

Michael Apkon, M.D., Ph.D. Assistant Professor, Department of Pediatrics and Cellular and Molecular Physiology, Yale University School of Medicine, New Haven, Connecticut

Ann M. Arvin, M.D. Lucile Packard Professor of Pediatrics and Microbiology/ Immunology, Stanford University School of Medicine, Stanford, California

Philip L. Ballard, M.D., Ph.D. Professor of Pediatrics, Division of Neonatology, University of Pennsylvania School of Medicine, and Children's Hospital of Philadelphia, Philadelphia, Pennsylvania

Roberta A. Ballard, M.D. Professor of Pediatrics and Obstetrics and Gynecology, Division of Neonatology, University of Pennsylvania School of Medicine, Children's Hospital of Philadelphia, Philadelphia, Pennsylvania

Eduardo Bancalari, M.D. Professor of Pediatrics, Division of Neonatology, Department of Pediatrics, University of Miami School of Medicine, Miami, Florida

William E. Benitz, M.D. Associate Professor, Divisions of Neonatal and Developmental Medicine, Department of Pediatrics, Stanford University School of Medicine, Stanford, California

William R. Berrington Research Associate, University of Alabama at Birmingham, Birmingham, Alabama

Richard D. Bland, M.D. Fields Professor of Pediatrics, University of Utah School of Medicine, Salt Lake City, Utah

John F. Bohnsack, M.D. Associate Professor, Department of Pediatrics, University of Utah Health Sciences Center, Salt Lake City, Utah

Shilpa Buch Assistant Professor of Pediatrics, University of Toronto, The Hospital for Sick Children, Toronto, Ontario, Canada

David P. Carlton, M.D. Associate Professor, Department of Pediatrics, University of Utah Health Sciences Center, Salt Lake City, Utah

Victor Chernick, M.D., F.R.C.P.C. Professor of Pediatrics, University of Manitoba, Winnipeg, Manitoba, Canada

Jacqueline J. Coalson, Ph.D. Professor, Department of Pathology, University of Texas Health Science Center, San Antonio, Texas

Peter Dargaville, M.D. Royal Children's Hospital, Victoria, Australia

Robert A. De Lemos* Hastings Professor of Pediatrics, University of Southern California, Los Angeles, California

David K. Edwards, M.D. Professor of Radiology and Pediatrics, University of California Medical School, San Diego, California

Eric C. Eichenwald, M.D. Assistant Professor, Harvard Medical School and Brigham and Women's Hospital, Boston, Massachusetts

*Deceased.

Leland L. Fan, M.D. Professor of Pediatrics, Baylor College of Medicine, Houston, Texas

Henry Jay Forman, Ph.D. Charles Krown Professor of Molecular Pharmacology and Toxicology, University of Southern California, Los Angeles, California

H. Lee Frank, M.D., Ph.D. Professor of Medicine and Pediatrics, Pulmonary Research Center, University of Miami School of Medicine, Miami, Florida

Bruce A. Freeman, Ph.D. Professor and Vice-Chair of Research, Department of Anesthesiology and Department of Biochemistry and Molecular Genetics, University of Alabama at Birmingham, Birmingham, Alabama

Michael R. Gomez, M.D. Assistant Professor of Pediatrics, Santa Rosa Children's Hospital, San Antonio, Texas

Alvaro Gonzalez, M.D. Instructor, Department of Pediatrics, University of Miami School of Medicine, Miami, Florida

Peter Groneck, M.D. Department of Pediatrics, Children's Hospital of the City of Cologne, Cologne, Germany

Imad Y. Haddad Department of Anesthesiology, University of Alabama at Birmingham, Birmingham, Alabama

Thomas N. Hansen, M.D. Professor and Chairman, Department of Pediatrics, Ohio State University, and Chief Executive Officer, Children's Hospital, Columbus, Ohio

Samuel Hawgood, M.B., B.S. Professor of Pediatrics, Pediatrics and Cardiovascular Research Foundation, University of California, San Francisco, California

Sheila G. Haworth, M.D., F.R.C.Path., F.R.C.P., F.A.C.C. British Heart Foundation Professor of Developmental Cardiology, Institute of Child Health, London, England

Thomas A. Hazinski, M.D. Professor and Vice-Chair, Department of Pediatrics, Vanderbilt University Medical Center, Nashville, Tennessee

W. Alan Hodson, M.D. Professor of Pediatrics, Division of Neonatal Biology, Department of Pediatrics, University of Washington, Seattle, Washington

John R. Hoidal, M.D. Professor, Department of Medicine, University of Utah, Salt Lake City, Utah

Mari K. Hoidal, M.S. Research Associate, Department of Medicine, University of Utah, Salt Lake City, Utah

Alan H. Jobe, M.D., Ph.D. Professor of Pediatrics, Division of Pulmonary Biology, Children's Hospital Medical Center, Cincinnati, Ohio

Richard J. King, Ph.D. Professor, Department of Physiology, University of Texas Health Science Center at San Antonio, San Antonio, Texas

Michael T. Kinter, Ph.D. Research Assistant Professor, Departments of Microbiology and Pathology, University of Virginia Health Science Center, Charlottesville, Virginia

Thomas R. Korfhagen Associate Professor, Department of Pediatrics, University of Cincinnati College of Medicine, and Children's Hospital Medical Center, Cincinnati, Ohio

George Lister, M.D. Professor, Departments of Pediatrics and Anesthesiology, Yale University School of Medicine, New Haven, Connecticut

Mingyao Liu University of Toronto, The Hospital for Sick Children, Toronto, Ontario, Canada

Diane E. Lorant Assistant Professor, Division of Neonatology, Department of Pediatrics, University of Utah Health Sciences Center, Salt Lake City, Utah

Alma Martinez, M.D., M.P.H. Assistant Professor, Department of Pediatrics, University of California, San Francisco, California

Donald J. Massaro, M.D. Cohen Professor of Pulmonary Research, Department of Medicine, Georgetown University School of Medicine, Washington, D.C.

Gloria D. Massaro, M.D. Professor, Department of Pediatrics, Georgetown University School of Medicine, Washington, D.C.

Sadis Matalon, Ph.D. Professor, Department of Anesthesiology, University of Alabama at Birmingham, Birmingham, Alabama

Rodrigo A. Nehgme, M.D. Assistant Professor, Department of Pediatrics, Yale University School of Medicine, New Haven, Connecticut

William H. Northway, Jr., M.D. Professor Emeritus of Radiology and Pediatrics, Lucile Packard Children's Hospital at Stanford, Palo Alto, California

Howard B. Panitch, M.D. Associate Professor of Pediatrics, University of Pennsylvania School of Medicine, and Division of Pulmonary Medicine, Children's Hospital of Philadelphia, Philadelphia, Pennsylvania

Bruce R. Pitt, Ph.D. Professor, Department of Pharmacology, University of Pittsburgh School of Medicine, Pittsburgh, Pennsylvania

Martin Post, Ph.D., D.V.M. Professor of Pediatrics, University of Toronto, The Hospital for Sick Children, Toronto, Ontario, Canada

Marlene Rabinovitch, M.D., R.F.C.P.(C) Professor, University of Toronto, and Director, Department of Cardiovascular Research, The Hospital for Sick Children, Toronto, Ontario, Canada

Scott H. Randell, Ph.D. Research Assistant Professor, Cystic Fibrosis/Pulmonary Research and Treatment Center, University of North Carolina, Chapel Hill, North Carolina

David J. Riley, M.D. Professor, Department of Medicine, University of Medicine and Dentistry of New Jersey—Robert Wood Johnson Medical School, Piscataway, New Jersey

Robert J. Roberts, M.D.* Professor and Chairman, Department of Pediatrics, University of Virginia Health Science Center, Charlottesville, Virginia

Timothy W. Robison, Ph.D. Food and Drug Administration, Bethesda, Maryland

Steven R. Seidner, M.D. Associate Professor, Department of Pediatrics, University of Texas Health Science Center, San Antonio, Texas

Thomas H. Shaffer, Ph.D. Professor, Departments of Physiology and Pediatrics, Temple University School of Medicine, Philadephia, Pennsylvania

---

*Deceased.

Michael P. Sherman, M.D. Professor and Chief, Division of Neonatology, Department of Pediatrics, University of California, Davis, California

Charles Vincent Smith, Ph.D. Professor, Department of Pediatrics, Baylor College of Medicine, Houston, Texas

Ilene R. S. Sosenko, M.D. Professor, Division of Neonatology, Department of Pediatrics, University of Miami School of Medicine, Miami, Florida

Christian P. Speer, M.D., F.R.C.P.(E) Professor, Department of Pediatrics, University of Würzburg, Würzburg, Germany

Mildred T. Stahlman, M.D. Professor, Department of Pediatrics, Vanderbilt University School of Medicine, Nashville, Tennessee

Ann R. Stark, M.D. Associate Professor, Department of Pediatrics, Harvard University, and Children's Hospital, Boston, Massachusetts

H. William Taeusch, M.D. Professor, Department of Pediatrics, University of California, San Francisco, California

A. Keith Tanswell, M.B., M.R.C.P.(UK), F.R.C.P.(C) Professor, University of Toronto, Division of Neonatology, The Hospital for Sick Children, Toronto, Ontario, Canada

Margaret M. Tarpey Associate Professor, Department of Anesthesiology, University of Alabama at Birmingham, Birmingham, Alabama

Michael J. Thomas, Ph.D. Professor of Biochemistry, Bowman Gray School of Medicine, Wake Forest University, Winston-Salem, North Carolina

Samuel J. Tilden, M.D. Professor, University of Alabama at Birmingham, Birmingham, Alabama

William E. Truog, M.D. Professor, Department of Pediatrics, University of Missouri, Kansas City, Missouri

Stephen E. Welty, M.D. Assistant Professor, Department of Pediatrics, Baylor College of Medicine, Houston, Texas

Carl W. White, M.D. Professor, Department of Pediatrics, University of Colorado Health Sciences Center, Denver, Colorado

Jeffrey A. Whitsett, M.D. Professor, Division of Pulmonary Biology, Department of Pediatrics, University of Cincinnati College of Medicine, and Children's Hospital Medical Center, Cincinnati, Ohio

Stephen L. Young, M.D. Professor, Department of Medicine, Duke University Medical Center, Durham, North Carolina

Sha Zhu Postdoctoral Fellow, University of Alabama at Birmingham, Birmingham, Alabama

CONTENTS

Part Four MECHANISMS OF LUNG INJURY AND REPAIR DURING DEVELOPMENT

1

Historical Perspective

Early Observations and Subsequent Evolution of Bronchopulmonary Dysplasia

WILLIAM H. NORTHWAY, Jr.

Lucile Packard Children's Hospital at Stanford
Palo Alto, California

I. Introduction and Background

Bronchopulmonary dysplasia (BPD) was first described in 1967 in a report documenting the clinical, radiologic, and pathological changes seen in prematurely born infants with severe respiratory distress syndrome (RDS) who had been treated with prolonged mechanical ventilation and warm, humidified 80–100% concentrations of oxygen (1). This report documented the appearance of a new, chronic pulmonary syndrome that was associated with the use of mechanical ventilation and supplemental oxygen treatment of these infants for longer than 6 days. In 1967, RDS was the leading cause of death in newborn infants. The natural course of RDS before the use of mechanical ventilation was either death by 4–5 days of age or complete recovery by 7 days of age, with a normal chest radiograph (2). The use of mechanical ventilation and supplemental oxygen treatment for respiratory failure secondary to RDS in the newborn infant was a continuation of the historical desire to decrease newborn infant mortality by employing improvements in medical care and applications of new technology.

II. Historical Perspective

A. Care of the Prematurely Born Infant

Modern care of the prematurely born infant began in the 19th century and was promoted in Paris by the obstetrician Stephane Tarnier and his pupil Pierre Constant Budin (3). Before the 19th century, high infant mortality was considered inevitable, and the death of prematurely born infants was only a minor part of the problem. An improvement in infant mortality by warming premature infants was first noted in 1829 by Villermé and Edwards (4). A closed incubator was first introduced at the Maternite at Port Royal in Paris where Tarnier was surgeon in chief in 1881 (5). The diagnosis of prematurity on the basis of birth weight was first described in 1872 (6). It was not until 1896 that a special hospital unit to prevent the spread of infection in premature infants was designed, which included hand washing and gowning of nurses before they handled the infants (7). Prematurity was still the most important cause of death in infants younger than 1 year of age in the 1930s and 1940s in the United States (3). Over half of the deaths caused by prematurity occurred in the first 24 hr of life (8,9). In the 1960s most pregnant women were being delivered in hospitals, rather than at home, and modern investigations of infant metabolism and feeding had begun (10,11). Penicillin and sulfonamides, as well as other antibiotics, had been developed and were used in caring for prematurely born infants. Even with all these advances, minimal handling and minimal treatment of sick premature infants remained the standard of care (12).

B. Hyaline Membrane Disease

Hyaline membranes in the lungs of newborn infants dying of respiratory failure were first described by Hochheim in 1903 (13). These membranes were attributed to aspiration of amniotic sac contents by Hochheim and others, and it was not until the critical review of this theory by Miller and Hamilton in 1949 that intensified investigation of this entity occurred (14). At about the same time it became apparent that hyaline membrane disease principally affected liveborn premature infants and infants of diabetic mothers, and there was an association of fetal anoxia with the disorder. Even as late as 1957, hyaline membrane disease, or respiratory distress syndrome (RDS) as it was subsequently named, was not included in the standard nomenclature of disease (15).

C. Diagnostic Radiology

The antemortem diagnosis of RDS could not be established until the development of modern chest radiographic techniques. Following the discovery of x-rays in December 1895 by Conrad Roentgen (16), their use for medical diagnosis spread rapidly throughout the world. Advances in this technology also occurred quickly, so that by the early 1950s, with improvements in x-ray tubes, film, intensifying screens, and equipment, it became possible to see fine anatomical detail in the lungs of newborn infants with RDS. Radiologic changes in the lungs of infants with RDS were described for the first time in 1953 by Donald and Lord (17). In the same year, Donald and Steiner, demonstrated the classic reticular granular pattern of density in the lungs with air bronchograms in infants with proven RDS (18). Peterson and Pendleton, 2 years later, differentiated the radiologic pattern of RDS from aspiration pneumonia, which allowed the establishment of a firm diagnoses of these disorders in nonfatal cases (2). They also described the radiologic course of RDS as being either progressive opacification of the lungs, with death in 3–5 days, or complete radiographic clearing in 7–10 days.

D. Mechanical Ventilation

The modern era of mechanical ventilation of newborn infants with respiratory failure began in 1953 when Donald and Lord described the use of a negative-pressure ventilator for prolonged artificial ventilation of the newborn infant (Fig. 1) (17,19). The history of resuscitation, however, extends back at least to 400 BC, with a description of cannulation of the trachea to support ventilation by Hippocrates (20). Chaussier, in 1806, developed the intralaryngeal tube for resuscitation of newborn infants (21). Truehead and Fell-O'Dwyer subsequently developed ventilating apparatuses for use in newborn infants (22), and Champneys, in 1882, characterized the pressures required to produce interstitial emphysema and pneumothorax in stillborn human infants (23).

E. Oxygen

Oxygen was first isolated by Joseph Priestley in 1771 (24), and was first used experimentally in newborn infants with respiratory difficulty in 1780 by Chaussier (25). Smith definitively described pulmonary oxygen toxicity in mice in 1899 (26). Although Bonnair published the first detailed clinical report of oxygen therapy in premature infants with cyanosis in 1891 (27), oxygen therapy did not become common practice in the care of premature infants until the 1930s and 1940s. It was not until the 1940s that perinatal asphyxia was appreciated as a major cause of neurological damage and death in the newborn (28). The high mortality rate from respiratory failure in premature infants contributed to the routine use of oxygen therapy in the care of all premature infants by the late 1940s. Use of supplemental oxygen was subsequently restricted when it was found that treatment with a high concentration of supplemental oxygen was associated with the appearance of retrolental fibroplasia (29). By 1962 it was recommended that no more than 40% oxygen be used in treating premature infants (30).

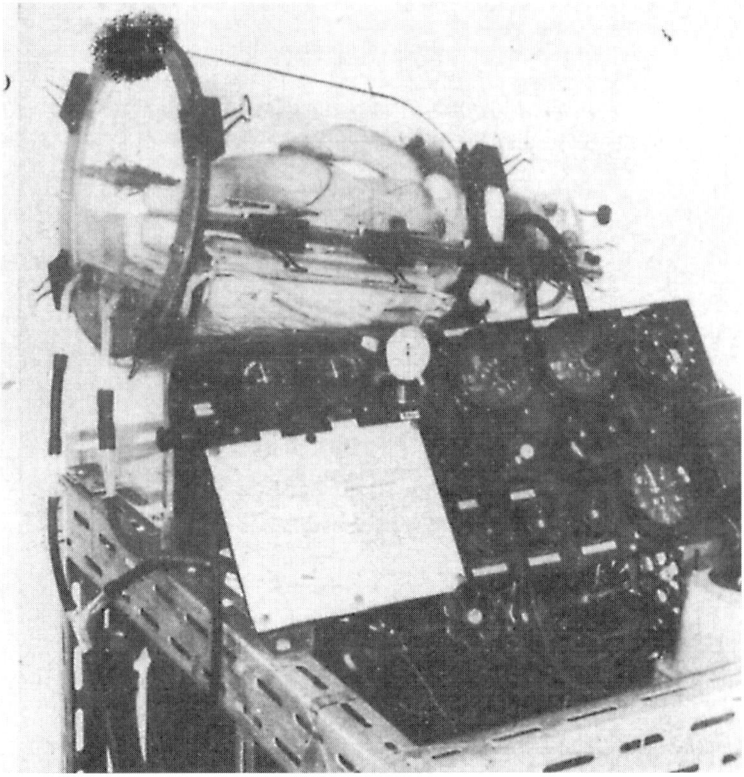

Figure 1 The modern era of prolonged mechanical ventilation of the newborn infant began with the "apparatus for amplifying natural respiration" used by Donald and Lord in 1953. (From Ref. 105.)

F. Prologue to BPD

A reevaluation of the therapy for RDS was stimulated by the demonstration by Avery and Mead in 1959 that the lungs of infants dying of RDS behaved as though they lacked surface-active material (31). Avery and Oppenheimer, in 1960 (32), found that deaths from RDS were increased when no or very little supplemental oxygen was used as treatment compared with an earlier period in which oxygen was used in higher concentration. These findings encouraged pediatricians to treat premature infants with RDS and respiratory failure with mechanical ventilation and concentrations of supplemental oxygen higher than 40% while monitoring arterial Po_2.

The first premature infant research center, sponsored by the National Institutes of Health (NIH), was established at Stanford University Medical Center in 1962. The first moribund infant with severe RDS was treated there with mechanical ventilation and supplemental oxygen therapy in 1963 by Drs. Vernon Thomas and Joe Daily, and the infant survived (33). The mechanical ventilator used had only two concentration settings for oxygen, 40% and 100%. The respiratory effectiveness of such treatment was measured, at that time, by the pH and the $Paco_2$ of arterialized capillary blood, and the infant's skin color.

Other newborn nurseries were having similar success with artificial ventilation and supplemental oxygen treatment of prematurely born infants with RDS. A series of 52 infants with RDS treated with negative-pressure ventilation and oxygen supplementation by Shepard and co-workers was reported in an abstract in 1964, in which 23 of the infants, when examined at ages 6 months to 6½ years, had radiographic findings said to be compatible with pulmonary fibrosis (34). Their findings were questioned in a discussion following the presentation, and a more complete presentation of the abstract was not published. That same year, Robertson and associates reported on the late stages of pulmonary hyaline membrane disease of the newborn (35). They demonstrated thickened alveolar walls, with an increase of fibroblasts and excess of reticulin or collagen fibers in three infants who died at 13, 21, and 23 days of life, and in one studied by lung biopsy in the eighth week of life. Two of these patients had received prolonged intermittent positive-pressure ventilation (IPPV) with high concentrations of oxygen. Emphysematous blebs and patchy infiltrate developed on early chest radiographs of their oldest living patient who had been treated with high positive pressure and 100% oxygen. These radiographic findings changed to small areas of atelectasis by 2 months of life. This infant had clinical signs of pulmonary disease at 2 months of age. This may have been the earliest clinical and radiographic description of BPD.

III. Early Observations

The original population of prematurely born infants with severe RDS in which BPD was recognized at Stanford University Medical Center were moribund and ventilated with intermittent positive-pressure ventilation and humidified 80–100% oxygen concentrations (high oxygen) (1). The use of intermittent positive-pressure ventilation was critical to the development of BPD because it proved to be a more effective artificial ventilation technique for small, severely ill, premature infants than negative-pressure ventilation and could keep these infants alive long enough to develop chronic lung disease. The prolongation of the usual clinical course of RDS for these moribund infants was dramatic as was the radiographic appearance of chronic lung disease.

A. Pathogenesis

High concentrations of supplemental oxygen were used initially with the hope that the oxygenation of these infants with RDS could be rapidly improved and the oxygen concentration rapidly decreased before pulmonary oxygen toxicity occurred. Unfortunately, this did not happen. Nine of the 13 infants treated with high oxygen concentrations for longer than 150 hr lived beyond 2 weeks of age and all demonstrated BPD; 5 died and 4 survived with BPD. Nine of the 19 infants treated for less than 150 hr with high oxygen concentrations survived and none had BPD. The initial data suggested that the etiology of BPD was related to pulmonary oxygen toxicity.

B. Radiology

The radiographic progression to chronic lung disease was originally divided into four stages (1). Stage I (2–3 days) (Fig. 2) was a period that clinically resembled acute RDS. All the infants reported had RDS as the cause of their respiratory

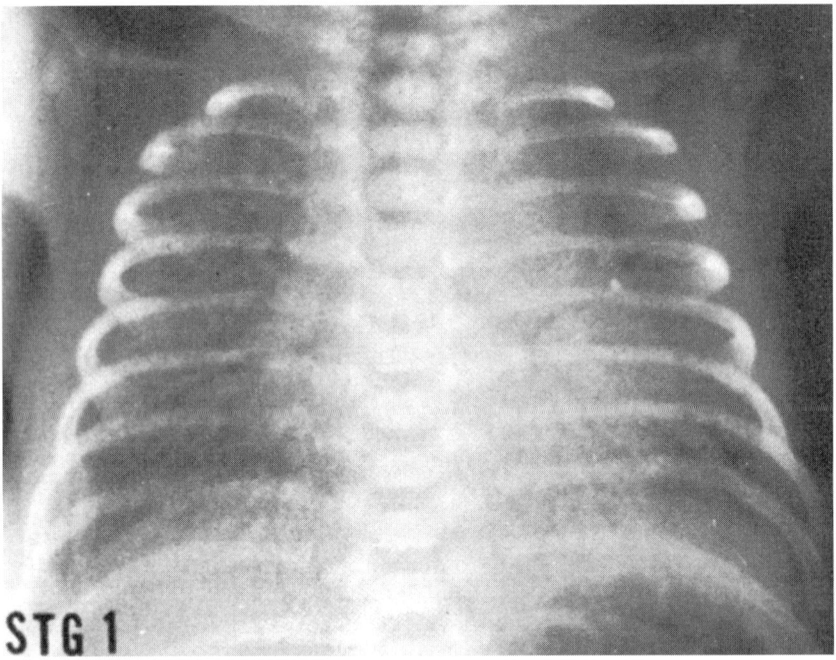

Figure 2 Chest radiograph of an infant from the original report of BPD with fine bilateral granularity and air bronchogram in the lungs characteristic of stage I disease. (From Ref. 1.)

failure. The early radiographic picture was indistinguishable from classic RDS. Stage II (4–10 days) had a chest radiograph that, in the severest cases, showed nearly complete opacification of both lungs. Stage III (10–20 days) was a period of transition to chronic disease, when the chest radiograph changed to a striking picture of small rounded areas of lucency distributed throughout both lungs. Stage IV (beyond 1 month) (Fig. 3) represented the beginning of chronic disease. The definition of chronic lung disease as beginning at 1 month of age was arbitrary and not manifested by any specific radiographic or clinical change that occurred at that time, but has proved to be a useful diagnostic criterion. Chest radiographs at this stage showed enlargement of the rounded lucent areas in the lungs that alternated with strands of radiodensity. The lungs were hyperexpanded and cardiomegaly could be present.

C. Pathology

The initial stage I pathological appearance of BPD reflected the pathology of the predisposing cause of respiratory failure—RDS with hyaline membranes and atelectasis. There was also patchy loss of ciliated cells, with metaplasia and necro-

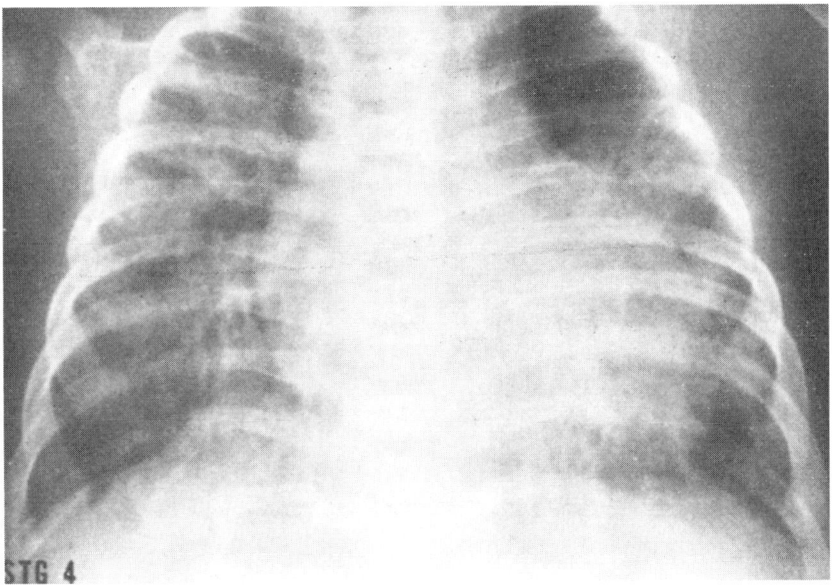

Figure 3 Chest radiograph of an infant from the original report of BPD with stage IV disease and persistence of irregular strands of density in the lungs, hyperexpansion, and cardiomegaly. (From Ref. 1.)

sis of the bronchiolar mucosa (1). During stage II, when the infants were usually weaned from the respirator, but might still be receiving high oxygen concentrations, histological examination showed necrosis and repair of alveolar epithelium, with emphysematous coalescence of alveoli; increased patchy bronchiolar necrosis, with patchy squamous metaplasia; and focal thickening of the capillary basement membranes. During stage III, the transition to chronic disease, there was widespread bronchial and bronchiolar mucosal metaplasia and hyperplasia and marked secretion of mucous and alveolar coalescence progressing to spherically circumscribed groups of emphysematous alveoli with atelectasis of surrounding alveoli. It was this pathological process that gave the chest radiograph its characteristic appearance with focal areas of radiolucency and radiodense stranding. In addition there was interstitial edema and focal thickening of the basement membranes and some interseptal collagen deposition. By stage IV, there was marked hypertrophy of peribronchiolar smooth muscle, with focally circumscribed groups of emphysematous alveoli and atelectatic alveolar areas. There was focal thickening of basement membranes, with separation of capillaries from alveolar epithelium. Vascular lesions of the pulmonary hypertensive type were seen, as well as marked heterotopia of alveolar epithelial cell types and widespread metaplasia of bronchiolar mucosa. Right-sided cardiomegaly might also be present. The progressive pathological changes in the immature lung affected both the parenchyma and airways and appeared to alter normal lung growth, suggesting the descriptive name *bronchopulmonary dysplasia*.

IV. The Evolution of BPD

Since its original description, BPD has been seen throughout the world when ever mechanical ventilation and supplemental oxygen therapy are used to treat prematurely born infants with respiratory failure. It is now as common as cystic fibrosis as a cause of chronic lung disease in children in the United States (36). Bronchopulmonary dysplasia clinics have been developed in many medical centers. Home care of patients with BPD is increasingly important (37,38). Parent support groups have been organized. The cost of care for patients with BPD both in and out of the hospital has become of concern (39). Bronchopulmonary dysplasia, however, is not only a clinical problem for neonatologists and pediatricians, but also for internists and general practitioners because it is now recognized that its sequelae may continue to affect the patient as an adult. Understanding BPD as it has evolved is basic to its future prevention and treatment.

A. Pathogenesis

The pathogenesis of BPD is now believed to be multifactorial. The four major etiologic factors are (1) respiratory failure, (2) lung immaturity, (3) pulmonary oxygen toxicity, and (4) volutrauma. Bronchopulmonary dysplasia can be best understood as an injury and repair process occurring in the immature lung secondary to pulmonary oxygen toxicity and pressure-induced trauma. The injury and repair process throughout its course may be mild, moderate, severe, or very severe (40). The clinical manifestations of BPD depend on the immaturity of the developing lung, the concentration of the supplemental oxygen, the level of airway pressure, and the duration of exposure to the oxygen and pressure.

Although BPD was originally described in infants with RDS, it is now recognized that treatment of respiratory failure from many causes, such as meconium aspiration pneumonia (41), neonatal pneumonia (42), congestive heart failure (43), the Wilson–Mikity syndrome (44), congenital diaphragmatic hernia (45), and marked degrees of prematurity with inadequate respiratory drive, can lead to BPD (46,47). Respiratory failure is critical to the pathogenesis of BPD because it requires treatment with supplemental oxygen and mechanical ventilation. Although pulmonary air leaks (pulmonary interstitial emphysema, pneumomediastinum, pneumothorax) (48), pulmonary edema (49), and pulmonary infection (50,52) are associated with an increased incidence of BPD, none of these factors have been shown to be essential to its development. Presumably these factors increase the risk of developing BPD by prolonging the need for mechanical ventilation and supplemental oxygen therapy.

The relation of the duration of high-concentration oxygen therapy to the development of BPD in the original population of infants with RDS strongly suggested that the etiology was related to pulmonary oxygen toxicity (1). Subsequent exposure of newborn guinea pigs to 95–100% oxygen produced pathological and radiographic changes in their lungs similar to the appearance of stage II BPD. These studies demonstrated, for the first time, that pulmonary oxygen toxicity could produce chest radiographic changes in a newborn animal model (52). Experiments with newborn C-57 black mice continuously exposed to 90–100% oxygen for up to 6 weeks produced a chronic lung disease that resembled all aspects of the pathology seen in human prematurely born infants with BPD (53). Tritiated thymidine uptake in these newborn mice demonstrated an inhibition of DNA synthesis—alteration in lung growth—relative to air-exposed controlled newborn mice (54), lending credence to the use of the term dysplasia in bronchopulmonary dysplasia. We now know that most newborn animals are relatively tolerant to hyperoxia compared with the adult of the same species (55). The ability of a newborn animal and probably the human newborn infant to survive a hyperoxic challenge that would kill an adult animal is related to its ability to increase its pulmonary antioxidant enzyme level in a hyperoxic environment, to produce fewer oxygen free radicals intracellularly, to have less inflammatory cell influx, to have fewer mature inflammatory cells with less effective oxidative bursts, to generate less inflammatory intermediaries, to have increased intracellular levels of polyunsaturated fatty acids (free oxygen radical scavengers), and to maintain cell proliferation when challenged by a hyperoxic exposure, to a greater extent than the adult animal (56). These features of the newborn animal response to oxygen injury in the lung are not present in the adult animal or human and may be reduced in the prematurely born human infant. The development of a BPD-like picture in the prematurely delivered primate or mammal requires both the presence of supplemental oxygen and mechanical ventilation; otherwise, the prematurely delivered animal will not survive long enough to develop BPD (57). As a result neither pressure-induced trauma nor pulmonary oxygen toxicity alone has been shown in any prematurely delivered animal model to produce the full range of pathology seen in BPD in the immature human infant. The level of oxygen concentration and peak ventilator pressure that is noninjurious to the very immature developing lung is unknown.

B. RDS Mortality

Improvements in management of the endotracheal tube, pulmonary toilet, the maintenance of the nutrition of the premature infant, accurate micromeasurement of blood gas tensions, establishment of normal physiological blood gas values for prematurely born infants in the first few hours of life, administration of more accurately measured concentrations of supplemental oxygen (58), improvements in the techniques of mechanical ventilation, including use of positive end-expiratory pressure (59), continuous positive-airway pressure (60), various types of jet ventilation, and the use of human and artificial surfactant, have resulted in a reduction in the mortality from RDS so that it is no longer the leading cause of death in live-born premature infants (61). Not only has the mortality from RDS decreased, but there have been significant modifications in BPD. These include a general decrease in the severity of the radiologic picture and changes in its epidemiology.

C. Incidence of BPD

With improvements in neonatal care and reduction in the use of high concentrations of oxygen and peak airway pressures, there has been a decrease in the incidence of BPD in the birth weight group who are heavier than 1500 g. The overall incidence in infants with RDS appears to have risen since 1962–1965, whereas the inhospital mortality for BPD has decreased. The overall incidence may have risen because there has been a concomitant increase in survival of very low birth weight infants (<1000 g) with BPD (62). In 1962–1965 intensive care techniques that would allow prolonged mechanical ventilation of these very low birthweight infants had not been developed. Infants as small as 280 g birthweight are now being successfully mechanically ventilated to survive (63). However, it is these very low birthweight infants that currently have the highest incidence of BPD and pose the greatest challenge to reducing its incidence (64).

D. Radiology

Modification of the original four-stage radiographic picture of development of BPD has accompanied the changes in birth–weight-specific incidence of BPD. These modifications are related to the mechanical ventilation of increasingly immature infants, utilization of lower concentrations of supplemental oxygen, and lower peak ventilator pressures. As a result the chest radiographic picture is usually less severe than originally described. Radiographic stage II, with complete opacification of both lungs, is seen infrequently. Radiographic stage IV disease or the chronic lung disease stage, with rounded lucencies and coarse radiodense stranding is still seen in the most severe cases, but more frequently there is a fine reticular increase in lung density that is prolonged beyond 28 days of age. In some cases, the lungs may only remain persistently hazy with some degree of hyperexpansion later than 28 days of age (65). The chronicity of these radiographic findings aids in establishing the diagnosis of BPD.

E. Diagnosis

As a result of these changes in the epidemiology and the radiographic picture of BPD, revised diagnostic criteria have been developed (66). The Bureau of Maternal and Child Health and Resources Development has put forward the following diagnostic criteria:

1. Positive-pressure ventilation during the first 2 weeks of life for a minimum of 3 days.
2. Clinical signs of respiratory compromise persisting beyond 28 days of age.
3. Requirement for supplemental oxygen longer than 28 days of age to maintain a Pa_{O_2} higher than 50 mmHg.
4. Chest radiograph with findings characteristic of BPD.

The use of mechanical ventilation is still considered a prerequisite for development of BPD even though BPD has been reported to have developed in an infant who was ventilated with only an Ambubag (67). Persistent respiratory distress requiring oxygen supplementation to maintain a Pa_{O_2} above 50 mmHg establishes the presence of lung disease beyond 28 days. The modified radiographic criteria allows for the changes from the original radiographic picture (68).

The clinical diagnosis of BPD remains difficult before 3–4 weeks of postnatal age. Tracheal aspiration with cytological analysis and radiologic correlation may provide earlier diagnosis (69). Biochemical analysis of bronchoalveolar lavage fluid has shed interesting information on the inflammatory response of the lung developing BPD (70–72), but has not yet been particularly useful clinically in establishing early diagnosis. It is unclear that early measurement of pulmonary mechanics will be helpful for prediction of infants at risk for BPD (73,74). Postponing the diagnosis to the equivalent of 36 weeks gestational age has been advocated as possibly providing a more useful prognosis relative to persistence of chronic lung disease, but the usefulness of this modification of diagnosis is still unclear (75). Toce and Edwards have developed a clinical–radiographic scoring system for judging the severity of BPD (76), and a new radiographic scoring system has been also been devised (77). The usefulness of these scoring systems in measuring the severity of BPD and providing prognostic information and measuring treatment efficiency is unclear.

F. Terminology

As a result of the changes in epidemiology and radiology of BPD, there has been increased use of the term *chronic lung disease of prematurity* to describe either the less severe form of BPD or the complete spectrum of BPD including the most severe form originally described (78). Regardless of the terminology, infants who die with chronic lung disease of prematurity or chronic lung disease of early infancy have the pathology of BPD (59).

G. Follow-Up

The surviving 1- to 2-year-old infants with BPD have persistent pulmonary dysfunction, including increased airways resistance, increased airway reactivity, low dynamic compliance, increased functional residual capacity, increased respiratory rate, high arterial carbon dioxide tension, low arterial oxygen tension, severe maldistribution of ventilation, right and sometimes left ventricular hypertrophy, pulmonary hypertension, and systemic hypertension (79–88). These abnormalities may improve, but do not necessarily resolve with age (89–91).

There is little information available on the histopathology of the lungs of older infants and young children who have previously had BPD. Margraf described the histopathology of the lung in a series of eight infants dying with persistent BPD (92). The oldest of these infants died 28 months after birth. There is one case report of an infant who died 34 months after birth, and this report included a description of the morphology and morphometry of the lungs (93). Both morphometric studies revealed that older infants with previous BPD had a decrease in the total alveolar number and internal alveolar surface area relative to control normal values. The study by Margraf showed an increase in bronchial smooth muscle and glands, and a decrease in bronchiolar diameter, with bronchiolar smooth-muscle hypertrophy in the patients with BPD. Children who undergo lung transplantation for persistent, severe BPD could provide additional information concerning the late pathological sequelae of this condition.

Although histopathological evidence of persistent lung damage is currently not available from children with BPD who are older than 34 months of age, persistent pulmonary dysfunction in older children and young adults with previous BPD has been demonstrated. Increased lung volumes, airway obstruction, and increased transcutaneous carbon dioxide tensions have been documented in a group of ten children with an average age of 10.5 years who had prior BPD (94). Other investigators have found persistent pulmonary dysfunction in infants with more recently diagnosed BPD (95) and in older children with BPD (90). The pulmonary dysfunction demonstrated in infants and in children with prior BPD often improves over time (90,91). Smythe noted increased airways resistance, air trapping, and blood gas and electrocardiographic abnormalities in nine patients with BPD with an average age of approximately 10 years (96). Methacholine challenge in these patients indicated the presence of persistent reactive airways disease.

Seventy-six percent of 25 young adults with prior BPD (mean age 18.3 years) showed increased airways resistance, air trapping, and increased reactive airways disease compared with a cohort of individuals who were matched for birth weight and a group of normal adults who were born at term gestation (97). Only 6 of these young adults had severe pulmonary dysfunction and only 6 suffered respiratory symptoms. Other investigators have reported similar late pulmonary dysfunction in young adults with previous BPD (98). It appears that many children and young adults with prior BPD can be expected to have some persistent pulmonary function abnormalities, but in most of these there are no symptoms of residual lung disease.

The chest radiograph of children with prior BPD tends to improve slowly over time and has been said to be normal by 2–3 years of age (99). However, permanent changes of BPD on chest radiographs may be seen in older children and young adults. These changes are typically subtle and consist primarily of peribronchial cuffing, focal and diffuse linear densities, hyperexpansion, pleural scarring, and occasional pectus carinatum or excavatum deformities (97,100). High-resolution computed tomography (CT) scans of the lungs of children and young adults with prior BPD can demonstrate septal thickening, areas of focal increased lucency that may represent either persistent emphysema or focal areas of air trapping, and vascular remodeling (101,102).

The persistent pulmonary dysfunction and radiographic changes seen in children and young adults with prior BPD may represent not only the sequelae of prior BPD but may also be related to intercurrent infection. Infants and children with BPD appear to have an increased risk of respiratory syncytial virus pneumonia (103) and greater severity of infection (104).

The persistent pulmonary dysfunction seen in infants and young children with more recently diagnosed BPD indicates that the radiographic and pulmonary dysfunction changes seen in young adults with prior BPD still occurs, even with the intervening improvements in neonatal intensive care. Although the use of high concentrations of oxygen and peak ventilator pressures has decreased since 1962–1965, supplemental oxygen and mechanical ventilation with increased airway pressure has been used to treat an increasingly immature lung and one that is possibly more susceptible to oxygen injury (56). Surfactant therapy, although correcting the surfactant deficiency, should not be expected to accelerate the anatomical maturity of the lung or the maturity of the antioxidant system.

Bronchopulmonary dysplasia or chronic lung disease of early infancy is unlikely to decrease in incidence or disappear until premature birth, respiratory failure in the newborn infant, pulmonary oxygen toxicity, and pressure-induced trauma are better understood and are prevented or more successfully treated.

References

1. Northway WH Jr, Rosan RC, Porter DY. Pulmonary disease following respirator-therapy of hyaline membrane disease: bronchopulmonary dysplasia. N Engl J Med 1967; 276:357–368.
2. Peterson HG Jr, Pendleton ME. Contrasting roentgenographic pulmonary patterns of the hyaline membrane and fetal aspiration syndromes. Am J Roentgen 1955; 74: 800–817.
3. Cone TE Jr. History of the Care and Feeding of the Premature Infant. Boston: Little, Brown, 1985.
4. Villermé MM, Milne-Edwards H. De l'influence de la temperature sur la mortalité des infants nouveau-nés. Ann Hyg Publique 1829; 2:291–307.
5. Auvard A. De la couveuse pour enfants. Arch Tocol 1883; 10:577–609.
6. Guéniot M. Sur la faiblesse congenitale et son traitement. Gaz Hôp (Paris) 1872; 45:1161–1162, 1171–1172.
7. Budin P. [The Nursing: The Feeding and Hygiene of Premature and Full-Term Infants.] Maloney WJ, trans. London: Caxton Publishing, 1907.
8. Hoch LA, Weymuller CA, James E. Reduction of mortality from premature birth: some practical measures. JAMA 1948; 136:217–221.
9. Hess JH. Experiences gained in a 30 year study of prematurely born infants. Pediatrics 1953; 11:425–434.
10. Rubner M, Heubner O. Die natürliche ernährung eines säuglings. Z Biol 1898; 36: 1–55.
11. Hess JH. Premature and Congenitally Diseased Infants. Philadelphia: Lea & Febiger, 1922.
12. Cone TE Jr. Perspectives in neonatology. In: Smith GF, Vidyasagar D, eds. Historical Review and Recent Advances in Neonatal and Perinatal Medicine. Vol. 1, Neonatal Medicine. Mead Johnson Nutritional Division, 1983:9–34.
13. Hochheim K. Ueber einige Befunde in den Lungen von Neugeborenen und die beziehung derselben zur aspiration von Fruchtwasser. Centralbl Pathol 1903; 14: 537–538.
14. Miller HC, Hamilton TR. The pathogenesis of "vernix membrane." Relationship to aspiration pneumonia in stillborn and newborn infants. Pediatrics 1949; 3:735–748.
15. Curtis P. Hyaline membrane disease. J Pediatr 1957; 51:726–741.

16. Röntgen WC. Ueber eine neue Art von Strahlen (Vorläugfige Mittheilung). Sitzber Phys Med Ges (Wurxb), December 1895; 9:132–141.
17. Donald I, Lord J. Augmented respiration. Studies in atelectasis neonatorum. Lancet 1953; 1:9–17.
18. Donald T, Steiner RE. Radiography in the diagnosis of hyaline membrane. Lancet 1953; 2:846–849.
19. Donald I, Young IM. An automatic respiratory amplifier. J Physiol 1952; 116:41P–43P.
20. Daily WJR, Smith PC. Mechanical ventilation of the newborn infant, I. Curr Probl Pediatr 1970; 1:1–29.
21. De Paul JAH. Bulletin De l'academie de medicine, September 4, 1977. Quoted in Matas R. Intralaryngeal insufflation. JAMA 1900; 34:1371–1375, 1468–1473.
22. Cited in Matas R. Intralaryngeal insufflation. JAMA 1900; 34:1271–1375, 1468–1473.
23. Champneys FH. Artificial respiration in stillborn children. Mediastinal emphysema and pneumothorax in connection with tracheostomy. An experimental inquiry. Med Chir Trans (Lond) 1882; 65:75–86.
24. Lavoisier AL. Recherches de M Priestly sur les differentes especes d'air, 1773. Reprinted in: Oeuvres de Lavoisier. Tome premier. Chapter 15. Paris: Imprimerie Imperiale, 1864:512–535.
25. Campbell A, Poulton EP. Oxygen and Carbon Dioxide Therapy. London: Oxford University Press, 1934:4.
26. Smith JL. The pathological effects due to increase of oxygen tension in the air breathed. J Physiol (Lond) 1899; 24:19–35.
27. Bonnaire E. Des inhalations d'oxygéne chez les nouveau-nés. J Med (Paris) 1891; 3(2nd ser):312–314.
28. Clifford SH, Cole WCC, Smith CA. Round table discussion of neonatal asphyxia. J Pediatr 1941; 19:258–273.
29. Kinsey VE. Retrolental fibroplasia: cooperative study of retrolental fibroplasia and the use of oxygen. Arch Ophthalmol 1956; 56:481–529.
30. Holt LE Jr, McIntosh R, eds. Pediatrics, 13th ed. New York: Appleton-Century-Crofts, 1962:159.
31. Avery ME, Mead J. Surface properties in relation to atelectasis and hyaline membrane disease. Am J Dis Child 1959; 97:517–523.
32. Avery ME, Oppenheimer EH. Recent increase in mortality from hyaline membrane disease. J Pediatr 1960; 57:533–559.
33. Thomas VD, Fletcher G, Sunshine P, Schafer IA, Klaus MH. Prolonged respirator use in pulmonary insufficiency of newborn. JAMA 1965; 193:183–190.
34. Shepard F, Gray J, Stahlman M. The occurrence of pulmonary fibrosis in children who had ideopathic respiratory distress syndrome. J Pediatr 1964; 65:1078–1079.
35. Robertson B, Tunell R, Rudhe U. Late stages of pulmonary hyaline membranes of newborn. Acta Paediatr 1964; 53:433–446.
36. Rozycki HJ, Kirkpatrick BV. New developments in bronchopulmonary dysplasia. Pediatr Ann 1993; 22:532–538.
37. Abman SH, Groothius JR. Pathophysiology and treatment of bronchopulmonary dysplasia. Pediatr Clin North Am 1994; 41:277–315.

38. Koops BL, Abman SH, Accurso FJ. Outpatient management and follow up of bronchopulmonary dysplasia. Clin Perinatol 1984; 11:101–122.
39. McAleese KA, Knapp MA, Rhodes TT. Financial and emotional cost of bronchopulmonary dysplasia. Clin Pediatr 1993; 32:393–400.
40. Bonikos DS, Bensch KG, Northway WH Jr, Edwards DK. Bronchopulmonary dysplasia: the pulmonary pathologic sequel of necrotizing bronchiolitis and pulmonary fibrosis. Hum Pathol 1976; 7:643–666.
41. Rhodes PG, Hall RT, Leonides JC. Chronic pulmonary disease in neonates with assisted ventilation. Pediatrics 1975; 55:788–796.
42. Campognose P, Singer DB. Neonatal sepsis due to nontypable *Haemophilus influenzae*. Am J Dis Child 1986; 40:117–121.
43. Mayes L, Perkett E, Stahlman MT. Severe bronchopulmonary dysplasia: a retrospective review. Acta Paediatr Scand 1983; 72:225–229.
44. Pusey VA, MacPherson RI, Chernick V. Pulmonary fibroplasia following prolonged artificial ventilation of newborn infants. Can Med Assoc J 1969; 100:451–457.
45. Bos AP, Hussain SM, Hazebrock FW, Tibboel, Meradji M, Molenaar JC. Radiographic evidence of bronchopulmonary dysplasia in high-risk congenital diaphragmatic hernia survivors. Pediatr Pulmonol 1993; 15:231–234.
46. Truog WE, Jackson JC, Badura RJ, Sorensen GK, Murphy JH, Woodrum JE. Bronchopulmonary dysplasia and pulmonary insufficiency of prematurity. Lack of correlation of outcome with gas exchange abnormalities at one month of life. Am J Dis Child 1985; 139:351–354.
47. Loeber NV, Morray JP, Kettrick RG, Downes JJ. Pulmonary function in chronic respiratory failure of infancy. Crit Care Med 1980; 8:596–601.
48. Moylan FMB, Walker AM, Krammer SS, et al. Alveolar rupture as an independent predictor of bronchopulmonary dyplasia. Crit Care Med 1978; 6:10–13.
49. Brown ER, Stark A, Sosenko IRS, et al. Bronchopulmonary dysplasia: possible relationship to pulmonary edema. J Pediatr 1978; 92:982–984.
50. Sawyer MH, Edwards DK, Spector SA. Cytomegalovirus infection and bronchopulmonary dyplasia in premature infants. Am J Dis Child 1987; 141:303–305.
51. Payne NR, Steinberg SS, Ackerman P, Chrenka BA, Sane SM, Anderson KT, Fangman JJ. New prospective studies of the association of *Ureaplasma urealyticum* colonization and chronic lung disease. Clin Infect Dis 1993 (suppl 1):S117–121.
52. Northway WH Jr, Rosan RC, Shahinian L Jr, Castellino RA, Gyepes MT, Durbridge T. Radiologic and histologic investigation of pulmonary oxygen toxicity in newborn guinea pigs. Invest Radiol 1969; 4:148–155.
53. Bonikos DS, Bensch KG, Northway WH Jr. Oxygen toxicity in the newborn. The effect of chronic continuous 100 percent oxygen exposure on the lungs of newborn mice. Am J Pathol 1976; 85:623–650.
54. Northway WH Jr, Rezeau L, Petriceks R, Bensch KG. Oxygen toxicity in the newborn lung: reversal of inhibition of DNA synthesis in the mouse. Pediatrics 1976; 57:41–46.
55. Frank L, Bucher JR, Roberts JR. Oxygen toxicity in neonatal and adult animals of various species. J App Physiol 1978; 45:699–704.

56. Frank L. Developmental aspects of experimental pulmonary oxygen toxicity. Free Radical Biol Med 1991; 11:463–494.
57. Coalson JJ, Kueth TJ, Escobedo MB, et al. A baboon model of bronchopulmonary dysplasia, II: pathologic features. Exp Med Pathol 1982; 37:335–350.
58. Hodson WA, Thomas K. Oliver and the growth of neonatology. J Pediatr 1988; 112:1030–1032.
59. Lewellyn MA, Swyer PR. Assisted and controlled ventilation in the newborn period on effect of oxygenation. Arch Dis Child 1973; 48:612–616.
60. Gregory GA, Kitterman JA, Phibbs RH, et al. Treatment of the ideopathic respiratory distress syndrome with continuous positive airway pressure. N Engl J Med 1971; 284:1333–1378.
61. Avery ME, Merritt TA. Surfactant-replacement therapy. N Engl J Med 1991; 324: 910–911.
62. Parker RA, Lindstrom DP, Cotton RB. Improved survival accounts for most, but not all, of the increase in bronchopulmonary dysplasia. Pediatrics 1992; 90:663–668.
63. Muraskas JK, Carlson NJ, Halsey C. Survival of a 280 gm infant. N Engl J Med 1991; 324:1598.
64. Northway WH Jr. Bronchopulmonary dysplasia: twenty five years later. Pediatrics 1992; 89:969–973.
65. Edwards DK. The radiology of bronchopulmonary dysplasia and its complications. In: Merritt TA, Northway WH Jr, Boynton BR, eds. Bronchopulmonary Dysplasia. Boston: Blackwell Scientific, 1988:185–234.
66. Bronchopulmonary dysplasia (BPD). In: Guidelines for the Care of Children with Chronic Lung Disease. Bureau of Maternal and Child Health and Resources Development. Pediatr Pulmonol 1989 (suppl 3):3.
67. Airede AK. Bronchopulmonary dysplasia: a case report. E Afr Med J 1993; 70: 57–60.
68. Heneghan MA, Sosulski R, Baquero JM. Persistent pulmonary abnormalities in newborns: the changing picture of bronchopulmonary dysplasia. Pediatr Radiol 1986; 16:180–184.
69. Noack G, Mortensson W, Robertson B, Nilsson R. Correlation between radiological and cytological findings in early development of bronchopulmonary dysplasia. Eur J Pediatr 1993; 152:1024–1029.
70. Rozycki HJ. Bronchoalveolar interleukin-1 beta in infants on day 1 of life. South Med J 1994; 87:991–996.
71. Watterberg KL, Carmichael DF, Gerdes JS, Werner S, Backstrom C, Murphy S. Secretory leukocyte to protease inhibitor and lung inflammation in developing bronchopulmonary dysplasia. J Pediatr 1994; 125:264–269.
72. Bagchi A, Viscardi RM, Taciak V, Ensor JE, McCrea KA, Hasday JD. Increased activity of interleukin-6 but not tumor necrosis factor-alpha in lung lavage of premature infants is associated with the development of bronchopulmonary dysplasia. Pediatr Res 1994; 36:244–252.
73. Van Lierde S, Smith J, Devlieger, Eggermont E. Pulmonary mechanics during respiratory distress syndrome in the prediction of outcome and differentiation of mild and severe bronchopulmonary dysplasia. Pediatr Pulmonol 1994; 17:218–224.

74. Farstad T, Bratlid D. Incidence and prediction of bronchopulmonary dysplasia in a cohort of premature infants. Acta Paediatr 1994; 83:19–24.
75. Shennan AT, Dunn MS, Ohlsson A, et al. Abnormal pulmonary outcomes in premature infants: prediction from oxygen requirement in the neonatal period. Pediatrics 1988; 82:527–532.
76. Toce SS, Farrell PM, Leavitt LA, Samuels DP, Edwards DK. Clinical and roentgenographic scoring systems for assessing bronchopulmonary dysplasia. Am J Dis Child 1984; 138:581–585.
77. Weinstein MR, Peters ME, Sadek M, et al, for the Newborn Lung Project. A new radiographic scoring system for bronchopulmonary dysplasia. Pediatr Pulmonol 1994; 18:284–289.
78. Hyde I, English RE, Williams JD. The changing pattern of chronic lung disease of prematurity. Arch Dis Child 1989; 64:448–451.
79. Loeber NV, Morray JP, Kettrick RG, Downes JJ. Pulmonary function in chronic respiratory failure of infancy. Crit Care Med 1980; 8:596–601.
80. Motoyama EK, Fort MD, Klesh KW, et al. Early onset of airway reactivity in premature infants with bronchopulmonary dysplasia. Am Rev Respir Dis 1987; 136:507.
81. Bryan MH, Hardie JJ, Reilly BJ, Swyer PR. Pulmonary function studies during the first year of life in infants recovering from the respiratory distress syndrome. Pediatrics 1973; 52:169–178.
82. Morray JP, Fox NW, Kettrick RG, Downes JJ. Improvement in lung mechanics as a function of age in the infant with severe bronchopulmonary dysplasia. Pediatr Res 1982; 16:290–294.
83. Gerhardt T, Hehre D, Feller R, et al. Serial determination of pulmonary function in infants with chronic lung disease. J Pediatr 1987; 110:448–456.
84. Watt JL, Ariagno RL, Brady JL. Chronic pulmonary disease in neonates after artifical ventilation: distribution of ventilation and pulmonary interstitial emphysema. Pediatrics 1977; 60:273–281.
85. Harrod JR, L'Heureux P, Wangensteen OD, Hunt CE. Longterm follow up of severe respiratory distress syndrome treated with IPPB. J Pediatr 1974; 84:277–286.
86. Melnick G, Pickoff AS, Ferrer PL, et al. Normal pulmonary vascular resistance and left ventricular hypertrophy in young infants with bronchopulmonary dysplasia: an echocardiographic and pathologic study. Pediatrics 1980; 66:589–596.
87. Berman W. Yabek SM, Dillon T, et al. Evaluation of infants with bronchopulmonary dysplasia using cardiac catheterization. Pediatrics 1982; 70:708–712.
88. Abman SH, Warady BA, Lum GM, Koops BL. Systemic hypertension in infants with bronchopulmonary dysplasia. J Pediatr 1984; 104:928–931.
89. Morray JP, Fox NW, Kettrick RG, Downes JJ. Improvement in lung mechanics as a function of age in the infant with severe bronchopulmonary dysplasia. Pediatr Res 1982; 16:290–294.
90. Gerhardt T, Hehre D, Feller R, Reifenberg L, Bancalari E. Serial determination of pulmonary function in infants with chronic lung disease. J Pediatr 1987; 110:448–456.
91. Blayney M, Eitan K, Whyte H, O'Brodovich H. Bronchopulmonary dysplasia im-

provement in lung function between 7 and 10 years of age. J Pediatr 1991; 18: 201–206.
92. Margraf LR, Tomashefski JF, Bruce MC, Dahms BB. Morphometric analysis of the lung in bronchopulmonary dysplasia. Am Rev Respir Dis 1991; 143:391–400.
93. Sobonya RE, Logvinoff MM, Taussig LM, Therrault A. Morphometric analysis of the lung in prolonged bronchopulmonary dysplasia. Pediatr Res 1982; 16:969–972.
94. Bader D, Ramos AD, Lew CD, et al. Childhood sequelae of infant lung disease: exercise and pulmonary function abnormalities after bronchopulmonary dysplasia. J Pediatr 1987; 110:693–699.
95. Tepper RS, Morgan WJ, Cota BS, Taussig LM. Expiratory flow limitation in infants with bronchopulmonary dysplasia. J Pediatr 1986; 109:1040–1046.
96. Smythe JA, Tabachnik E, Duncan WJ, et al. Pulmonary function and bronchial hyperreactivity in long-term survivors of bronchopulmonary dysplasia. Pediatrics 1981; 68:336–340.
97. Northway WH Jr, Moss RB, Carlisle KB, et al. Late pulmonary sequelae of bronchopulmonary dysplasia. N Engl J Med 1990; 323:1793–1799.
98. Ater D, Garver R, Kim YC, Wohl MEB. Long term follow up lung function in adults following bronchopulmonary dysplasia (BPD). Respir Crit Care Med 1995; 151:A664.
99. Mortensson W, Lindroth M. The course of bronchopulmonary dysplasia. A radiographic follow-up. Acta Radiol Diagn 1986; 27:19–22.
100. Griscom NT, Wheeler WB, Sweezey NB, Kim YC, Lindsey JC, Wohl ME. Bronchopulmonary dysplasia: radiographic appearance in middle childhood. Radiology 1989; 171:811–814.
101. Oppenheim C, Mamouman T, Sayegh N, Deblic J, Sheinmann P, Lalleman D. Bronchopulmonary dysplasia—value of CT in identifying sequelae. Am J Roentgenol 1994; 163:169–172.
102. Northway WH Jr. Unpublished observations.
103. Groothuis JR, Salbenblatt CK, Lauer BA. Severe respiratory syncytial virus infection in older children. Am J Dis Child 1990; 144:346–348.
104. Meert K, Heideman S, Lieh-Lai M. Sarnaik AP. Clinical characteristics of respiratory syncytial virus infections in healthy versus previously compromised host. Pediatr Pulmonol 1989; 7:167–170.
105. Donald I, Lord J. Augemented respiration: studies in atelectasis neonatorum. Lancet 1953; 1:13.

2

Epidemiology of Bronchopulmonary Dysplasia

Clinical Risk Factors and Associated Clinical Conditions

ALMA MARTINEZ and H. WILLIAM TAEUSCH

University of California
San Francisco, California

PETER DARGAVILLE

Royal Children's Hospital
Victoria, Australia

I. Introduction

Why does bronchopulmonary dysplasia (BPD) develop in some premature infants with respiratory distress syndrome (RDS) and not in others? Described throughout this volume are the many influences that are responsible for progression, cessation, or resolution of the disease. During the course of BPD, growth, maturation, continuing injury, and repair are simultaneously occurring in the lung. At the same time, other organs affect, and are affected by, the disease status in the lung. For example, high pulmonary vascular resistance leads to hypoxemia that exacerbates the respiratory failure characteristic of BPD, and in severe cases results in cor pulmonale.

Many other diseases that are seen by neonatologists also are associated with immaturity at birth. It follows that BPD frequently coexists with other such diseases. In this chapter, we discuss clinical risk factors for BPD, as well as other conditions with which it frequently coexists.

II. Major Perinatal Clinical Risk Factors for BPD

A. Effects of Obstetric and Maternal Factors

Abruptio Placentae, Asphyxia

Whether maternal obstetrical problems represent independent risk factors for the development of BPD in the neonate is unclear. An association between abruptio placentae at birth and BPD has been reported (1); another report, however, did not corroborate this association in a smaller number of patients (2). Additionally, these same authors could find no association between BPD and other maternal clinical conditions, including maternal diabetes, pregnancy-induced hypertension, eclampsia, maternal fever at delivery, prolonged rupture of membranes (> 24 hr), placenta previa, cesarean section, or breech delivery. Results from animal studies suggest that fetal asphyxia affects risk and severity of respiratory distress syndrome (RDS) in newborns (3) and, as described later, severity of RDS and its pulmonary complications is the most important determinant of BPD.

Intrauterine Fetal Growth

An association between poor intrauterine growth and BPD has been described (4). When comparing preterm neonates of the same gestational age, those who had poor intrauterine weight gain and lower birth weight had an increased risk of acquiring BPD.

Level of Care in Hospital of Birth

Although Parker and co-workers (5) found an increased association between the nursery level of care in hospital of birth and neonatal mortality, they were unable to find any association with the incidence of BPD. Likewise, other investigators have found no increased risk for BPD associated with place of birth (6–8).

Prenatal Steroid Therapy

The relation between maternal antenatal steroid treatment and subsequent BPD has been examined in a few studies, with an overall favorable effect. In a randomized clinical trial of phenobarbital prophylaxis for neonatal intracranial hemorrhage, the effect of antenatal steroid treatment on neonatal outcomes was studied in a group of 223 intubated infants weighing less than 1751g (9). Seventy-six infants with BPD (defined as oxygen requirement at 28 days and with abnormal chest radiographs) and 147 control infants were studied. After controlling for potential confounding variables, infants whose mothers did not receive antenatal steroids had an increased risk of acquiring BPD (odds ratio of 3:95% confidence intervals approximately 1:8) when compared with the infants of women who received a complete course of steroids. Partial treatment with antenatal steroids was associated with an intermediate effect. After controlling for gender and birth weight, a benefit was shown in all groups except for extremely low birth weight male infants. Among male infants, the beneficial effects of steroids on reduction of BPD was evident only in those whose birth weight was more than 1 kg. There was no loss of protective effect in infants delivered beyond 7 days after steroid treatment. In another study, the effect of antenatal steroid administration in 244 infants was compared with 434 control infants (10). After adjusting for potentially confounding obstetrical variables and birth weight, the treated group showed significantly decreased mortality rates. Additionally, the treated infants required less ventilatory support, had fewer days receiving supplemental oxygen, and had a significantly decreased incidence of BPD and patent ductus arteriosus. In contrast, a separate study failed to show a beneficial effect of antenatal steroids on the incidence of BPD (11). This study restricted entry to infants with a birth weight of less than 1 kg, and did not adjust for clinical variables that previously have been shown to affect morbidity. Review of these results by an NIH Child Health and Human Development (NICHD) work group has led to recently published guidelines that markedly expand the indications for prenatal steroid use by obstetricians (12).

The usefulness of steroids, not only for prevention of RDS, but also for amelioration of BPD, suggests that some premature infants may be suffering from relative corticosteroid deficiency. When premature infants received ACTH injections 5–7 days after birth, the cortisol response was significantly less in infants who later acquired BPD compared with the response of premature infants who did not subsequently acquire BPD (13–15). The authors speculated that infants with relative cortisol deficiency cannot blunt the early postnatal pulmonary inflammation associated with RDS. Therefore, these infants are at increased risk of BPD precipitated by events, analogous to those that often predispose adults to adult respiratory distress syndrome (ARDS).

Indomethacin

In a randomized study of the effects of prenatal indomethacin treatment for women in preterm labor, investigators reported an increased risk of BPD in infants whose mothers received indomethacin when compared with infants whose mothers received a β-adrenergic agonist alone for the prevention of preterm labor (16). Infants who were exposed to indomethacin also had a higher incidence of RDS and necrotizing enterocolitis. The authors hypothesized that indomethacin, used to reduce uterine contractility and risk of premature birth, also caused significant effects in the fetus. The pathophysiology of this interesting association between antenatal indomethacin and risk of BPD is unclear. Possible mechanisms include pulmonary hypertension and resultant lung edema from inhibition of prostacyclin production and failure of the ductus arteriosus to constrict, or from adverse effects on surfactant physiology (16). The outcome measures presented in this report, however, were not analyzed according to birth weight or gestational age; therefore, comparisons of the incidence of BPD cannot be made with other studies.

Ethnic Differences

Variation in the risk and severity of RDS related to ethnic differences has been observed in premature infants for many years. Worldwide, there are differences in rates of RDS. In the United States, several studies of low birth weight infants have demonstrated that white preterm infants are more likely to have RDS than African American infants (5,6,17,18). Two studies that controlled for the severity of initial RDS found ethnicity to be an independent variable predictive of the risk of BPD (5,18). Palta et al. (6) found that white preterm infants were more likely than infants of other races to acquire BPD, with an odds ratio of 2.2. Other investigators have shown that among preterm infants weighing less than 1500 g at birth, the risk of acquiring BPD is 10% less in African American newborns than in others (18,19). This association between ethnicity and risk for BPD, however, was not seen in all studies (7,19).

It is unclear why ethnic differences might influence the risk of lung disease in premature infants, but associated poverty and other related maternal stress might be contributory. It is possible that such stress might evoke hormonal signals that in turn may increase the risk of premature birth. On the other hand, such stress might induce more rapid fetal maturation, thereby inhibiting development of lung disease. The influence of socioeconomic status and related conditions, such as maternal nutrition, maternal use of drugs, alcohol, and tobacco, and the need to work throughout pregnancy, are not well defined relative to the risk of BPD.

Genetic Influences

There may be other genetic factors that influence the risk of neonatal lung disease. Variability within certain loci in the SP-A gene among ethnic groups has recently been described (20). The investigators found a higher incidence of the SP-A allelic variant 6A in Nigerians, and hypothesized that this variant is protective against RDS in prematurely born infants. The authors suggested that this might explain the low incidence of RDS in Nigerian infants (20). This variant, however, is not frequent in African Americans and, therefore, cannot explain the difference in RDS risk seen in this country. A study of the racial differences in lecithin/sphingomyelin (L/S) ratios in this country concluded that protection against RDS cannot be explained by early maturation of lecithin synthesis, and the authors proposed that advanced maturity of other surfactant components, or anatomical differences in alveolar size or structure might explain the difference in RDS risk

(21). Further study will be required to define the possible reasons for differences in the risk of newborn lung disease as a function of ethnic variation.

In a study of human leukocyte antigens (HLA) in 101 newborn infants, Hafez et al. (22) found that carriage of HLA-A3 and B14 was associated with greater risk of RDS. Twin studies have demonstrated a greater concordance for RDS in monozygotic than in dyzygotic twins, although obstetrical factors may confound this association (23). Several studies examining the role of familial factors in predispositon to RDS have noted a higher incidence of RDS in siblings of an index case than in siblings of an infant with no lung disease (24–26).

There is some evidence that a family history of atopy may predispose to the development of BPD in infants with RDS. Nickerson and Taussig (27) obtained a family history of asthma in 13 of 17 infants with BPD, compared with 7 of 21 infants who had RDS that did not progress to BPD. They concluded that infants with a genetic predisposition to airway reactivity are more likely to have RDS after an acute lung insult. Other investigators have failed to confirm this association (28), but the few infants involved in both studies directly assessing the relation between familial atopy and BPD risk do not allow a firm conclusion to be drawn.

Variation and mutation within the gene for surfactant protein B (SP-B) are now known to be associated with RDS (29,30). The most extreme example of genetic determination of neonatal lung disease is that seen in infants with congenital deficiency of SP-B (30). These infants present soon after birth with severe, progressive respiratory failure from a condition that was previously termed congenital alveolar proteinosis (see Chap. 21).

B. Effects of Neonatal Factors

Apgar Scores

The Apgar score is a method of assessing an infant's clinical condition during the transition to extrauterine life. Various authors have reported associations between the Apgar score at 1 or 5 min after birth and subsequent development of BPD (5,6,31). Other investigators confirmed the value of the 5-min Apgar score to predict the development of BPD (8,32).

Birth Weight and Gestation

Despite reported differences in the incidence of BPD from center to center (17,18,33), and despite differences in the manner in which BPD is defined (18,19,34), studies consistently show the highest incidence of BPD in the most immature and smallest of survivors. Table 1 lists the incidence of BPD for low birth weight infants from a number of studies, as well as the definition of BPD used in each study. Other investigators have reported an inverse relation between

Table 1 Incidence of BPD (%) Reported by Birth Weight Distribution

Ref.	Weight (g)[a]					Definition of BPD[b]
	500–750	*751–1000*	*1001–1250*	*1251–1500*		
33	96	70	48	25		Mechanical ventilation > 48 hr, ventilatory assistance or supplemental oxygen at 30 days after birth
41	100	50	29	6		Mechanical ventilation in first week, supplemental oxygen 28 days after birth, abnormal chest radiograph
	700–800	*801–900*	*901–1000*	*1001–1250*	*1250–1500*	
17	76	68	46	26	13	Supplemental oxygen at 28 days after birth
18	89	80	60	38	15	Supplemental oxygen at 28 days after birth
	< 1000	*1001–1500*	*1001–2000*	*> 1500*	*> 2000*	
8(?)	67	—	56	—	6	Supplemental oxygen at 28 days after birth
50	48	18	—	1	—	Supplemental oxygen at 28 days after birth, and Northway classification stage III or IV BPD (51)

[a]Data are shown as the percentage of surviving infants with disease.
[b]The definition of BPD, as used by each author.

gestational age and the incidence of BPD (4,35). Additionally, many investigators have found that birth weight and gestational age are useful in predicting variables in the development of BPD in neonates (5–8,32,36–38), as well as for predicting mortality risk of infants with BPD (39). Even among infants of identical gestational ages, infants with very low birth weights have the greater risk for BPD (4).

Gender

Respiratory distress syndrome is more prevalent and more severe in male than in female preterm infants (6,7,17,18). Several recent studies of low birth weight infants have reported an association between male gender and development of BPD that is independent of the severity of the initial lung disease. In a multivariate assessment of risk factors for chronic lung disease in 581 infants with birth weights less than 1500 g, male gender was an independent risk factor for chronic lung disease, with an odds ratio of 1.9 (6). These data suggest that not only is the male preterm infant more likely to have RDS, but he is also at greater risk for subsequent development of BPD. Even when the increased risk of early mortality for male preterm infants is taken into account, BPD is more likely to develop in male than in female infants. With rare exceptions (8), most epidemiological studies of infants with BPD, in which gender has been considered, have demonstrated a male preponderance (7).

It is unclear why male infants are at greater risk for lung disease. One possible contributing variable is that there may be fewer pulmonary receptors for epithelial growth factor in the developing male fetus (40). This apparent male propensity for BPD merits further study.

Effects of RDS Severity

Early studies of infants with lung disease showed that the largest, most mature infants had less severe RDS (reflected by Apgar score, radiographic severity, duration of assisted ventilation, and peak inspiratory pressure) and tended to survive without development of BPD (2). Conversely, the smallest, least mature, and most ill infants had the highest mortality rates from RDS. Therefore, the infants who acquired BPD were mostly of intermediate weight, maturity, and severity of RDS. Despite the paucity of patients in some of the subgroups, the authors speculated that birth weight, maturity, and severity of RDS helped to identify susceptibility to BPD.

In a more recent, multicenter study, multivariate analysis was used to assess risk factors for BPD among 361 newborn infants with birth weights less than 1500 g (6). The authors concluded that extremely premature infants were at increased risk for BPD, regardless of the baseline severity of acute respiratory disease. Factors associated with increased risk of BPD in the multivariate model included very low birth weight and gestational age, low Apgar score 1 min after birth, male infant, white race, as well as greater severity of acute disease. After adjusting for these baseline factors, clinical conditions that identified more severely ill neonates, such as the presence of a patent ductus arteriosus, high peak inspiratory pressures, need for high concentrations of inspired oxygen 96 hr after birth, and high fluid intake, were associated with subsequent development of BPD.

Other investigators measured the severity of acute illness in 60 infants who required mechanical ventilation during the first week after birth (41). Measures of severity of acute illness in infants with subsequent BPD were compared with infants who survived without BPD. Infants whose respiratory distress evolved into BPD had significantly higher maximum peak inspiratory and mean airway pressure, higher oxygen requirements, and greater alveolar–arterial oxygen gradients in the first week after birth (41). Other investigators have used clinical respiratory variables present as early as 6 hr after birth as indicators of risk for subsequent BPD (31). In a prospective, longitudinal study of 56 infants with RDS, the severity of acute respiratory disease (assessed by ventilator rate and maximal inspiratory pressure) on the third day after birth, combined with gestational age, were highly associated with subsequent severe BPD or death (38). Others also have shown BPD to be associated with more severe acute atelectasis, higher ventilation rate at 96 hr, and lower Pa_{CO_2} at 48 hr after birth (7,31). The severity of RDS, as determined by scoring of chest radiographs in infants with acute RDS, has been reportedly associated with subsequent development of BPD (2,5).

Investigators continue to question the association between severity of acute illness and subsequent risk of BPD. There is continuing controversy over the relative importance of the severity of acute lung disease versus the medical and ventilatory management of the preterm infant as contributing factors in the development of BPD.

Other Neonatal Pulmonary Conditions That May Contribute to BPD

Whereas more than 90% of BPD develops in the aftermath of premature birth and RDS, BPD can follow any severe neonatal lung disease that requires prolonged supplemental oxygen and ventilatory therapy. For example, BPD is a consequence of ventilation and oxygen therapy of hypoplastic lungs in about 33% of surviving infants who are born with congenital diaphragmatic hernia, most of whom are born at term (42). Pulmonary function testing at age 11 years in survivors of congenital diaphragmatic hernia showed abnormalities of minor clinical significance (43). Some of the worst cases of BPD since the introduction of surfactant have developed in premature infants who have been born between 24 and 28 weeks gestation after many weeks of oligohydramnios, often associated with ruptured amniotic membranes. When this scenario is duplicated experimentally in animals, lung hypoplasia results. Therefore, the combination of lung hypoplasia with lung immaturity, and possibly the additive effect of pulmonary infection may result in lungs that are barely able to sustain gas exchange despite high supplemental oxygen and ventilator pressures. Vergani and co-workers have suggested that lung hypoplasia associated with oligohydramnios, may be prevented by amnioinfusion (44).

Meconium aspiration pneumonia is another frequent neonatal lung disease (3:1000 live births) that is commonly associated with prolonged respiratory morbidity; this condition, however, is rarely associated with severe BPD. Yuksel et al. (45) found that 8 of 35 infants with severe meconium aspiration pneumonia required long-term bronchodilator therapy for up to 6 months after birth.

III. Clinical Risk Scoring Systems

Various scoring systems incorporating clinical and radiographic criteria have been reported for assessing the severity of BPD (2,37,46). Several investigators have reported the use of such methods for predicting the risk of BPD (4,6,8,19,36,38,47–49) and mortality from BPD (38,39), and for predicting morbidities among infants with BPD (20,48,50). As improved therapies for reducing risk of BPD become available, these prognostic algorithms may become useful for assessing therapeutic efficacy.

A. Radiographic Scoring Systems to Assess the Severity of Disease

Application of the radiologic scoring system, first proposed by Northway and colleagues (51), showed a strong correlation between radiographic abnormalities and lung pathological findings among patients with fatal BPD (52). Subsequently, other investigators tested a scoring system using both radiologic and clinical pulmonary disease scores and showed a significant correlation between clinical and radiologic scores at 21 days after birth (37). With use of multiple regression analysis, these investigators found that the best predictors of clinical scores were birth weight, gestational age, and radiologic score 21 days after birth. The authors cautioned that because radiologic distinction between early BPD and resolving RDS may not be possible in the first few weeks after birth, this proposed scoring system was intended to be used 21 days after birth to assess severity of BPD. Modifications of this radiologic scoring system have been proposed and evaluated in a large series of infants (37). These radiographic scoring systems continue to play an important role in quantifying the severity of BPD (see Chap. 4).

B. Scoring Systems To Predict the Risk of BPD

Various methods have been proposed to predict the risk of BPD developing in infants who are born prematurely. Clearly, accurate prediction of the risk for development of BPD can be beneficial for conducting clinical research. Accurate predictions would help identify those infants at highest risk for the outcome of interest (BPD, or death from BPD), so that improved clinical intervention studies could be designed. Additionally, accurate predictor variables would enable investigators to compare the different incidences of BPD from different nurseries and institutions.

Several methods that are based almost exclusively on clinical perinatal factors to predict the occurrence of BPD have been proposed. An early description used a simple screening procedure 48 hr after birth (36). These investigators used birth weight (600–1250 g) and need for mechanical ventilation within 48 hr of birth to predict poor outcomes. With these criteria, the authors identified infants with a 61% risk of subsequent BPD. A separate high-risk group of infants was defined as infants receiving more than 60% supplemental oxygen for longer than 2 hr within the 48-hr period. These infants had an 81% risk of subsequent BPD. With regression-modeling methods, other investigators found that, after controlling for a number of variables, male sex, and low $Paco_2$ 48 hr after birth were the best predictors of BPD (7). Hakulinen et al. (4) found that the best predictors of development of BPD were prolonged need for 100% oxygen (> 24 hr), presence of pneumonia, and 5-min Apgar score less than 7. Other investigators have shown that birth weight, gestational age, antenatal steroid treatment, intubation in the delivery room, and maternal toxemia were significant predictors in a multivariate model (49). These variables were used to determine a risk score that comprised characteristics that were present before initiation of intensive care. This method controls for important perinatal factors in infants when comparing the incidence of BPD between centers. Sinkin et al. (8) described two separate regression equations that can be used to identify risk of BPD either at 12 hr or 10 days after birth. These equations rely on birth weight, gestational age, Apgar score 5 min after birth, and ventilatory data to derive risk scores for each infant at the distinct time points. These risk scores can be used to derive the probability of subsequent BPD in preterm infants. Ehrenkranz et al. (47) have described a logistic regression model to identify infants at high risk of subsequent BPD or death associated with BPD. This report concluded that the most important predictors of poor outcome were the fraction of inspired oxygen on the tenth postnatal day, mean airway pressure on the fifth day of life, and gestational age at birth. The authors reported that this model had 81% sensitivity and 72% specificity for predicting development of BPD.

Various studies have combined radiologic scoring systems with clinical variables to predict outcomes (4,38). In one study, chest radiographs were used to determine the presence and severity of lung disease and its severity at postnatal day 28. Gestational age and respiratory status 3 days after birth were useful in predicting poor outcome, defined either as BPD diagnosed by characteristic radiographs, or death (38). Palta et al. (32) presented a method for deriving a baseline severity index score for infants with respiratory distress. This approach uses clinical determinants (birth weight, 5-min Apgar score, respiratory variables) and a radiologic score (32). The method represents a way to control for severity of baseline disease when comparing the incidence of BPD between different centers. In a subsequent paper, these same authors used this baseline risk score to control for baseline severity of disease in infants, and found that the presence of a patent ductus arteriosus, the magnitude of ventilator pressures, the need for supplemental oxygen 96 hr after birth, and fluid intake were significant predictors of BPD (6).

Infants with BPD have various pulmonary function abnormalities. Goldman et al. (52) hypothesized that the presence of early pulmonary function abnormalities in infants could be used to predict subsequent development of BPD. These investigators measured lung mechanics in a group of infants with RDS whose birth weight was more than 750 g, and who required mechanical ventilation. The infants who progressed to BPD had higher pulmonary resistance than the control group in the first 4–5 days after birth.

C. Scoring Systems to Predict Mortality Risk with BPD

Several investigators have attempted to predict the risk of mortality in infants with BPD (39,47). Shaw et al. (39) showed that the incidence of death during initial hospitalization correlated with the number of days of mechanical ventilation, male sex, inspired oxygen concentration at postnatal day 28, and inversely correlated with gestation. An equation using these parameters was derived and then validated on a separate group of infants. This equation was most useful at the extremes of the calculated probability; that is, when the probability was either high or low: it tended to overpredict death in the middle range. These authors cautioned that, although these results were helpful in guiding clinicians in counseling parents on the prognosis for their infants, it was impossible to accurately predict the outcome for individual cases (54). Others, using multicenter data for infants with a birth weight less than 1000 g, have developed a logistic regression model to predict poor outcome at 36 weeks postconceptional age (47). This model, using the fraction of inspired oxygen on postnatal day 10, the mean airway pressure on postnatal day 5, and gestational age, was predictive of mortality or oxygen dependence at 36 weeks postconceptional age, with a sensitivity of almost 75% and specificity of 56%.

D. Scoring Systems to Predict Morbidity with BPD

By using combined clinical and radiologic assessment at postnatal days 21 and 27, Ariagno and co-workers (50) were unable to predict which infants would require use of supplemental oxygen at home, or which infants would have growth retardation 1 year after birth. These investigators reported that the number of hours an infant breathed more than 80% oxygen correlated with both outcome measures. Other investigators found that respiratory measurements (inspired oxygen and ventilator dependence) on day 28 significantly correlated with a prolonged need for supplemental oxygen (48). Another study showed that in infants weighing less than 1500 g, there was only a weak correlation between oxygen requirement at 28 days and subsequent abnormal pulmonary outcomes. Only 38% of infants who required supplemental oxygen at postnatal day 28 had abnormal outcomes (19). These authors reported that a better predictor of pulmonary morbidity was continued oxygen requirement at 36 weeks corrected postnatal age. With this endpoint, the positive predictive value for subsequent abnormal pulmonary outcomes increased to 63%.

Thus, multiple prenatal and postnatal factors, such as obstetrical management, gestational age, birth weight, gender, ethnicity, and severity of RDS, influence the risk of subsequent BPD. However, predicting risk for an individual infant remains problematic. Quite apart from the factors that lead to individual variations in the development of RDS (e.g., obstetrical circumstances, gender, race, genetic factors), there is considerable variability among infants in their responses to lung injury and their rates of lung repair.

IV. Postnatal Factors That Affect BPD

A. Surfactant Treatment

Because of the influence of surfactant on severity of RDS, and because severity of RDS influences development of BPD, clinical factors that may affect the incidence of BPD need to be discussed in the context of their role in the pre- and postsurfactant era. Although surfactant was first approved for clinical use in the United States in the spring of 1991, the full influence of surfactant on BPD is not yet clear. Many of the randomized trials that assessed the efficacy of surfactant treatment for RDS found minimal effect on the incidence of BPD. A widespread clinical impression is that BPD is now generally less severe, with fewer infants reaching endstage lung disease. This view was commonly held even before surfactant therapy came into use (5). Surfactant treatment and prenatal steroid treatment have lessened the severity of RDS, thereby reducing the amount of supplemental oxygen used, the magnitude of ventilator pressures used, the duration of high ventilator pressures used, and the duration of intubation—all of which are well-accepted risk factors for BPD (55). Surfactant helps to save the lives of extremely low birth weight infants, who in previous years would have died at an early age before manifesting BPD. These infants now contribute heavily to the numbers of patients with BPD. The importance of the severity of the initial RDS as a primary risk factor for BPD is now giving ground to prenatal or postnatal infection and patent ductus arteriosus as major associated clinical conditions (56). Because of these changes, more of the smallest infants are surviving, with the risk of BPD remaining about the same in this group.

B. Respiratory Practices

Despite long-standing use of high concentrations of inspired oxygen to treat infants with RDS, with the first description of BPD appearing in 1967 (51), BPD as a frequent and serious problem for premature infants was not appreciated until after 1970. ''Persistent pulmonary dysfunction,'' with no mention of the term bronchopulmonary dysplasia, received only two pages of text in the third edition of Avery's *The Lung and Its Disorders in the Newborn Infant* that was published in 1974 (57). Mayes and co-workers (58) reported that from 1974 to 1978, only 2.5% of over 900 infants who were mechanically ventilated at Vanderbilt hospitals had severe BPD. This history implies that ventilators were required to allow infants with lung disease to survive long enough for BPD to become manifest. It was not until the late 1970s that ventilator support of tiny infants was commonplace.

The ways in which damage to the lung by oxygen and ventilator support can be caused and minimized are discussed in other chapters. Although these factors may not ''cause'' BPD, their overuse, may increase the risk of BPD; therefore, these practices contribute to risk and severity of BPD in the same way that fluid therapy does: enough is essential, too much is detrimental.

C. Patent Ductus Arteriosus

During fetal life, most blood from the heart bypasses the lungs, as blood flows from the pulmonary artery to the aorta through the ductus arteriosus. Healthy newborn infants have marked decreases in pulmonary vascular resistance concomitant with closure of the ductus arteriosus soon after birth. Premature infants recovering from RDS often have persistent patency of the ductus arteriosus, and as pulmonary vascular resistance falls postnatally increased blood flow to the lungs may result in interstitial and alveolar edema (see Chap. 29). A patent ductus arteriosus complicates recovery from RDS, and many believe it predisposes to BPD. As with many manifestations of immaturity, risk factors for patent ductus arteriosus are also risk factors for BPD, making it difficult to understand whether a PDA influences the risk of BPD. Knight (59) reviewed 12 studies that assessed whether closure of the ductus arteriosus, either surgically or medically with indomethacin, reduces the risk of BPD. In only three of these studies, during which ductal closure was carried out early, was there a suggestion of a reduction of BPD (relative risk close to 1.5). Knight concluded that the ductus arteriosus is a marker for, rather than a contributor to, the development of BPD.

Rojas and co-workers (56) carried out extensive retrospective logistic regression analyses to study which clinical factors were most important antecedents of BPD after mild RDS. The study identified 119 infants with a birth weight of less than 1000 g who required only minimal ventilatory support or oxygen in the immediate newborn period. Of these infants, 37% acquired BPD, defined as need for supplemental oxygen for more than 28 of the first 60 postnatal days, coupled with characteristic radiographic findings. In this group of very immature infants, with only mild or no initial RDS, the odds ratio for BPD was 6 if a PDA was present, 4 if sepsis occurred, and 48 if the combination of sepsis and PDA was diagnosed. Thus, a PDA is associated with an increased risk of subsequent BPD. Although animal and clinical evidence indicates that the left-to-right shunt associated with a PDA contributes to the pathogenesis of BPD, it is unclear if its closure mitigates this risk.

D. Fluid Management

High fluid intake over the first 4–8 weeks after birth is considered to increase risk and severity of BPD through several mechanisms. First, it has been thought that increased fluids contribute to an increased left-to-right flow through the PDA, thereby ''flooding'' the lungs. Second, increased fluid intake contributes to interstitial and alveolar edema which, in turn, may decrease lung compliance, increase oxygen and ventilator requirements, interfere with enteral nutrition, and perhaps predispose to infection.

Investigators have approached this conundrum in imaginative retrospective and prospective studies. In a retrospective study, Van Marter (60) examined a group of 147 premature infants at risk for BPD. Those diagnosed with BPD received on average 17% more total fluid, 10% more crystalloid fluid, and 193% more colloid per day than did control infants. Those with BPD had net weight gain in the first 4 days after birth, in contrast with the weight loss that normally occurs during this interval. Those with BPD had a greater likelihood of having a clinical diagnosis of PDA, and they were more likely to have received furosemide on the third and fourth postnatal days.

Was high fluid intake a marker for severity of illness? To test this possibility, the investigators examined the lowest mean blood pressures in the first week and the lowest pH values. Low blood pressures were not associated with increased risk of BPD in the analysis, which was stratified according to birth weight, but the lowest pH values were associated with increased risk for BPD. Additionally, the rate of colloid administration had a significant dose–response relation with the degree of respiratory support, including the magnitude of maximum inspired oxygen concentration, peak inspiratory pressure, end-expiratory pressure, and ventilator rate.

In a prospective, randomized trial of 100 consecutive infants with a birth weight less than 1751 g, Tammela and Koivisto (61) randomized infants to a high fluid intake or a ''dry'' fluid intake regimen over the first 28 days after birth. By 14 days, the high-intake group had an average intake of about 185 mL kg^{-1} d^{-1}, and the dry group had an average intake of about 145 mL kg^{-1} d^{-1}. All of the outcome measures tended to favor the dry group. At 40 weeks postconception, the dry group had twice as many infants with a normal chest radiograph and no clinical signs of BPD as did the high fluid intake group. This controlled study, in addition to other reports, indicates that excess fluid can predispose to BPD.

D. Air Leak

The presence of an extrapulmonary air leak (e.g., pneumothorax, pneumomediastinum, subcutaneous emphysema, or pulmonary interstitial emphysema) is a consequence of the magnitude and duration of inspiratory pressures applied during mechanical ventilation, heterogeneous lung volumes, and rupture of fragile, immature lung units. Air leaks provide clear-cut evidence that immature lungs have been damaged in the attempt to drive oxygen into and CO_2 out of the underdeveloped gas exchange organ. Berg et al. (62) were among the earliest to report the association between air leak and chronic lung disease. Pulmonary interstitial emphysema often represents severe injury that occurs in the most immature lungs (63). Such injury may trigger an unusually severe inflammatory response, which probably accounts for the importance of air leak as a predisposing factor for BPD (64). Air leak was one of the major risk factors for BPD in the presurfactant era. With the widespread use of surfactant therapy, air leak complications in infants with RDS have decreased from 30% to less than 10%.

E. Infection

Prenatal (e.g., chorioamnionitis) and postnatal infections may play a role in the pathogenesis of a subset of infants in whom BPD develops. Interleukin (IL)-8 and granulocyte elastase are both found in higher concentrations in tracheal aspirates of infants born to mothers with evidence of chorioamnionitis, and these infants have a higher risk of BPD compared with gestation-matched control infants (65). BPD also increases susceptibility to certain infections, such as respiratory syncytial virus (see Chap. 8), that may exacerbate the progression of BPD.

V. Summary

The following represent current premises about clinical trends relative to BPD.

1. BPD is caused by injury from mechanical ventilator and oxygen applied to or hypoplastic lungs.
2. The trend in the last 10 years (before and after the advent of surfactant therapy for RDS in conjunction with prenatal glucocorticoids) has been a reduction in the severest forms of BPD. End-stage lung disease from BPD is becoming much less common than it was previously.
3. BPD now is more often associated with infection and PDA in premature infants, rather than being a consequence of severe RDS alone.

There are still unanswered questions concerning the epidemiology of BPD. Further studies are needed to identify antecedents of this condition.

References

1. Palta M, Gabbert D. Pregnancy complications and chronic lung disease in the premature neonate. Am J Epidemiol 1990; 132:759.
2. Edwards D, Dyer W, Northway W. Twelve years' experience with bronchopulmonary dysplasia. Pediatrics 1977; 59:839–845.
3. Orzalesi MM, Mtotayama E, Jacobson HN, et al. The development of the lungs of lambs. Pediatrics 1965; 35:373.
4. Hakulinen A, Heinonen K, Jokela V, Kiekara O. Occurrence, predictive factors and associated morbidity of bronchopulmonary dysplasia in a preterm birth cohort. J Perinat Med 1988; 16:437–446.
5. Parker R, Lindstrom D, Cotton R. Improved survival accounts for most, but not all, of the increase in bronchopulmonary dysplasia. Pediatrics 1992; 90:663–668.
6. Palta M, Gabbert D, Weinstein M, Peters M. Multivariate assessment of traditional risk factors for chronic lung disease in very low birth neonates. J Pediatr 1991; 119: 285–292.
7. Kraybill E, Runyan D, Bose C, Khan J. Risk factors for chronic lung disease in infants with birth weights of 751 to 1000 grams. J Pediatr 1989; 115:115–120.
8. Sinkin R, Cox C, Phelps D. Predicting risk for bronchopulmonary dysplasia: selection criteria for clinical trials. Pediatrics 1990; 86:728–736.
9. Van Marter L, Leviton A, Kuban K, Pagano M, Allred E. Maternal glucocorticoid therapy and reduced risk of bronchopulmonary dysplasia. Pediatrics 1990; 86:331–336.
10. Doyle L, Kitchen W, Ford G, Rickards A, Lissenden J, Ryan M. Effects of antenatal steroid therapy on mortality and morbidity in very low birth weight infants. J Pediatr 1986; 108:287–292.
11. Papageorgiou A, Doray J, Ardila R, Kunos I. Reduction of mortality, morbidity and respiratory distress syndrome in infants weighing less than 1000 g by treatment with betamethasone and ritodrine. Pediatrics 1989; 83:493–497.

12. National Institutes of Health (NIH) Consensus Conference. Effects of corticosteroids for fetal maturation. JAMA 1995; 273:413–418.
13. Groneck P, Gotze-Speer B, Oppermann M, Eiffert H, Speer CP. Association of pulmonary inflammation and increased microvascular permeability during the development of bronchopulmonary dysplasia: sequential analysis of inflammatory mediators in respiratory fluids of high-risk preterm neonates. Pediatrics 1994; 93:712–718.
14. Watterberg KL, Scott SM. Evidence of early adrenal insufficiency in babies who develop bronchopulmonary dysplasia. Pediatrics 1995; 95:120–125.
15. Watterberg KL, Scott SM. Babies who develop bronchopulmonary dysplasia and chronic lung disease have decreased serum cortisol in the first week of life. Pediatr Res 1995; 37:2116A.
16. Eronen M, Pesonen E, Kurki T, Teramo K, Hylikorkala O, Hallman M. Increased incidence of bronchopulmonary dysplasia after antenatal administration of indomethacin to prevent preterm labor. J Pediatr 1994; 124:782–788.
17. Avery M, Tooley W, Keller J, Hurd S, Bryan H, Cotton R, Epstein M, Fitzhardinge P, Hansen C, Hansen T, Hodson A, James L, Kitterman J, Nielsen H, Poirier T, Truog W, Wung J. Is chronic lung disease in low birth weight infants preventable? A survey of eight centers. Pediatrics 1987; 79:26–30.
18. Horbar J, McAuliffe T, Adler S, Albersheim S, Cassady G, Edwards W, Jones R, Kattwinkel J, Kraybill E, Krishnan V, Raschko P, Wilkinson A. Variability in 28-day outcomes for very low birth weight infants: an analysis of 11 neonatal intensive care units. Pediatrics 1988; 82:554–559.
19. Shennan A, Dunn M, Ohlsson A, Lennox K, Hoskins E. Abnormal pulmonary outcomes in premature infants: prediction from oxygen requirement in the neonatal period. Pediatrics 1988; 82:527–532.
20. Rishi A, Hatzis D, McAlmon K, Floros J. An allelic variant of the 6A gene for human surfactant protein A. Am J Physiol 1992; 262(5 pt 1):L566–L573.
21. Richardson D, Torday J. Racial differences in predictive value of the lecithin/sphingomyelin ratio. Am J Obstet Gynecol 1994; 170:1273–1277.
22. Hafez M, el-Sallab S, Khashaba M, Risk M, el-Morsy A, Bassiony M, el-Kenawy F, Zaghloul W. Evidence of HLA-linked susceptibility gene(s) in respiratory distress syndrome. Dis Markers 1989; 7:201–208.
23. Myrianthopoulos NC, Churchill JA, Baszynski AJ. Respiratory distress syndrome in twins. Acta Genet Med Gemellol 1971; 20:199–204.
24. Lankenau HM. A genetic and statistical study of the respiratory distress syndrome. Eur J Pediatr 1976; 123:167–177.
25. Graven S, Mesenheimer H. Respiratory distress syndrome and the high risk mother. Am J Dis Child 1965; 109:489–494.
26. Nagourney B, Usher R, Kramer M. Is there a familial tendency in the etiology of respiratory distress syndrome? Pediatr Res 1990; 27:1288.
27. Nickerson BF, Taussig LM. Family history of asthma in infants with bronchopulmonary dysplasia. Pediatrics 1980; 65:1140–1145.
28. Smith J, Tabachnik E, Duncan W, Reilly B, Levison H. Pulmonary function and bronchial hyperreactivity in long-term survivors of bronchopulmonary dysplasia. Pediatrics 1981; 68:336–340.
29. Floros J, Veletza V, Kotikalapudi P, Krizkova L, Karinch A, Friedman C, Buchter

S, Marks K. Dinucleotide repeats in the human surfactant protein B gene and respiratory distress syndrome. Biochem J 1995; 305:583–590.

30. Nogee L, deMello D, Dehner L, Colten H. Deficiency of pulmonary surfactant protein B in congenital alveolar proteinosis. N Engl J Med 1993; 328:406–410.
31. Garland J, Buck R, Allred E, Leviton A. Hypocarbia before surfactant therapy appears to increase bronchopulmonary dysplasia risk in infants with respiratory distress syndrome. Arch Pediatr Adolesc Med 1995; 149:617–622.
32. Palta M, Gabbert D, Fryback D, Widjaja I, Peters M, Farrell P, Johnson J. Development and validation of an index for scoring baseline respiratory disease in the very low birth weight neonate. Pediatrics 1990; 86:714–721.
33. Kraybill E, Bose C, D'Ercole A. Chronic lung disease in infants with very low birth weight. A population-based study. Am J Dis Child 1987; 141:784–788.
34. Bancalari E, Sosenko I. Pathogenesis and prevention of neonatal chronic lung disease: recent developments. Pediatr Pulmonol 1990; 8:109–116.
35. Bardin C, Papageorgiou A. Outcome of infants born between 22 and 25 weeks gestation. Clin Invest Med 1995; 18:a45.
36. Cohen A, Taeusch H. Prediction of risk of bronchopulmonary dysplasia. Am J Perinatol 1983; 1:21–22.
37. Toce S, Farrell P, Leavitt L, Samuels D, Edwards D. Clinical and roentgenographic scoring systems for assessing bronchopulmonary dysplasia. Am J Dis Child 1984; 138:581–585.
38. Van Lierde S, Smith J, Devlieger H, Eggermont E. Outcome of respiratory distress syndrome at 28 days: a prospective longitudinal study. Eur Respir J 1992; 5:1243–1248.
39. Shaw N, Ruggins N, Cooke R. Infants with chronic lung disease: predictors of mortality at day 28. J Perinatol 1993; 13:464–467.
40. Klein J, Nielsen H. Androgen regulation of epidermal growth factor receptor binding activity during fetal rabbit lung development. J Clin Invest 1993; 91:425–431.
41. Yip Y, Tan K. Bronchopulmonary dysplasia in very low birth weight infants. J Pediatr Child Health 1991; 27:34–38.
42. Bos AP, Hussain SM, Hazebroek FW, Tibboel D, Meradji M, Molenaar JC. Radiographic evidence of bronchopulmonary dysplasia in survivors of congenital diaphragmatic hernia. Pediatr Pulmonol 1993; 15:231–234.
43. Ijsselstijn H, Tibboel D, Hop WJ, Molenaar JC, de Jongste JC. Long-term pulmonary sequelae in children with congenital diaphragmatic hernia. Am J Respir Crit Care Med 1997; 155:174–180.
44. Vergani P, Locatelli A, Strobelt N, Mariani S, Cavallone M, Arosio P, Ghidini A. Amnioinfusion for prevention of pulmonary hypoplasia in second-trimester rupture of membranes. Am J Perinatol 1997; 14(6):325–329.
45. Yuksel B, Greenoough A, Gamsu HR. Neonatal meconium aspiration syndrome and respiratory morbidity during infancy. Pediatr Pulmonol 1993; 16:358–361.
46. Weinstein M, Peters M, Sadek M, Palta M. A new radiographic scoring system for bronchopulmonary dysplasia. Pediatr Pulmonol 1994; 18:284–289.
47. Ehrenkranz R, Verter J, Fanaroff A, Wright L, Stevenson D, Shankaran S, Papile L, Donovan E. Predicting BPD and oxygen dependence at 36 weeks post-conceptional age. Pediatr Res 1995; 37:330*A*.

48. Hansen T, Wallack M, Dey A, Boivin P, Vohr B, Oh W. Prognostic value of clinical and radiological status on day 28 of life for subsequent course in very low birthweight (< 1500 g) babies with bronchopulmonary dysplasia. Pediatr Pulmonol 1993; 15:327–331.
49. Van Marter L, Pagano M, Allred E, Leviton A, Kuban K. Rate of bronchopulmonary dysplasia as a function of neonatal intensive care practices. J Pediatr 1992; 120:938–946.
50. Ariagno R, Fulroth R, Baldwin R, Glotzbach S. Incidence of bronchopulmonary dysplasia, growth failures, and pulmonary dysfunction assessed by clinical scoring. J Perinatol 1991; 11:311–314.
51. Northway W, Rosan R, Porter D. Pulmonary disease following respirator therapy of hyaline membrane disease. N Engl J Med 1967; 276:357–368.
52. Edwards D, Colby T, Northway W. Radiographic–pathologic correlation in bronchopulmonary dysplasia. J Pediatr 1979; 95:834–836.
53. Goldman S, Gerhardt T, Sonni R, Feller R, Hehre D, Tapia J, Bancalari E. Early prediction of chronic lung disease by pulmonary function testing. J Pediatr 1983; 102:613–616.
54. Shaw N. On prognostication of bronchopulmonary dysplasia. Pediatr Pulmonol 1994; 18:122.
55. Robertson B, Taeusch HW, eds. Surfactant Therapy for Lung Disease. New York: Marcel Dekker, 1995.
56. Rojas M, Gonzalez A, Bancalari E, Claure N, Poole C, Silva-Neta, G. Changing trends in the epidemiology and pathogenesis of neonatal chronic lung disease. J Pediatr 1995; 126:605–610.
57. Avery M, Fletcher B. The Lung and Its Disorders in the Newborn Infant, Vol. 1. Philadelphia: WB Saunders, 1974.
58. Mayes L, Perkett E, Stahlman M. Severe bronchopulmonary dysplasia: a retrospective review. Acta Paediatr Scand 1983; 72:225–229.
59. Knight DB. Patent ductus arteriosus: how important to which babies? Early Hum Dev 1992; 29:287–292.
60. Van Marter L, Leviton A, Allred E, Pagano M, Kuban K. Hydration during the first days of life and the risk of bronchopulmonary dysplasia in low birth weight infants. J Pediatr 1990; 116:942–949.
61. Tammela O, Koivisto ME. Fluid restriction for preventing bronchopulmonary dysplasia? Reduced fluid intake during the first weeks of life improves the outcome of low-birth-weight infants. Acta Paediatr 1992; 81:207–212.
62. Berg TJ, Pagtakhan RD, Reed MH. BPD and lung rupture in hyaline membrane disease: influence of continuing distending pressure. Pediatrics 1975; 75:80–84.
63. Gaylord MS, Thieme RE, Woodall DL, Quissell BJ. Predicting mortality in low birth weight infants with pulmonary interstitial emphysema. Pediatrics 1985; 76:219–224.
64. Stahlman M, Cheatham W, Gray ME. The role of air dissection in bronchopulmonary dysplasia. J Pediatr 1979; 95:878–880.
65. Takasaki J, Ogawa Y. Interleukin 8 and granulocyte elastase alpha 1 proteinase inhibitor complex in the tracheobronchial aspirate of infants with chronic lung disease following intrauterine infection. Acta Paediatr Jpn 1996; 38:132–136.

3

Clinical Course and Lung Function Abnormalities During Development of Neonatal Chronic Lung Disease

EDUARDO BANCALARI and ALVARO GONZALEZ

University of Miami School of Medicine
Miami, Florida

I. Introduction

Despite the considerable advances in the prevention and management of respiratory distress syndrome (RDS), neonatal chronic lung disease (CLD) persists as one of the major complications in premature infants who require prolonged mechanical ventilation (1–3). Moreover, the increasing survival of very immature infants has produced an increase in the number of infants with CLD, with variations in incidence among institutions that range from 15 to 50% in infants with birth weights lower than 1500 g (4–8).

Described originally by Northway and colleagues in 1967 (9), bronchopulmonary dysplasia (BPD) is the chronic lung damage that results from multiple injuries to the immature lung. The clinical presentation and severity of BPD varies widely, ranging from the small premature infant who needs low levels of supplemental oxygen and mechanical ventilation for a few weeks, to more severely affected infants who remain ventilator-dependent for months or years, or who die of severe cardiopulmonary failure.

The "classic" or original form of BPD was observed primarily in preterm infants who had severe RDS and received high inspired oxygen concentration and prolonged mechanical ventilation with very high positive-airway pressures.

Their clinical and roentgenographic course was described in four stages, ending with the severe chronic lung damage characterized by persistent respiratory failure and a chest radiograph that reveals areas of increased density owing to fibrosis and collapse, surrounded by areas of marked hyperinflation and emphysema. In recent years, however, with improvements in respiratory care and the introduction of exogenous surfactant, this form of severe CLD is becoming less common and has been replaced by less severe forms of lung disease that are observed more frequently in small premature infants who survive after prolonged mechanical ventilation (7,10–12). A large proportion of infants who acquire this milder form of chronic lung damage have had no RDS, or mild RDS that improves quickly after surfactant administration, and that requires mechanical ventilation because of apnea and poor respiratory effort. These infants, therefore, are not being exposed to high airway pressures or inspired oxygen concentrations, but they often are adversely influenced by nosocomial infections and a patent ductus arteriosus (PDA), both of which have been identified as important pathogenic factors in the development of CLD (12).

Because the term BPD is usually associated with the more severe forms of lung damage, and most infants today have the milder forms, we prefer to use the term neonatal chronic lung disease to include all forms and leave the term BPD to describe only the more severe cases that fit the stage IV criteria originally described by Northway (9). This chapter describes the clinical characteristics, evolution, and initial lung function abnormalities of these two forms of chronic lung disease.

II. Definition and Incidence

The reported incidence of CLD varies widely. This is due not only to differences in patient populations and in management, but also to different criteria used to define CLD. Some authors include only patients with a clinical and roentgenographic evolution that fits the original description by Northway et al. (9). Most clinicians are using a more liberal definition of *CLD*, which includes *all patients who after mechanical ventilation remain oxygen dependent for more than 28 days and who have persistent abnormal changes on their chest radiographs* (13). Some authors have simplified this definition to the need of oxygen supplementation for more than 28 days or at the 28th day of postnatal age, without specifying radiographic changes. These definitions, although simpler, are more likely to include infants without clear-cut CLD. Another proposed definition is persistent oxygen requirement up to 36 weeks postconceptional age (14). The problem with this definition is that it excludes an appreciable number of extremely immature infants (23–26 weeks gestation) who require prolonged mechanical ventilation and oxygen supplementation (2–3 months) and have persistent radiographic changes, whereas it inappropriately includes larger infants (33–35 weeks gestation) who may be considered to have CLD after only 1–3 weeks of oxygen exposure. Consequently, we prefer to use the definition of oxygen dependency for 28 days or more, with persistent radiographic changes, because it is more representative of the presence of chronic lung damage in premature infants. The data from our center, presented later in this chapter, are based on this definition.

There are also several differences in the base population, such as race, proportion of males, proportion of inborn infants, altitude, or others, that may affect the incidence of CLD. Differences in management, such as the indications for intermittent positive-pressure ventilation (IPPV) and fluid management, and the survival rate of ventilated infants also influence the incidence of CLD.

The incidence of CLD in mechanically ventilated infants with RDS and a birth weight of 1500 g or less who survive ranges between 15 and 50%. This incidence is closely related to the gestational age and birth weight. Although CLD can occur in full-term infants, it is uncommon in infants born after 32–34 weeks of gestation. The incidence of CLD at the University of Miami/Jackson Memorial Medical Center in recent years is 22% in the survivors with birth weight between 500 and 1500 g who received mechanical ventilation. Most cases occur in extreme premature infants who weigh less than 1000 g at birth, who have an incidence of 33%, whereas among those infants who weigh between 1000 and 1500 g at birth, the incidence is close to 2%. Figure 1 illustrates the incidence of CLD in infants less than 1500 g born in our institution in years 1995 and 1996.

III. Clinical Presentation

The diagnosis of CLD is based on the clinical and roentgenographic manifestations, but these are nonspecific. With rare exceptions, the development of CLD occurs in a premature infant and follows the use of mechanical ventilation with intermittent positive-pressure during the first weeks after birth. Mechanical ventilation is usually indicated for respiratory failure resulting from RDS, but also may be required for other causes of respiratory failure. The development of CLD is often suspected when mechanical ventilation and oxygen dependence extend beyond 10–14 days. Nonetheless, definitive roentgenographic features do not typically develop until later in the course, usually close to the third or fourth week postnatally. Although the clinical presentation varies widely, there are two major forms that differ not only in their manifestations, but may also have different pathogenic mechanisms.

A. "Classic" or Severe Form of CLD

This classic form of CLD was more common before the introduction of exogenous surfactant therapy, and it is usually seen after severe respiratory distress

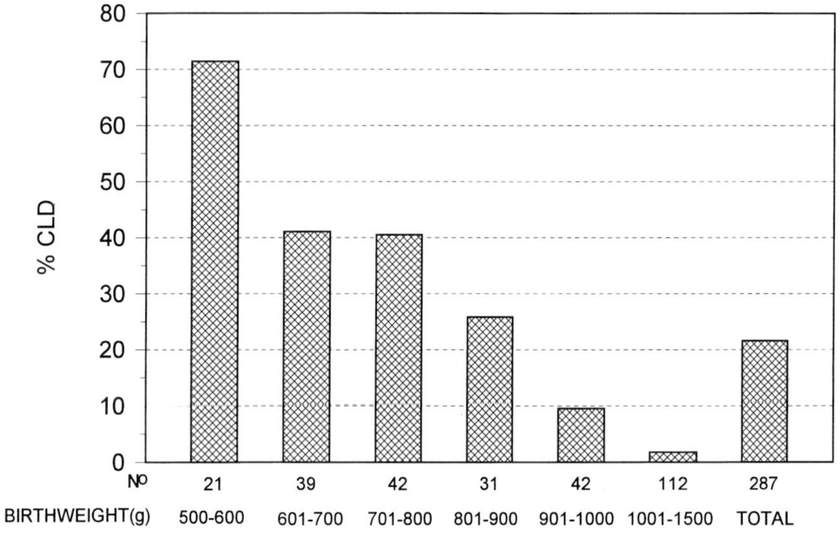

Figure 1 Incidence of CLD by birth weight in infants weighing less than 1500 g born in years 1995–1996 at the University of Miami/Jackson Memorial Medical Center. All infants received mechanical ventilation and survived more than 28 days.

syndrome (RDS). These infants require mechanical ventilation with high airway pressures and inspired oxygen concentrations during the first week of life, and not infrequently, the course is complicated by a pneumothorax or pulmonary interstitial emphysema (PIE). These complications require increases in ventilatory support and inspired oxygen concentration, which further aggravate the lung damage. Other complications, such as persistent patency of a ductus arteriosus, with associated heart failure and pulmonary edema, as well as nosocomial infections frequently develop in these patients and contribute to the progression in severity of chronic lung damage.

Despite all therapeutic efforts, these infants remain ventilator-dependent beyond 14 days and chronic radiographic changes, such as densities, linear–reticular opacities, and occasionally cystic changes begin to appear at this stage. These infants usually remain oxygen-dependent and acquire pulmonary radiographic changes that are characterized by hyperinflation and patchy atelectasis (Fig. 2). The roentgenographic progression of BPD through the sequence of four stages, originally described by Northway et al. (9), is now infrequent. The roentgenographic appearance of stage I is essentially indistinguishable from that of uncomplicated RDS. Dense parenchymal opacification, as described in stage II BPD, is commonly due to other processes, such as congestive heart failure from a patent

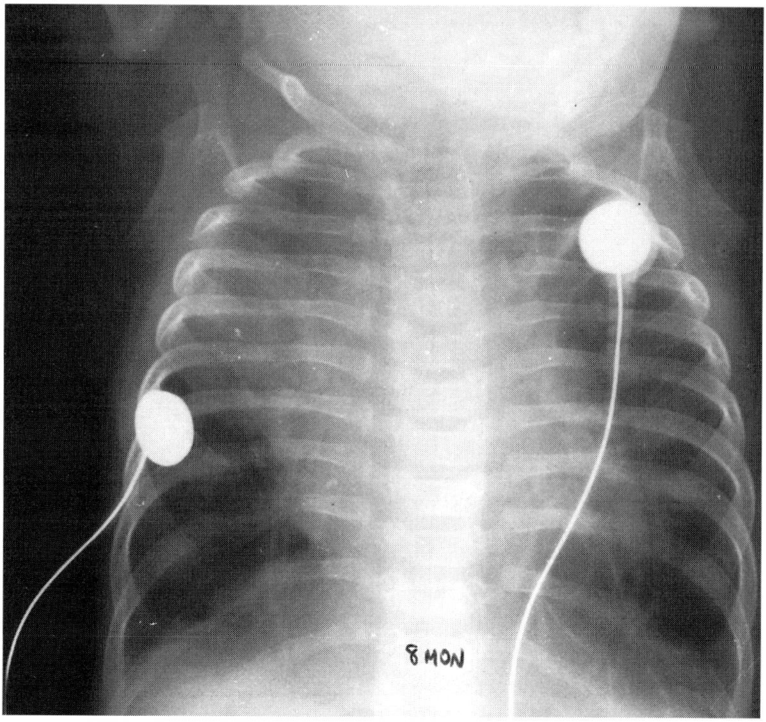

Figure 2 Chest radiograph of an infant with a severe form of CLD.

ductus arteriosus (PDA), fluid overload, or pulmonary hemorrhage. The bubble-like pattern of stage III BPD is not always seen, and when it does occur, it does not always follow a period of parenchymal opacity. Finally, the roentgenographic development of the more advanced form of BPD (stage IV) may be more insidious than originally described, and it usually appears after 3–4 weeks of positive-pressure ventilation. The major features of stage IV BPD include hyperinflation and nonhomogeneity of pulmonary tissue, with multiple fine or coarser densities extending to the periphery (see Fig. 2).

Despite surfactant administration, severe RDS sometimes can progress to severe lung damage, especially if there is a delay in administration of surfactant, or if an insufficient dose is given. The use of surfactant is not always harmless; occasionally it is associated with complications that can aggravate the respiratory course. In most instances, however, surfactant administration produces rapid improvement in oxygenation and lung function, especially in lung volume of infants with RDS (15–17). Accordingly, infants receiving exogenous surfactant should be closely monitored, and the ventilatory settings decreased as soon as there are signs of improvement. Failure to do this may result in lung overdistention, which may lead to pneumothorax or PIE. This can further aggravate the respiratory failure and require increases in the ventilatory and oxygen support, thereby increasing lung damage from excessive parenchymal stretch and oxygen toxicity. Pulmonary hemorrhage is another complication of exogenous surfactant therapy, which is more frequent in the more immature infants (18,19). When the hemorrhage is severe, blood enters the air spaces and inactivates surfactant, with resultant worsening of respiratory failure and increased need for ventilatory support.

Other causes of initial severe respiratory failure are also associated with the development of CLD, such as pneumonia, lung hypoplasia, and meconium aspiration syndrome. Among these, pneumonia is the most important, and group B streptococci (GBS) is the most frequent organism isolated in early neonatal sepsis. GBS infection often leads to failure of multiple organ systems, and respiratory failure, in particular, may be life-threatening. Radiographically, GBS pneumonia cannot be distinguished from a severe RDS, but the response to surfactant replacement is usually short-lived or absent, requiring a high degree of ventilatory support for prolonged periods. Frequently, GBS pneumonia is complicated by air leaks, shock, and persistent pulmonary hypertension. These infants may die early of cardiorespiratory failure, and among those who survive, particularly those who are extremely premature, a substantial number become afflicted with CLD. Although less common, nosocomial pneumonia caused by other microorganisms such as gram-negative bacteria, may produce a similar pattern of lung damage (see Chap. 8).

With the introduction of surfactant replacement and improvements in ventilator management, the incidence of this severe form of CLD decreased considerably. Table 1 shows the effect of the introduction of surfactant treatment in the

Table 1 Influence of the Introduction of Exogenous Surfactant in the Incidence of Severe RDS and CLD in Infants ≤ 1000 g born at UM/JMH between 1989 and 1994

	Presurfactant (89–90) $n = 57$	Postsurfactant (92–94) $n = 243$
Severe RDS	17/57 (30%)	26/243 (11%)
Mild or no RDS	40/57 (70%)	217/243 (89%)
CLD in severe RDS	13/17 (76%)	20/26 (77%)
CLD in mild or no RDS	13/40 (32%)	76/217 (35%)
Total CLD	26/47 (46%)	96/243 (39%)
CLD from severe RDS	13/26 (50%)	20/96 (21%)
CLD from mild RDS	13/26 (50%)	76/96 (79%)

incidence of severe RDS and CLD in our institution. The incidence of severe initial respiratory failure decreased from 30 to 11%, and consequently the proportion of infants with CLD and who initially presented with severe respiratory distress has declined considerably. Currently, this pattern of disease progression accounts for less than one-fourth of all the infants who acquire CLD in our institution.

Severe forms of RDS are more common in boys and in whites, and are inversely related to the gestational age of the infant (20–22). All these characteristics are also important risk factors for the development of CLD. The ultimate factors that produce the lung injury are the exposure to high positive airway pressures and high inspired oxygen concentration in an infant with an immature lung. The role of each of these variables in the development of lung injury is discussed in detail in other sections of this book.

Evolution of Severe CLD

As a result of the severe lung damage, these infants present signs of chronic respiratory failure, such as tachypnea, chest retractions, and frequent episodes of cyanosis (hypoxemia), especially with agitation and nursing procedures. Blood gas measurements usually reveal persistent CO_2 retention. Figure 3 illustrates the typical pattern of the oxygen requirement of these infants during the first month of life. Oxygen need starts high because of the severe initial respiratory failure, and then remains moderately elevated over time, usually for several weeks. Pulmonary edema frequently develops in these infants, complicating their respiratory course. This can be associated with reopening of the ductus arteriosus, or it may be a manifestation of the lung damage, with associated capillary leak of protein-rich fluid. The patients frequently have rales on auscultation, and chest radiographs reveal lung opacification. Fluid restriction, diuretics, and prompt intervention to close the PDA usually improve this condition. CLD is also characterized by an increased airway resistance (23,24), which manifests clinically with tachypnea, wheezing with scattered or diffuse rhonchi on auscultation, overexpansion of the lungs on the chest radiograph, and hypercapnia. The cause of this increased resistance is multifactorial, including airway inflammation, with hyperplasia and metaplasia of bronchial epithelium, increased production of mucus from glandular hyperplasia, mucosal edema, localized infections, and bronchial hyperreactivity. These infants may also develop large-airway damage, with bronchomalacia that can lead to severe dynamic airway obstruction, especially during episodes of agitation and increased intrathoracic pressure (25,26). Many infants with CLD have lobar or segmental atelectasis resulting from retained secretions and airway obstruction.

Acute pulmonary infection, either bacterial or viral, frequently complicates the course of the disease, sometimes resulting in respiratory failure and even death in infants with severe lung damage (27).

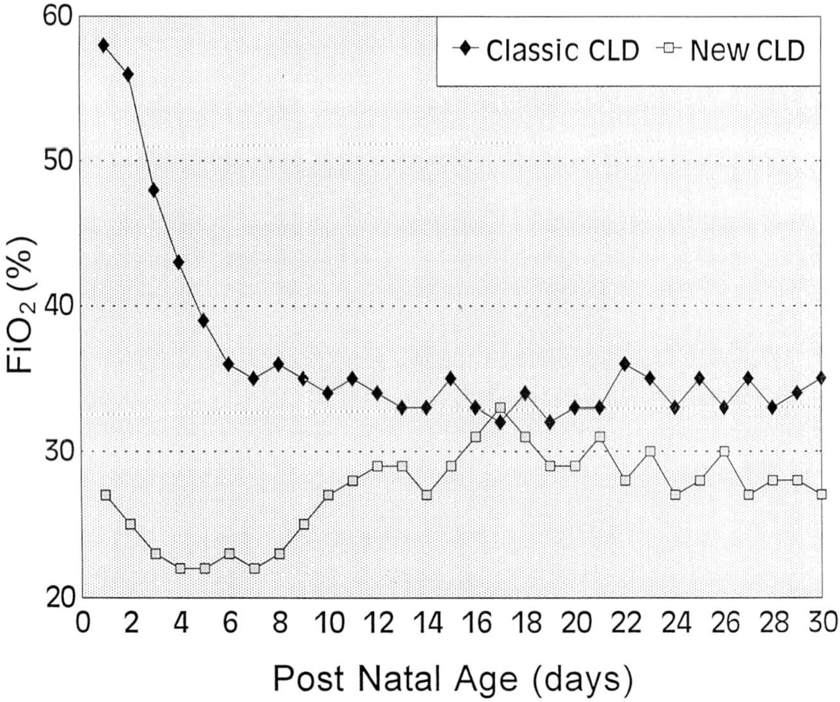

Figure 3 Evolution of oxygen requirement in the two forms of CLD.

Infants with more severe disease frequently display signs of right ventricular failure secondary to pulmonary hypertension, with cardiomegaly, hepatomegaly, and fluid retention (28). The electrocardiogram (ECG) shows signs of right ventricular hypertrophy, which can be confirmed by echocardiography. In some infants anastomoses may develop between the systemic and pulmonary circulations, which may further aggravate pulmonary hypertension (28). Cor pulmonale is less common now, as CLD is usually less severe than it was two decades ago, and there is greater emphasis on maintaining normal arterial oxygenation.

Outcome of Severe CLD

Once lung damage has developed, these infants require mechanical ventilation and increased inspired oxygen concentrations for several weeks, months, or sometimes years. Infants with more severe lung damage may die of progressive respiratory failure, cor pulmonale, or acute complications, especially intercurrent infections. Mortality rates of about 30–40% have been reported in infants with severe CLD, and most of them occur during the first year of life, secondary to respiratory failure, sepsis, or intractable cor pulmonale (28,29).

Most survivors show slow but steady improvement in their lung function (24) and roentgenographic pictures, and after variable time periods they can be weaned from the ventilator and oxygen therapy. After extubation, most infants continue to have chest wall retractions and tachypnea, and they frequently have rales and bronchial sounds on auscultation.

Because of the respiratory failure, infants with CLD take oral feedings with difficulty, and frequently require nasogastric or orogastric feeding. Although weight gain is usually below the expected normal for their age, children who receive adequate oxygen supplementation and appropriate nutritional support may achieve consistent rates of growth (30,31). The lower weight gain is multifactorial, and among the mechanisms that may limit growth are a higher energy expenditure required by the increased work of breathing, increased oxygen consumption, inadequate caloric intake, and chronic hypoxemia (32–34). Adequate nutrition is important for lung growth and repair, and nutritional deficits may impair recovery and adversely affect the outcome of these infants (35). With adequate nutrition, oxygen therapy, and control of infections and heart failure, gradual improvement in pulmonary function may be accompanied by resolution of cor pulmonale and roentgenographic evidence of healing.

Among the survivors with CLD, lower respiratory tract infections are common during the first 2 years of life (36). Although their exact incidence is difficult to ascertain from the literature, not infrequently they require hospitalization for prolonged periods. Frequently, no specific organisms are isolated, suggesting a viral etiology. Episodes of wheezing and airway obstruction are also common during the first 2 years of life, and infection with respiratory syncytial virus can be life-threatening (27). Acute roentgenographic evidence of hyperinflation may be difficult to appreciate in infants with severe BPD because their baseline radiograph often shows lung overexpansion. Such acute episodes of airway obstruction may be accompanied by the radiographic appearance of focal, segmental, and transient atelectasis.

Pulmonary function studies in infants with severe CLD have shown that pulmonary function may remain abnormal for many years, even though the infants may be asymptomatic (37). A high incidence of obstructive airway disease has been observed at 8 years of age in a small group of survivors with BPD (38). Northway and associates have recently reevaluated pulmonary function in their original cohort of infants with severe BPD reported in 1967 (39). At an age ranging between 14 and 23 years, these adolescents and young adults still exhibited some evidence of pulmonary dysfunction, characterized by airway obstruction, airway hyperreactivity, and hyperinflation. The ultimate clinical consequences of these findings remain to be determined, but most long-term studies suggest that, with growth, pulmonary function tends to improve.

Infants with severe CLD also have more neurodevelopmental sequelae when compared with control groups, and they exhibit impaired growth curves (40–44). Although data from longer-term studies are not yet available, it is apparent that neurodevelopmental prognosis also depends on the severity of the CLD and on the presence of other risk factors for developmental delays that occur frequently in infants with CLD, such as intracranial hemorrhage, hearing impairment, and retinopathy of prematurity. Infants with CLD have also been reported to have an increased risk for sudden infant death but the evidence for this is not conclusive (45,46).

B. "New" or Mild Form of CLD

Most small premature infants who acquire CLD at present have a mild initial respiratory course and require ventilatory support for management of apnea and poor respiratory effort. These infants represent 79% of all infants diagnosed with CLD in our institution (see Table 1). In contrast with infants with severe CLD, these infants require mechanical ventilation with low pressures and oxygen concentration; therefore, they are not exposed to pressure-induced trauma and oxygen toxicity. The typical oxygen requirement for these infants is illustrated in Figure 3. These infants require low or moderate initial concentrations of oxygen for treatment of mild RDS that usually responds favorably to exogenous surfactant. This is often followed by a few days with minimal or no supplemental oxygen need (''honeymoon''). Many of these infants, however, have a progressive deterioration in their lung function over time, wherein their ventilatory and oxygen requirements increase, accompanied by signs of respiratory failure (tachypnea, retractions, and such). This deterioration is frequently triggered by bacterial or viral infections or heart failure secondary to a PDA. In these patients, the functional and roentgenographic lung changes are usually mild, sometimes showing only diffuse haziness that persists over time, without the more coarse changes of nonuniform inflation and cystic nature that is often observed in the classic severe form CLD (Fig. 4).

We have recently reported an epidemiological study to identify the main risk factors that predispose these infants to CLD (12). The results revealed that after prematurity, the presence of episodes of symptomatic PDA and infections were associated with a significantly higher risk for the development of CLD (Fig. 5). Furthermore, when both complications (PDA and infection) occurred at the same time, they produced a synergistic interaction, further increasing their effect on the development of CLD. As a consequence of the left-to-right shunting through the PDA, pulmonary blood flow and lung fluid increase, negatively affecting lung function and gas exchange and, thereby, increasing the risk for CLD (47–49). There is also compelling evidence that supports the role of infection and inflammation in the pathogenesis of CLD (50). Prolonged neutrophil influx

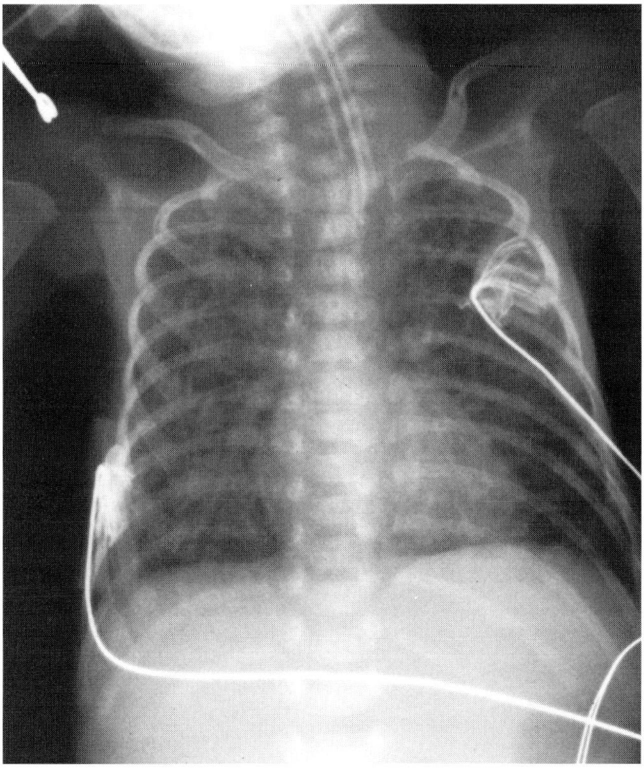

Figure 4 Chest radiograph of an infant with mild or new form of CLD.

and increased cytokine activity in bronchoalveolar lavage (BAL) fluid have been associated with an increased likelihood of CLD in ventilator-dependent premature infants (51,52). Colonization with specific microorganisms, such as cytomegalovirus and *Ureaplasma urealyticum* have also been associated with increased risk for CLD (53–55). Searching for an explanation for this interaction between PDA and infections, we have demonstrated that the presence of infection in the premature infant adversely affects permanent closure of the ductus, often inducing late ductal opening and failure to respond to medical treatment with indomethacin (56). One possible mechanism for this interaction is the elevated serum level of prostaglandins and tumor necrosis factor (TNF) observed in infants with infections. In addition, infants with infections frequently have complications that delay or impede the treatment of the PDA. As a result, the ductus remains open for prolonged periods, maintaining an increased pulmonary blood flow, high capillary pressure, and pulmonary edema.

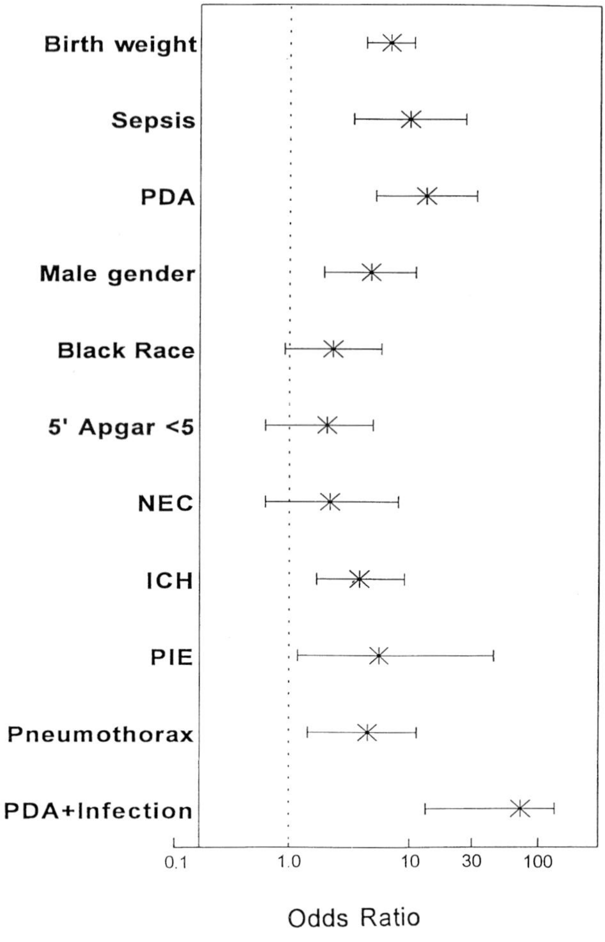

Figure 5 Odds ratios (*) and their 95% confidence intervals for predicting development of CLD, as assessed by logistic regression analysis of 119 infants with mild or no initial respiratory failure. Birthweight was analyzed per 100-g decrement.

Evolution of Mild CLD

As in infants with severe CLD, but to a lesser degree, infants with mild CLD also show signs of chronic respiratory failure, such as tachypnea, chest wall retractions, and frequent episodes of cyanosis (hypoxemia), especially with agitation, and mild hypercapnia. As observed in Figure 3, the oxygen dependence of these infants is moderate. Chronic pulmonary edema occurs frequently and is manifest by rales on auscultation and a chest radiograph revealing diffuse lung opacification. These infants also may have signs of increased airway resistance (tachypnea, wheezing, with scattered or diffuse rhonchi on auscultation, overexpanded lungs in the chest radiograph, and hypercapnia), but this is usually not as pronounced as in the infants with classic CLD. Some infants with mild CLD may also have lobar or segmental atelectasis resulting from retained secretions and airway obstruction. Signs of right ventricular failure secondary to pulmonary hypertension are uncommon in this milder form of CLD. Acute pulmonary infections, either bacterial or viral, may also complicate the course of these infants, but when they do occur, they are better tolerated with less lung dysfunction.

Outcome of Mild CLD

These infants also require mechanical ventilation and elevated inspired oxygen concentration for prolonged periods, usually several weeks or months. Occasionally, they may progress to more severe lung damage and die of progressive respiratory failure or acute complications, especially intercurrent infections. Most infants survive and show slow but steady improvement in their lung function and radiographic changes and, after variable periods, can be extubated and weaned from oxygen therapy.

Infants with this form of CLD are often difficult to feed, tolerate fluids poorly, and their growth is usually less than the expected rate of growth for infants of similar gestational ages.

With adequate nutrition, oxygen supplementation, and control of infections and heart failure, gradual improvement in pulmonary function is accompanied by roentgenographic evidence of healing. Lower respiratory tract infections are common during the first 2 years of life, and some infants require hospitalizations for episodes of acute airway obstruction and respiratory failure. There is limited follow-up data of pulmonary function in these infants, but the abnormalities are less pronounced and tend to improve during the first 3 years of life (24).

IV. Differential Diagnosis of CLD

The diagnosis of neonatal CLD is based on the clinical and roentgenographic course described earlier, but these signs are not specific for any given etiology. Although the pathogenesis of CLD is not conclusively established, it is accepted that the lung damage usually results from the interaction of a variety of factors, among which the most important are prematurity, mechanical ventilation with high airway pressures and increased inspired oxygen concentrations, PDA, and infections. Other factors that may lead to chronic lung damage and must be investigated before concluding that the infant has CLD are specific viral, fungal, or bacterial perinatal infections; congenital heart disease, such as total anomalous pulmonary venous drainage; pulmonary lymphangiectasia; chemical pneumonitis, resulting from recurrent aspiration; cystic fibrosis; and idiopathic pulmonary fibrosis.

Of all differential diagnostic possibilities, Wilson–Mikity syndrome has probably engendered the greatest confusion with BPD (57). The roentgenographic similarities have caused some investigators to associate the two conditions, although differences appear to exist in terms of their clinical course. Patients with Wilson–Mikity syndrome generally have an initially benign course, with an insidious onset of respiratory failure and roentgenographic abnormalities. In contrast, most patients with the severe form of CLD initially have a greater degree of acute respiratory failure and greater need for increased inspired oxygen concentrations and assisted ventilation. Thus, even though the final roentgenographic appearance of the two conditions can be indistinguishable, the characteristic clinical histories usually permit easy distinction of these two conditions. In recent years, for unknown reasons, there has been a notable decline in the incidence of this syndrome, which is rarely diagnosed today. It is likely that the cases described by Wilson and Mikity correspond to the milder form of CLD seen today in the smaller infants.

V. Lung Function During Development of CLD

The transition from a normal immature lung to CLD can occur at different postnatal ages, but usually occurs gradually during the first weeks of life. In infants with severe RDS, the acute lung injury usually occurs shortly after birth and is produced by mechanical ventilation with high airway pressures and inspired oxygen concentrations. In these infants, lung function remains abnormal, with sustained impairment of pulmonary compliance and gradual development of increased airway resistance, which characterizes lung function in CLD. This classic evolution from severe RDS to CLD has become less common with the use of prenatal steroids and the administration of exogenous surfactant. In infants with uncomplicated RDS, surfactant treatment results in a normalization of lung function within 12–24 hr (15–17). Most infants with CLD today have a later deterioration in lung function that is usually secondary to complications, such as a PDA or nosocomial infections (12,56). These triggering events produce progressive respiratory failure, prolonging the need for mechanical ventilation and oxygen therapy, which contribute to the progression of disease.

It is clear that the risk for acquiring CLD is related to the severity of the initial respiratory failure. Consequently, several investigators have attempted to develop predictive models for CLD by relating the severity of the respiratory failure during the first days of life with the risk for CLD. These models are useful to identify populations at risk of CLD to be enrolled in preventive or therapeutic clinical trials. These studies have identified factors, such as low birth weight and gestational age, low Apgar score, male gender, and white race, as characteristics that increase the risk for CLD (5,58,59) (see Chap. 2).

A. Pulmonary Resistance

The availability of pulmonary function testing in critically ill neonates has afforded the possibility of using these measurements as a more accurate marker of lung damage and better predictor of CLD. With these tests, Goldman et al. (23) showed that infants who eventually acquired CLD had an increased airway resistance during the first week of life when compared with infants who recovered without lung sequelae (Fig. 6). Similar findings were reported by Motoyama et al. (60), who found increased airway reactivity during the first 3 weeks of life in infants with subsequent CLD, and by Gerhardt et al. (24), who measured decreased pulmonary conductance during the first year in infants with CLD (Fig. 7a). The underlying changes that explain this increased airway resistance in infants with evolving CLD include edema, hyperplasia and metaplasia of the airway epithelium, increased mucus secretion, with decreased clearance, and hypertrophy of airway smooth muscle. Release of inflammatory mediators also contribute to airway edema and bronchoconstriction in these infants (50,61).

B. Pulmonary Compliance

Pulmonary compliance is reduced during the early stages of CLD (see Fig. 7b). Several investigators have demonstrated that measured lung compliance in the

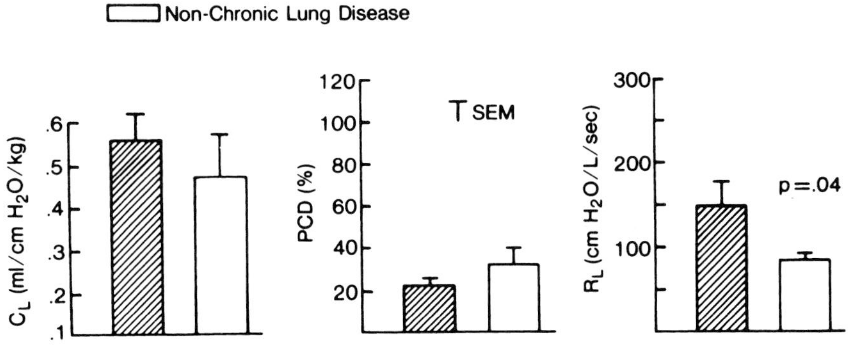

Figure 6 Mean values for compliance (C_L), pulmonary clearance delay (PCD), and resistance (R_L) are compared in infants who later acquired CLD and those who did not. The difference in resistance is statistically significant. (From Ref. 23.)

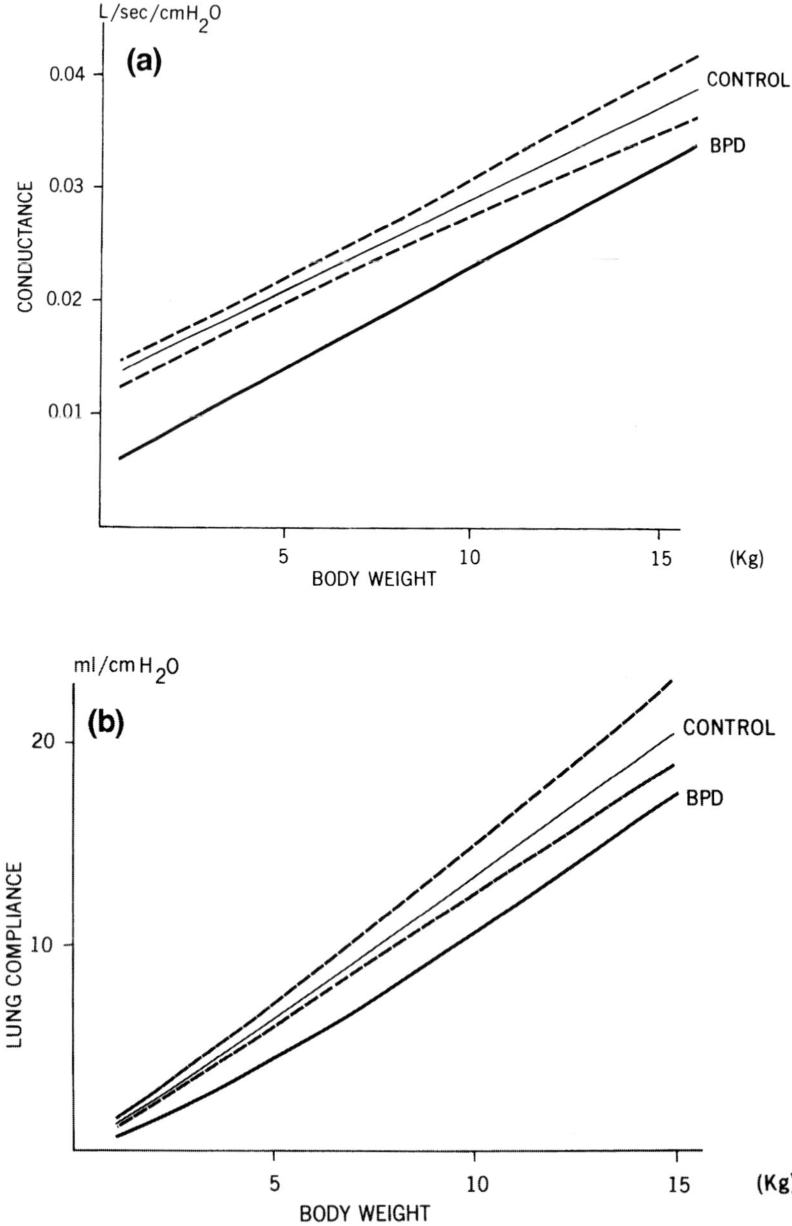

Figure 7 Relation of (a) pulmonary conductance and (b) lung compliance to body weight in infants with chronic lung disease (heavy line) and control infants (thin line and its 95% confidence limits). Both values tend to normalize as the infants grow during the first 3 years after birth. (From Ref. 24.)

first few days after birth has a strong predictive value for later development of CLD (17,62,63). Freezer and collaborators demonstrated that dynamic compliance measured on the first day of life in infants with RDS was a better independent predictor for the development of CLD than gestational age or birthweight (63). In contrast with this, other groups of investigators have been unable to correlate early measurements of pulmonary compliance with the subsequent development of CLD (23,64,65).

The reduction in lung compliance observed during early CLD is probably due to loss of lung volume and to the changes in elastic properties of the lung tissue secondary to edema and fibrosis. Dynamic compliance is further reduced because it becomes frequency-dependent as a result of increased airway resistance. Pulmonary hypertension, when severe, may also contribute to stiffening of the lungs (66).

C. Lung Volume

Measurements of lung volume during the early stages of CLD have shown a reduced functional residual capacity (FRC) that gradually increases to become normal or even higher than normal after several months of life (24) (Fig. 8). This increase in FRC may reflect the normalization of lung function in some infants, but in infants with severe CLD, it may reflect overinflation from severe airway obstruction and gas trapping.

VI. Therapeutic Interventions and Lung Function During Development of CLD

Several therapeutic interventions can modify lung function during the early stages of CLD. This is important because by ameliorating some of the early abnormalities in lung function it may be possible to change the course of the disease. The more basic and simplest intervention is to provide an inspired oxygen concentration sufficient to maintain normal oxygenation, as this can alleviate the severe bronchoconstriction that occurs in response to hypoxia in these infants (67). Bronchodilators can also help alleviate elevated airway resistance and decreased dynamic compliance in infants with CLD. (68–73).

The administration of diuretics also increases lung compliance and decrease airway resistance in these infants (74,75). The beneficial effects of diuretics are mediated not only by their renal effects, but also seem to be related to the direct influence that these drugs have on lung fluid balance (74,76–79). Despite the short-term beneficial effects of diuretics on lung function, they do not appear to modify the final outcome of the disease (80,81).

Because of the increasing evidence that inflammation plays a crucial role in the pathogenesis of CLD, various studies have been performed to evaluate the

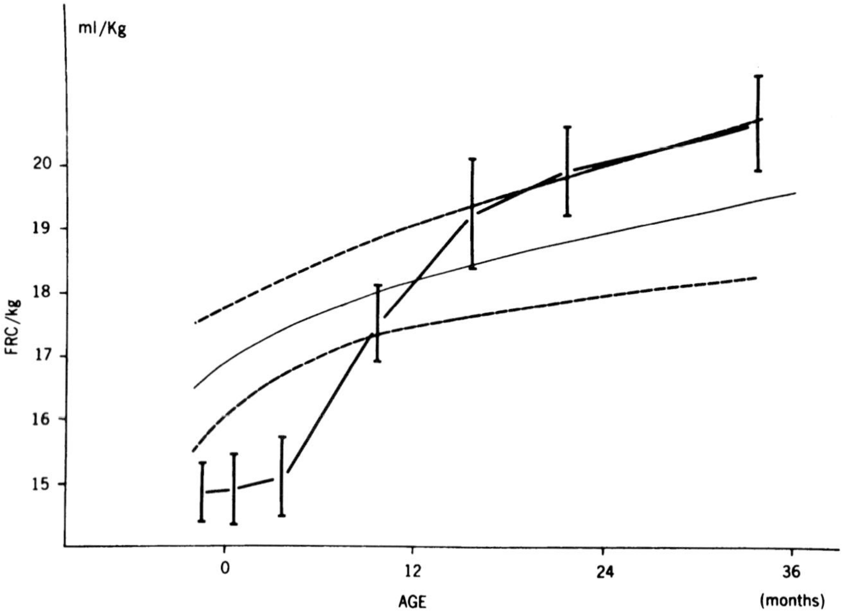

Figure 8 Sequential measurements of FRC per kilogram in infants with chronic lung disease (mean ± SE, heavy line). Measurements were shifted to left to correct for lower gestational age. For comparison, curves for normal infants (thin line) and its 95% confidence limits (dashed lines) are shown. (From Ref. 24.)

effects of systemic steroid administration during early stages of CLD (82–85). In most of these studies, systemic steroid administration has rapidly improved lung function, with an increase in compliance, decrease in airway resistance, and reduction in oxygen and ventilatory requirements. This facilitates weaning these infants from mechanical ventilation, thereby shortening the duration of mechanical ventilation.

In an attempt to minimize the side effects of these drugs, diuretics and steroids have been administered directly into the lungs by nebulization (86,87). Both drugs produced some improvement in lung compliance and resistance, with no noticeable side effects.

All these therapeutic interventions improve lung function and can accelerate the process of weaning ventilator-dependent infants. Although one would expect that faster weaning from high inspired oxygen levels and positive-pressure ventilation would result in less pulmonary damage and a lower incidence of CLD, there is still no conclusive evidence that intervention with any of these drugs modifies the overall incidence or severity of the disorder. Despite this lack of evidence of long-term beneficial effects, these pharmacological interventions have become part of the routine management of these infants because of the immediate improvement in lung function that they produce (see Chap. 12).

Looking into the future, it is likely that gentler ventilation strategies and pharmacological interventions to modulate the inflammatory process in the lung will lead to further reduction in the incidence and severity of CLD. Whether early measurements of pulmonary function will be useful in determining which ventilator strategies or pharmacological interventions are more effective needs to be evaluated. The predictive value of early measurements of pulmonary function for the development of CLD also needs to be reassessed now that the pathogenesis of CLD has changed and the severity of the lung damage is considerably milder than a few years ago. It will also be important to determine what the influence of these milder forms of CLD is on long-term pulmonary function of these children as they became adults.

References

1. Hack M, Horbar JD, Malloy MH, et al. Very low birth weight outcome of National Institute of Child Health and Human Development Neonatal Network. Pediatrics 1991; 87:587–597.
2. Horbar J, Soll RF, Sutherland JM, et al. A multicenter randomized, placebo-controlled trial of surfactant therapy for respiratory distress syndrome. N Engl J Med 1989; 320:959–965.
3. Truog WE, Prueitt JL, Woodrum DE. Unchanged incidence of bronchopulmonary dysplasia in survivors of hyaline membrane disease. J Pediatr 1978; 92:261–264.
4. Avery ME, Tooley WH, Keller JB, et al. Is chronic lung disease in low birth weight infants preventable? A survey of eight centers. Pediatrics 1987; 79:26–30.
5. Palta M, Gabbert D, Weinstein MR, et al. Multivariate assessment of traditional risk factors for chronic lung disease in very low birth weight neonates. J Pediatr 1991; 119:285–292.
6. Van Marter LJ, Gabbert D, Weinstein MR, et al. Rate of bronchopulmonary dysplasia as a function of neonatal intensive care practices. J Pediatr 1992; 120:938–946.
7. Parker RA, Pagano M, Allred EN. Improved survival accounts for most, but not all, of the increase in bronchopulmonary dysplasia. Pediatrics 1992; 90:663–668.
8. Horbar JD, McAuliffe TL, Adler SM, et al. Variability in 28-day outcomes for very low birth weight infants: an analysis of 11 neonatal intensive care units. Pediatrics 1988; 82:554–559.
9. Northway WH, Rosan RC, Porter DY. Pulmonary disease following respiratory therapy of hyaline membrane disease. Bronchopulmonary dysplasia. N Engl J Med 1967; 276:357–368.
10. Wung JT, Koons AH, Driscoll JM, James LS. Changing incidence of bronchopulmonary dysplasia. J Pediatr 1979; 95:845–847.
11. Heneghan MA, Sosulski R, Baquero JM. Persistent pulmonary abnormalities in new-

borns: the changing picture of bronchopulmonary dysplasia. Pediatr Radiol 1986; 16:180–184.
12. Rojas MA, Gonzalez A, Bancalari E, et al. Changing trends in the epidemiology and pathogenesis of neonatal chronic lung disease. J Pediatr 1995; 126:605–610.
13. Bancalari E, Abdenour GE, Feller R, Gannon J. Bronchopulmonary dysplasia: clinical presentation. J Pediatr 1979; 95:819–823.
14. Shennan AT, Dunn MS, Ohlsson A, et al. Abnormal pulmonary outcomes in premature infants: prediction from oxygen requirements in the neonatal period. Pediatrics 1988; 82:527–532.
15. Davis JM, Veness-Meehan K, Notter RH, et al. Changes in pulmonary mechanics after the administration of surfactant to infants with respiratory distress syndrome. N Engl J Med 1988; 319:476–479.
16. Goldsmith LS, Greenspan JS, Rubenstein SD, et al. Immediate improvement in lung volume after exogenous surfactant: alveolar recruitment versus increased distension. J Pediatr 1991; 119:750–755.
17. Bhutani VK, Abbasi S, Long W, et al. Pulmonary mechanics and energetics in preterm infants who had respiratory distress syndrome treated with synthetic surfactant. J Pediatr 1992; 120:S18–24.
18. Raju TNK, Langenber P. Pulmonary hemorrhage and exogenous surfactant therapy: a metaanalysis. J Pediatr 1993; 123:603–610.
19. Pappin A, Shenker N, Hack M. Extensive intraalveolar pulmonary hemorrhage in infants dying after surfactant therapy. J Pediatr 1994; 124:621–626.
20. Miller HC, Futrakul P. Birth weight, gestational age, and sex as determining factors in the incidence of respiratory distress syndrome of prematurely born infants. J Pediatr 1968; 72:628–635.
21. Farrell PM, Avery ME. Hyaline membrane disease. Am Rev Respir Dis 1975; 111: 657–687.
22. Perelman RH, Palta M, Kirby R, Farrell PM. Discordance between male and female deaths due to the respiratory distress syndrome. Pediatrics 1986; 78:238–244.
23. Goldman SL, Gerhardt T, Sonni R, et al. Early prediction of chronic lung disease by pulmonary function testing. J Pediatr 1983; 102:613–617.
24. Gerhardt T, Hehre D, Feller R, et al. Serial determination of pulmonary function in infants with chronic lung disease. J Pediatr 1987; 110:448–456.
25. Miller RW, Woo P, Kellman RK, Slagle TS. Tracheobronchial abnormalities in infants with bronchopulmonary dysplasia. J Pediatr 1987; 111:779–782.
26. McCubbin M, Frey EE, Wagener JS, et al. Large airway collapse in bronchopulmonary dysplasia. J Pediatr 1989; 114:304–307.
27. Groothuis JR, Gutierrez KM, Lauer BA. Respiratory syncytial virus infection in children with bronchopulmonary dysplasia. Pediatrics 1988; 82:199–203.
28. Goodman G, Perkin RM, Anas NG, et al. Pulmonary hypertension in infants with bronchopulmonary dysplasia. J Pediatr 1988; 112:67–72.
29. Shankaran S, Szego E, Eizert D, et al. Severe BPD: predictors of survival and outcome. Chest 1984; 88:607–610.
30. Abman SH, Accurso FJ, Koops BL. Experience with home oxygen in the management of infants with BPD. Clin Pediatr 1984; 23:471–476.

31. Groothuis JR, Rosenberg AA. Home oxygen promotes weight gain in infants with BPD. Pediatrics 1988; 82:199–203.
32. Kurzner SI, Garg M, Batista M, et al. Growth failure in BPD: elevated metabolic rates and pulmonary mechanics. J Pediatr 1988; 112:73–80.
33. Weinstein MR, Oh W. Oxygen consumption in infants with BPD. J Pediatr 1981; 99:958–961.
34. Koops BL, Abman SH, Accurso FJ. Outpatient management and follow-up of BPD. Clin Perinatol 1984; 11:101–122.
35. Sosenko IRS, Frank L. Nutritional influences on lung development and protection against chronic lung disease. Semin Perinatol 1991; 15:462–168.
36. Cunningham CK, McMillan JA, Gross SJ. Rehospitalization for respiratory illness in infants less than 32 weeks gestation. Pediatrics 1991; 88:527–533.
37. Blayney M, Kerem E, Whyte H, et al. BPD: improvement in lung function between 7 and 10 years of age. J Pediatr 1991; 118:201–206.
38. Smyth JA, Tabachnik E, Duncan WJ, et al. Pulmonary function and bronchial hyperreactivity in long-term survivors of bronchopulmonary dysplasia. Pediatrics 1981; 68:336–340.
39. Northway WH, Moss RB, Carlisle KB, et al. Late pulmonary sequelae of bronchopulmonary dysplasia. N Engl J Med 1990; 323:1793–1799.
40. Vohr BR, Bell EF, Oh W. Infants with bronchopulmonary dysplasia: growth pattern and neurologic and developmental outcome. Am J Dis Child 1982; 136:443–447.
41. Markestad T, Fitzhardinge PM. Growth and development in children recovering from bronchopulmonary dysplasia. J Pediatr 1981; 98:597–602.
42. Meisels SJ, Rivers A, Hack M. Growth and development of preterm infants with respiratory distress syndrome and bronchopulmonary dysplasia. Pediatrics 1986; 77: 345–352.
43. Bozynski MEA, Brown ER, Neff RK, et al. Bronchopulmonary dysplasia and postnatal growth in extremely premature black infants. Early Hum Dev 1990; 21:83–92.
44. Skidmore MD, Rivers A, Hack M. Increased risk of cerebral palsy among very low-birthweight infants with chronic lung disease. Dev Med Child Neurol 1990; 32:325–332.
45. Werthammer J, Brown ER, Neff RK, et al. Sudden infant death syndrome in infants with bronchopulmonary dysplasia. Pediatrics 1982; 69:301–304.
46. Abman SH, Burchell MF, Shaffer MS, et al. Late sudden unexpected deaths in hospitalized infants with bronchopulmonary dysplasia. Am J Dis Child 1989; 143:815–819.
47. Gerhardt T, Bancalari E. Lung compliance in newborns with patent ductus arteriosus before and after surgical ligation. Biol Neonate 1980; 38:96–105.
48. Stefano JL, Abbasi S, Pearlman SA, et al. Closure of the ductus arteriosus with indomethacin in ventilated neonates with respiratory distress syndrome. Effects on pulmonary compliance and ventilation. Am Rev Respir Dis 1991; 143:236–239.
49. Brown ER. Increased risk of bronchopulmonary dysplasia in infant with patent ductus arteriosus. J Pediatr 1979; 95:865–866.
50. Pierce MR, Bancalari E. The role of inflammation in the pathogenesis of bronchopulmonary dysplasia. Pediatr Pulmonol 1995; 19:371–378.

51. Ogden BE, Murphy S, Saunders GC, Johnson JD. Lung lavage of newborns with respiratory distress syndrome: prolonged neutrophil influx is associated with bronchopulmonary dysplasia. Chest 1983; 83:31S–33S.
52. Bagghi A, Viscardi RM, Taciak V, et al. Increased activity of interleukin-6 but not tumor necrosis factor-α in lung lavage of premature infants is associated with the development of bronchopulmonary dysplasia. Pediatr Res 1994; 36:244–252.
53. Sawyer MH, Edwards DK, Spector SA. Cytomegalovirus infection and bronchopulmonary dysplasia in premature infants. Am J Dis Child 1987; 141:303–305.
54. Cassell GH, Crouse DT, Cannup KC, et al. Association of *Ureaplasma urealyticum* infection of the lower respiratory tract with chronic lung disease and death in very low birth weight infants. Lancet 1988; 2:240–244.
55. Wang EEL, Ohlsson A, Kellner JD. Association of *Ureaplasma urealyticum* colonization with chronic lung disease of prematurity: results of a metaanalysis. J Pediatr 1995; 127:640–644.
56. Gonzalez A, Sosenko IRS, Chandar J, et al. Influence of infection on patent ductus arteriosus and chronic lung disease in premature infants $\leq$ 1000 g. J Pediatr 1996; 128:470–478.
57. Wilson MG, et al. A new form of respiratory disease in premature infants. Am J Dis Child 1960; 99:489–499.
58. Sinkin RA, Cox C, Phelps DL. Predicting risk for bronchopulmonary dysplasia: selection criteria for clinical trials. Pediatrics 1990; 86:728–736.
59. Ryan SW, Wild NJ, Arthur RJ, Shaw BNJ. Prediction of chronic neonatal lung disease in very low birthweight neonates using clinical and radiological variables. Arch Dis Child 1994; 71:F36–F39.
60. Motoyama EK, Fort MD, Klesh KW, et al. Early onset of airway reactivity in premature infants with bronchopulmonary dysplasia. Am Rev Respir Dis 1987; 136:50–57.
61. Mirro R, Armstead W, Leffler C. Increased airway leukotriene levels in infants with severe bronchopulmonary dysplasia. Am J Dis Child 1990; 144:160–161.
62. Graff MA, Novo RP, Diaz M, et al. Compliance measurement in respiratory distress syndrome: the prediction of outcome. Pediatr Pulmonol 1986; 2:332–336.
63. Freezer NJ, Sly PD. Predictive value of measurements of respiratory mechanics in preterm infants with HMD. Pediatr Pulmonol 1993; 16:116–123.
64. Van Lierde S, Smith J, Devlieger H, Eggermont E. Pulmonary mechanics during respiratory distress syndrome in the prediction of outcome and differentiation of mild and severe bronchopulmonary dysplasia. Pediatr Pulmonol 1994; 17:218–224.
65. Kirpalani H, Schmit B, Gaston S, et al. Birthweight, early passive respiratory system mechanics, and ventilator requirements as predictors of outcome in premature infants with respiratory failure. Pediatr Pulmonol 1991; 10:195–198.
66. Bancalari E, Jesse MJ, Gelband H, Garcia O. Lung mechanics in congenital heart disease with increased and decreased pulmonary blood flow. J Pediatr 1977; 90:192–195.
67. Tay-Uyboco JS, Kwiatkowski K, Cates DB, et al. Hypoxic airway constriction in infants of very low birth weight recovering from moderate to severe bronchopulmonary dysplasia. J Pediatr 1989; 115:456–459.
68. Gomez-Del-Rio M, Gerhardt T, Hehre D, et al. Effect of a beta agonist nebulization

on lung function in neonates with increased pulmonary resistance. Pediatr Pulmonol 1986; 2:287–291.
69. Brundage KL, Mohsini KG, Froese AB, Fisher JT. Bronchodilator response to ipratropium bromide in infants with bronchopulmonary dysplasia. Am Rev Respir Dis 1992; 12:162–169.
70. Rotschild A, Solimano A, Puterman M, et al. Increased compliance in response to salbutamol in premature infants with developing bronchopulmonary dysplasia. J Pediatr 1989; 115:984–991.
71. Stefano JL, Bhutani VK, Fox W. A randomized placebo-controlled study to evaluate the effects of oral albuterol on pulmonary mechanics in ventilator-dependent infants at risk of developing BPD. Pediatr Pulmonol 1991; 10:183–190.
72. Kao LC, Warburton D. Effects of isoproterenol inhalation on airway resistance in chronic bronchopulmonary dysplasia. Pediatrics 1984; 73:509–513.
73. Kao L, Durand D, Nickerson B. Effects of metaproterenol and atropine on the pulmonary mechanics of infants with bronchopulmonary dysplasia. Pediatr Pulmonol 1989; 6:74–80.
74. McCann EM, Lewis K, Deming DD, et al. Controlled trial of furosemide therapy in infants with chronic lung disease. J Pediatr 1985; 106:957–961.
75. Englehardt B, Elliott S, Hazinski TA. Short- and long-term effects of furosemide on lung function in infants with bronchopulmonary dysplasia. J Pediatr 1986; 109: 1034–1039.
76. Bland RD, McMillan DD, Bressack MA. Decreased pulmonary transvascular fluid filtration in awake newborn lambs after intravenous furosemide. J Clin Invest 1978; 62:601–609.
77. Demling BH, Will JA. The effect of furosemide on the pulmonary transvascular fluid filtration rate. Crit Care Med 1978; 6:317–319.
78. O'Donovan BH, Bell EF. Effects of furosemide on body water compartments in infants with bronchopulmonary dysplasia. Pediatr Res 1989; 26:121–124.
79. Berner ME, Teague WG Jr, Scheerer RG, Bland RD. Furosemide reduces lung fluid filtration in lambs with lung microvascular injury from air emboli. J Appl Physiol 1989; 67:1990–1996.
80. Rush MG, Engelhardt B, Parker RA, Hazinski TA. Double-blind, placebo-controlled trial of alternate-day furosemide therapy in infants with chronic bronchopulmonary dysplasia. J Pediatr 1990; 117:112–118.
81. Kao LC, Durand DJ, McCrea RC, et al. Randomized trial of long-term diuretic therapy for infants with oxygen-dependent bronchopulmonary dysplasia. J Pediatr 1994; 124:772–781.
82. Avery GB, Fletcher AB, Kaplan M, Brudno DS. Controlled trial of dexamethasone in respirator-dependent infants with bronchopulmonary dysplasia. Pediatrics 1985; 74:106–111.
83. Yoder MC Jr, Chua R, Tepper R. Effect of dexamethasone on pulmonary inflammation and pulmonary function of ventilator-dependent infants with bronchopulmonary dysplasia. Am Rev Respir Dis 1991; 143:1044–1048.
84. Gladstone IM, Ehrenkranz RA, Jacobs HC. Pulmonary function tests and fluid balance in neonates with chronic lung disease during dexamethasone treatment. Pediatrics 1989; 84:1072–1076.

85. Durand M, Sardesai S, McEvoy C. Effects of early dexamethasone therapy on pulmonary mechanics and chronic lung disease in very low birth weight infants: a randomized, controlled trial. Pediatrics 1995; 95:584–590.
86. Rastogi A, Luayon M, Ajayi OA, Pildes RS. Nebulized furosemide in infants with bronchopulmonary dysplasia. J Pediatr 1994; 125:976–979.
87. LaForce WR, Brudno S. Controlled trial of beclomethasone dipropionate by nebulization in oxygen- and ventilator-dependent infants. J Pediatr 1993; 122:285–288.

4

Radiographic Features of BPD and Potential Application of New Imaging Techniques

DAVID K. EDWARDS

University of California Medical School
San Diego, California

WILLIAM H. NORTHWAY, Jr.

Lucile Packard Children's Hospital at Stanford
Palo Alto, California

I. Introduction

This chapter is composed of two parts. The first part (Secs. II–III) discusses the conventional radiology of bronchopulmonary dysplasia (BPD), emphasizing plain-film radiographic findings. The second part (Secs. IV and V) delineates the technical advances that have occurred in diagnostic radiology during the past decade, and reflects on how these changes may be applicable to the clinical and scientific evaluation of BPD.

II. The Radiographic Progression of BPD

A. Progression Through Radiographic Stages

As BPD was initially described (1), the plain chest radiographic findings progressed as a function of time through a series of appearances that were descriptively summarized as stages. These stages were pathologically reflected by the progression of injury and repair in the immature lung. Stage I was the initial appearance of uncomplicated respiratory distress syndrome (RDS); stage II presented a period of relative radiopacity of the lung that subsequently cleared to a bubbly appearance (stage III). Stage IV was the final appearance of chronic lung disease, with enlarged, rounded lucencies and radiodense strands in the lungs that persisted beyond 1 month of age.

That the patients initially described with stage IV BPD usually progressed predictably through these stages (2) probably reflects the relative homogeneity of the patient population and therapies that pertained in the early days of oxygenation and assisted ventilation of preterm newborns with RDS. Respiratory support was primarily intermittent positive-pressure ventilation and negative-pressure ventilation, with high inspired oxygen tensions. Survivors who acquired BPD had severe initial lung disease that was mild enough to permit survival, but severe enough to require extensive respiratory support. Therapeutic emphasis was properly on survival and, secondarily, on the reduction of lung injury.

With the recognition of BPD, therapeutic endeavors increasingly included efforts to mitigate lung damage. Simultaneous medical advances also permitted survival of increasingly immature infants, and of infants with relatively more severe underlying lung disease. As the variety of the therapeutic modalities increased, the treatment for respiratory failure in the neonate became more variable. The population of survivors who acquired BPD following respiratory failure broadened and became less homogeneous than those described initially.

One result of this change in disease pattern is that the radiographic progression of BPD through identifiable stages has become less common than in the past (3,4). Thus, the final radiographic appearance of BPD is an endpoint that develops by way of a variety of radiographic pathways. Furthermore, the radiographic appearance of this endpoint—chronic or stage IV BPD—varies from patient to patient. In addition, the initial description of BPD was limited to chronic disease arising in the setting of RDS. Since then, BPD has been shown to develop not just in this setting, but also after a wide variety of underlying neonatal diseases for which respiratory assistance is required (5). In such conditions, the initial radiographic findings reflect the underlying disease, and the early stages, as described in the RDS setting, are largely inapplicable.

B. Modification of the Progression of BPD

It is clear that the radiographic progression of BPD had been modified by the aforementioned factors, so that clearly defined stages are commonly not identifiable (6). A much more common progression is an insidious appearance of BPD. The affected patient's early chest radiographs reflect the underlying disease, usually RDS. Often the initial radiographic severity is ameliorated by exogenous surfactant administration (7). Complications of prematurity and of respiratory therapy, such as left-to-right shunting through a patent ductus arteriosus (PDA) or intrathoracic air leaks (pulmonary interstitial emphysema, pneumothorax, and such), often dominate the radiographic findings during the first to 1–2 weeks after birth.

As the infant's course becomes stable, the lungs may simply heal, permitting timely discharge from the hospital, but infants with evolving BPD commonly remain ventilator-dependent. Radiographic abnormalities that are often subtle appear initially at 2–3 weeks postnatally; these abnormalities persist and commonly worsen. Eventually, the persistence and progression of these abnormalities suggest a radiographic diagnosis of BPD. It is often difficult, even with retrospective examination of sequential radiographs, to assign an unequivocal time of onset of BPD. This difficulty is further confounded by superimposed processes, such as air leaks, pulmonary edema from fluid overload, focal atelectasis from mucous plugging, and pneumonia, all of which may mask underlying chronic changes for varying lengths of time.

A progression that is relatively uncommon, but particularly insidious, is the development of BPD in the setting of chronic pulmonary interstitial emphysema (PIE). On a single radiograph, diffuse PIE itself can camouflage the changes of BPD. In infants whose PIE becomes chronic, it is virtually impossible to distinguish the changes of BPD from the radiographic appearance of interstitial air (5).

C. The Problem of Early Radiographic Diagnosis of BPD

It may be advantageous to diagnose BPD as early as possible to enable appropriate initiation of therapy, such as glucocorticoids (8) or surfactant (9) administration. Because the radiographic picture of BPD is often insidious, however, chest radiographs may be of little value in establishing an early diagnosis. Many entities that are generally transient (Table 1) can simulate the radiographic changes of BPD, including fluid overload, interstitial edema from other causes, PIE, and viral pneumonia. The most reliable finding of BPD is its chronicity; its radiographic abnormalities do not appear and disappear as do those of most other processes. The necessity of waiting to see if an abnormality is or is not chronic therefore may prevent early diagnosis.

There are other long-standing conditions that may simulate BPD, but most of these conditions arise within a clinical setting distinct from neonatal respiratory

Table 1 Radiographic Differential Diagnosis of BPD

Entities, usually transient, that may simulate developing BPD

1. Interstitial edema (usually reflecting fluid overload or PDA)
2. Pulmonary interstitial emphysema
3. Viral pneumonia

Entities that may simulate chronic BPD

1. Long-lived viral pneumonia, especially cytomegalovirus
2. Wilson–Mikity syndrome
3. Chronic pulmonary interstitial emphysema

insufficiency and ventilatory assistance. Viral pneumonia, most notably from cytomegalovirus infection, often leads to persistent respiratory distress in infants at risk for BPD, accompanied by radiographs that closely simulate BPD (10–12). Thus, chronicity does not invariably establish a diagnosis of BPD.

D. Radiologic–Pathological Correlation in BPD

The value of the chest radiograph in BPD depends largely on the accuracy with which radiographic findings reflect specific lung pathology. The few studies of BPD that have attempted to correlate autopsy data with radiographs have employed the radiologic- and pathological-staging categories I through IV. This radiographic progression has become uncommon in recent years. Previous correlations studies suggest that the abnormalities observed in chest radiographs tend to underestimate the severity of lung pathology. In more than one half of published cases, radiographic stage lagged behind the pathological stage; in 40% of cases, there was radiographic–pathological agreement (13–15). Thus, the radiographic findings probably should be considered an optimistic assessment of the true pathological state of the lungs, at least in those infants who die and whose lungs undergo postmortem examination.

III. BPD as a Chronic Lung Disease

A. Radiographic Appearance of Chronic BPD

The radiographic appearance of long-standing BPD varies considerably along a spectrum of mild to severe. Radiographic severity closely parallels the degree of respiratory compromise (16,17), and severe radiographic changes are associated with increased likelihood of death (18).

Mild BPD (Fig. 1) may radiographically reveal only a faint accentuation of line shadows, presumably reflecting interstitial disease. There may be a normal level of inflation, or mild hyperinflation. The lungs appear homogeneously involved. The radiographic picture in severe BPD (Figs. 2 and 3) is more clearly abnormal, with evidence of extreme hyperinflation and disordered pulmonary architecture. Dense line shadows are often visible, presumably representing fibrosis, atelectasis, or pleural fissures. Regions of emphysema alternate with these line shadows and with areas of apparent consolidation or atelectasis. Although the lungs are globally involved, the appearance is usually nonuniform from region to region. Cardiomegaly and a prominent main pulmonary artery may indicate the presence of cor pulmonale (see Fig. 2). Patients with moderate BPD (Fig. 4) show findings between these extremes. Commonly, there is a pattern of lacy abnormal densities that obscure vascular shadows and extend peripherally from the hilum of the lungs (3,4).

The important radiographic hallmarks of chronic BPD are (1) an interstitial

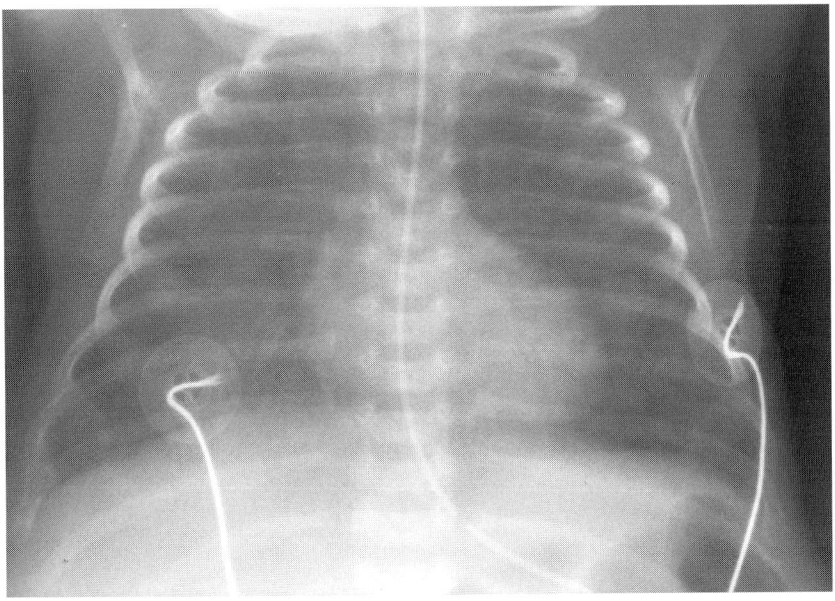

Figure 1 Radiographically and clinically mild BPD, in an 30-day-old infant. The lungs show faint, lacy abnormal markings bilaterally and homogeneously.

pattern, rather than a fluffy, or alveolar pattern, or an airway disease pattern with fine peribronchial thickening; (2) hyperinflation, except in mildly affected infants who may be normally inflated; (3) equal or similar involvement of both lungs, with no marked upper- or lower-lobe accentuation; (4) gradual, as opposed to abrupt, onset of findings; and (5) chronicity. A tendency for the thorax to be relatively flat in the anteroposterior dimension has also been noted (20,21).

B. Radiographic Differential Diagnosis of BPD

Each of the radiographic hallmarks of BPD has its own differential diagnosis. For example, hyperinflation characteristically occurs in other chronic ailments, such as cystic fibrosis, asthma, and acyanotic congenital heart disease with large left-to-right intracardiac shunts. These disorders, however, have other distinctive radiographic findings that do no occur in BPD, such as marked peribronchial thickening in cystic fibrosis and enlarged pulmonary arteries in shunt lesions. Whereas a single chest radiograph, by itself, may convincingly simulate developing or chronic BPD, there are relatively few situations in which the clinical setting leaves any doubt about the diagnosis of BPD (Table 1).

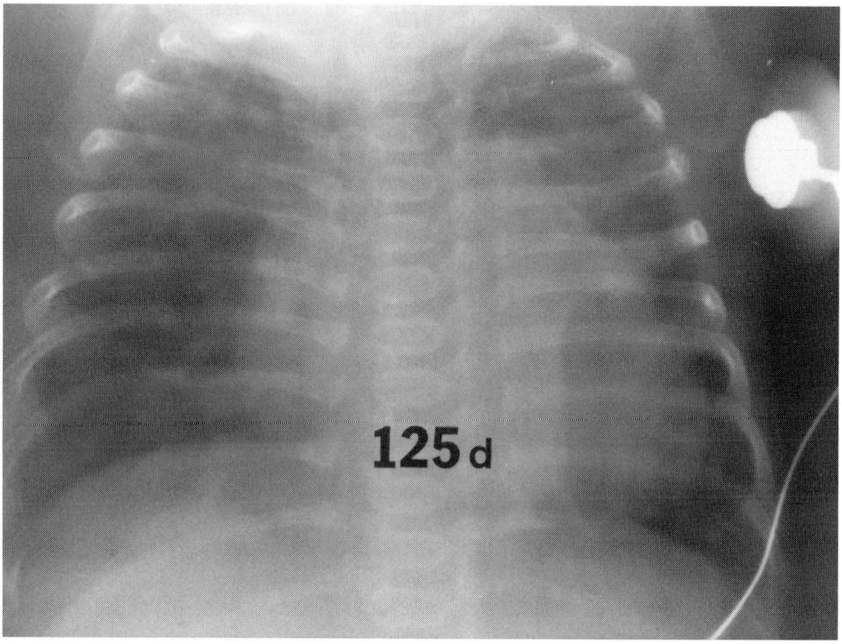

Figure 2 Radiographically and clinically severe BPD, in a 4-month-old infant. Streaks of abnormal density are seen in both lungs; the heart is enlarged, and the left lower lobe is persistently collapsed, probably secondary to cardiomegaly. The main pulmonary artery is enlarged, reflecting pulmonary hypertension.

C. Uncommon Radiographic Appearances of Chronic BPD

Asymmetrical involvement of the lungs in BPD has been reported following collapse of the less affected lung (22). Focal emphysema of the right lower and middle lobes may occur, evidently as a result of focal airway damage from suctioning catheters (19). Occasionally, prolonged radiopacity, presumably reflecting pulmonary edema, may occur for several weeks, usually in ventilator-dependent infants with moderate to severe BPD (5).

D. Grading the Severity of Chronic BPD

At least two systems have been devised that attempt to summarize the radiographic findings in chronic BPD with a single integer (23,24). These systems assign numerical values to various findings on a representative film, and a score is formed by summing these values. Such scores seem to correlate fairly well with clinical indices of respiratory function (16) and provide at least a semiquantitative

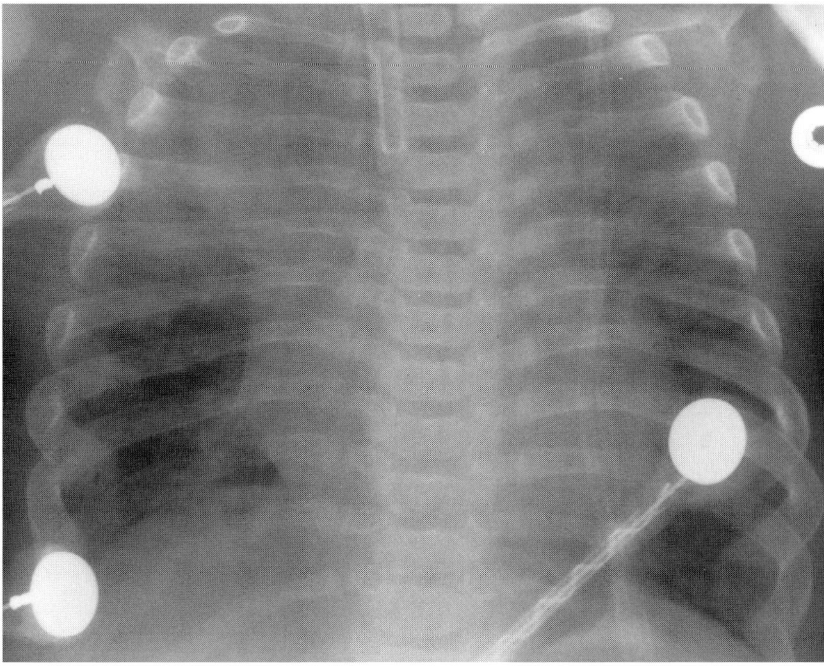

Figure 3 Radiographically severe chronic BPD in an 8-month-old infant on continuing assisted ventilation. There is cardiomegaly and substantial hyperinflation; abnormal markings are notable in both lungs.

method of assessing the severity of radiographic changes for statistical analyses and comparison and for standardization of results between institutions. Notably, these systems attempt to assess the radiographic severity of BPD in infants using both the clinical and the radiographic findings of BPD.

E. The Radiographic Evolution of Chronic BPD

Once an individual patient no longer requires respiratory support and is able to breathe room air, the radiographic and lung function abnormalities tend to improve over time (25,26). By school age or even earlier, the chest radiograph may become entirely normal (27), although chronic abnormalities may persist, such as line shadows that probably represent strands of fibrosis or prominent pleural fissures (21). Computed tomographic (CT) scans of the chest of children with BPD have shown these persistent abnormalities better than have chest radiographs (28). Complications and conditions associated with chronic BPD, other than those of prematurity per se, are listed in Table 2.

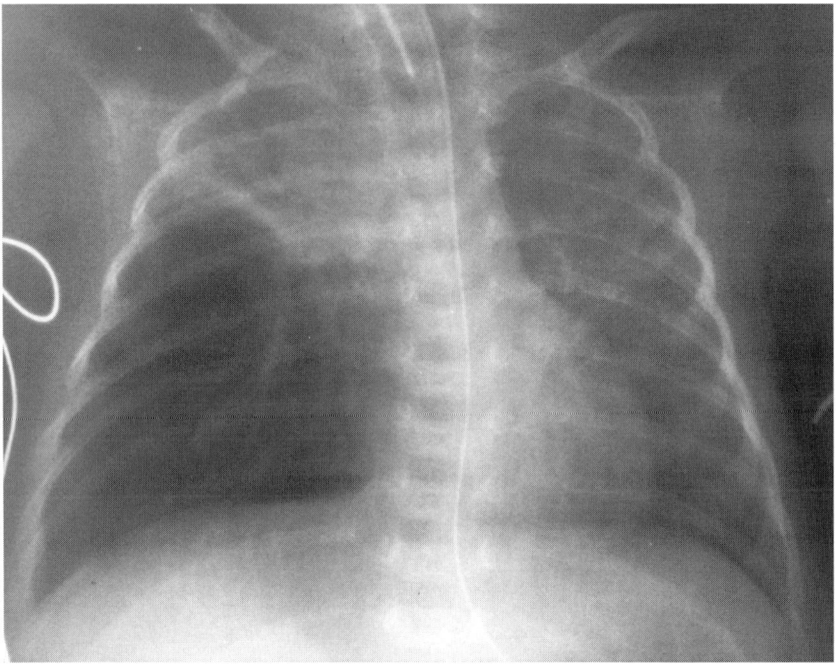

Figure 4 Radiographically moderate BPD in a 36-day-old infant. Diffuse abnormal markings are best appreciated in the left lung. The right lower and middle lobes are hyperinflated secondary to obstructing granulomas caused by suctioning catheters irritating the bronchus intermedius. (From Ref. 19.)

IV. New Imaging Techniques

During the past decade new technologies to image and evaluate the lung have been developed, including computed tomographic (CT) scanning, magnetic resonance imaging (MRI), and radionuclide imaging. These techniques offer the possibility to not only improve imaging of organ structure, but also to evaluate some aspects of organ physiology. All may be able to provide answers to pertinent questions on the structural and physiological changes that occur during the development and progression of BPD. The very small premature infant, in whom BPD is most likely to develop, presents a challenge to the use of these diagnostic techniques, particularly early in the course of the disease when these infants are most fragile and unstable on ventilatory assistance. Although diagnostic ultrasound can be used portably in the nursery to evaluate cardiac structure and function in infants with BPD, it has limitations for lung imaging, as sonic waves in

Table 2 Complications and Associations of Chronic BPD

Disorder	Probable etiology	Imaging	Ref.
Congestive heart failure	Lung disease	Chest radiograph	29
Right ventricular hypertrophy	Lung disease	Echocardiogram	30
Left ventricular hypertrophy	Unknown; hypertension?	Echocardiogram	31, 32
Recurrent pneumonias; focal atelectasis	Poor clearance of secretions	Chest radiograph	3, 33, 34
Central airway obstructions	Intubation; suction catheters	Airways radiographs; assisted expiration radiography; CT	19, 35
Demineralization; rickets	Diuretic therapy	Wrist or knee radiographs; bone densitometry	36, 37
Pathological fractures	Diuretic therapy	Plain radiographs of affected areas	38
"Flat chest"	Unknown; soft bones?	Chest radiograph	20
Renal calcifications	Calciuria (diuretic therapy)	Renal sonography	39
Cholelithiasis	Hyperalimentation?	Sonography; abdominal radiograph	40

the diagnostic range do not traverse air-filled organs, such as the lung. Other imaging techniques such as CT and MRI scanning, require that infants be transported to the imaging facilities, a formidable challenge in the setting of intensive care and mechanical ventilation of tiny, sick infants.

A. Computed Tomography

Computed tomographic scanning of the lung includes such techniques as rapid helical CT scanning (41), high-resolution CT scanning (42), dynamic CT scanning, with inspiration and expiration imaging (43), CT scanning with three-dimensional (3-D) reconstruction, which can provide bronchogram-like images of the airways and mapping of the vascular bed (41), and electron beam CT scanning, which can provide scan slices in 100 msec or less and, frequently, obviate the need for sedation of the uncooperative infant or child. The greatly increased speed of image acquisition and enhanced image resolution ($<$1-mm range), of the newer CT scanners has improved our ability to visualize the parenchyma, airways, and vessels in the lung, but requires the use of x-irradiation.

Efforts are being made to lower the radiation dose from CT scanning of the chest (32).

B. Magnetic Resonance Imaging

The same improvement in speed of image acquisition and improved resolution has also occurred in MRI. Although MRI is more motion-sensitive than CT scanning, various sophisticated techniques have been developed to minimize the effect of cardiac and respiratory motion on lung imaging. Magnetic resonance imaging can provide quantitative oxygenation measurements of blood (44), visualization and measurement of flow in pulmonary vessels (45–47), and visualization of pulmonary parenchyma (48). The lung presents special challenges to the use of all these techniques because of physiological motion, low proton density and resultant weak signal intensity, and magnetic field inhomogeneity owing to numerous tissue–air interfaces. Relative inhomogeneity, which causes a shortening of T2 and T2*, also presents problems in the use of magnetic resonance spectroscopy, MRI diffusion imaging, and other rapid-imaging methods. A recent development in MRI is imaging of highly magnetized noble gases (He and Xe; 49). These gases can be extremely polarized to produce a very sharp MRI signal. These methods, which are still in an early research stage, may provide a means of studying lung ventilation and function.

C. Radionuclide Imaging

Radionuclide imaging can measure distribution of ventilation with a radiolabeled gas, ^{133}Xe (50), pulmonary perfusion with macroaggregated albumin (51), and the relation of ventilation and perfusion (52) with $C^{15}O_2$. It is possible that the site and extent of inflammation in BPD could be detected by gallium 67 citrate imaging (53) or newer experimental techniques using either radiolabeled human polyclonal IgG labeled with ^{111}In (54,55), or chemotactic peptides labeled with technetium-99m (56). These agents all concentrate to a significant degree in zones of inflammation. Acute processes are readily detected with peptides, whereas more chronic processes are better detected with IgG or gallium imaging.

D. Diagnostic Ultrasound

Although diagnostic ultrasound has limited imaging ability in the lung, Doppler ultrasound may be helpful in detection of pulmonary hypertension by measurement of pulmonary regurgitation (57).

V. Potential Applications

The new imaging techniques have potential application to those infants in whom BPD is developing, to those in whom it has already developed, and to children and adults with prior BPD. In the research setting, these methods, along with more conventional counterparts, may improve our understanding of the origin and pathophysiology of BPD. The clinical use of these newer techniques will depend largely on their ability to provide answers to questions that will result in different or earlier therapeutic interventions, provide evaluation of the efficacy of such interventions, or provide additional information that can be used prognostically.

Their use is not without cost and risk. Use of these technologies with the very small premature infant in whom BPD is developing may require transporting the infant to an MRI or CT scanner suite while the infant is being mechanically ventilated, oxygen supplemented, and receiving parenteral nutrition. CT scanning requires radiation exposures that are higher than those needed for a chest radiograph. Radionuclide studies also involve exposure to ionizing radiation and may require moving the infant. Magnetic resonance imaging requires the exclusion of all ferromagnetic devices or accessories from the area of the infant in the magnet. Computed tomographic and MRI scanning and radionuclide studies of the child before the age of cooperation may require the use of sedation or even general anesthesia, although the need for sedation is reduced with faster imaging methods.

A. Early Diagnosis, Pathophysiology, and Treatment Effectiveness

The diagnosis of early BPD may be made histologically, based on cell injury, toward the end of the first postnatal week of life (1). It is possible that new imaging techniques could provide insight into the pathophysiology of BPD and an earlier clinical diagnosis than is currently provided by the clinical status of the patient and chest radiography. However, because the lungs of the very low birth weight, prematurely born infant are so small, resolution of fine tissue detail will be a problem for all of these techniques. Moreover, it is not clear that an earlier diagnosis of BPD by any imaging technique will result in a significant change in therapy or in prognosis. Earlier diagnosis of BPD is more likely to come from improved knowledge of the biochemical markers of the early injury and repair process in the lung. Intervention with antioxidants, or specific anti-inflammatory treatment, may not be dependent on earlier diagnosis of the development of BPD either by biochemical markers or by new imaging technology. Such therapy is often used prophylactically in the appropriate clinical setting. However, new and more accurate imaging methods could be important in documenting the efficacy of new treatments.

B. Severity and Prognosis

Infants with BPD have increased airways resistance, increased airways reactivity, air trapping, and may have pulmonary hypertension, as well as a decrease in the area of the pulmonary vascular bed (58–67). Early evaluation of the physiological and anatomical changes in the lung could be both prognostically significant and helpful in evaluating effectiveness of treatment.

Inspiration and expiration spiral CT scanning of the lung and electron beam CT scanning of the lung can identify areas of air trapping and demonstrate alterations in the distribution of pulmonary vasculature (Fig. 5). These techniques could be applied even to the very young infant because of the rapidity of the scan rate. In the older infant and child, these techniques may help determine the diameter of the airway lumen, as small as 2 mm, and to evaluate the thickness of the airway wall, both of which may be altered in BPD. MRI flow techniques may help determine redistribution of blood flow in the lung, and measure regional changes in oxygenation. MRI techniques for visualization of the pulmonary parenchyma may improve detection of prior lung injury and ongoing repair without the need for ionizing radiation. Nuclear medicine ventilation–perfusion scanning techniques may be helpful in defining mismatches of ventilation and perfusion. Doppler ultrasound studies may help detect persistent pulmonary hypertension. More aggressive use of newer-imaging technologies could contribute not only to our understanding of the pathophysiology of BPD but also to an enhanced severity scoring system for BPD, that could have prognostic significance.

The natural course of BPD is poorly understood, and its consequences in the older adult with prior BPD have yet to be determined. The newer-imaging techniques provide the opportunity to evaluate in serial studies lung inflammation, anatomical changes in the lung, and physiological changes, including changes in pulmonary blood flow and air trapping in a relatively noninvasive manner. The higher-speed acquisition techniques with CT or MRI scanning should allow their use, either with less or no sedation, in the child who is too young to cooperate. CT scanning is already being used to evaluate the bronchiectasis, lung destruction, and air trapping of children and adults with cystic fibrosis (68). It could also be used to evaluate and follow children and young adults with

Figure 5 (a and b) A 9-year-old former prematurely born infant with BPD and severe reactive airway disease. (FVC = 52% predicted; FEV_1 = 48% predicted; $FEF_{25-75\%}$ = 17% predicted). Posteroanterior and lateral radiographs of the chest show lung hyperexpansion and scattered strands of parenchymal density. (c and d) High-resolution CT scan slice (1-mm–thick section) of the chest obtained during (c) inspiration and (d) expiration at the same examination at a level below the carina. The scan during expiration shows increased density in the more normal areas of lung and increased lucency in areas of air trapping, compared with the scan during inspiration. There is an abnormal distribution of the pulmonary vessels. (Courtesy of Eric Effmann, M.D.)

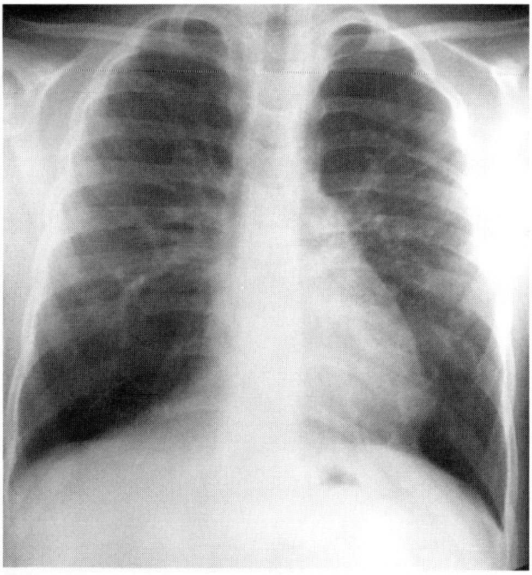

(a)

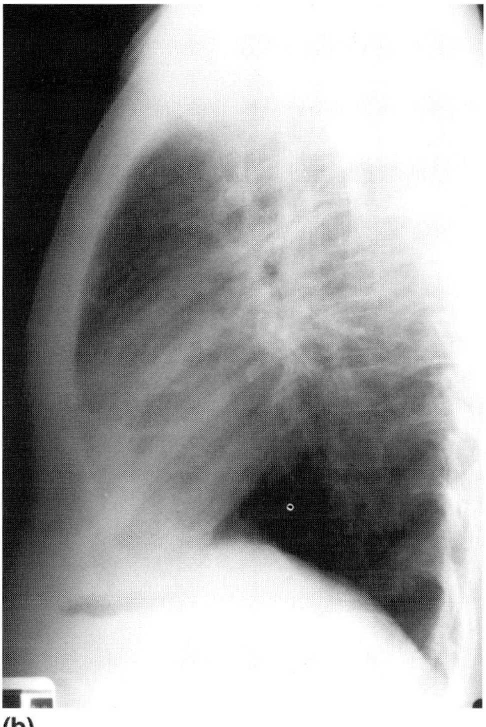

(b)

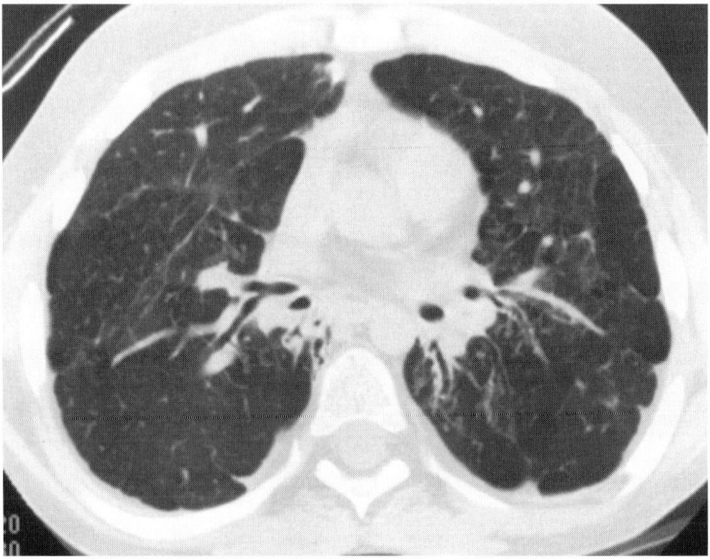

(c)

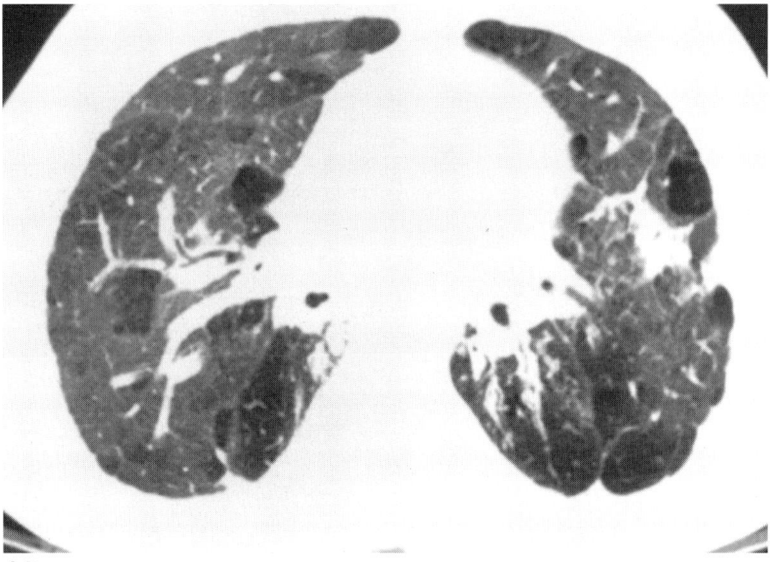

(d)

Figure 5 Continued

previous BPD. Particular attention will need to be paid to dose reduction with CT scanning so that it can be safely used in both male and female children without fear of injury to developing reproductive organs (69). In the young female, immature breast tissue poses a particular problem for radiation sensitivity. MRI techniques for measurement of blood flow and oxygenation could provide insights into those long-term consequences of injury and repair that affect the pulmonary vascular bed.

Thoughtful use of the newer imaging technologies can enhance our understanding of the basic pulmonary pathophysiology of BPD, define the consequences of injury and repair in the developing lung, and help evaluate the efficacy of therapeutic interventions on the sequelae of BPD.

Acknowledgments

The authors gratefully acknowledge the contribution of Ann Leung, Sandy A. Napel, Norbert J. Pelc, and H. William Strauss, to the section on application of new imaging techniques.

References

1. Northway WH Jr, Rosan RC. Radiographic features of pulmonary oxygen toxicity in the newborn: bronchopulmonary dysplasia. Radiology 1968; 91:49–58.
2. Edwards DK, Dyer WM, Northway WH Jr. Twelve years' experience with bronchopulmonary dysplasia. Pediatrics 1977; 59:839–846.
3. Edwards DK. Radiographic aspects of bronchopulmonary dysplasia. J Pediatr 1979; 95:823–829.
4. Singleton EB. Radiologic considerations of intensive care in the premature infant. Radiology 1981; 140:291–300.
5. Edwards DK III. The radiology of bronchopulmonary dysplasia and its complications. In: Merritt TA, Northway WH Jr, Boynton BR, eds. Bronchopulmonary Dysplasia. Boston: Blackwell Scientific 1988:185–234.
6. Heneghan MA, Sosulski R, Baquero JM. Persistent pulmonary abnormalities in newborns: the changing picture of bronchopulmonary dysplasia. Pediatr Radiol 1986; 16:180–184.
7. Edwards DK, Hilton SvW, Merritt TA, Hallman M, Mannino F, Boynton BR. Respiratory distress syndrome treated with human surfactant: radiographic findings. Radiology 1985; 157:329–334.
8. LaForce WR, Brudno DS. Controlled trial of beclomethasone dipropionate by nebulization in oxygen- and ventilator-dependent infants. J Pediatr 1993; 122:285–288.
9. Pandit PB, Dunn MS, Kelly EN, Perlman M. Surfactant replacement in neonates with early chronic lung disease. Pediatrics 1995; 95:851–854.

10. Whitley RJ, Brasfield D, Reynolds DW, Stagno S, Tiller RE, Alford CA. Protracted pneumonitis in young infants associated with perinatally acquired cytomegaloviral infection. J Pediatr 1976; 89:16–22.
11. Paryani SG, Yeager AS, Hosford-Dunn H, et al. Sequelae of acquired cytomegalovirus infection in premature and sick term infants. J Pediatr 1985; 107:451–456.
12. Sawyer MH, Edwards DK, Spector SA. Cytomegalovirus infection and bronchopulmonary dysplasia in premature infants. Am J Dis Child 1987; 141:303–305.
13. Oppermann HC, Wille L, Bleyl U, Obladen M. Bronchopulmonary dysplasia in premature infants. A radiological and pathological correlation. Pediatr Radiol 1977; 5: 137–141.
14. Edwards DK, Colby TV, Northway WH Jr. Radiographic–pathologic correlation in bronchopulmonary dysplasia. J Pediatr 1979; 95:834–836.
15. Kwok-Liu JP, Zylak CJ, deSa DJ. Bronchopulmonary dysplasia. A radiologic–pathologic correlation. J Can Assoc Radiol 1980; 31:238–241.
16. Toce SS, Farrell PM, Leavitt LA, Samuels DP, Edwards DK. Clinical and roentgenographic scoring systems for assessing bronchopulmonary dysplasia. Am J Dis Child 1984; 138:581–585.
17. Ahrens P, Zielen S, Stover B, von Loewenich V, Hofmann D. Pulmonary sequelae of long-term ventilation of very low birth weight premature infants. Results of a follow-up study of 6- to 9-year-old children. Klin Padiatr 1991; 203:366–371 [German].
18. Gray PH, Grice JF, Lee MS, Ritchie BH, Williams G. Prediction of outcome of preterm infants with severe bronchopulmonary dysplasia. J Paediatr Child Health 1993; 29:107–112.
19. Miller KE, Edwards DK, Hilton S, Collins D, Lynch F, Williams R. Acquired lobar emphysema in premature infants with bronchopulmonary dysplasia: an iatrogenic disease? Radiology 1981; 138:589–592.
20. Edwards DK, Hilton SvW. Flat chest in chronic bronchopulmonary dysplasia. Am J Roentgenol 1987; 149:1213–1216.
21. Griscom NT, Wheeler WB, Sweezey NB, Kim YC, Lindsey JC, Wohl ME. Bronchopulmonary dysplasia: radiographic appearance in middle childhood. Radiology 1989; 171:811–814.
22. Sickles EA, Gooding CA. Asymmetric lung involvement in bronchopulmonary dysplasia. Radiology 1976; 118:379–383.
23. Edwards DK. Radiology of hyaline membrane disease, transient tachypnea of the newborn, and bronchopulmonary dysplasia. In: Farrell PM, ed. Lung Development: Biological and Clinical Perspectives. Vol. II. New York: Academic Press, 1982:47–89.
24. Weinstein MR, Peters ME, Sadek M, Palta M. A new radiographic scoring system for bronchopulmonary dysplasia. Pediatr Pulmonol 1994; 18:284–289.
25. Nickerson BG. Bronchopulmonary dysplasia. Chronic pulmonary disease following neonatal respiratory failure. Chest 1985; 87:528–535.
26. Mortensson W, Lindroth M. The course of bronchopulmonary dysplasia. A radiographic follow-up. Acta Radiol Diagn 1986; 27:19–22.
27. Tammela OKT, Lanning FP, Koivisto ME. The relationship of fluid restriction dur-

ing the 1st month of life to the occurrence and severity of bronchopulmonary dysplasia in low birth weight infants: a 1-year radiological follow up. Eur J Pediatr 1992; 151:367–371.
28. Oppenheim C, Mamou-Mani T, Sayegh N, de Blic J, Scheinmann P, Lallemand D. Bronchopulmonary dysplasia: value of CT in identifying pulmonary sequelae. Am J Roentgenol 1994; 163:169–172.
29. Fouron J-C, Le Guennec J-C, Villemant D, Bard H, Perreault G, Davignon A. Value of echocardiography in assessing the outcome of bronchopulmonary dysplasia of the newborn. Pediatrics 1980; 65:529–535.
30. Stocker JT. Pathologic features of long-standing ''healed'' bronchopulmonary dysplasia: a study of 28 3- to 40-month old infants. Hum Pathol 1986; 17:943–961.
31. Melnick G, Pickoff AS, Ferrer PL, Peyser J, Bancalari E, Gelband H. Normal pulmonary vascular resistance and left ventricular hypertrophy in young infants with bronchopulmonary dysplasia: an echocardiographic and pathologic study. Pediatrics 1980; 66:589–596.
32. Abman SH, Warady BA, Lum GM, Koops BL. Systemic hypertension in infants with bronchopulmonary dysplasia. J Pediatr 1984; 104:928–931.
33. Hakulinen A, Heinonen K, Jokela V, Kiekara O. Occurrence, predictive factors and associated morbidity of bronchopulmonary dysplasia in a preterm birth cohort. J Perinat Med 1988; 16:437–446.
34. Lindroth M, Jonson B, Svenningsen NW, Mortensson W. Pulmonary mechanics, chest x-ray and lung disease after mechanical ventilation in low birth weight infants. Acta Paediatr Scand 1980; 69:761–770.
35. Joshi VV, Mandavia SG, Stern L, Wiglesworth FW. Acute lesions induced by endotracheal intubation. Occurrence in the upper respiratory tract of newborn infants with respiratory distress syndrome. Am J Dis Child 1972; 124:646–649.
36. Steichen JJ, Gratton TL, Tsang RC. Osteopenia of prematurity: the cause and possible treatment. J Pediatr 1980; 96:528–534.
37. Venkataraman PS, Han BK, Tsang RC, Daugherty CC. Secondary hyperparathyroidism and bone disease in infants receiving long-term furosemide therapy. Am J Dis Child 1983; 137:1157–1161.
38. Gefter WB, Epstein DM, Anday EK, Dalinka MK. Rickets presenting as multiple fractures in premature infants on hyperalimentation. Radiology 1982; 142:371–374.
39. Hufnagle KG, Khan SN, Penn D, Cacciarelli A, Williams P. Renal calcifications: a complication of long-term furosemide therapy in preterm infants. Pediatrics 1982; 70:360–363.
40. Callahan J, Haller JO, Cacciarelli AA, Slovis TL, Friedman AP. Cholelithiasis in infants: association with total parenteral nutrition and furosemide. Radiology 1982; 143:437–439.
41. Rubin GD, Dake MD, Semba CP. Current status of 3 dimensional CT scanning for imaging the vasculature. Radiat Clin North Am 1995; 33:51–70.
42. Mayo JR, Webb RW, Gould R, Stein MG, Bass I, Gamsu G, Goldberg HI. High resolution CT of the lungs: an optimal approach. Radiology 1987; 163:507–510.
43. Sern EJ, Webb RW, Gamsu G, Goldberg HI. Dynamic quantitative computed tomograph. A predictor of pulmonary function in obstructive lung disease. Invest Radiol 1994; 29:564–569.

44. Wright GA, Hu BS, Macovski A. Estimating oxygen saturation of blood in vivo with MR imaging at 1.5 T. J MRI 1991; 1:275–283.
45. Pelc NJ, Sommer FG, Li KPC, Brosnan, TJ, Herfkens RJ, Enzmann DR. Quantitative MR flow imaging. Magn Reson Q 1994; 3:125–147.
46. Silverman JM, Julien PM, Herfkens RJ, Pelc NJ. Quantitative differential pulmonary perfusion: MR versus radionuclide lung scanning. Radiology 1993; 189:699–701.
47. Rubin GD, Herfkens RJ, Pelc NJ, Foo TKF, Napel SA, Shimakawa A, Steiner RM, Bergin CJ. Single breath-hold pulmonary MR angiography: optimization and comparison of three imaging strategies. Invest Radiol 1994; 29:766–772.
48. Bergin CJ, Glover GH, Pauly JM. Lung parenchyma: magnetic susceptibility in MR imaging. Radiology 1991; 180:845–848.
49. Middleton H, Black RD, Saam B, Cates GD, Cofer GP, Guenther R, Happer W, Hedlund LW, Johnson GA, Juvan K, Swartz J. MR imaging with hyperpolarized ^{3}He gas. Magn Reson Med 1995; 33:271–275.
50. Pityn PJ, King ME, Chamberlain MJ. A simple method for studying lung ventilation. Nucl Med Commun 1993; 14:1079–1083.
51. Susskind H, Acevedo JC, Iwai J, Rasmussen DL, Heydinger DK, Pate HR, Harold WH, Brill AB. Heterogeneous ventilation and perfusion: a sensitive indicator of lung impairment in nonsmoking coal miners. Eur Respir J 1988; 1:232–241.
52. Nichols AB, Beller GA, Cachavi S, McKusick KA, Strauss HW. Detection of pulmonary emboli by positron imaging of inhaled 15-O-labeled carbon dioxide. Semin Nucl Med 1980; 10:252–258.
53. Susskind H, Rom WH. Lung inflammation in coal miners assessed by uptake of ^{67}Ga-citrate and clearance of inhaled^{99m} Tc-labeled diethylenetriamine pentaacetate aerosol. Am Rev Respir Dis 1992; 146:47–52.
54. Fishman JA, Strauss HW, Fischman AJ, Nedelman M, Callahan R, Khaw BA, Rubin RH. Imaging of *Pneumocystis carinii* pneumonia with ^{111}In-labelled non-specific polyclonal IgG: an experimental study in rats. Nucl Med Commun 1991; 12:175–187.
55. Buscombe JR, Oyen WJ, Grant A, Claessens RA, van der Meer J, Corstens FH, Ell PJ, Miller RF. Indium-111–labeled polyclonal human immunoglobulin: identifying focal infection in patients positive for human immunodeficiency virus. J Nucl Med 1993; 34:1621–1625.
56. Fischman AJ, Babich JW, Rubin RH. Infection imaging with technetium-99m–labeled chemotactic peptide analogs. Semin Nucl Med 1994; 24:154–168.
57. Matsuyama T, Kodama K, Kitabake A, Sato H, Nanto S, Inoue M. Continuous wave Doppler echocardiographic detection of pulmonary regurgitation and its application to noninvasive estimation of pulmonary artery pressure. Circulation 1986; 74:484–492.
58. Loeber NV, Morray JP, Kettrick RG, Downes JJ. Pulmonary function in chronic respiratory failure of infancy. Crit Care Med 1980; 8:596–601.
59. Motoyama EK, Fort MD, Klesh KW, et al. Early onset of airway reactivity in premature infants with bronchopulmonary dysplasia. Am Rev Respir Dis 1987; 136:50–57.
60. Bryan MH, Hardie JJ, Reilly BJ, Swyer PR. Pulmonary function studies during the

first year of life in infants recovering from the respiratory distress syndrome. Pediatrics 1973; 52:169–178.
61. Morray JP, Fox NW, Kettrick RG, Downes JJ. Improvement in lung mechanics as a function of age in the infant with severe bronchopulmonary dysplasia. Pediatr Res 1982; 16:290–294.
62. Gerhardt T, Hehre D, Feller R, et al. Serial determination of pulmonary function in infants with chronic lung disease. J Pediatr 1987; 110:448–456.
63. Watt JL, Ariagno RL, Brady JL. Chronic pulmonary disease in neonates after artificial ventilation: distribution of ventilation and pulmonary interstitial emphysema. Pediatrics 1977; 60:273–281.
64. Harrod JR, L'Heureux P, Wangensteen OD, Hunt CE. Long term follow up of severe respiratory distress syndrome treated with IPPB. J Pediatr 1974; 84:277–286.
65. Melnick G, Pickoff AS, Ferrer PL, et al. Normal pulmonary vascular resistance and left ventricular hypertrophy in young infants with bronchopulmonary dysplasia: an echocardiographic and pathologic study. Pediatrics 1980; 66:589–596.
66. Berman W, Yabek SM, Dillon T, et al. Evaluation of infants with bronchopulmonary dysplasia using cardiac catheterization. Pediatrics 1982; 70:708–712.
67. Abman SH, Warady BA, Lum GM, Koops BL. Systemic hypertension in infants with bronchopulmonary dysplasia. J Pediatr 1984; 104:928–931.
68. Nathanson T, Conboy K, Murphy S, Afshani E, Kuhn JP. Ultrafast computerized tomography of the chest in cystic fibrosis: a new scoring system. Pediatr Pulmonol 1991; 11:81–86.
69. Ambosino MM, Genieser NB, Roche KJ, Lawerence RM. Feasibility of high-resolution, low dose chest CT in evaluating the pediatric chest. Pediatr Radiol 1994; 24: 6–10.

5

Pathology of Chronic Lung Disease of Early Infancy

JACQUELINE J. COALSON

University of Texas Health Science Center
San Antonio, Texas

I. Introduction

The decade of the 1960s heralded the era when assisted ventilation was used to treat respiratory failure in this country. The development of techniques to prevent patients from dying of cardiovascular collapse following World War II, and renal failure following the Korean War, allowed the lung to emerge as the "failing" organ during the Vietnam War (1). During this time, intensive care units became abundant and the technology of artificial ventilation advanced in infants and adults. The culmination of this progress in medical management and equipment development gave rise to two diseases, one affecting infants, the other adults: namely, bronchopulmonary dysplasia (BPD) and adult respiratory distress syndrome (ARDS), both described in the February 16, 1967 issue of the *New England Journal of Medicine*. At the time, oxygen was not widely recognized to be a severe cellular injurant, and the consequences of tissue barotrauma induced by high airway pressures were not well defined.

Northway and associates (2) described a distinctive radiographic pattern of chronic lung disease (CLD) and accompanying pathological changes in 32 premature infants who had respiratory distress syndrome (RDS) and were treated in a neonatal intensive care unit. The average gestational age and birth weight of the infants were 32 weeks and 1893 g, respectively. They speculated that BPD's pathogenesis was a prolongation of the healing phase of severe hyaline membrane disease (HMD), combined with generalized pulmonary oxygen toxicity, and recognized that endotracheal intubation and mechanical ventilation might have contributed to the disease development.

We now know that the pathology described by Northway and his associates, and augmented by additional investigators in following years (3–10), reflected primarily the consequences of elevated oxygen and ventilator-induced injury on a relatively immature and surfactant-deficient lung. The advent of positive end-expiratory pressure (PEEP) and continuous positive-airway pressure (CPAP), lower oxygen tensions, and better ventilatory strategies in the 1970s probably influenced the pathology of BPD, but this was not documented in any pathological study. Other advances in management, such as regionalization of care and better-nursing techniques, augmented the technological progress, and an increase of surviving infants with lower birth weights was evident in the BPD population even before the introduction of exogenous surfactant therapy during the 1980s (11–14).

BPD is now a disease that is seen primarily in preterm newborns who weigh less than 1000 g and are born at 24–26 weeks gestation. The use of exogenous surfactant, coupled with the advances in critical care management that have led to less barotrauma and oxygen injury, has resulted in the present pattern of injury, which reflects an extremely immature lung with impaired alveolar growth and development owing to developmental arrest, and subsequent abnormal reparative processes. Its pathogenesis involves extreme lung immaturity, treatment-induced oxygen and volutrauma injury, and an inflammatory response that elicits host autoinjury and disorganized repair.

II. Comparison of Classic BPD Pathology with BPD Pathology in the 1990s

Unfortunately, the histopathological changes currently described in most articles and textbooks for infants with BPD derive from infants who died without the benefit of newer treatment modalities and who were autopsied during the 1960s and 1970s (3–10). Also, as O'Brodovich and Mellins suggested, autopsy findings represent the most severe end of the disease spectrum (15). A review of the older pathology is presented, however, for historical interest and for a better understanding of how the new technologies and treatments have altered the disease.

A. Classic BPD Pathology

From clinical, radiographic, and autopsy data, Northway et al. (2) originally described four stages of disease development. Stage I was seen in infants 2–3 days of age who had classic acute respiratory distress syndrome. A patchy loss of ciliated cells and sites of metaplasia and necrosis of the bronchiolar mucosa were seen associated with the typical findings of hyaline membranes: hyperemia and atelectasis. Stage II was described in infants 4–10 days of age and was called the period of regeneration. Regeneration of alveolar epithelium, with persistence of hyaline membranes and emphysematous coalescence of alveoli were the pathological findings. Airway changes included patchy bronchiolar necrosis, with overlying hyaline membranes and sites of squamous metaplasia. Stage III was manifest in 10- to 20-day-old infants and was called the period of transition to chronic disease. Fewer hyaline membranes were present, and the alveolar epithelium still showed regenerative activity. Macrophages were present, and widespread bronchial and bronchiolar mucosal metaplasia was evident. Spherical, circumscribed groups of emphysematous alveoli, with surrounding atelectatic alveoli, were described. An increase in interseptal collagen was seen. Stage IV was found in infants older than 1 month and was called the period of chronic disease. Within the circumscribed areas of emphysematous alveoli, bronchioles showed peribronchiolar smooth-muscle hypertrophy, whereas in areas of atelectasis, normal bronchioles were present. Increased connective tissue deposition and pulmonary hypertensive vascular changes of periarteriolar thickening, right ventricular hypertrophy, and cardiomegaly with cor pulmonale were present in infants with stage IV disease. This stage of chronic disease occurred in 28% of the infants and was associated with 80–100% oxygen concentrations and positive-pressure ventilation for more than 150 hr. No doubt the primary factors involved in the pathogenesis of these lesions involved oxygen injury acting through production of free radicals and lipid peroxidation products and pulmonary barotrauma, superimposed on a relatively immature, surfactant-deficient lung.

Bonikos and co-workers (10) studied 21 infants who died during 1970–1974 following treatment with high oxygen concentrations and positive-pressure ventilation with PEEP. Only one of these infants was less than 30 weeks gestation and none weighed less than 1000 g. They graded the histopathological changes into mild, moderate, severe, and very severe, and presented a lengthy list of findings for each grade. No vascular lesions were evident in mild-to-moderate cases, but endothelial proliferation, degeneration of elastica, medial muscular hypertrophy, and adventitial fibrosis were evident in severe cases. This detailed study became and remains the frequently quoted reference for the pathology of BPD. Tracheal aspirates from BPD infants were evaluated cytologically and correlated using Bonikos et al.'s classification (16,17), and several additional studies substantiated, expanded, or negated some of the described histopathological features of BPD. For example, in a series of papers, several investigators evaluated the fibroproliferative airway disease, and its causal relation to the emphysematous or atelectatic sites of lung injury (5,7,9,18,19); one of these studies did not substantiate vascular changes of pulmonary hypertension (5). However, the distillation of all these reports yielded a collection of pathological findings that were generally accepted for BPD: an altered inflation pattern, with zones of overdistended, fibrotic alveoli, alternating with atelectatic or fibrotic zones (Figs. 1–3); squamous metaplasia of airway epithelium (Fig. 4a,b); obliterative bronchiolitis, peribronchial fibrosis, airway smooth-muscle hypertrophy, and vascular hypertensive lesions (see Fig. 4a,b).

The aforementioned pathological findings were derived primarily from infants who died a few weeks to several months after birth. Several investigators had included a few long-term survivors in their patient series (2,7,10,19,20), but it was Stocker, in 1986, who reported on the pathological features of 28 infants

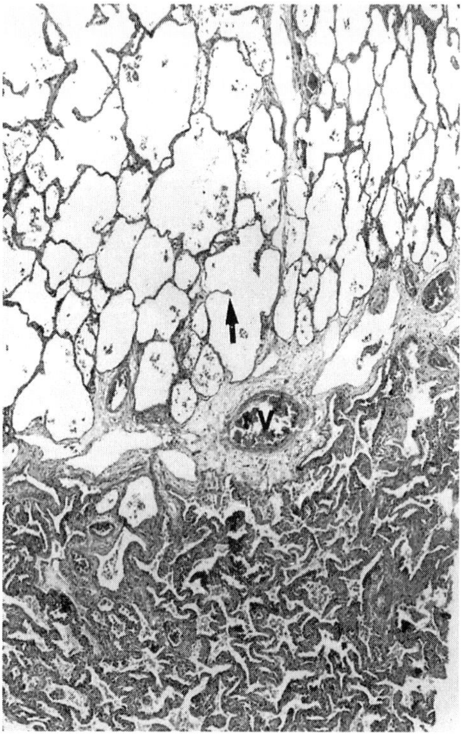

Figure 1 Lung tissue section (autopsy) from an infant with BPD who was born at 34 weeks gestation and died 4 months after birth. The section shows an altered inflation pattern of overexpanded, thinned saccular walls, separated from the atelectatic, thickened saccular walls by an interlobular septum that contains a vein (v). In a few of the overexpanded air spaces, rare alveolar duct septae are seen (arrow) (H & E; ×46).

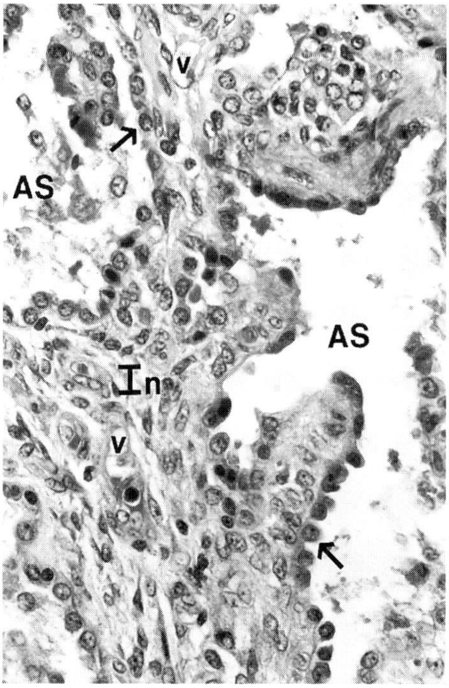

Figure 2 Lung tissue section (autopsy) from an infant with BPD who was born at 34 weeks gestation and died 4 months after birth. In the atelectatic portion of the altered inflation pattern, the saccular walls, although collapsed, show increased interstitial cellularity and fibroproliferation (In). The walls show type 2 cell hyperplasia (arrows). There are scattered small vessels (v), most of which are centrally located. As = airspaces (H & E; ×210).

who died at 3–40 months of age with long-standing ''healed'' BPD (21). These children had been treated between 1974 and 1984, and 4 of the 28 weighed less than 1000 g at birth. Enlarged hearts were present in 25 of the 28 infants. Gross examination of lungs showed retention of the alternating areas of hyperexpansion and atelectasis. Prevalent microscopic features that persisted in the patients with healed BPD included submucosal fibrosis and muscular hyperplasia of bronchi (50%); bronchial submucosal inflammation (86%); bronchiolar mild submucosal fibrosis and muscular hyperplasia (79%); alveolar septal fibrosis of variable severity (100%); increased alveolar macrophages (79%); adventitial fibrosis in parabronchial pulmonary arteries (79%), parabronchial arteries (82%); and arterioles (71%); and medial hypertrophy in parabronchiolar pulmonary vessels (64%).

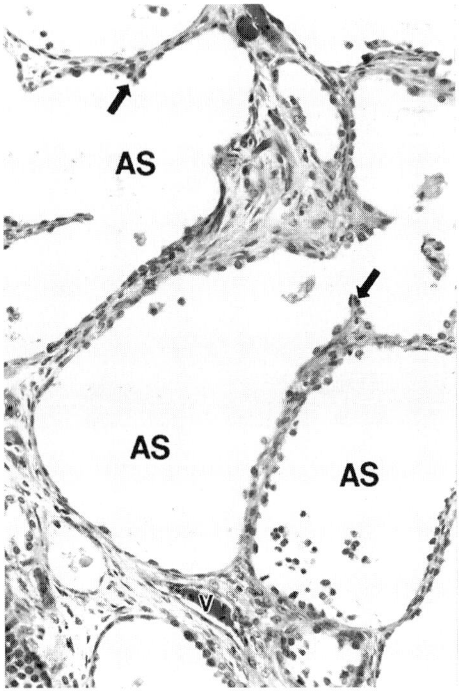

Figure 3 Lung tissue section (autopsy) from an infant with CLD who was born at 34 weeks gestation and died 4 months after birth. The overexpanded airspaces (AS) show saccular walls that are thinned and fibrotic, with few capillaries. There are a few short secondary crest/alveolar eruptions along the fibrotic walls (arrows), as well as scattered blood-filled precapillary vessels (v) (H & E; ×106).

B. "Transition" BPD Pathology Reports

During the 1980s, several papers appeared in which a number of low-birthweight, early-gestation babies with BPD were included among groups of patients with BPD that also included infants with gestations of 30 weeks or more, and weights of more than 1000 g (22–25). One of these reports included several study groups, one of which consisted of nine "very premature infants," seven of whom weighed 1000 g or less (22). This paper described a retention of a "premature lung pattern," which showed a "tubular alveolar structure" in these very small, immature infants. Erickson et al. (23) examined the lungs of 46 patients who were autopsied at The Johns Hopkins Hospital, and found that regardless of birthweight or gestational age, two morphological patterns and three patient groups emerged. One group had interstitial fibrosis, another had marked enlarge-

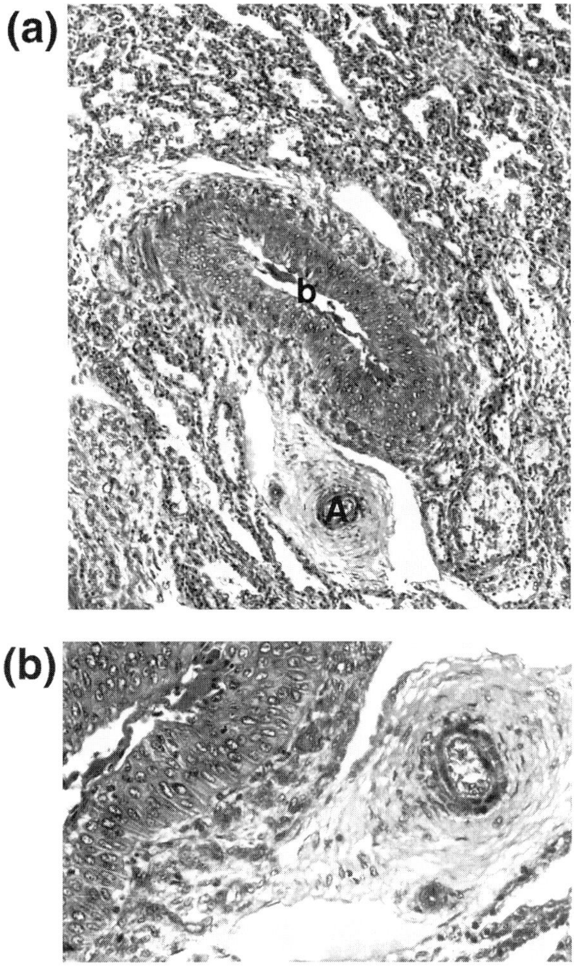

Figure 4 Lung tissue section (autopsy) from an infant with BPD who was born at 34 weeks gestation and died 4 months after birth. (a) The terminal bronchiole (b) shows squamous metaplasia, and the muscular wall of the pulmonary artery (A) is markedly thickened; (b) stratified squamous epithelium lines the bronchiole, and the artery shows severe adventitial fibrosis and a narrow lumen (H & E; ×115 and 230, respectively).

ment of distal airspaces, and a third group had a combination of the two patterns. These authors suggested that the lesions were age-related and reflected a progression from early interstitial fibrosis, which with prolonged survival and continued lung growth evolved into a picture of enlarged distal airspaces. In 1987, Hislop et al. (25) quantitated alveolar development in premature infants who required ventilation, one group of whom had HMD. The 20 infants (birth weights not given) with HMD were born at 25–33 weeks gestation, were mechanically ventilated from 3 days to 11 weeks duration, and died between 4 days and 14 months after birth. In infants who died between 32 and 40 weeks postconceptional age, shallow alveoli were present, but the alveolar walls had not thinned or projected into the alveolar ducts. Two cases showed proliferative BPD pathology. Those infants who died at more than 55 weeks postconceptional age had alveoli that were variable in shape, both within the same lung and between cases. Some were thin-walled, enlarged, and simple in outline; others were small, thick-walled, and had extra elastic in their walls. The authors specifically stated that there was an increase in muscle in the airway walls, and that tracts of interstitial fibrosis were not present. Airway epithelial pathology, however, was not discussed. Of interest, children who had received mechanical ventilation, either with or without a history of HMD, had reduced alveolar number and decreased internal surface area measurements. The lungs of control premature infants, who did not receive assisted ventilation, had normal alveolar counts and internal surface areas at death. These findings led Hislop and co-workers (25) to speculate that the changes seen in BPD could, in part, be a response of the immature lung to conventional mechanical ventilation.

Tomashefski and colleagues (26) quantitated the vascular changes in eight patients with BPD, with gestational ages of 27–32 weeks (five more than 30 weeks gestation), who died 2–8 weeks after birth. They described the internal diameter of axial arteries as a variable, being excessively wide in two patients and diffusely narrowed in three others; and the percentage medial thickness of muscular preacinar and intra-acinar pulmonary arteries was reduced compared with fetal values. However, there was an increased number of intra-acinar arteries, and some were fully muscularized. These findings led the authors to conclude that the vascular changes represented an adaptive response to injury in a hypoplastic and immature lung.

In a larger group of infants, with gestational ages from 25 to 34 weeks (6 more than 30 weeks gestation), Hislop and Haworth (27) used quantitative morphometric techniques to study the lungs of 17 premature infants who had HMD and died with CLD at ages varying between 2 weeks and 3.5 years. Irrespective of the age at death, the lungs of all infants showed an increase in pulmonary arterial medial thickening, whether or not they had cor pulmonale. The lesions in the youngest age group (2–13 weeks postnatal) appeared to reflect retention of the fetal vascular state. In infants who died between 4 and 15 months and between 6 months and 3½ years, there was further extension of muscle into smaller arteries. In the oldest group (6 months to 3½ years), there was a marked increase of muscularity in vessels within the alveolar wall, and it was this group who died with cor pulmonale. In all infants, the alveolar/arterial ratio was normal, but alveolar number was reduced, as was the total number of arteries. This same study called attention to reduced postnatal alveolar growth and absence of extensive fibrosis.

C. Recent BPD Autopsy Pathology

Very Immature Extremely Low-Birth-Weight Infants Without Surfactant Treatment

Three papers have addressed the pathological findings in very premature, extremely low-birth-weight infants of gestational ages 24–30 weeks (26–28). The infants reported in these studies did not receive prenatal steroids and were not treated with exogenous surfactant. In the Chambers and van Velzen study (28), 83 infants who died between 1983 and 1987 with birth weights ranging from 520 to 1658 g and gestational ages ranging from 23.5 to 30 weeks were autopsied. All were initially ventilated with 100% oxygen, but some had stabilized at concentrations of 70–80% before death. All infants who died after 10 days or more of mechanical ventilation had persistence of simple, evenly distributed terminal airspaces, lined by undifferentiated cuboidal epithelium, and separated by evenly widened septa, with hypercellular fibrous stroma and increased amounts of subepithelial elastic tissue. Arrested alveolar development was documented quantitatively by low Emery counts of the terminal respiratory units. In those infants who lived 17–156 days, airway changes, such as squamous metaplasia and peribronchial fibrosis, were infrequent and negligible. The only consistent bronchial change was smooth-muscle hyperplasia and a mild increase in mucin secretion. Vascular changes were consistently present, but consisted of endothelial edema, mild medial thickening, some increase in elastic tissue, and an occasional thrombus. A high proportion of infants with evolving disease were noted to have severe acute pulmonary interstitial emphysema of relatively late onset, suggesting that the immature alveolar wall with abundant mesenchyme was more susceptible to barotrauma.

Van Lierde et al.'s study (29) from Belgium included autopsied infants born between 1980 and 1988. Two major variants were described. One was a bronchiolitic form, similar to that originally described by Northway et al. (2). Seen primarily in infants weighing 820–1075 g, with gestational ages of 27–29 weeks, the pathology of this form included squamous metaplasia of the trachea, major bronchi and airways, and connective tissue proliferation, and varying amounts of atelectasis. The other variant was called an interstitial form, and was characterized by arrested development of terminal airspaces, which were evenly thickened and fibrosed and not alveolarized. Infants in this group had birth weights of 880–1165 g (mean, 1060 g) and gestational ages of 25.5–29 weeks (mean, 26 weeks). The median age at death was 23 days, with a range of 15–52 days in the interstitial group; and 11 days, with a range of 4–21 days in the bronchiolar group. Vascular lesions were not discussed in this study.

Margraf et al. (30) examined autopsy specimens of eight infants who were born at gestational ages of 24–30 weeks (birth weights were not given), and who died at postnatal ages of 2–28 months. All the infants had had HMD. Their lungs showed varying amounts of bronchial and bronchiolar squamous metaplasia, marked simplification of acinar structure, variable but constant alveolar septal fibrosis, and abnormalities in elastic fiber architecture and arrangement. When compared with the lungs of six control infants, mean linear intercept determinations showed that total alveolar number was decreased, and lung internal surface area was reduced. Little evidence of age-related compensatory alveolar development was evident. Bronchiolar smooth-muscle hypertrophy was seen in seven patients. They also found increased quantities of smooth-muscle and submucosal gland tissue in large airways, similar to the earlier observations of Hislop and Haworth (31). Increased musculature in airway walls persists as a finding in BPD, and significant increases of bronchiolar neuroendocrine cells have also been reported (32,33).

A summary of the newer pathological findings in CLD of infants who have been born at less than 30 weeks gestation and with birth weights less than 1000 g would include less airway epithelial disease than previously described, less severe vascular disease, varying degrees of interstitial fibrosis, increased elastic fiber deposition in the saccular walls, and an abundance of large, simplified airspaces (i.e., minimal alveolization), rather than alternating zones of fibrosis–atelectasis and overinflation. Figures 5–10 show examples of the histopathological features of lungs from non–surfactant-treated infants who were treated and died with BPD during the last decade. All the infants were less than 30 weeks gestation. The figures show the pathological features that were present at varying ages during disease progression (e.g., 2-weeks and 1-, 2.5-, 6.5-, 7-, and 8-month specimens).

Very Immature Extremely Low-Birth-Weight Infants with Surfactant Treatment

Husain et al. (34) examined autopsy specimens from 14 surfactant-treated infants with BPD, 8 non–surfactant-treated BPD patients, and 15 age-matched controls who were autopsied from 1988 through 1994. The infants were treated with three doses of exogenous surfactant (either Survanta or Exosurf), given by intratracheal aerosolization during the first 24 hr. No history of prenatal steroid treatment was given. Gestational ages of the non–surfactant-treated BPD patients ranged from

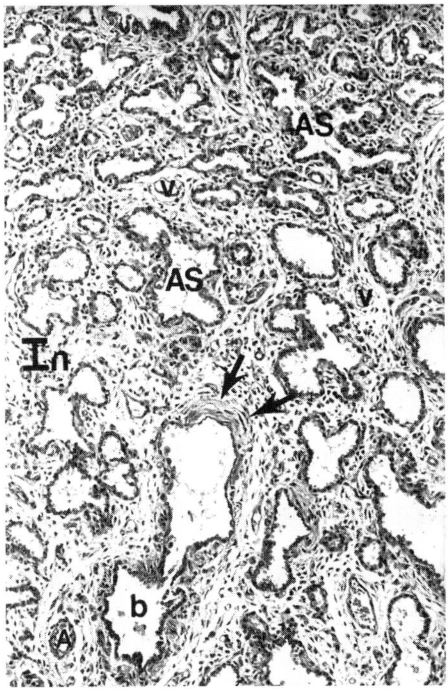

Figure 5 Lung tissue section (autopsy) from an infant who was born at 25 weeks gestation and died 2 weeks after birth. Considerable fibroproliferation is present throughout the interstitium (In) of the distal lung. The terminal bronchiole (b) opens into an ectatic airway, the wall of which contains some condensed connective tissue (arrows). The saccules are lined with cuboidal epithelium and show little secondary crest formation. A few small vessels (v) are centrally placed in the thickened saccular walls. AS = airspace (H & E; ×110).

24 to 30 weeks, birth weights were not stated. Gestational ages of the nonsurfactant-treated BPD group ranged from 27 to 29 weeks. Of the 14 surfactant-treated infants, 8 lived for 1–6 weeks, whereas the other 6 survived for 12–413 weeks. Length of life in the nonsurfactant-treated BPD group ranged from 2 to 71 weeks. Mild to moderate alveolar septal fibrosis was evident in 5 of the 14 surfactant-treated study group, whereas 7 of the 8 nonsurfactant-treated infants had moderate to severe alveolar septal fibrosis of the type associated with the long-standing healed BPD changes described by Stocker in 1986 (21). No necrotizing bronchiolitis was evident in the surfactant group, and in most infants, a normal-appearing capillary bed was noted. When mean linear intercepts and radial alveolar counts were used to evaluate the degree of alveolization and alveolar size,

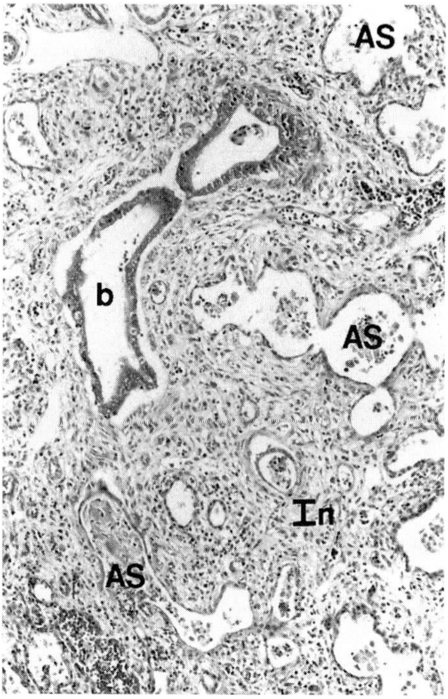

Figure 6 Lung tissue section (autopsy) from an infant who was born at 26 weeks gestation and died 1 month after birth. The bronchiolar epithelium is artifactually lifted from its thickened and fibrotic wall (b). The surrounding airspaces (AS) contain proteinaceous debris and scattered inflammatory cells. The saccular walls show interstitial widening (In) and no evidence of alveolarization (H & E; ×110).

and then expressed as a ratio, an ''acinar arrest'' was noted in the BPD patient specimens, with a postconceptual age older than 40 weeks, when compared with control specimens without BPD. They concluded that the use of postnatal surfactant therapy did not alter the inhibition of acinar development that occurs in BPD infants.

D. Recent BPD Biopsy Pathology: Very Immature, Extremely Low-Birth-Weight Infants

As stated earlier, autopsy findings represent the severe end of the spectrum in BPD. Thus, it is useful to review the pathology of lung biopsy specimens obtained from infants with severe, but not necessarily lethal, disease. I have examined such specimens obtained surgically from infants with BPD at Wilford Hall USAF

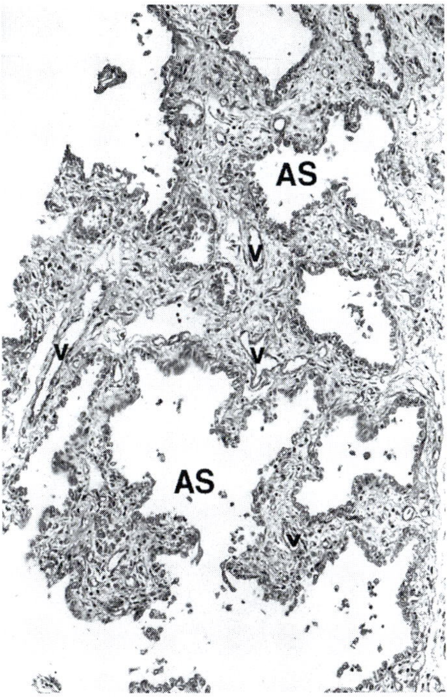

Figure 7 Lung tissue section (autopsy) from an infant who was born at 25 weeks gestation and died 2½ months after birth. The saccular walls show considerable interstitial fibroproliferation and many centrally placed dilated vessels (v). The unevenly sized airspaces (AS) show no alveoli (H & E; ×110).

Medical Center and area hospitals, only one of whom received exogenous surfactant treatment. Ten open-lung biopsies were obtained from low birth weight infants on ventilatory support at postnatal ages ranging from 2 weeks to 7 months. The gestational ages at birth ranged from 24 to 28 weeks (mean, 26 weeks), and birth weights ranged from 570 to 1100 g (mean 809 g). There were no complications following the open-lung biopsy, and 50% of the infants survived. The histopathological findings in the open-lung biopsies at 2 weeks, 1 month, 2.5 months, and 7 months are illustrated in Figures 11–15.

Airway epithelial changes of metaplasia and hyperplasia were negligible at all stages of the disease that were studied (see Figs. 11–15). The altered inflation pattern of emphysema and severe atelectasis–fibrosis was seen inconsistently, but there were dilated saccules or terminal airspaces that varied in size in all of the specimens (see Figs. 11–14). A simplified distal lung acinus and *a*

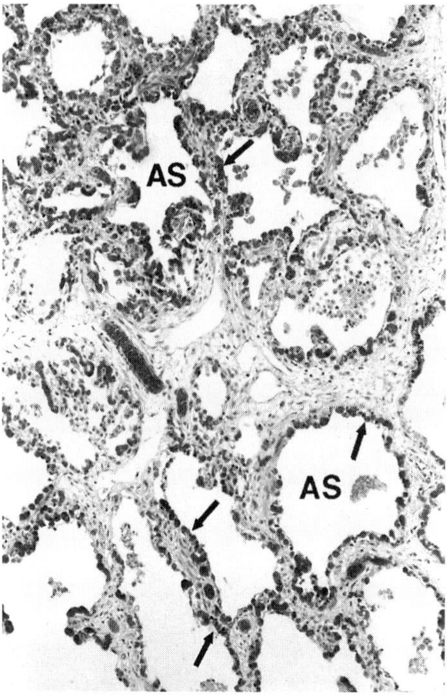

Figure 8 Lung tissue section (autopsy) from an infant who was born at 26 weeks gestation and died 6½ months after birth. Dilated airspaces (AS), with no evidence of alveolarization, are evident. The interstitium is thickened. Note the placement of the blood-filled capillaries beneath the epithelial lining (arrows), similar to that described by McKay et al. (105) as festooning of the capillary bed. A few larger vessels are in the thickened interstitium (H & E; ×110).

consistent lack of significant alveolarization (i.e., alveolar hypoplasia,) were the primary findings, even in the biopsy specimen obtained at postnatal age 7 months (see Figs. 11–14). The most variable finding was the degree of cellularity and fibrosis in the terminal respiratory units (see Figs. 11–14), but this variability was less notable than it was in most autopsy specimens of lung (e.g., Figs. 2, 5–7). The two biopsies obtained at 2 weeks showed a widened cellular interstitium and poorly formed secondary crests, both by light and electron microscopy (Figs. 11 and 16). Thereafter, in the 1- and 2.5-month–biopsy specimens, there was variability in the degree of interstitial thickening: in some cases, there were thin saccular walls only; in others, thin saccular walls were interspersed among focal, widened septae, or more diffusely widened septae (see Figs. 12 and 13). The

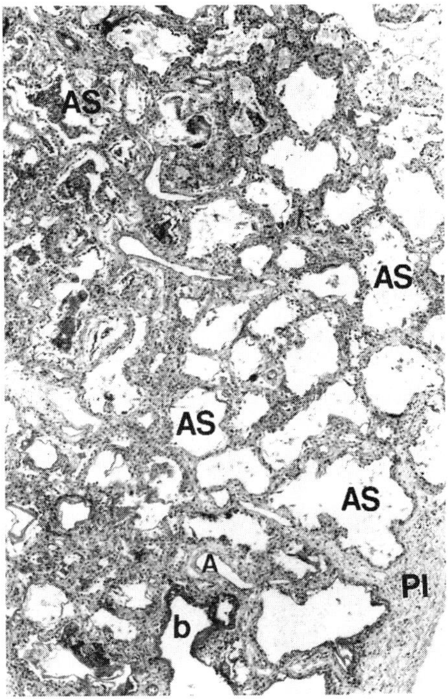

Figure 9 Lung tissue section (autopsy) from an infant who was born at 28 weeks gestation and died 7 months after birth. Many of the airspaces (AS) contain protein and red blood cells. The ectatic airspaces are not alveolarized. The pleura (Pl) is thickened and fibrotic. b = bronchiole; A = pulmonary artery (H & E; ×46).

specimen obtained at 7 months had thinned, more fibrotic saccular walls (see Fig. 14), with focal accumulation of elastic fibers (not shown). In most cases, the smooth-muscle content in the walls of bronchioles appeared normal (see Fig. 15). However, these specimens were from the distal lung, and sampling may be too limited to fully assess vascular muscle content or fibrointimal or medial arterial changes in vessels accompanying small bronchi. A few pulmonary arteries accompanying the terminal and respiratory bronchioles did appear to have thickened smooth-muscle medias (see Fig. 15).

The most striking finding was an abnormal capillary configuration. A subepithelial position of the capillaries was frequently seen in the sites of fibroproliferation, and the microvessels were dilated focally. Other areas of fibroproliferation showed more centrally placed capillaries. Platelet endothelial cell adhesion molecule (PECAM; CD31), a marker for endothelial cells, was used to immuno-

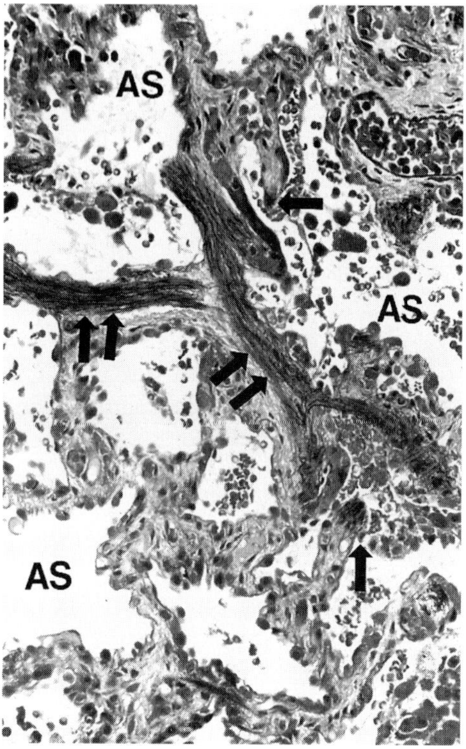

Figure 10 Lung tissue section (biopsy) from an infant who was born at less than 30 weeks gestation and underwent a lung biopsy 8 months later. The section was stained with van Gieson elastica stain and shows layered elastic fibers within thickened saccular walls (double arrows). Elastic fiber deposition is also seen in the tips of alveolar ducts (arrows). There is decreased overall cellularity within the interstitium and more connective tissue deposition. AS = airspace (H & E; ×230).

stain these lung specimens and those of gestational controls. An adaptive dysmorphic pattern of vascular organization was seen in the diseased lungs (Figs. 17 and 18). There were prominent ''corner'' vessels, plus adjacent dilated vessels, and the capillaries were extremely sparse in the thinned saccular walls (not shown), and dilated and more abundant in other sites (see Figs. 17 and 18). The 7-month-biopsy specimen showed type I collagen staining on the trichrome–elastica-stained preparation. The histopathological changes that have evolved in the pathology of BPD are summarized in Table 1.

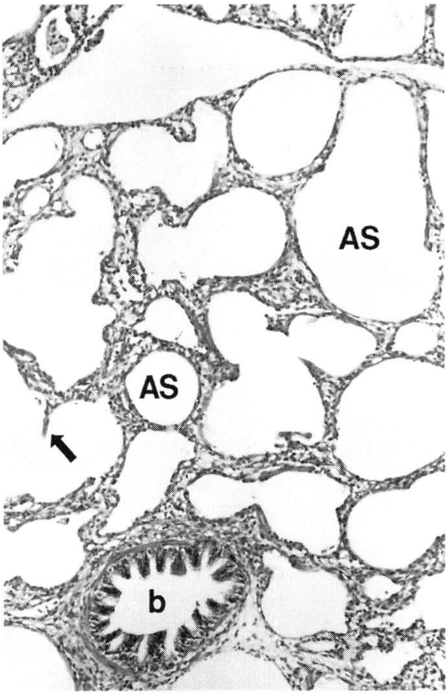

Figure 11 Lung tissue section (biopsy) from an infant who was born at 28 weeks gestation and had a lung biopsy performed 2 weeks later. The terminal bronchiole (b) shows epithelial infolding, but no squamous metaplasia, and a thin muscular layer. The surrounding saccules (AS) are unevenly expanded and show little secondary crest formation (arrows) (H & E; ×110).

III. Major Differences in "Old" BPD Versus "New" BPD Pathology: Airway and Interstitial Disease

In the immature infant, the widespread deficiency of surfactant at the saccular or alveolar level results in a lung with a potentially more compliant compartment: the noncartilaginous airways. Almost four decades ago, Gruenwald (35) determined that pressure–volume recordings from human lungs with HMD had abnormally high opening pressures and poor stability on deflation. The portion of the lung that expanded with application of high pressure was the terminal bronchiole and its several generations of respiratory bronchioles, with resultant tissue injury. In an elegant series of experiments, Robertson (36,37) demonstrated that, during

(a)

(b)

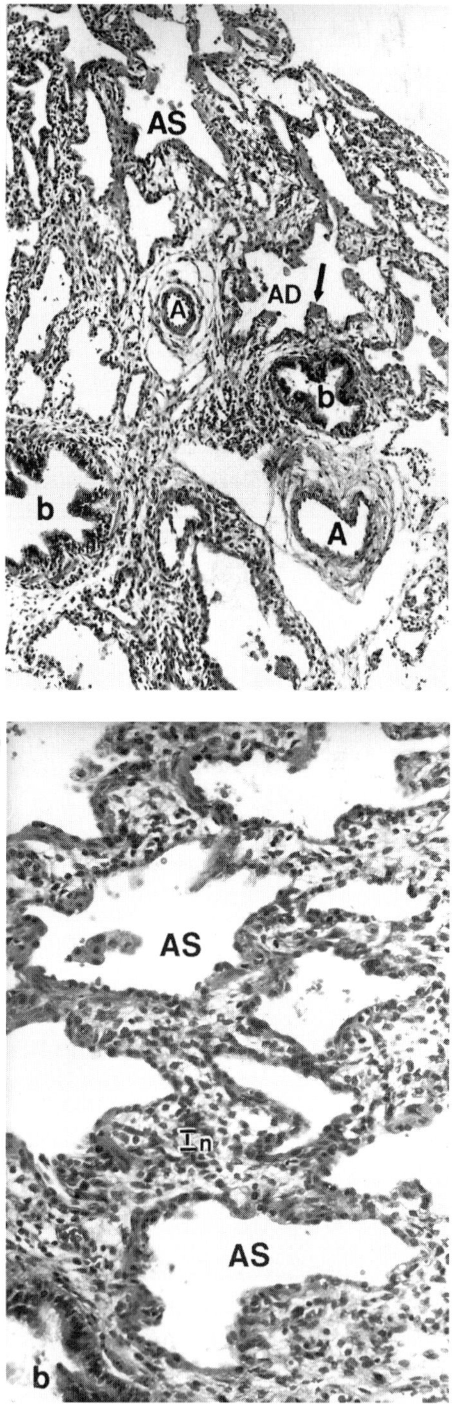

the first few minutes of spontaneous or ventilator-assisted breathing, the bronchiolar epithelium overstretches and then lifts from the underlying basement membrane. Epithelial lifting in terminal airways was noted in very early autopsy reports of human infants with HMD, but was thought to be artifactual, secondary to autolysis (38).

Experimental evidence indicated that elevated oxygen levels and sustained effects of positive-pressure ventilation were both causative injurious agents that induced the squamous metaplasia of airways seen in early BPD. It was reported in several animal species exposed to elevated oxygen levels in chambers without ventilator-induced injury. Ludwin et al. (39) found that airway squamous metaplasia occurred even in the absence of high ventilatory peak pressures in airways of 100% oxygen-treated mice. Retrospective studies of autopsy cases, however, have implied that the severity of airway lesions correlated better with the peak airway pressures associated with mechanical ventilation than with the total dose of oxygen delivered (4,9,40,41). Robertson et al. (37) described squamous metaplasia of bronchiolar epithelium in infants older than 1 month of age, who were ventilated with peak inflation pressures higher than 50 cmH_2O. The recognition by investigators, during the 1970s, that high levels of inspired oxygen and peak inflation pressure were injurious to the lung led to the more judicious use of both, and perhaps this accounts for the marked reduction in airway epithelial lesions now reported in autopsies of infants with BPD.

The lack of severe airway epithelial lesions may also help explain the apparent difference of the altered inflation pattern noted at autopsy in recent reports, compared with earlier descriptions of lung pathology in BPD. Early experiments in animal models showed that a static inflation pressure of 35 cmH_2O caused an irregular pattern of alveolar expansion in immature rabbits (42). Those airways supplying atelectatic and less compliant distal parenchyma were believed to undergo more severe ventilator-induced injury. Many investigators surmised that obstruction of the terminal airways resulted from hyaline membrane formation that, within 2–3 days following birth, coalesced and formed plugs, leading to

Figure 12 Lung tissue section (biopsy) from an infant who was born at 24–25 weeks gestation and had a lung biopsy performed 1 month later. (a) Several bronchioles are present [b], accompanied by pulmonary artery branches (A). An interstitial mononuclear inflammatory infiltrate is in the bronchiolar wall and throughout the interstitium. The distal airspaces (AS) are unevenly inflated, with little evidence of secondary crest formation except in alveolar duct (AD) areas, where they are widened and have prominent distal tips of connective tissue (arrows). (b) The saccular walls are lined with cuboidal epithelium and the interstitium (In) contains many mononuclear cells (H & E; ×110 and 220, respectively).

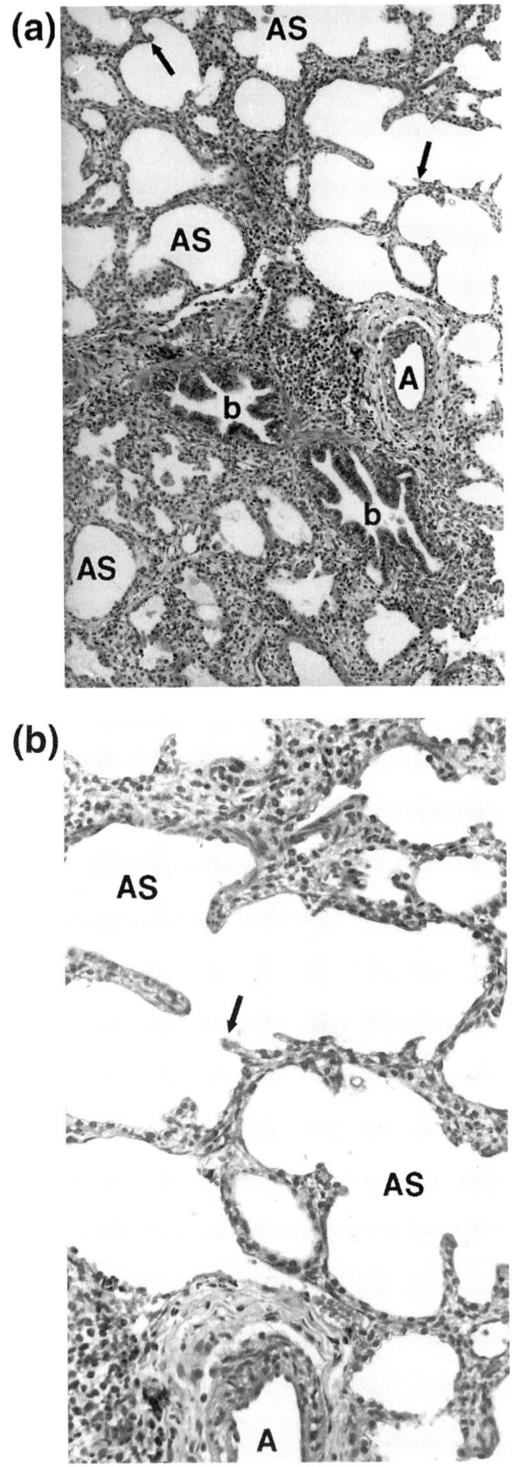
(a)
AS
AS
A
b
b
AS
(b)
AS
AS
A

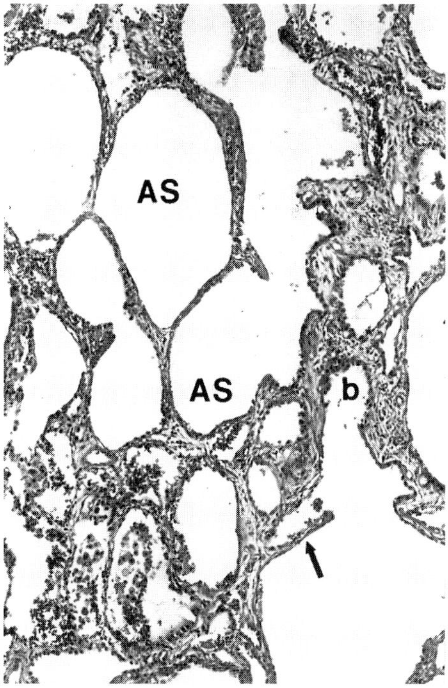

Figure 14 Lung tissue section (biopsy) from an infant who was born at 26–27 weeks gestation and underwent an open-lung biopsy 7 months after birth. There is considerable thinning of the distal airspaces (AS), but a lack of overall alveolarization persists. Note the variation in the interstitial fibroproliferation and the unevenly expanded airspaces. The bronchiole (b) branches into the alveolar duct area that shows a thickened alveolar septum (arrow) (H & E; ×110).

Figure 13 Lung tissue section (biopsy) from an infant who was born at 26 weeks gestation and underwent an open-lung biopsy 2½ months after birth. Two patterns are evident in the distal parenchyma. (a) The saccular walls are thickened and hypercellular in the lower portion. An interstitial inflammatory infiltrate of mononuclear cells is dispersed around the partially muscularized bronchioles [b] and the slightly thickened pulmonary artery (A). (b) The distal parenchyma (AS) is unevenly inflated with a few alveolar duct septae and some blunted alveolar structures (arrows), better seen in panel b. A = pulmonary artery (H & E; ×110 and 230, respectively).

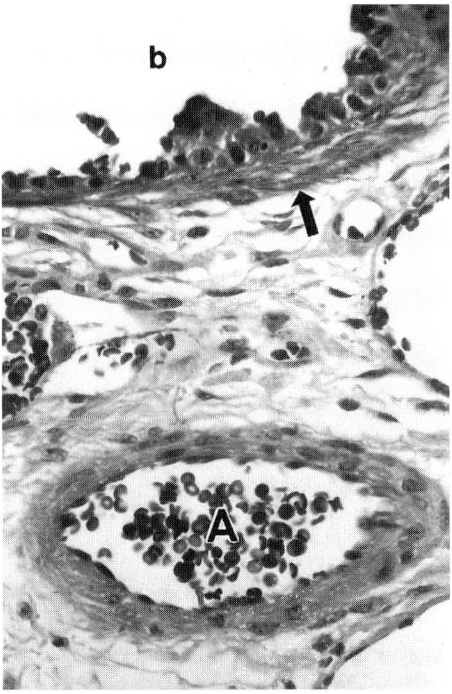

Figure 15 Lung tissue section (biopsy) from an infant who was born at 26–27 weeks gestation and underwent an open-lung biopsy 7 months after birth. The bronchiolar wall contains little muscle (arrow), and the pulmonary artery (A) has minimal, if any, medial hypertrophy. b = bronchiole (trichrome connective tissue stain; ×460).

obstruction. In his study of long-standing healed BPD, Stocker (21) claimed that necrotizing bronchiolitis functioned to protect parenchyma distal to the occlusion from high ventilatory pressures and the direct toxic effects of elevated oxygen, and resulted in the hyperexpanded portion of the altered inflation pattern.

It is likely that the judicious use of less oxygen and lower peak airway pressures and tidal volumes has decreased the severity of the interstitial fibrosis in patients with BPD and CLD. Interstitial fibrosis was the main residual feature that Stocker (21) defined in the healed stage of BPD, and was consistently found in his study group of 24 infants who died at 3–40 months of age with moderate to severe BPD. He suggested that the septal fibrosis and pulmonary scarring resulted directly from barotrauma-induced stretching of the alveolar wall during ventilatory therapy. Perhaps the reduction of barotrauma-induced interstitial pulmonary emphysema, a primary factor in the pathogenesis of BPD (43,44), also has influ-

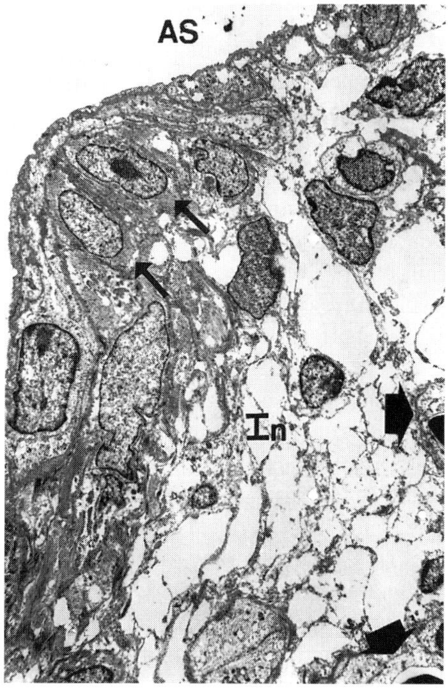

Figure 16 Lung tissue section (biopsy) from an infant who was born at 28 weeks gestation and underwent an open-lung biopsy 2 weeks after birth. Ultrastructurally, increased connective fibers are layered below the epithelial lining. Two mesenchymal cells are aligned at a different angle beneath the lifted epithelium (early secondary crest formation?; arrows). The interstitium (In) shows increased matrix or edema, and portions of two vessels are seen (arrow tips). AS = airspace (lead citrate and uranyl acetate; ×2800).

enced the decrease in fibroproliferation in more recent pathological findings of BPD.

Experimental studies of ventilator-induced lung injury show that microvascular permeability, recruitment of neutrophils, and activation of mediators result in distal lung tissue injury and interstitial and alveolar edema (reviewed in Ref. 45), but none of the acute studies in immature lungs have yielded fibroproliferation (46–51). With a series of lung markers for injury in a neonatal pig model, Davis et al. (50) found less atelectasis, edema formation, fibrinous exudate, and inflammation in ventilator-induced lung disease compared with injury associated with hyperoxia alone. In experimental models, prolonged oxygen exposure induces increased interstitial cellularity, and the pathological lesions that are associ-

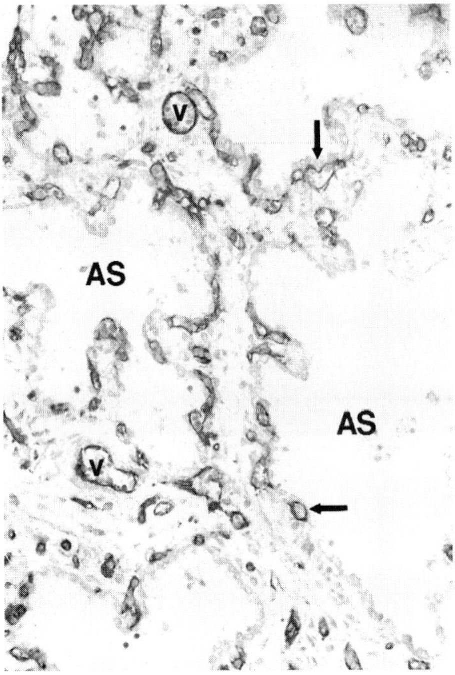

Figure 17 Lung tissue section (autopsy) from an infant with CLD who was born at 25 weeks gestation and died 2 weeks after birth. The capillaries (arrows) and corner vessels (v) are immunostained for platelet endothelial cell adhesion molecule (CD31; PECAM). Note the double layer of capillaries and some centrally positioned small vessels. AS = airspaces (×230).

ated with experimentally induced oxygen toxicity are similar to those in BPD, especially the classic type (39,52–58).

IV. Alveolar Hypoplasia and Vascular Dysmorphic Changes: The Consistent Findings in New BPD

A review of human lung development focuses and defines the problem of current BPD in low birth weight infants (59,60). The stages and accompanying developmental events of lung development are reviewed in Table 2. The extent of lung development between 24–26 weeks gestation and 30–32 weeks gestation is considerable (Figs. 19 and 20). The lung at 24 weeks is in the canalicular stage of

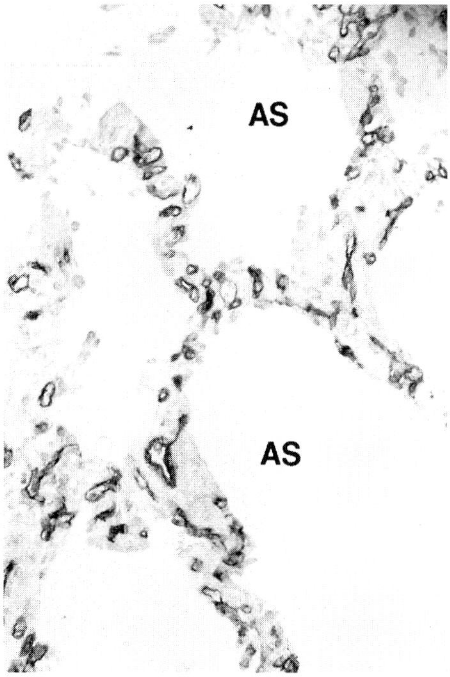

Figure 18 Lung tissue section (biopsy) from an infant who was born at 26–27 weeks gestation and underwent an open-lung biopsy 7 months after birth. The corner vessels and capillaries show considerable variation in size and appearance in this preparation that is immunostained for PECAM. This represents an adaptive, dysmorphic pattern. AS = airspaces (×230).

development (see Fig. 19), and at 30 weeks the lung is in the saccular stage. Although alveoli are present in some infants at 32 weeks gestation (see Fig. 20), they are not uniformly present until 36 weeks. Thus, premature birth and initiation of pulmonary gas exchange interrupts normal alveolar development, thereby triggering the production of a major feature of BPD. A decrease in alveolarization, however, is not unique to the extremely immature survivors with BPD. In spite of the fact that gestationally older infants at least have saccules and a few alveoli, premature delivery and treatment with supplemental oxygen and positive-pressure mechanical ventilation leads to a reduced number of alveoli, a decrease in internal surface area, and an increase in mean linear intercepts in human infants (20,25,30) and in preterm baboons (61) with BPD. Now that less oxygen and smaller tidal volumes are being used to manage immature infants with lung dis-

Table 1 Evolution of Pathology in BPD

Late 1960s to early 1970s
Altered inflation pattern of atelectasis and overinflation
Severe airway epithelial lesions (hyperplasia, squamous metaplasia)
Airway smooth-muscle hyperplasia
Extensive fibroproliferation
Prominent vascular hypertensive lesions
Late 1970s to 1980s
Retention of simplified terminal respiratory unit
Negligible airway epithelial lesions
Airway smooth-muscle hyperplasia
More variable fibroproliferation
Less severe preacinar vascular lesions
Adaptive dysmorphic changes in distal vasculature
Antenatal steroids and postnatal surfactant treatment era: can the lung restart arrested maturational processes
Unknown pathology

ease, future studies need to determine if normal alveolar development can resume in the face of new treatments that blunt or prevent inflammatory autoinjury and resultant dysregulated fibroproliferative responses.

The hallmark of the canalicular phase is vasculogenesis, during which capillaries form from mesenchymal progenitors and fuse in the interstitium (57,58,62). Some of the vessels in the primitive airspace walls that are destined to become saccules and then alveoli are still dispersed and situated centrally within the interstitium at 24–26 weeks gestation, although some of the microvessels are subepithelial. Much more information is available about growth and response to injury of vessels the size of precapillary and larger arterioles, whereas very little is known about the capillaries. Their dysmorphic adaptation to an extrauterine environment needs additional study. The presence of an adequate vasculature in the lung may be the critical determinant of successful respiratory gas exchange and survival of extremely immature infants.

Thinning of the interstitium also starts in the canalicular phase, and elastin is deposited in the saccular walls in preparation for secondary crest formation (63). Loosli and Potter (64) determined, four decades ago, that elastic fiber deposition in the developing lung served as the stimulus for alveolar formation. Several studies (11,19,21,22) have documented that the elastic fiber configuration in BPD is abnormal (e.g., areas of elastic fiber condensation, fragmentation, and twisting), especially at the level of the alveolar duct (see Fig. 10). There are only a few studies that have examined the interstitial cellular, connective tissue fiber, and extracellular matrix responses to injury in premature lungs (65–67). The

Table 2 Stages of Human Lung Development

Embryonal
First 7 weeks of gestation
Airways to level of bronchopulmonary segments develop
Lining epithelium is multilayered collection of spindle cells
Pseudoglandular
Extends from 7 to 16 weeks gestation
Dichotomous branching of 16–25 generations of airways occurs to the level of the acinus
Differentiation of respiratory epithelial cells and cartilage
Angiogenetic development of preacinar vasculature completed
Canalicular
Extends from approximately 16 to 26–28 weeks gestation
Peripheral lining cells become cuboidal and distinct from bronchiolar epithelium
Differentiation of type 2 epithelial cells begins
Development of distal pulmonary circulation by vasculogenesis with capillaries present at 20 weeks
Interstitial tissue decreases with thinning of the future gas-exchanging units
Saccular
Extends from 26–28 to 32–36 weeks gestation
Marked decrease in interstitial space of saccular walls
Cylindrical saccules are subdivided by secondary crests (tissue projections into the airspace)
Crests contain a double-capillary layer
Alveolar
Extends from 32–36 weeks to term gestation
Thinning of the secondary crests and fusion of capillaries form alveoli

Source: Refs. 58, 59, 61.

repair process is thought to resemble wound healing, and collagen type I/type III ratios are decreased in lungs that are undergoing repair and cell proliferation in infants with BPD when compared with control lungs (67). The infant lung, compared with the adult, has less intramural organization, a specific type of healing response in which fibroblasts, myofibroblasts, and endothelial cells migrate into a fibrin-rich matrix in the alveolar space (68). Idell and Viscardi and their co-workers (69,70) demonstrated increased fibrinolytic activity in human and baboon neonates with BPD, which likely enhanced the dissolution of the intra-alveolar proteinaceous exudate (hyaline membranes) that formed during the exudative phase of BPD.

As gestational development continues, the cylindrical saccules are subdivided by secondary crests (Fig. 21), which have a double-capillary layer during the saccular phase. This double capillary undergoes fusion as the lung matures

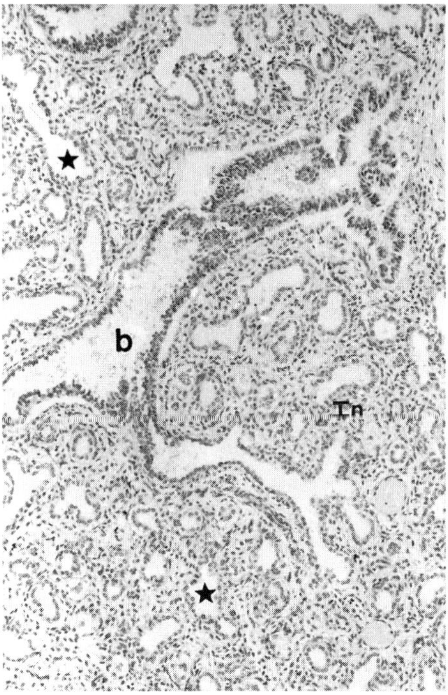

Figure 19 Lung tissue section (autopsy) from an infant who was stillborn at 24 weeks gestation. The immersion-fixed lung specimen shows a terminal bronchiole (b) and its branches in the respiratory portion of the lung. The distal airspaces (★) have rounded airspaces separated by intervening mesenchyme (In) (H & E; ×110).

and alveoli form. The secondary crests become alveoli; thin-walled structures the depth of which exceeds their width when viewed microscopically. The human lung at term contains alveoli (Fig. 22), and alveolarization continues postnatally for about 2 years (71).

The ''new'' pathology of BPD does not include infants who are treated with antenatal steroids and postnatal surfactant and go on to acquire the ''BPD'' of this era, better termed chronic lung disease (CLD) of early infancy. However, as noted earlier, postnatal exogenous surfactant treatment alone did not enhance alveolarization in BPD survivors (34). As predicted by an early experimental study (72), a beneficial effect of exogenous surfactant treatment was documented by Pinar et al. (73) in the pathology of humans with HMD. These authors graded and compared several different histopathological features known to exist in infants who did and did not receive calf lung surfactant (Survanta). They demon-

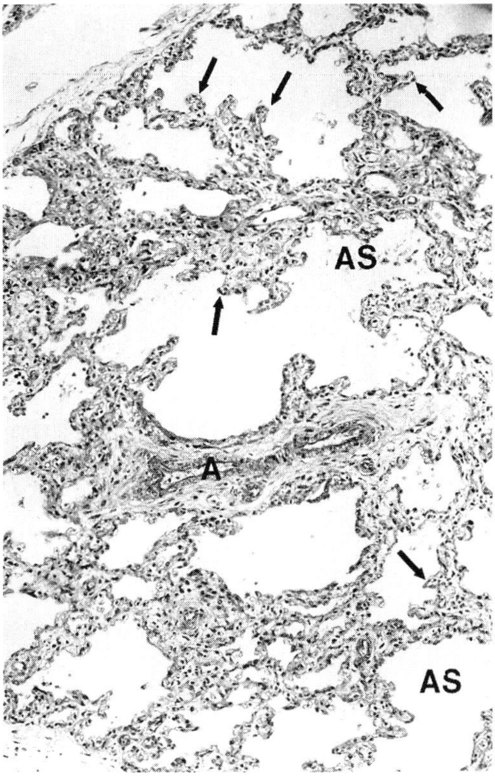

Figure 20 Lung tissue section (autopsy) from an infant who was born at 32–33 weeks gestation and died 5 days after birth. The immersion-fixed specimen shows considerable thinning of the interstitial compartment when compared with that of the 24-week gestation specimen. The large saccular spaces (AS) show secondary crest eruptions (arrows), the progenitors of the alveoli. A = pulmonary artery (H & E; ×110).

strated that there were significantly fewer hyaline membranes, less epithelial necrosis, and pulmonary interstitial emphysema in surfactant-treated infants, whereas pulmonary hemorrhage was comparable in both groups.

We recently described a baboon model of borderline viability in which antenatal steroid and postnatal surfactant treatment are used in conjunction with appropriate oxygenation and ventilatory strategies to mimic human CLD (see Chap. 38) (74,75). Following 1–2 months of ventilatory support, data show that in spite of appropriate treatment modalities, the lesions of alveolar hypoplasia and vascular developmental arrest and adaptive dysmorphic changes are not prevented in extremely immature lungs. These infant baboons are difficult to wean

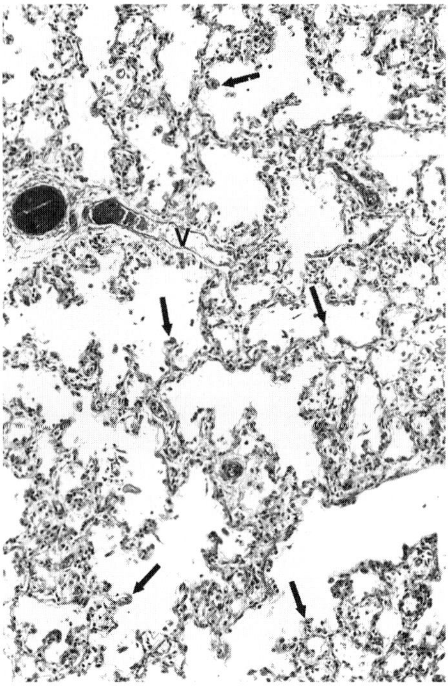

Figure 21 Lung tissue section (autopsy) from an infant who was stillborn at 38 weeks. The lung specimen depicts the alveolar phase of lung development. Considerable thinning of the secondary crests (arrows) and a more thinned interstitium are evident throughout the lung. V = vessel (H & E; ×106).

from ventilatory support, and the possibility of a delayed spurt of alveolar and vascular growth in long-term survivors following successful weaning merits further inquiry.

V. Pathogenesis of BPD in the 1990s

The etiology of BPD classically included the factors of oxygen toxicity, barotrauma, and immaturity, which over time led to the disease and its manifestations. The debate concerning the relative roles of oxygen and positive-pressure ventilation is still ongoing. During fetal development, the lung exists in an hypoxic environment, with arterial oxygen tensions of 20–25 mmHg; therefore, air itself could represent hyperoxia to an immature lung (76,77). The need for high airway pressures, with resultant lung injury, is substantially less with the use of exoge-

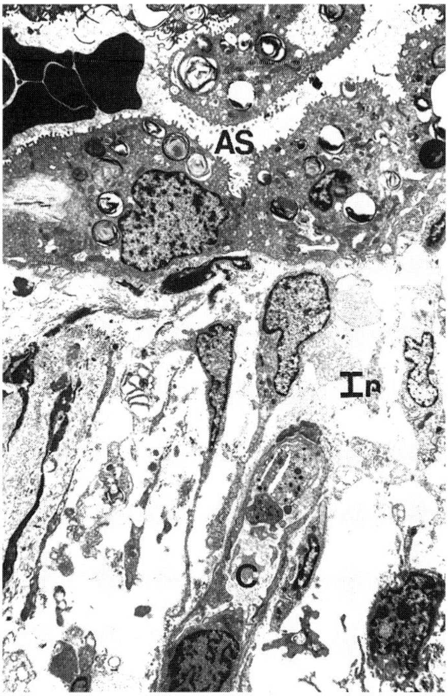

Figure 22 Lung tissue section (biopsy) from an infant who was born at 33 weeks gestation and underwent a lung biopsy 3 weeks later. Hyperplastic type 2 cells are seen lining the airspace (AS). The underlying interstitium (In) shows abundant extracellular matrix, mesenchymal cells, and some connective tissue fibers. Platelets and a mononuclear cell are evident in a capillary (C) (lead citrate and uranyl acetate; ×2800).

nous surfactant treatment, but the immature lung does not have the structural framework to withstand forced-air breathing without incurring injury. An inflammatory response results when the pulmonary bronchoalveolar (saccular) epithelial and endothelial structural framework is disrupted (reviewed in 78,79). This inflammatory response mediates an autoinjury in the host and elicits the subsequent repair responses in the immature lung (see Figs. 22 and 23). Lung injury also can occur when intrauterine infection antedates the delivery of premature infants. Maternal chorioamnionitis can result in an active inflammatory response that directly or indirectly triggers a response in the fetus (80–83). Such infants probably have a heightened inflammatory response at birth, when compared with infants who are delivered without associated chorioamnionitis. The lung injury induces increased vascular permeability, leading to leakage of protein-rich fluid in the saccular spaces. O'Brodovich and his colleagues have shown in

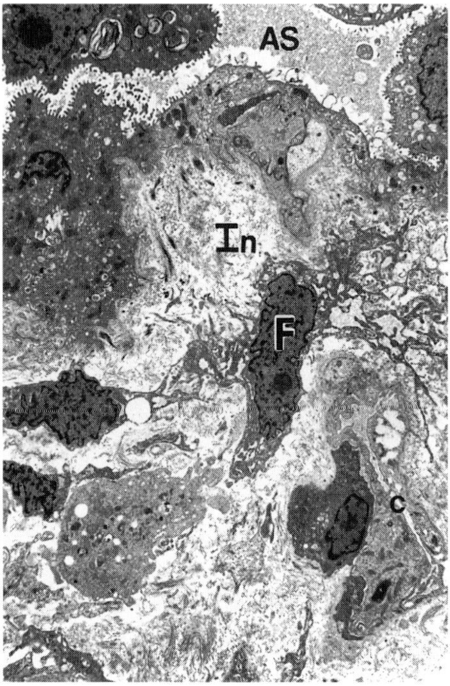

Figure 23 Lung tissue section (biopsy) from an infant who was born at 32 weeks gestation and underwent a lung biopsy 3 months later. Two of the alveolar epithelial lining cells have cytoplasmic microvilli and very few cytoplasmic lamellar inclusion bodies. The capillary (c) is centrally located in the interstitium (In), which contains fibroblasts (F) with many cytoplasmic extensions, and other cells. Edema is present in the airspace (AS) (lead citrate and uranyl acetate; ×2800).

separate studies that increased epithelial permeability is manifest in the lungs of infants with HMD and BPD (84,85). Many blood cells, including platelets, neutrophils, and monocytes, react to the injury, and a cascade of other cells and mediators then contributes to the ongoing process (86,87). Several studies now document that increased numbers of neutrophils, high elastase levels, activated alveolar macrophages, increased inflammatory markers, including proinflammatory cytokines and chemokines, and several lipid mediators are present in samples of airway lavage from infants with BPD (reviewed in Refs. 78,79).

Alveolar macrophages, by virtue of their chemotactive properties, and the production and release of cytokines and growth factors, probably contribute to the onset of inflammation and the disordered repair of the immature lung. Immature lungs contain few, if any, alveolar macrophages before birth; they are recruited into the alveoli near birth (88,89). In both the nonhuman primate models of HMD (89) and BPD (90), alveolar macrophages and neutrophils are recruited from the vasculature into the alveolar space within a few days after birth. In the premature monkey model of HMD, Jacobs and colleagues (91) showed that increased numbers of alveolar macrophages were related to the presence of surface-active material in lavage fluid and the absence of HMD. Neutrophils increase in the airways of infants with BPD (16,86,87,92) in response to chemoattractants. The inflammatory cell populations in immature infants lack functional characteristics, such as phagocytosis and chemotaxis, when compared with mature counterparts (93). Under comparable hyperoxic conditions, premature animals do not succumb as quickly as adult animals that receive a comparable hyperoxic insult (94,95), probably partly related to the relative paucity of alveolar macrophages and other inflammatory cells that would participate in mediator release.

The inflammatory autoinjury in BPD can be augmented by an inflammatory reaction that is induced by microbial agents. Elastase was present in tracheal aspirates of infants who were ventilated with more than 60% oxygen for 5 days, and its presence was more often associated with positive bacterial or viral cultures (96). Histopathologically, autopsy specimens of infants with BPD frequently have a terminal inflammatory process, with increased numbers of alveolar macrophages and polymorphonuclear neutrophils (PMNs) (97) and intramural organization of intra-alveolar exudates. Infection, especially bronchopneumonia, was the common cause of death in a study of infants with BPD who died between 4 weeks and 4 months after birth (98). Mechanically ventilated baboons with hyperoxia-induced BPD had more severe lung injury when they became colonized and acquired pneumonia from *Pseudomonas aeruginosa*, rather than from coagulase-negative staphylococcal organisms (99). Cordero and Ayers (100) showed that severe BPD developed in mechanically ventilated infants who were colonized with gram-negative bacteria. Epidemiological data also show a strong association between systemic infections and the development of CLD (101).

VI. Summary

As the technical advances in respiratory care, equipment, and methods (monitoring arterial oxygen, use of PEEP, and such) were instituted in the 1970s, more infants with HMD survived, and the incidence of BPD in such infants who weighed more than 1000 was 40%. Now the widespread use of antenatal corticosteroids, exogenous surfactant therapy, and better clinical management of immature neonates has resulted in increased survival rates of infants who are born prematurely at less than 28 weeks gestation, with birth weights less than 1000 g. Exogenous surfactant therapy has not prevented BPD in these newborns, despite reducing oxygen requirements and severity of RDS. CLD develops in up to 90% of very low birth weight survivors, even after they receive only minimal amounts of assisted ventilation (102–104). Thus, the *immature state* of the lung is very likely the major factor in the pathogenesis of BPD in the 1990s.

The extent of lung development at different gestational time points has influenced the pathology of BPD. The lung at 24–26 weeks is still in the canalicular stage of development and is just beginning to enter the saccular (primitive alveolar) stage. Alveoli are present as early as 32 weeks, but alveolization is not observed consistently until 36 weeks.

At the present time, there is a spectrum of clinical BPD and of pathological findings: the very low birth weight infant who is treated early with surfactant; other very low birth weight infants who are not given surfactant at birth, especially those who are outborn; or those who are rescued with surfactant following birth. The pathological findings in the lungs of low birth weight infants include alveolar hypoplasia, vascular arrest and adaptive dysmorphic changes, and variable interstitial proliferation in response to its premature adaptation to the extrauterine environment. Much work is needed to determine if the inflammatory autoinjury and resultant impairment of lung healing and growth can be prevented in an immature lung. The pathological findings underscore the impression that BPD in this low birth weight group, with greater pulmonary immaturity, may have as many crippling sequelae in older children and adults as in those infants who acquired BPD in the 1960s and early 1970s. This current spectrum of disease, which is dependent on so many factors, requires extensive research efforts.

References

1. Baue AE. Multiple organ or systems failure. In: Haimovici H, ed. Vascular Emergencies. New York: Appleton-Century-Crofts, 1982:125–132.
2. Northway WH Jr, Rosan RC, Porter DY. Pulmonary disease following respirator therapy of hyaline-membrane disease: bronchopulmonary dysplasia. N Engl J Med 1967; 276:357–368.
3. Becker MJ, Koppe JG. Pulmonary structural changes in neonatal hyaline membrane disease treated with high pressure artificial respiration. Thorax 1969; 24:689–994.
4. Pusey VA, MacPherson R, Chernick V. Pulmonary fibroplasia following prolonged artificial ventilation of newborn infants. Can Med Assoc J 1969; 100:451–457.
5. Anderson WR, Strickland MB. Pulmonary complications of oxygen therapy in the neonate. Postmortem study of bronchopulmonary dysplasia with emphasis on fibroproliferative obliterative bronchitis and bronchiolitis. Arch Pathol 1971; 91: 506–514.
6. Banerjee CK, Girling DJ, Wigglesworth JS. Pulmonary fibroplasia in newborn babies treated with oxygen and artificial ventilation. Arch Dis Child 1972; 47:509–518.

7. Anderson WR, Strickland MB, Tsai SH, Haglin JJ. Light microscopic and ultrastructural study of the adverse effects of oxygen therapy on the neonate lung. Am J Pathol 1973; 73:327–348.
8. Rosan RC. Hyaline membrane disease and related spectrum of neonatal pneumopathies. In: Rosenberg HS, Bolande W, eds. Perspectives in Pediatric Pathology, Vol 2. Chicago: Year Book Publishers, 1975:15–60.
9. Taghizadeh A, Reynolds EOR. Pathogenesis of bronchopulmonary dysplasia following hyaline membrane disease. Am J Pathol 1976; 82:241–264.
10. Bonikos DS, Bensch KG, Northway WH Jr, Edwards DK. Bronchopulmonary dysplasia: the pulmonary pathologic sequel of necrotizing bronchiolitis and pulmonary fibrosis. Hum Pathol 1976; 7:643–666.
11. Reynolds EOR, Taghizadeh A. Improved prognosis of infants mechanically ventilated for hyaline membrane disease. Arch Dis Child 1974; 49:505–515.
12. Wung J-T, Koons AH, Driscoll JM, James LS. Changing incidence of bronchopulmonary dysplasia. J Pediatr 1979; 95:845–847.
13. Edwards DK. Radiographic aspects of bronchopulmonary dysplasia. J Pediatr 1979; 95:823–829.
14. Northway WH. Observations on bronchopulmonary dysplasia. J Pediatr 1979; 95: 815–818.
15. O'Brodovich HM, Mellins RB. Bronchopulmonary dysplasia. Unresolved neonatal acute lung injury. Am Rev Respir Dis 1985; 132:694–709.
16. Merritt TA, Puccia JM, Stuard ID. Cytologic evaluation of pulmonary effluent in neonates with respiratory distress syndrome and bronchopulmonary dysplasia. Acta Cytol 1981; 25:631–639.
17. Merritt TA, Stuard ID, Puccia J, Wood B, Edward DK, Finkelstein J, Shapiro DL. Newborn tracheal aspirate cytology: classification during respiratory distress syndrome and bronchopulmonary dysplasia. J Pediatr 1981; 98:949–956.
18. Takemura T. Histopathological study of the adverse effects of prolonged respirator therapy of the neonate lung. Acta Pathol Jpn 1981; 31:199–210.
19. Anderson WR, Engel RR. Cardiopulmonary sequelae of reparative stages of bronchopulmonary dysplasia. Arch Pathol Lab Med 1983; 107:603–608.
20. Sobonya RE, Logvinoff MM, Taussig LM, Theriault A. Morphometric analysis of the lung in prolonged bronchopulmonary dysplasia. Pediatr Res 1982; 16:969–972.
21. Stocker JT. Pathologic features of long-standing ''healed'' bronchopulmonary dysplasia. Hum Pathol 1986; 17:943–961.
22. Nakamura Y, Hosokawa Y, Nakashima T, Komatsu Y, Nakashima H, Kuyama M, Fukuda S, Hashimoto T. Pulmonary complications of long-term respiratory care in infants. Relationship to bronchopulmonary dysplasia. Acta Pathol Jpn 1981; 31: 75–84.
23. Erickson AM, de la Monte SM, Moore GW, Hutchins GM. The progression of morphologic changes in bronchopulmonary dysplasia. Am J Pathol 1987; 127:474–487.
24. Takemura T, Akamatsu H. Ultrastructural study on the pulmonary parenchyma of the neonate following prolonged mechanical ventilation. Acta Pathol Jpn 1987; 37: 1115–1126.

25. Hislop AA, Wigglesworth JS, Desai R, Aber V. The effects of preterm delivery and mechanical ventilation on human lung growth. Early Hum Dev 1987; 15:147–164.
26. Tomashefski JF, Oppermam HC, Vawter GF. BPD: a morphometric study with emphasis on the pulmonary vasculature. Pediatr Pathol 1984; 2:469–487.
27. Hislop AA, Haworth SG. Pulmonary vascular damage and the development of cor pulmonale following hyaline membrane disease. Pediatr Pulmonol 1990; 9:152–161.
28. Chambers HM, Van Velzen D. Ventilator-related pathology in the extremely immature lung. Pathology 1989; 21:79–83.
29. Van Lierde S, Cornelis A, Devlieger H, Moerman P, Lauweryns J, Eggermont E. Different patterns of pulmonary sequelae after hyaline membrane disease: heterogeneity of bronchopulmonary dysplasia? Biol Neonate 1991; 60:152–162.
30. Margraf LR, Tomashefski JF, Bruce MC, Dahms BB. Morphometric analysis of the lung in bronchopulmonary dysplasia. Am Rev Respir Dis 1991; 143:391–400.
31. Hislop AA, Haworth SG. Airway size and structure in the normal fetal and infant lung and the effect of premature delivery and artificial ventilation. Am Rev Respir Dis 1990; 410:1717–1726.
32. Johnson DE, Anderson WR, Burke BA. Pulmonary neuroendocrine cells in pediatric lung disease: alterations in airway structure in infants with bronchopulmonary dysplasia. Anat Rec 1993; 236:115–119.
33. Cutz E, Gillan JE, Perrin DG. Pulmonary neuroendocrine cell system: an overview of cell biology and pathology with emphasis on pediatric lung disease. Perspect Pediatr Pathol 1995; 18:32–70.
34. Husain AN, Siddiqui NH, Stocker JT. Pathology of arrested acinar development in postsurfactant bronchopulmonary dysplasia. Hum Pathol 1998; 29:710–717.
35. Gruenwald P. Normal and abnormal expansion of the lungs of newborn infants obtained at autopsy. II. Opening pressure, maximal volume, and stability of expansion. Lab Invest 1963; 12:563–576.
36. Robertson B. The evolution of neonatal respiratory distress syndrome into chronic lung disease. Eur Respir J 1989; 3(suppl 2):33S–37S.
37. Robertson B. Pathology of neonatal surfactant deficiency. Perspect Pediatr Pathol 1987; 11:6–46.
38. Barter RA, Maddison TG. The nature of the neonatal pulmonary hyaline membrane. Arch Dis Child 1960; 35:460–464.
39. Ludwin SK, Northway WH, Bensch KG. Oxygen toxicity in the newborn. Necrotizing bronchiolitis in mice exposed to 100 percent oxygen. Lab Invest 1974; 31:425–435.
40. Stocks J, Godfrey S, Reynolds EOR. Airway resistance in infants after various treatments for hyaline membrane disease: special emphasis on prolonged high levels of inspired oxygen. Pediatrics 1978; 61:178–183.
41. Stocks J, Godfrey S. The role of artificial ventilation, oxygen and CPAP in the pathogenesis of lung damage in neonates. Pediatrics 1976; 57:352–362.
42. Grossman G. Expansion pattern of terminal airspaces in the premature rabbit lung after tracheal deposition of surfactant. Pflugers Arch 1977; 367:205–209.

43. Watts JL, Ariagno RL, Brady JP. Chronic pulmonary disease in neonates after artificial ventilation: distribution of ventilation and pulmonary interstitial emphysema. Pediatrics 1977; 60:273–281.
44. Moylan FMB, Walker AM, Krammer SS, Todres ID, Shannon DC. Alveolar rupture as an independent predictor of BPD. Crit Care Med 1978; 6:10–13.
45. Dreyfuss D, Saumon G. Ventilator-induced lung injury. Am J Respir Crit Care Med 1998; 157:294–323.
46. Nilsson R. The artificially ventilated preterm rabbit neonate as experimental model of hyaline membrane disease. Acta Anaesthesiol Scand 1982; 26:89–103.
47. Gerstmann DR, deLemos RA, Coalson JJ, Clark RH, Wiswell TE, Winter DC, Kuehl TJ, Meredith KS, Null DM. Influence of ventilatory technique on pulmonary baroinjury in baboons with HMD. Pediatr Pulmonol 1988; 5:82–91.
48. Meredith KS, deLemos RA, Coalson JJ, King RJ, Gerstmann DR, Kumar R, Kuehl TJ, Winter DV, Taylor A, Clark RH, Null DM. Role of lung injury in the pathogenesis of hyaline membrane disease in premature baboons. J Appl Physiol 1989; 66: 2150–2158.
49. Carlton DP, Cummings JJ, Scheerer RS, Poulain FR, Bland RD. Lung overexpansion increases pulmonary microvascular protein permeability in young lambs. J Appl Physiol 1990; 69:577–583.
50. Davis JM, Dickerson B, Metlay L, Penney DP. Differential effects of oxygen and barotrauma on lung injury in the neonatal piglet. Pediatr Pulmonol 1991; 10:157–163.
51. Troug WE, Jackson JC. Alternative modes of ventilation in the prevention and treatment of BPD. Clin Perinatol 1992; 19:621–647.
52. Pratt PC. Pathology of pulmonary oxygen toxicity. Am Rev Respir Dis 1974; 110(suppl):51–57.
53. Jones R, Zapol WM, Reid LM. Oxygen toxcity and restructuring of pulmonary arteries: a morphometric study. Am J Pathol 1985; 121:212–223.
54. Fox RB, Hoidal JR, Brown DM, Repine JE. Pulmonary inflammation due to O_2 toxicity: involvement of chemotactic factors and PMNs. Am Rev Respir Dis 1982; 123:521–523.
55. Crapo JD. Morphologic changes in pulmonary oxygen toxicity. Annu Rev Physiol 1986; 48:721–731.
56. Coalson JJ, Kuehl TJ, Prihoda TJ, deLemos RA. Diffuse alveolar damage in the evolution of bronchopulmonary dysplasia in the baboon. Pediatr Res 1988; 24:357–366.
57. Coalson JJ, King RJ, Winter VT, Prihoda TJ, Anzueto AR, Peters JI, Johanson WG. O_2 and pneumonia-induced lung injury. I Pathological and morphometric studies. J Appl Physiol 1989; 67:346–356.
58. Randell SH, Mercer RR, Young SL. Neonatal hyperoxia alters the pulmonary alveolar and capillary structure of 40-day-old rats. Am J Pathol 1990; 136:1259–1266.
59. Langston C, Kida K, Reed M, Thurlbeck WM. Human lung growth in late gestation and in the neonate. Am Rev Respir Dis 1984; 129:607–613.
60. Langston C, Thurlbeck WM. Lung growth and development in late gestation and early postnatal life. Perspect Pediatr Pathol 1982; 7:203–235.

61. Coalson JJ, Winter V, deLemos RA. Decreased alveolarization in baboon survivors with bronchopulmonary dysplasia. Am J Respir Crit Care Med 1995; 152:640–646.
62. Roman J. Cell–cell and Cell–matrix interactions in development of the lung vasculature. In: McDonald JA, ed. Lung Growth and Development. New York: Marcel Dekker, 1997:355–389.
63. Crouch EC, Mecham RB, Davila RM, Noguchi A. Collagens and elastic fiber proteins in lung development. In: McDonald JA, ed. Lung Growth and Development. New York: Marcel Dekker, 1997:327–364.
64. Loosli CG, Potter EL. Pre and postnatal development of the respiratory portion of the human lung with reference to elastic fibers. Am Rev Respir Dis (suppl) 1959; 80:5–23.
65. Bateman E, Turner-Warwick M, Adelmann-Grill BC. Immunohistochemical study of collagen types in human fetal lung and fibrotic disease. Thorax 1981; 36:645–653.
66. Wigglesworth JS, Desai R, Aber B. Quantitative aspects of perinatal lung growth. Early Hum Dev 1987; 15:203–212.
67. Cherukupalli K, Larson JE, Rotschild A, Thurlbeck WM. Biochemical, clinical, and morphologic studies on lungs of infants with bronchopulmonary dysplasia. Pediatr Pulmonol 1996; 215–229.
68. Coalson JJ. Pathophysiologic features of respiratory distress in the infant and adult. In: Ayres S, A. Grenvik A, Holbrook PR, Shoemaker WC Jr, eds. Textbook of Critical Care. 3rd ed. Philadelphia: WB Saunders, 1995:797–805.
69. Viscardi RM, Broderick K, Sun C-CJ, Yale-Loehr AJ, Hessamfar A, Taciak V, Burke KC, Koenig KB, Idell S. Disordered pathways of fibrin turnover in lung lavage of premature infants with respiratory distress syndrome. Am Rev Respir Dis 1992; 146:492–499.
70. Idell S, Kumar A, Koenig KB, Coalson JJ. Pathways of fibrin turnover in lavage of premature baboons with hyperoxic lung injury. Am J Respir Crit Care Med 1994; 149:767–775.
71. Thurlbeck WM. Postnatal human lung growth. Thorax 1979; 37:564–571.
72. Cutz E, Enhorning G, Robertson B, Sherwood WG, Hill DE. Hyaline membrane disease: effect of surfactant prophylaxis on lung morphology in premature primates. Am J Pathol 1978; 92:581–590.
73. Pinar H, Makarova N, Rubin LP, Singer DB. Pathology of the lung in surfactant-treated neonates. Pediatr Pathol 1994; 14:627–636.
74. Coalson JJ, Winter V, Yoder B. Decreased alveoli and surface area in premature baboons with long term bronchopulmonary dysplasia. Am J Respir Crit Care Med 1998; 157:A373.
75. Coalson JJ, Winter V, Yoder B. Dysmorphic vascular development in premature baboons with bronchopulmonary dysplasia. Am J Respir Crit Care Med 1997; 155:A262.
76. Dejours P. Principles in Comparative Respiratory Physiology. 2nd ed. Amsterdam: Elsevier/North Holland, 1981.
77. Towell ME, Johanson J, Smedstadk K, Andrew M, Wu TL. Fetal blood and tissue PO_2 during maternal oxygen breathing. J Dev Physiol 1984; 5:177–185.

78. Zimmerman JJ. Bronchoalveolar inflammatory pathophysiology of bronchopulmonary dysplasia. Clin Perinatol 1995; 22:429–456.
79. Pierce MR, Bancalari E. The role of inflammation in the pathogenesis of bronchopulmonary dysplasia. Pediatr Pulmonol 1995; 19:371–378.
80. Gibbs RS, Romero R, Hillier SL, Eschenbach DA, Sweet RL. A review of premature birth and subclinical infection. Am J Obstet Gynecol 1992; 166:1515–1528.
81. Hillier SL, Witkin SS, Krohn MA, Watts DH, Kiviat NB, Eschenbach DA. The relationship of amniotic fluid cytokines and preterm delivery, amniotic fluid infection, histologic chorioamnionitis, and chorioamnion infection. Obstet Gynecol 1993; 81:941–948.
82. Mazor M, Chaim W, Horowitz S, Romero R, Glezerman M. The biomolecular mechanisms of preterm labor in women with intrauterine infection. Isr J Med Sci 1994; 30:317–322.
83. Watterberg KL, Demers LM, Scott SM, Murphy S. Chorioamnionitis and early lung inflammation in infants in whom bronchopulmonary dysplasia develops. Pediatrics 1996; 97:210–215.
84. Jefferies AL, Coates G, O'Brodovich H. Pulmonary epithelial permeability in hyaline-membrane disease. N Engl J Med 1984; 311:1075–1080.
85. O'Brodovich H, Coates G. Pulmonary clearance of ^{99m}Tc:DTPA in infants who subsequently develop bronchopulmonary dysplasia. Am Rev Respir Dis 1988; 137: 210–212.
86. Ogden BE, Murphy SA, Saunders GC, Pathak D, Johnson JD. Neonatal lung neutrophils and elastase/proteinase inhibitor imbalance. Am Rev Respir Dis 1984; 130: 817–821.
87. Merritt TA, Cochrane CG, Holcomb K, Bohl B, Hallman M, Strayer D, Edwards DK, Gluck, L Elastase and alpha 1-proteinase inhibitor activity in tracheal aspirates during respiratory distress syndrome: role of inflammation in the pathogenesis of bronchopulmonary dysplasia. J Clin Invest 1983; 172:656–666.
88. Alenghat E, Esterly JR. Alveolar macrophages in perinatal infants. Pediatrics 1984; 74:221–223.
89. Jackson JC, Chi EY, Wilson CB, Truog WE, Teh EC, Hodson WA. Sequence of inflammatory cell migration into lung during recovery from hyaline membrane disease in premature newborn monkeys. Am Rev Respir Dis 1987; 135:937–940.
90. Jenkinson SG, Roberts RJ, de Lemos RA, Lawrence RA, Coalson JJ, King RJ, Null DM Jr, Gerstmann DR. Allopurinol-induced effects in premature baboons with respiratory distress syndrome. J Appl Physiol 1991; 70:1160–1167.
91. Jacobs RF, Wilson CB, Palmer S, Springmeyer SC, Henderson WR, Glover DM, Kessler DL, Murphy JH, Hughes JP, van Belle G, Chi EY, Hodson WA. Factors related to the appearance of alveolar macrophages in the developing lung. Am Rev Respir Dis 1985; 131:548–553.
92. Groneck P, Gotze-Speer B, Opperman M, Effert H, Speer CP. Association of pulmonary inflammation and increased microvascular permeability during the development of BPD: a sequential analysis of inflammatory mediators in respiratory fluids of high-risk preterm neonates. Pediatrics 1994; 93:712–718.
93. Kurland G, Cheung ATW, Miller ME, Ayin SA, Cho MM, Ford EW. The ontogeny

of pulmonary defenses: alveolar macrophage function in neonatal and juvenile rhesus monkeys. Pediatr Res 1988; 23:293–297.
94. Frank L, Bucher JR, Roberts, RJ. O_2 toxicity in neonatal and adult animals of various species. J Appl Physiol 1979; 45:699–704.
95. Coalson J, Tiffee J, Winter V, Allred C. Apoptosis in hyperoxia-treated premature and adult baboons. Am J Respir Crit Care Med 1996; 153:A1389.
96. Bruce MC, Schuyler M, Martin RJ, Starcher BC, Tomashefski JF, Wedig KE. Risk factors for the degradation of lung elastic fibers in the ventilated neonate—implications for impaired lung development in bronchopulmonary dysplasia. Am Rev Respir Dis 1992; 146:204–212.
97. Vapaavuori EK, Krohn K. Intensive care of small premature infants. II. Postmortem findings. Acta Paediatr Scand 1971; 60:49–58.
98. Turkel SB, Sims ME, Guttenberg ME. Postponed neonatal death in the premature infant. Am J Dis Child 1986; 140:576–579.
99. Coalson JJ, Gerstmann DR, Winter VT, deLemos RA. Bacterial colonization and infection studies in the premature baboon with bronchopulmonary dysplasia. Am Rev Respir Dis 1991; 144:1140–1146.
100. Cordero L, Ayers LW, Davis K. Neonatal airway colonization with gram-negative bacilli: association with severity of bronchopulmonary dysplasia. Pediatr Infect Dis J 1997; 16:18–23.
101. Rojas M, Gonzalez A, Bancalari E, Claure N, Poole C, Silva-Neto G. Changing trends in the epidemiology and pathogenesis of neonatal chronic lung disease. J Pediatr 1995; 126:605–610.
102. Tooley WH. Epidemiology of bronchopulmonary dysplasia. J Pediatr 1979; 95: 851–858.
103. Hazinski TA. BPD. In: Chernick V, ed. Kendig's Disorders of the Respiratory Tract in Children. 5th ed. Philadelphia: WB Saunders, 1990:300–320.
104. Hudak BB, Egan EA. Impact of lung surfactant therapy on chronic lung disease in premature infants. Clin Perinatol 1992; 19:591–602.
105. McKay CA, Faulkner CS, Edwards WH. Unusual pulmonary reaction to respiratory therapy in a premature newborn. Hum Pathol 1985; 16:629–631.

6

The Usefulness of Bronchoalveolar Lavage in Infants with Evolving Chronic Lung Disease

CARL W. WHITE

University of Colorado Health Sciences Center
Denver, Colorado

LELAND L. FAN

Baylor College of Medicine
Houston, Texas

I. Introduction

Studies of the mechanisms of disease pathogenesis and progression in human infants are hampered by the lack of availability of pulmonary tissue for study. Obtaining bronchoalveolar lavage (BAL) fluid to reach pulmonary cells and epithelial lining fluid has been used to overcome this shortcoming. Problems that complicate the use of these materials include (1) the use of suboptimal and nonstandardized techniques for obtaining fluids, (2) lack of adequate reference indices, (3) lack of normal control data from healthy premature infants, and (4) safety issues. Because of these concerns, each study involving use of BAL must be examined critically, and results should be considered to be only semiquantitative. Despite these difficulties, useful concepts concerning bronchopulmonary dysplasia (BPD) pathogenesis have been suggested and supported through human clinical studies that have depended on BAL fluids. Through use of lavage or pulmonary effluent fluids, considerable information has been reported on tracheobronchial–alveolar cellularity, inflammatory cytokines, and other mediators, proteases and antiproteases, and surfactant components, during the progression of BPD. Less information has been presented about oxidants and antioxidants and about infectious agents obtained from BAL. In this chapter we discuss various aspects of the airway lavage procedure as it is used in infants, and we describe a few specific examples in which BAL materials have helped provide insight into the pathogenesis of BPD.

II. General Considerations

A. Definition

Bronchoalveolar lavage has been used primarily as a research tool, initially in adults and more recently in infants and children (reviewed in 1–3). Material derived from BAL in infants, however, can also be useful in evaluating new pulmonary infiltrates, possible lung infection, and other disorders. BAL in older children and adults is typically performed using a wedged fiberoptic bronchoscope that is advanced to a subsegmental bronchus, followed by instillation and retrieval of isotonic saline. Because the smallest pediatric bronchoscope with a directable tip, which has a suction channel, is rather large (3.6 mm in diameter), its use in this procedure is not possible in the human premature infant. Thus, a variety of nonbronchoscopic techniques have been used in an attempt to study the epithelial lining fluids from these infants.

B. Techniques

Although most studies of lung epithelial lining fluids in human infants have not used true BAL, there are at least a couple of exceptions to this generalization. Alpert and associates (4) used a wedge pressure catheter that was 60 cm long, with a 1.35-mm diameter (4-F) and an inflatable balloon just proximate to its tip, which he advanced through the airway by an endotracheal tube in 20 sedated, ventilated infants and children, ages 1–77 months (median: 9 months) The smallest infant weighed 950 g. Electrocardiography (ECG), pulse oximetry, chest inspection, and auscultation were used to monitor the patients, but neither radiographs nor fluoroscopy were routinely employed. With the balloon inflated, five aliquots of isotonic saline, 0.75 mL/kg each, were infused and aspirated sequentially, followed by balloon deflation and catheter removal. The use of such an inflated balloon might provide more reliable sampling of distal respiratory units than would the use of a ''wedged'' bronchoscope. The report of this study did not include detailed cytological information, but it was stated that alveolar macrophages were abundant in all samples. Diagnostic information was provided in 5 of the 20 patients and contributory findings were provided in an additional 12 patients. Neither oxygen need nor ventilatory status changed, nor was there detectable airway obstruction or other complications in any patient during this rather lengthy procedure (10–20 min).

Koumbourlis and Kurland extended the nonbronchoscopic technique in ventilated infants (5). In this study, 15 patients, aged 0.5–18 months, were studied. All were intubated (size 3.5- to 4.0-mm endotracheal tubes) and mechanically ventilated. In addition, all patients had received sedation (fentanyl citrate) and muscle relaxants (vecuronium). The principal difference between this study and the preceding one of Alpert et al. was that a larger and more rigid catheter, an 8-Fr feeding tube with an external diameter of 2.55 mm, was used in these larger and older patients. The suction channel of this catheter was considerably larger than that of the pediatric fiberoptic bronchoscope, and this catheter also is firmer than the one that was used by Alpert. Although alveolar macrophages were retrieved in all specimens, many neutrophils were also obtained. As in the study of Alpert, however, absolute and differential cell counts of the lavage fluid were not reported. Hence, it is difficult to be certain which technique provided better samplings of material from the distal airspaces. The latter technique, however, did yield a return of about 70% of lavage fluid, and diagnostic information was obtained from 9 of the 15 patients. Other than a transient decrease in oxygen saturation, there were no detectable complications of the procedure.

Both of the aforementioned studies included primarily larger infants and toddlers. Use of bronchoscopic techniques for BAL in premature humans remains experimental and is still at a very early stage of development. Two small pilot studies of this technique will be presented later in this discussion. One can assume, however, that the technical problems of wedging a catheter to obtain authentic BAL fluid will be even greater, and the potential for multiple complications will be considerably higher in the small premature infant than it is in older, larger infants. Several related issues, most of which have been addressed in previous studies with adults and older children, have not yet been studied in premature or even in term infants. Some of these issues are (1) which lobe or lobes are most appropriate to lavage (upper, middle, or lower; right vs. left); (2) what is the optimal dwell time (the amount of time after instillation that the lavage fluid is allowed to remain in the lung before it is removed); (3) how many aliquots of fluid should be instilled, and what volume of each aliquot; and (4) should first aliquot be discarded or be pooled with subsequent aliquots (fractional processing vs. pooling)? Another consideration is whether or not to filter the sample through gauze to remove mucus. Because of small-volume yields in the premature infant, filtering the fluid might further limit the amount of material available for study.

Because of anatomical limitations, the term BAL may be misleading when it is applied to previous studies of newborn infants. Virtually all studies of premature infants with respiratory distress have used what could be called most accurately *tracheal effluent* as a source of pulmonary epithelial lining fluid. These materials may have been obtained either by direct aspiration or following instillation of one or a few aliquots of saline, followed by ventilation and suctioning at the distal end of the endotracheal tube. It is likely, therefore, that the cellular and biochemical materials obtained in this way derive primarily from the central airways, rather than the distal air spaces. Thus, these samples may just reflect the composition of liquid contained in the terminal respiratory units. For example, insertion of a tube into the trachea elicits a neutrophilic inflammatory response within hours in adult rabbits (6). Although several studies have demonstrated an association between neutrophilic inflammation, as indicated in the tracheal effluent, and the eventual development of BPD in human infants, the extent to which early inflammation is present in the distal airspaces of such patients is unclear.

C. Comparison of Cellular Elements Obtained in Tracheal Effluents Compared with Histopathology of Lung Parenchyma

Relatively little information is available on the relation between cellular elements found in tracheal effluent fluid versus cellular elements in distal lung tissue. In the premature baboon model of BPD, however, such comparative information is available (7). Infant baboons that were mechanically ventilated for 3 weeks with sufficient oxygen to yield normal arterial oxygenation (''PRN oxygen'') did not acquire BPD, whereas infant baboons that were mechanically ventilated with 100% oxygen for 3 weeks had clear-cut evidence of BPD. Tracheal aspirates obtained from these two groups of baboons, however, showed no significant differences in absolute quantities of neutrophils or mononuclear cells over the 3 weeks of study. Indeed, there was a trend for greater absolute numbers of both neutrophils and mononuclear cells in tracheal aspirates from PRN than in those from 100% oxygen-treated animals. These findings might have been related to a lack of homogeneity of ventilation and to poor communication between distal respiratory units and central airways. At autopsy, however, there was a substantial increase in macrophages (about eightfold greater) in atelectatic sections from BPD lungs compared with PRN lungs. Even overexpanded sections of lung from animals with BPD showed a similar trend, with threefold or more mononuclear cells than from the lungs of animals without BPD. Postmortem numbers of neutrophils were similar in the lungs of baboons with and without BPD. These results may indicate that cellular events differ in the distal portions of the lung compared with what is detected in tracheal aspirates. The cumulative nature of the tracheal aspirate data presented in this study may have obscured true correlations with morphometric studies obtained at autopsy.

A more recent study (8) reported that in intubated human premature infants, the absolute quantities and percentages of mononuclear cells and neutrophils measured in simultaneously obtained tracheal aspirates and deep pulmonary lavage (BAL) samples are infrequently correlated. Again, this study suggests that cellular and cytokine findings in central and distal airways may be dissimilar. This contention is certainly supported by the findings of Grigg and co-workers (9), who used ''blind'' placement of a 5-Fr suction catheter into the distal airways of intubated infants of less than 32 weeks gestation. In sequential BAL aliquots (1 mL/kg), they found a marked decrease in the numbers of neutrophils obtained, both in absolute numbers (declining from 0.22 to 0.02 million cells) and as a percentage of total cells (declining from 65 to 18% of cells between the first and second aliquots; $p = 0.004$). Likewise, the percentage of total cells that were alveolar macrophages increased from 35 to 82% ($p = 0.004$) between the first and second aliquots, although the absolute quantities of macrophages obtained in the two samples were not different. Because the wedged catheter or bronchoscope is usually located at about the fourth branching of the airways, the first aliquot contains cells that are much more representative of central than of distal airways, whereas subsequent aliquots are more representative of distal units. Hence, samples obtained from central airways may exaggerate the degree of inflammation in distal lung units in premature newborns. The extent of early inflammation in distal airways and lung parenchyma of infants who subsequently acquire BPD remains unknown. Several reports have shown that increased numbers of inflammatory cells and their secretory products in tracheal aspirates of human infants may correlate with eventual development of BPD. Although the principal airway lesions associated with BPD are considered to be at the bronchiolar level (7), sampling from such areas requires more invasive techniques than are commonly used. Central airways inflammation also may contribute to, or at least correlate with, the development of BPD.

D. Reference Proteins and Measurement

Because tracheal aspirate and BAL samples frequently are obtained after prior instillation of saline, and because alterations in airway fluid compositions may occur in evolving BPD, the choice of a suitable biochemical reference, such as a protein, to be used as a denominator in normalizing BAL biochemical measurements, is critical. Substances that have been used as reference standards, either exogenous or endogenous, have included potassium, methylene blue, inulin, urea, total protein, and most commonly, albumin (10). Detailed methods for determining the yield of authentic epithelial lining fluid (ELF) in BAL using urea have been presented (11). However, because urea is a small diffusable molecule, such calculations will be affected by numerous factors, including regional lung perfusion, dwell time, and alveolar–capillary permeability. Use of even larger molecules, such as albumin, can also be influenced by these factors. Because albumin enters lung secretions by leaking across the epithelium, use of this protein as a reference index may be problematic. Recently, Watts and Bruce (10) suggested that the secretory component of immunoglobulin A (IgA) may be a more appropriate reference standard than albumin in studies of tracheal aspirates in premature infants because secretory component is less influenced by changes in alveolar–capillary membrane permeability. Secretory component (SC) of IgA is a large (78-kDa) glycoprotein. It is secreted by bronchial and bronchiolar epithelium, and it is minimally present in blood plasma. There is little or no change in the concentration of SC of IgA in plasma with advancing gestational or chronologic age. Thus, there are numerous theoretical advantages to its use. In septic infants, tracheal aspirate albumin concentration increased by more than 50%, whereas SC concentration was unchanged. SC is regulated independently of IgA secretion. Therefore, SC is unlikely to change appreciably in response to acute or chronic infection. The reported findings in infants with sepsis appear to confirm this notion. Likewise, anti-inflammatory therapy with dexamethasone did not change absolute SC levels in tracheal aspirate, nor was the tracheal aspirate/plasma ratio for SC altered. In contrast, both the concentration of albumin in tracheal aspirate and the tracheal aspirate/plasma ratio for albumin decreased significantly as the concentration of albumin in plasma increased during dexamethasone therapy for BPD (10).

E. Safety

Safety is an extremely important consideration in clinical application of a procedure, such as BAL, in human infants. Airway suctioning to obtain tracheal effluent secretions is relatively noninvasive and adds little or no risk to that which exists with routine maintenance of endotracheal tube patency. The use of side arm adapters allow continued effective positive-pressure ventilation in infants with respiratory distress, provided that the seal between catheter and adapter is adequate (12). No serious complications of the more invasive lavage procedures were observed in either of the aforementioned studies that employed nonbronchoscopic lavage in infants and older children (4,5). In a study by LoMonaco et al. (8), ''deep pulmonary lavage'' of preterm infants was associated with only transient oxygen desaturation and increased oxygen requirement (8). Alpert et al. (4) did not observe decreased oxygenation or changes in ECG, oxygen requirement, or ventilatory status during or after airway suctioning. Likewise, Koumbourlis and Kurland (5) saw no radiographic deterioration with nonbronchoscopic airway lavage, and none of the patients required increased ventilatory support. These investigators, however, did observe transient decreases in oxyhemoglobin saturation during lavage in several patients, with resolution following the procedure. Arterial blood gas values obtained up to 3 hr after the procedure showed no deterioration in pH or carbon dioxide elimination. However, these studies did not include sick premature infants, and it would seem that any technique that uses extensive airway lavage might compromise respiratory gas exchange and increase ventilatory requirements in small, premature infants. Studies by Grigg and co-workers (9) indicate that hypoxemia and increased blood pressure lasting more than 3 min are common in preterm infants who undergo BAL. Such side effects also may occur during the course of routine airway suctioning to maintain endotracheal tube patency. The only reported fatality associated with pediatric fiberoptic bronchoscopy occurred in the setting of the critically ill, intubated, and mechanically ventilated child (13). Hence, it would seem prudent to continue to limit the use of the procedure, both for clinical and research purposes, to removal of tracheal effluent secretions, especially in critically ill newborns.

F. Normal Indices

Normal values for cell retrieval from BAL in children have been published (14). Eighteen patients, ages 3 months to 10 years, were studied using standard techniques. Three aliquots of saline, 1 mL/kg each, were instilled through the fiberoptic bronchoscope into the right middle lobe. The pooled second and third aliquots yielded an average of 1.55×10^5/mL (range $0.75–2.57 \times 10^5$), with 91% (range 84–94%) alveolar macrophages, 7.5% (range 4.7–12.8%) lymphocytes, 1.7% (range 0.6–3.5%) neutrophils, and 0.15% (0–0.3%) eosinophils. The helper/cytotoxic T-cell ratio was 0.58 (range 0.4–1.0). These values, with the exception of the helper/cytotoxic T-cell ratio, are similar to normal values for adults. Helper/cytotoxic T-cell ratios for normal adults have been reported in the 1.8–2.7 range (14). This difference in T-cell ratios relative to adults has been confirmed in other BAL studies in children. Hence, Ratjen et al. found a mean CD4/CD8 lymphocyte ratio of 0.68 (48 children; ages 3–16 years; 15), and Clement and co-workers measured a CD4/CD8 ratio of 0.8 ± 0.1 (mean $\pm$ SEM) in 11 children (16).

The data for BAL differential cell counts reported by Riedler et al. (14) are consistent with other reports, although there are some minor differences. Ratjen et al. (15) observed a relatively higher percentage of lymphocytes and lower percentage of alveolar macrophages (mean, 78.9% macrophages). However, almost half of the patients in this study were undergoing elective surgery for removal of hypertrophic lymphoid tissue in the upper airway (tonsils, adenoids). Another study showed a relative increase in the percentage of neutrophils recovered by BAL fluid (mean values: 86% macrophages, 8.7% lymphocytes, 5.5% neutrophils, 0.2% eosinophils) of 16 children, ages 2–32 months (17). These children were undergoing fiberoptic bronchoscopy for either (1) evaluation of previous foreign body removal, or (2) persistent stridor. Thus, it is likely that some of these children did not have normal airways (17). The differential cell count values of the study by Riedler et al. (14) were similar to those reported by Clement et al. (16), although the numbers of recovered cells in this study were almost double those reported by Riedler et al. In the study of Riedler et al. (14), patients with documented viral or bacterial infections were excluded from analysis. Therefore, the latter study may provide the most representative sample of ''healthy'' children. Although term and preterm infants may differ significantly for some of the cell values, nonetheless, these are the closest thing to normal BAL values that are available in babies.

The study of Midulla et al. (17) also provided information about potential age-related differences in BAL constituents of children. Specifically, there was a decline in BAL neutrophils in toddlers (13–36 months) relative to infants (1–12 months) from 7.6 ± 1.8% to 2.9 ± 1% ($p = 0.04$) with increased age. There was also a tendency for the concentration of several macromolecules including total protein, albumin, fibronectin, and hyaluronic acid, to decrease in BAL with advancing age, despite similar recovery of both fluid (43%) and cells (56×10^4 to 60×10^4/mL) for both groups of children. In a small subseries within this study, interesting data were presented indicating that the site of lavage can have substantial effect on the concentrations of various proteins measured. Hence, there was a great deal of variability in the mean concentrations of total protein, albumin, and fibronectin measured between the right middle lobe and the lingula, with all concentrations being markedly higher at the latter site. This occurred despite the existence of no variation in the concentration of hyaluronic acid at both sites (19–20 μg/L for both; 17). These findings have great implications for the possibility of substantial variations in measured concentrations of cytokines and other proteins related to site of lavage in studies of human newborns when "deep" or distal samples are collected. It is possible that this interpatient variability could be, at least partly related to the fact that the sampling of various lobes is random in newborns. This problem is unique to this age group, because a directable-tip bronchoscope is used in older children and adults.

Although abundant new data have recently become available pertinent to BAL in older infants and children, values for BAL constituents in healthy premature, or even term, infants is still unavailable. When control infants have been studied, they generally have been term or near-term infants who have required airway intubation and ventilator support for nonpulmonary conditions (18). Alternative means of controlling BAL studies in premature infants have also been used. Most commonly, statistical comparisons have been made between data from groups of infants who subsequently acquired BPD and those who did not. Likewise, prospective comparisons have been made between groups of patients who received therapeutic interventions, such as dexamethasone, and those who did not. Hence, comparative information from normal infants of comparable gestational and chronologic age is generally unavailable.

III. Inflammation: Marker or Protagonist of Injury?

A. Inflammatory Cells: Neutrophils and Macrophages

Despite the aforementioned limitations of BAL studies in premature infants, useful information has been gained relative to BPD pathogenesis. Knowledge about inflammatory cells and their products, proteases and antiproteases, and, to a lesser extent, oxidants and antioxidants, in evolving BPD has been garnered. Merritt and colleagues initially described the inflammatory progression of BAL cytology in BPD (18). This study demonstrated that a persistence of acute and chronic inflammatory cells in tracheal secretions is strongly associated with subsequent development of BPD. The Papanicolaou method was used for staining the cells. The study showed that the cytopathological picture of acute and chronic inflammation reverses in patients who do not go on to acquire BPD, whereas 70% of those with subsequent BPD manifest what was called "class III" cytopathology. This consisted of persistent and prominent polymorphonuclear (PMN) neutrophils and macrophages, as well as the presence of multinucleated histiocytes in several patients. The latter cell type was seen in 11 of 13 patients who had pulmonary air leaks. The class III cytologies were associated with ongoing exposure to hyperoxia and aggressive ventilatory support. Class III findings were not usually present until after 10 days of ventilator therapy.

The persistence and prominence of neutrophilic inflammation in infants who acquire BPD has been confirmed by other investigators (19–21). One prospective study showed that the percentage of neutrophils did not increase in lavage fluids obtained from central airways of BPD infants when compared with infants with respiratory distress syndrome (RDS; non-BPD) and ventilated control infants during the first 5 days of life (22). This study, however, varied only in the timing of the neutrophil influx; all studies have confirmed that such an influx ultimately occurs in infants who later have BPD. Nonetheless, the pathogenesis of BPD probably reflects much more than a simple dependence on early infiltration of neutrophils and release of inflammatory mediators. What incites inflammation and triggers its resolution has been the basis for considerable investigation and speculation. Of particular interest has been the recent description of neutrophils undergoing apoptosis in the airways of the premature newborn (23). These cells were obtained from distal airways using a wedged catheter. Ingestion of neutrophils by macrophages was also observed in these eight patients. Whether these neutrophils had undergone apoptotic or necrotic cell death could not be discerned, but there was no evidence to support the latter. It could be speculated that failure of neutrophilic apoptosis might lead to persistence of inflammation in BPD. Unfortunately, data pertinent to the outcome of the original eight patients studied are unavailable, and studies that address this possibility have not yet been published.

What is certain is that, during resolution of pulmonary inflammation after RDS, elevated numbers of macrophages, rather than neutrophils, predominate. Jackson and colleagues (24) showed, in morphometric studies of lungs of primates with resolving hyaline membrane disease (HMD), that there was a tenfold increase in the percentage of macrophages among lung tissue inflammatory cells as the percentage of polymorphonuclear cells decreased.

Recently, another cell type, the eosinophil, has been suggested to play a role during the acquisition of BPD (25). In this study, lavage levels of eosinophilic cationic protein (ECP) were elevated, as were lavage PMN elastase levels and peripheral blood eosinophils, in BPD, relative to non-BPD, patients. In addition, in two BPD patients, eosinophil-derived major basic protein (MBP) was demonstrated in lung biopsy tissue obtained during surgical closure of the ductus arteriosus.

B. Proinflammatory Substances: Cytokines and Eicosanoids

Inflammation in the airways can be provoked by diverse stimuli, including endotracheal intubation (6) and exposure to hyperoxia (26). In addition, the procedure of bronchoalveolar lavage itself can lead to acute neutrophilic inflammation in the lungs of adult humans (27). The issue of whether or not neutrophilic inflammation causes acute hyperoxic lung injury has been debated for some time, and there are now at least as many papers that do not support this contention as those that do. Indeed, there are several well-documented oxidant-mediated biochemical and histopathological features of oxygen toxicity, as well as increased alveolar–capillary membrane permeability of the lung, that precede, by hours to days, any detectable neutrophilic infiltration (28–31). However, even though these arguments are quite pertinent to acute, lethal hyperoxic lung injury in animal models, they may be less relevant to the chronic sublethal pulmonary injury that characterizes BPD. Hence, questions of cause and effect related to neutrophilic inflammation and BPD are germane, and they should be carefully explored. Even if inflammation does not itself deliver the initial insult, it may be a major contributor to its propagation.

Role of Cytokines

Cytokines, such as interleukin-8 (IL-8) and others, and eicosanoids, such as leukotriene B_4 (LTB_4), typically have been considered to have a potential role in the inflammation that ensues as pulmonary oxygen toxicity progresses. Evidence for increased IL-8 expression has been found in chronic inflammatory lung disorders of both children (32) and adults (33,34) at both early and advanced stages of the disease. In a recent study (8), IL-8 mRNA expression was present in airway cells from all six infants who were studied from 1 to 28 days postnatally. The infants ranged from 25 to 31 weeks gestational age, and their birth weights ranged from 650 to 1050 g. In each infant both deep pulmonary lavage and tracheal effluent secretions were studied. No differences in IL-8 message expression were detected between samples taken from central and distal airways. There was, however, no attempt at quantitation of IL-8 mRNA in this study. Nonetheless, it is clear that IL-8 was ubiquitously expressed throughout the respiratory tract, with message for IL-8 being found in every lavage cell sample in which β-actin was also detected (n = 12). In the same study, mRNA for IL-1α was detected in 10 of 12 samples, IL-1β in 6 of 12 samples, IL-6 in 8 of 12 samples, and tumor necrosis factor-alpha (TNF-α) in 5 of 11 samples. There were no correlations between the presence or absence of various cytokines within each pair of samples obtained from central and distal airways. Thus, with the exception of IL-8, there is no apparent relation between the mRNA expression of various inflammatory cytokines in proximal and distal airways. Information on protein abundance of the various cytokines within proximal and distal airways will also be useful. This report (8) did not describe how many of the six infants studied subsequently had BPD.

In another, more extensive, study of inflammatory cytokines and BPD, there was a strong association between development of BPD and the presence of IL-6 bioactivity in tracheal secretions of 30 patients (22). With the standard (7TD1) bioassay, IL-6 activity in this fluid on the first day of life was 15-fold higher in the 19 infants who eventually acquired BPD, compared with 10 control infants. These control infants required ventilatory support for various cardiac and gastrointestinal disorders, and none had detectable infection. Infants with subsequent BPD also had 6.6-fold higher IL-6 activity in tracheal secretions than did 11 infants who had RDS without subsequent BPD. However, there were no detectable differences of antigenic IL-6 measured by enzyme-limited immunosorbent assay (ELISA) at any time point. Nonetheless, IL-6 activity in tracheal secretions on day 1 of life was significantly higher (by almost fourfold) in patients who died than it was in patients who survived. Increased IL-6 activity in tracheal secretions persisted in the BPD group through age 14 days and then decreased. The two patients with RDS without subsequent BPD who were studied on day 14 of life also showed substantial IL-6 activity in their airway secretions. Developmental factors probably contributed to the outcome of this study, for average gestational ages were 26.2 ± 1.5, 28.9 ± 1.7, and 34.7 ± 5.1 weeks (mean ± SD), respectively, in the BPD, RDS, and control groups. Late onset sepsis tended to be more common in the BPD group than it was in the RDS and control groups, although differences in the incidence of sepsis between groups was not statistically significant. The reason for the discrepancy between measurements of IL-6 antigen and activity is unclear. Likewise, the potential role that IL-6 might play in BPD pathogenesis is unclear.

These findings for infants with RDS and BPD are similar to the observations that have been reported for IL-6 in adult patients with respiratory distress syndrome (ARDS) (reviewed in Ref. 35). IL-6 might play a direct role in the pathogenesis of BPD, or its production might reflect simply the presence of other inflammatory cytokines, such as IL-1, which may increase the production of IL-6. Both TNF and IL-1 can induce production and the release of IL-6. Induction by TNF seems an unlikely stimulus in this instance, for TNF bioactivity and antigen were not significantly greater in lavage specimens of patients with subsequent BPD, when compared with patients with RDS alone. Indeed, TNF activity in lavage specimens of patients with RDS tended to exceed TNF activity in fluids from patients with subsequent BPD during that interval. TNF activity in lavage fluid increased later, on days 14 and 28, in patients who acquired BPD. Hence, TNF did not appear to drive IL-6 production. Concentrations of IL-1, which may be less available for detection in biological fluids because of cell binding (36), were not examined in this study. TNF also can be highly cell-bound under certain conditions; therefore, its presence might have gone undetected. It also is possible that IL-6 is a marker for bacterial exposure or infection. Hence, Grigg et al. (37) reported increased antigenic IL-6 in distal pulmonary lavage specimens in day 1 premature infants after prolonged rupture of membranes. Amniotic fluid IL-6 antigen generally is elevated in association with acute chorioamnionitis and frequently predicts neonatal morbidity or mortality (38). Nonetheless, Bagchi et al. did not observe an increase of IL-6 antigen or activity in tracheal lavage samples from newborns who were delivered in the presence of chorioamnionitis compared with infants without associated infection, although maternal antibiotic therapy may have influenced their results. Apparent discrepancies between studies also may reflect differences in the site at which lavage fluids were obtained in the various studies.

Murch et al. (39) found very low levels of TNF in tracheal effluent samples obtained on postnatal days 1–3 in 20 preterm infants whose gestation was 24–31 weeks. TNF concentrations increased with increasing postnatal age. TNF levels did not differ in those infants who later acquired BPD compared with those who did not. Concentrations of TNF in tracheal lavage specimens of all 6 infants decreased after treatment with dexamethasone. These changes in TNF were accompanied by impressive clinical improvement of all steroid-treated infants. There was no association between concentrations of TNF measured in tracheal lavage fluids and serum obtained from these patients

In another study that included measurement of IL-1β in tracheal lavage in infants with BPD, the concentration of IL-1β in lavage fluid from four infants with BPD was higher than it was in infants who had less need for supplemental oxygen (40). In infants who still required ventilatory support on day 14, concentrations of IL-1β in lavage specimens were higher than they had been on postnatal day 1. On day 1, IL-1β was directly related to lavage neutrophil count and inversely related to gestational age. IL-1β was present in lavage fluids from most intubated infants on day 1 or day 14 (40). Two additional studies (41,42) also have suggested that early elevation in lavage IL-1β activity is associated with subsequent BPD. Another cytokine the elevation of which in lavage may be associated with subsequent BPD is macrophage inflammatory protein-1α (MIP-1α). The concentrations of these (IL-1β and MIP-1α), TNFα, and of other inflammatory markers and cells may be decreased following dexamethasone therapy (42).

Effect of Dexamethasone on Cytokines, Eicosanoids, and Other Markers of Inflammation

Several investigations have documented a clinically beneficial effect of dexamethasone in established BPD (43–48). Various studies have documented a decrease in lavage neutrophils and different inflammatory mediators after initiation of dexamethasone therapy. Dexamethasone therapy also decreases the concentration of a variety of other proteins in lavage fluid, consistent with a decrease in alveolar–capillary membrane permeability in association with diminished inflammation. Beneficial effects of dexamethasone may include decreased inflammation, changes in the surfactant system, altered capillary or epithelial permeability or epithelial protein clearance, movement of ions and water, or a combination of factors.

In a double-blind, placebo-controlled study on the effects of a 3-day treatment with dexamethasone for preterm infants with BPD, tracheal lavage neutrophil counts, albumin, elastase/2x α_1–antitrypsin, and fibronectin concentrations, all were decreased in association with improved pulmonary function (49). Treated infants also required less inspired oxygen and ventilator support than did control infants. In another study, dexamethasone therapy was associated with both a decrease in LTB_4 concentration in tracheal lavage fluid, as well as a decreased chemotactic response of neutrophils to tracheal secretions (50). The same investigators reported increases in neutrophil chemotactic activity, LTB_4, IL-8, complement component C5-derived anaphylotoxin, elastase α_1–protease complex, α_1–protease inhibitor activity, neutrophil counts, and albumin, each referenced to secretory component for IgA, in tracheal aspirates from neonates with prolonged respiratory distress and subsequent BPD, when compared with neonates without BPD (51). Dexamethasone may also decrease TNF concentrations in tracheal lavage secretions of patients with established BPD (39). Dexamethasone therapy also decreased hydrogen peroxide release from stimulated alveolar macrophages (52). In another study of potential mechanisms by which dexamethasone therapy may benefit patients with BPD, tracheal effluents from dexamethasone-treated infants had decreased concentrations of nonsedimentable proteins within 3 days after initiation of treatment compared with tracheal effluents from placebo-treated infants. At a constant protein concentration, the tracheobronchial fluids from placebo-treated infants caused greater in vitro inhibition of the surface activity of surfactant than did such fluids from treated infants. Surfactant protein A (SP-A) concentrations in tracheal effluents were elevated transiently in the treated group. However, there was no demonstrable effect on phosphatidylcholine or disaturated phosphatidylcholine. Likewise, dexamethasone treatment had no effect on the surface activity of the sedimentable surfactant complexes in these fluids. Therefore, it was inferred that there was little effect on functional quantities of SP-B and SP-C. There was also no effect of dexamethasone therapy on tracheal lavage concentrations of IL-1β, lactoferrin, or myeloperoxidase, a marker for neutrophils (53). Hence, this study supports a role for dexamethasone therapy in decreasing protein concentrations in the lung's epithelial lining fluid, either by decreasing alveolar–capillary membrane permeability or by increasing reuptake of protein. However, this study suggests that such an effect may have occurred independently of any influence on inflammatory cells or mediators or on surfactant components. Perhaps other indirect mechanisms influencing permeability, such as induction of lipocortins, could play a role (discussed in Ref. 54).

C. Protease–Antiprotease Imbalance

The possibility of a protease–antiprotease imbalance in the lungs of patients with BPD was first suggested by Merritt and co-workers (19). This study found that elastase inhibitory capacity, which is primarily a result of α_1-antitrypsin activity, decreased progressively on postnatal days 1–3 in infants who subsequently acquired BPD. On days 4, 5, and 8, this activity remained less in lavages from infants who subsequently had BPD compared with tracheal lavages from infants without subsequent BPD. This decline in elastase inhibitory capacity occurred despite similar concentrations of antigenic α_1-antitrypsin in the BPD group compared with the other two groups. The authors attributed these findings to inactivation of α_1-antitrypsin, possibly by oxidants; such inactivation occurs through oxidation of a methionine residue in α_1-antitrypsin. In addition, free elastase activities in tracheal lavage specimens were substantially elevated after postnatal day 3. The increase in elastase relative to α_1-antitrypsin activity, as well as a persistence of neutrophilic inflammation in BPD patients, was confirmed (10,20). The former study (10) also showed that α_2-macroglobulin, a high molecular weight antiprotease that is not normally found in healthy adult lung, appeared in the tracheal lavage fluid of newborns who required prolonged ventilation. Merritt et al. showed that the excess elastase in tracheal lavage specimens from BPD patients was of neutrophil origin. Its biochemical pattern of inhibition was consistent with neutrophil, rather than macrophage, elastase (55). The latter investigation again confirmed the overall elastase–antiprotease imbalance in BPD, and also demonstrated that this imbalance is profoundly exaggerated (about three to fourfold) in lavages from BPD patients with associated bacterial pneumonia. A more recent study confirmed the presence of excess elastase activity and of neutrophils in infants with BPD compared with infants without BPD, but found no difference in the concentration of another potent endogenous elastase inhibitor—secretory leukocyte protease inhibitor (SLPI)—between infants with and without BPD (21). This study suggests one reasonable potential therapy: SLPI, which may counter a deleterious effect of inflammation without likely harm to host defenses. The effect of various therapies, including dexamethasone, indomethacin, and synthetic and human surfactants, on elastase–antiprotease imbalance have also been studied in evolving BPD (18,56,57).

Whereas studies demonstrating loss of α_1-antitrypsin activity, despite detection of the antigenic protein, have suggested excessive oxidant production within the lungs of patients with evolving BPD (19), there have been relatively few additional studies that have done so (58,59). It appears likely, however, that reactive oxygen metabolites, most likely derived from inflammatory cells, may be involved in the inactivation of α_1-antitrypsin. The specific oxygen metabolite involved in this inactivation is unclear. Demonstration of the presence of reactive oxygen species is difficult because of their rapid metabolism. Molecular oxygen itself may be an important oxidizing substance for critical targets of hyperoxia in the lung (26,60); hence, other defensive strategies to circumvent such direct oxidation may have an as yet undetermined role in antioxidative defense. Indeed, there is compelling evidence to suggest a deficiency of *intracellular* antioxidants within premature lungs. However, the status of extracellular antioxidants, such as those present in the lung's extracellular lining fluid is less well known. Such extracellular antioxidants, however, may have a significant modulatory role in pulmonary oxidant injury, and studies of these antioxidants in human infants with BPD are also needed.

Although cytokines, chemotaxins, adhesion molecules, and oxygen radicals are inviting targets for potential therapeutic interventions, it must be remembered that (1) the premature newborn is a particularly impaired host relative to antibacterial defenses, and (2) even in adults with respiratory distress, there is a fine line between beneficial and excessive (i.e., harmful) therapy to curb the potentially toxic effects of an exuberant antibacterial inflammatory response (reviewed in Ref. 35).

IV. Clinical Usefulness of BAL in BPD

In addition to the wide range of research applications described in the foregoing, BAL may be useful in clinical management of infants after exogenous surfactant therapy. Lavage fluids may also provide a useful means of monitoring for potential adverse biochemical or cellular effects of new therapies, such as nitric oxide and liquid ventilation. In addition, BAL may be helpful in obtaining diagnostic materials when evaluating an interstitial lung process that may be mistaken for BPD (1,2,61). BAL may also provide a useful means for diagnosing infection with bacteria, viruses, chlamydia, pneumocystis, fungi, or other organisms in infants, with and without BPD. Finally, BAL can be useful in diagnosing other intercurrent pulmonary conditions, such as aspiration of gastric or oropharyngeal contents, that may complicate the course of infants with BPD (62). Infants with BPD may be vulnerable to gastroesophageal reflux and aspiration because of possible lung hyperinflation, associated central nervous system dysfunction, or vocal cord paresis or injury (63–66). The use of the lipid index, a score based on the percentage of macrophages staining positively for lipid and on the intensity of that staining in cytological preparations from BAL, to quantify lipid-laden macrophages can be a useful tool in assessing lavage fluids from these infants (62,67,68).

Besides being useful for diagnosing complications of BPD, lavage fluid may also be useful for measuring biochemical markers of disease severity. Among these are the elevation of the basement membrane protein laminin (69) and the depression of tracheal aspirate fibrinolytic activity (decreased plasminogen activator–plasmin activity) (70).

V. Conclusion

In summary, bronchoalveolar lavage is a more difficult, potentially more dangerous and less well-standardized procedure for use in premature infants than it is in older children and adults. Studies of tracheal effluent secretions from infants with respiratory distress have provided useful clues for the pathogenesis of BPD. Analysis of the composition of tracheal lavage specimens to assess mechanisms of disease is problematic; however, animal models may provide a means for clarifying the extent to which events occurring in the distal lung are reflected in pooled secretions from proximal airways. Such investigations are now needed. As modern treatment continues to improve, human pathological materials will continue to become even more scarce than they are at present. Hence, strategies for optimally using lavage material need to be further refined.

The use of tracheal lavage or BAL in premature newborns with evolving BPD can provide limited information on the presence or absence of complicating lung infection, aspiration, or other processes (71). Associations have been found between acquisition of BPD and the presence or absence of various inflammatory cell types or mediators. However, such associations generally can realize cause–effect importance only when such causation is established through pharmacological or genetic manipulation of reliable animal models. In human trials, the effectiveness of various interventions, such as anti-inflammatory, antiprotease, or antioxidant interventions, or alternate modes of ventilation, for example, may be monitored in part through measurement of various markers in tracheal lavage fluid.

There are numerous questions remaining about BPD pathogenesis. Among these is, "What are the mechanisms that lead to resolution of inflammation?" Here, data from human infants who do not later acquire BPD may be more valuable than that from those who do. For example, subtraction analyses or other rapid methods for surveying expressed mRNAs might be employed to identify markers for those with resolving illness. Perhaps cytokines or other factors that lead to resolution of inflammation could be better clarified through such an approach. In addition, a better understanding is needed of what mechanisms are involved in prevention of normal alveolar and vascular growth and development during the evolution of BPD. Perhaps factors that stimulate reepithelialization or that inhibit fibroblast proliferation or collagen production could also be identified and used therapeutically. Besides these, the potential emerging roles of surfactant proteins A and D in modulating infection, possibly a very important factor in BPD pathogenesis, may warrant additional attention in clinical studies.

However, perhaps the greatest need for additional study is in the earliest events in RDS, which then progresses to BPD. Specifically, we need a better understanding of what causes the formation and removal of alveolar edema in the premature newborn so that its resolution can be accelerated or augmented. Such work will include exploration of the ontogeny and regulation of various ion and water channels, pores and pumps, various ATPases, and the pathways that provide energy for these systems. Through appropriate modulation of these systems, the demand for mechanical ventilation and oxygen might be minimized. Although tracheal lavage specimens may provide only ''tip of the iceberg'' information, it is conceivable that they also could be useful in such studies.

Acknowledgments

This work was supported by grants from the National Institutes of Health RO-1 HL52732, U10 HL 56263, and SCOR P50 HL 46481 (C.W.). The authors are grateful to Jacque Guthrie for technical assistance during preparation of the manuscript.

References

1. Fan LL. Evaluation and therapy of chronic interstitial pneumonitis in children. Curr Opin Pediatr 1994; 6:248–254.
2. Fan LL, Langston C. Chronic interstitial lung disease in children. Pediatr Pulmonol 1993; 16:184–196.
3. Boat TF, Tepper R, Stecenko A, et al. Assessment of lung function and dysfunction in studies of infants and children. Am Rev Respir Dis 1993; 148:1105–1108.
4. Alpert BE, O'Sullivan BP, Panitch HB. Nonbronchoscopic approach to bronchoalveolar lavage in children with artificial airways. Pediatr Pulmonol 1992; 13:38–41.
5. Koumbourlis AC, Kurland G. Nonbronchoscopic bronchoalveolar lavage in mechanically ventilated infants: technique, efficacy, and applications. Pediatr Pulmonol 1993; 15:257–262.
6. Larsen GL, Webster RO, Worthen GS, Gumbay RS, Henson PM. The additive effect of intravascular complement activation and brief episodes of hypoxia in producing increased permeability in the rabbit lung. J Clin Invest 1985; 75:902–910.
7. Coalson JJ, Winter VT, Gerstmann DR, Idell S, King RJ, Delemos RA. Pathophysiologic, morphometric and biochemical studies of the premature baboon with bronchopulmonary dysplasia. Am Rev Respir Dis 1992; 145:872–881.
8. LoMonaco MB, Barber CM, Sinkin RA. Differential cytokine mRNA expression by neonatal pulmonary cells. Pediatr Res 1996; 39:247–251.

9. Grigg J, Arnon S, Silverman M. Fractional processing of sequential bronchoalveolar lavage fluid from intubated babies. Eur Respir J 1992; 5:727–732.
10. Watts CL, Bruce MC. Comparison of secretory component for immunoglobulin A with albumin as reference proteins in tracheal aspirate from preterm infants. J Pediatr 1995; 127:113–122.
11. Rennard SI, Martin PG, Crystal RG. Estimation of volume of epithelial lining fluid recovered by lavage using urea as marker of dilution. J Appl Physiol 1986; 60:532–538.
12. Zmora E, Merritt TA. Use of side-hold endotracheal tube adapter for tracheal aspiration. Am J Dis Child 1980; 134:250–254.
13. Wagener JS. Fatality following fiberoptic bronchoscopy in a two-year-old child. Pediatr Pulmonol 1987; 3:197–199.
14. Reidler J, Grigg J, Robertson CF. Bronchoalveolar lavage cellularity in healthy children. Am J Respir Crit Care Med 1995; 152:163–168.
15. Ratjen AF, Bredendiek M, Zheng L, Brendel M, Costabel U. Lymphocyte subsets in bronchoalveolar lavage fluid of children without bronchopulmonary disease. Am J Respir Crit Care 1995; 152:174–178.
16. Clement A, Chadelat K, Masliah J, Housset B, Sardet A, Grimfeld A, Tournier G. A controlled study of oxygen metabolite release by alveolar macrophages from children with interstitial lung disease. Am Rev Respir Dis 1987; 136:1424–1428.
17. Midulla F, Villani A, Ronchetti R. Bronchoalveolar lavage studies in children without lung parenchymal disease: cellular constituents and protein levels. Pediatr Pulmonol 1995; 20:112–118.
18. Merritt TA, Stuard ID, Puccia J, et al. Newborn tracheal aspirate cytology: classification during respiratory distress syndrome and bronchopulmonary dysplasia. J Pediatr 1981; 98:949–956.
19. Merritt TA, Cochrane CG, Holcomb K, et al. Elastase and alpha-1-proteinase inhibitor activity in tracheal aspirates during RDS. Role of inflammation in the pathogenesis of bronchopulmonary dysplasia. J Clin Invest 1983; 72:656–662.
20. Ogden BE, Murphy SA, Saunders GC, Pathak D, Johnson JD. Neonatal lung neutrophils and elastase/proteinase inhibitor imbalance. Am Rev Respir Dis 1984; 130: 817–821.
21. Watterberg KL, Carmichael DF, Gerdes JS, Werner S, Backstrom C, Murphy S. Secretory leukocyte protease inhibitor and lung inflammation in developing bronchopulmonary dysplasia. J Pediatr 1994; 125:264–269.
22. Bagchi A, Viscardi RM, Tacia KV, Ensor JE, McCrea KA, Hesday JD. Increased activity interleukin-6 but not tumor necrosis factor-α in lung lavage of premature infants is associated with the development of bronchopulmonary dysplasia. Pediatr Res 1994; 36:244–252.
23. Grigg JM, Savill JS, Sarraf C, Haslett C, Silverman M. Neutrophil apoptosis and clearance from neonatal lungs. Lancet 1991; 338:720–722.
24. Jackson JC, Chi EY, Wilson CB, Truog WE, Teh EC, Hodson WA. Sequence of inflammatory cell migration into lung during recovery from hyaline membrane disease in premature newborn monkeys. Am Rev Respir Dis 1987; 135:937–940.
25. Yamamoto C, Kojima T, Hattori K, Nogi S, Imamura H, Tsubura A, Kobayashi Y.

Eosinophilia in premature infants: correlation with chronic lung disease. Acta Paediatr 1996; 85:1232–1235.
26. Fox RB, Hoidal JR, Brown DM, Repine JE. Pulmonary inflammation due to oxygen toxicity: involvement of chemotactic factors and polymorphonuclear leukocytes. Am Rev Respir Dis 1981; 123:521–523.
27. Von Essen SG, Robbins RA, Spurzem JR, Thompson AB, McGranaghan SS, Rennard SL. Bronchoscopy with bronchoalveolar lavage causes neutrophil recruitment to the lower respiratory tract. Am Rev Respir Dis 1991; 144:848–854.
28. Gardner PR, Nguyen DH, White CW. Aconitase is a sensitive and critical target of oxygen poisoning in cultured mammalian cells and in rat lungs. Proc Natl Acad Sci USA 1994; 91:12248–12252.
29. Freeman BA, Crapo JD. Biology of disease: free radicals and tissue injury. Lab Invest 1982;47:412–426.
30. Barry BE, Crapo JD. Patterns of accumulation of platelets and neutrophils in rat lung during exposure to 100% and 85% oxygen. Am Rev Respir Dis 1985; 132: 548–555.
31. Davis WB, Rennard SI, Bitterman PB, Crystal RG. Pulmonary oxygen toxicity. Early reversible changes in human alveolar structures induced by hyperoxia. N Engl J Med 1983; 309:878–883.
32. Khan TZ, Wagener JS, Accurso FA, Riches DWH. Early inflammation in infants with cystic fibrosis. Am J Respir Crit Care Med 1995; 151:1075–1108.
33. Carre PC, Mortenson RL, King TE Jr, Noble PW, Sable CL, Riches DW. Increased expression of the interleukin-8 gene by alveolar macrophages in idiopathic pulmonary fibrosis. A potential mechanism for the recruitment and activation of neutrophils in lung fibrosis. J Clin Invest 1991; 88:1802–1810.
34. Carre PC, King TE Jr, Mortensen R, Riches DW. Cryptogenic organizing pneumonia: increased expression of interleukin-8 and fibronectin genes by alveolar macrophages. Am J Respir Cell Mol Biol 1994; 10:100–105.
35. White CW, Das KC. Role of cytokines in acute lung injury. In: Crystal R, West J, Weibel E, Barnes P, eds. The Lung. Scientific Foundations. 2nd ed. Philadelphia: Lippincott–Raven Publications, 1996:188.1–188.14.
36. Ghezzi P, Dinarello CA, Bianchi M, Rosandich ME, Repine JE, White CW. Hypoxia increases production of cytokines IL-1 and TNF by human mononuclear cells. Cytokine 1991; 3:189–194.
37. Grigg JM, Barber A, Silverman M. Increased levels of interleukin-6 in preterm ventilated infants after prolonged rupture of membranes. Am Rev Respir Dis 1992; 145: 782–786.
38. Yoon BH, Romero R, Kim CJ, et al. Amniotic fluid interleukin-6: a sensitive test for antenatal diagnosis of acute inflammatory lesions of preterm placenta and prediction of perinatal morbidity. Am J Obstet Gynecol 1995; 172:960–970.
39. Murch SH, MacDonald TT, Wood CBS, Costeloe KL. Tumor necrosis factor in the bronchoalveolar secretions of infants with the respiratory distress syndrome and the effect of dexamethasone treatment. Thorax 1992; 47:44–47.
40. Rozycki HL. Bronchoalveolar interleukin-1 beta in infants on day 1 of life. South Med J 1994; 87:991–996.
41. Rindfleisch MS, Hasday JD, Taciak V, Broderick K, Viscardi RM. Potential role of

interleukin-1 in the development of bronchopulmonary dysplasia. J Interferon Cytokine Res 1996; 16:365–373.
42. Murch SH, Costeloe K, Klein NJ, MacDonald TT. Early production of macrophage inflammatory protein-1 alpha occurs in respiratory distress syndrome and is associated with poor outcome. Pediatr Res 1996; 40:490–497.
43. Mammel MC, Green TP, Johnson DA, Thompson TR. Controlled trial of dexamethasone therapy in infants with bronchopulmonary dysplasia. Lancet 1983; 1:1356–1358.
44. Avery GB, Fletcher AB, Kaplan M, Brudno S. Controlled trial of dexamethasone in respirator-dependent infants with bronchopulmonary dysplasia. Pediatrics 1984; 75:106–111.
45. Barrington K, Finer NN. Evaluation of the efficacy of dexamethasone in prevention of severe bronchopulmonary dysplasia. J Perinatol 1985; 5:26–32.
46. Cummings JJ, D'Eugenio DB, Grooss SJ. A controlled trial of dexamethasone in preterm infants at high risk for bronchopulmonary dysplasia. N Engl J Med 1989; 320:1505–1510.
47. Harkavy KL, Scanlon JW, Chowdhry PK, Grylack LJ. Dexamethasone therapy in ventilator-and-oxygen-dependent infants: a controlled study. J Pediatr 1989; 115: 979–983.
48. Collaborative Dexamethasone Trial Group. Dexamethasone in neonatal chronic lung disease: an international placebo-controlled trial. Pediatrics 1991; 88:421–427.
49. Yoder MCJ, Chua R, Tepper R. Effect of dexamethasone on pulmonary inflammation and pulmonary function of ventilator-dependent infants with bronchopulmonary dysplasia. Am Rev Respir Dis 1991; 143(5 pt 1):1044–1048.
50. Groneck P, Reuss D, Götze-Speer B, Speer CP. Effects of dexamethasone on chemotactic activity and inflammatory mediators in tracheobronchial aspirates of preterm infants at risk for chronic lung disease. J Pediatr 1993; 122:938–944.
51. Groneck P, Götze-Speer B, Opperman M, Effert H, Speer CP. Association of pulmonary inflammation and increased microvascular permeability during the development of BPD: a sequential analysis of inflammatory mediators in respiratory fluids of high-risk preterm neonates. Pediatrics 1994; 93:712–718.
52. Clement A, Chadelat K, Sardet A, Grimfield A, Tournier G. Alveolar macrophage status in bronchopulmonary dysplasia. Pediatr Res 1988; 23:470–473.
53. Kari MA, Raivio KO, Venge P, Hallman M. Dexamethasone treatment of infants at risk for chronic lung disease: surfactant components and inflammatory parameters in airway specimens. Pediatr Res 1994; 36:387–393.
54. Stelzner TJ, O'Brien RF, Sato K, Weil JV. Hypoxia-induced increases in pulmonary transvascular protein escape in rats. Modulation by glucocorticoids. J Clin Invest 1988; 82:1840–1847.
55. Walti H, Tordet C, Gerbaut L, Saugier P, Moriette G, Relier JP. Persistant elastase/proteinase inhibitor imbalance during prolonged ventilation of infants with BPD: evidence for the role of nosocomial infections. Pediatr Res 1989; 26:351–355.
56. Gerdes JS, Harris MC, Polin RA. Effect of dexamethasone and indomethacin on elastase, $alpha_1$-proteinase inhibitor, and fibronectin in bronchoalveolar lavage fluid from neonates. J Pediatr 1988; 113:727–731.
57. Gerdes J, Whitsett J, Long W. Elastase activity and surfactant protein concentration

in tracheal aspirates from neonates receiving synthetic surfactant. J Pediatr 1992; 120:S34–S39.

58. Varsila E, Pesonen E, Andersson S. Early protein oxidation in the neonatal lung is related to development of chronic lung disease. Acta Paediatr 1995; 84:1296–1299.
59. Contreras M, Hariharan N, Lewandoski JR, Ciesielski W, Koscik R, Zimmerman JJ. Bronchoalveolar oxyradical inflammatory elements herald bronchopulmonary dysplasia. Crit Care Med 1996; 24:29–37.
60. Gardner PR, Raineri I, Epstein LB, White CW. Superoxide radical and iron modulate aconitase activity in mammalian cells. J Biol Chem 1995; 270:13399–13405.
61. Fan LL, Mullen AL, Brugman SM, Inscore SC, Parks DP, White CW. Clinical spectrum of chronic interstitial lung disease in children. J Pediatr 1992; 121:867–872.
62. Radford PJ, Stillwell PC, Blue B, Hertel G. Aspiration complicating bronchopulmonary dysplasia. Chest 1995; 107:185–188.
63. Fan LL, Flynn JW, Pathak DR, et al. Predictive value of stridor in detecting larygneal injury in extubated neonates. Crit Care Med 1982; 10:453–455.
64. Fan LL, Flynn JW, Pathak DR. Risk factors predicting laryngeal injury in intubated neonates. Crit Care Med 1983; 11:431–433.
65. Fan LL, Flynn JW. Laryngoscopy in neonates and infants: experience with the flexible fiberoptic bronchoscope. Laryngoscope 1981; 91:451–456.
66. Fan LL, Sparks LM, Dulinski JP. Applications of an ultrathin flexible bronchoscope for neonatal and pediatric airway problems. Chest 1986; 89:673–676.
67. Colombo JL, Halberg TK, Sammut PH. Time course of lipid-laden macrophages with acute and recurrent milk aspiration in rabbits. Pediatr Pulmonol 1992; 12:95–98.
68. Colombo JL, Halberg TK. Recurrent aspiration in children: lipid-laden alveolar macrophage quantitation. Pediatr Pulmonol 1987; 3:86–89.
69. Alnahhas MH, Karathanasis P, Martich Kriss V, Pauly TH, Bruce MC. Elevated lamin concentrations in lung secretions of preterm infants supported by mechanical ventilation are correlated with radiographic abnormalities. J Pediatr 1997; 131:555–560.
70. Singhal KK, Parton LA. Plasminogen activator activity in preterm infants with respiratory distress syndrome: relationship to the development of bronchopulmonary dysplasia. Pediatr Res 1996; 39:229–235.
71. Fan LL, Lum Lung MC, Wagener JS. The diagnostic value of bronchoalveolar lavage in immunocompetent children with chronic diffuse pulmonary infiltrates. Pediatr Pulmonol 1997; 23:8–13.

7

Inflammatory Mediators in Neonatal Lung Disease

CHRISTIAN P. SPEER

University of Würzburg
Würzburg, Germany

PETER GRONECK

Children's Hospital of the City of Cologne
Cologne, Germany

I. Introduction

Despite the array of recent improvements in neonatal intensive care, chronic lung disease (CLD) of early infancy, which is often referred to as bronchopulmonary dysplasia (BPD), is still a significant cause of long-term morbidity and mortality in extremely low-birth-weight infants, many of whom have had early respiratory distress syndrome (RDS), sometimes despite prenatal steroid and postnatal surfactant treatments. CLD has a multifactorial etiology. The principal risk factors that have been identified are lung immaturity, barotrauma, and overdistended airspaces from positive-pressure ventilation, and oxygen administration. Nevertheless, the exact mechanisms that lead to lung injury and hinder healing are incompletely understood. There is growing evidence, however, that repetitive positive-pressure inflation and oxygen toxicity induce a complex inflammatory reaction in the airways and the interstitium of the immature lungs of infants with RDS and CLD (reviewed in Refs. 1–5). This pulmonary inflammation is characterized by an accumulation of various cells and associated release of inflammatory mediators that contribute to increased lung microvascular permeability and tissue injury, with resultant chronic respiratory failure.

II. Neutrophils and Macrophages

Merritt and co-workers (6) were the first to demonstrate that preterm infants at an early stage of RDS had high numbers of inflammatory cells present in their airways when compared with controls infants who were ventilated for nonpulmonary reasons. By postnatal day 3 or 4, however, preterm infants who subsequently acquired BPD had many more inflammatory cells in their airways compared with infants who recovered from RDS. The predominant cell that was identified in the airway secretions at the early stage of inflammation was the neutrophil. These findings have been confirmed by other investigators who have evaluated the inflammatory cells in the airway lavage specimens of infants with early evolving BPD (7–10). Moreover, a similar increase of neutrophil numbers has been observed in premature monkeys with RDS (11). With resolution of RDS, the neutrophil count in specimens of tracheobronchial fluid decreased, but it remained abnormally high in those infants who went on to have CLD. Thus, it has been suggested that the persistence of neutrophils is associated with the development of CLD (4).

Alveolar macrophages increase substantially in airway sections of infants with RDS by approximately 4 days after birth, after which macrophages are the predominant inflammatory cell within the lungs of infants with BPD (7,12). By 4 months after birth alveolar macrophages account for about 90% of the total population of inflammatory cells within the airspaces of infants with BPD (13). Recently, Murch and colleagues (14) demonstrated that macrophages and neutrophils were abundant in bronchoalveolar lavage (BAL) specimens of infants with evolving RDS. In another study, the same group of investigators used immunohistochemical techniques to assess inflammatory changes in lung tissue of 40 infants who had died with acute RDS (15). The interstitial density of CD-68–positive macrophages was at least 15-fold greater, and neutrophils were 10-fold greater in lungs of infants who died at 2–3 days after birth with RDS compared with stillborn infants of equivalent gestation (15).

Although the role of neutrophils and macrophages in lung injury of preterm infants remains incompletely defined, recent observations suggest that these cells have various harmful effects on epithelial and endothelial cell integrity, and also contribute to other types of lung damage. Both neutrophils and macrophages have essential roles in host defense mechanisms of newborn infants. Despite some quantitative and functional deficiencies of the neonatal neutrophil, such as decreased adherence, deformability, and chemotaxis (16), the phagocytic properties of these cells and various mediators that they generate and release participate in the complex interactions that characterize pulmonary inflammation. However, impaired neutrophil functions, combined with deficits in humoral host defense mechanisms, may contribute to the increased susceptibility of preterm infants to pulmonary and systemic nosocomial infections (17). Host defense properties of neonatal and adult macrophages, in contrast with those of neutrophils, are very similar (18).

III. Neutrophil and Macrophage Recruitment

Airway secretions of infants with RDS have a high chemotactic activity. Moreover, the airway secretions of infants who later acquired CLD exhibited even greater chemotactic activity at postnatal day 5 when compared with patients without subsequent CLD (9). The anaphylatoxin C5a (19), leukotriene B_4 (LTB_4), and interleukin-8 (IL-8), which are important chemoattractants for human neutrophils, have been detected in the bronchoalveolar fluid of these infants. After recovery from RDS, the concentrations of C5a and LTB_4 were significantly higher in those infants who later acquired CLD compared with babies with RDS without subsequent CLD. In addition, high concentrations of these chemoattractants have been found in the late stages of CLD (20). These data are consistent with the notion that C5a and LTB_4 contribute to neutrophil influx in both the early and later stages of CLD. LTB_4 is produced mainly by neutrophils and alveolar macrophages. Both in vivo and in vitro experiments have indicated that C5a is most likely synthesized and activated by enzymatic cleavage within the airspaces of the lung (6). The same holds true for IL-8, which is locally produced by alveolar macrophages, fibroblasts, type II epithelial cells, and endothelial cells when they are stimulated by hypoxia, hyperoxia, endotoxin, or other noxious substances. IL-8, which is probably the most important chemotactic factor in the lung (21), was present in high concentrations in samples of airway lavage fluid obtained from infants with evolving CLD 2 weeks after birth (9). These data have been confirmed in studies conducted by several investigators (10,22–26). Moreover, Munshi et al. (24) recently reported that the concentration of IL-8 in tracheal aspirates of infants with evolving CLD increased before the marked neutrophil influx into the lungs of these infants occurred. Besides C5a, LTB_4, and IL-8, other substances with chemotactic properties, such as platelet activating factor, intercellular adhesion molecule-1 (ICAM-1), 5-hydroxyeicosatetraenoic acid (5-HETE), and elastin degradation products (22), have been identified in the airways of infants with CLD (20).

Before migrating from the circulation into the lungs, the neutrophil must adhere to the vascular endothelium. Endothelial cells express various adhesion molecules, or selectins (i.e., E-selectin), which bind to complementary sites on the neutrophils (see Chap. 32) and IL-8 plays an important role in the increased expression of neutrophil cell surface receptors (β_2-integrins), such as CD11b/CD18. IL-8 also is thought to help regulate expression of adhesion molecules, such as ICAM-1, on pulmonary endothelial cells (27).

Infants with CLD, when compared with control infants, have increased concentrations of ICAM-1 in their tracheal aspirates (10,28). In addition, increased plasma concentrations of soluble ICAM-1 have been detected in infants with CLD at postnatal age 10–14 days (22). A recent report indicates that serum concentrations of E-selectin are significantly higher during the first week of life in infants who later will acquire BPD than in patients without subsequent BPD (29). These studies provide indirect evidence for the recruitment of neutrophils during the evolution of CLD.

Two potent β-chemokines have been detected in bronchoalveolar lavage fluid of infants with RDS and BPD, macrophage inflammatory protein-1α (MIP-1α) and RANTES (regulated on activation, normal T-cell expressed and secreted). These chemokines induce chemotaxis of monocytes and macrophages. A recent report showed that the concentration of MIP-1α in airway lavage fluid of infants was associated with later development of pulmonary fibrosis (15).

IV. Cytokines

Besides IL-8, other proinflammatory cytokines, such as tumor necrosis factor-α (TNF-α), interleukin-1 (IL-1), and interleukin-6 (IL-6), may be important contributors to the early inflammatory response by recruiting and activating inflammatory cells. Several investigators have measured increased concentrations of TNF-α, IL-1, and IL-6 in bronchoalveolar lavage fluid obtained from infants who subsequently acquired CLD (26,30–32). The concentration of IL-1β_2 and activities of IL-1 and IL-6 were significantly greater during the first week of life in lung lavage fluids obtained from infants who later had BPD than in those of infants with uncomplicated RDS or control infants without lung disease (12,31,33). In lung lavage fluid of infants who later acquired BPD, the concentration and activity of TNF-α were not increased compared with relevant control infants on the first postnatal day, but subsequently increased, reaching peak concentrations on day 14 (31). Interestingly, increased TNF-α levels in amniotic fluid during amnionitis were associated with a higher incidence of neonatal RDS, suggesting that there might be an association between perinatal appearance of TNF-α and loss of barrier function within terminal respiratory units of the immature lung (34). The time sequence of the appearance of these cytokines in bronchoalveolar lavage suggests that IL-1β might contribute to the postnatal pulmonary increases of TNF-α and IL-8. In addition, IL-1β may play a pivotal role in the host response to infection and inflammation. Many of the proinflammatory actions of IL-1β and TNF-α are similar (33); however, systemic administration of TNF-α in dogs induced more severe lung injury than did IL-1 (35). The pulmonary response to IL-1 administration has been characterized by neutrophil infiltration and generation of oxygen metabolites, which appear to mediate the leak of protein-rich fluid into the lungs in a rat model of ARDS (36). Treatment of surfactant-depleted rabbits with aerolized IL-1 receptor antagonist before induction of experimental lung injury with oxygen and positive-pressure ventilation decreased inflammation and lung microvascular permeability to protein (37).

Various investigators have used reverse transcriptase polymerase chain reaction (RT-PCR) to detect mRNA for IL-1α, IL-1β, IL-6, IL-8, and TNF-α in bronchoalveolar cells of infants with RDS and CLD (23,32,38). These data indicate that mRNA of various cytokines is expressed by alveolar macrophages, neutrophils, epithelial, and endothelial cells, and perhaps other cells within the lungs during the inflammatory process. In a recent study, Jones and co-workers (23) set out to determine if premature birth would alter the expression of anti-inflammatory cytokines that modulate lung inflammation. Production of several proinflammatory cytokines, including TNF-α, IL-1β, and IL-8, is regulated in part by the anti-inflammatory cytokine IL-10. The investigators compared the mRNA expression and protein abundance of pro- and anti-inflammatory cytokines in the lungs of preterm infants with RDS and term newborn infants with meconium aspiration syndrome. Pulmonary expression of mRNA or protein for proinflammatory cytokines was present in all patients from both groups. In contrast, IL-10 mRNA was undetectable in most of the samples from preterm infants, but was present in samples obtained from term infants. These results suggest that preterm infants with pulmonary inflammation may be unable to express the anti-inflammatory cytokine IL-10, in contrast to infants who are born at term. The authors speculated that IL-10 gene expression could be developmentally regulated, and that the susceptibility of the preterm infant to CLD may partly reflect an inability to regulate inflammation through the expression of the anti-inflammatory cytokine IL-10 (23).

In addition, preterm neonates who are exposed to inflammatory stimuli within the airways may have a decreased ability to generate endogenous anti-inflammatory steroids. In a recent study, up to 40% of infants who later acquired BPD had evidence of impaired adrenal function, as indicated by a blunted cortisol response to injection of corticotropin (adrenocorticotropin; ACTH) during the first week of life (39). Moreover, low serum cortisol levels were correlated with increased pulmonary protein leak and increased concentrations of inflammatory mediators in tracheal secretions (40). An insufficient inflammatory response to lung trauma or airway infection also could be an important factor in the development of BPD.

Murch and colleagues (15) used immunohistochemistry to study the interstitial inflammatory response in lungs of preterm infants who died of acute RDS in the week after birth. These studies showed a rapid postnatal increase in the mucosal density of CD68^{+} macrophages and cells that were immunoreactive for TNF-α: the signal for these cells was maximal in lungs of infants who died within 72 hr after birth. When using a cationic probe specific for sulfated glycosaminoglycans (GAGs), the inflammatory infiltration was associated with striking loss of endothelial basement membrane and interstitial GAGs, a process that was almost complete by postnatal day 3. The temporal relation of these findings suggests that degradation of sulfated GAGs may be mediated by the macrophage-derived cytokines, TNF-α, and IL-1 (41), or by other inflammatory products that are released by neutrophils and macrophages.

V. Elastolytic Damage

During the past 15 years several investigators have evaluated the possible role of elastase, a powerful neutral protease that is stored in the azurophilic granules of neutrophils, in the pathogenesis of acute and chronic lung disease of preterm infants. Neutrophils that have entered the airways release elastase during the process of phagocytosis or following cell death. Pulmonary tissue elastin is the primary substrate of neutrophil elastase. Under normal circumstances, elastase is rapidly bound and inactivated by α_1-protease-inhibitor (α_1-PI), which protects the alveolar–capillary unit from proteolytic damage by forming an elastase–α_1-PI complex. This complex is highly stable and can be identified in high concentrations in the plasma of newborns with neonatal septicemia (42). In tracheobronchial secretions of infants with RDS and BPD, increased concentrations of neutrophil elastase and low activities of α_1-PI have been detected (6,43–45). An imbalance between elastase and α_1-PI within the airways may be a hallmark of lung injury in preterm infants (46). Merritt and co-workers (46) reported that α_1-PI was inactivated by proteolytic cleavage of oxidized α_1-PI in the pulmonary tissue and by complex formation of elastase with α_1-PI in infants with RDS. The authors speculated that toxic oxygen radicals, which are released by inflammatory cells or by other oxidizing systems, could contribute to the subsequent inactivation of α_1-PI, thereby resulting in the inability to neutralize neutrophil-mediated release of elastase (6).

Despite this intriguing hypothesis, clinical data on the presence of free elastase in tracheobronchial fluid of infants with RDS and BPD are somewhat contradictory. Some investigators have detected free elastase levels in nearly all infants with RDS who later acquired BPD (6,7,47), whereas other investigators detected increased concentrations of free elastase in airway secretions of only a few infants with RDS. In most infants with RDS, neutrophil elastase is largely inactivated by α_1-PI (9,48–50). One recent study showed that free elastase was present in bronchoalveolar secretions of approximately 30% of infants with severe RDS during the first three postnatal days, but none of these infants had evidence of protection from α_1-PI, so that the presence of free elastase in the airways was associated with an increased risk of acute air leak syndrome (48). In addition, prenatal infections are associated with increased elastolytic damage and development of pulmonary emphysema (51). High concentrations of free elastase also have been found in infants with proven bacterial colonization of airway secretions (52). These inconsistencies in clinical findings and the detection of free elastase at various time points during the evolution of RDS and BPD in the evaluated groups of patients most likely reflect differences in their disease severity and different etiologies of the inflammation process, and in the different assay procedures that have been used. There is, however, considerable evidence that free elastase within the lung, when unabated by α_1-proteinase inhibition, contributes to the development of acute and chronic lung injury.

The unopposed action of free elastase in the lungs of mechanically ventilated preterm infants may lead to elastin degradation in evolving BPD (53). Increased urinary excretion of desmosine, an elastolytic degradation product of mature cross-linked elastin, was identified in infants who had free elastase in their tracheobronchial secretions. The authors concluded that both hyperoxia and infection may place ventilated infants at risk for degradation of lung elastic fibers, and that this may lead to impaired alveolar septation. This notion is particularly noteworthy in light of reports that alveolar septation is markedly reduced in lungs of infants with severe BPD (54). Moreover, disruption of sulfated glycosaminoglycans and changes in hyaluronan deposition have been attributed to elastin degradation in both intestinal inflammation and in RDS of preterm monkeys (55,56). There seem to be at least two critical periods in which the protease–antiprotease imbalance may be detected in infants with RDS and CLD: one period immediately after birth, which possibly reflects the degree of lung injury, hyperoxia, and prenatal infection; and a later period, which is apparently associated with colonization or infection of the airways.

VI. Inflammatory Mediators and Pulmonary Infections

Recent epidemiological data support an association between chorioamnionitis, systemic infections, colonization of the airways, and the development of CLD, especially in very low birth weight infants with a history of mild or no RDS (57). In this population, persistent patency of the ductus arteriosus (PDA), usually associated with a nosocomial infection, was identified as an important predisposing factor in the pathogenesis of CLD (58,59). The same group of investigators detected increased serum concentrations of 6-ketoprostaglandin-$F_{1\alpha}$ in infants with nosocomial infections. These vasoactive mediators, which most likely are produced by inflammatory cells, may help prevent the closure of the ductus arteriosus which, in turn, may contribute to the development of CLD (60).

In a recent metanalysis, *Ureaplasma urealyticum* colonization was clearly associated with an increased risk for preterm infants to acquire CLD (61). Airway colonization with *U. urealyticum* or various bacterial microorganisms at birth was associated with a significant inflammatory response on the first day of life in infants with RDS (62). Chemotactic activity, numbers of neutrophils, and concentrations of IL-1, LTB_4, and elastase were increased in tracheobronchial secretions of colonized infants compared with noncolonized neonates. Concentrations of C5a and IL-8, however, were not different between the groups (62). These data suggest that the secretion of only some cytokines and inflammatory mediators is amplified by the presence of microorganisms or microbial products. High concentrations of IL-1 have been detected in bronchoalveolar lavage fluid obtained from infants with perinatal colonization of the airways on the first postnatal day (62). In animal studies, intratracheal instillation of endotoxin induced an intra-alveolar inflammatory response that was characterized by a sequential influx of neutrophils, monocytes, and lymphocytes. The kinetics and magnitude of this inflammatory response were reproduced by intratracheal instillation of IL-1 (63), and it was blocked by administration of an IL-1 receptor antagonist (64).

Increased concentrations of various inflammatory mediators have been detected in infants with bacterial colonization or infection of the airways (65) and in children with pneumonia (66,67). It is unclear, however, if there are differences in the profile of inflammatory mediators or in the sequence of inflammatory events between infants with colonized airways and those with proven pulmonary infection. Moreover, there is no clear evidence that a difference exists between the inflammatory reaction evoked by microbes compared with that of nonspecific stimuli, such as hyperoxia or excessive stretch in the immature lung of preterm infants. Studies are needed to examine the role of pulmonary infection in the development of CLD to help provide new insights into the pathogenesis and possible presentation of this condition.

VII. Pulmonary Protein Leaks

One of the most important pathophysiological features in RDS is increased alveolar capillary permeability (68). Preterm infants with RDS have increased concentrations of albumin in their lung secretions. At postnatal day 10–14, albumin concentrations in bronchoalveolar secretions of infants who later had CLD exceeded albumin concentrations that were measured in infants who recovered from RDS (9). This abnormal lung protein leak, which presumably reflects increased permeability of the respiratory epithelium, is pathognomonic for the early stage of CLD, and it is clearly associated with a deterioration of lung function and a worsening of the clinical situation. The possible role of increased pulmonary vascular filtration pressure in edema formation associated with CLD is discussed in Chapter 29.

During the inflammatory process, several factors may have detrimental effects on lung protein leaks: direct effects of inflammatory cells and various mediators, including oxygen metabolites and proteolytic enzymes; increased blood flow, in some cases through a patent ductus arteriosus; and respiratory tract infection (58). A variety of lipid mediators, including leukotrienes, prostacyclin, platelet-activating factor, and endothelin-1, all of which may affect the pulmonary circulation, have been detected in airway secretions of infants with BPD (20,69–71). In addition, elevated urinary levels of leukotriene E_4 have been measured in infants with CLD (72). It seems likely that TNF-α, I1-8, and other cytokines also may affect the pulmonary microcirculation by activating inflammatory cells and, thereby, releasing proteolytic enzymes (elastase, collagenase, cathepsin, and other granule constituents, such as defensins) or toxic oxygen radicals. Thus, it is likely that CLD is mediated, at least partly, by an arsenal of both cellular and humoral mediators (3). The significance of individual mediators, or of the inflammatory sequence that lead to protein leaks in the lung, has yet to be defined.

VIII. Oxygen Toxicity

The possible role of oxidative stress in the development of CLD and BPD was recently reviewed by Saugstad (73), who previously introduced the hypothesis that oxygen free radicals may play a significant role in the pathogenesis of CLD (74). These toxic oxygen radicals are either produced by neutrophils and macrophages or by the tissue-bound hypoxanthine–xanthine oxidase system, especially under hyperoxic conditions. Neutrophils, monocytes, and macrophages from preterm and newborn infants are as capable as those of adult phagocytes of generating toxic oxygen metabolites through activation of the NADPH oxidase system (O_2^-, H_2O_2, $\cdot OH$); 16,75). Furthermore, resting and stimulated alveolar macrophages of infants with BPD produce increased amounts of hydrogen peroxide (H_2O_2) when compared with cells from control infants (13). There is ample documentation that free neutrophil elastase in respiratory tract secretions may prime monocytes and macrophages for greater release of toxic oxygen radicals (76). A similar phenomenon has been observed with endothelin-1, a potent endothelium-derived vasoconstrictor peptide. Airway epithelial cells, as well as endothelial cells, synthesize and secrete endothelin-1 which, in turn, stimulates alveolar macrophages to generate greater amounts of oxygen metabolites that could contribute to pulmonary oxidative damage (71).

Several reports have emphasized the detrimental effects of toxic oxygen metabolites in causing peroxidation of lung tissue and associated development of CLD. A Finnish group of researchers convincingly demonstrated lipid peroxidation in very low-birth-weight infants by measuring the concentration of ethane and pentane in the expired air (77); considerably higher concentrations of lipid peroxidation products were detected in infants with a poor outcome, compared with measurements made in infants who had a good outcome. In addition, the same group of investigators demonstrated that infants with high expired ethane and pentane concentrations during the first week of life had an increased risk of dying or acquiring BPD (78). Direct measurements of protein carbonyl content, a marker of oxidation, in bronchoalveolar secretions revealed increased concentrations of these oxidation products in infants with RDS and in patients who later had BPD (78,79). Similar results have been obtained by investigators who have analyzed malonedialdehyde-thiobarbituric acid (MDA-TBA) as a measure of lipid peroxidation (80), and by those who have measured allantoin, a possibly stable marker of free radical generation in vivo (81). Contradictory results were recently reported by Dutch scientists, who did not detect increased plasma or erythrocyte concentrations of various markers of lipid peroxidation in preterm infants (30–35 weeks gestation) with RDS compared with control infants (82). These infants, who were relatively more mature than those who were included in other studies, would be considered as low-risk patients for subsequent development of CLD (82).

IX. Conclusions and Outlook

The studies reviewed in this chapter provide considerable evidence that development of chronic lung disease in infants is associated with release of cytokines

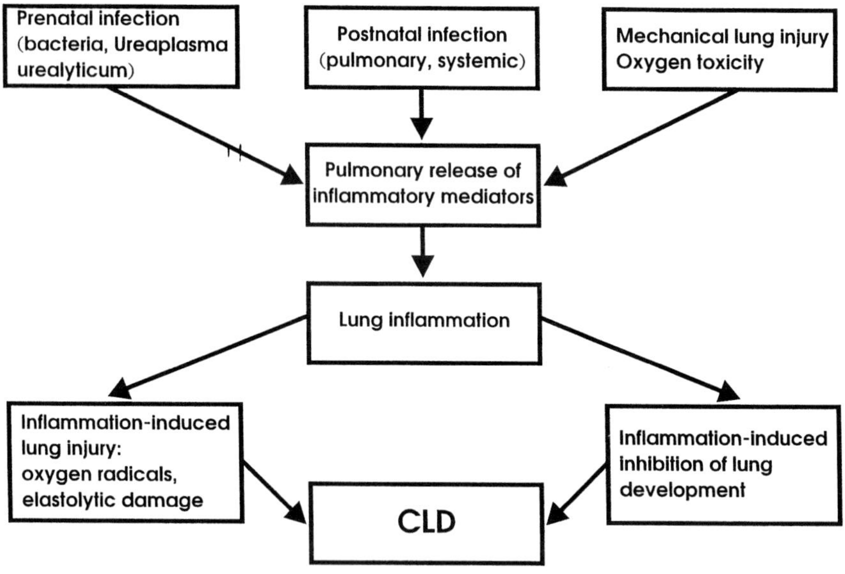

Figure 1 Possible prenatal and postnatal factors contributing to the inflammation component of chronic lung disease (CLD) of infancy.

and other inflammatory mediators within the lung. Increased concentrations of inflammatory mediators may derive from prenatal infection, local or systemic postnatal infection, or from lung injury caused by mechanical ventilation and oxygen toxicity (Fig. 1). The mechanisms by which these conditions induce release of cytokines within the lung have yet to be defined.

Pulmonary inflammation occurs during a stage of incomplete lung development. Little is known about the progression from inflammation to pulmonary fibrosis and, moreover, about the adverse effect of the inflammatory process on alveolar formation in early CLD. Knowledge is lacking on how pulmonary inflammation may interfere with postnatal lung development in extremely immature infants. Studies using transgenic mice have provided some insight on the regulation of lung development by autocrine–paracrine interactions of several polypeptide growth factors and their associated receptors (83). Effects of proinflammatory cytokines on the sequential release of growth factors and on receptor expression in the developing lung may help clarify the molecular mechanisms that lead to BPD. Knowledge of this sort is needed to help formulate strategies to prevent BPD, perhaps by inhibiting specific proinflammatory cytokines.

References

1. Groneck P, Speer CP. Inflammatory mediators and bronchopulmonary dysplasia. Arch Dis Child 1995; 73:F1–F3.
2. Pierce MR, Bancalari E. The role of inflammation in the pathogenesis of bronchopulmonary dysplasia. Pediatr Pulmonol 1995; 19:371–378.
3. Zimmermann JJ. Bronchoalveolar inflammatory pathophysiology of bronchopulmonary dysplasia. Clin Perinatol 1995; 22:429–456.
4. Kotecha S. Cytokines in chronic lung disease of prematurity. Eur J Pediatr 1996; 155 (suppl 2):S14–S17.
5. Özdemir A, Brown MA, Morgan WJ. Markers and mediators of inflammation in neonatal lung disease. Pediatr Pulmonol 1997; 23:292–306.
6. Merritt TA, Cochrane CG, Holcomb K, Bohl B, Hallman M, Strayer D, Edwards DK, Gluck L. Elastase and α_1-proteinase inhibitor activity in tracheal aspirates during respiratory distress syndrome. J Clin Invest 1983; 72:656–666.
7. Ogden BE, Murphy SA, Saunders GC, Pathak D, Johnson JD. Neonatal lung neutrophils and elastase/proteinase inhibitor imbalance. Am Rev Respir Dis 1984; 130: 817–821.
8. Arnon S, Grigg J, Silverman M. Pulmonary inflammatory cells in ventilated preterm infants: effect of surfactant treatment. Arch Dis Child 1993; 69:44–48.
9. Groneck P, Goetze-Speer B, Oppermann M, Eiffert H, Speer CP. Association of pulmonary inflammation and increased microvascular permeability during the development of bronchopulmonary dysplasia: a sequential analysis of inflammatory mediators in respiratory fluids of high risk preterm infants. Pediatrics 1994; 93:712–718.
10. Kotecha S, Chan B, Azam N, Silverman M, Shaw RJ. Increase in interleukin-8 and

soluble intercellular adhesion molecule-1 in bronchoalveolar lavage of premature infants with chronic lung disease. Arch Dis Child 1995; 72:F90–F96.
11. Jackson JC, MacKenzie AP, Chi EY, Standaert TA, Truog WE, Hodson WA. Mechanisms for reduced total lung capacity at birth and during hyaline membrane disease in premature newborn monkeys. Am Rev Respir Dis 1990; 142:413–419.
12. Rindfleisch MS, Hasday JD, Taciak V, Broderick K, Viscardi RM. Potential role of interleukin-1 in the development of bronchopulmonary dysplasia. J Interferon Cytokine Res 1996; 16:365–373.
13. Clement A, Chadelat K, Sardet A, Grimfeld A, Tournier G. Alveolar macrophage status in bronchopulmonary dysplasia. Pediatr Res 1988; 23:470–473.
14. Murch SH, Costeloe K, Klein NJ, MacDonald TT. Early production of macrophage inflammatory protein 1α occurs in respiratory distress syndrome and is associated with poor outcome. Pediatr Res 1996; 40:490–497.
15. Murch SH, Costeloe K, Klein NJ, Rees H, McIntosh N, Keeling JW, MacDonald TT. Mucosal tumor necrosis factor-α production and extensive disruption of sulfated glycosaminglycans begin within hours of birth in neonatal respiratory distress syndrome. Pediatr Res 1996; 40:484–489.
16. Speer CP, Johnston RB. Neutrophil function in newborn infants. In: Polin RA, Fox WW, eds. Fetal and Neonatal Physiology. Philadelphia: WB Saunders, 1998:1954–1960.
17. Stoll BJ, Gordon T, Korones SB, Shankaran S, Tyson JE, Bauer CR, Fanaroff AA, Lemons JA, Donovan EF, Oh W, Stevenson DK, Ehrenkranz RA, Papile LA, Verter J, Wright L. Early-onset sepsis in very low birth weight neonates: a report from the National Institute of Child Health and Human Development Neonatal Research Network. J Pediatr 1996; 129:72–80.
18. Speer CP, Gahr M, Wieland M, Eber S. Phagocytosis associated functions in neonatal macrophages. Pediatr Res 1988; 24:213–216.
19. Groneck P, Oppermann M, Speer CP. Levels of complement anaphylatoxin C5a in pulmonary effluent fluid of infants at risk for chronic lung disease and effects of dexamethasone treatment. Pediatr Res 1993; 34:586–590.
20. Stenmark KR, Eyzaguirre M, Westcott JY, Henson PM, Murphy RC. Potential role of eicosanoids and PAF in the pathophysiology of bronchopulmonary dysplasia. Am Rev Respir Dis 1987; 136:770–772.
21. Kunkel SL, Standiford T, Kasahara K, Strieter RM. Interleukin-8 (IL-8): the major neutrophil chemotactic factor in the lung. Exp Lung Res 1991; 17:17–23.
22. Little S, Dean T, Bevin S, Hall M, Ashton M, Church M, Warner J, Shute J. Role of elevated plasma soluble ICAM-1 and bronchial lavage fluid IL-8 levels as markers of chronic lung disease in premature infants. Thorax 1995; 50:1073–1079.
23. Jones CA, Cayabyab RG, Kwong KY, Stotts C, Wong B, Hamdan H, Minoo P, DeLemos RA. Undetectable interleukin (IL)-10 and persistent IL-8 expression early in hyaline membrane disease: a possible developmental basis for the predisposition to chronic lung inflammation in preterm newborns. Pediatr Res 1996; 39:966–975.
24. Munshi UK, Niu JO, Siddiq MM, Parton LA. Elevation of interleukin-8 and interleukin-6 precedes the influx of neutrophils in tracheal aspirates from preterm infants who develop bronchopulmonary dysplasia. Pediatr Pulmonol 1997; 24:331–336.
25. Takasaki J, Ogawa Y. Interleukin 8 and granulocyte elastase in the tracheobronchial

aspirate of infants without respiratory distress syndrome or intrauterine infection and development of chronic lung disease. Acta Paediatr Jpn 1997; 39:437–441.

26. Jónsson B, Tullus K, Brauner A, Lu Y, Noack G. Early increase of TNFα and IL-6 in tracheobronchial aspirate fluid indicator of subsequent chronic lung disease in preterm infants. Arch Dis Child 1997; 77:F198–F201.
27. Rocker GM. Ischaemia/reperfusion, inflammatory response and acute lung injury. Thorax 1997; 52:841–842.
28. Kojima T, Sasai M, Kobayashi Y. Increased soluble ICAM-1 in tracheal aspirates of infants with bronchopulmonary dysplasia. Lancet 1993; 342:1023–1024.
29. Ramsay PL, Hegemier SE, Welty SE. An early clinical marker for the development of bronchopulmonary dysplasia: soluble E-selectin. Pediatrics 1997; 100:(suppl)499A.
30. Murch SH, MacDonald TT, Wood CBS, Costeloe KL. Tumour necrosis in the bronchoalveolar secretions of infants with the respiratory distress syndrome and the effect of dexamethasone treatment. Thorax 1992; 47:44–47.
31. Bagchi A, Viscardi RM, Taciak V, Ensor JE, McCrea KA, Hasday JD. Increased activity of interleukin-6 but not tumor necrosis factor-α in lung lavage of premature infants is associated with the development of bronchopulmonary dysplasia. Pediatr Res 1994; 36:244–252.
32. Kotecha S, Wilson L, Wangoo A, Silverman M, Shaw RJ. Increase in interleukin (IL)-1α and IL-6 in bronchoalveolar lavage fluid obtained from infants with chronic lung disease of prematurity. Pediatr Res 1996; 40:250–256.
33. Viscardi RM, Hasday JD, Gumpper KF, Taciak V, Campbell AB, Palmer TW. Cromolyn sodium prophylaxis inhibits pulmonary proinflammatory cytokines in infants at high risk for bronchopulmonary dysplasia. Am J Respir Crit Care Med 1997; 156:1523–1529.
34. Hitti J, Krohn MA, Patton DL, Tarcy-Hornoch P, Hillier SL, Cassen EM, Eschenbach DA. Amniotic fluid tumor necrosis factor-α and the risk of respiratory distress syndrome among preterm infants. Am J Obstet Gynecol 1997; 177:50–56.
35. Eichhacker PQ, Hoffman WD, Farese A. TNF but not IL-1 in dogs causes lethal lung injury and multiple organ dysfunction similar to human sepsis. J Appl Physiol 1991; 71:1979–1989.
36. Leff JA, Baer JW, Bodman ME, Kirkman JM, Shanley PF, Patton LM, Beehler CJ, McCord JM, Repine JE. Interleukin-1-induced lung neutrophil accumulation and oxygen metabolite-mediated lung leak in rats. Am J Physiol 1994; 266:L2–L8.
37. Narimanbekov IO, Rozyiki HL. Effect of IL-1 blockade on inflammatory manifestations of acute ventilator-induced lung injury in a rabbit model. Exp Lung Res 1995; 21:239–254.
38. LoMonaco MB, Barber CM, Sinkin RA. Differential cytokine mRNA expression by neonatal pulmonary cells. Pediatr Res 1996; 39:248–251.
39. Watterberg KL, Scott SM. Evidence of early adrenal insufficiency in babies who develop bronchopulmonary dysplasia. Pediatrics 1995; 95:120–125.
40. Watterberg KL, Scott SM. Lower serum cortisol correlates with increased protein leak and evidence of inflammation in tracheal lavage fluid in very low birth weight infants. Pediatrics 1997; 100 (suppl):495A.
41. Klein NJ, Shennan GI, Heyderman RS, Levin M. Alteration in glycosaminoglycan

metabolism and surface charge on human umbilical vein endothelial cells induced by cytokines, endotoxin and neutrophils. J Cell Sci 1992; 102:821–832.
42. Speer CP, Ninjo O, Gahr M. Elastase-alpha-1-proteinase inhibitor in early diagnosis of neonatal septicemia. J Pediatr 1986; 108:987–990.
43. Gerdes JS, Harris MC, Polin RA. Effects of dexamethasone and indomethacin on elastase, α_1-proteinase inhibitor, and fibronectin in bronchoalveolar lavage fluid from neonates. J Pediatr 1988; 113:732–737.
44. Yoder MC, Chua R, Tepper R. Effect of dexamethasone on pulmonary inflammation and pulmonary function of ventilator-dependent infants with bronchopulmonary dysplasia. Am Rev Respir Dis 1991; 143:1044–1048.
45. Ohlsson K. Sveger T, Svenningsen N. Protease inhibitors in bronchoalveolar lavage fluid from neonates with special references to secretory leukocyte protease inhibitor. Acta Paediatr 1992; 81:757–759.
46. Merritt TA, Stuard ID, Puccia J, Edwards DK, Finkelstein J, Shapiro DL. Newborn tracheal aspirate cytology: classification during respiratory distress syndrome and bronchopulmonary dysplasia. J Pediatr 1986; 98:949–956.
47. Watterberg KL, Carmichael DF, Gerdes JS, Werner S, Backstrom C, Murphy S. Secretory leukocyte protease inhibitor and lung inflammation in developing bronchopulmonary dysplasia. J Pediatr 1994; 125:264–269.
48. Speer CP, Reuss D, Harms K, Herting E. Gefeller O. Neutrophil elastase and acute pulmonary damage in infants with severe respiratory distress syndrome. Pediatrics 1993; 91:794–799.
49. Tegtmeyer FK, Moller J, Richter A, Wilken B, Fischer T. Plasma concentration of elastase–α_1-proteinase inhibitor complex in surfactant-treated preterm neonates with respiratory distress syndrome. Eur Respir J 1994; 7:260–264.
50. Sluis KB, Darlow BA, Vissers MC, Winterburn CC. Proteinase–antiproteinase balance in tracheal aspirates from neonates. Eur Respir J 1994; 7:251–259.
51. Fujimura M, Kitajima H, Nakayama M. Increased leucocyte elastase of the tracheal aspirate at birth and neonatal pulmonary emphysema. Pediatrics 1993; 92:564–569.
52. Walti H, Tordet C, Gerbaut L, Saugier P, Moriette G, Relier JP. Persistent elastase/proteinase inhibitor imbalance during prolonged ventilation of infants with bronchopulmonary dysplasia: evidence for the role of nosocomial infections. Pediatr Res 1989; 26:351–355.
53. Bruce MC, Wedig KE, Jentoft N, Martin RJ, Cheng PW, Boat TF, Fanaroff AA. Altered urinary excretion of elastin cross-links in premature infants who develop bronchopulmonary dysplasia. Am Rev Respir Dis 1985; 131:568–572.
54. Margraf LR, Tomashefiski JF Jr, Bruce MC, Dahms BB. Morphometric analysis of the lung in BPD. Am Rev Respir Dis 1991; 143:391–400.
55. Murch SH, MacDonald TT, Walker-Smith JA, Levin M, Lionetti P, Klein NJ. Disruption of sulphated glycosaminoglycans in intestinal inflammation. Lancet 1993; 341:711–714.
56. Juul SE, Kinsella MG, Jackson JC, Truog WE, Standaert TA, Hodson WA. Changes in hyaluronan deposition during early respiratory distress syndrome in premature monkeys. Pediatr Res 1994; 35:238–243.
57. Watterberg KL, Demers LM, Scott SM, Murphy S. Chorioamnionitis and early lung

inflammation in infants in whom bronchopulmonary dysplasia develops. Pediatrics 1996; 97:210–215.
58. Rojas MA, Gonzalez A, Bancalari E, Claure N, Poole C, Silva-Neto G. Changing trends in the edpidemiology and pathogenesis of neonatal chronic lung disease. J Pediatr 1995; 126:605–610.
59. Cordero L, Ayers LW, Davis K. Neonatal airway colonization with gram-negative bacilli: association with severity of bronchopulmonary dysplasia. Pediatr Infect Dis J 1997; 16:18–23.
60. Gonzales A, Sosenko IRS, Chandar J, Hummler H, Claure N, Bancalari E. Influence of infection on patent ductus arteriosus and chronic lung disease in premature infants weighing 1000 grams or less. J Pediatr 1996; 128:470–478.
61. Wang EEL, Matlow AG, Ohlsson A, Nelson SC. *Ureaplasma urealyticum* infections in the perinatal period. Clin Perinatol 1997; 24:91–105.
62. Groneck P, Götze-Speer B, Speer CP. Inflammatory bronchopulmonary response of preterm infants with microbial colonisation of the airways at birth. Arch Dis Child 1996; 74:F51–F55.
63. Ulich TR, Watson LR, Yin S, et al. The intratracheal administration of endotoxin and cytokines. I. Characterisation of LPS-induces IL-1 and TNF mRNA expression and the LPS-, IL-1-, and TNF induced inflammatory exudate. Am J Pathol 1991; 138:1485–1496.
64. Ulich TR, Yin S, Guo K, delCastillo J, Eisenberg SP, Thompson RC. The intratracheal administration of endotoxin and cytokines. III: The interleukin-1 receptor antagonist inhibits endotoxin- and IL-1 induced acute inflammation. Am J Pathol 1991; 138:521–524.
65. Grigg J, Barber A, Silverman M. Increased levels of bronchoalveolar fluid interleukin-6 in preterm ventilated infants after prolonged rupture of membranes. Am Rev Respir Dis 1992; 145:782–786.
66. Willmot RW, Kassab JT, Kilian PL, Benjamin WR, Douglas SD, Wood RE. Increased levels of interleukin-1 in bronchoalveolar washings from children with bacterial pulmonary infections. Am Rev Respir Dis 1990; 142:365–368.
67. Buck C, Gallati H, Pohlandt F, Bartmann P. Increased levels of tumor necrosis factor alpha (TNF-alpha) and interleukin 1 beta (IL-1 beta) in tracheal aspirates of newborns with pneumonia. Infection 1994; 22:238–241.
68. Jefferies AL, Coates G, O'Brodovich H. Pulmonary epithelial permeability in hyaline-membrane disease. N Engl J Med 1984; 311:1075–1080.
69. Mirro R, Armstead W, Leffler C. Increased airway leukotriene levels in infants with severe bronchopulmonary dysplasia. Am J Dis Child 1990; 144:160–161.
70. Gaylord MS, Smith ZL, Lorch V, Blank ML, Snyder H. Altered platelet-activating factor levels and acetylhydrolase activities are associated with increasing severity of bronchopulmonary dysplasia. Am J Med Sci 1996; 312:149–154.
71. Kojima T, Hattori K, Hirata Y, Aoki T, Sasai-Takedatsu M, Kino M, Kobyashi Y. Endothelin-1 has a priming effect on production of superoxide anion by alveolar macrophages: its possible correlation with bronchopulmonary dysplasia. Pediatr Res 1996; 39:112–116.
72. Davidson D, Drafta D, Wilkens BA. Elevated urinary leukotriene E_4 in chronic lung disease of extreme prematurity. Am J Respir Crit Care Med 1995; 151:841–845

73. Saugstad OD. Bronchopulmonary dysplasia and oxidative stress: are we closer to an understanding of the pathogenesis of BPD? Acta Paediatr 1997; 86:1277–1282.
74. Saugstadt OD. Oxygen radicals and pulmonary damage. Pediatr Pulmonol 1985; 1: 167–175.
75. Speer CP, Ambruso DR, Grimsley JA, Johnston RB. Oxidative metabolism in cord blood monocytes and monocyte-derived macrophages. Infect Immun 1985; 50:191–192.
76. Speer CP, Pabst M, Hedegaard HB, Rest RF, Johnston RB. Enhanced release of oxygen metabolites by monocyte-derived macrophages exposed to proteolytic enzymes: activity of neutrophil elastase and cathepsin G. J Immunol 1984; 133:2151–2156.
77. Pitkanen OM, Hallman M, Andersson SM. Correlation of free oxygen radical-induced lipid peroxidation with outcome in very low birth-weight infants. J Pediatr 1990; 116:760–764.
78. Varsila E. Pitkanen O, Hallman M, Andersson S. Immaturity-dependent free radical activity in premature infants. Pediatr Res 1994; 36:55–59.
79. Gladstone IM, Levine RL. Oxidation of proteins in neonatal lungs. Pediatrics 1994; 93:764–768.
80. Inder TE, Darlow BA, Sluis KB, Winterbourn CC, Graham P, Sanderson KJ, Taylor BJ. The correlation of elevated levels of an index of lipid peroxidation (MDA-TBA) with adverse outcome in the very low birthweight infant. Acta Paediatr 1996; 85: 1116–1122.
81. Ogihara T, Okamoto R, Kim H-S, et al. New evidence for the involvement of oxygen radicals in triggering neonatal chronic lung disease. Pediatr Res 1996; 39:117–119.
82. van Zoeren-Grobben D, Lindeman JHN, Houdkamp E, Moison RMW, Wijnen JT, Berger HM. Markers of oxidative stress and antioxidant activity in plasma and erythrocytes in neonatal respiratory distress syndrome. Acta Paediatr 1997; 86:1356–1362.
83. Whitsett JA, Zhou L. Use of transgenic mice to study autocrine–paracrine signaling in lung morphogenesis and differentiation. Clin Perinatol 1996; 23:753–769.

8

Infection in the Pathogenesis of Bronchopulmonary Dysplasia

WILLIAM E. BENITZ and ANN M. ARVIN

Stanford University School of Medicine
Stanford, California

I. Introduction

Improvements in strategies for care of preterm infants with respiratory distress over the past decade have changed the major clinical conditions associated with development of chronic pulmonary disease, as reflected by a requirement for oxygen support at 28 days of age or a gestational age of 36 weeks. Two decades ago, the factors most strongly related to development of bronchopulmonary dysplasia (BPD) were prolonged exposure to high inspired oxygen concentrations and barotrauma, as indicated by high peak inspiratory and mean airway pressures, particularly in preterm infants. As antenatal induction of lung maturation by maternal steroid therapy, reduction of supplemental oxygen, and positive-pressure ventilation requirements by surfactant replacement therapy, and refinement of conventional and high-frequency ventilation strategies to minimize barotrauma have reduced the mortality and morbidity of chronic lung disease among premature infants, pulmonary infection appears to have become a more significant contributor to the pathogenesis of chronic oxygen dependency in infancy. The goal of this chapter is to review the epidemiological and pathogenetic observations that may illuminate this relation.

II. Epidemiological Correlations

In a recent analysis, Rojas et al. found that sepsis was a significant independent risk factor for development of chronic lung disease (CLD) in preterm infants (1). Among 119 infants of birth weight 500–1000 g who survived more than 28 days and required a fraction of inspired oxygen greater than 0.25 for fewer than 3 of the first 5 days after birth, 64 were diagnosed with sepsis, documented by at least one positive blood culture in the first month after birth. Infants also had clinical signs of sepsis, such as lethargy, hypotension, poor skin perfusion, hypothermia, or apnea, and they frequently had an abnormal leukocyte count, with an increased proportion of immature granulocytes (immature/mature granulocyte ratio >0.3). Most episodes of infection were caused by *Staphylococcus epidermidis* (46%) or *Candida albicans* (32%). Forty-four infants required supplemental oxygen for at least 28 days during the first 2 months after birth, and their chest radiographs showed either persistent hazy opacification or a pattern of cyst-like lucency and density of the lungs. Chronic lung disease developed in 35 of the 64 infants with sepsis, but in only 9 of the 55 who were not infected (crude odds ratio 6.2, 95% confidence interval [CI], 2.6–14.5). In a logistic regression model that adjusted for effects of other variables, but included no interaction terms, the odds ratio for chronic lung disease was 4.4 (95% CI, 1.3–14.5) for infants with sepsis. Birth weight and patent ductus arteriosus (PDA) were also significantly associated with CLD in this study. Inclusion of these variables in a logistic regression that included interaction terms showed that the odds of CLD were markedly increased (odds ratio 48.3; 95% CI, 6.3 → 100) when sepsis occurred in concert with a patent ductus arteriosus, but neither of these diagnoses alone was significantly associated with CLD (odds ratio 1.5; 95% CI, 0.2–10.1 for sepsis alone; odds ratio 4.5; 95% CI, 0.8–24.7 for PDA alone). Although these data provide compelling evidence for an *association* between the combination of sepsis and patent ductus arteriosus and subsequent development of CLD in preterm infants, they do not establish a causal relation between infection and CLD.

Yeager et al. noted a similar relation between cytomegalovirus (CMV) infection and CLD in infants with birth weights less than 1500 g (2). Persistence of an oxygen requirement for more than 7 weeks after birth was observed in 6 of 18 CMV excretors and in 15 of 88 nonexcretors (odds ratio 2.4; 95% CI, 0.8–7.3). Infants who began to excrete CMV in their urine before 6 weeks of age were at particularly high risk, with 4 of 6 such infants requiring oxygen for more than 7 weeks, compared with only 1 of 7 with a later onset of CMV excretion ($p = 0.10$ by Fisher exact test) or to infants who did not excrete CMV ($p = 0.02$ by Fisher exact test). Sawyer et al. observed that infants with CMV infection were more likely to develop radiographic changes consistent with BPD, had a more prolonged requirement for oxygen supplementation, and remained in the hospital for longer than infants who did not have CMV infection (3). Although these data suggest a higher risk of BPD in CMV-infected infants, these authors did not describe the effects of CMV infection on the prevalence of a persistent oxygen requirement at 28 days of age or 36 weeks postconceptional age.

Among term infants, the prevalence of CLD as a sequela of bacterial pneumonia has not been well delineated. The prevalence of this complication was not described in recently published series of 74 infants with neonatal pneumonia (4) and 146 infants with group B streptococcal infection (5), for example. However, infants with severe infection appear to be at substantial risk for CLD, in that 30% of infants with sepsis who were treated with extracorporeal membrane oxygenation (ECMO) require supplemental oxygen for more than 1 month (6). In contrast, only 12% of infants treated with ECMO for other conditions had a prolonged oxygen requirement, suggesting that the inflammation associated with sepsis increased the risk of acquiring CLD. This apparent difference in risk, however, was not statistically significant ($p = 0.15$ by Fisher exact test), so these observations do not provide strong evidence of a relation between bacterial infection and BPD.

Abzug et al. reported persistence of an oxygen requirement after hospital discharge in 27% of 40 patients who had culture-proved viral pneumonia in the first 30 days after birth (7). The most commonly isolated viruses in this series were respiratory syncytial virus (RSV; 55%), enterovirus (15%), rhinovirus (15%), and parainfluenza virus (8%). Because fewer than 25% of these patients were premature, this complication rate may be higher than would be expected in the absence of infection. However, the number of these infants who had persistent oxygen requirements for more than 28 days after the onset of illness or persistent abnormalities on chest radiographs was not reported. The contribution of viral pneumonia to development of CLD in infancy, therefore, remains uncertain.

The relation between infection with *Ureaplasma urealyticum* and BPD has been more extensively studied than that for any other infection. Since the initial report of a putative association by Cassell et al. in 1988 (8), nearly two dozen additional studies of this association have been reported (9–30). From a meta-analysis of studies published through 1994, Wang et al. concluded that the relative risk of BPD was significantly greater in infants who have been colonized with *U. urealyticum* (31). Analysis of studies published since 1994 (25–30), in addition to the earlier studies included in the analysis of Wang et al., confirms that this is a statistically significant association (Mantel-Haenszel pooled odds ratio 3.5; 95% CI, 2.8–4.4). Few of these studies, however, attempted to control for covariance of *Ureaplasma* colonization with other factors that may predispose to development of BPD. With stepwise logistic regression, Sanchez and Regan developed a model incorporating birth weight, need for intubation, and *Ureaplasma* colonization that correctly predicted the presence or absence of CLD in 94% of their study sample (9), suggesting that *Ureaplasma* colonization may be a significant independent risk factor for BPD even after controlling for the effects of birth weight. These authors, however, did not explicitly describe significance testing for the regression variables. Recently, Pacifico et al. reported that a persistent oxygen requirement at 36 weeks gestation is independently associated with *Ureaplasma* colonization ($p = 0.0001$) in multivariate analysis that controlled for gestational age and the presence of a patent ductus arteriosus (30). In contrast, Payne et al. (16) and van Waarde et al. (27) have reported that *Ureaplasma* colonization is not associated with an increased risk for BPD in multivariate regressions that control for the effects of gestational age alone, or gestational age coupled with birth weight, sex, and patent ductus arteriosus. da Silva et al. demonstrated no increased risk for CLD, either at 28 days after birth or 36 weeks postconceptional age, for infants with *Ureaplasma* colonization detected either by culture or polymerase chain reaction (PCR) (29), even without multivariate regression. In their stepwise multiple logistic regression, only gestational age and bacterial colonization of the endotracheal tube were significantly associated with persistence of an oxygen requirement at 28 days after birth, and only birth weight, patent ductus arteriosus, and bacterial colonization of the endotracheal tube were significantly associated with persistence of an oxygen requirement at 36 weeks postconceptional age. Although most individual studies and metaanalyses of pooled data from multiple studies do support an association between *Ureaplasma* colonization of the respiratory tract and subsequent development of BPD in preterm infants, the implication that this association is independent of prematurity or low birth weight remains controversial.

In a premature baboon model of *Ureaplasma* infection (32), the pathological findings are characterized by a mild acute inflammation that is much less severe than that observed in human infants with this infection (33,34). The report also described a specific pattern of bronchiolitis, with epithelial ulcerations that are not seen in human infants with BPD. Although these observations confirm that *Ureaplasma* can cause respiratory infection in premature primates, it does not appear that this model reproduces the pathology of BPD. This discrepancy could be the result of species-specific differences in the inflammatory response, lack of specific maternal antibody in the experimental animals, or less pathogenicity of the organism that was used in the model. If the typical response to this infection does not include a marked neutrophilic infiltrate, as suggested by the model, subtle damage to the lungs caused by this infection would appear to contribute only modestly to the pathogenesis of BPD (32).

Whether the organism causes BPD or is simply a marker for other associated variables will be difficult to resolve until randomized, blinded clinical trials of antibiotics that effectively inhibit growth of the organism demonstrate a reduction in the prevalence of CLD. Further evaluation of the potential contributions of *U. urealyticum* to CLD in infancy will require targeted research efforts. Although the organisms can be detected in cultures of clinical specimens within 1–7 days, special laboratory methods are required, but are not widely available.

Serological methods are not useful for diagnosis because infants have transplacentally acquired IgG antibodies to *Mycoplasma hominis* and *U. urealyticum*, and the IgM response has not been characterized. Direct detection can be accomplished by antigen, DNA probe, and PCR methods, but experience with these methods for diagnosis of infection in infants is scant. In most circumstances, colonization is difficult to distinguish from infection when specimens are obtained from mucosal sites or as endotracheal aspirates. Correlations with pulmonary morbidity using these methods are likely to encounter the same obstacles that are associated with studies based on culture.

In summary, these observations suggest an association between bacterial, fungal, viral, or mycoplasmal infection and subsequent CLD, but the data are not conclusive and no causal relation has been established. Until better epidemiological correlations become available, evaluation of the role of infection in the pathogenesis of BPD will depend on elucidation of the mechanisms by which infections elicit inflammation and the relation between inflammatory processes and development of BPD.

III. Pathogenetic Mechanisms

The cascade of cytokine release, white cell activation, oxygen radical production, and proteolytic enzyme activity may lead to injury to the epithelium and matrix, disordered healing, and abnormal progression of parenchymal growth and differentiation (35). Because microorganisms may initiate this inflammatory cascade, pathogenesis of BPD following pulmonary infections may not be fundamentally different from that which is associated with pulmonary immaturity. As examples of this process, the inflammatory responses to infection with group B streptococci or RSV are summarized in the following.

Animal models of group B β-hemolytic streptococcal (GBS) sepsis have permitted identification of two phases of this disease (36). The initial phase is characterized by hypoxemia, pulmonary hypertension, and reduced cardiac output associated with increased plasma concentrations of thromboxane B_2, presumably reflecting increased release of the potent vasoconstrictor thromboxane A_2 (36,37). This phase is followed by a further decline in cardiac output, systemic hypotension, increased pulmonary vascular permeability, neutropenia, pulmonary sequestration of neutrophils, associated with increased levels of thromboxane B_2, 6-ketoprostaglandin $F_{2\alpha}$, and tumor necrosis factor-alpha (TNF-α) (36–38). Oxygen radical production is essential for killing group B streptococci, which predominantly localize in the lung (39). Scavengers for hydroxyl free radicals ameliorate the pulmonary edema, pulmonary hypertension, and hypoxemia induced by group B streptococci, suggesting that production of these radicals is also an important component of the pathogenesis of respiratory failure (40). Oxidant injury from release of free radicals, therefore, is a likely consequence of GBS sepsis and pneumonia.

A consideration of how RSV infection may lead to chronic lung disease illustrates the complexity of the research that is required to elucidate such basic pathogenic mechanisms. Taking just a few examples from the extensive literature, it is apparent that the inflammatory response is as important as the lysis and destruction of respiratory tract cells that is caused directly by virus infection of these cells. In vitro experiments demonstrate that RSV induces release of proinflammatory cytokines, such as interleukin-8 (IL-8), by human peripheral blood mononuclear cells; these effects are observed in early phase after exposure to the virus, and occur with minimal or no virus replication (41). In addition, RSV infection induces secretion of IL-6 and IL-8 by pulmonary epithelial cells (42). The pathway for these effects must be defined through mechanisms of basic cell biology. For example, induction of IL-11 in pulmonary epithelial cells requires infectious RSV and occurs through activation of NF-κB by the virus (43). The broad, interactive connections that culminate in the inflammatory effects of RSV are also evident from experiments showing that RSV elicits production of RANTES by respiratory epithelial cells production, which then mediates the activation of eosinophils and basophils (44). RSV infection of alveolar macrophages induces production of IL-10, which has the capacity to inhibit the induction of virus-specific T-cell immune responses and delay the clearance of virus from lung sites (45). Current evidence links the pathogenicity of RSV to its capacity to favor induction of Th2 rather than Th1 responses (46,47). The effort to understand the connection between RSV and lung disease also requires analysis of the viral gene products and identification of virulence genes. For RSV and other respiratory pathogens, such as influenza A and B, virus strains that have been cold-adapted have decreased infectivity for lower respiratory tract. This phenotype for RSV has now been traced to mutations in the fusion and L proteins. The change in lung pathogenicity is related to differences in four nucleotides within the viral genome (48). These subtle sequence differences can be considered essential for the virus to cause acute lung disease and induce the cascade of proinflammatory and virus-specific, immune-mediated responses that result in chronic lung damage. To date, most of the analysis of the basic pathways that are involved depends on in vitro and animal model experiments. In some reports, these observations are being extended to studies of infants with RSV disease, as illustrated by the report that macrophages obtained by bronchoalveolar lavage (BAL) contain infectious virus and that TNF and IL-1 expression is detected (49).

Recent investigations have demonstrated that levels of inflammatory mediators, including IL-6 (50), complement component C5-derived anaphylotoxin (51), leukotriene B_4 (51), and IL-8 (50,51), are elevated in tracheal fluids early in the course of infants who are destined to acquire BPD. Neutrophil chemoattractants and a large number of neutrophils also appear in the airways of infants who acquire BPD (35). The mechanisms by which neutrophil activation, cytokine release, and oxidant radicals may contribute to development of BPD are reviewed in detail elsewhere in this volume. There is no reason to expect that the consequences of activation of the inflammatory cascade are dependent on the nature of the inflammatory stimulus. In addition to these direct effects of infection, the hypoxemia, pulmonary edema, pulmonary hypertension, and systemic hypotension that characterize these illnesses typically evoke an aggressive therapeutic response, including administration of oxygen in high concentrations, assisted ventilation at high inspiratory and mean airway pressures, and often large tidal volumes. Adverse effects of these interventions on immature lungs can be anticipated whether respiratory insufficiency is caused by infection or by immaturity.

References

1. Rojas MA, Gonzalez A, Bancalari E, Claure N, Poole C, Silva-Neto G. Changing trends in the epidemiology and pathogenesis of neonatal chronic lung disease. J Pediatr 1995; 126:605–610.
2. Yeager AS, Palumbo PE, Malachowski N, Ariagno RL, Stevenson DK. Sequelae of maternally derived cytomegalovirus infections in premature infants. J Pediatr 1983; 102:918–922.
3. Sawyer MH, Edwards DK, Spector SA. Cytomegalovirus infection and bronchopulmonary dysplasia in premature infants. Am J Dis Child 1987; 141:303–305.
4. Webber S, Wilkinson AR, Lindsell D, Hope PL, Dobson SR, Isaacs D. Neonatal pneumonia. Arch Dis Child 1990; 65:207–211.
5. Yagupsky P, Menegus MA, Powell KR. The changing spectrum of group B streptococcal disease in infants: an eleven-year experience in a tertiary care hospital. Pediatr Infect Dis J 1991; 10:801–808.
6. McCune S, Short BL, Miller MK, Lotze A, Anderson KD. Extracorporeal membrane oxygenation therapy in neonates with septic shock. J Pediatr Surg 1990; 25:479–482.
7. Abzug MJ, Beam AC, Gyorkos EA, Levin MJ. Viral pneumonia in the first month of life. Pediatr Infect Dis J 1990; 9:881–885.
8. Cassell GH, Waites KB, Crouse DT, et al. Association of *Ureaplasma urealyticum* infection of the lower respiratory tract with chronic lung disease and death in very-low-birth-weight infants. Lancet 1988; 2:240–245.
9. Sanchez PJ, Regan JA. *Ureaplasma urealyticum* colonization and chronic lung disease in low birth weight infants. Pediatr Infect Dis J 1988; 7:542–546.
10. Wang EE, Frayha H, Watts J, et al. Role of *Ureaplasma urealyticum* and other pathogens in the development of chronic lung disease of prematurity. Pediatr Infect Dis J 1988; 7:547–551.
11. Witman MN, Johnson GM, Holman M, Scorza WE. Pulmonary effects of the genital mycoplasmas in extremely low birth weight infants [abstr]. 1991.
12. Izraeli S, Samra Z, Sirota L, Merlob P, Davidson S. Genital mycoplasmas in preterm infants: prevalence and clinical significance. Eur J Pediatr 1991; 150:804–807.

13. Horowitz S, Landau D, Shinwell ES, Zmora E, Dagan R. Respiratory tract colonization with *Ureaplasma urealyticum* and bronchopulmonary dysplasia in neonates in southern Israel. Pediatr Infect Dis J 1992; 11:847–851.
14. Abele-Horn M, Hentschel J. [*Ureaplasma urealyticum* in newborn and premature infants. Its association with bronchopulmonary dysplasia]. Dtsch Med Wochenschr 1992; 117:408–414.
15. Sanchez PJ, Hall M, Diaz N, Defazio P. *Ureaplasma urealyticum* (Uu) and chronic lung disease (CLD) in premature infants [abstr]. Pediatr Res 1992; 29:336A.
16. Payne NR, Steinberg SS, Ackerman P, et al. New prospective studies of the association of *Ureaplasma urealyticum* colonization and chronic lung disease. Clin Infect Dis 1993; 17 (suppl 1):S117–S121.
17. Dyke MP, Grauaug A, Kohan R, Ott K, Andrews R. *Ureaplasma urealyticum* in a neonatal intensive care population. J Paediatr Child Health 1993; 29:295–297.
18. Valencia GB, Banzon F, Cummings M, McCormack WM, Glass L, Hammerschlag MR. *Mycoplasma hominis* and *Ureaplasma urealyticum* in neonates with suspected infection. Pediatr Infect Dis J 1993; 12:571–573.
19. Saxen H, Hakkarainen K, Pohjavuori M, Miettinen A. Chronic lung disease of preterm infants in Finland is not associated with *Ureaplasma urealyticum* colonization. Acta Paediatr 1993; 82:198–201.
20. Smyth AR, Shaw NJ, Pratt BC, Weindling AM. *Ureaplasma urealyticum* and chronic lung disease. Eur J Pediatr 1993; 152:931–932.
21. Heggie AD, Jacobs MR, Butler VT, Baley JE, Boxerbaum B. Frequency and significance of isolation of *Ureaplasma urealyticum* and *Mycoplasma hominis* from cerebrospinal fluid and tracheal aspirate specimens from low birth weight infants. J Pediatr 1994; 124:956–961.
22. Jonsson B, Karell AC, Ringertz S, Rylander M, Faxelius G. Neonatal *Ureaplasma urealyticum* colonization and chronic lung disease. Acta Paediatr 1994; 83:927–930.
23. Cordero L, Coley BD, Miller RL, Mueller CF. Bacterial and *Ureaplasma* colonization of the airway: radiologic findings in infants with bronchopulmonary dysplasia. J Perinatol 1997; 17:428–433.
24. Photopoulos S, Fanariotis D, Anatolitou F, et al. Colonization of neonates in intensive care with genital mycoplasmas [abstr]. Pediatr Res 1994; 36:60A.
25. Alfa MJ, Embree JE, Degagne P, et al. Transmission of *Ureaplasma urealyticum* from mothers to full and preterm infants. Pediatr Infect Dis J 1995; 14:341–345.
26. Garland SM, Bowman ED. Role of *Ureaplasma urealyticum* and *Chlamydia trachomatis* in lung disease in low birth weight infants. Pathology 1996; 28:266–269.
27. van Waarde WM, Brus F, Okken A, Kimpen JL. *Ureaplasma urealyticum* colonization, prematurity and bronchopulmonary dysplasia. Eur Respir J 1997; 10:886–890.
28. Abele-Horn M, Peters J, Genzel-Boroviczeny O, Wolff C, Zimmermann A, Gottschling W. Vaginal *Ureaplasma urealyticum* colonization: influence on pregnancy outcome and neonatal morbidity. Infection 1997; 25:286–291.
29. Da Silva O, Gregson D, Hammerberg O. Role of *Ureaplasma urealyticum* and *Chlamydia trachomatis* in development of bronchopulmonary dysplasia in very low birth weight infants. Pediatr Infect Dis J 1997; 16:364–369.
30. Pacifico L, Panero A, Roggini M, Rossi N, Bucci G, Chiesa C. *Ureaplasma urealyti-*

cum and pulmonary outcome in a neonatal intensive care population. Pediatr Infect Dis J 1997; 16:579–586.
31. Wang EE, Ohlsson A, Kellner JD. Association of *Ureaplasma urealyticum* colonization with chronic lung disease of prematurity: results of a metaanalysis. J Pediatr 1995; 127:640–644.
32. Walsh WF, Butler J, Coalson J, Hensley D, Cassell GH, deLemos RA. A primate model of *Ureaplasma urealyticum* infection in the premature infant with hyaline membrane disease. Clin Infect Dis 1993; 17 (suppl 1):S158–S162.
33. Quinn PA, Gillan JE, Markestad T, et al. Intrauterine infection with *Ureaplasma urealyticum* as a cause of fatal neonatal pneumonia. Pediatr Infect Dis 1985; 4:538–543.
34. Waites KB, Crouse DT, Philips JBD, Canupp KC, Cassell GH. Ureaplasmal pneumonia and sepsis associated with persistent pulmonary hypertension of the newborn. Pediatrics 1989; 83:79–85.
35. Pierce MR, Bancalari E. The role of inflammation in the pathogenesis of bronchopulmonary dysplasia. Pediatr Pulmonol 1995; 19:371–378.
36. Rojas J, Larsson LE, Hellerqvist CG, Brigham KL, Gray ME, Stahlman MT. Pulmonary hemodynamic and ultrastructural changes associated with group B streptococcal toxemia in adult sheep and newborn lambs. Pediatr Res 1983; 17:1002–1008.
37. Rojas J, Larsson LE, Ogletree ML, Brigham KL, Stahlman MT. Effects of cyclooxygenase inhibition on the response to group B streptococcal toxin in sheep. Pediatr Res 1983; 17:107–110.
38. Gibson RL, Redding GJ, Henderson WR, Truog WE. Group B *Streptococcus* induces tumor necrosis factor in neonatal piglets. Effect of the tumor necrosis factor inhibitor pentoxifylline on hemodynamics and gas exchange. Am Rev Respir Dis 1991; 143: 598–604.
39. Bowdy BD, Marple SL, Pauly TH, Coonrod JD, Gillespie MN. Oxygen radical-dependent bacterial killing and pulmonary hypertension in piglets infected with group B streptococci. Am Rev Respir Dis 1990; 141:648–653.
40. Pauly TH, Bowdy BD, Haven CA, Barr SB, Gillespie MN. Evidence for hydroxyl radical involvement in group B *Streptococcus*-induced pulmonary hypertension and arterial hypoxemia in young piglets. Pediatr Res 1988; 24:735–739.
41. Arnold R, Konig B, Galatti H, Werchau H, Konig W. Cytokine (IL-8, IL-6, TNF-alpha) and soluble TNF receptor-I release from human peripheral blood mononuclear cells after respiratory syncytial virus infection. Immunology 1995; 85:364–372.
42. Arnold R, Humbert B, Werchau H, Gallati H, Konig W. Interleukin-8, interleukin-6, and soluble tumour necrosis factor receptor type I release from a human pulmonary epithelial cell line (A549) exposed to respiratory syncytial virus. Immunology 1994; 82:126–133.
43. Bitko V, Velazquez A, Yang L, Yang YC, Barik S. Transcriptional induction of multiple cytokines by human respiratory syncytial virus requires activation of NF-kappa B and is inhibited by sodium salicylate and aspirin. Virology 1997; 232:369–378.
44. Saito T, Deskin RW, Casola A, et al. Respiratory syncytial virus induces selective production of the chemokine RANTES by upper airway epithelial cells. J Infect Dis 1997; 175:497–504.

45. Panuska JR, Merolla R, Rebert NA, et al. Respiratory syncytial virus induces interleukin-10 by human alveolar macrophages. Suppression of early cytokine production and implications for incomplete immunity. J Clin Invest 1995; 96:2445–2453.
46. Graham B. Immunological determinants of disease caused by respiratory syncytial virus. Trends Microbiol 1996; 4:290–293.
47. Hussell T, Spender LC, Georgiou A, O'Garra A, Openshaw PJ. Th 1 and Th 2 cytokine induction in pulmonary T cells during infection with respiratory syncytial virus. J Gen Virol 1996; 77:2447–2455.
48. Connors M, Crowe J, Firestone C, Murphy B, Collins P. A cold-passaged, attenuated strain of human respiratory syncytial virus contains mutations in the F and L genes. Virology 1995; 208:478–484.
49. Midulla F, Villani A, Panuska JR, et al. Respiratory syncytial virus lung infection in infants: immunoregulatory role of infected alveolar macrophages. J Infect Dis 1993; 168:1515–1519.
50. Munshi UK, Niu JO, Siddiq MM, Parton LA. Elevation of interleukin-8 and interleukin-6 precedes the influx of neutrophils in tracheal aspirates from preterm infants who develop bronchopulmonary dysplasia. Pediatr Pulmonol 1997; 24:331–336.
51. Groneck P, Gotze-Speer B, Oppermann M, Eiffert H, Speer CP. Association of pulmonary inflammation and increased microvascular permeability during the development of bronchopulmonary dysplasia: a sequential analysis of inflammatory mediators in respiratory fluids of high-risk preterm neonates. Pediatrics 1994; 93:712–718.

9

Ventilation Strategies and Bronchopulmonary Dysplasia

W. ALAN HODSON

University of Washington
Seattle, Washington

I. Introduction

Mechanical ventilation is considered to be one of the most important of the many putative etiologic factors in bronchopulmonary dysplasia (BPD). Is this blame justified, and if so, what is the rationale for the various ventilatory strategies that have been proposed to minimize lung injury? There has been much research, as well as speculation, on the optimal means of mechanical ventilation. The quest for a noninjurious mode of ventilatory support continues. Current innovations include permissive hypercapnia, avoidance of mechanical ventilation, ''gentler'' respirators (e.g., high-frequency oscillation), and various forms of noninvasive ventilation. Improvement in gas exchange was once the single major goal of mechanical ventilation, whether the cause of respiratory failure was neuromuscular or pulmonary. As this goal has become more easily obtainable with adjunctive treatment, such as exogenous surfactant, the focus has been on obtaining acceptable gas exchange with the least possible amount of inspired oxygen and applied pressure. Several chapters in this volume address various aspects of the causal relation of mechanical ventilation to BPD; the pathology of ''barotrauma''; the role of different mechanical ventilatory patterns; lung injury from overexpansion; and the effects of various respiratory care practices on BPD. Until there is more clear-cut evidence of a decidedly superior respirator or pattern of ventilation, various strategies will continue to be proposed and championed.

A discussion of ventilation strategies needs to include, in addition to issues of lung mechanics, the possible influence of mechanical ventilation on other cofactors of morbidity, such as oxygen injury, infection, nutrition, inflammation (cytokines), and pulmonary blood flow. In formulating an optimal strategy, many variables need to be considered, including the anatomical site within the lungs that is affected by changes in mechanical ventilation, the degree of pulmonary maturation, the use of adjunctive therapy, and the stage of disease, and the postnatal age of the baby. Ventilatory strategies may result in different effects at different sites in the lung. Will a particular strategy have an effect on the alveoli or airways, large or small airways, lobar or total lung pathophysiology? All of these variables have complicated the search for the ideal or optimal ventilatory strategy. Therefore, a vast amount of literature has resulted from this ''pick your poison'' approach. The unavailability of a satisfactory, inexpensive animal model of BPD has retarded research progress and has led to more fancy than fact. As long as the precise mechanism and site of injury resulting from intermittent positive-pressure ventilation (IPPV) is not well understood, it is difficult to devise a strategy of innocuous mechanical ventilation. Also, it is most likely that there are multiple pathways leading to lung injury. Therefore, one strategy is probably not appropriate for all situations, and no one factor can be singled out to guide a strategy for all. Assessment of individual situations, including consideration of temporal changes, is important. The degree of immaturity of the lung is probably the most important variable influencing susceptibility to injury secondary to mechanical ventilation. Even with a focus on the most immature infants, there is no single homogeneous group of babies wherein a single ventilatory strategy is suitable for all.

II. Barotrauma Versus Volutrauma

Of the many factors that may contribute to BPD, ''barotrauma'' is perceived as the major culprit. Simply put, too much pressure within the lung will result in tearing of fragile alveolar walls or disruption of terminal airway epithelium if alveoli are collapsed. Dissection of air along the terminal and small airways often leads to pneumothorax and pneumomediastinum. This dissection presumably occurs along the perivascular and peribronchial sheaths toward the hilum and toward the periphery. The physical trauma that results in stretching or tearing of tissues and disruption of epithelial layers and their basement membranes then can lead to cellular responses of repair and inflammation with release of growth factors and cytokines, thus increasing the vulnerability to oxygen toxicity. Disordered or unregulated growth may occur, as well as ischemia of some tissues from a compromised vascular supply.

Is pressure really the critical factor, or does overdistension result from excess volume, so-called volutrauma? Other abnormalities are attributed to barotrauma in addition to stretching or overdistension. These include sheer forces, fluctuating pressures resulting in repeated opening and closing of alveoli, and sustained pressure resulting in decreased venous return and cardiac output. A pressure that is too low will lead to alveolar collapse, increasing right-to-left shunt through the lungs, and worsening hypoxemia. To some, barotrauma is equated strictly with air leak syndromes. What level of distending pressure is too high? Is the end-expiratory volume the major concern or is it excessive cyclic movements? The volume versus pressure issue is a semantic one, because transpulmonary pressure, not intra-alveolar pressure, determines alveolar volume. Owing to the heterogeneity of pathological changes in the immature lung, there is a propensity for uneven gas distribution. Normal or healthy units of the lung may sustain transpulmonary pressures of 35 cmH_2O; however, this may place undue traction forces on adjacent collapsed areas of the lung, resulting in tearing. Other areas of the lung may have abnormal or immature structural support within the interstitium, such as collagen and elastin, or the elastic axial network from the hilum to the pleura has not fully developed, leading to intolerance of seemingly harmless distending pressures or volumes.

The physical forces that are applied to the lung should be referred to in more scientific terms, rather than made-up terms, such as barotrauma or volutrauma. Appropriate terms in physics include: stress, strain, and sheer stress. *Stress* is force per unit area; *strain* is change in length divided by initial length; and *sheer* stress is force per unit surface area in the direction of the prevailing flow. Boyle's law states that, for a given mass of gas, the product of its volume and pressure remains constant. As Nelson lightheartedly suggests (1), the problem is one of too much gas in the lung—''gasmasstrauma.'' How is it possible for the clinician to quantitate these specific forces acting at multiple sites in the lung? This is a difficult, if not impossible, task. Therefore, terms such as ''stretch,'' ''tear,'' or ''deformation'' have much more clinical significance and relevance. Regardless of the terms used, mechanical respirators can transmit forces related to volume and pressure to all parts of the lung. The beneficial or adverse effects of these forces are determined by several ventilator variables, such as pressure, flow, volume, and time, acting in synchrony or adversely with lung variables, such as compliance, resistance, and resulting time constants in various parts of the lung. It is a daunting task indeed, to second-guess the right balance between biology and machine under the influence of so many variables. Yet, that is the goal of optimal ventilator management; complicated further by the possibility that settings that produce optimal gas exchange may be the very ones that are inflicting lung damage. The combinations and permutations of choices of respirator settings to increase or decrease the arterial oxygen and carbon dioxide tensions are too numerous to arrive at a practical or simple algorithm. Can an appropriate strategy be devised?

III. Site of Pathology and Ventilatory Strategy

It is useful, if not necessary, to consider the potential pathology of BPD at various sites within the lung, and how mechanical ventilation might enhance or ameliorate these lesions at various anatomical locations (Fig. 1). The pathology and, therefore, the strategy, will continue to change over time in each part of the lung as recovery or worsening of the clinical situation occurs.

A. Site of Pathology

Trachea

The endotracheal tube contributes to some of the tracheal damage. Initially, there is likely to be epithelial damage from direct trauma from the endotracheal tube, with secondary epithelial dysplasia and altered mucociliary transport distal to the endotracheal tube (2–4). There may be increased pooling of secretions within the trachea owing to poor mucociliary transport and increased susceptibility to oxygen toxicity. Strategies are limited to removing the tube or developing techniques of noninvasive ventilation (e.g., nasopharyngeal synchronized mechanical ventilation).

Large Airways

The major bronchii are probably not abnormal during the early stages of mechanical ventilation in the susceptible premature infant either with or without hyaline membrane disease (HMD). Later, the large airways may suffer epithelial dysplasia, inflammation, and smooth-muscle hypertrophy. Because cartilage development is incomplete, large airways may collapse or close temporarily. It is hypothesized that large airway collapse is responsible for recurrent episodes of transient hypoxemia commonly seen in respirator-dependent infants who usually weigh less than 800 g at birth (5). Maintaining a constant minimum airway pressure throughout the respiratory cycle may help prevent airway closure. The presence of the endotracheal tube in combination with assisted ventilation often results in disorganization and damage to the ciliated epithelium distal to the endotracheal tube (6,7). Possible injurious factors include jets of gas, desiccation from inspired gas, and oxygen toxicity. Ciliary defects associated with BPD have been described, and ciliated cells appear to detach more easily than goblet cells (8), resulting in subsequent impairment of mucociliary transport (9).

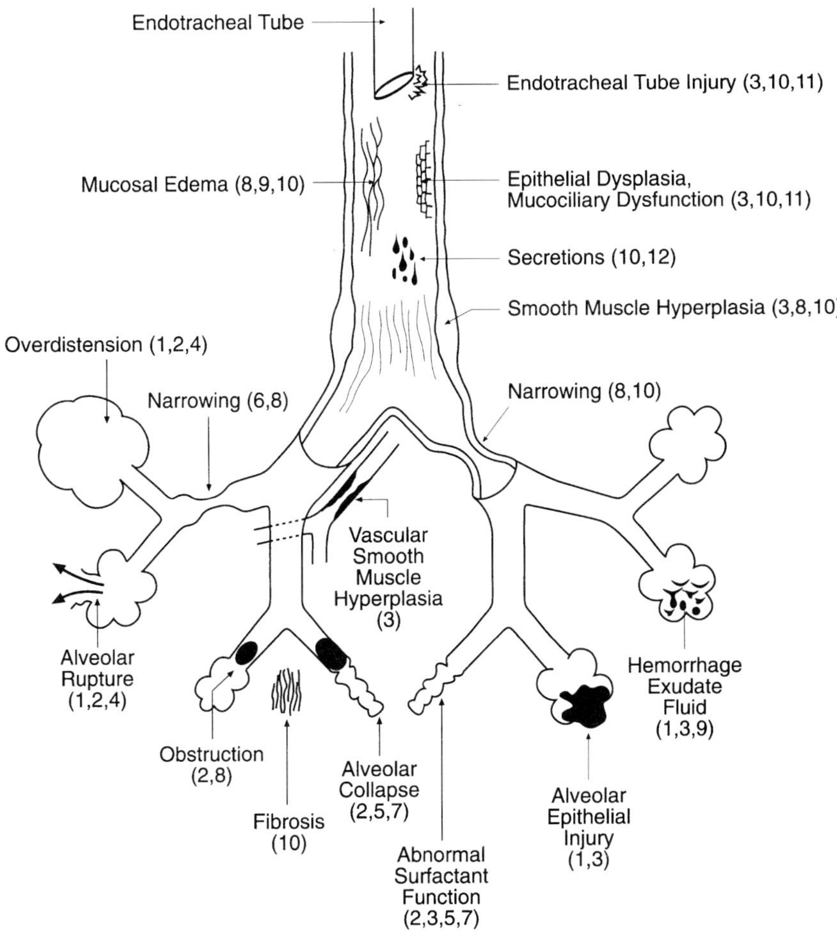

Strategies:

1. Minimize PIP	5. Increase MAP	9. Diuretics
2. Optimal PEEP	6. Decrease rate	10. Corticosteroids
3. Minimize F_iO_2	7. Surfactant admin.	11. Extubate
4. Decrease MAP	8. Bronchodilators	12. Suction

Figure 1 Ventilatory strategies and lung injury.

Small Airways

Resistance to inflation of collapsed alveoli can lead to overdistension and damage of respiratory bronchioles. Coalson et al. (10) have described pathological abnormalities in 10–25% of airways in their hyperoxia-induced baboon model of BPD. There is primary damage to bronchiolar ciliary function and mucous membranes, resulting in severe bronchiolitis and alveolar fibrosis (7). There is secondary regeneration and hyperplasia of bronchiolar airway epithelium after 5–15 days (11) and extensive evidence for the toxic effects of oxygen on small airways (12,13). Epithelial dysplasia, poor mucociliary clearance, and abnormalities of the Clara cells probably result in extreme narrowing of the most peripheral airways, sometimes with complete airway obstruction. Smooth-muscle hyperplasia occurs in airways larger than 1500 mm in circumference, making it possible for BPD infants to have bronchospasm early in the course of their illness (14).

Alveoli

Alveolar damage in HMD is well described (15). The progression of this alveolar damage during early and late stages of BPD is less clear. This is due to a lack of animal models of BPD other than the subhuman primate. In the baboon model of BPD, Coalson et al. (16) have described distended alveolar ducts and diffuse alveolar damage. This injury is attributed to a combination of mechanical ventilation and oxygen toxicity. Early pathology in the monkey model of HMD indicates extensive alveolar damage, including epithelial necrosis, denudation of basement membranes, endothelial damage, and filling of alveoli with fluid and debris (15). These effects occur within a few hours of birth and are probably not attributable to oxygen toxicity, but more likely are due to mechanical injury to primitive alveoli and alveolar ducts, as well as terminal bronchioles. Injury of the respiratory bronchioles from sheer forces and overdistension secondary to collapsed alveoli has been described by Nilson et al. (17).

Interstitium

Lung pathology of human infants who have died with BPD demonstrates marked changes within the interstitium, including distension, increased numbers of inflammatory cells, thickening of the interstitium with disrupted collagen and elastin formation, and an increased number of fibroblasts, leading to fibrosis after approximately 2 months of age (18). Animal models of BPD and HMD indicate an increased amount of interstitial fluid and some interstitial hemorrhage, as well as disordered elastin deposition (19).

Vascular Injury

Postmortem studies of human infants with BPD demonstrate vascular smooth-muscle hyperplasia (20,21). During the first few weeks of life there is abnormal persistence of the fetal state, followed by an abnormal muscularization of peripheral arteries. Both overexpansion of alveoli and oxygen toxicity increase lung microvascular permeability, with interstitial protein leak and edema (22–25). Alveolar cell damage may disrupt regulation of vascular growth. Messenger RNA and protein for vascular endothelial growth factor (VEGF) are decreased by alveolar epithelial cell injury (26), with the potential for impaired postnatal microvascular development. An increase in pulmonary vascular resistance and altered pulmonary blood flow can result. These abnormalities are important considerations, as too little or too much oxygen can aggravate the vascular injury. It is relevant to balance mechanical respirator variables with oxygen administration.

B. Modes of Ventilation

Ventilator Variables

There are many commercially available mechanical ventilators that are suitable for neonates, including the extremely low birth weight infant. All of these devices apply positive pressure at the proximal airway. The few devices that employ negative extrathoracic pressure have been applied without success, primarily because of technical difficulties in application to infants who weigh less than 1000 g. Positive-pressure devices permit time cycling, flow regulation, pressure limitation, and synchronized assistance to spontaneous respiration (Table 1).

A brief summary of these variables and alternate modes of ventilation is examined here, as well as the ventilatory strategies that have evolved from attempts to minimize the putative effects of each of them to the pathogenesis of BPD.

Peak Inspiratory Pressure

The peak inspiratory pressure (PIP) is the major determinant of how much pressure and gas volume reach the distal parts of the lung. Positive-pressure ventila-

Table 1 Respirator Variables

Peak inspiratory pressure (PIP; cmH_2O)
Positive end-expiratory pressure (PEEP; cmH_2O)
Mean airway pressure (MAP; cmH_2O)
Frequency or rate per minute (f)
Inspiratory time (T_I; sec)
Expiratory time (T_E; sec)
Inspiratory/expiratory ratio (I/E)
Inflation volume (V; mL)
Flow rate ($\dot{V}$; L/min)

tors are designed to discontinue inspiratory flow once a predetermined pressure has been reached. This pressure is usually sensed at the proximal end of the endotracheal tube. A normal, excised lung brought to airlessness will usually require 30–35 cmH_2O to achieve maximum inflation, with opening of alveoli from the collapsed state occurring between 9 and 12 cmH_2O pressure (27). The *inflection point* is defined as the point on the pressure–volume curve at which there is an increase in the slope of the inflation curve associated with the opening of most alveoli. The inflection point and pressure–volume characteristics of the abnormal lung, as in HMD, are considerably different from the normal lung, and an inspiratory pressure sufficient to fully inflate the normal lung will result in considerably less distension of the diseased lung.

Positive End-Expiratory Pressure

The spontaneously breathing infant maintains a ''physiological'' amount of pressure within the airways at the end of expiration by closure of the larynx (28). This pressure is probably close to 2 cmH_2O. Hence, ''grunting'' sounds during expiration in infants with HMD reflect an effort by the infant to increase end-expiratory pressure by retarding or braking expiratory flow with early narrowing or closure of the larynx. Intubation eliminates this protective mechanism, and a constant pressure of at least 3–4 cmH_2O should be maintained, except when the lung is overinflated. Without applied positive end-expiratory pressure (PEEP), alveolar pressure drops to zero, and alveolar volume falls below functional residual capacity (FRC). In abnormal lungs (e.g., with surfactant deficiency), alveoli may collapse and require a high pressure to reopen them.

Continuous Positive Airway Pressure

The application of steady pressure on the nose or nasopharynx to prevent expiratory nasal pressure from falling to zero is usually set at 4–6 cmH_2O. The rationale is the same as with PEEP (i.e., to prevent alveolar collapse). It also may prevent small airways from collapsing. Continuous positive airway pressure (CPAP) may overdistend airways, thus increasing anatomical dead space and possibly causing CO_2 retention.

Mean Airway Pressure

The mean airway pressure (MAP) is the average pressure in the lung throughout the respiratory cycle and is derived from integrating the area under the pressure curve. This integrated area will be affected by pressure-waveform, PIP, PEEP, inspiratory time, and frequency.

Rate and Inspiratory/Expiratory Ratio

The ventilatory rate influences minute ventilation and alveolar ventilation. There has been an arbitrary assignment of *rapid ventilation* as more than 60 breaths per minute, while *slow* is considered fewer than 40 breaths per minute. Inspiratory

(I) and expiratory (E) times, hence, the I/E ratio, can be adjusted on most ventilators. The time constant of the lung (compliance times resistance) is the most important physiological variable affecting distribution of applied volume and, hence, barotrauma. The *single time constant* is defined as the time required for that region of the lung to expire 63% of its tidal volume, and three times this duration is required to expire 99% of the volume. Different regions of the lung may have different time constants. The effects of changing frequency, therefore, the I/E ratio, will depend on the various time constants within different regions of the lung which, in turn, may vary with the stage of pulmonary abnormality.

IV. Modes of Conventional Ventilators

Each year more sophisticated neonatal respirators appear on the market. Many now incorporate microprocessors that permit automatic adjustment to variations in flow, volume, or pressure and allow the patient to have more autonomy (patient-triggered ventilation). Available ventilatory strategies require knowledge of the many variables that can result in markedly different respiratory patterns with possible adverse or beneficial effects on the lung. Conventional ventilators have several options.

A. Time-Cycled, Pressure-Limited Ventilators

The time-cycled, pressure-limited type is the most common neonatal ventilator in use. Pressure limitation is predetermined and the volume delivered before this pressure limit will vary depending on the set flow rate and inspiratory time (T_I). Once set, the flow rate remains constant. The pressure limitation prevents sudden changes in PIP as lung compliance changes, and tidal volume (V_T) may be suboptimal if there is a sudden decrease in lung compliance (C_L). Conversely, excess volume may result from a sudden improvement in C_L, (e.g., following surfactant administration). Alveolar ventilation and CO_2 removal are increased by an increase in PIP, respirator rate (f) and T_I. MAP is increased by increasing any one of several variables, including PIP, f, T_I, gas flow, or PEEP. If there is poor oxygenation, F_{IO_2} is increased.

Intermittent Mandatory Ventilation

The ventilator delivers a constant number of breaths per minute with a preset pressure limit. The spontaneously breathing infant may breathe at an independent rate, and at times, ventilator and infant will have opposite intentions for the direction of airflow. With constant flow ventilators, fresh gas is always available for spontaneous breaths. Occasionally, particularly in extremely small infants, the infant's spontaneous breathing may be entrained to that of the ventilator, and this usually requires a ventilatory rate of more than 40–50 breaths per minute. When spontaneous ventilatory efforts are counterproductive to intermittent mandatory ventilation (IMV), sedation or muscular paralysis is necessary if no other options are available.

Synchronized Intermittent Mandatory Ventilation

The infant's inspiratory effort triggers the onset of a mechanical breath through a pressure or flow sensor in the respirator or through impedance changes in the abdominal or chest wall as a result of movement. The machine response time is 50–60 msec, and sensitivity has been increased to detect a change in airway flow of 0.2 L/min. The infant may breathe at any frequency in synchrony with the respirator. However, a preset backup rate will ensure a minimum number of breaths per minute. The rationale is to eliminate asynchronous breaths and minimize distending pressure. Further refinements now permit partial or full support of each breath. The improvements in response times in triggering sensitivity make this machine more feasible for use with extremely small infants, although not yet failsafe. A large trial is underway in Europe to determine if patient-triggered ventilation has an effect on reducing chronic lung disease.

Pressure-Support Mode

The pressure-support mode permits the infant to receive a set pressure support for each spontaneous breath. The preset pressure (e.g., 10 cmH_2O) is sustained until the cessation of inspiratory effort, which depends on an expiratory trigger mechanism. A level of PEEP can be maintained throughout the respiratory cycle. The inspiratory flow rate can be varied to produce a square pressure wave or a more gradual, prolonged inspiratory rise.

Assist–Control Mode

In the assist–control mode, the respirator is synchronized with the infant's spontaneous breaths and provides a full assist to each spontaneous breath (pressure-regulated). If there is failure to breathe or a spontaneous effort is insufficient to trigger the respirator, a mechanical control breath is delivered. This control rate is set at a minimum frequency to ensure adequate ventilation in the event of apnea. A more complex addition to the assist–control mode is "proportional assist." Proportional assist allows different proportions of the breath to be assisted depending on the combination of the flow rate and volume delivered for that particular inspiration.

B. Time-Cycled, Volume-Regulated Ventilation

Volume-controlled respirators have been less popular for ventilating small premature infants. The newer ventilators provide a choice between pressure limitation or volume limitation modes, and at times, volume-controlled ventilation would be preferable. The volume control mode can be used in conjunction with pressure support. Pressure-regulated, volume-controlled devices (e.g., SV 300, Siemens-Elema, Solna, Sweden) permit the achievement of an adequate V_T at variably lower pressures than the maximum or "set" peak inspiratory pressure.

V. High-Frequency Ventilation

A. Rapid Conventional Ventilation

Past efforts to reduce barotrauma led to low-volume, pressure-limited ventilation at rates up to the maximal capacity of a conventional ventilator (29). Ventilatory rates varied between 60 and 160/min and required shortening of T_I to avoid air trapping. This mode is referred to as high-frequency positive-pressure ventilation (HFPPV) and has proved successful during the acute stages of HMD (30–33). However, the rapid rate can lead to gas trapping or altered mechanics if there is insufficient time for expiration (34,35). At later stages of lung disease, likely associated with unequal time constants, HFPPV may aggravate lung injury, increasing the risk of subsequent BPD. The risk of adverse effects from this pattern may be increased if there is radiologic evidence of hyperinflation or localized cystic areas in the lung.

Over the past 15 years there has been extensive interest in the use of different types of high-frequency ventilators (HFV) utilizing jet, flow interruption, or oscillation devices. Most of the initial studies were concerned with prevention or treatment of air leak syndromes or for rescue from failed conventional mechanical ventilation, including the avoidance of extracorporeal membrane oxygenation (ECMO). More recently, it has been recommended as a strategy for preventing BPD. No studies on human infants have compared the different types of HFV in a controlled trial with comparable types and stages of lung disease.

High-Frequency Jet Ventilation

Jet ventilators usually cycle at frequencies between 3 and 10 Hz (180–600 cycles/min) and require a specialized triple-lumen endotracheal tube or a specially designed endotracheal tube circuit adapter. This form of ventilation delivers a low-volume, high-velocity jet of gas and was initially proposed for use primarily in infants with air leak syndromes. There is a background of gas flow from a respirator that permits conventional tidal breathing. Again, the rationale has been the avoidance of high peak and mean airway pressures. Two controlled trials (36,37) have demonstrated efficacy of gas exchange, but neither trial demonstrated a decreased incidence of BPD. No advantages to this form of ventilation have yet been documented to recommend this as a strategy to prevent or ameliorate BPD.

Flow Interruption Devices

These devices produce a rapid interruption of gas flow that results in an inspiratory jet at frequencies of 10–15 Hz. A unique hybrid ventilator (Infrasonics, San Diego, CA) permits the infant to breathe spontaneously, and can provide high-frequency flow-interrupted ventilation during expiration, thereby combining conventional with high-frequency ventilation. This option presents more flexibility to optimize gas exchange. The strategy is to avoid high, distending pressures. No clear-cut advantage has been demonstrated for this mode of ventilation in the prevention of BPD. Adverse outcomes and poor neurological outcome in infants studied under this treatment regimen are reported (38–40).

High-Frequency Oscillatory Ventilation

Many studies have demonstrated that high-frequency oscillatory ventilation (HFOV) provides effective gas exchange in infants with severe lung disease and in various animal models of neonatal lung disease (41–47). A small tidal volume of 1–2 mL delivered at frequencies of 8–16 Hz permits a low mean airway pressure and reduces the development of air leak syndrome (48). The Sensormedics apparatus (Sensormedics, Anaheim, CA) has an active expiratory phase and the *T*I can be adjusted. Several controlled trials have been reported, the first of which was the HiFi Study (49–52). Four of these have been subjected to a metaanalysis (53). The HiFi study (49) did not demonstrate a reduced incidence of BPD. The trend from the other three studies was toward a reduced incidence of BPD at 28–30 days of age, but the difference was not statistically significant. Initial studies of this ventilation strategy did not include use of exogenous surfactant (49,50). A criticism of the HiFi study was that it may not have included sufficient PIP to cause recruitment of terminal respiratory units, thereby resulting in inadequate lung gas volume (54,55). Subsequently, other studies have employed a so-called high-volume strategy (56,57). Lung volume assessment is provided by serial chest radiographs, and mean airway pressure is increased if lung inflation appears inadequate.

B. Rationale

As HFPPV delivers exceedingly small tidal volumes, and MAP is not significantly different than it is during conventional mechanical ventilation (CMV), alveolar pressure, hence, alveolar volume changes should be minimized, thereby reducing the risk of barotrauma. With a sustained higher mean lung volume, high peak inspiratory pressures are avoidable. It is possible for the alveolar pressure to be considerably higher than the mean airway pressure, so that there is some risk of alveolar overinflation when it is not suspected (58–61). The optimal settings of frequency, MAP, and amplitude should be derived from estimating the influence of the mechanical properties of the lung. Frequency, tidal volume, and mean airway pressure strategies have been modeled by Venegas and Fredburg (62). Combinations of frequency and pressure that result in a desired peak alveolar-distending pressure may vary as a function of lung compliance. In an infant with HMD and alveolar collapse, relatively high frequencies will be required compared with what may be used to optimize respiratory gas exchange in lungs of normal infants.

The aim is to open terminal airway units as gently as possible and maintain the pressure above the closing pressure of the airspace. Elimination of CO_2 is rarely a problem, and increasing the amplitude of the oscillatory wave generally improves alveolar ventilation. Hypoxemia, mostly from intrapulmonary shunting of blood without oxygenation, should be alleviated by increasing mean airway pressure, with a resultant increase in FRC through recruitment of collapsed alveoli. It is possible, but unproved, that a constant mean airway pressure may afford benefit by maintaining patency of the smallest airways, thereby preventing alveolar collapse.

HFOV appears to be the most logical strategy for effective ventilation, while minimizing stretch injury. The evidence of its benefits as protective in decreasing the incidence or severity of BPD, however, is not compelling.

C. Possible Adverse Effects

Intracranial Hemorrhage

There was a small but significant increase in severe intracranial hemorrhage in infants on HFV that were enrolled in the HiFi study (49). A metaanalysis of nine studies (63) compared HFV with conventional ventilation to determine the risk for intracranial hemorrhage. Variables that were examined included gestational age, birth weight, surfactant administration and age of entry into each of the studies. The results of the HiFi study were excluded, and there were no significant differences in the occurrence or severity of intracranial hemorrhage. There was a wide variation in occurrence, probably owing to multiple factors in each of the studies, including changes in MAP and cardiac output. With greater use of all modes of ventilation, there has been increased attention given to possible hemodynamic changes, and the incidence of intracranial hemorrhage appears to be reduced. A study by Patel and Kline (64) that compared CMV and HFV by flow interruption showed a 50% reduction in severe intracranial hemorrhage (grade 3 or 4) with CMV, although this difference was not significant. Other studies have examined the incidence of neurological abnormalities associated with HFJV (39,40). There was an increased incidence of severe intracranial hemorrhage and periventricular leukomalacia. The latter may be related to hypocarbia, perhaps associated with low cerebral blood flow (39,65,66). The common use of surfactant therapy and antenatal corticosteroids may result in a decreased risk of intracranial hemorrhage regardless of the mode of ventilation.

Air Leaks

Analysis of published results (53) reveals a similar incidence of air leak syndrome with HFV compared with other modes of ventilation. In those studies, which also included treatment with surfactant, there was a trend toward a reduced incidence of air leak with HFOV. The use of decreased PIP should reduce the risk. However, unsuspected and inadvertent high alveolar pressure can result in gas trapping and an increased risk for pneumothorax or interstitial emphysema.

Airway Injury

Several studies have examined tracheobronchial injury following various modes of high-frequency ventilation (38,67–72). No differences were found between CMV and HFOV. However, HFJV has been associated with mucosal damage, particularly in the upper trachea. These effects may be from turbulence and sheer forces that result from the high-velocity jet of gas, especially if humidification of the gas is not adequate (38).

Hemodynamic Effects

Very few animal studies have addressed the effects of HFOV on cardiac output, venous return, pulmonary blood flow, or cerebral blood flow. Mild but constant impairment in cardiovascular function has been described in septic piglets (73). Studies on human infants suggest that left ventricular output is reduced, affecting blood pressure or heart rate when changing from conventional to HFOV (74). Comparable levels of mean airway pressure, however, were not evaluated.

VI. Strategies to Minimize Barotrauma

Now that patient variables and machine variables have been reviewed, how does one manage an optimal alignment between these two sets of variables with the goal of minimizing lung injury? How does a specific strategy affect a suspected injury at a specific site in the lung? How do the postnatal age and degree of severity of clinical illness influence strategy? The strategies that have been advocated to minimize barotrauma include: minimizing PIP, decreasing MAP, shortening T_I, reversing the I/E ratio, muscular paralysis, altering the mechanics of the lungs, as with surfactant replacement therapy, synchronizing the respirator, and changing to nonconventional ventilation. When all of these methods fail, it is unlikely that further lung injury will be prevented. However, newer strategies, such as nitric oxide inhalation, liquid ventilation, and less invasive forms of ventilation are being considered. How does one assess the appropriate PIP? How helpful are serial chest radiographs? Is permissive hypercapnia an acceptable risk? Other nonrespirator strategies need to be considered, such as inflammatory agents, corticosteroids, diuretics, bronchodilators, sedatives, analgesics, and ways to minimize oxidant injury to the lung. If both oxygen toxicity and barotrauma are equally injurious to the lung, how does one decide, for example, whether an oxygen concentration of more than 50% is more harmful than a PIP of greater than 25 cmH_2O? The relative contribution from these risks will vary with individual patients and with various stages of the disease process. Therefore, each strategy must be designed around individual clinical circumstances and stage of illness.

A. CPAP and PEEP

End-expiratory pressure may be applied with or without a ventilator. The strategies involved in both modes will be discussed together because of their comparable physiological effects. The high appeal of CPAP is that it may obviate the need for mechanical ventilation. A large part of the stimulus for the use of CPAP instead of mechanical ventilation comes from the attempt to discern which ventilatory care strategies may result in a decreased incidence of BPD. A review of eight centers (75) suggested that the practice of early use of nasal CPAP (at Columbia Presbyterian Medical Center) was beneficial, and additional evidence from a subsequent survey of 11 centers reaffirmed this impression (76). The avoidance of endotracheal intubation should decrease the likelihood of damage to the tracheal mucosa, altered mucociliary function, and increased risk of infection. In addition, CPAP avoids application of high peak inflation pressures. The target population of extremely low-birth-weight infants (less than 1000 g), with an expected need for prolonged mechanical ventilation owing to concurrent lung disease (HMD) or recurrent severe apnea, is at greatest risk for development of BPD. Does the use of CPAP avoid intubation? Does it permit earlier extubation, and does it maintain alveolar patency in a spontaneously breathing infant? End-expiratory pressure should prevent alveolar collapse in the surfactant-deficient state. The indications for the use of CPAP in a spontaneously breathing infant have been set rather arbitrarily and are related to concerns for oxygen toxicity when inspired oxygen is over 60%. More recently, however, infants with mild lung disease and minimal oxygen needs have been treated with nasal CPAP, presumably to prevent alveolar collapse and to maintain a satisfactory lung volume. Infants who are born at 24–27 weeks gestation have few, if any, alveoli. Therefore, alveolar duct distension may occur. Also, CPAP may help maintain patency of extremely small terminal airways. It has not been possible to study these effects in the distal lung in human infants, other than inferences from changes in gas exchange. Alveoli that are already open may become further distended, with an overall decrease in lung compliance because of a shift to the flatter portion of the pressure–volume curve. Collapsed alveoli require an inspiratory pressure of 12–15 cmH_2O, well above the pressures that are generally applied with CPAP or PEEP (27). If the infant does not generate sufficient inspiratory pressures to open distal lung units, overdistension and unequal ventilation may follow. An increase in FRC has been measured in infants who were treated with CPAP (77).

Theoretically, the use of exogenous surfactant, administered with positive pressure followed by CPAP, might result in more alveoli remaining open. If, however, surfactant restores a lower minimum surface tension, then subsequent CPAP should not be necessary. Because of abnormal mechanical properties of the immature lung, or changes associated with HMD or intra-alveolar fluid, peripheral airways may have traction forces that cause collapse, in which event CPAP might help prevent small-airway closure. There is evidence that CPAP distends proximal airways, with a resultant decrease in supraglottic airway resistance (78). The beneficial effects of CPAP have been reviewed by Bancalari and Sinclair (79). There is no published evidence from a controlled study showing that prophylactic CPAP prevents BPD. Four trials evaluated the efficacy of CPAP in infants with HMD and demonstrated an increase in Po_2, a decrease in Fio_2, and a decrease in death rate, with no significant effect on the incidence of BPD (80–83). A subsequent study of early versus delayed use of CPAP was conducted to determine the optimum time of treatment for infants with HMD; this study showed a reduced need for subsequent mechanical ventilation when CPAP was applied early, rather than late (79). The effect on the incidence or severity of BPD was not evaluated.

CPAP by nasal prongs can result in air leakage through the mouth and leak around the nares, resulting in a requirement for increased airflow which, in turn, may result in airway pressure variations. A newer device has been constructed (Aladdin) to overcome this problem by adding a variable jet of gas at the nasal prongs to create a fluidic jet which, in turn, maintains a constant flow of air. Hence, there is a constant pressure throughout the respiratory cycle (84). The device also incorporates a fluidic jet during exhalation to reduce resistance to flow.

CPAP/PEEP may result in airway distension which, in turn, causes an increase of anatomical dead space that may contribute to CO_2 retention and an increased risk of air leak and air trapping (77,85). Nasal irritation and increased work of breathing, gastric distension, and even gastric rupture have been reported to complicate attempts at gastric feedings during CPAP. Thus, a constant orogastric tube is usually employed in conjunction with nasal CPAP. Also, excessive mean airway pressure may reduce cardiac output and decrease pulmonary blood flow.

The use of CPAP is now widespread. Its popularity probably derives from the belief that intubation and mechanical ventilation might be avoided. In infants without significant lung disease, this may be warranted. In infants weighing less than 1000 g with lung disease, it is unclear whether mechanical ventilation can be avoided or delayed. Minimization of barotrauma and a decrease in FIO_2 are worthy goals. It is difficult to prove the efficacy of NCPAP in reducing the incidence or severity of BPD because of the many variables that need to be controlled in a randomized trial. As refinements in commercial devices and application of CPAP improve, harmful effects should be minimized as we await evidence of its role in ameliorating BPD.

B. Optimal Distending Pressure

Most of the various strategics for the least harmful pattern of ventilation focus on decreasing barotrauma by decreasing PIP and MAP. The major reason for initiating mechanical ventilation is to maintain appropriate distension, and hence ventilation, of the lung while maintaining patency of alveoli to decrease right-to-left shunting and improve oxygenation. There is, therefore, a delicate balance between the optimum pressure to alleviate this problem vis-à-vis the pressure that causes trauma—a double-edged sword. The more immature the infant, the more susceptible he or she is likely to be to pressure-induced injury. Another dilemma relates to the balance between the effects of oxygen toxicity versus those of airway pressure, and how to strike an appropriate balance when both oxygen and distending pressure are needed.

The degree of distension from peak inspiratory pressure depends on the regional compliance of the lung which, in turn, influences the amount of volume delivered to that part of the lung. If compliance is low, then a sufficient peak pressure is required to result in a tidal volume that is sufficient for gas exchange.

Assessment

The stimulus for changing distending pressure comes from the assessment of blood gas values. However, changes in FIO_2 or respirator rate, or improving synchrony may be as effective. Air entry comparisons between right and left sides of the chest should be done by auscultation and by observing motion of the chest wall and abdomen during mechanical breaths. A chest radiograph taken at end-inspiration helps determine whether there is sufficient lung volume. Mechanical ventilators now come equipped with accessories to measure pulmonary function nearly continuously. Pulmonary function data may be displayed by continuous graphic analysis of pressure–volume loops, pressure–flow loops, and individual values for pressure, volume, and flow. Being able to observe a measured change in V_T following a change in PIP should facilitate respirator management. A major problem is the inaccuracy of some of the measurements owing to their dynamic nature, the problem of air leak around the endotracheal tube, and the site of measuring pressure and flow proximal to the lung. If the measurements were indeed reliable, then it would be a tremendous asset to have measurements of lung compliance, resistance, and tidal volume associated with changes in delivered gas volume, flow, airway pressure, and rate.

Strategies

As most ventilators are time-cycled, pressure-limited, and flow-variable, the potential to limit injury to the lung is controlled by PIP, PEEP, and MAP. A common-sense strategy is to use the lowest PIP and MAP that will result in acceptable gas exchange without requiring excessively high levels of inspired oxygen. The strategy needs to be reevaluated with each improvement or deterioration in gas exchange throughout the entire course of mechanical ventilation.

Once thought to be a consequence of HMD, BPD now frequently develops after an initial period (approximately 1 week) of minimal, if any, lung disease. This phenomenon is most common in infants of less than 27 weeks gestation, who often receive mechanical ventilation and surfactant shortly after birth and are not extubated because of poor respiratory drive or recurrent apnea. These extremely premature infants are perhaps the most vulnerable to acquire stretch-induced lung injury; hence, the popularity of using nasal CPAP rather than CMV. Many infants initially require mechanical ventilation with minimal supplemental oxygen, and later require progressively more oxygen. Can this sequence be prevented or ameliorated by altering ventilatory strategies? Very little evidence has come forth to evaluate different strategies of management in these very small infants in a controlled fashion.

Initial PIP and MAP requirements are determined by the presence and severity of early lung disease, and the efficacy of surfactant treatment in accomplishing alveolar patency. Ideally, PIP will be kept below 25 cmH_2O and may be reduced to 16 cmH_2O or less before considering extubation. With severe HMD, atelectasis and resultant marked intrapulmonary shunting of blood may increase demands for ventilator support, sometimes leading to a PIP of 30 cmH_2O or higher. If compliance is uniformly decreased throughout the lung, 30 cmH_2O may not cause as much overdistension as 16 cmH_2O in a lung that already has some overexpansion. The duration of the applied pressure becomes another important variable. At an increased flow rate, a prolonged inspiratory time may increase the risk of lung injury. There have been many studies on the strategy of altering inspiratory flow rate and time of inspiration to adjust the mean airway pressure (86–92). An increase in inspiratory flow rate will increase mean airway pressure and may be advantageous in recruiting collapsed lung, but it may be disadvantageous if there is increased airway resistance or airway obstruction.

As HMD progresses through its reparative stages, and as radiologic evidence of BPD appears, associated with an inability to wean from mechanical ventilation or supplemental oxygen, the underlying changes in pulmonary pathology require constant attention to changing the ventilatory strategy. Interstitial edema, alveolar exudates, bronchiolar narrowing, and airway mucosal inflammation may change compliance and resistance considerably. Resulting alterations in time constants within different parts of the lung may make it exceedingly difficult to optimize the relation between applied pressure and inspiratory time. Therefore, there is an increased likelihood of respirator-induced damage, as the heterogeneity of lung pathology becomes more marked (see Fig. 1). This, in turn, will result in more disorganized repair. Overexpanded or ruptured alveoli form cystic, emphysematous-like areas that may be subtended by one small or partially obstructed terminal bronchiole that tends to trap gas. Another part of the lung with interstitial and alveolar edema may lead to collapse and require an increase in pressure and volume to result in effective ventilation. The different time constants within different regions of the same lung make selection of a suitable ventilation strategy a challenge. However, maintaining the lowest possible peak and mean airway pressures is desirable even if inspired oxygen needs increase or hypercapnia develops. HFOV may be advantageous under these circumstances.

Permissive Hypercapnia

The efforts to minimize barotrauma have led to lower-volume and lower-pressure ventilation, with resultant hypercapnia (93). The possible benefits and adverse effects of accepting an elevated $Paco_2$, often referred to as permissive hypercapnia, have been reevaluated, and this approach has become popular in the ventilator management of both infants and adults with respiratory failure. Several studies have examined this approach in adults with ARDS (94–96) and saline-lavaged rabbits (97), and results have not been conclusive. The interest in permissive hypercapnia in low-birth-weight infants, stimulated by the proposals of Wung (93) and others (80,98), has been long-standing. Much interest in the acceptance of hypercapnia also stems from efforts to avoid intubation and mechanical ventilation (93,99). Additionally, there are increasing concerns over the possible adverse effects of hypocapnia, including decreased cerebral blood flow, periventricular leukomalacia, and decreased cerebral oxygenation (65,66,100–102). There has been no uniform definition of permissive hypercapnia, and CO_2 values ranging from 55–120 mmHg have been advocated. The usual range in infants, however, varies between 55 and 70 mmHg.

What are the adverse consequences of allowing the Pco_2 to rise above 55 mmHg? If the Pco_2 is consistently between 55 and 60 mmHg, pH will gradually approach 7.40 in response to renal retention of bicarbonate. Theoretically, the increase in Pco_2 and the associated decrease in pH could increase pulmonary vascular resistance. In the steady state, however, there is minimal evidence to support this concern. Acute elevations in Pco_2 will transiently affect intracellular pH, but with continued elevation of Pco_2, intracellular buffering should occur rapidly. Until compensation occurs, however, there may be adverse effects from the transient increase in pulmonary vascular resistance.

No definitive studies in infants have clarified the role of permissive hypercapnia in preventing BPD. Claims that decreased intubation rates have been associated with a decreased incidence of BPD (75,99) need prospective study. Preliminary observations by Mariani et al. (103) who compared $Paco_2$ values of 35–45 mmHg versus 45–55 mmHg during the first 4 days after birth, reportedly resulted in decreased ventilator days when infants were allowed to have the higher $Paco_2$ values, but there was no difference in the incidence of BPD.

Patient-Triggered Ventilation

One of the most important strategies in minimizing barotrauma is to allow the infant to synchronize respiratory efforts with the ventilator whenever possible. Asynchrony between patient and respirator can result in inefficient gas exchange, inadequate tidal volumes, gas trapping, patient anxiety, and the need to increase applied PIP. The risk of air leak is increased, and there may be fluctuations in cardiac function and blood flow owing to variations in intrathoracic pressure. Often the adverse effects of asynchrony may lead to adjustments in respirator frequency and I/E ratio, sometimes eliciting attempts at analgesia or muscular paralysis. Patient-triggered respiration requires a machine with a rapid and sensitive response time, and it also demands sufficient inspiratory effort by the infant (104–110). Abdominally triggered techniques have been less satisfactory than airway sensors (109–116). Hyperventilation can occur when the ventilator is kept in the assist–control mode if the triggering device is too sensitive.

The most commonly used system to mechanically ventilate the lungs of tiny infants is SIMV, and modifications permit flow synchrony or passive support, with pressure limitations depending on the infant's stage of illness or recovery and spontaneous respiratory effort. More sophisticated systems deliver a pressure proportional to the infant's inspiratory effort, which can vary with each breath. The optimal triggering system and mode of inspiratory support, needs further study. No data are yet available from which to assess the effects of these strategies on subsequent BPD.

VII. Liquid Ventilation

Liquid ventilation with perfluorocarbon fluid (PFC) has been demonstrated to provide effective ventilation in animal models of newborn respiratory diseases (117–121) and in preliminary trials conducted with human infants (122,123). Ventilation with PFC should lower interfacial tension, permit opening of collapsed alveoli, and improve gas exchange. Perfluorochemicals have high solubility for O_2 and CO_2, low surface tension, and are biologically inert.

With full liquid ventilation, surface forces are reduced to that of the PFC lung interface, but not to the same degree as existing in the surfactant replete lung. The lung is first filled with liquid, and a liquid tidal volume must then be cycled. A precise, volume-controlled, pressure-limited, and time-cycled delivery is required, as well as extracorporeal membrane oxygenation and CO_2 removal from the liquid. Respiratory frequencies, therefore, must be slow (i.e., about 5–8 cycles/min).

Partial liquid ventilation (PLV), or perfluorocarbon-associated gas exchange (PAGE) was first proposed by Fuhrman et al. (124,125). With this technique, an amount of PFC equivalent to the normal FRC (approximately 30 mL/kg) is instilled in the trachea, and respiratory gas exchange occurs by conventional mechanical ventilation. This method has the practical advantage of not requiring extracorporeal gas exchange. Oxygen and carbon dioxide are constantly exchanged with the intrapulmonary PFC through each ventilator breath.

A. Clinical Trials

Greenspan et al. (122) were the first to describe the use of full tidal liquid ventilation (TLV) of humans using a gravity-assisted approach. The infants were terminally ill, but had a transient improvement in respiratory gas exchange. Additional clinical trials utilizing partial liquid ventilation (PLV) are in progress. Two completed studies (122,123) demonstrated short-term safety, improvement in lung volumes and gas exchange in infants who were failing mechanical ventilation. Other trials of PLV are being conducted in children and adults with ARDS. Three collaborative controlled clinical trials are underway involving (1) infants with severe respiratory failure; (2) full-term infants with a variety of forms of severe respiratory failure; and (3) infants with congenital diaphragmatic hernia. Thus far, these studies have not provided sufficient data to permit assessment of the possible role of PLV in the prevention of BPD. The evaluation of full liquid ventilation is awaiting the development of a system for reliably delivering a cyclic tidal volume of liquid.

B. Animal Studies

Experimental studies on animal models of both newborn and adult lung injury have provided extensive physiological information on the effects of partial and total liquid ventilation (124–133). Most have been short-term studies and have demonstrated less injury to respiratory epithelium following TLV (118,133). Preliminary studies of premature monkeys treated with total liquid ventilation from birth in our laboratory have demonstrated less lung injury compared with CMV during the first 3 hr of life. Animal studies indicate successful oxygenation, CO_2

removal, and the ability to revert back to gas ventilation with subsequent long-term survival (134). Successful recovery from full tidal liquid ventilation led to the concept of partial liquid ventilation (124,125), and long-term PLV has been successful in near-term baboons (135).

C. Effects of Liquid Ventilation

The major rationale for liquid ventilation has been to minimize surface tension. In the surfactant-deficient lung, compliance improves, and a lower PIP is required because of the lower interfacial tension between PFC and the lung. Changes in interfacial tension with PFC have been examined in the preterm lamb lung, in addition to the effects of adding exogenous surfactant (136,137). Liquid filling results in less airway pressure required during inflation and more pressure during deflation than with exogenous surfactant alone. The combination of surfactant pretreatment and liquid ventilation has the greatest effect of increasing pressure–volume stability. Other physiological consequences include possible differences in volume expansion between upper and lower lobes owing to the effects of gravity, slower diffusion rates of oxygen through the liquid, and adverse effects on the distribution of pulmonary blood flow. These effects will differ depending on whether full or partial liquid ventilation is applied.

D. Safety and Efficacy

Before the acceptance of any form of liquid ventilation, considerably more research is needed. Which patients are likely to benefit? Are there specific lung abnormalities that might be worsened? The large number of animal studies and the limited number of clinical trials provide strong evidence for its efficacy in providing gas exchange, and demonstrate that more uniform inflation with less distending pressure is possible. Preliminary studies suggest that lung injury may be less than with gas ventilation of premature animals. Many issues of safety need to be resolved and will require longer periods of study. The use of PFC as a blood substitute and for various imaging and radiologic procedures has demonstrated that it is an inert substance. Long-term toxicity following prolonged liquid ventilation, however, has not been excluded, and PFC has not yet received FDA approval. Because of the high specific gravity of PFC (twice as dense as lung tissue), the dependent part of the adult lung can be overdistended during TLV, and during PLV overdistension of the upper lung has led to lung rupture. These effects of gravity are probably minimal in the newborn lung. The approval for use of full tidal liquid ventilation will depend on the development of a safe and effective liquid ventilator that would allow extensive clinical trials, first in premature animals with respiratory failure, and then in premature human infants with respiratory failure.

E. Research Challenges

In addition to the foregoing concerns, there are many unresolved questions related to optimal methods of delivery, dosage, timing, and duration of treatment for both TLV and PLV. How important is gravity in the distribution of PFC in the neonatal lung? There are at least theoretical concerns that PLV may cause overdistension of the upper parts of the lung, whereas greater distribution of TLV to lower parts of the lung may adversely affect local pulmonary blood flow. The high evaporative loss of PFC poses the problem of how to determine the appropriate volume and rate of replacement during both modes of ventilation. PLV is the most practical method to apply at present, yet the optimal volume required to alter surface properties or promote uniform inflation is unknown. With PLV, does PFC form a thin lining layer or does the liquid puddle? The interfacial forces between PFC and the alveolar lining layer may determine whether there is layering or droplet formation (137). Studies are needed on the efficacy of very small volumes, perhaps in combination with exogenous surfactant. Surfactant mixed with PFC may distribute throughout the lung better than surfactant alone. Because PFC is imiscible, mucus may accumulate and form a thick layer along the lining of the airways. If PFC enters the lung tissue, will it impair function? How much time is required for its elimination from the lung? Does PFC affect the secretion or function of surfactant? Does PFC interfere with macrophage function and increase the risk of infection or inflammation? Would liquid ventilation for the first minutes or hours of life reduce the risk of initial barotrauma? Would intermittent use (i.e., once or twice a day) alleviate mechanical problems in the abnormal lung? Would a combination of HFOV and PLV be less injurious to the lung than PLV applied with CMV? There are many more questions than answers, and much more research is needed before this mode of ventilation will gain clinical acceptance. At present, there is no evidence demonstrating a protective effect against the development of BPD.

VIII. Weaning from Mechanical Ventilation

Strategies for weaning from mechanical ventilation require assessment of the infant's ability to maintain adequate gas exchange with spontaneous breathing. In spite of careful clinical assessment of the appropriate timing for extubation, the infant often decides this by self-extubation. There is a lack of sensitive and specific indicators to allow accurate prediction of tolerance for extubation (114,115,138). Efforts to measure lung mechanics, self-generated inspiratory pressure, minimal oxygen needs, or minimal ventilator settings have yet to result in a satisfactory algorithm for successful extubation. Techniques for the reduction of PIP, MAP, or frequency, and their temporal sequencing, depend on clinical judgment. Gradual reduction in ventilator settings, with close observation of clinical respiratory effort, gas exchange assessment, and radiologic evidence of lung volume helps in this clinical judgment. "Training" of the respiratory muscles may be needed (139). Often the chest wall muscles and diaphragm have been minimally stressed, raising the question of disuse atrophy. Use of "pressure support" ventilation provides a less strenuous trial for the infant and may facilitate muscle strengthening. The use of SIMV, with a minimum preset mandatory rate, also helps to determine the infant's spontaneous ventilatory pattern (114,115,140). Gradual reduction in distending pressure should be the first goal of weaning, followed by reduction of inspired oxygen and, subsequently, a reduction in ventilator rate. End-tidal P_{CO_2} and oxygen saturation monitoring, as well as transcutaneous P_{O_2} and P_{CO_2} measurements are helpful in determining the magnitude and rate of change of ventilatory support. Assessment of pulmonary function before extubation has not proved helpful (141).

Most infants who are less than 32 weeks of postconceptional age are likely to manifest recurrent apnea following extubation. Respiratory stimulants, such as caffeine or theophylline, are often helpful in reducing the frequency and severity of apnea, and in situations for which extubation is anticipated, such treatment needs to be initiated before assisted ventilation is stopped.

Weaning to CPAP remains controversial. There is evidence that the requirement for reintubation is reduced in infants who have recurrent apneic episodes (142), although other studies have not shown efficacy (143). The Aladdin device appears to be better tolerated than conventional CPAP devices. The overall goal of both weaning and extubation should be to minimize lung injury from excessive pressure and stretch, and to reduce the risks that exist when an endotracheal tube is in place (mechanical trauma, increased secretions, obstruction, increased requirement for suction, and increased infection).

IX. Other Forms of Respiratory Support

Because there have been no studies addressing the practicality or efficacy of newer or noninvasive forms of ventilatory assistance in the prevention of BPD, only a brief summary will be given here. There will be experimentation with some of these methods in the continuing quest for noninjurious means to assist ventilation.

A. Continuous Negative-Pressure Ventilation

Continuous negative pressure has been applied to infants with respiratory failure at a number of centers (81,144–148). Intermittent negative-pressure ventilation has been effective in infants with respiratory failure and associated with a lower incidence of pneumothorax when compared with CMV (149). Improvement in oxygenation also has occurred in studies following failure with positive-pressure ventilation (146,150). The primary reason why this technique has not gained popular acceptance relates to the marked technical difficulties associated with its use in infants who weigh less than 1000 g. Negative pressure has not been widely used in infants, and is not readily adapted to routine care. Moreover, there is no evidence that negative-pressure ventilation can be used for most of the infants who are especially vulnerable to the development of BPD. Thus, this approach is not presently part of a preventive ventilatory strategy.

B. External Chest Wall Vibration

External high-frequency oscillation can be applied to the chest wall by high-frequency negative-pressure ventilation or by air compression within a plethysmograph utilizing positive chest wall pressure (32,151,152). This method avoids endotracheal intubation yet uses the same principles of HFOV delivered through an ET tube. The Hayek oscillator is a chest wall cuirass system, which at 1–3 Hz is effective in ventilating adult humans (153) and provides optimal gas exchange in rabbits at frequencies of 6–9 Hz (154). Although a small chest cuirass has been manufactured, there have been no clinical trials to evaluate its effectiveness to support small infants with lung disease, let alone any ameliorating effects on the incidence of BPD.

C. Positive-Pressure Ventilation by Nasal Mask BiPAP and NCPAP

Positive pressure can be administered via face or nasal mask using a volume or pressure controlled respirator and by a bilevel positive ventilator (BiPAP). The latter device provides continuous flow of positive pressure, which cycles between a preset high and low positive pressure. This device has had extensive use with adults. It is triggered by the patient's respiratory efforts and flow continues for a fixed time or until it falls below a set threshold. The nasal mask is extremely flexible to permit a tight seal and minimize leaks. A nasopharyngeal tube may be necessary in small infants to avoid airleaks. Although it has not yet been adapted for neonatal use, it is conceivable that this system, with a sensitive synchronized trigger device, may prevent intubation of extremely low-birth-weight infants with minimal lung disease. It also might facilitate earlier extubation or weaning of infants who are receiving CMV.

D. Extracorporeal Membrane Oxygenation

The use of ECMO is not technically feasible in infants with a weight of less than approximately 2 kg. These infants, who are at greatest risk for BPD, therefore, are not suitable candidates for ECMO.

E. Adjunctive Therapy

All ventilatory strategies need to consider the role of adjunctive therapy in modifying mechanical variables of ventilation. There is as much controversy over the relative contribution of many pharmacological treatments as there is over the optimum mode of ventilation. Adjunctive therapies, such as corticosteroids, bronchodilators, indomethacin, and diuretics are considered elsewhere in this volume (see Chap. 12). Assessment of the cause and site of pathology should determine the rationale for the use of such treatment. Most drug therapy is intended to modify lung pathology; hence, the mechanics of breathing may be affected, thus necessitating appropriate ventilator changes.

X. Future Needs

The incidence of pulmonary air leak has appeared to decrease over the past few years. This is generally attributed to advances in ventilator strategies, although no specific change can be proved. Close attention to the risks of lung distension from excessive pressure and volume, along with adjunctive therapy, appear to have led to a reduction in the severity of BPD. The tolerance threshold for barotrauma, however, needs better definition. It is not yet clear that the incidence of BPD has decreased as a result of new ventilatory strategies. Advances in treatment directed at oxygen toxicity, inflammation, infection, nutrition, fluid balance, and closure of the ductus arteriosus make the analysis of the contribution of any one management strategy extremely difficult. There is further need for research to understand respirator-related lung injury. What determines the threshold for barotrauma in individual patients? Does any cyclic movement with gas, including spontaneous breathing, in the extremely immature infant act as a stimulus to redirect the growth patterns preexisting in the fetal lung? Is this stimulus sufficient to redirect lung growth from cell multiplication to differentiation? Does this cyclic movement, for which the lung is not yet programmed, signal an abnormal cellular response, which initiates the BPD process? What are the signals resulting from lung distension? The search for the most gentle type of mechanical ventilation should lead to less lung injury and optimal gas exchange, but most likely will be insufficient for prevention of BPD. Would liquid ventilation more nearly mimic in utero conditions and decrease mechanically induced injury? Does mechanical ventilation contribute to BPD by damaging alveoli, interstitium, small airways, large airways, or all components? What is the relative contribution of each? Are mechanical stimuli alone able to stimulate smooth-muscle hypertrophy, fibroblast proliferation, alveolar epithelial cell dysplasia, airway epithelial cell dysplasia, or do these responses result from actual physical damage or destruction of particular cells? How important to tolerance of mechanical ventilation is the maturational status of the matrix structure of collagen and elastin? Is the risk for barotrauma highest with the first few breaths after birth? Does damage result from an unequal distribution of initial breaths, unequal clearance of lung liquid, and nonuniformity of the establishment of a stable air–liquid interface? Is it possible that injuries sustained in the first minutes or hours after birth could result in a delayed cellular response that requires several days or even weeks to manifest itself? How much of a contribution to this potential injury comes from the sudden and marked increase in oxygen exposure?

The baboon models of BPD provide an opportunity to gain some insight into the maturational differences in the response to putative adverse stimuli (10,16,155–157). The baboon delivered at 140 days gestation (77% gestation), and mechanically ventilated following surfactant administration does not develop evidence of BPD if oxygen exposure is minimal, whereas the baboon infant delivered at 69% of gestation (equivalent to 27–28 weeks of human gestation) often acquires BPD even when oxygen and trauma from mechanical ventilation are minimized (156,157). What is the contribution, if any, from patency of the ductus arteriosus? Is there any preventative role for the use of indomethacin or diuretics? What is the mechanism by which corticosteroids improve the pathophysiology? What is the site of action for the beneficial effects of corticosteroids? When should they be administered?

Further studies are needed to determine the efficacy of HFOV. Would the use of HFOV begun soon after birth, combined with surfactant treatment in extremely low-birth-weight infants, provide protection against BPD? Studies of combinations of ventilatory strategies are needed, such as intermittent partial liquid ventilation (with close attention to the risks of uneven distribution of ventilation), HFOV, and surfactant from the outset (158), with the goal of opening and sustaining patency of alveoli and alveolar ducts.

Controlled studies are needed to evaluate noninvasive respiratory support, such as CPAP or perhaps nasal BiPAP, in avoiding mechanical ventilation.

XI. Summary

Further refinements in ventilatory techniques should help reduce the severity of chronic lung injury. However, the incidence of BPD may not be altered. A greater emphasis should be placed on understanding the temporal changes in the cellular and physiological response to the underlying disease process, and how the degree of lung immaturity influences this response. Basic mechanisms of the immature lung's response to injury and repair are needed. It is important to know if altered growth mechanisms have a lifelong effect on the number and size of alveoli, as well as subsequent airway structures. Improved techniques and strategies of ventilatory support are important to minimize lung injury. Many other contributing factors need better understanding to improve the overall strategy for treating or preventing BPD.

References

1. Nelson MN. J'accuse! M. LeComte de La Place a prohibe le recruitment des alveoles du poumon. Pediatrics 1996; 98:1196–1197.
2. Deoras KS, et al. Structural changes in the trachea in preterm lambs induced by ventilation. Pediatr Res 1989; 26:434–437.
3. Joshi VV, et al. Acute lesions induced by endotracheal intubation. Am J Dis Child 1972; 124:646–649.
4. Gau GS, et al. Iatrogenic epithelial change caused by endotracheal intubations of neonates. Early Hum Dev 1987; 15:221–229.
5. Bolivar JM, et al. Mechanisms for episodes of hypoxemia in preterm infants undergoing mechanical ventilation. J Pediatr 1995; 127:767–773.
6. Lee RMKW, O'Brodovich H. Airway epithelial damage in premature infants with respiratory failure. Am Rev Respir Dis 1988; 137:450–457.
7. Bonikos DS, et al. Bronchopulmonary dysplasia: the pulmonary pathologic sequel of necrotizing bronchiolitis and pulmonary fibrosis. Hum Pathol 1976; 7:643–666.
8. Lee RMKW, et al. Ciliary defects associated with the development of bronchopulmonary dysplasia, ciliary motility and ultrastructure. Am Rev Respir Dis 1984; 129:190–193.
9. Rasche RFH, Kuhns LR. Histopathologic changes in airway mucosa of infants after endotracheal intubation. Pediatrics 1972; 50:632–637.
10. Coalson JJ, et al. A baboon model of bronchopulmonary dysplasia. II. Pathologic features. Exp Mol Pathol 1982; 37:335–350.
11. Taghizadeh A, Reynolds EOR. Pathogenesis of bronchopulmonary dysplasia following hyaline membrane disease. Am J Pathol 1976; 82:241–264.
12. Harrison G, et al. Bronchiolitis induced by experimental acute and chronic oxygen intoxication in young rats. J Pathol 1970; 102:115–122.
13. Boat TF. Studies of oxygen toxicity in cultured human neonatal respiratory epithelium. J Pediatr 1979; 95:916–919.
14. Sward-Comunelli SL, et al. Airway muscle in preterm infants: changes during development. J Pediatr 1997; 130:570–576.
15. Jackson JC, et al. Mechanisms for reduced total lung capacity at birth and during hyaline membrane disease in premature newborn monkeys. Am Rev Respir Dis 1990; 142:413–419.
16. Coalson JJ, et al. Diffuse alveolar damage in the evolution of bronchopulmonary dysplasia in the baboon. Pediatr Res 1988; 24:357–366.
17. Nilsson R, et al. Pathogenesis of neonatal lung lesions induced by artifical ventilation: evidence against the role of barotrauma. Respiration 1980; 40:218–225.
18. Bruce MC, et al. Risk factors for the degradation of lung elastic fibers in the ventilated neonate. Implications for impaired lung development in bronchopulmonary dysplasia. Am Rev Respir Dis 1992; 146:204–212.

19. Pierce RA, et al. Chronic lung injury in preterm lambs: disordered pulmonary elastin deposition. Am J Physiol 1997; 272:452–460.
20. Tomashefski JF, et al. Bronchopulmonary dysplasia: a morphometric study with emphasis on the pulmonary vasculature. Pediatr Pathol 1984; 2:469–487.
21. Hislop AA, Haworth SG. Pulmonary vascular damage and the development of cor pulmonale following hyaline membrane disease. Pediatr Pulmonol 1990; 9:152–161.
22. Bressack MA, et al. Pulmonary oxygen toxicity: increased microvascular permeability to protein in unanesthetized lambs. Lymphology 1979; 12:133–139.
23. Carlton DP, et al. Lung overexpansion increases pulmonary microvascular protein permeability in young lambs. J Appl Physiol 1990; 69:577–583.
24. Carlton DP, et al. Lung vascular protein permeability in preterm fetal and mature newborn sheep. J Appl Physiol 1994; 77:782–788.
25. Bland RD, et al. Lung fluid balance in lambs before and after premature birth. J Clin Invest 1989; 84:568–576.
26. Maniscalco WM, et al. Hyperoxic injury decreases alveolar epithelial cell expression of vascular endothelial growth factor (VEGF) in neonatal rabbit lung. Am J Respir Cell Mol Biol 1997; 16:557–567.
27. Palmer S, et al. Lung development in the fetal primate *Macacca nemestrina*: II. Pressure–volume and phospholipid changes. Pediatr Res 1977; 11:1051–1056.
28. Harrison VC, et al. The significance of grunting in hyaline membrane disease. Pediatrics 1968; 41:549–559.
29. Sjostrand U. Review of the physiological rationale for and development of high-frequency positive pressure ventilation HFPV. Acta Anaesthesiol Scand Suppl 1977; 64:7–27.
30. Bland RD, et al. High frequency mechanical ventilation in severe hyaline membrane disease an alternative treatment? Crit Care Med 1980; 8:275–280.
31. Heicher DA, et al. Prospective clinical comparison of two methods for mechanical ventilation of neonates: rapid rate and short inspiratory time versus slow rate and long inspiratory time. J Pediatr 1981; 98:957–961.
32. Eyal FG, et al. High frequency positive-pressure ventilation in neonates. Crit Care Med 1984; 12:793–797.
33. Boros SJ, et al. Using conventional ventilators at unconventional rates. Pediatrics 1984; 74:487–492.
34. Gonzalez F, et al. Rapid mechanical ventilation effects on tracheal airway pressure, lung volume and blood gases of rabbits. Am J Perinatol 1986; 3:347–351.
35. Hird M, et al. Gas trapping during high frequency positive pressure ventilation using conventional ventilators. Early Hum Dev 1990; 22:51–56.
36. Keszler M, et al. Multicenter controlled trial comparing high-frequency jet ventilation and conventional mechanical ventilation in newborn infants with pulmonary interstitial emphysema. J Pediatr 1991; 119:85–93.
37. Carlo WA, et al. Early randomized intervention with high-frequency jet ventilation in respiratory distress syndrome. J Pediatr 1990; 117:765–770.
38. Wiswell TE, et al. Different high-frequency ventilator strategies: effect on the propagation of tracheobronchial histopathologic changes. Pediatrics 1990; 85:70–78.
39. Wiswell TE, et al. Effects of hypocarbia on the development of cystic periventricu-

lar leukomalacia in premature infants treated with high-frequency jet ventilation. Pediatrics 1996; 98:918–924.
40. Wiswell TE, et al. High-frequency jet ventilation in the early management of respiratory distress syndrome is associated with a greater risk for adverse outcomes. Pediatrics 1996; 98:1035–1043.
41. Truog WE, et al. Effect of high-frequency oscillation on gas exchange and pulmonary phospholipids in experimental hyaline membrane disease. Am Rev Respir Dis 1983; 127:585–589.
42. Truog WE, et al. Effects of prolonged high-frequency oscillatory ventilation in premature primates with experimental hyaline membrane disease. Am Rev Respir Dis 1984; 130:76–80.
43. Truog WE, Jackson JC. Alternative modes of ventilation in the prevention and treatment of bronchopulmonary dysplasia. Clin Perinatol 1992; 19:621–647.
44. Bell RE, et al. High-frequency ventilation compared to conventional positive-pressure ventilation in the treatment of hyaline membrane disease in primates. Crit Care Med 1984; 12:764–768.
45. de Lemos RA, et al. Ventilatory management of infant baboons with hyaline membrane disease: the use of high frequency ventilation. Pediatr Res 1987; 21:594–602.
46. de Lemos RA, et al. A comparison of ventilation strategies for the use of high-frequency oscillatory ventilation in the treatment of hyaline membrane disease. Acta Anaesthesiol Scand Suppl 1989; 90:102–107.
47. Gertsmann DR, et al. Influence of ventilatory technique on pulmonary baroinjury in baboons with hyaline membrane disease. Pediatr Pulmonol 1988; 5:82–91.
48. The HFO Study Group. Randomized study of high-frequency oscillatory ventilation in infants with severe respiratory distress syndrome. J Pediatr 1993; 122:609–619.
49. The HIFI Study Group. High-frequency oscillatory ventilation compared with conventional ventilation in the treatment of respiratory failure in preterm infants. N Engl J Med 1989; 370:88–93.
50. Clark RH, et al. Prospective randomized comparison of high-frequency oscillatory and conventional ventilation in respiratory distress syndrome. Pediatrics 1992; 89: 5–12.
51. Ogawa Y, et al. A multicenter randomized trial of high-frequency oscillatory ventilation as compared with conventional mechanical ventilation in preterm infants with respiratory failure. Early Hum Dev 1993; 32:1–10.
52. Gertsmann DR, et al. The Provo multicenter early HFOV trial: improved pulmonary and clinical outcome in respiratory distress syndrome. Pediatrics 1996; 98:1044–1057.
53. Bhuta T, Henderson-Smart DJ. Elective high-frequency oscillatory ventilation versus conventional ventilation in preterm infants with pulmonary dysfunction: systemic review and meta-analysis. Pediatrics 1997; 100:e6–e13.
54. Bond DM, Froese AB. Volume recruitment maneuvers are less deleterious than persistent low lung volumes in the atelectasis-prone rabbit lung during high-frequency oscillation. Crit Care Med 1993; 21:402–412.
55. Bryan AC, Froese AB. Reflections on the HIFI trial. Pediatrics 1991; 87:565–567.
56. Bond DM, et al. Sustained inflations improve respiratory compliance during high-

frequency oscillatory ventilation but not during large tidal volume positive-pressure ventilation in rabbits. Crit Care Med 1994; 22:1269–1277.

57. Dimitriou G, Greenough A. Measurement of lung volume and optimal oxygenation during high frequency oscillation. Arch Dis Child 1995; 72:F180–F183.
58. Fredberg JJ, et al. Alveolar pressure nonhomogeneity during small-amplitude high frequency ventilation. J Appl Physiol 1984; 57:788–800.
59. Fredberg JJ, et al. Factors influencing mechanical performance of neonatal high-frequency ventilation. J Appl Physiol 1987; 62:2485–2490.
60. Franz ID, Close RH. Alveolar pressure swings during high frequency ventilation in rabbits. Pediatr Res 1985; 19:162–166.
61. Allen JL, et al. Alveolar pressures magnitude and asynchrony during high frequency oscillations of excised rabbit lung. Am Rev Respir Dis 1985; 132:343–349.
62. Venegas JG, Fredberg JJ. Understanding the pressure cost of ventilation: why does high-frequency ventilation work? Crit Care Med 1994; 22 (suppl 9):S49–S57.
63. Clark RH, et al. Intraventricular hemorrhage and high-frequency ventilation: a meta-analysis of prospective clinical trials. Pediatrics 1996; 98:1058–1061.
64. Patel CA, Klein JM. Outcome of infants with birth weight less than 1000 grams with respiratory distress syndrome treated with high-frequency ventilation and surfactant therapy. Arch Pediatr Adolesc Med 1995; 149:317–321.
65. Wilson DF, et al. Effect of hyperventilation on oxygenation of the brain cortex of newborn piglets. J Appl Physiol 1991; 70:2691–2696.
66. Vanucci RC, et al. Carbon dioxide protects the brain from hypoxic-ischemic damage: an experimental study in the immature rat. Pediatrics 1995; 95:868–874.
67. Kirpilani H, et al. Diagnosis and therapy of necrotizing tracheobronchitis in ventilated neonates. Crit Care Med 1985; 13:792–797.
68. Boros SJ, et al. Necrotizing tracheobronchitis: a complication of high-frequency ventilation. J Pediatr 1986; 109:95–100.
69. Mammel MC, et al. High frequency ventilation and tracheal injuries. Pediatrics 1986; 77:608–613.
70. Clark RH, et al. Tracheal and bronchial injury in high-frequency oscillatory ventilation compared with conventional positive pressure ventilation. J Pediatr 1987; 111: 114–118.
71. Wiswell TE, et al. Tracheal and bronchial injury with high frequency oscillatory and high frequency flow interruption compared with conventional positive pressure ventilation. Pediatr Pulmonol 1987; 3:376.
72. Wiswell TE, et al. Tracheal and bronchial injury in high-frequency oscillatory ventilation compared with conventional positive pressure ventilation. J Pediatr 1988; 112:249–256.
73. Osiovich HC, et al. Hemodynamic effects of conventional and high frequency oscillatory ventilation in normal and septic piglets. Biol Neonate 1991; 59:244–252.
74. Laubscher B, et al. Hemodynamic changes during high frequency oscillation for respiratory distress syndrome. Arch Dis Child 1996; 74:F172–F176.
75. Avery ME, et al. Is chronic lung disease in low birthweight infants preventable? A survey of eight centers. Pediatrics 1987; 79:26–30.
76. Horbar JD, et al. Variability in 28-day outcomes for very low birthweight infants: an analysis of neonatal intensive care units. Pediatrics 1988; 82:554–559.

77. Saunders RA, et al. The effects of continuous positive airway pressure on lung mechanics and lung volumes in the neonate. Biol Neonate 1976; 29:178–186.
78. Miller MJ, et al. Effects of nasal CPAP on supraglottic and total pulmonary resistance in preterm infants. J Appl Physiol 1990; 56:141–146.
79. Bancalari E, Sinclair JC. Mechanical ventilation. In: Sinclair JC, et al., eds. Effective Care of the Newborn Infant. New York: Oxford University Press, 1992:200–220.
80. Rhodes PG, et al. Minimizing pneumothorax and bronchopulmonary dysplasia in ventilated infants with hyaline membrane disease. J Pediatr 1983; 103:634–637.
81. Fanaroff AA, et al. Controlled trial of continuous negative external pressure in the treatment of severe respiratory distress syndrome. J Pediatr 1973; 82:921–928.
82. Belenky DA, et al. Is continuous transpulmonary pressure better than conventional respiratory management of hyaline membrane disease? A controlled study. Pediatrics 1976; 58:800–808.
83. Durbin GM, et al. Controlled trial of continuous inflating pressure for hyaline membrane disease. Arch Dis Child 1976; 51:163–169.
84. Moa G, et al. A new device for administration of nasal continuous positive airway pressure in the newborn: an experimental study. Crit Care Med 1988; 16:1238–1242.
85. Locke RG, et al. Inadvertent administration of positive end-distending pressure during nasal cannula flow. Pediatrics 1993; 91:135–138.
86. Boros SJ, Orgill AA. Mortality and morbidity associated with pressure and volume-limited infant ventilators. Am J Dis Child 1978; 132:865–869.
87. Boros SJ. Variations in inspiratory:expiratory ratio and airway pressure wave form during mechanical ventilation: the significance of mean airway pressure. J Pediatr 1979; 94:114–117.
88. Chan V, Greenough A. Inspiratory and expiratory times for infants ventilator-dependent beyond the first week. Acta Paediatr 1994; 83:1022–1024.
89. Edberg KE, et al. Lung volume, gas mixing and mechanics of breathing in mechanically ventilated very low birthweight infants with idiopathic respiratory distress syndrome. Pediatr Res 1991; 30:496–500.
90. Hird M, Greenough A. Inflation time in mechanical ventilation of preterm neonates. Eur J Pediatr 1991; 150:440–443.
91. Ramsden CA, Reynolds EOR. Ventilator settings for newborn infants. Arch Dis Child 1987; 62:529–538.
92. Stewart AR, et al. Effects of alterations of inspiratory and expiratory pressures and inspiratory/expiratory ratios on mean airway pressure, blood gases, and intracranial pressure. Pediatrics 1981; 67:474–481.
93. Wung J, et al. Management of infants with severe respiratory failure and persistence of the fetal circulation, without hyperventilation. Pediatrics 1985; 76:488–494.
94. Bidani A, et al. Permissive hypercapnia in acute respiratory failure. JAMA 1994; 272:957–962.
95. Hickling KG, et al. Low mortality rate in adult respiratory distress syndrome using

low-volume pressure-limited ventilation with permissive hypercapnia: a prospective study. Crit Care Med 1994; 22:1568–1578.
96. Hickling KG, Joyce C. Permissive hypercapnia in ARDS and its effect on tissue oxygenation. Acta Anaesthesiol Scand Suppl 1995; 107:201–218.
97. Hickling KG, et al. Pressure-limited ventilation with permissive hypercapnia and minimum PEEP in saline-lavaged rabbits allows progressive improvement in oxygenation, but does not avoid ventilation-induced lung injury. Intensive Care Med 1996; 22:1445–1452.
98. Kraybill EN, et al. Risk factors for chronic lung disease in infants with birthweights of 751–1000 grams. J Pediatr 1989; 115:115–120.
99. Poets CF, Sens B. Changes in intubation rates and outcome of very low birth weight infants: a population-based study. Pediatrics 1996; 98:24–27.
100. Garland JS, et al. Hypocarbia before surfactant therapy appears to increase bronchopulmonary dysplasia risk in infants with respiratory distress syndrome. Arch Pediatr Adolesc Med 1995; 149:617–622.
101. Wyatt JS, et al. Response of cerebral blood volume to changes in arterial carbon dioxide tension in preterm and term infants. Pediatr Res 1991; 29:553–557.
102. Hansen N, et al. The effects of variations in $Paco_2$ on brain blood flow and cardiac output in the newborn piglet. Pediatr Res 1984; 18:1132–1136.
103. Mariani G, et al. Randomized trial of permissive hypercapnia in preterm infants: a pilot study. Pediatr Res 1997; 41:163A.
104. Donn SM, et al. Flow-synchronized ventilation of preterm infants with respiratory distress syndrome. J Perinatol 1994; 14:90–94.
105. Donn SM, Nicks JJ. Special ventilatory technologies and modalities. I. Patient-triggered ventilation. In: Goldsmith JP, Karatkin SH, eds. Assisted Ventilation of the Neonate. 3rd ed. Philadelphia: WB Saunders, 1996:215–228.
106. DeBoer DF, et al. Long-term trigger ventilation in neonatal respiratory distress syndrome. Arch Dis Child 1993; 68:308–311.
107. Chan V, et al. Influence of lung infection and reflex activity on the success of patient-triggered ventilation. Early Hum Dev 1994; 37:9–14.
108. Greenough A, et al. Airway pressure triggered ventilation for preterm neonates. J Perinat Med 1991; 19:471–476.
109. Greenough A, Milner AD. Respiratory support using patient triggered ventilation in the neonatal period. Arch Dis Child 1992; 67:69–71.
110. Greenough A. Patient-triggered ventilation. Pediatr Pulmonol Suppl 1995; 11P:98–99.
111. Bernstein G, et al. Response time and reliability of three neonatal patient-triggered ventilators. Am Rev Respir Dis 1993; 148:358–364.
112. Hird MF, Greenough A. Causes of failure of neonatal patient triggered ventilation. Early Hum Dev 1990; 23:101–108.
113. Hird MF, Greenough A. Comparison of triggering systems for neonatal patient triggered ventilation. Arch Dis Child 1991; 66:426–428.
114. Chan G, Greenough A. Comparison of weaning by patient triggered ventilation or synchronous intermittent mandatory ventilation in preterm infants. Acta Paediatr 1994; 83:335–337.

115. Chan V, Greenough A. Randomised controlled trial of weaning by patient triggered ventilation or conventional ventilation. Eur J Pediatr 1993; 152:51–54.
116. Hummler HD, et al. Patient-triggered ventilation in neonates: comparison of a flow and impedance triggered system. Am J Respir Crit Care Med 1996; 154:1049–1054.
117. Shaffer TH, Wolfson MR. Liquid ventilation: an alternative ventilation strategy for management of neonatal respiratory distress. Eur J Pediatr 1996; 155 (suppl 2P): S30–S34.
118. Wolfson MR, et al. Comparison of gas and liquid ventilation: clinical, physiological and histological correlates. J Appl Physiol 1992; 72:1024–1031.
119. Jackson JC, et al. Full-tidal liquid ventilation with perfluorocarbon for prevention of lung injury in newborn non-human primates. Artif Cells Blood Substit Immobil Biotechnol 1994; 22:1121–1132.
120. Leach CL, et al. Partial liquid ventilation in premature lambs with respiratory distress syndrome: efficacy and compatibility with exogenous surfactant. J Pediatr 1995; 126:412–420.
121. Leach CL, et al. Partial liquid ventilation with perflubron in premature infants with severe respiratory distress syndrome. The Liqui Vent Study Group. N Engl J Med 1996; 335:761–767.
122. Greenspan JS, et al. Liquid ventilation of human preterm neonates. J Pediatr 1990; 117:5–11.
123. Leach CL, et al. Perfluorocarbon-associated gas exchange (partial liquid ventilation) in respiratory distress syndrome: a prospective, randomized, controlled study. Crit Care Med 1993; 21:1270–1278.
124. Fuhrman BP, et al. Perfluorocarbon associated gas exchange. Crit Care Med 1991; 19:712–722.
125. Fuhrman BP, et al. Perfluorocarbon-associated gas exchange (PAGE): gas ventilation of the perfluorocarbon filled lung. Artif Cells Blood Subst Immobil Biotechnol 1994; 22:1133–1139.
126. Schweiler GH, Robertson B. Liquid ventilation in immature newborn rabbits. Biol Neonate 1976; 29:343–353.
127. Rufer R, Spitzer HL. Liquid ventilation in the respiratory distress syndrome. Chest 1974; 66:295–305.
128. Shaffer TH, Moskowitz GD. Demand-controlled liquid ventilation of the lungs. J Appl Physiol 1974; 36:208–213.
129. Shaffer TH, et al. Liquid ventilation. Pediatr Pulmonol 1992; 14:102–109.
130. Shaffer TH, et al. Liquid ventilation in premature lambs: uptake, biodistribution and elimination of perfluorodecalin liquid. Reprod Fertil Dev 1996; 8:409–416.
131. Mates EA, et al. Gas exchange during gas and liquid ventilation. J Intensive Care Med 1996; 11:313–325.
132. Hirschl RB, et al. Development and application of a simplified liquid ventilator. Crit Care Med 1995; 23:157–163.
133. Varani J, et al. Perfluorocarbon protects lung epithelial cells from neutrophil-mediated injury in an in vitro model of liquid ventilation therapy. Shock 1996; 6:339–344.
134. Salman NH, et al. Prolonged studies of perfluorocarbon associated gas exchange

and of the resumption of conventional mechanical ventilation. Crit Care Med 1995; 23:919–924.
135. Sekins KM, et al. Long-term partial liquid ventilation (PLV) with perflubron in the near-term baboon neonate. Artif Cells Blood Substi Immobil Biotechnol 1994; 22: 1381–1387.
136. Tarczy-Hornoch P, et al. Effects of exogenous surfactant on lung pressure–volume characteristics during liquid ventilation. J Appl Physiol 1996; 80:1764–1771.
137. Tarczy-Hornoch P, et al. Surfactant replacement increases compliance in premature lambs during partial liquid ventilation in situ. J Appl Physiol 1998; 84:1316–1322.
138. Chan V, Greenough A. Randomised trial of methods of extubation in acute and chronic respiratory distress. Arch Dis Child 1993; 68:570–572.
139. Tan S, et al. The effects of respiratory training with inspiratory flow resistive loads in premature infants. Pediatr Res 1992; 31:613–618.
140. Dimitriou G, et al. Synchronous intermittent mandatory ventilation modes compared with patient triggered ventilation during weaning. Arch Dis Child 1995; 72: F188–F190.
141. Veness-Meehan KA, et al. Pulmonary function testing prior to extubation in infants with respiratory distress syndrome. Pediatr Pulmonol 1990; 9:2–6.
142. So BH, et al. Application of nasal continuous positive airway pressure to early extubation in very low birthweight infants. Arch Dis Child 1995; 72:F191–F193.
143. Annibale DJ, et al. Randomized, controlled trial of nasopharyngeal continuous positive airway pressure in the extubation of very low birth weight infants. J Pediatr 1994; 124:455–460.
144. Chernick V. Continuous negative chest wall pressure therapy for hyaline membrane disease. Pediatr Clin North Am 1973; 20:407–417.
145. Outerbridge EW, et al. Continuous negative pressure in the management of severe respiratory distress syndrome. J Pediatr 1972; 81:384–391.
146. Samuels MP, Southall DP. Negative extrathoracic pressure in treatment of respiratory failure in infants and young children. Br Med J 1989; 299:1253–1257.
147. Samuels MP, et al. Continuous negative extrathoracic pressure in neonatal respiratory failure. Pediatrics 1996; 98:1154–1160.
148. Mockrin LD, Bancalari EH. Early versus delayed initiation of continuous negative pressure in infants with hyaline membrane disease. Anesthesiology 1975; 87:596–600.
149. Monin PJP, et al. Assisted ventilation in the neonate—comparison between positive and negative respirators. Pediatr Res 1976; 10:464.
150. Cvetnic WG, et al. Reintroduction of continuous negative pressure ventilation in neonates: two year experience. Pediatr Pulmonol 1990; 8:245–253.
151. Zidulka A, et al. Ventilation by high-frequency chest wall compression in dogs with normal lungs. Am Rev Respir Dis 1983; 127:709–713.
152. Harf A, et al. Ventilation by high-frequency oscillation of thorax or trachea in rats. J Appl Physiol 1984; 56:155–160.
153. al-Saady NM, et al. External high frequency oscillation in normal subjects and in patients with acute respiratory failure. Anaesthesia 1995; 50:1031–1035.
154. Chartrand DA, et al. Lung and chest wall mechanics in rabbits during high-frequency body-surface oscillation. J Appl Physiol 1990; 68:1722–1726.

155. Coalson JJ, et al. Pathophysiologic, morphometric, and biochemical studies of the premature baboon with bronchopulmonary dysplasia. Am Rev Respir Dis 1992; 145:872–881.
156. Coalson JJ, et al. Decreased alveolarization in baboon survivors with bronchopulmonary dysplasia. Am J Respir Crit Care Med 1995; 152:640–646.
157. Coalson JJ. Experimental models of bronchopulmonary dysplasia. Biol Neonate 1997; 71:35–38.
158. Jackson JC, et al. Reduction in lung injury after combined surfactant and high-frequency ventilation. Am J Dis Child 1994; 124:646–649.

10

Effect of Respiratory Care Practices on the Development of Bronchopulmonary Dysplasia

MICHAEL R. GOMEZ

Santa Rosa Children's Hospital
San Antonio, Texas

THOMAS N. HANSEN

Ohio State University
and Children's Hospital
Columbus, Ohio

I. Introduction

Some reports in the literature have suggested that endotracheal intubation may increase the risk for chronic lung disease (CLD) in preterm infants. Stern and co-workers noted that bronchopulmonary dysplasia (BPD) was rare in infants ventilated using negative-pressure respirators and concluded that, in addition to exposure to high oxygen, chronic lung disease in infants required exposure to positive pressure or an endotracheal tube (1). More recently, in a retrospective study of nursery practices, Avery and co-workers found that the incidence of chronic lung disease appeared to be lowest in intensive care units that relied on nasal application of continuous positive airway pressure (NCPAP), rather than endotracheal intubation (2). Although there are multiple ways in which endotracheal intubation might contribute to chronic lung disease in infants, this chapter will concentrate on two:

1. Interference with normal warming and humidification of inspired gas by the nose and upper pharynx
2. Increased risk of aspiration

Because there is a considerable amount of information about the first of these, warming and humidifying inspired gas, much of this chapter focuses on this important issue.

II. Gas Temperature and Humidity

Endotracheal intubation bypasses the normal heating and humidifying functions of the nasopharynx. This section will discuss how the nasopharynx carries out these functions and what the effect of bypassing the nasopharynx might be.

A. Background

Definitions of Important Terms

Humidity is water in the form of its individual molecules in the gaseous state and, as such, can be expressed in terms of a partial pressure. As with any gas, the partial pressure of water in its gaseous state increases with increasing temperature (Fig. 1; 3). The *absolute humidity* of a mixture of gases is expressed as weight of water per unit volume of gas (most commonly mgH_2O/L gas). Absolute humidity is measured by extracting all of the water from a given volume of gas and measuring the weight of the water removed. The partial pressure of water

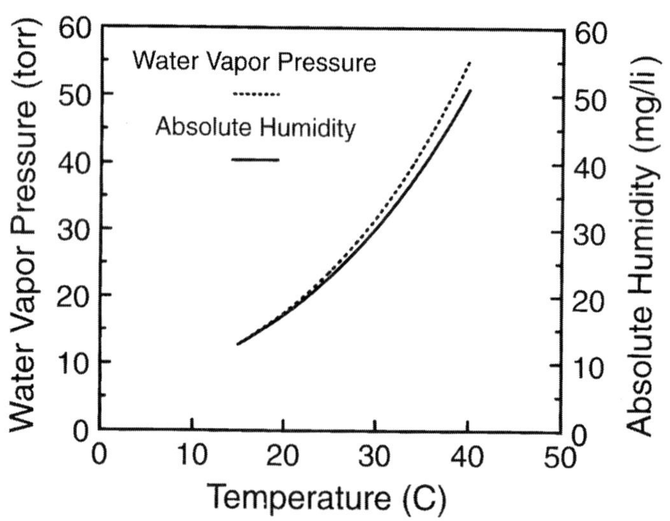

Figure 1 Vapor pressure and absolute humidity of gas fully saturated with water. (Data from Ref. 3.)

vapor increases with increasing temperature. Therefore, if sufficient water is available to a mixture of gases, the water content (absolute humidity) of that mixture will increase as temperature increases. The maximum amount of water that a mixture of gases can hold at any given temperature (maximum capacity) is calculated from tables or graphs (see Fig. 1) relating water vapor pressure to temperature:

$$\text{Maximum capacity} = P_{H_2O} \cdot T^{-1} \cdot 288 \text{ mg} \cdot \text{K} \cdot \text{Torr}^{-1} \cdot \text{L}^{-1} \quad (1)$$

where T is the gas temperature in degrees Kelvin (K), P_{H_2O} is the vapor pressure of water in torr at that temperature and the constant (288 mg $\cdot$ K$\cdot$torr^{-1} $\cdot$ L^{-1}) converts pressure per Kelvin to mgH_2O/L gas.

The water content of a gas is commonly expressed as *relative humidity*, the actual water content of a gas divided by the maximum capacity at that temperature:

$$\text{Relative humidity} = \text{absolute humidity} \cdot \text{maximum capacity}^{-1} \cdot 100\% \quad (2)$$

In many of the studies reviewed in this chapter, relative humidity is measured using a hygrometer, and absolute humidity (AH) is calculated from Eqs. (1) and (2) as:

$$\begin{aligned} \text{Absolute humidity} &= \text{relative humidity} \cdot P_{H_2O} \cdot T^{-1} \cdot 100\%^{-1} \\ &\quad \times 288 \text{ mg} \cdot \text{K} \cdot \text{torr}^{-1} \cdot \text{L}^{-1} \end{aligned} \quad (3)$$

An *aerosol* is a mixture of extremely small particles and gas. The particles may be liquid droplets, or tiny bits of solid material, and are distributed throughout the gas. If water is present in a mixture of gases in its gaseous state, it is termed humidity. However, if water is present in its liquid state in the form of small particles, it is then referred to as an aerosol. Aerosols are produced by nebulizers, devices that shatter water into small particles and mix these small particles into the gas stream.

Warming and Humidifying Inspired Gas During Normal Breathing

The water content and temperature of inspired gas can vary considerably; alveolar gas is fully saturated with water at body temperature (4). The process of heating and humidifying inspired gas is accomplished by the upper and lower airways. During inspiration, the airway epithelium loses heat and water to the inspired gas until the gas reaches a point in the tracheobronchial tree where it is heated to body temperature and is fully saturated with water. This point is referred to as the *isothermal saturation boundary* (ISB). Dery (5) measured inspired and expired gas temperatures and relative humidities at various points in the tracheobronchial tree of adults who had tracheostomies in place before neck irradiation.

Inspired gas temperature and relative humidity increased as the gas moved down the tracheobronchial tree and reached body temperature and a relative humidity of 100% at a point 5 cm below the tracheal bifurcation, thus defined as the ISB (Table 1). McFadden and co-workers (6) used catheters with thermistors imbedded in them to measure temperatures simultaneously at seven different locations from the glottis to the first subsegmental bronchi of adult volunteers (see Table 1). Their results were qualitatively similar to those of Dery, but gas temperatures were 1°–2°C lower at comparable sites in the tracheobronchial tree. The ISB was just distal to the third subsegmental bronchi. These studies showed that increases in minute ventilation and decreases in inspired gas temperature and humidity shifted the ISB more distally in the tracheobronchial tree. In a later study, Dery (4) measured temperature and humidity of alveolar gas in anesthetized, intubated, and ventilated dogs and found that even under conditions of extreme hyperventilation with room air, the ISB remained above the level of the alveolus.

During expiration, gas temperature remains constant until it moves past the ISB, at which point gas temperature progressively decreases as it contacts mucosa that was cooled during inspiration. As the temperature of gas exiting the body is greater than that of gas entering the body, respiration results in a net loss of both heat and water. The specific heat of air is low, and most heat is lost from the respiratory tract as latent heat of vaporization. A normal man breathing room air loses about 10 g of water per hour (5).

Warming and Humidifying Inspired Gas with Endotracheal Intubation

Endotracheal intubation bypasses the nose and upper airway, removes their contribution to heating and humidification of gas, and moves the ISB toward the lung periphery. Dery (5) used a thermistor and a dew-point hygrometer to measure gas temperature and relative humidity at points in the respiratory tract of intubated and ventilated patients (Table 2). The increase in gas temperature and relative humidity occurred at points lower in the tracheobronchial tree than in spontane-

Table 1 Gas Temperature and Relative Humidity at Various Sites in the Respiratory Tract in Spontaneously Breathing Adults

	T°C inspiration Dery (5)	RH (%) Dery (5)	T°C inspiration McFadden (6)	T°C expiration McFadden (6)
Nasopharynx	32	65	—	—
Glottis	33.2	70	32	33
Distal trachea	35.3	88	33	34
Carina	36.8	95	33	34.2
Bronchi	37	100	34.8	35.2

Table 2 Gas Temperature and Relative Humidity at Various Sites in the Respiratory Tract in Intubated Adults

	Inspiratory gas T°C	Relative humidity (%)	Expiratory gas T°C
Endotracheal tube	25	55	29
Distal trachea	32	75	33.2
Carina	33.5	87	33.8
3rd subsegmental bronchi	37	100	37

Source: Ref. 5.

ously breathing adults, and the ISB moved distally to the level of the third subsegmental bronchi. He estimated that the intubated patient breathing dry gas loses roughly 12 g/hr of water—almost all of which must derive from the tracheobronchial tree. If ventilator gas is cold and dry, this problem is amplified. On the other hand, if inspired gas is warmed and humidified, the ISB will move centrally toward the tip of the endotracheal tube.

B. Methods for Altering Inspired Gas Temperature and Humidity

Because of concerns about delivering dry, cold gas to the airways, a number of devices have been developed to both heat and humidify inspired gas in intubated and ventilated neonates (7). These devices can be broadly classified by whether they add only gaseous water to inspired gas, *humidifiers*, or whether they also add particulate water, *nebulizers*.

Humidifiers

The amount of gaseous water that a humidifier can add to a mixture of gases is limited by duration of contact between gas and water, the surface area of the point of contact, and the temperature. The temperature determines the maximum capacity of the gas for accommodating water vapor and, ultimately, determines the absolute humidity that can be delivered. The time of contact between the gas and water and the surface area available for exchange of water vapor determine how much water vapor is transferred to the gas. There are three general types of humidifiers: (1) simple, (2) heated, and (3) heated with heated wire circuits.

Simple Humidifiers. Simple humidifiers (Table 3) do not employ heat, and although some can deliver gas with a relative humidity of 100%, the total amount of water added to inspired gas (AH) is not adequate for intubated patients. For example, calculations show that a simple humidifier operating at 20°C and 100% relative humidity, will deliver only 17 mg of water per liter of gas. Gas

Table 3 Simple Humidifiers

Type	Method of humidification	Efficiency
Pass-over	Gas flows over the surface of the water and then to the patient.	Low
Bubble	Gas flows through a diffuser into water, generating bubbles that increase the surface area for humidification; gas then flows to the patient.	Moderate
Jet	Gas flow produces an aerosol that disperses water particles into the gas stream, increasing the surface area for humidification. Baffles prevent delivery of particulate water to the patient.	High

Source: Ref. 7.

in the distal trachea is normally 100% humidified at a temperature of 34°C and should contain approximately 37 mg of water per liter of inspired gas. The difference in water content must be supplied by the airway epithelium, resulting in loss of heat and water and potential drying of airway secretions.

Heated Humidifiers. Heated humidifiers (Table 4) deliver more water to the airways by heating the inspired gas to increase the total amount of water added to the inspired gas or absolute humidity. The temperature of the gas that is delivered to the patient is regulated by a servodevice that measures gas temperature at the airway and adjusts the heater output of the humidifier.

Table 4 Heated Humidifiers

Type	Method of humidification	Efficiency
Cascade	Gas is forced through a grid that is covered by a film of heated water. The froth that is generated humidifies the stream of gas to the patient. Gas temperature delivered to the patient can be regulated by a servo.	High
Bubble	Gas flows through a diffuser into heated water generating bubbles that increase surface area for humidification. The heated and humidified gas then flows to the patient.	High
Wick	Gas flows past wick (blotting paper or sponge) that remains saturated with water by capillary action. The wick is surrounded by heaters. Wick humidifiers do not bubble gas through water or grids and have a very low resistance to flow.	High

Source: Ref. 7.

Heated Wire Circuits. Gas that is heated and humidified in the humidifier begins to cool as it flows through the ventilator tubing to the patient. Cooling causes the relative humidity of the gas to increase to 100% and gas condenses in the ventilator tubing (*rainout*). Condensation in the ventilator tubing increases the risk of the infant receiving a dump of water from the ventilator circuit and may increase the risk of bacterial contamination (8). Most circuits that are used with neonatal ventilators incorporate heating wires in the inspiratory and expiratory tubing to prevent cooling of gas and associated condensation. The heating wires regulate the gas temperature within the airway, while the humidifier temperature is regulated separately and, depending on the device, can be as much as 3°C lower or higher than the airway temperature. If humidifier temperature is lower than airway temperature, relative humidity will decrease, and there will be less condensation or rainout. If humidifier temperature is greater than airway temperature, relative humidity will exceed 100% and rainout will occur.

Condensing Humidifiers (HME). These humidifiers are placed between the airway adapter and the endotracheal tube, and they function as ''artificial noses'' (9). They provide a large surface for heat and water exchange and usually contain a hygroscopic material. During exhalation gas cools as it passes through the HME, water condenses on the internal surfaces, and the surfaces are heated by the latent heat released as the water vapor condenses. During inspiration, water evaporates from these surfaces, inspired gas is humidified, and latent heat of vaporization is released to the gas. Overall these devices can return as much as 70% of expired heat and humidity to inspired gas. Concerns about whether these devices provide adequate humidity for continuously ventilated infants have limited their use in pediatrics (10). Initial concerns about excessive dead space and resistance imposed by these devices appear to be unfounded, for studies have shown that neither dead space nor resistance is greater than with other anesthesia equipment (11).

Nebulizers

Nebulizers generate aerosols and can produce inspired gas humidities at or above 100%. They may increase the risk of infection, however (12,13), or as we will discuss later, they may contribute to additional ling injury.

Most nebulizers use Bernoulli's principle of lowering the lateral pressure around a jet of gas. Gas is forced through a jet creating a negative pressure at the orifice of a capillary tube that draws water from a reservoir into the jet stream, where it is shattered into small particles. Nebulizers may contain a baffle to reduce the size of the particles that enter the gas stream. The reservoir may be heated to increase the temperature of the aerosolized water.

Ultrasonic nebulizers use sound waves to break water into small particles that enter the inspired gas stream. These nebulizers produce very small particles, approximately 3–6 μm in diameter, and are very effective at delivering particulate water to the airways, thereby increasing the risk of water intoxication.

C. Consequences of Altering Inspired Gas Temperature and Humidity

Ventilation with Gases with Low Temperature and Humidity

If the upper airway has been bypassed, the inspired gas must be heated and humidified before delivery. If this is not accomplished, the difference in heat and water content must be supplied by the airway epithelium, resulting in loss of both heat and water, and potential drying of airway secretions (7). Over the last 30 years several adverse consequences of ventilation with gas at low temperature and humidity have been described.

Loss of Heat

The specific heat of inspired gas is low, so that most of the heat that is lost by the respiratory tract is lost as latent heat of vaporization, as water leaves the respiratory epithelium to humidify the inspired gas. Ventilation of rabbits with dry gas for 6 hr resulted in a 2% decrease in body weight and 4°C decrease in rectal temperature, whereas ventilation with saturated gas at 22°C resulted in no weight loss and only a 2°C decrease in rectal temperature (14). In human infants undergoing major operations, those who were ventilated with dry gas had an average rectal temperature 1.2°C lower than those infants who were ventilated with fully saturated gases (15). It has been estimated that 33% of basal heat production in neonates may be required to heat and humidify dry inspired gases (14).

Loss of Water and Airway Plugging

Water lost to humidify inspired gas comes from moisture lining the respiratory epithelium and from secretions in the endotracheal tube. In dogs, a decrease in the humidity of inspired gas results in increased osmolality of tracheal mucus, increased viscosity of secretions, and plugging of airways (16). Theoretically, these thick secretions could also lead to plugging of mucus-secreting glands and decreased secretion of mucus. In neonates undergoing major surgical operations, postoperative atelectasis was more common in those infants who were ventilated with dry anesthetic gases than in those who were ventilated with humidified gases (15). Such atelectasis might derive from mucus-plugging of airways.

Impaired Mucociliary Clearance

Ventilation with dry gas substantially decreases mucociliary clearance. Burton (17) measured the rate of clearance of India ink placed on the mucus layer of the trachea of anesthetized dogs and found that 3–5 hr of ventilation with dry anesthesia gas (19°C, absolute humidity [AH] < 5 mg H_2O/L) grossly reduced mucociliary clearance. This effect was prevented by ventilation with anesthesia gas that was fully saturated (AH, 39–44 mgH_2O/L) and heated to 35–37°C. Baetjer and co-workers (18) measured the rate of clearance of Na^{131} I droplets injected into the lower trachea of chicks and found greater rates of clearance when ventilation was provided with warm moist air (temperature 35°C, AH 37 mgH_2O/L), rather than cold, dry air (temperature 4°C, AH <5 mgH_2O/L). In similar experiments, Forbes (19) measured the clearance of lycopodium powder from the tracheal epithelium of intubated greyhounds that breathed air at 37°C. Breathing air at relative humidities of 75 and 100% (AH 33 and 44 mgH_2O/L, respectively) had no effect on tracheal mucus flow, whereas decreasing humidity to 50% and 25% (AH 22 and 11 mgH_2O/L, respectively) caused flow to cease within 30 min in the majority of animals. Fonkalsrud and co-workers (20) intubated dogs with double-lumen Carlen's tubes to ventilate the left lung with gas at 37°C that was humidified to 100% (AH, 44 mgH_2O/L) or 130% (AH, 56.8 mgH_2O/L) and to simultaneously ventilate the right lung with gas at 20°C and 20% relative humidity (AH, 3.9 mgH_2O/L). The rate of clearance of tantalum dust remained near normal in the left lung during the 6-hr experiment, but particle clearance was markedly reduced in the right lung. Mucus secretions in the right lung were described as profuse and voluminous. Finally, Hirsch and colleagues (21) measured the movement of Teflon disks up the trachea in dogs that breathed air that was 100% humidified and heated to 38°C (AH, 46 mgH_2O/L) for 4 hr versus air that was dried and at room temperature 23°C (AH, <5 mgH_2O/L). Breathing dry air decreased tracheal mucus velocity by 50% after 1 hr and to near zero after 3 hr. Rehumidification restored mucus velocity to about 50% of control.

Damage to Airways

The reduction in mucociliary clearance results, at least in part, from injury of ciliated cells, with subsequent loss of function. After 6 hr of ventilation with dry gas, scanning electron microscopy reveals granular, stringy material clinging to individual cilia, and is associated with matting and tangling of cilia and the development of pores on the cilia rug (20). Chalon and associates (22) found that ciliated epithelial cells that were recovered by bronchoalveolar lavage (BAL) from adult patients who were undergoing general anesthesia were extensively damaged by ventilation with dry gas at 22–26°C (AH = 0). Cell injury included damage to endplates, loss of the nuclear chromatin network and nuclear pyknocytosis. Patients who were ventilated with gas at 22–26°C and 60% relative humidity (AH, 19–24 mgH_2O/L) or fully saturated gas at 37°C (AH = 44 mgH_2O/L) had no evidence of injury to ciliated cells. Studies using isolated tracheobronchial trees from adult rats found that at a constant temperature of 37°C, changes in absolute humidity markedly affected ciliary beat frequency (23). Water contents above 24 mgH_2O/L had no effect, whereas exposure to AH of 8.77 $mgH_2O/$

L for 1 min decreased beat frequency by 35%. This decrease was reversible if the exposure time was 1 min, but it was irreversible if exposure time was increased to 8 min. Exposure to an absolute humidity of 2.19 mgH_2O/L for 30 sec resulted in an 80% reduction in beat frequency that was reversible, whereas exposure for 2–5 min resulted in irreversible ciliostasis.

Ventilation of dogs with cold dry gas for as little as 3 hr may result in acute inflammatory changes in the airways, including ulceration and erosion of the tracheal epithelium, with leukocyte infiltration into the lamina propria (21). These lesions were not ameliorated by rehumidification. In similar studies, ventilation of rabbits with dry anesthetic gas slowed clearance of secretions and caused destruction of cilia and mucus glands. In addition, the epithelium was disorganized and flattened, and the basement membranes were disorganized, leading to loss of elasticity and ultimate collapse of bronchioles. Finally, there was desquamation of cells into the lumen and ulceration of the epithelium, with debris demonstrable in the airways for as long as 3 weeks. Ventilation with gases fully saturated with water at 22°C (AH, 19 mgH_2O/L) prevented all of these changes (14). In studies of intubated lambs that received continuous positive airway pressure breathing, conventional mechanical ventilation, or high-frequency ventilation for 6 hr, the major determinant of lung injury was relative humidity of inspired gas (24). Lambs that breathed gas at 36°C and a relative humidity of 90% (AH, 37.0 mgH_2O/L) had little injury to the airway, whereas lambs that breathed gas at 36°C and 30% relative humidity (AH, 12.5 mgH_2O/L) had marked tracheal damage 5 mm below the tip of the endotracheal tube. This included severe erosion, blistering and necrosis of the tracheal epithelium.

Ventilation with dry gas even for relatively short time periods can affect measurements of lung function. Minute ventilation and oxygen uptake were both reduced in dog lungs that were ventilated with dry gas for 6 hr (20), and ventilation with dry air (AH, 3.1 mgH_2O/L) for 5 hr decreased static lung compliance by 25% (25). These studies found different effects on surfactant function: one noted no effect and concluded that the changes in lung function were the result of atelectasis (25), whereas the other study found that ventilation with dry gas impaired surfactant function (20).

Studies in Ventilated Infants

Two groups of investigators have reported that ventilation of human infants with gas that is cold or dry may result in lung injury. Tarnow-Mordi and co-workers (26) analyzed 3705 measurements of inspired gas temperature in 149 ventilated infants during the first 96 hr after birth. In their study, all infants were ventilated with a standard ventilator, and inspired gas was humidified using a wick type heated humidifier. Infants were divided into two groups, based on temperature of the inspired gas measured at the proximal airway: 34.5°–36.5°C and 36.6°–37.6°C. There was no difference in mortality between groups. Among infants weighing less than 1500 g ($n = 88$), however, those who breathed gas at higher temperature had less respiratory morbidity than those who breathed gas at lower temperature (Table 5).

In another study of ventilator-dependent preterm infants (27), ventilation for 10 min with gas at 24°C and 50% relative humidity (AH, 11.5 mgH_2O/Liter) resulted in a 50% increase in the resistive work of breathing. In infants with BPD, cold air (0°–5°C) administered by face mask increased total pulmonary resistance by 77% (28).

Studies of infants who were ventilated with high-frequency jet ventilators (HFJV) examined the effects of dry gas ventilation on the development of necrotizing tracheobronchitis (NTB; 29,30). NTB is characterized by necrosis of the tracheal mucosa, resulting in airway obstruction caused by sloughed mucosal cells and mucus (31–35). It is difficult to adequately humidify the pulsed jet that is delivered with HFJV, and inadequate humidification is likely to contribute to the development of NTB (30,36–38). In several studies with animals HFJV resulted in tracheal injury when only the entrained gas was humidified; this injury was reduced by also humidifying the pulsed jet of gas (39,40). It is not surprising, therefore, that NTB was reported initially in neonates who were ventilated with HFJV with humidification of only the entrained gas (29,30). Although adequate humidification of inspired gas probably does play a role in NTB, recent data suggest that pressure-induced tracheal ischemia also contributes to this injury (41,42).

Ventilation with Gases with High Temperature and Humidity

Gas delivered to the airway at excessive temperature and water content also can produce injury, especially if the gas contains particles of water (aerosols). Exposure to aerosolized saline for 72 hr resulted in severe bronchopneumonia in puppies (43). In intubated, anesthetized, spontaneously breathing rats, exposure to gas containing nebulized water at contents above 15 mgH_2O/Liter resulted in a progressive increase in airway resistance (44), presumably secondary to mucosal

Table 5 Respiratory Morbidity in Infants <1500 g Ventilated with Different Inspired Gas Temperatures

Group	n	Deaths	Pneumothorax	F_{IO_2} at 29 days
34.5–36.5°C	28	27%	43%	37 ± 21
36.6–37.6°C	60	16%	13%	28 ± 9
p value		NS	0.006	0.001

Source: Ref. 26.

swelling, accumulation of mucus, and ciliary dysfunction that led to narrowing of airway diameter.

To determine the most appropriate water content for inspired gas Noguchi and co-workers (45) measured alveolar ventilation, functional residual capacity (FRC), lung compliance, alveolar–arterial (A–a)Po_2 difference, pulmonary shunt ratio, cardiac output, and oxygen consumption in tracheotomized adult dogs that breathed dry air (RH 40%) at 15°C, followed by fully saturated air that was delivered at temperatures between 20° and 40°C (Table 6). FRC and lung compliance appeared optimal when inspired gas temperature was between 25° and 35°C (AH, 22–30 mgH_2O/L air). As temperature increased above 35°C (AH greater than 39 mgH_2O/L air) or below 20°C (AH less than 17 mg H_2O/L air), FRC and lung compliance decreased significantly. Their results suggested that satisfactory lung function could be maintained in adult dogs by delivering fully saturated air between 25° and 30°C. Their finding that lung function decreased as AH decreased is not surprising, but the finding that lung function also declined with temperatures above 35°C was unexpected and may relate to the design of their bubble humidifier, which did not eliminate the possibility of particulate water entering the airway.

Tsuda and co-workers (46) determined the optimal inspired gas temperature and humidity for 32 anesthetized adult dogs that breathed dry air (15°C and RH <40%) or fully saturated air at 25°–40°C for 6 hr through a tracheotomy. Airway histology was normal in the two groups that breathed air at 25° and 30°C (AH, 23 and 30 mgH_2O/L), but histology was distinctly abnormal in all other groups. For those that breathed dry air, cilia in the trachea were matted, twisted, and stuck together. For those that breathed air at 35° and 40°C (AH, 40 and 51 mgH_2O/L), the regular array of cilia in secondary and tertiary bronchi was also disrupted, with apparent adhesion and matting of cilia. In addition, the dogs that breathed either dry gas or fully saturated gas at 40°C had evidence of surfactant inactiva-

Table 6 Effects of Inspired Gas Temperature and Water Content on Lung Volume (FRC) and Dynamic Lung Compliance

Temperature (°C)	15	20	25	30	35	40
n	8	4	4	4	5	5
AH (mgH_2O/L)	5	17	23	30	40	51
ΔFRC (%)[a]	-27 ± 3^b	-11 ± 5	-2.5 ± 18	5.6 ± 6	-12 ± 2^b	-14 ± 2.3^b
ΔCompliance (%)[a]	-27 ± 4^b	-2.5 ± 3.2	5 ± 1	6 ± 7.3	-7.2 ± 2.3^b	-13 ± 4.4^b

[a]Calculated as percentage change (Δ) from baseline after 6 hr.
[b]Different from baseline $p < 0.05$.
AH, absolute humidity.
Source: Ref. 45.

tion. In these experiments, no attempt was made to heat the tubing, so that particulate water may have been present in the inspiratory limb, especially as gas temperature was increased.

The particularly damaging effects of particulate water on the lung were underscored in experiments by John and colleagues (47; Table 7), who ventilated rabbits for 6 hr through a tracheotomy. The inspired gas flowed through a nebulizer at room temperature (22°C), or it was heated to produce a proximal airway temperature of 36°C (cold- and warmed-nebulized groups). In both of these groups of rabbits, particulate water was present in the gas stream. Another group of rabbits was ventilated with air that was nebulized at room temperature and then heated to 36°C (warmed, humidified air). All three groups were compared with rabbits that did not have tracheostomies and that breathed room air spontaneously (controls).

All of the rabbits in the control and warmed humidified groups survived, whereas 9 of 22 rabbits in the nebulized groups died before the end of the study. Animals that received air containing particulate water became hypotensive and acidotic during the course of the experiments, and they had interstitial and intra-alveolar edema at postmortem examination (Fig. 2). Average pulmonary arterial wall thickness was significantly greater in the rabbits that received air containing particulate water than in the control rabbits or the rabbits that received warmed, humidified air. In later experiments, Todd and John (48) studied three different mechanisms for providing humidity to rabbits that had tracheotomies and that were either mechanically ventilated or breathed spontaneously with CPAP:

1. Standard wick-type humidifier, with a heated wire in the inspiratory limb.
2. Standard wick-type humidifier, plus instillation of water into the airway by continuous infusion.
3. Standard wick-type humidifier, with heated wires in the inspiratory and expiratory limbs.

Table 7 Temperature and Water Content of Groups of Rabbits That Were Ventilated with Nebulized or Humidified Air

Gas conditions	Temperature (°C)	Relative humidity[a] (%)	Absolute humidity (mgH_2O/L)
Cold nebulized	22	>120	~31
Warmed nebulized	36	120	50
Warmed humidified	36	75	31

[a]Relative humidity exceeds 100% because of the presence of particulate water in the inspired gas.
Source: Ref. 47.

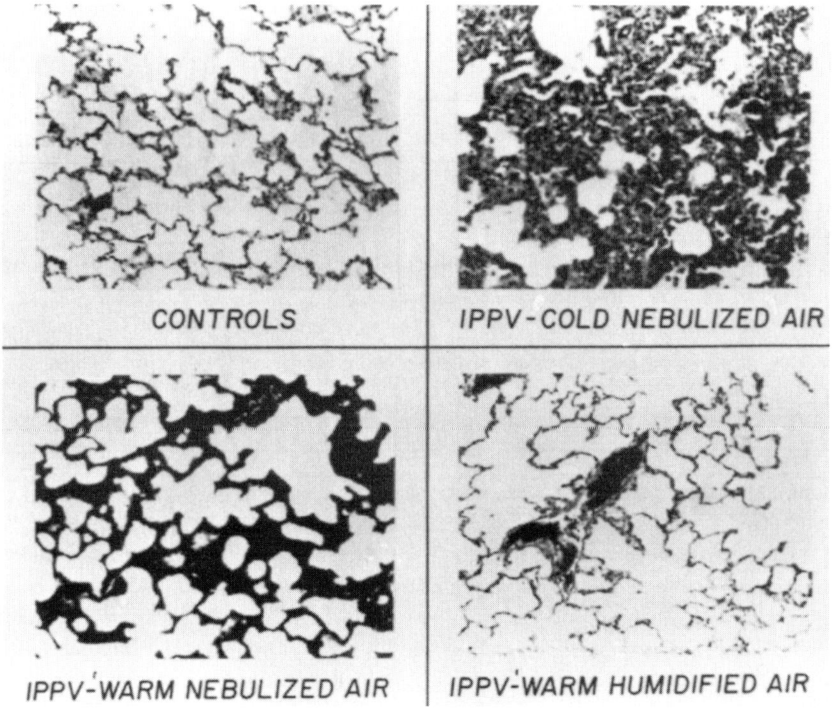

Figure 2 Histological sections of lung obtained from rabbits that were ventilated with different means of gas humidification: Note the interstitial widening after ventilation with warm, nebulized air, and interstitial widening and intra-alveolar edema after ventilation with cold nebulized air. (From Ref. 47.)

In groups 1 and 2, particulate water was always present in the inspiratory limb of the ventilator circuit. In group 3 the humidifier temperature was set 2.5°C lower than airway temperature to prevent condensation in the ventilator tubing. Relative humidity was approximately 86% and absolute humidity was 36 mgH_2O/L. Animals that had water instilled into their airways all had evidence of pulmonary edema at postmortem examination. Rabbits in groups 1 and 2 had structural and ultrastructural lesions that included increased vascular wall thickness, perivascular edema, and increased collagen deposition. In both studies (47,48) the presence of particulate water was associated with the development of lung injury.

In another study that examined airway resistance in humans who breathed air that was passed through an ultrasonic nebulizer containing normal saline, ½ normal saline, or distilled water, for 15 min, airway resistance was increased, and this increase was blocked by prior inhalation of isoproterenol (49). In another study of human volunteers, breathing aerosolized water at AH of >28.8 mgH_2O/L (temperature 30–38°C) doubled specific airway resistance at 6 hr (50). In intubated, neurosurgical patients with normal lungs, 1 hr of breathing gas nebulized at 31°C increased the A–a gradient for oxygen (51). The authors of this study proposed four possible complications of aerosol therapy: (1) swelling of retained secretions, (2) precipitation of bronchospasm, (3) fluid overload, and (4) contamination with other particulate material.

Summary

In summary, ventilation with gas that is too cold or too dry can cause significant lung injury. Likewise, ventilation with gas that is too hot or that contains too much water, especially if that gas contains particulate water (Table 8), can damage the lung.

D. Problems with Delivery of Heated and Humidified Gas

The data showing that ventilation with cold, dry air causes lung damage provides strong rationale for the standard practice of heating and humidifying the inspired gas that is delivered to infants who require mechanical ventilation. The American National Standards Institute (ANSI) requires that inspired gas have an AH of 30 mgH_2O/L if the upper airway has been bypassed, whereas the British Standards Institute requires 33 mgH_2O/L. Despite these recommendations and convincing data showing that gas in the trachea normally is only 33°–35°C at 88% humidity (AH, 31–35 mgH_2O/L), there is a strong sentiment in the literature for delivering inspired gas that is fully saturated at body temperature (37°C and 44 mgH_2O/L; 52). This standard is seldom met. In 1986, a survey of neonatal units in the British Isles found that none of the commonly used humidifiers provided fully to the airways, saturated gas at body temperature, and fewer than half of the units surveyed used humidifiers and settings that provided gas at an absolute humidity of 33 mgH_2O/L (53). In another study, 396 measurements of inspired gas temperature and humidity were made in 14 intubated mechanically ventilated neonates (54). Sixty-three percent of the measurements of absolute humidity were less than 33 mgH_2O/L—the minimum acceptable standard for intubated patients recommended by the British Standards Institution; only two of the measurements yielded values for absolute humidity greater than 40 mgH_2O/L. If inspired gas temperature was 36°C, most of the measurements of AH were more than 33 mgH_2O/L, whereas if gas temperature was 34°C, most of the measurements were less than 33 mgH_2O/L (55). These data indicate that it is very difficult to predict the water content of inspired gas. As noted in the following section, there are several nursery practices that may contribute to this difficulty (56).

Table 8 Effects of Gas Temperature and Humidity on the Lung

Consequences of ventilation with gases with low temperature and humidity	Consequences of ventilation with gases with high temperature and humidity
Studies using animals	
Decrease in core temperature (14,15).	Adhesion and matting of cilia (46)
Drying of airway secretions (7,16)	Severe bronchopneumonia (43)
Endotracheal tube and airway plugging with atelectasis (14,15).	Interstitial and intraalveolar edema (47,48)
Impaired mucociliary clearance (17–21)	Increased pulmonary arterial wall thickness (47,49)
Injury to ciliated epithelial cells (14,20,22,23,46)	Increased mean minimum surface tension (46)
Ulceration and erosion of the trachea (14,21,24)	Increased airway resistance (44)
Impaired surfactant function (20)	Decreased lung volume and compliance (45)
Decreased minute ventilation and oxygen uptake (20)	Hypotension, acidosis, and death (47)
Decreased static lung compliance (25)	
Studies in humans	
Increased incidence of pneumothorax and chronic lung disease (26)	Alveolar flooding with microatelectasis (51)
Increased total pulmonary resistance (27)	Increased airway resistance (49,50)
Necrotizing tracheobronchitis (29,30,36–39)	Increased A–a gradient (51)

Incubators and Radiant Warmers

Management of inspired gas humidity is more complex when infants are ventilated inside incubators or under radiant warmers. If the temperature probe controlling the heated wire circuit is inside the incubator and if the incubator temperature is high (36.5°C), then the temperature in the humidifier and in the heated wire circuit will be lower than the incubator temperature. As a result, the absolute humidity of gas delivered to the infant will be low. Additionally, as the inspired gas is heated within the segment of tubing inside the incubator, the relative humidity may also be low. Locating the temperature probe for the heated wire circuit outside of the incubator alleviates this problem, but if incubator temperature is greater than circuit temperature, relative humidity of the gas delivered to the infant's airway will still be less than expected, based on humidifier and circuit temperatures. Similar phenomena would be expected if the infant were nursed under a radiant warmer and the temperature probe were unshielded.

O'Hagan and co-workers (56) measured inspired gas temperature and humidity in mechanically ventilated infants under a variety of nursery conditions. In their study, gas flow rate and room temperature remained constant. The humidifier temperature probe was located 50 cm from the proximal airway, and for infants who were nursed in incubators, the probe was outside the incubator. For infants nursed on radiant warmers, the probe was not shielded. When incubator temperature was moderate (34.1 ± 1.3°C), absolute humidity varied linearly with humidifier temperature. However, there was considerable scatter in absolute humidity at any given incubator temperature. For a humidifier temperature of 36°C, absolute humidity ranged from 17 to 43 mgH_2O/L. Even when the humidifier temperature was greater than 35°C, absolute humidity was less than 30 mgH_2O/L on 35 of 479 measurements. When incubator temperature was lower (32.9 ± 1.8°C), absolute humidity varied inversely with humidifier temperature. This phenomenon probably occurred because gas was cooled as it entered the tubing in the incubator, with resultant condensation, thereby lowering the absolute water content of the gas. Thus, the final water content of the gas was determined by the incubator, rather than the temperature of the humidifier. Attempts to inhibit condensation by shielding the tubing within the incubator reduced water accumulation within the tubing by about 15%. The inspired gas for infants nursed under radiant warmers had absolute humidities that were less than those for infants who were nursed in isolettes. Presumably this occurred because the radiant warmer heated the unshielded humidifier probe, thereby causing the humidifier temperature and absolute humidity of inspired gas to decrease.

Heated Wires

Condensation of water in the ventilator tubing is an important problem associated with delivery of heated, humidified gas to infants who receive mechanical ventilation. Once gas leaves the humidifier, it loses heat and moisture to the cooler ventilator tubing in the form of condensation or rainout (55). Water in the ventilator tubing may be dumped inadvertently into the patient's airway. This may be a source of particulate water, similar to that described earlier by Todd and Johns (48), or it may act as a reservoir for nosocomial infection (8).

To prevent condensation, manufacturers have placed heating wires inside the ventilator tubing to reduce loss of heat and water to the tubing (55). Although this modification is often effective in preventing condensation, heated circuits make the regulation of inspired gas humidity more complex. If, for example, circuit temperature is greater than humidifier temperature, relative humidity of delivered gas will decrease, and unsaturated gas will be delivered to the airway

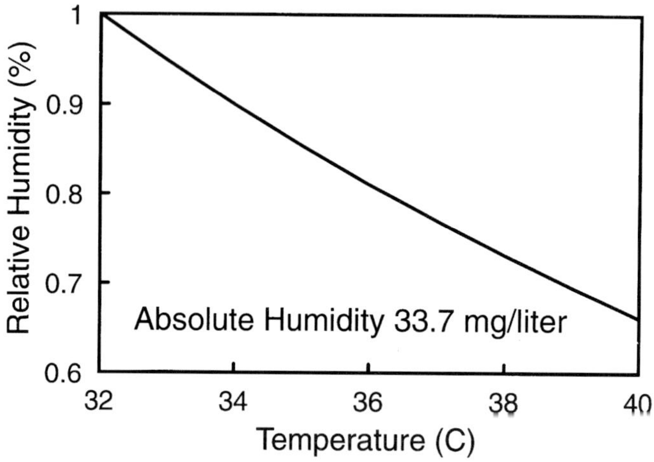

Figure 3 For a constant absolute humidity, relative humidity decreases as inspired gas temperature increases: The graph was plotted using data from Ref. 3 and Eq. (1)–(3) in Section I.

(Fig. 3). As relative humidity is not monitored, this decrease may not be recognized until airway obstruction or some other complication occurs.

Miyao and co-workers (57) noted a greater incidence of endotracheal tube plugging when they used heated wire circuits to prevent condensation of water in the ventilator tubing. Because heated wires often lower relative humidity, they reasoned that relative humidity was important in preventing dry secretions from accumulating in the upper airway and endotracheal tube (Fig. 4).

Miyao and co-workers (57) studied the effects of varying inspired gas temperature on water removal from the upper airway by flowing gas from a humidifier through a simulated trachea (Table 9). Water removal was measured by placing a preweighed wet piece of filter paper in the simulated trachea. When absolute humidity was held constant, more water was removed from the trachea when the inspired gas was heated with heating wires and the relative humidity of the gas was reduced.

Gilmour and associates also measured relative humidity of gases delivered through circuits with and without heating wires (58). They uniformly found that relative humidity was lower in circuits with heated wires than in those without. In their studies, distal circuit temperature was held constant, so humidifier temperature was greater in the circuits without heated wires, and therefore absolute humidity of the gas was also greater in the absence of heating wires.

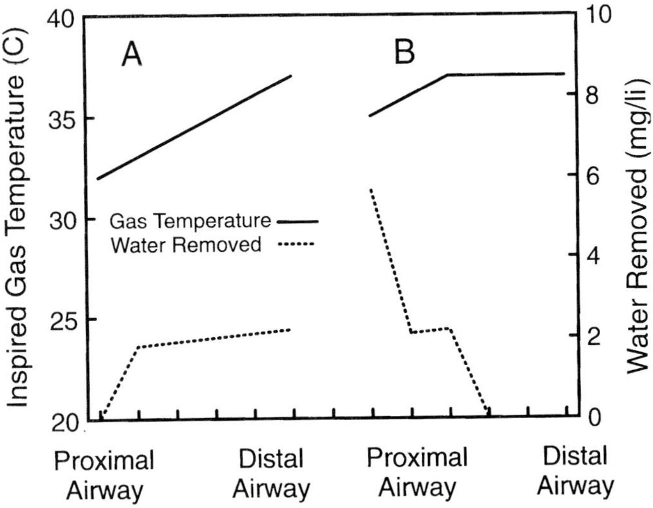

Figure 4 A qualitative model showing the effects of varying inspired gas temperature, hence, relative humidity, on water removal from the airway epithelium when humidifier temperature and absolute humidity remain constant (32°C and 33.7 mgH_2O/L): (A) Inspired gas temperature is 32°C and relative humidity is 100%. As the gas progresses down the tracheobronchial tree it is progressively warmed and humidified until it reaches 100% saturation at body temperature in the distal airways. In this example, water is gradually removed from the respiratory epithelium as the gas temperature gradually increases. Although a total of 10 mgH_2O/L of water is removed from the epithelium, this removal occurs over a relatively large portion of the tracheobronchial tree. (B) Inspired gas temperature is 35°C and relative humidity is 86%. In this instance, the high thermal energy of inspired gas results in removal of a large amount of water from the endotracheal tube and proximal trachea, with distal airways contributing little to the overall humidification of inspired gas. This disproportionate removal of water from the upper trachea and endotracheal tube may result in drying of secretions and secondary airway plugging, or in damage to the tracheal epithelium. (Data from Ref. 57.)

E. Clinical Implications and Future Research

Methods of ventilatory support that do not interfere with the gas humidification and warming functions of the upper airway appear to result in less chronic lung disease than methods that bypass the upper airway (1,2). It is also clear that delivery of inspired gas with too little or too much water can injure the lung. Therefore, it is reasonable to think that delivering inspired gas at an optimum temperature and humidity might decrease the incidence of chronic lung disease

Table 9 Effect of Relative Humidity on Removal of Water from a Simulated Upper Airway

Absolute humidity (mgH_2O/L)	Heating wire	Temperature (°C)	Relative humidity (%)	Water removed (g/30 min)
19	+	35	48	5.9 ± 0.2
19	−	24	87	2.9 ± 0.4

Source: Ref. 57.

in ventilated infants. Unfortunately, the optimum temperature and humidity of inspired gas is not known. Chatburn has suggested the solution of matching the output of any therapeutic gas delivery system to the inspiratory conditions that prevail at the point of entry into the respiratory system (55). For the ventilated infant, this would mean delivering gas at a temperature between 33° and 35°C, with a relative humidity of 88–100% (AH ranging from 31 to 39 mgH_2O/L). Actual delivery of gas at this temperature and humidity is complicated by nursery practices, such as temperature probe placement (inside versus outside the incubator, or on versus off the warmer), and the use of heated wire circuits. Depending on these practices, gas may be delivered with a low relative humidity and result in drying of tracheal secretions, or particulate water may enter the airway and cause additional lung injury. Moreover, the data of Tarnow-Mordi (26) suggest that ventilation of infants with gas temperatures less than 36.6°C increases respiratory morbidity.

Another approach might be to deliver the gas at body temperature fully saturated with water (AH, 44 mgH_2O/L). This would get around the problems associated with drying of secretions throughout the tracheobronchial tree and would eliminate respiratory water loss. Nursery practices, however, pose considerable problems in delivery of gas at this temperature and humidity. In addition, studies with animals suggest that provision of fully saturated gas at temperatures greater than 35°C can cause airway damage.

The solution to this clinical problem demands additional research. Studies should be performed in animals under simulated nursery conditions to determine the optimal temperature and water content for inspired gas. These studies must correlate inspired gas conditions with measurements of lung function and tissue injury. After obtaining this data, a randomized clinical trial should be performed to determine optimum inspired gas temperature and absolute humidity. This trial must measure and control the water content of inspired gas and must control for all of the nursery practices that can affect relative humidity, absolute humidity, and delivery of particular water.

In the meantime, we recommend that inspired gas temperature should be maintained at about 34°–36°C, and that relative humidity should be greater than

90%. In the absence of the ability to measure relative humidity, the gas temperature in the circuit at the level of the patient's airway should be as close to the humidifier temperature as possiblc, for relative humidity decreases by 5% for each degree centigrade that humidifier temperature is below airway temperature (see Fig. 3.).

III. Aspiration

Bypassing the upper airway with an endotracheal tube also may increase the risk of lung injury by increasing the potential for aspiration of oral or gastric secretions.

A. Aspiration in Intubated Infants

Because of size limitations and concerns about airway tissue damage and subsequent tracheal stenosis, the standard of practice in newborn medicine is to manage premature infants with endotracheal tubes that do not fit snugly within the trachea. As a result, the space between the endotracheal tube and the airway of the intubated infant presents a risk for passage of oral or gastric contents into the lungs. A common approach for detecting aspiration in intubated infants is to apply a solution of Evans blue dye to the back of the tongue and then look for blue staining of secretions suctioned from the endotracheal tube. Among the first to apply this technique to infants and children were Browning and Graves, who noted that infants and young children who were intubated with uncuffed endotracheal tubes had an incidence of aspiration of 77% (59). They noted that infants with suspected aspiration became agitated soon after dye was applied. Goitein and co-workers noted a much lower incidence of aspiration (16%) in a similar study, but found that the risk of aspiration increased as age decreased (60). They noted that one-third of episodes of aspiration were accompanied by a decrease in oxygenation. Finally, Goodwin and co-workers recovered blue dye from the tracheal secretions of 16 of 20 preterm infants within 10 min of intraoral instillation (61). They also noted a small, but significant, decrease in arterial oxygenation in the infants who aspirated dye. In premature baboons that are continuously ventilated and subsequently acquire BPD, the progression to lower airway infection consistently begins with colonization of the upper airways, an observation that led these investigators to conclude that aspiration of infected upper airway secretions plays a major role in nosocomial pulmonary infections (62).

Contamination of lower airways by upper airway secretions is also being recognized as a problem during mechanical ventilation of adults. In one study, an intracuff pressure in the endotracheal tube of less than 20 cmH_2O yielded a fourfold increase in the risk of nosocomial pneumonia (63). These authors concluded that leakage of colonized subglottic secretions around the cuff of the endotracheal tube is the most important risk factor for pneumonia during the first 8 days of intubation and mechanical ventilation.

B. Lung Injury Secondary to Aspiration

Evidence That Repeated Aspiration Leads to Lung Injury

Animal Studies. Injection of gastric juice, hydrochloric acid, pepsin, or steapsin into the lungs of rabbits produces three distinct patterns of lung injury: an acute fatal pulmonary edema, a subacute hemorrhagic pneumonia, and chronic lung injury with interstitial fibrosis and areas of emphysema, bronchiolar regeneration, and vasculitis. The latter pattern of injury is quite similar to that noted in infants with stage 4 BPD. The first pattern of lung injury has been reproduced by instilling 0.1 N hydrochloric acid (2 mL/kg) into the lungs of dogs (64,65). This acute, florid pulmonary edema is secondary to damage to the alveolar–capillary membrane, and in some respects is similar to the lesion noted by Jefferies and co-workers (66).

Clinical Studies. In studies of adult humans with fibrotic lung disease, Mays and Dubois (1976) noted that the incidence of hiatal hernia and demonstrable gastroesophageal reflux was much higher in patients with idiopathic pulmonary fibrosis than in controls or in patients with pulmonary fibrosis from known causes (Table 10; 67). They concluded that chronic reflux may play a role in idiopathic pulmonary fibrosis.

Older children with recurrent pneumonia, bronchitis, and asthma frequently have gastroesophageal reflux (68–71) and often show dramatic symptomatic improvement with medical or surgical treatment of their reflux (69,70).

Relation Between Chronic Aspiration and BPD

Herbst and co-workers identified 14 oxygen-dependent infants who were less than 4 weeks old and had chest radiographs compatible with BPD. These infants

Table 10 Incidence of Gastroesophageal Reflux Complicating Pulmonary Fibrosis in Adults

		Hiatal hernia		Reflux	
Underlying disorders	*N*	No.	%	No.	%
Controls	270	76	28	23	9
Idiopathic pulmonary fibrosis	48	41	85	26	54
Immune-mediated pulmonary fibrosis	15	5	33	4	27
Pulmonary fibrosis, other causes	23	11	48	5	22

had recurrent apnea and evidence of chronic reflux by barium swallow and esophageal pH testing. Antireflux treatment decreased the number of episodes of apnea and resulted in a prompt reduction in oxygen requirement. In many cases, there was also gradual improvement in their chest radiographs (72). These results led Herbst to conclude in a later review that the respiratory symptoms and radiographic changes associated with gastroesophageal reflux in premature infants closely mimic the changes seen in BPD (73). Giuffre and co-workers reported on nine ventilator-dependent infants with BPD and gastroesophageal reflux. Symptoms of BPD improved markedly in seven of the nine after surgical interventions to inhibit reflux.

C. Prevention of Aspiration

If aspiration around the endotracheal tube plays a role in the development of BPD, there are two possible solutions to the problem: (1) extubate the infant earlier, perhaps using other forms of positive airway pressure support, such as nasal CPAP, or (2) develop a safe endotracheal tube that protects the airway from aspiration.

Nasal CPAP

Since the paper by Avery and associates described a lower incidence of chronic lung disease in a center relying extensively on nasal CPAP rather than endotracheal intubation (2), there has been considerable interest in the role of nasal CPAP in facilitating early weaning of infants from endotracheal intubation, or in eliminating the need for intubation. Several studies have examined the use of nasal CPAP in promoting early extubation.

Higgens and co-workers (74) found that for infants with respiratory distress syndrome who weighed less than 1000 g, the success rate for extubation was 76% when infants were extubated to nasal CPAP, compared with 21% when they were extubated without immediate application of CPAP. Their results were similar to those of Engelke and colleagues (75), who found that nasal CPAP facilitated extubation in somewhat larger infants recovering from respiratory distress syndrome. In contrast, Annibale and co-workers (76) found no advantage from extubation to nasal CPAP compared with extubation to oxygen alone in a group of infants who weighed between 600 and 1500 g. In their study, however, most of the infants received surfactant replacement, and not all infants had respiratory distress syndrome. Hence, the average age at time of extubation was considerably less than that noted in the study by Higgens et al. (74). It is noteworthy that the success rate of extubation to oxygen alone among infants who weighed less than 1000 g (47%) was less than that noted by Higgens et al. for extubation to nasal CPAP (76%) in infants of similar size. It is also of interest that the two studies used different techniques for the application of continuous positive airway pressure. Annibale and associates used a single nasopharyngeal tube, whereas Higgens and co-workers used nasal prongs. As a result, the resistance to gas flow may have been greater in the study of Annibale. As both studies used roughly the same amount of positive airway pressure (6 cmH_2O), the delivered pressure to the posterior pharynx may have been greater in the Higgens trial, perhaps accounting for the difference in effectiveness. This potential difference emphasizes the importance of titrating the level of nasal CPAP to the patient's clinical status.

Subsequent to the report by Avery (2), another study has suggested that it is possible to manage small preterm infants ($<$1500 g) with nasal CPAP alone (77). In this study, 80% of infants were eventually discharged home, and none acquired BPD. These results seemed compelling, but as Roberton pointed out in an accompanying editorial (78), the population studied was fundamentally healthy, with a low incidence of asphyxia and a high incidence of antenatal corticosteroid use to prevent respiratory distress syndrome. In this era of increased use of antenatal corticosteroids and surfactant prophylaxis to prevent hyaline membrane disease, however, there is growing interest in the potential use of nasal CPAP after administration of surfactant. It is important to remember that even if early CPAP is effective in reducing the risk of BPD, loss of ventilatory control and subsequent apnea might increase other complications of prematurity, such as intraventricular hemorrhage (78), or even overall mortality (79).

Redesigned Endotracheal Tube

Recently, Kolobow and co-workers (80) designed an endotracheal tube, using the same wire reinforcement technologies that have allowed the development of nonkinking catheters with thin walls for use in extracorporeal membrane oxygenation. The wall thickness of these tubes is considerably less than the wall thickness of conventional endotracheal tubes. Thus, the resistance to gas flow through these tubes is less when compared with conventional tubes of similar external diameters. These tubes also may incorporate flexible plastic "gills" that collapse as the tube is inserted or withdrawn, but that expand in the presence of a positive airway pressure to seal the airway and prevent leak around the tube while minimizing pressure applied to the walls of the trachea. Whether these tubes could prevent aspiration in intubated infants and reduce the chance of lung injury remains to be determined.

IV. Conclusions

There is strong evidence that both temperature and humidity of inspired gas are important factors in respiratory management of preterm infants. Ventilation with gas that is cold and dry clearly results in significant lung injury, as does ventilation with gas containing particulate water. To further complicate matters, the published data about the upper limit for inspired gas temperature are confusing and somewhat contradictory. More research is needed before optimal conditions for inspired gas temperature and humidity can be defined.

Likewise, the potential for aspiration of upper airway and gastric contents into the lungs of intubated infants is an important concern. The role that aspiration plays in the genesis of chronic lung disease in premature infants, however, is unclear. With the widespread use of antenatal corticosteroids and surfactant prophylaxis, studies should be performed to determine whether long-term intubation and ventilation is still necessary for most small preterm infants. In addition, redesigned endotracheal tubes may help lower the risk of aspiration and perhaps of chronic lung disease in those infants who are receiving mechanical ventilation.

References

1. Stern L, et al. Negative pressure artificial respiration: use in treatment of respiratory failure of the newborn. Can Med Assoc J 1970; 102:595–601.
2. Avery ME, et al. Is chronic lung disease in low birth weight infants preventable: a survey of eight centers. Pediatrics 1987; 79:26–30.
3. Handbook of Chemistry and Physics. 41st ed. Cleveland: Chemical Rubber, 1960: 2327.
4. Dery R. Humidity in anesthesiology IV: determination of the alveolar humidity and temperature in the dog. Can Anaesth Soc J 1971; 18:145–151.
5. Dery R. The evolution of heat and moisture in the respiratory tract during anaesthesia with a non-rebreathing system. Can Anaesth Soc J 1973; 20:296–309.
6. McFadden ER, et al. Thermal mapping of the airways in humans. J Appl Physiol 1985; 58:564–570.
7. McPherson SP, Spearman CB. Humidifiers and nebulizers. In: Respiratory Therapy Equipment. 3rd ed. St Louis: CV Mosby, 1985:119–162.
8. Craven DE, et al. Contaminated condensate in mechanical ventilator circuits. Am Rev Respir Dis 1984; 129:625–628.
9. Heat and Moisture Exchangers. Emergency Care Research Institute, 1983:155–167.
10. Hanssler L, et al. Membrane humidification—a new method for humidification of respiratory gases in ventilator treatment of neonates. Arch Dis Child 1992; 67:1182–1184.
11. Wilkinson KA, et al. Assessment of a hygroscopic heat and moisture exchanger for paediatric use. Anaesthesia 1991; 46:296–299.
12. Pierce AK, Sanford JP. Bacterial contamination of aerosols. Arch Intern Med 1973; 131:156–9.
13. Vesley D, et al. Bacterial output from three respiratory therapy humidifying devices. Respir Care 1979; 24:228–234.
14. Marfatia S, et al. Effect of dry and humidified gases on the respiratory epithelium of rabbits. J Pediatr Surg 1975; 10:583–592.

15. Fonkalsrud EW, et al. Reduction of operative heat loss and pulmonary secretions in neonates by use of heated and humidified anesthetic gases. J Thorac Cardiovasc Surg 1980; 80:718–723.
16. Man SFP, et al. Effects of temperature, relative humidity, and mode of breathing on canine airway secretions. J Appl Physiol 1979; 46:205–210.
17. Burton JDK. Effects of dry anaesthetic gases on the respiratory mucous membrane. Lancet 1962; 1:235–238.
18. Baetjer AM. Effect of ambient temperature and vapor pressure on cilia–mucus clearance rate. J Appl Physiol 1967; 23:498–504.
19. Forbes AR. Humidification and mucus flow in the intubated trachea. Br J Anaesth 1973; 45:874–878.
20. Fonkalsrud EW, et al. A comparative study of the effects of dry vs. humidified ventilation on canine lungs. Surgery 1975; 78:373–380.
21. Hirsch JA, et al. Effects of dry air and subsequent humidification on tracheal mucous velocity in dogs. J Appl Physiol 1975; 39:242–246.
22. Chalon J, et al. Effects of dry anesthetic gases on tracheobronchial ciliated epithelium. Anesthesiology 1972; 37:338–343.
23. Horstmann G, et al. Influence of temperature and decreased water content of inspired air on the ciliated bronchial epithelium: a physiological and electron microscopical study. Acta Otolaryngol 1977; 84:124–131.
24. Todd DA, et al. Tracheal damage following conventional and high-frequency ventilation at low and high humidity. Crit Care Med 1991; 19:1310–1316.
25. Rashad K, et al. Effect of humidification of anesthetic gases on static compliance. Anesth Analg 1967; 46:127–133.
26. Tarnow-Mordi WO, et al. Low inspired gas temperature and respiratory complications in very low birth weight infants. J Pediatr 1989; 114:438–442.
27. Greenspan JS, et al. Airway responsiveness to low inspired gas temperature in preterm neonates. J Pediatr 1991; 118:443–445.
28. Greenspan JS, et al. Airway reactivity as determined by a cold air challenge in infants with bronchopulmonary dysplasia. J Pediatr 1989; 114:452–454.
29. Pokora T, et al. Neonatal high-frequency jet ventilation. Pediatrics 1983; 72:27–32.
30. Carlon GC, et al. Clinical experience with high frequency jet ventilation. Crit Care Med 1981; 9:1–6.
31. Pietsch JB, et al. Necrotizing tracheobronchitis: a new indication for emergency bronchoscopy in the neonate. J Pediatr Surg 1985; 20:391–393.
32. Kirpalani H, et al. Necrotizing tracheobronchitis. Pediatrics 1986; 78:1167–1168.
33. Kirpalani H, et al. Diagnosis and therapy of necrotizing tracheobronchitis in ventilated neonates. Crit Care Med 1985; 13:792–797.
34. Mimouni F, et al. Necrotizing tracheobronchitis: case report. Pediatrics 1986; 77: 366–368.
35. Metlay LA, et al. A new iatrogenous lesion in newborns requiring assisted ventilation. N Engl J Med 1983; 309:111–112.
36. Boros SJ, et al. Necrotizing tracheobronchitis: a complication of high-frequency ventilation. J Pediatr 1986; 109:95–100.
37. Froese AB, Bryan AC. High frequency ventilation. Am Rev Respir Dis 1987; 135: 1363–1374.

38. Clark RH. High frequency ventilation. J Pediatr 1994; 124:661–670.
39. Ophoven JP, et al. Tracheobronchial histopathology associated with high-frequency jet ventilation. Crit Care Med 1984; 12:829–832.
40. Doyle HJ, et al. Different humidification systems for high-frequency jet ventilation. Crit Care Med 1984; 12:815–819.
41. Wiswell TE, et al. Different high-frequency ventilator strategies: effect on the propagation of tracheobronchial histopathologic changes. Pediatrics 1990; 85:70–78.
42. Wiswell TE, et al. Determinants of tracheal bronchial histologic alterations during conventional mechanical ventilation. Pediatrics 1989; 84:304–311.
43. Modell JH, et al. Effect of chronic exposure to ultrasonic aerosols on the lung. Anesthesiology 1967; 28:680–688.
44. Melville GN. Water content level in inspired air on specific airway resistance in rats. Respiration 1972; 29:127–134.
45. Noguchi H, et al. A study of humidification in tracheostomized dogs. Br J Anaesth 1973; 45:844–848.
46. Tsuda T, et al. Optimum humidification of air administered to a tracheostomy in dogs: scanning electron microscopy and surfactant studies. Br J Anaesth 1977; 49: 965–977.
47. John E, et al. Effects of gas temperature and particulate water on rabbit lungs during ventilation. Pediatr Res 1980; 14:1186–1191.
48. Todd DA, John E. Lung injury and repair in rabbits from ventilation with moist air. Br J Exp Pathol 1989; 70:637–645.
49. Cheney FWJ, Butler J. The effects of ultrasonically-produced aerosols on airway resistance in man. Anesthesiology 1968; 29:1099–1106.
50. Melville GN, et al. Changes in specific airway resistance during prolonged breathing of moist air. Can J Physiol Pharmacol 1968; 48:592–597.
51. Kuo CD, et al. Aerosol, humidity and oxygenation. Chest 1991; 99:1352–1356.
52. Chatburn RL, Primiano FPJ. A rational basis for humidity therapy. Respir Care 1987; 32:249–253.
53. Tarnow-Mordi WO, et al. Evidence of inadequate humidification on inspired gas during artificial ventilation of newborn babies in the British Isles. Lancet 1986; 2: 909–910.
54. Tarnow-Mordi WO, et al. Inadequate humidification of respiratory gases during mechanical ventilation of the newborn. Arch Dis Child 1986; 61:698–700.
55. Chatburn RL. Physiologic and methodologic issues regarding humidity therapy. J Pediatr 1989; 114:416–420.
56. O'Hagan M, et al. Is neonatal inspired gas humidity accurately controlled by humidifier temperature? Crit Care Med 1991; 19:1370–1373.
57. Miyao H, et al. Relative humidity, not absolute humidity, is of great importance when using a humidificr with a heating wire. Crit Care Med 1992; 20:674–679.
58. Gilmour IJ, et al. The effect of heated wire circuits on humidification of inspired gases. Anesth Analg 1994; 79:160–164.
59. Browning DJ, Graves SA. Incidence of aspiration with endotracheal tubes in children. J Pediatr 1983; 102:582–584.
60. Goitein KJ, et al. Incidence of aspiration in endotracheally intubated infants and children. Crit Care Med 1984; 12:19–21.

61. Goodwin SR, et al. Aspiration in intubated premature infants. Pediatrics 1985; 75: 85–88.
62. Coalson JJ, et al. Bacterial cononization and infection studies in the premature baboon with bronchopulmonary dysplasia. Am Rev Respir Dis 1991; 144:1140–1146.
63. Rello J, et al. Pneumonia in intubated patients: role of the respiratory airway care. Am J Respir Crit Care Med 1996; 154:111–115.
64. Grimbert FA, et al. Increased pulmonary vascular permeability following acid aspiration. J Appl Physiol 1981; 51:335–345.
65. Nanjo S, et al. Concentrated albumin does not affect lung edema formation after acid instillation in the dog. Am Rev Respir Dis 1983; 128:884–889.
66. Jefferies AL, et al. Pulmonary epithelial permeability in hyaline-membrane disease. N Engl J Med 1984; 311:1075–1080.
67. Mays EE, Dubois JJ. Pulmonary fibrosis associated with tracheobronchial aspiration: a study of the frequency of hiatal hernia and gastroesophageal reflux in interstitial pulmonary fibrosis of obscure etiology. Chest 1976; 69:512–515.
68. Euler AR, et al. Recurrent pulmonary disease in children: a complication of gastroesophageal reflux. Pediatrics 1979; 63:47–51.
69. Berquist WE, et al. Gastroesophageal reflux-associated recurrent pneumonia and chronic asthma in children. Pediatrics 1981; 68:29–35.
70. Danus O, et al. Esophageal reflux—an unrecognized cause of recurrent obstructive bronchitis in children. J Pediatr 1976; 89:220–224.
71. Christie DL. Pulmonary complications of esophageal disease. Pediatr Clin North Am 1984; 31:835–849.
72. Herbst JJ, et al. Gastroesophageal reflux causing respiratory distress and apnea in newborn infants. J Pediatr 1979; 95:763–768.
73. Herbst JJ. Gastroesophageal reflux. J Pediatr 1981; 98:859–870.
74. Higgins RD, et al. Nasal continuous positive airway pressure facilitates extubation of very low birth weight neonates. Pediatrics 1991; 88:999–1003.
75. Engelke SC, et al. Postextubation nasal continuous positive airway pressure. Am J Dis Child 1982; 136:359–361.
76. Annibale DJ, et al. Randomized, controlled trial of nasopharyngeal continuous positive airway pressure in the extubation of very low birth weight infants. J Pediatr 1994; 124:455–460.
77. Kamper J, et al. Early treatment with nasal continuous positive airway pressure in very low-birth-weight infants. Acta Paediatr Scand 1993; 82:193–197.
78. Roberton NRC. Does CPAP work when it really matters? Acta Paediatr Scand 1993; 82:206–207.
79. Drew JH. Immediate intubation at birth of the very-low-birth-weight infant. Am J Dis Child 1982; 136:207–210.
80. Kolobow T, et al. A new ultrathin-walled, non-kinking, low-resistance endotracheal tube for neonatal use: preliminary studies of a new no-pressure cuff. Biomed Instrum Technol 1994; 28:123–129.

11

Influence of Surfactant Replacement on Development of Bronchopulmonary Dysplasia

ALAN H. JOBE

Children's Hospital Medical Center
Cincinnati, Ohio

I. Statement of the Question

This book is about the description, pathogenesis, treatment, prevention, and outcomes of infants with bronchopulmonary dysplasia (BPD). The single most important new therapy available for the highest-risk infants (small and immature) is surfactant treatment for respiratory distress syndrome (RDS). Surfactant treatments are the most thoroughly studied therapy in neonatology. The results of over 40 excellent randomized, controlled trails that include thousands of infants have been published. It would seem to be straightforward to answer the question if surfactant prevents BPD because this outcome was consistently recorded as a primary outcome variable in the clinical trials. However, several factors complicate a simple answer to the question. My goals are to present the clinical data, develop the arguments why surfactant therapy should decrease BPD, ask why surfactant might not decrease BPD, and finally, try to answer the question. This chapter is written from the perspective of a commentary or editorial because there is no consensus on the effects of surfactant on BPD.

II. Review of the Clinical Data

The overall incidence of BPD has increased or decreased since about 1980, depending on the database (1,2). The incidence of BPD depends primarily on the size distribution of infants and death rates for infants who weigh less than 1000 g (3). Parker and associates (2) used logistic regression models to conclude that 83% of the increase in incidence of BPD at Vanderbilt University between 1976 and 1990 was explained by increased survival of tiny infants. However, there remained a part of the increased incidence of BPD that could not be explained by averted neonatal death.

The target populations for the clinical trials randomizing infants to surfactant or placebo were the very preterm infants at high risk of respiratory distress syndrome (RDS), BPD, and death. The primary outcome variables for most of the large studies were death and BPD. Individual trials demonstrated increased BPD, no difference in the incidence of BPD, or decreased BPD with surfactant treatment. However, the extensive databases from the multiple controlled trials allow estimates of the effect of surfactant treatment on BPD by metanalyses of the trials provided by Roger Soll (4–8). The odds ratios and 95% confidence intervals (CI) are given in Figure 1. Three of the four strategies approved for clinical use of surfactant for RDS (delivery room treatment of infants at risk of RDS or the treatment of established RDS with lung source surfactants) had no effect on the incidences of BPD. In these metanalyses, the incidence of BPD ranged from about 20 to 40% in the control groups. The significant decrease in BPD found with the use of synthetic surfactants to treat RDS resulted from a very large trial in larger infants where the incidence of BPD was 5.5% in the placebo group and 2.5% in the control group (9). Although this difference was significant, the finding has little effect on the overall epidemiology of BPD because the affected population includes very few of the infants with severe BPD. Therefore, surfactant does not decrease the incidence of BPD based on a direct comparison of surfactant treatment with placebo controls.

Different surfactant treatment strategies also have been evaluated. These trials do not include a placebo group, but they could provide insight if differences in BPD rates occurred. A metanalysis of the comparison trials of delivery room to subsequent treatment of RDS does not demonstrate any differential effect of these strategies on the incidence of BPD (8; see Fig. 1).

The OSIRIS trial that compared early mandatory surfactant treatment versus later selective treatment also demonstrated no effect on the incidence of BPD (10). A multicenter European trial comparing 50 mg/kg and 100 mg/kg Alveofact (a surfactant from bovine lung) reported that the incidence of BPD was 33% with low-dose and 24% with high-dose surfactant (11). High- versus low-dose Curosurf (a surfactant from pig lung) resulted in the same incidence of BPD (12). Another multicenter European trial evaluated single versus multiple doses

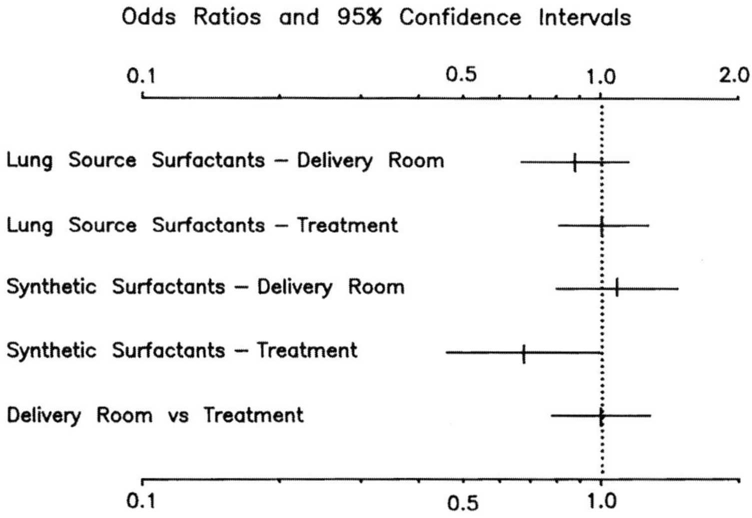

Figure 1 Effect of surfactant treatment on the incidence of BPD in randomized controlled trials: Surfactant given either in the delivery room to prevent RDS or to treat RDS had no effect on the incidence of BPD. The exception was the decrease in BPD after treatment of RDS with synthetic surfactant; however, this result is not representative of the outcomes for tiny infants (see text). A comparison of delivery room treatment versus treatment of RDS did not result in a difference in the incidence of BPD. Odds ratios and 95% confidence limits from the metanalyses Soll. (From Refs. 4–8.)

of Curosurf (13). The odds ratio for multidose treatment decreasing BPD relative to single-dose treatment was 1.12 (95% CI, 0.57–2.23), indicating no beneficial effect of multiple doses. There is also no evidence that a synthetic surfactant influences the incidence of BPD differently from a lung source surfactant (14). The overall odds ratio for BPD for four comparison trials of Survanta (a surfactant from bovine lung) relative to Exosurf (a synthetic surfactant) was 0.95 (95% CI, 0.83–1.08). However, an interpretation of the equivalence of BPD is complicated by significantly fewer deaths in infants receiving the natural surfactant. Recent trials comparing another natural surfactant, Infasurf, and the synthetic surfactant, Exosurf, also found no difference in the incidence of BPD (15,16). Therefore, the clinical data involving different treatment strategies do not show differential effects on the incidence of BPD.

The question can be approached from the epidemiological perspective by asking how the introduction of surfactant into routine clinical care influenced

BPD and other outcomes. A report from the National Institute of Child Health and Human Development (NICHD) Neonatal Network categorized outcomes for the 2 years before and 1 year after the introduction of surfactant therapy for all infants weighing between 601 and 1300 g (17). Forty percent of the infants received surfactant, and death decreased from 28% before to 20% after surfactant was introduced (adjusted odds ratio for death 0.73; 95% CI, 0.55–0.95). The odds ratio for BPD adjusted for infant characteristics was 1.05 (95% CI, 0.81–1.36), indicating no effect of the introduction of surfactant on the incidence of BPD. The adjusted odds ratio for BPD in those infants surviving for 28 days also was not significant. A similar study by Schwartz et al. (18) reported a 30% decrease in the death rate of infants with birth weights of 500–1500 g after the introduction of surfactant. The death rate declined 40% in infants with BPD, although the overall incidence of BPD did not change with the advent of surfactant therapy when compared with the presurfactant time period (adjusted odds ratio 1.1; 95% CI, 1.0–1.3). A third epidemiological report of infants, who weighed less than 1500 g from Palta et al. (19) analyzed three time periods: before surfactant therapy, during the period of investigational new drug use, and after approval of the synthetic surfactant Exosurf. Although death rates decreased, the incidence of BPD initially increased from 21 to 36% and then decreased to 27% for the period after approval of Exosurf. These data indicate that surfactant has not reduced the incidence of BPD for very low birth weight infants.

Several issues need to be considered before concluding that surfactant therapy does not reduce the incidence of BPD. The major issue is the effect of surfactant on death rates. In both the randomized trials and the epidemiological studies, surfactant treatment consistently has been associated with a 30–40% decrease in death of the infants at highest risk for BPD. Most of the analyses report BPD incidences relative to infants randomized. Egberts and deWinter (20) make the point that if the denominator is surviving infants rather than randomized infants, surfactant treatment can be shown to significantly decrease BPD among survivors. A survivor analysis did not reach significance in the epidemiological study of Horbar et al. (17). Nevertheless, the impressive decrease in death means that surfactant treatment has "rescued" many tiny infants from death. The logical conclusion is that these infants should be at the highest risk for BPD. Viewed from this perspective, no change in the incidence of BPD indicates that surfactant has decreased BPD from what it would have been if this group of marginal infants had survived without surfactant therapy.

A second major factor of clinical importance is the severity of BPD. Unfortunately, the surfactant efficacy trials did not categorize BPD beyond the definition of oxygen need at 28 days (often without correlative chest radiographs). Epidemiological data characterizing severity and duration of BPD are not available. It is my clinical impression that the incidence of severe, prolonged, and debilitating BPD has dramatically decreased. The observation by Schwartz et al.

(18) that death in infants with BPD decreased after the introduction of surfactant is consistent with that conclusion. Surfactant treatments do not change the incidence of BPD based on the minimal definition of supplemental oxygen use at 28 days (with or without characteristic radiographic changes). However, surfactant treatments in conjunction with other improvements in neonatal care, such as the increased use of antenatal glucocorticoids and new approaches to neonatal ventilation almost certainly have decreased the severity of BPD. Decreased severity, together with a decreased death rate, indicate indirectly that surfactant treatments have had a major effect on BPD.

This conclusion is supported by the limited amount of follow-up information that is available. Exosurf-treated infants had lower airway resistance and overall better pulmonary mechanics than did control infants at a postnatal age of 1 year (21). Randomization to Survanta resulted in less oxygen need and a lower incidence in cerebral palsy at 6-months adjusted age (22). The surfactant-treated infants had less wheezing at 1 and 2 years than did control infants. These outcomes are consistent with a decrease in severity of BPD resulting from surfactant treatment.

III. Why Should Surfactant Treatments Decrease BPD?

A. Surfactant Effects on Lung Mechanics

Surfactant has several effects on the preterm, surfactant-deficient lung that result in improved lung function. These effects should decrease the need for mechanical ventilation and supplemental oxygen (23). Treatment of the surfactant-deficient lung with either a natural surfactant that contains all surfactant components or a clinical surfactant changes the pressure–volume relations of the lung (24; see Fig. 2). The lung fills with more gas at a lower pressure and is more stable on deflation to low transpulmonary pressures. Because dead space is changed very little, the increased gas volume is being accommodated by the recruitment of parenchymal gas volume with the potential for improved gas exchange. The increased volume stability translates to an increased functional residual capacity. The primary clinical outcome of increased lung gas volume and functional residual capacity is improved arterial oxygenation (23). Surfactant treatment of the surfactant-deficient lung will decrease the inspiratory time constant (the lung is easier to inflate) and increase the expiratory time constant (the lung deflates more slowly; 25). The lengthening of the expiratory time constant can result in air trapping and overinflation if short expiratory times are used with mechanical ventilation.

Compliance may improve immediately after surfactant therapy if a natural surfactant is used. However, compliance changes have not been reported by all investigators. A reason for the inconsistent compliance responses is the interac-

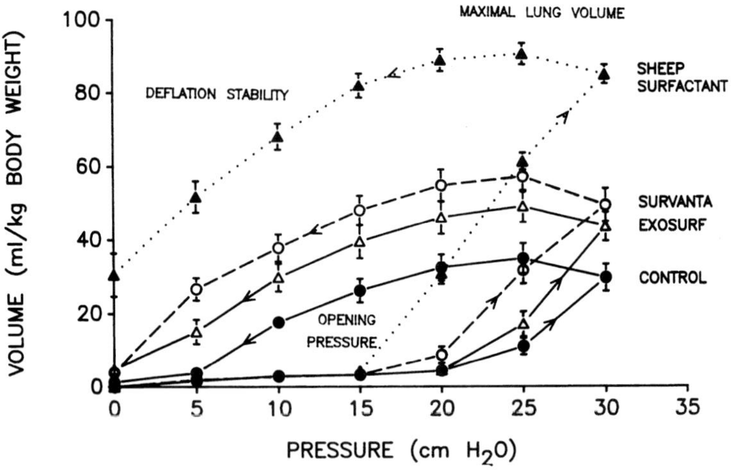

Figure 2 Quasistatic pressure–volume curves for preterm rabbit lungs after treatment with the three surfactants and ventilation for 15 min: The surfactants increased lung volumes and volume stability relative to control lungs. (From Ref. 23.)

tion between the surfactant effects on lung volumes and the style of ventilatory support selected. For example, Davis et al. (26) reported that surfactant treatment caused no change in compliance with mechanical ventilation, but compliance improved when spontaneous breaths were measured. Kelly et al. (27) found that if ventilator pressures were lowered after surfactant treatment, both static and dynamic compliance improved. This result underscores the possibility that lung overinflation may occur after surfactant treatment.

B. Uniformity of Inflation

The measurements of lung volumes from pressure–volume curves or clinical assessments of functional residual capacity and tidal volume do not identify where the gas is located in the lungs. The characteristic histopathology of RDS is atelectasis intermingled with overdistended alveoli, small airways, and alveolar ducts (28). Atelectasis and overdistention are the net effects of the lack of surfactant and high transpulmonary pressures. Because of the La Place relation (the retractive force of surface tension is greater for small-diameter alveoli and airways than for larger-diameter alveoli and airways), the more compliant lung regions become overdistended and the less compliant lung regions collapse in lungs of infants with RDS. Either result is potentially harmful and may contribute to the development of chronic lung injury. If atelectasis persists, inflammation and fibrosis can occur. Overdistension of regional lung units may lead to stretch-related injury (29).

A uniform distribution of a treatment dose of surfactant should facilitate uniform lung expansion and reestablish the interdependence of alveoli for the maintenance of uniform alveolar expansion (20). Figure 3 is a sketch of alveolar size distributions with and without surfactant treatment. In the surfactant-deficient lung, most of the alveoli are underinflated. If surfactant distribution were perfectly uniform throughout the lung, then alveolar diameters would have a normal size distribution appropriate for the stage of alveolar development for that infant. This uniformity of alveolar size after effective surfactant treatment implies increased airspace volume without overdistention or alveolar collapse. The third curve is a sketch of what would happen if the surfactant distribution were nonuniform. Many of the alveoli remain uninflated and the alveoli that received the surfactant overinflate, with the risk of stretch-induced lung injury. If ventilator pressures were decreased in the latter situation, overinflation would be decreased, but collapse of the untreated alveoli also would become more severe.

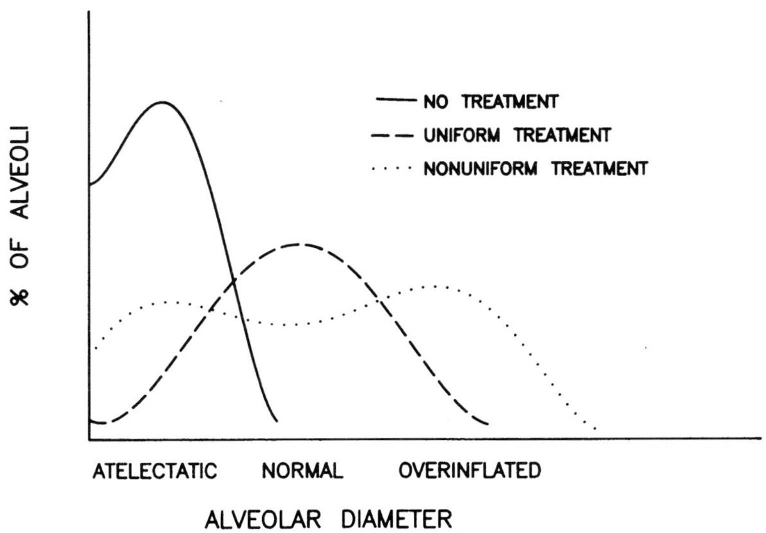

Figure 3 Idealized representation of alveolar size distributions: Alveoli in the surfactant-deficient lung will be atelectatic or very small unless very high ventilatory pressures are used. Following a uniformly distributed surfactant treatment, alveoli will expand uniformly to a larger mean diameter. If a surfactant treatment were not uniform, the alveoli not receiving surfactant would not expand and the alveoli that receive surfactant may overexpand with mechanical ventilation. (From Ref. 30.)

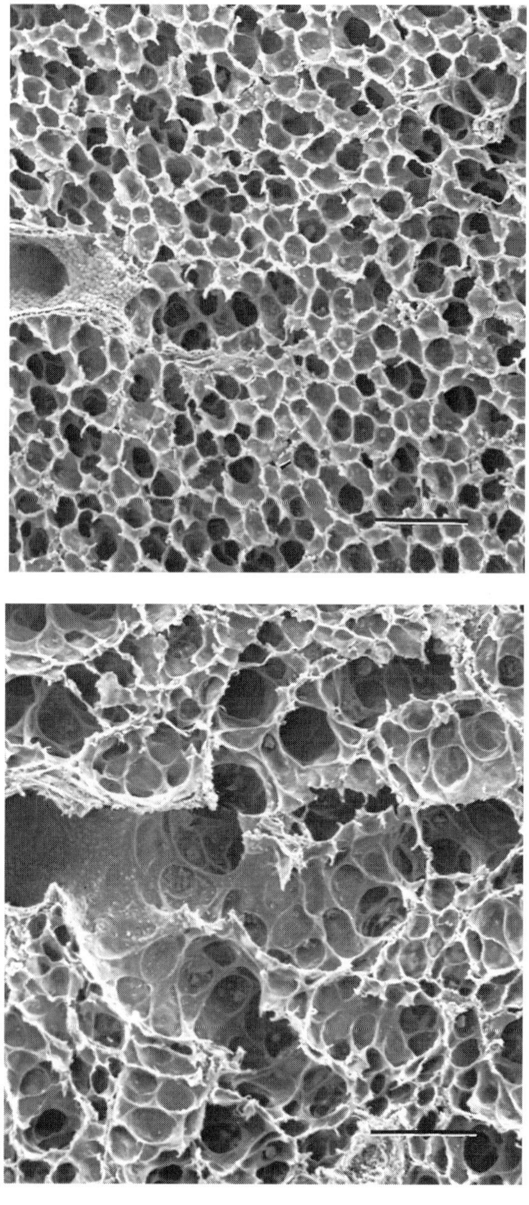

(a) (b)

Figure 4 Scanning electron micrographs of preterm lamb lungs: (a) The fetal lung that has never been ventilated has uniform alveolar sizes without distortion, and (b) the lung ventilated for 24 hr demonstrates dilation of alveolar ducts with alveolar size heterogeneity and compression atelectasis. (c) At higher magnification, alveoli are flattened and tissue crests are prominent. Bar, 100 μm in A and B and 20 μm in C. (From Ref. 31.)

(c) 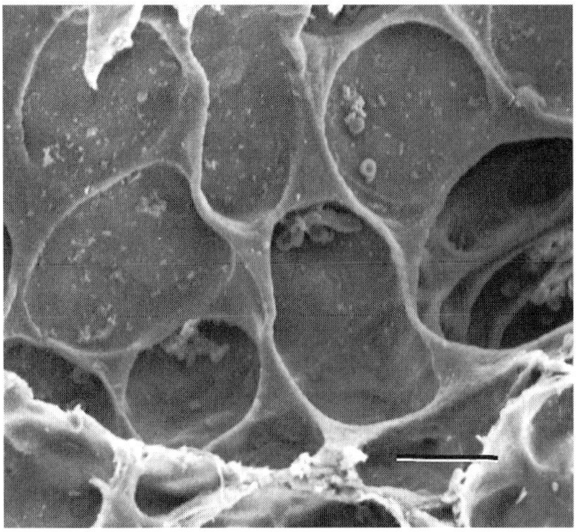

In preterm ventilated lambs treated with natural surfactant at birth to achieve an optimum distribution, there was more uniformity of alveolar inflation, together with a decrease in compression atelectasis at the margins of the overinflated zones at 24 hr relative to lambs not treated with surfactant (31; Fig. 4). In a subsequent anatomical study with less mature lambs, a comparison of lung regions treated with surfactant and regions not treated with surfactant in the same animal showed much more atelectasis, stretch, and distortion in regions that did not receive surfactant (32). These considerations of alveolar size may relate to the incidence of BPD in surfactant-treated infants. Treatment with surfactant might improve lung volumes and oxygenation, but if surfactant distribution is not uniform or if ventilator pressures are excessive, overdistention and lung injury with the therapy might contribute to the development of BPD.

C. Surfactant and Pulmonary Edema

Ventilation of the surfactant-deficient lung results in disruption of the epithelium of the small airways (28). Treatment of preterm rabbits with surfactant prevents this injury, even if the lungs are overinflated (33). Development of edema in the preterm lung increases as gestational age decreases (34,35). This relation is probably partly related to maturation of the lung because the amount of edema can be decreased by prenatal corticosteroid treatment (36). Surfactant treatment of preterm rabbits decreases the leak of radiolabeled albumin from the vasculature to the lung tissue and alveoli (34). Surfactant treatment of preterm lambs also decreases edema formation, as well as vascular injury (35,37). The mechanisms for decreasing pulmonary injury and edema with surfactant therapy could be the maintenance of a more uniformly inflated lung (less stretch); decreased surface tensions that change the balance of interstitial and alveolar pressures, thereby minimizing fluid movement into the alveoli (38); or a specific effect of surfactant on the alveolar and airway epithelium. The effect probably is primarily a result of minimizing stretch-related injury, because very preterm lambs can be ventilated without the development of edema if small tidal volumes are used (39).

IV. Why Surfactant Treatment Might Not Affect the Incidence of BPD

A. Lung Injury Progressing to BPD

The major hypothesis for the pathogenesis of BPD is that the lung is injured by the combination of supplemental oxygen and pressure–volume effects of mechanical ventilation. Injury provokes inflammatory and healing responses that result in progressive injury. This sequence is consistent with models of lung injury in preterm animals (40–42). These concepts are thoroughly reviewed elsewhere in this volume. Surfactant should tend to mitigate this injury sequence because most infants treated with surfactant require lower pressures on mechanical ventilation and less supplemental oxygen. However, there is a flaw in this argument based on the epidemiology of BPD in tiny infants without severe RDS. In a recent report of 119 ventilator-supported infants with birth weights between 500 and 1000 g who required fewer than 3 days of supplemental oxygen higher than 25% during the first 5 days of life, chronic lung disease developed in 37% of the infants (43). This incidence of chronic lung disease is the same as that reported in the surfactant trials. Therefore, infants who are at highest risk for BPD tend to acquire BPD somewhat independently of their initial disease severity. Certainly prolonged use of high-ventilatory pressures and supplemental oxygen can cause BPD, but such therapy is not necessary for the development of BPD in tiny infants who do not have surfactant deficiency at birth (43). It is noteworthy that many (up to 40%) of those infants who are at risk for RDS and who are treated with surfactant in the delivery room would not acquire RDS even if they were not treated with surfactant. The incidence of BPD is about the same for weight-matched infants independent of surfactant treatment strategy (8,10). A number of the infants who acquired BPD probably would not have had RDS and, therefore, did not need surfactant treatment. From this logic, it is possible to conclude that most cases of BPD are not caused by surfactant deficiency and, therefore, surfactant treatment should have little effect on the incidence of BPD. This conclusion ignores the effects of surfactant on death and the less severe nature of BPD in many of the tiny infants. However, surfactant probably is not central to the pathophysiology initiating the development of BPD, other than in a secondary role to minimize the use of mechanical ventilation and supplemental oxygen.

B. Surfactant and the Inflammatory Response

The airspaces of the preterm lung at birth contain very few macrophages or granulocytes provided there is no congenital infection. Macrophages normally increase after birth, but granulocytes are prominent only if an inflammatory response is present (44). If surfactant has anti-inflammatory properties, then its use might moderate the inflammation that is associated with the development of BPD. Endogenous surfactant in the normal lung presumably is not proinflammatory. In fact, many host defense roles have been proposed for the lipid and protein components of surfactant (45). Most of the recent work on inflammatory mediators in airway samples from infants have included surfactant-treated infants (46,47). The presence of elastase in airway samples did not correlate with the time of surfactant treatment with Curosurf or with the initial severity of lung injury (46). The use of Curosurf also did not correlate with indicators of increased microvascular permeability and inflammatory mediators in airway samples of infants at risk for BPD (47). Bagchi et al. (48) found that interleukin-6 but not tumor necrosis factor-α was associated with the development of BPD. However, there were no differences in interleukin-6 activity in airway samples for those infants who were treated with surfactant relative to the untreated infants. Although limited information is available, there is no indication that surfactant treatment is anti-inflammatory in the preterm lung at risk for BPD.

There is another mechanism by which surfactant treatment could mitigate the inflammatory response. In adult animals made surfactant deficient by saline lung lavage, subsequent ventilation results in severe respiratory failure if conventional ventilation techniques are used (49). The animals have massive accumulations of granulocytes in the lungs, together with pulmonary edema and hyaline membrane formation. Granulocyte depletion with cytotoxic agents before saline lavage and conventional ventilation minimizes the injury and the subsequent respiratory failure (50). High-frequency oscillation, or other strategies designed to increase lung volumes and recruit alveoli after the saline lavage, also prevents white blood cell recruitment to the lungs, inhibits the development of pulmonary edema, and enhances the effectiveness of surfactant therapy (51). Although this work has been done primarily in the saline lavaged adult lung, the results are likely to be important for the preterm lung. If the lung is ventilated at low lung volumes, injury mediated by white cell migration to the lungs occurs. Surfactant treatments can increase functional residual capacity and facilitate lung volume recruitment (23). Therefore, surfactant treatments should result in a decreased inflammatory response, if appropriate assisted ventilation is used after surfactant treatment. In support of this concept, Gerstman et al. (52) report that high-frequency oscillation, using a high lung volume strategy, decreased chronic lung disease in infants treated with surfactant relative to conventionally ventilated infants.

C. Surfactant, Style of Ventilation, and BPD

Another hypothesis in the surfactant–BPD relation is that BPD is caused in many infants by neonatal care practices that result in lung injury or that do not optimize the effects of surfactant on RDS. This hypothesis is controversial and potentially threatening to neonatal caregivers because most neonatologists are confident in their approach to ventilating infants. However, there are epidemiological and experimental data to support the hypothesis. The investigators in the Vermont–Oxford Trials Network reported in 1993 that the incidence of BPD in infants with birth weights between 501 and 1500 g varied between neonatal units from about 15 to 70% (53). This range of incidences is unlikely to be explained by differences in patient population alone. Avery ct al. (54) reported variable rates of BPD between neonatal units, with the unit having the lowest rate using a type of respiratory support that emphasized continuous positive airway pressure without intubation. This style of treatment resulted in high P_{CO_2} values in the infants. Kraybill et al. (55) noted that lower P_{CO_2} values at 48 hr of age correlated with the development of BPD in ventilated preterm infants. Furthermore, the BPD rates by center were inversely related to P_{CO_2} levels at 48 and 96 hr. This counterintuitive notion that low P_{CO_2} values correlate with subsequent lung injury was also reported for infants for the interval between birth and surfactant treatment (56). The incidence of BPD correlated with P_{CO_2} levels before surfactant treatment, with the highest incidence in infants with P_{CO_2} values less than 30 mmHg. This correlation was valid, even for infants who had mild lung disease. An explanation for these observations is that ventilation of the very premature lung (independent of surfactant status) to low systemic P_{CO_2} values may result in stretch-induced injury and begin the sequence resulting in BPD (57). The injury that initiates the development of BPD may occur in the delivery room. Preterm lambs that are ventilated with high tidal volumes immediately following delivery had decreased responses to surfactant treatments and pulmonary edema (58,59).

Other care practices may also affect the incidence of BPD independently of surfactant treatment. Van Marter et al. (60) used multivariant analysis to try to explain different incidences of BPD between neonatal units. They found that part of the difference could be explained by fluid management during the first days of life. In an interesting study comparing responses of infants with RDS to surfactant treatment between two neonatal units, Hallman et al. (61) found decreased severity of RDS and increased survival without BPD in one unit, but not in the other. A multivariant analysis suggested that fluid and ventilator management influenced the efficacy of surfactant treatment. If management indeed influenced the incidence of both BPD and the clinical responses to surfactant, it would not be surprising if surfactant treatment alone had little or no effect on the incidence of BPD.

Also there are experimental data indicating that surfactant and injury responses are dependent on ventilation style. In the foregoing section, it was pointed out that ventilation at low lung volumes can cause white blood cell migration into the lungs, inflammation, and pulmonary edema (50,51). The improved respiratory status of preterm primates supported with high-frequency ventilation using a high lung volume strategy is probably partly explained by avoiding ventilation at low lung volumes (51,62). With a high-frequency ventilation strategy and surfactant treatment lung injury in preterm primates can be minimized (63). The same concepts apply to conventional ventilation of the preterm lung. The data in Figure 5 demonstrate that the ventilatory pressure values that accompanied different ventilatory strategies designed to achieve comparable P_{CO_2} values in preterm rabbits depended on the type of surfactant that was used to treat the animals (64,65). A ventilation strategy using no positive end-expiratory pressure and a tidal volume of 10 mL/kg required higher pressures for all surfactants than did a strategy of 3 cmH_2O positive end-expiratory pressure and 7 mL/kg tidal volumes. The effect on pulmonary edema, measured as the recovery of intravascular radiolabeled albumin from the alveoli and airways, also depended strikingly on the surfactant used to treat the animals. The low tidal volume strategy uniformly decreased pulmonary edema.

There are no clinical studies comparing ventilation strategies and short-term surfactant responses. The effects of different ventilation strategies and the choice of surfactant on the incidence of BPD remains untested. Different surfactants may require different ventilation strategies to optimize outcomes in clinical practice. The definition of an optimal outcome should not be a low P_{CO_2} after surfactant treatment. A low P_{CO_2} may predict an increased incidence of BPD (57).

D. Surfactant Abnormalities in BPD

The possibility that surfactant is abnormal in infants with BPD has been studied only superficially. Infants with RDS have a surfactant that contains more phosphatidylinositol and less phosphatidglycerol, and this "immature" phospholipid pattern remains for much longer in infants developing BPD than for infants that resolve RDS without BPD (66). Surfactant protein levels have not been evaluated systematically in infants with BPD. Infants recovering from RDS have increasing amounts of SP-A in airway samples over the first few days of life (67,68). In contrast, in a primate model of BPD, Coalson et al. (69) found that the low levels of SP-A present at birth did not increase with the development of BPD. The potential importance of SP-A in the progression to BPD is indicated by Figure

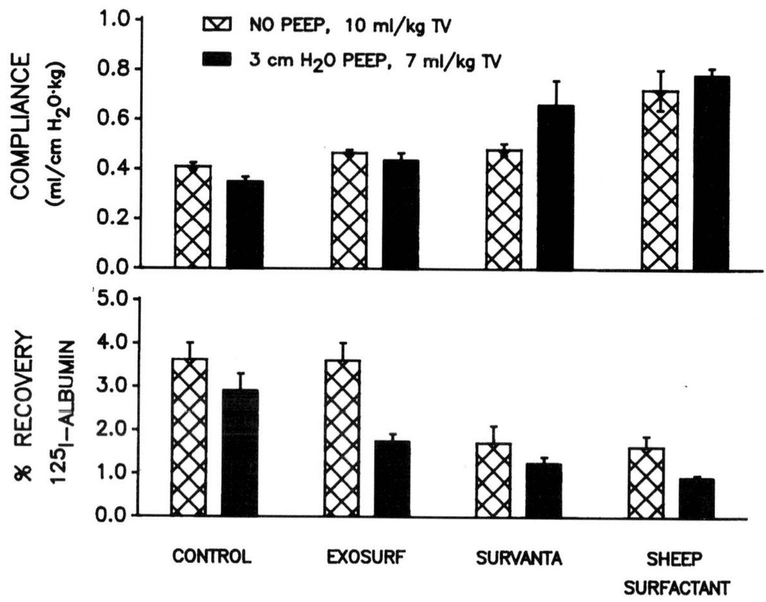

Figure 5 Effect of ventilation style on compliance and development of pulmonary edema in ventilated preterm rabbits: A ventilation strategy of no positive end-expiratory pressure (PEEP) and 10 mL/kg tidal volume (TV) resulted in minimal improvement in compliance with Exosurf and Survanta treatment. The 3 cmH_2O PEEP and 7 mL/kg TV strategy improved compliance for rabbits treated with Survanta. Sheep surfactant improved compliances with either strategy. In the lower frame, pulmonary edema was estimated by the amount of ^{125}I-albumin given by intravascular injection at birth that was recovered in alveolar washes at 30 min of age. The use of PEEP decreased albumin recovery for each surfactant treatment. (Data from Ref. 64.)

6. Infants who weighed less than 1000 g who died or developed BPD had very low SP-A/saturated phosphatidylcholine ratios in samples from the airspaces relative to infants without these poor outcomes (69). This outcome indicator was independent of surfactant treatment. SP-A can enhance the function of surfactants that lack SP-A, can protect surfactant from inactivation by edema fluid, and is a host defense protein. However, mice deficient in SP-A have normal lung function and surfactant metabolism (70). SP-A may be only an indicator of the stages of lung development or it may be important in the pathogenesis of BPD.

Other than composition changes in surfactant phospholipids, the characteristics of surfactant in BPD have received minimal attention. An indication that surfactant function may be abnormal is suggested by a small clinical trial of surfactant treatment of ten infants with early BPD (71). The infants required less

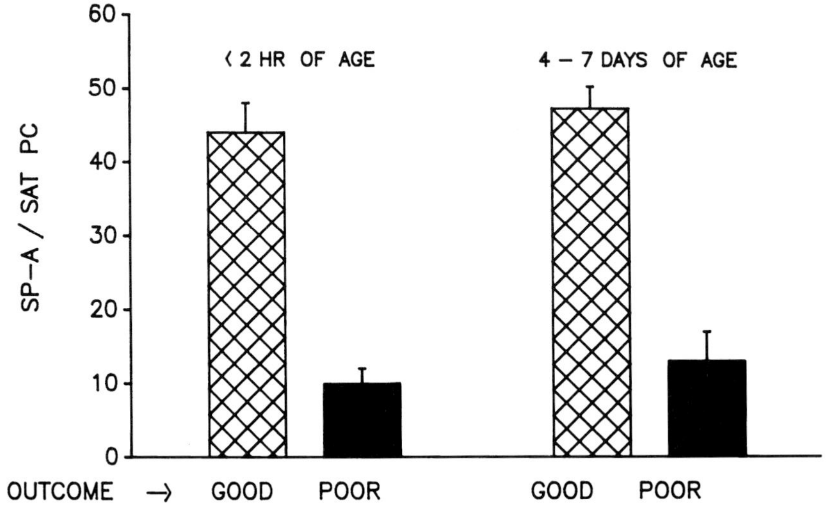

Figure 6 Outcomes of infants smaller than 1 kg in relation to SP-A to saturated phosphatidylcholine ratios (SP-A/Sat PC) in airway samples: A good outcome was defined as survival without BPD, and a poor outcome was death or BPD. The SP-A/Sat PC ratios in airway samples collected either before 2 hr of age or at 4–7 days of age were predictive of outcome. The interval between 2 hr and 4 days included surfactant treatment. (Data from Ref. 68.)

supplemental oxygen for 72 hr after a single dose of surfactant. Preterm baboons that are delivered at 125 days gestation that are ventilated and subsequently have BPD, by 6 days of age accumulate lung tissue pools of surfactant equivalent to those of term baboons (72). However, alveolar pools remain small, and the alveolar surfactant has decreased function. The mechanisms responsible for these changes remain to be characterized. The endogenous surfactant pools in infants with BPD may be abnormal and may contribute to the abnormal lung mechanics.

V. Summary

Although the clinical data do not directly support the hypothesis that surfactant treatments decrease BPD, the increased survival of surfactant-treated infants without an increase in the incidence of BPD, and the decreased severity of BPD, are consistent with the notion that surfactant treatments decrease the incidence and severity of BPD in very low birth weight infants who survive. There are several mechanisms by which surfactant might decrease BPD. These include a decreased need for ventilatory support and supplemental oxygen, improved lung mechanics, the potential for more homogeneous lung inflation, and decreased pulmonary edema. However, counterbalancing these beneficial effects may be the pathophysiology of BPD and inflammation in the very preterm lung. The frequent occurrence of BPD in infants without RDS suggests that surfactant treatments may not interrupt those processes. Clinical management styles have not been evaluated to optimize surfactant effects and may mitigate against any benefit resulting from surfactant treatment. Finally, abnormalities in endogenous surfactant may contribute to the pathophysiology of BPD. Just as surfactant treatments do not decrease other complications of prematurity, such as patent ductus arteriosis, intraventricular hemorrhage, and necrotizing enterocolitis (4–8), surfactant is not a panacea that prevents BPD.

References

1. Corcoran JD, Patterson CC, Thomas PS, Halliday HL. Reduction in the risk of bronchopulmonary dysplasia from 1980–1990: results of a multivariate logistic regression analysis. Eur J Pediatr 1993; 152:677–681.
2. Parker RA, Lindstrom DP, Cotton RB. Improved survival accounts for most, but not all, of the increase in bronchopulmonary dysplasia. Pediatrics 1992; 90:663–668.
3. Hack M, Horbar JD, Malloy MH, Tyson JE, Wright E, Wright L. Very low birth weight outcomes of the National Institute of Child Health and Human Development Neonatal Network. Pediatrics 1991; 87:587–597.
4. Soll RF. Synthetic surfactant treatment of RDS, Oct. 1994. In: Sinclair JL, Bracken MB, Soll RF, Horbar JD, eds. The Cochrane Neonatal Database. Published through Cochrane updates on disk.
5. Soll RF. Natural surfactant extract treatment of RDS, Oct. 1994. In: Sinclair JL, Bracken MB, Soll RF, Horbar JD, eds. The Cochrane Neonatal Database. Published through Cochrane updates on disk.
6. Soll RF. Prophylactic administration of synthetic surfactant, Oct. 1994. In: Sinclair JL, Bracken MB, Soll RF, Horbar JD, eds. The Cochrane Neonatal Database. Published through Cochrane updates on disk.
7. Soll RF. Prophylactic administration of natural surfactant, Sept. 1994. In: Sinclair JL, Bracken MD, Soll RF, Horbar JD, eds. The Cochrane Neonatal Database. Published through Cochrane updates on disk.
8. Soll RF. Prophylactic surfactant versus treatment with surfactant, Sept. 1994. In: Sinclair JL, Bracken MD, Soll RF, Horbar JD, eds. The Cochrane Neonatal Database. Published through Cochrane updates on disk.
9. Long W, Corbet A, Cotton R, et al. A controlled trial of synthetic surfactant in infants weighing 1250 g or more with respiratory distress syndrome. N Engl J Med 1991; 325:1696–1703.
10. OSIRIS Collaborative Group. Early versus delayed neonatal administration of a synthetic surfactant—the judgment of OSIRIS. Lancet 1992; 340:1363–1369.

11. Gortner L, Pohlandt F, Bartmann P, et al. High-dose versus low-dose bovine surfactant treatment in very premature infants. Acta Pediatr 1994; 83:135–141.
12. Halliday HL, Tarnow-Mordi WO, Corcoran JD, Patterson CC. Multicenter randomized trial comparing high and low dose surfactant regimens for the treatment of respiratory distress syndrome (the Curosurf 4 trial). Arch Dis Child 1993; 69:276–280.
13. Speer CP, Robertson B, Cursted T, et al. Randomized European multicenter trial of surfactant replacement therapy for severe neonatal respiratory distress syndrome: single versus multiple doses of Curosurf. Pediatrics 1992; 89:13–20.
14. Halliday HL. Natural vs. synthetic surfactant in neonatal respiratory distress syndrome. Drugs 1996; 51:226–237.
15. Hudak ML, Farrell EE, Rosenberg AA, et al. A multicenter randomized, masked comparison trial of natural versus synthetic surfactant for the treatment of respiratory distress syndrome. J Pediatr 1995; 128:396–406.
16. Hudak ML, Martin DJ, Egan EA, et al. A multicenter randomized masked comparison trial of synthetic surfactant versus calf lung surfactant extract in the prevention of neonatal respiratory distress syndrome. Pediatrics 1997; 100:39–50.
17. Horbar JD, Wright EC, Onstad L, et al. Decreasing mortality associated with the introduction of surfactant therapy: an observational study of neonates weighing 601 to 1300 grams at birth. Pediatrics 1993; 92:191–196.
18. Schwartz RM, Luby AM, Scanlon JW, Kellogg RJ. Effect of surfactant on morbidity, mortality, and resource use in newborn infants weighing 500 to 1500 g. N Engl J Med 1994; 330:1476–1480.
19. Palta M, Weinstein MR, McGuinness G, Gabbert D, Brady W, Peters ME. Morality and morbidity after availability of surfactant therapy. Arch Pediatr Adolesc Med 1994; 148:1295–1301.
20. Egberts J, de Winter JP. Meta-analyses of surfactant and bronchopulmonary dysplasia revisited. Lancet 1994; 344:882.
21. Abbasi S, Bhutani VK, Gerdes JS. Long-term pulmonary consequences of respiratory distress syndrome in preterm infants treated with exogenous surfactant. J Pediatr 1993; 122:446–452.
22. Survanta Multidose Study Group. Two-year follow-up of infants treated for neonatal respiratory distress syndrome with bovine surfactant. J Pediatr 1994; 124:962–967.
23. Jobe AH. Pulmonary surfactant therapy. N Engl J Med 1993; 328:861–868.
24. Fujiwara T. Surfactant replacement in neonatal RDS. In: Robertson B, Van Golde LMG, Batenburg JJ, eds. Pulmonary Surfactant. Amsterdam: Elsevier Science, 1984: 479–503.
25. Noack G, Curstedt T, Grossmann G, Nilsson R, Robertson B. Passive expiratory flow–volume recordings in immature newborn rabbits. Respiration 1990; 57:1–5.
26. Davis JM, Veness-Meehan K, Notter RH, Bhutani VK, Kendig JW, Shapiro DL. Changes in pulmonary mechanics after the administration of surfactant to infants with respiratory distress syndrome. N Engl J Med 1988; 319:476–479.
27. Kelly E, Bryan H, Possmayer F, Frndova H, Bryan C. Compliance of the respiratory system in newborn infants pre- and post surfactant replacement therapy. Pediatr Pulmonol 1993; 15:225–230.

28. Robertson B. Pathology and pathophysiology of neonatal surfactant deficiency. In: Robertson B, Van Golde LMG, Batenburg JJ, eds. Pulmonary Surfactant. Amsterdam: Elsevier Science, 1984:383–418.
29. Dreyfuss D, Saumon G. Role of tidal volume, FRC, and end-inspiratory volume in the development of pulmonary edema following mechanical ventilation. Am Rev Respir Dis 1993; 148:1194–1203.
30. Jobe AH. Techniques for administering surfactant. In: Robertson B, Taeusch HW, eds. Surfactant Therapy for Lung Disease. New York: Marcel Dekker, 1995:309–324.
31. Pinkerton KE, Lewis JF, Rider ED, et al. Lung parenchyma and type II cell morphometrics: effect of surfactant treatment on preterm ventilated lamb lungs. J Appl Physiol 1994; 77:1953–1960.
32. Pinkerton KE, Woods E, Rider E, Ikegami M, Jobe AH. Effects of unilateral surfactant instillation on ventilated preterm sheep lung structure. Am J Respir Crit Care Med 1994; 149:A97.
33. Nilsson R, Grossmann G, Robertson B. Bronchiolar epithelial lesions induced in the premature rabbit neonate by short periods of artificial ventilation. Acta Pathol Microbiol Scand 1980; 88:359–367.
34. Ikegami M, Jobe AH, Seidner S, Yamada T. Gestational effects of corticosteroids and surfactant in ventilated rabbits. Pediatr Res 1989; 25:32–37.
35. Jobe AH, Jacobs H, Ikegami M, Berry D. Lung protein leaks in ventilated lambs: effect of gestational age. J Appl Physiol 1985; 58:1246–1251.
36. Ikegami M, Berry D, Elkady T, Pettenazzo A, Seidner S, Jobe AH. Corticosteroids and surfactant change lung function and protein leaks in the lungs of ventilated premature rabbits. J Clin Invest 1987; 79:1371–1378.
37. Carlton DP, Cho SC, Davis P, Lont M, Bland RD. Surfactant treatment at birth reduces lung vascular injury and edema in preterm lambs. Pediatr Res 1995; 37: 265–270.
38. Raj JU. Alveolar liquid pressure by micropuncture in isolated lungs of mature and immature fetal rabbits. J Clin Invest 1987; 79:1579–1588.
39. Ikegami M, Rebello CM, Jobe AH. Surfactant inhibition by plasma: gestational age and surfactant treatment effects in preterm lambs. J Appl Physiol 1997; 81:2517–2522.
40. Escobedo MB, Hilliard JL, Smith F, et al. A baboon model of bronchopulmonary dysplasia. Exp Mol Pathol 1982; 37:323–334.
41. Coalson JJ, Winter VT, Gerstmann DR, Idell S, King RJ, Delemos RA. Pathophysiologic, morphometric, and biochemical studies of the premature baboon with bronchopulmonary dysplasia. Am Rev Respir Dis 1992; 145:872–881.
42. Tsuno K, Miura K, Takeya M, Kolobow T, Morioka T. Histopathologic pulmonary changes from mechanical ventilation at high peak airway pressures. Am Rev Respir Dis 1991; 143:1115–1120.
43. Rojas MA, Gonzalez A, Bancalari E, Claure N, Poole C, Silva-Neto G. Changing trends in the epidemiology and pathogenesis of neonatal chronic lung disease. J Pediatr 1995; 126:605–610.
44. Ogden BE, Murphy SA, Saunders GC, et al. Neonatal lung neutrophils and elastase/proteinase inhibitor imbalance. Am Rev Respir Dis 1984; 130:817–821.

45. Sherman MP, Ganz T. Host defense in pulmonary alveoli. Annu Rev Physiol 1992; 54:331–350.
46. Speer CP, Ruess D, Harms K, Hertin E, Gefeller O. Neutrophil elastase and acute pulmonary damage in neonates with severe respiratory distress syndrome. Pediatrics 1993; 91:794–799.
47. Groneck P, Gotze-Speer B, Oppermann M, Eiffert H, Speer CP. Association of pulmonary inflammation and increased microvascular permeability during the development of bronchopulmonary dysplasia: a sequential analysis of inflammatory mediators in respiratory fluids of high-risk preterm neonates. Pediatrics 1994; 93:712–718.
48. Bagchi A, Viscardi RM, Taciak V, Ensor JE, McCrea KA, Hasday JD. Increased activity of interleukin-6 but not tumor necrosis factor-α in lung lavage of premature infants is associated with the development of bronchopulmonary dysplasia. Pediatr Res 1994; 36:244–252.
49. Hamilton PP, Onayemi A, Smyth JA, et al. Comparison of conventional and high-frequency ventilation: oxygenation and lung pathology. J Appl Physiol 1983; 55: 131–138.
50. Kawano T, Mori S, Cybulsky M, et al. Effect of granulocyte depletion in a ventilated surfactant-depleted lung. J Appl Physiol 1987; 62:27–33.
51. Froese AB, McCulloch PR, Sugiura M, Vaclavik S, Possmayer F, Moller F. Optimizing alveolar expansion prolongs the effectiveness of exogenous surfactant therapy in the adult rabbit. Am Rev Respir Dis 1993; 148:569–577.
52. Gerstmann DR, Minton SD, Stoddard RA, et al. The Provo multicenter early high-frequency oscillatory ventilation trial: improved pulmonary and clinical outcome in respiratory distress syndrome. Pediatrics 1996; 98:1044–1056.
53. The Investigators of the Vermont–Oxford Trials Network Database Project. The Vermont–Oxford Trials Network: very low birth weight outcomes for 1990. Pediatrics 1993; 91:540–545.
54. Avery ME, Tooley W, Keller J, et al. Is chronic lung disease in prematurely born infants preventable? Pediatrics 1987; 79:26–30.
55. Kraybill EN, Runyan DK, Bose CL, Khan JH. Risk factors for chronic lung disease in infants with birth weights of 751 to 1000 grams. J Pediatr 1989; 115:115–120.
56. Garland JS, Buck RK, Allred EN, Leviton A. Hypocarbia prior to surfactant therapy appears to increase bronchopulmonary dysplasia risk in infants with respiratory distress syndrome. Arch Pediatr Adolesc Med 1995; 149:617–622.
57. Jobe AH. Hypocarbia and bronchopulmonary dysplasia. Arch Pediatr Adolesc Med 1995; 149:615–616.
58. Ingimarsson J, Björklund T, Curstedt JJ, Robertson B, Werner O, Vilstrup CT. Neonatal resuscitation with a few large breaths compromises the effect of subsequent surfactant replacement in immature lambs. Acta Anaethesiol Scand 1995; 39(suppl 105):153.
59. Wada K, Ikegami M, Jobe AH. Tidal volume effects on surfactant treatment responses with initiation of ventilation in preterm lambs. J Appl Physiol 1997; 83: 1054–1061.
60. Van Marter LJ, Pagano M, Allred EN, Leviton A, Kuban KCK. Rate of bronchopul-

monary dysplasia as a function of neonatal intensive care practices. J Pediatr 1992; 120:938–946.
61. Hallman M, Merritt TA, Bry K, Berry C. Association between neonatal care practices and efficacy of exogenous human surfactant: results of a bicenter randomized trial. Pediatrics 1993; 91:552–560.
62. Gerstmann DR, deLemos RA, Coalson JJ, et al. Influence of ventilatory technique on pulmonary baroinjury in baboons with hyaline membrane disease. Pediatr Pulmonol 1988; 5:82–91.
63. Jackson JC, Truog WE, Standaert TA, et al. Reduction in lung injury after combined surfactant and high-frequency ventilation. Am J Respir Crit Care Med 1994; 150: 534–539.
64. Rider ED, Ikegami M, Whitsett JA, Hull W, Absolom D, Jobe AH. Treatment responses to surfactant containing natural surfactant proteins in preterm rabbits. Am Rev Respir Dis 1993; 147:669–676.
65. Rider ED, Jobe AH, Ikegami M, Sun B. Different ventilation strategies alter surfactant responses in preterm rabbits. J Appl Physiol 1992; 73:2089–2096.
66. Obladen M. Alterations in surfactant composition. In: Menitt TA, Northway WH, Boynton BR, eds. Bronchopulmonary Dysplasia. Boston: Blackwell Scientific 1988: 131–141.
67. Moya FR, Montes HF, Thomas VL, Mouzinho AM, Smith JF, Rosenfeld CR. Surfactant protein A and saturated phosphatidylcholine in respiratory distress syndrome. Am J Respir Crit Care Med 1994; 150:1672–1677.
68. Hallman M, Merritt TA, Akino T, Bry K. Surfactant protein A, phosphatidylcholine, and surfactant inhibitors in epithelial lining fluid. Am Rev Respir Dis 1991; 144: 1376–1384.
69. Coalson JJ, King RJ, Yang F, et al. SP-A deficiency in primate model of bronchopulmonary dysplasia with infection. Am J Respir Crit Care Med 1995; 151:854–866.
70. Ikegami M, Korfhagen TR, Bruno MD, Whitsett JA, Jobe AH. Surfactant metabolism in surfactant protein A-deficient mice. Am J Physiol 1997; 272:L479–L485.
71. Pandit PB, Dunn MS, Kelly EN, Perlman M. Surfactant replacement in neonates with early chronic lung disease. Pediatrics 1995; 95:851–854.
72. Seidner SR, Jobe AH, Coalson JJ, Ikegami M. Abnormal surfactant metabolism and function in preterm ventilated baboons. Am J Respir Crit Care Med 1998; 158:1982–1989.

12

Drug Treatment for Established BPD

THOMAS A. HAZINSKI

Vanderbilt University Medical School
Nashville, Tennessee

I. Introduction

The treatment of infants with established bronchopulmonary dysplasia (BPD) remains a common, frustrating, and expensive problem in neonatology, pediatric pulmonology, pediatric critical care, and general pediatrics. Although some believe that BPD prevalence is falling, partly owing to maternal corticosteroid use, and that BPD infants have less severe disease than in the past, these opinions have not yet been documented. BPD follow-up programs remain active in most pediatric centers, and are as busy as ever. Much progress has been made recently in understanding the antecedents of BPD, and risk factors for its development are well known (1,2). In the past decade, the use of surfactant replacement, high-frequency ventilation, and perhaps some modes of corticosteroid therapy have improved the survival rates of very low birth weight (VLBW) infants, but have not reduced the prevalence of BPD. In addition, several biologically plausible therapies have been developed. These include prenatal treatment with glucocorticoid and thyrotropin-releasing hormone (TRH), which showed substantial promise (3), and early treatment of infants at risk with corticosteroids (4,5), inositol (6), superoxide dismutase (7), and α_1-protease inhibitor (8,9). Unfortunately, recent clinical trials have shown that neither prenatal TRH–glucocorticoid therapy (10) nor postnatal α_1-protease inhibitor (11) significantly reduced the incidence or severity of BPD. It is possible that newer forms of mechanical ventilation, including perfluorocarbon-assisted (12) and patient-triggered (13,14), may reduce the incidence or severity of BPD. However, there is still no scientifically proved and widely accepted method to prevent BPD.

Despite these advances and exciting prospects, today in most newborn intensive care units (NICUs), pediatric wards, and outpatient centers in most countries, infants will be encountered with established BPD who are still receiving high-dose oxygen therapy or mechanical ventilation (or both), or who have been readmitted for the treatment of a pulmonary exacerbation. During their evaluation, there probably will be discussions about therapeutic options, including oxygen, diuretics and fluid balance (15), bronchodilators, corticosteroids, and nutrition. The discussion may itself be frustrating, because few of these therapies have been rigorously tested for long-term efficacy in randomized, controlled trials. Moreover, it is uncertain whether drugs of proved short-term efficacy in moderately premature infants will also be effective in the extremely low birth weight infants, who now constitute the most infants with BPD. As a result, the clinician must continue to be guided by an understanding of the complex pathophysiology of BPD, by a knowledge of drug effects and interactions, and by careful clinical assessment of individual therapeutic responses.

This chapter will briefly review the scientific rationale, use, and potential pitfalls of some of the aforementioned drugs for the treatment of abnormal lung mechanics and gas exchange that are present in infants with established BPD. Although much has been learned from animal models and from in vitro studies, this chapter will focus primarily on clinical studies in infants with BPD. Several other reviews of this subject have been published recently, and this chapter should be considered complementary to these other works (16–19). We will not discuss in detail the use of drugs to *prevent* BPD because, as of this writing, no postnatal therapy or combination of therapies has been unequivocally shown to reduce the incidence or severity of BPD. The ventilator management of infants with BPD and chronic respiratory failure is also beyond the scope of this chapter. Finally, we will speculate about the gaps that exist in our understanding of drug therapy for BPD and future directions in BPD research that should be explored. Our hope is that the physician–scientist will find this chapter useful, both in making decisions about therapy in infants with BPD and in planning future investigative efforts.

At the outset, one must first deal with a vexing question: When can an infant be said to have established BPD? In this chapter, we will use the term *BPD* to mean the persistence of oxygen-dependence and abnormal respiratory symptoms beyond postnatal day 28. This definition identifies a subset of infants with unresolved lung injury using oxygenation and clinical examination as objective criteria. Other definitions of BPD, which employ chest radiographs and clinical scoring systems, are somewhat subjective and are rarely used to make individual treatment decisions. However, this definition also has limitations, for it can legitimately be argued that the pathophysiological abnormalities termed BPD are established in the first weeks of life, as suggested by data from animal models, human lung histology, and lung lavage data. However, much of the data supporting the use of many BPD drugs have been obtained from studies that enrolled infants with this commonly accepted definition.

II. Oxygen Therapy

Supplemental oxygen therapy remains the mainstay of BPD care, for chronic alveolar hypoxemia, secondary to ventilation–perfusion inequalities, is usually present in infants with established BPD. The serious implications of chronic *alveolar* hypoxemia of BPD must be differentiated from the more benign form of systemic hypoxemia that is present in infants with cyanotic congenital heart disease (CCHD). In infants with CCHD without lung injury, alveolar and lung perivascular Po_2 levels are normal, but venous admixture and shunt result in a low Po_2 level in arterial blood. This low Po_2 level in arterial blood is partially offset by increased cardiac output, which can maintain systemic oxygen delivery. By contrast, in infants with BPD and untreated or unrecognized alveolar hypoxemia, the lung perivascular Po_2 level is reduced, leading to complex and poorly understood effects. These include hypoxia-associated effects on the expression of genes that influence lung vascular development (20,21), on functional responses to vasoactive agents (22), and alterations in lung structure that can lead to an irreversible increase in pulmonary vascular resistance (23). Therefore, although both CCHD and BPD infants have systemic hypoxemia, only the BPD infant has alveolar hypoxemia which, if untreated, can lead to fatal pulmonary hypertension.

Oxygen can be considered both a nutrient and a drug, and although never subjected to randomized controlled trials, oxygen has the strongest scientific rationale and widest margin of safety. The hazards of chronic alveolar hypoxemia are well known, and most have been demonstrated in infants with BPD: pulmonary hypertension and right ventricular failure (24), and slow somatic and brain growth (25). In animal models, chronic hypoxemia causes gastrointestinal malabsorption and delayed maturation of digestive enzymes (26). By contrast, hazardous side effects of low-flow supplemental oxygen therapy sufficient to achieve a near-normal oxygen saturation, have never been described in infants with BPD or in animal models of lung injury or development. In our experience, it is the rapid downward adjustment of oxygen therapy, rather than oxygen therapy per se, that has led to adverse clinical consequences.

Our current practice is to provide supplemental oxygen by nasal cannula to maintain hemoglobin saturation higher than 92% and lower than 95% (i.e., a

Pa_{O_2} between 65 and 90 mmHg at normal pH) when the infant is both awake and asleep. If there is clinical or echocardiographic evidence of pulmonary hypertension, we maintain oxygen saturation in the 95–96% range. Pulse oximetry is used to measure oxygen saturation while the infant is quiet and awake. We also measure and record oxygen saturation after 10 min of room air breathing every 2–3 weeks, as infants who receive low-flow oxygen may sometimes have a substantial degree of desaturation while breathing room air. Commercially available pulse oximeters are accurate within $\pm 2\%$ when the oximeter is reading in the 90–96% range; hence, it is unlikely that hyperoxia will occur at the prescribed oxygen flow rate (27,28). Moreover, oxygen therapy by nasal prongs rarely achieves inspired oxygen concentrations much higher than 35% (29); thus, concerns about additional oxygen-mediated lung injury are unwarranted.

Oxygen therapy is discontinued only after diuretics (and supplemental KCl), fluid restriction, and corticosteroids have been discontinued. If somatic growth rate (measured in grams per day) stops or slows by more than 20% in the weeks following the discontinuation of oxygen therapy and despite adequate caloric intake, this is considered to be strong evidence of significant intermittent hypoxemia, for which we restart supplemental oxygen therapy. If the need for supplemental oxygen increases or fails to decrease during the first 2 or 3 months after discharge from intensive care, a search is made for coexisting conditions that might mimic BPD or delay lung repair (see later).

We do not recommend transient increases in supplemental oxygen therapy for feeding or agitation. These common infant activities rarely, if ever, cause sustained hypoxemia, and if they do, it is likely that the maintenance dose of oxygen is too low or the infant has pulmonary hypertension with episodic increases in intrapulmonary or interatrial shunting of blood. In either event, the dose of oxygen should be increased.

It is also important to recognize that many instances of ''transient hypoxemia'' usually are caused by inappropriate application of the oximeter probe or to misunderstanding of the oximeter device itself. Studies have clearly documented the inability of both hospital and home caretakers to use oximeters and to interpret oximetry data correctly (30,31). In our view, pulse oximetry should be used to assess oxygen saturation during precisely defined steady-state conditions, or it should be used to confirm a clinical impression that hypoxemia is present.

Although most centers use nasal cannulas to deliver supplemental oxygen, some centers use nasopharyngeal catheters, citing more reliable oxygen delivery with the latter method (32,33), but either method yields acceptable results.

III. Diuretic Therapy

The use of drugs with diuretic properties to improve lung mechanics and respiratory gas exchange is now fairly well accepted, and in some NICUs diuretics have become the standard of care for most infants with established BPD. In infants with BPD, pulmonary edema is present and is manifest as rales (crackles) or wheezing, probably secondary to interstitial and peribronchiolar puddling of water in the lung's interstitial spaces. The rationale for diuretic therapy in infants with established BPD has been presented in other monographs (15–19), but rests largely on the finding of increased microvascular permeability and pulmonary edema in neonates with respiratory failure and in animal models of acute lung injury (34). It is likely that fluid balance in the first days of life is a risk factor for subsequent BPD, and one single-center clinical trial of fluid restriction in LBW infants with respiratory failure found a 40% reduction in the incidence of BPD (35). This single-center study, performed before the widespread use of surfactant replacement therapy, is provocative and deserves further exploration.

Both daily (36) and alternate-day (37) short-term use of furosemide improves lung mechanics and gas exchange in infants with established BPD. Thiazide-type diuretics, alone or in combination with spironolactone, have improved lung function in some studies (38), but not in others (39). The alleged advantage of using thiazides because they cause less hypercalciuria is poorly documented and probably should not be used as the sole rationale for their use.

The efficacy of long-term diuretic therapy is unproved. One randomized trial lasting 6 weeks concluded that daily thiazide therapy was beneficial (40), but a large excess of boys in the placebo group may have biased the results in favor of the drug. A trial of long-term daily thiazide–spironolactone therapy detected no ultimate clinical benefit, although oxygen therapy was reduced more rapidly in the treated group (41). In this latter study, both groups received furosemide intermittently, so the true effect of diuretic therapy is somewhat uncertain.

The mechanisms by which drugs with diuretic properties improve lung function are unknown, but there is evidence that neither direct nor indirect effects of simple diuresis (i.e., a renal effect) can completely explain the beneficial effect (reviewed in Ref. 16). For example, in infants with BPD, furosemide quickly increases urine volume and decreases extracellular fluid volume, but after a few days the diuretic effect is abolished, but lung function remains improved (36,37,42). The mechanism responsible for this tachyphylaxis is unknown. It is possible that furosemide exerts a direct effect on lung fluid balance independently of its renal and systemic vascular effects by altering surfactant function, ion–water transport, or pulmonary vascular tone (16).

Recently, on the basis of reports in adults who *inhaled* furosemide (in doses that do not provoke a diuresis) showing that it prevents but does not reverse, allergen- and exercise-induced bronchospasm in asthmatics, the efficacy of aerosolized furosemide has been examined in infants with BPD. The possible benefit has been transient, variable, or explained by systemic absorption of the inhaled drug (43). This form of diuretic therapy cannot be recommended.

Most infants with established BPD do not require diuretics. In our practice, less than 20% of all oxygen-dependent infants are receiving long-term diuretic therapy. If diuretic therapy is begun, supplemental KCl must also be administered to prevent diuretic-induced metabolic alkalosis (see later discussion). As gas exchange improves, diuretic therapy is reduced to alternate day for 2–4 weeks and then discontinued entirely. When diuretic therapy has been discontinued entirely, we then reduce oxygen therapy. We do not use thiazide-type diuretics either alone or in combination with spironolactone.

Short-term diuretic therapy may be useful in infants with established BPD and acute fluid overload, such as might occur following blood transfusion, intravenous administration of immunoglobulin, or inadvertent overhydration.

Two side effects of prolonged diuretic therapy warrant attention: (1) diuretic-induced hypokalemia–alkalosis–hypoventilation and (2) hypercalciuria, with secondary hyperparathyroidism and nephrocalcinosis.

Diuretic-induced hypokalemia and alkalosis can be diagnosed by finding a blood pH (not base deficit) that is inappropriate for the infant's clinical state. For example, the *hypercarbic* infant with established BPD should have a compensated respiratory acidosis; that is, the blood pH should be 7.3–7.35, and the serum bicarbonate should be slightly elevated (Fig. 1A). However, if salt intake is low

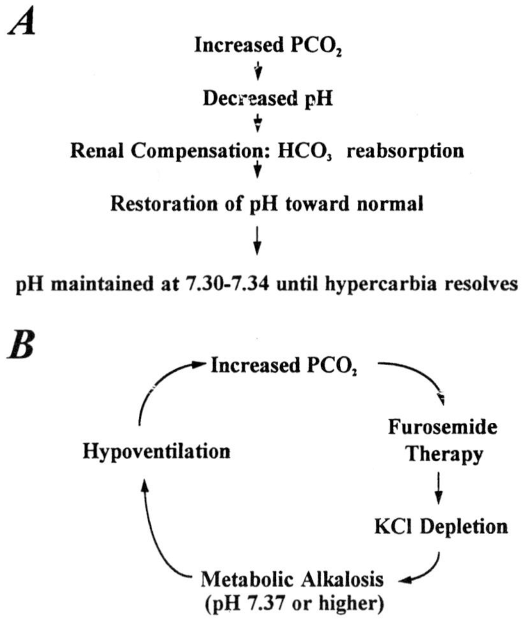

Figure 1 (A) Compensated respiratory acidosis in BPD. (B) Diuretic-induced metabolic alkalosis in BPD.

(e.g., in fluid-restricted infants or in infants who are fed breast milk with its low salt content, or fed diluted formula), if diuretic therapy is excessive, or if supplemental KCl is not administered, losses of potassium and chloride can lead to a *primary metabolic alkalosis*. In this situation, the blood pH will be in the high-normal range or even elevated, and the $Paco_2$ may also increase as the infant hypoventilates to reduce blood pH to normal, creating an unfavorable inhibition of ventilation (see Fig. 1B). Sometimes only the rising Pco_2 and not the rising pH is noted, and the furosemide dose is further increased, as the clinician believes that the hypercarbia is due to worsening lung function; in fact, the hypercarbia is a normal physiological response to an iatrogenic metabolic alkalosis. This latter situation can be identified only by the measurement of blood pH, as infants with both physiological and iatrogenic hypercarbia will have elevated bicarbonate, Pco_2, and calculated base excess. The important point to remember is this: if a hypercarbic infant with BPD is receiving diuretic therapy, blood pH should be between 7.30 and 7.35. A normal or elevated blood pH value suggests a diuretic-induced alkalosis. If iatrogenic metabolic alkalosis is present, the treatment is to reduce the furosemide dose or to provide additional KCl.

The second complication of long-term diuretic therapy is hypercalciuria with secondary hyperparathyroidism and calcium deposition in the renal interstitium, termed nephrocalcinosis (44). The diagnosis of nephrocalcinosis is established by the finding of echogenic areas during renal ultrasonography. This condition is poorly understood and its incidence is quite variable, presumably owing to the lack of precise ultrasonographic criteria. Moreover, the association between nephrocalcinosis and furosemide therapy is somewhat weak. For example; very low birth weight infants with no history of furosemide therapy have nephrocalcinosis by renal ultrasound (45). Therefore, although furosemide causes nephrocalcinosis in infants without BPD (46), the infant with established BPD has many other risk factors for renal damage and nephrocalcinosis, including white race, family history of renal calculi, parenteral nutrition, and episodes of hypoxemia and hypotension (44,45,47,48). Rarely, nephrocalcinosis can lead to renal calculi, hematuria, and to renal insufficiency. A recent study has indicated that furosemide-induced nephrocalcinosis can lead to abnormalities in urinary acidification and mild reductions in creatinine clearance at 1–2 years of age even after nephrocalcinosis resolves (49). The long-term consequences of these furosemide-associated abnormalities in both glomerular and tubular dysfunction are unknown. However, this potential complication serves to emphasize that long-term furosemide therapy should be reserved for those infants with severe established BPD who have clear-cut evidence of diuretic-responsive pulmonary disease.

What is the future of diuretic therapy in infants with BPD? Because the renal effect of diuretic drugs may not be responsible for the beneficial pulmonary effect, new classes of lung-specific agents might be developed based on a better understanding of the mechanisms of lung water and solute transport in the lung.

IV. Inhaled Bronchodilator Therapy

Premature infants can respond to bronchoconstrictor stimuli, and some infants who were born prematurely, regardless of whether or not they have BPD, have bronchial smooth-muscle hypertrophy and airway hyperresponsiveness (16–18,50). In addition, clinical assessment of infants with BPD indicate that they sometimes have persistent or intermittent wheezing, and pulmonary function testing reveals expiratory airflow limitation similar to that observed in infants with asthma. Because the inhalation of β_2-adrenergic agonist drugs improve lung function in infants with asthma, several studies of short-term inhaled and parenteral β_2-adrenergic agonist therapy have shown transient improvement in lung mechanics and gas exchange (16,51); however, no long-term studies have been reported. A family history of asthma may (52) or may not (53) be a risk factor for the development of BPD and for long-term oxygen dependency in infants with established BPD, prompting further speculation that asthma and BPD may share similar pathophysiological mechanisms.

These observations form the scientific rationale for the use of drugs with bronchodilator properties in infants with BPD. If such infants demonstrate persistent or intermittent clinical evidence of reversible airway obstruction, intermittent inhaled β-agonist therapy may be indicated. If chronic cough, wheezing, or congestion persists despite bronchodilator therapy, and other pulmonary disorders can be ruled out, long-term inhaled anti-inflammatory therapy with either inhaled cromolyn sodium or inhaled corticosteroids should be strongly considered. To administer these medications, we use a compressed air nebulizer and rarely employ the metered-dose inhaler (MDI) with spacer method, for the latter technique is difficult and compliance is poor. In addition, we do not use oral β-agonist therapy because of its high incidence of side effects and narrow therapeutic index. Because of concerns about the development of tachyphylaxis, intermittent β-agonist therapy is most often employed, although some patients appear to require daily therapy to maintain long symptom-free intervals.

Two pitfalls in the use of β_2-agonist drugs (albuterol, terbutaline, and metaproteronol) should be mentioned: (1) β-agonist-induced *vaso*dilation leading to hypoxemia, and (2) β-agonist-induced augmentation of airway instability in the infant with both BPD and tracheomalacia. Both pitfalls are related to the complex and focal pathological features of BPD at both the acinar and preacinar levels, leading to complex ventilation–perfusion $\dot{V}/\dot{Q}$ relations (54).

The first pitfall is fairly straightforward and is similar to the problem seen frequently in patients with $\dot{V}/\dot{Q}$ mismatch caused by status asthmaticus and atelectasis. The reasoning is as follows: Some infants with BPD have focal distal airway obstruction that is not due to bronchoconstriction, but is due to airway metaplasia and mucus plugging. These infants will have poorly ventilated and appropriately underperfused lung units (i.e., they have appropriate $\dot{V}/\dot{Q}$ matching) and may not respond to β-agonist therapy with bronchodilation. However, in very high doses or with prolonged use, β-agonist therapy will increase pulmonary blood flow through these underventilated lung units, leading to severe $\dot{V}/\dot{Q}$ mismatch, an increase in venous admixture (shunt), and hypoxemia that is poorly responsive to oxygen therapy.

The second pitfall of β-agonist therapy is seen in BPD infants with tracheomalacia, which has been observed in up to 50% of infants with BPD who are discharged from the neonatal intensive care unit (55,56). It has been demonstrated that infants with tracheomalacia maintain the stability of large airways by an increase in airway smooth-muscle tone (57). In such infants, β-agonist therapy will *increase* airway resistance by further reducing airway stability, and drugs with bronchoconstrictor properties will *improve* airflow limitation in these infants (Fig. 2). This phenomenon probably explains why inhaled bronchodilator therapy has variable effects on lung mechanics in infants with BPD (58). Tracheomalacia should be suspected in any infant with BPD who has signs or symptoms of airway obstruction and whose clinical status is worsened by inhaled bronchodilator therapy.

These two undesirable effects of β-agonist therapy are unpredictable and emphasize the need to individualize therapy. In infants with established bronchial hyperreactivity who require daily treatment, the β-agonist is diluted with cromolyn sodium, saline, or in countries where it is available, budesonide. Inhaled anticholinergic agents, such as ipratroprium bromide, have been used to treat airflow limitation in infants with BPD (59). Its proponents advocate using this agent instead of saline or cromolyn sodium as a diluent for inhaled β-agonist therapy. In animals there is basal cholinergic tone in airway smooth muscle, but the role of cholinergic pathways in the airways of infants with BPD has not been systematically examined. If tracheomalacia is present, anticholinergic drugs may have variable effects on airflow resistance.

Methylxanthines such as theophylline are not currently used in the treatment of bronchial hyperreactivity in infants with BPD. Theophylline's erratic pharmacokinetics and multiple side effects, including seizures and relaxation of the gastroesophageal junction, multiple drug interactions with antibiotics and prokinetic agents, and lack of efficacy by the inhaled route, render it less valuable as a first-line drug for this population.

What is the future of bronchodilator therapy for infants with BPD? There is no convincing evidence that one β_2-agonist agent is superior to any other, except perhaps in onset and duration of action. These inhaled drugs are best employed in the treatment of episodes of expiratory airflow limitation associated with respiratory infections. Newer agents that cause bronchodilation by nonadrenergic mechanisms, such as the new class of oral leukotriene receptor antagonists, might be considered for efficacy studies in infants with BPD.

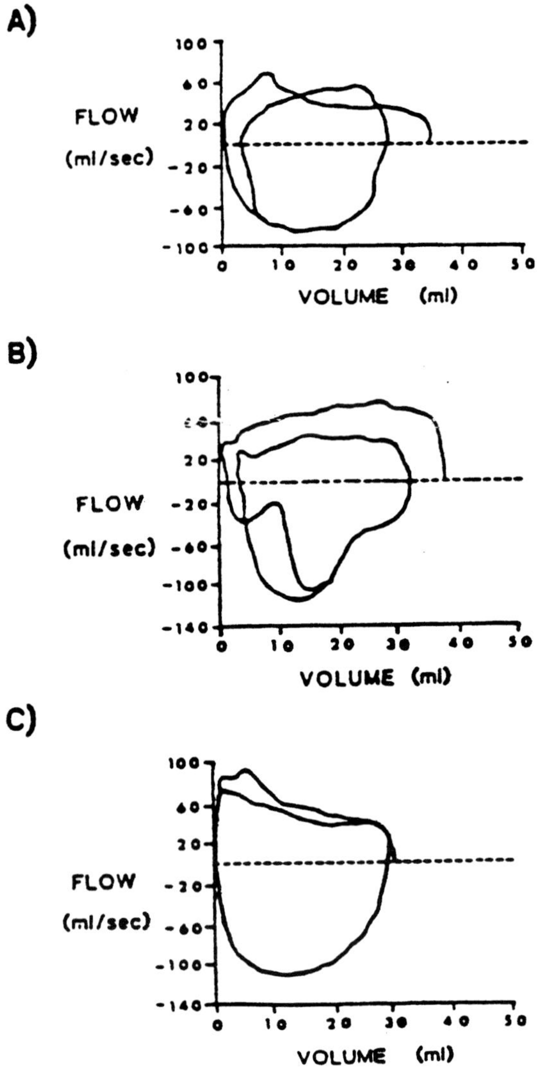

Figure 2 Beta-agonist inhalation reduces expiratory flow in infants with tacheomalacia. Depicted are three tidal flow-volume (small loop) and forced expiratory flow-volume curves from an infant with tracheomlacia. In panel A (top), forced expiratory flow is 37 mL/s, actually below tidal flow rate. Albuterol inhalation (panel C on bottom) reduced airflow by 11%, but methacholine inhalation (panel B in middle) increased expiratory flow by 88% (From Panitch, 1990, with permission).

V. Anti-Inflammatory Therapy

The scientific rationale for the development and use of anti-inflammatory drugs in the treatment of BPD is based on four considerations: (1) pathological evidence of lung inflammation seen in postmortem lung specimens from infants with BPD (54,60); (2) studies of the role of inflammation in young pediatric patients with chronic asthma (61) and cystic fibrosis (62), which have yielded new insights into the molecular mechanisms of inflammation in patients with these chronic lung diseases; (3) the observations that perinatal infections (2,63,64) are risk factors for the subsequent acquisition of BPD; and (4) the finding of cytokines, signaling molecules, and activated inflammatory cells in the tracheal lavage fluid of infants with established BPD and in infants destined to acquire BPD (60,65–67).

The pathological evidence of lung inflammation in fatal BPD is perhaps not surprising, for most deaths of BPD infants are attributable to infection. The recent finding that lung inflammation may begin prenatally in infants destined to acquire BPD (63,64) is startling in its implications, because it suggests that BPD may be the inevitable result of inflammatory lung injury already established before birth. When one considers the data from lung lavage studies that link inflammation to BPD, it must be recognized that these studies are based on obtaining tracheal aspirates or lung lavage fluid. Such studies require the infant to be intubated, so that babies who die or who are extubated are not available for repeated sampling. Moreover, tracheal aspirates from cohort-matched infants without BPD or with non-BPD respiratory illnesses have not been sampled to serve as control groups in these studies. As a result, it is still uncertain which of these cytokines and signaling factors are in the causal pathway to BPD and which are harmless markers of lung inflammation or repair. Future studies should focus on the identification of those mediators for which abundance or activity can be modulated to yield beneficial clinical effects in infants with BPD.

Drugs that inhibit specific inflammatory mediators have been developed for patients with asthma, but have not yet been tested in infants with BPD. For example, leukotriene receptor antagonists, including zileuton, montelukast, and zafirlukast, have both bronchodilator and anti-inflammatory properties in patients with asthma (68). These agents primarily target the receptor for leukotriene D_4 and provide evidence that blockade of a single signal transduction pathway has yielded beneficial effects in a disease that, similar to BPD, is multifactorial, but is almost certain to involve abnormalities of multiple inflammatory mediators.

In infants with BPD, only nonspecific anti-inflammatory agents have been evaluated. This class of drug includes cromolyn sodium, nedocromil, and corticosteroids. Cromolyn sodium has no proved effectiveness in infants with BPD, perhaps because it is administered only by inhalation, and its bioavailability is markedly reduced when delivered to mechanically ventilated infants (69). However, one recent randomized, controlled trial found that cromolyn therapy reduced the levels of several cytokines in tracheal aspirates of infants with BPD, but BPD incidence and severity were unaffected (70). There are no published studies that have examined the effects of nedocromil, another broad-spectrum inhaled anti-inflammatory agent, in infants with BPD.

The most thoroughly tested anti-inflammatory agent used in the treatment of infants with BPD is corticosteroids therapy, which remains one of the most controversial aspects of BPD treatment. As based on an early report of efficacy in small trials, two large multicenter, randomized controlled trials were unable to detect any beneficial effect of daily corticosteroid therapy begun 14–38 days after birth (71,72), and recent trials of steroid therapy begun in the first days of life have ranged from promising (4,73) to negative (74). The rationale for immediate postnatal corticosteroid therapy has been bolstered somewhat by the finding of relative adrenal unresponsiveness and low corticol levels in BPD-prone neonates (75,76). A reported metanalysis of five early steroid regimens found no effect on NICU death or sepsis rates and a small reduction in BPD incidence (77). Unfortunately, few clinical trials have proposed or tested a mechanism of action that might explain its effects.

It has been demonstrated repeatedly that a short course of parenteral dexamethasone will hasten extubation and transiently improve lung mechanics in infants with established BPD, but these short-term benefits have not resulted in long-term beneficial effects on morbidity, mortality, or cost. Several studies have reported transient cessation of somatic and brain growth during dexamethasone therapy (71,72). The mechanisms and long-term consequences of this catabolic effect are unknown, but should strengthen further the search for mediator-specific anti-inflammatory therapies.

Despite these repeated observations of limited long-term effectiveness of corticosteroid therapy, daily or alternate-date dexamethasone therapy has become a standard of care in many NICUs. After almost two decades of use, it is still uncertain who, when, and for how long to treat, and how to deliver the drug. This widespread use of dexamethasone in the face of so many negative trials is quite remarkable, and is probably explained by the often dramatic response of some infants to initial corticosteroid therapy. However, equally noteworthy are the infants who are clearly unresponsive to large doses of corticosteroids (78). In addition, some infants with BPD acquire a form of corticosteroid-dependency, and their lung function deteriorates when corticosteroid therapy is reduced. Such steroid-resistent and steroid-dependent infants may provide clues to the pathogenesis of BPD. It is likely that the variability in corticosteroid response is partly explained by there being multiple pathways to BPD, and that some of these pathways are active in individual infants and can be attenuated, at least temporarily, by corticosteroid therapy.

Given the successful use of inhaled corticosteroid therapy for asthma, there are recent reports of the use of inhaled corticosteroids in infants with BPD. One study detected no benefit of aerosolized budesonide therapy (79), but bioavailability of this drug may have influenced the outcome. Several groups have defined the critical parameters to consider when planning to use inhaled steroids (80,81), and large randomized trials are underway.

What is the future of anti-inflammatory therapy for infants with BPD? Unique cytokine abnormalities in the lavage fluid of infants with BPD confirm that inflammation plays a key role in its pathogenesis. In addition, recent evidence suggests that proinflammatory cytokines are present in lung fluid even before birth, suggesting that prenatal therapy with drugs directed against specific proinflammatory pathways should be considered. Although the technique of lung lavage has intrinsic limitations, the identification of mediators of etiologic importance will require more comprehensive analysis of both proinflammatory and anti-inflammatory mediators in lung fluid. Such investigations are often considered as descriptive and not hypothesis-driven, but they can also be viewed as a necessary first step in the identification of clinically relevant therapies. It is also hoped that insights gained from the study of inflammatory mechanisms in asthma and cystic fibrosis can be applied to infants with BPD. Further progress in this area will require the formulation and testing of mechanistic hypotheses either in clinical trials or in well-characterized animal models of BPD.

VI. Nutrition Therapy

It is logical to believe that perinatal malnutrition leads to BPD by augmenting postnatal lung injury and delaying lung repair (82). Even in immature infants without respiratory failure, postnatal caloric and nutrient intake cannot duplicate in utero accretion rates. As a result, the sick, VLBW infant is properly viewed as vulnerable to the adverse effects of caloric and specific nutrient deficiency. All available forms of neonatal nutrition are poor substitutes for intrauterine nutrient delivery, even though advances in the safety of both enteral and parenteral nutrients have been substantial. However, a randomized trial of early intravenous hyperalimentation was stopped prematurely because of excess morbidity in the hyperalimented group (83). This lack of apparent beneficial effect may have been due to the adverse effects of arachidonic acid and other lipids in the intravenous nutrition mixture, or to the amino acid profile used in the intravenous nutrition solutions, which is partially restricted by solubility limitation of individual nutrients and not by the nutritional requirements of the infant.

There is much evidence that premature neonates are born with the need for specific nutrients, the abundance of which was inadequate in early enteral formulas. More than a decade ago, it was demonstrated that deficiencies of specific nutrients, such as vitamin E (84) and vitamin A (85), can lead to BPD, and commercial infant formulas and vitamin supplements were adjusted accordingly. Recently, however, a large multicenter study confirmed that supplementation with vitamin A was associated with a small, but significant, reduction in the incidence of BPD (85). The powerful effects of retinoids in animal models of lung injury and lung development suggest that vitamin A and related compounds should be explored further in preventing BPD (see Sec. VIII).

Another nutrient which is deficient in the premature neonate is inositol, a lipid that is a precursor for the synthesis of pulmonary surfactant. On the basis of studies suggesting that premature infants had low concentrations of inositol in serum, a multicenter, randomized, controlled trial of inositol supplementation was performed (6). This meticulous study demonstrated a reduction in the incidence of BPD, but curiously, this finding has not been pursued.

Infants with severe BPD are at risk for ongoing malnutrition and failure to thrive and for delayed lung repair. There is some evidence that some of these infants have defective vitamin A kinetics (87), limited capacity for fat absorption (88), gastroesophageal reflux, oral aversiveness, and increased energy expenditure that cannot be totally explained by abnormal lung mechanics (89,90). The optimal composition of caloric intake in terms of protein, fat, and carbohydrate is unknown. Infants with BPD produce more carbon dioxide when fed high-carbohydrate diets, but this increase in CO_2 load is probably negligible (90,91). No randomized trials can guide the clinician in this area, but some observations can provide the basis for general recommendations for nutrition in BPD infants.

What is the desired caloric intake in infants with established BPD? From observations in our center, we no longer emphasize caloric intake targets, but instead, seek to maintain an average growth rate between 15 and 30 g/day for all infants with established BPD. This is based on our unpublished observations that growth rates in this range can be maintained at caloric intakes of 90–150 cal/kg per day; this range probably partly reflects the wide range of resting energy expenditure in BPD infants (87,91). In any event, we believe that an infant with BPD is making excellent progress if that infant can sustain this growth rate, with a stable or declining requirement for supplemental oxygen.

Another observation we have made in our center is that augmentation of commercial infant formula with unsaturated oils, medium-chain triglycerides, and glucose polymers is of unproved and limited effectiveness to improve weight gain. Many of the recipes that are used in the NICU are too complex and cumbersome for home use, and many of these recipes produce unstable emulsions that separate during feeding even after vigorous blending. If a 30-cal/oz formula is necessary, we do not supplement lower density formulas, but use commercially available infant formulas, such as Pediasure or Alimentum. Formulas with caloric densities greater than 30 cal/oz are not used. If an infant cannot maintain a growth rate between 15 and 30 g/day on an intake of 135 cal/kg per day, a search is made for coexisting conditions that are interfering with lung repair. This next section discusses some of these conditions.

When infants with established BPD fail to sustain a growth rate of 15–30 g/day, at least four possibilities should be considered: (1) The infant is hypoxemic because of premature termination or excessive reduction of supplemental oxygen therapy; (2) maternal–child interaction difficulties leading to decreased caloric intake; (3) gastroesophageal reflux; and (4) other coexisting diseases that cause lung injury or delay repair such as asthma, cystic fibrosis, acyanotic congenital heart disease, tracheal stenosis or malacia, tracheoesophageal malformation, vascular rings, or aspiration owing to swallowing dysfunction.

For the first possibility, the adverse effects of chronic hypoxemia on somatic growth has been well documented in BPD infants (25). In these situations, restarting or increasing supplemental oxygen therapy usually will improve weight gain, and caretakers must be convinced of the essential role of oxygen as a nutrient. The second possibility, maternal–child interaction difficulties, is a broad category and can include everything from infant oral-aversiveness, improper formula preparation, inadvertent underfeeding or overfeeding, poverty, inadequate parenting skills, the presence of environmental inhalant hazards, or neglect. The use of formulas with caloric densities greater than 30 cal/oz in BPD infants has no evidence to support it.

The third possibility, gastroesophageal reflux (GER), deserves separate consideration because left untreated, GER can lead to malnutrition, reflex bronchospasm, and airway inflammation caused by aspiration of gastric acid, and delayed lung repair. In infants with GER, three abnormalities are present: (1) delayed gastric emptying leading to early satiety and decreased oral intake, (2) increased stomach volume, and (3) episodic relaxation of the gastroesophageal junction permitting flow of acidic stomach contents toward the larynx. GER remains a clinical diagnosis, supported if necessary by esophageal pH monitoring. Barium esophagography is often performed to exclude tracheoesophageal malformations and vascular rings, and not to diagnose GER (94).

A fourth explanation for failure to thrive in BPD infants is the coexistence of other disorders. It must also be emphasized that these coexistent disorders may delay lung repair, prompt rehospitalization, or predispose the infant to frequent respiratory exacerbations. For this reason, the rehospitalization of a BPD infant for a pulmonary exacerbation of presumably infectious origin should prompt consideration of the possibility that factors other than infection are working in concert with BPD to cause or worsen respiratory distress.

Asthma has already been discussed previously. Infants with reversible airway obstruction should be considered for long-term anti-inflammatory therapy and have compressed-air nebulizers available for use at home. Caretakers should be counseled about the ill effects of environmental tobacco smoke exposure. It is not yet known whether asthma and BPD share common pathophysiological mechanisms, but if such links were found, it could have important implications for the treatment of both conditions. Such links require further exploration.

Acyanotic congenital heart disease also can cause pulmonary edema, pulmonary hypertension, or cardiac dysfunction that may be difficult to detect in infants with BPD. In one study, 50% of infants with pulmonary hypertension and severe BPD had a left-to-right cardiac shunt that could be detected only by angiography (24). In our experience, the most severe and persistent failure to thrive has been seen in BPD infants with ''small'' intracardiac shunts owing to atrial or ventricular septal defects. Infants with BPD who are suspected to have a patent foramen ovale or septal defects and whose failure to thrive is unexplained, despite thorough evaluation, should be considered for early surgical repair.

Tracheomalacia can lead to airway instability, stridor, wheezing, and chronic respiratory distress. Tracheomalacia may be suspected clinically or diagnosed by flexible fiberoptic bronchoscopy. Another clue to the presence of tracheomalacia is that their airflow limitation may be *worsened* by inhaled bronchodilator therapy, presumably because these infants maintain large-airway caliber and stability by constriction of airway smooth muscle (57). Malacia is usually self-limiting, but may require therapy with oxygen and continuous positive airway pressure. *Tracheal stenosis* is a rare complication of neonatal lung injury and may present early with signs and symptoms of airway obstruction, or it may present with growth failure or recurrent croup long after BPD has resolved.

Vascular rings and *H-type tracheoesophageal fistulas* can cause respiratory symptoms and growth failure in BPD infants by causing tracheal compression, choking spells, cough, or vomiting. Barium esophogography can exclude these possibilities.

Finally, *swallowing dysfunction* may cause chronic respiratory distress, atelectasis, recurrent pneumonia, wheezing, and failure to thrive. It should be considered especially in BPD infants with neurological injury. This entity is important to distinguish from GER, because neither antireflux medications nor surgery will effectively treat aspiration. Although thickened feedings are occasionally successful in preventing aspiration in infants with swallowing dysfunction, gastrostomy tube feedings may be necessary and can be discontinued when neurological status improves.

VII. Other Drug Treatments for BPD

In some centers, systemic hypertension has been identified in infants with established BPD (95). It has been identified in infants with the most severe lung disease and those treated with corticosteroid therapy, and resolves with time or with treatment with furosemide or other conventional antihypertensive agents. The use of inhaled bronchodilators may increase the risk. In our center, we have not observed this feature of chronic BPD (96).

Given anecdotal reports of low growth hormone levels in BPD infants, growth hormone therapy has also been tested in limited open trials and was ineffective. In addition, recent reports indicate that growth hormone therapy does not prevent the corticosteroid-induced weight loss and protein catabolism in infants with BPD (97).

Infants with established or recently resolved BPD are three times more likely than term infants to require rehospitalization for the treatment of respiratory infections in the first 2 years of life (98). Environmental and familial factors, such as tobacco smoke exposure, family history of asthma, and crowded living conditions, also increase the risk. Therefore, part of the treatment of BPD infants is to educate their families about avoidable risk factors, immunize their siblings and household contacts against respiratory infections, and minimize office visits and elective surgery during the fall and winter months. In some regions, respiratory syncytial virus (RSV) bronchiolitis is an important pathogen leading to substantial morbidity. Monthly infusions of an immunoglobulin preparation enriched with anti-RSV antibodies have demonstrated a significant reduction in the risk of hospitalization in infants with BPD, although the prophylactic regimen is expensive and has no effect on mortality (99). Neither conventional immunoglobulin preparations nor RSV-enriched immunoglobulin preparations are effective as treatment for established bronchiolitis. Recently, monthly injections of a monoclonal antibody directed against RSV has had effects similar to anti-RSV antibody-enriched immunoglobulin infusions (100). RSV vaccines have also been developed and are undergoing clinical trials. Although many viruses can cause acute bronchiolitis in BPD infants, the elimination of RSV bronchiolitis with either active or passive immunization would be an important advance in post-NICU care.

VIII. Future Research Directions

It is evident that more must be learned about the metabolic and molecular mechanisms that lead to the acquisition of BPD and slow its repair. At this writing, prospects for prevention or attenuation of BPD with new neonatal therapies seem promising, but will require a better understanding of how the immature lung develops ex utero and how it responds to injury by oxidant stress, altered pulmonary vascular reactivity, inflammation, and mechanical stress. A few examples are given in the following.

Lung Development

The recent demonstration by Massaro and Massaro of the potent effects of retinoids on both normal (101) and abnormal (102) ex utero lung acinar development suggests potential therapeutic roles for compounds that modulate development of distal respiratory units. A recent multicenter clinical trial of vitamin A supplementation in VLBW infants demonstrated a small but significant reduction in BPD incidence (84). These data are given added importance by recent reports from both human infants with BPD (54) and animal models of BPD (103) that indicate that abnormal alveolar septation and capillary invasion, and not metaplasia of proximal airway epithelium, are the most prominent anatomical features of BPD in VLBW infants.

Oxidant Stress

There is substantial, albeit indirect, evidence that oxygen therapy and other factors increase lung oxidant stress in infants with BPD (104). This general hypothesis has been tested for decades in the laboratory, and is now being examined in clinical trials. For example, the results of studies of inhaled antioxidant therapy, such as recombinant human superoxide dismutase, should be reported soon (105). Moreover, based on the rationale that cytochrome P450-derived metabolites are present in the hyperoxic neonatal lung, a randomized controlled trial of P450 inhibition is also underway (106). Other strategies directed at sources of oxidant production, such as the generation of hydroxyl radical in free–iron-catalyzed reactions, also deserve further study.

In therapeutic trials designed to reduce lung oxidant stress, it will be important to link clinical outcomes with concomitant changes in in vivo markers of oxidant stress. The recent finding of elevated F_2-isoprostane levels (107) and 3-nitrotyrosine (108) in tracheal aspirate fluid in oxygen-exposed infants at risk for BPD may provide a much-needed in vivo marker of oxidant stress. Further advances in our understanding of the role of oxidant stress in the pathogenesis of BPD will require a better knowledge of the sites and mechanisms of lung oxidant production in the developing lung, and on the regulation of constitutive enzymatic and nonenzymatic antioxidant pool sizes in specific lung cell populations. This information will permit the design and testing of other strategies to either increase antioxidant production or decrease oxidant production at the most important sites of oxidant stress.

Altered Pulmonary Vascular Reactivity

Another therapeutic strategy worth considering is based on the rationale that pulmonary vascular responsiveness is impaired in infants with BPD and, in particular, that the kinetics of endogenous nitric oxide production may be impaired in the BPD lung (109). If this is true, the use of inhaled nitric oxide (iNO), especially in view of its potential antioxidant (110) and anti-inflammatory (106) effects, are being explored in animal models (111) and in early trials in infants with BPD.

Lung Inflammation

Worldwide experience with corticosteroid therapy seems to have provided some proof that inflammatory pathways are involved. However, it is equally clear that broad-spectrum anti-inflammatory therapy with corticosteroids has no proved long-term benefit, and that more specific anti-inflammatory agents need to be developed. For example, in the neonate, oxygen breathing appears to increase the production of cytochrome P450-derived metabolites of arachidonic acid which, as proinflammatory agents, might cause further lung injury (112). If this is true, therapies based on reducing the lung pool size of these metabolites might be beneficial. This possibility is now undergoing clinical trials. In addition, much needs to be learned about the role of endogenous anti-inflammatory compounds, such as IL-10 and IL-13 (113,114) because it is likely that the ultimate treatment of lung inflammation in BPD will require the restoration of the balance between proinflammatory and anti-inflammatory molecules at specific sites.

Mechanical Stretch

The adverse effects of stretching the immature lung with mechanical ventilation have been recognized for decades; it leads to airleaks and to the transudation of interstitial fluids and serum into alveoli. Moreover, lung cell stretch modulates the production of endogenous signaling molecules, such as nitric oxide (115).

IX. Summary

Early hopes that advances in the treatment of neonatal respiratory failure in VLBW infants would reduce BPD have not yet been realized. The past decade has not seen major advances in the development or testing of new drugs to treat established BPD, but clinical trials of novel therapies are underway, and the negative results of large-scale clinical trials are prompting the formulation of new hypotheses to test at bench and bedside. At present, the clinician is left with a rational, but limited, array of drugs to treat infants with established BPD. The use of *supplemental oxygen therapy* to maintain oxygen saturation in the physiological range has the strongest rationale and the widest margin of safety, and remains the mainstay of BPD care. In the context of BPD, oxygen should be considered both a nutrient and a drug, and closely monitored with properly performed and interpreted oximetry. Drugs with diuretic properties, most notably *oral furosemide with KCl supplementation*, are useful for a small subset of BPD infants who demonstrate a beneficial response to a therapeutic trial. Diuretic-induced metabolic alkalosis must be avoided. *Inhaled β-agonists* are useful to treat acute episodes of wheezing, but if an infant develops persistent or recurrent wheezing, other coexisting conditions should be considered and excluded before embarking on long-term therapy with bronchodilator drugs. Undesirable side effects of β-agonists, such as worsening $\dot{V}/\dot{Q}$ matching and further destabilizing unstable airways, should be avoided. Infants with clear-cut evidence of recurrent reversible airway obstruction should be considered for combined inhaled anti-inflammatory and bronchodilator therapy. *Corticosteroid therapy* is often used to treat established BPD, despite an enormous amount of negative or equivocal data. Very early corticosteroid therapy, begun shortly after birth to prevent the development of BPD, is biologically plausible, but results have been mixed. *Good nutrition* should be an important goal, but conventional formulas should be used. Expensive, unproved, homemade concoctions should be avoided. A growth rate of 15–30 g/day is a reasonable expectation. Infants who fail to maintain that growth rate should be evaluated for hypoxemia, maternal–child interaction difficulties, or for coexisting medical conditions such as reflux, aspiration, tracheal stenosis, or congenital heart disease.

Future research efforts should be directed at the identification and testing of agents that reverse alterations in lung structure associated with premature birth and acute lung injury, and agents that reduce inflammation and oxidant stress. Recent evidence indicates that these treatments may require initiation before or shortly after birth to be most effective. In the ultimate clinical evaluation of any BPD treatment strategy, care must be taken to assure that experimental groups are properly stratified for the strongest risk factors for BPD, such as birth weight, gestational age, maternal steroid therapy, male gender, white race, and perhaps sepsis and the presence of a symptomatic patent ductus arteriosus.

Acknowledgment

This work was supported by HL 56636.

References

1. Sinkin RA, Cox C, Phelps DL. Predicting risk for bronchopulmonary dysplasia: selection criteria for clinical trials. Pediatrics 1990; 86:728–736.
2. Rojas MA, Gonzalez A, Bancalari E, Claure N, Poole C, Silva-Neto G. Changing trends in the epidemiology and pathogenesis of neonatal chronic lung disease. J Pediatr 1995; 126:605–610.
3. Ballard RA, Ballard PL, Creasy RK, Padbury J, Polk DH, Bracken M, Moya FR, Gross I, TRH Study Group. Respiratory disease in very-low-birthweight infants after prenatal thyrotropin-releasing hormone and glucocorticoid. Lancet 1992; 339: 510–515.

4. Durand M, Sardesai S, McEvoy C. Effects of early dexamethasone therapy on pulmonary mechanics and chronic lung disease in very low birth weight infants: a randomized, controlled trial. Pediatrics 1995; 95:584–590.
5. Rastogi A, Akintorin SM, Bez ML, Morales P, Pildes RS. A controlled trial of dexamethasone to prevent bronchopulmonary dysplasia in surfactant-treated infants. Pediatrics 1996; 98:204–210.
6. Hallman M, Bry K, Hoppu K, Lappi M, Pohjavuori M. Inositol supplementation in premature infants with respiratory distress syndrome. N Engl J Med 1992; 326: 1233–1239.
7. Rosenfeld WN, Davis JM, Parton L, Richter SE, Price A, Flaster E, Kassem N. Safety and pharmacokinetics of recombinant human superoxide dismutase administered intratracheally to premature neonates with respiratory distress syndrome. Pediatrics 1996; 97:811–817.
8. Koppel R, Han RN, Cox D, Tanswell AK, Rabinovitch M. alpha l-Antirypsin protects neonatal rats from pulmonary vascular and parenchymal effects of oxygen toxicity. Pediatr Res 1994; 36:763–770.
9. Stiskal J, Dunn M, O'Brien K, Shennan A, Kelly E, Longley T, Chappel L, Koppel R, Rabinovitch M. $alpha_1$-Proteinase inhibitor (A_1PI) therapy for the prevention of bronchopulmonary dysplasia (BPD) in premature infants. Pediatr Res 1996; 39:247A.
10. Ballard RA, Ballard PL, Cnaan A, Pinto-Martin J, Davis DJ, Padbury JF, Phibbs RH, Parer JT, Hart MC, Mannino FL, Sawai SK. Antenatal thyrotropin-releasing hormone to prevent lung disease in preterm infants. North American Thyrotropin-Releasing Hormone Study Group. N Engl J Med 1998; 338:493–498.
11. O'Brien K, Wyile G, Kelly E, Wylie L, Stiskal J, Shennan A, Rabinovitch M, Dunn M. Efficacy of α-1 proteinase inhibitor (AIPI) therapy for the prevention of chronic lung disease of prematurity (CLD) is supported by supplementary statistical analyses. Pediatr Res 1998; 43:186A.
12. Leach CL, Greenspan JS, Rubenstein SD, Shaffer TH, Wolfson MR, Jackson JC, DeLemos R, Fuhrman BP, for the Liquivent Study Group. Partial liquid ventilation with perflubron in premature infants with severe respiratory distress syndrome. N Engl J Med 1996; 335:761–815.
13. Nikischin W, Gerhardt T, Everett R, Gonzalez A, Hummler H, Bancalari E. Patient-triggered ventilation: a comparison of tidal volume and chestwall and abdominal motion as trigger signals Pediatr Pulmonol 1996; 22:28–34.
14. Cleary JP, Berstein G, Mannino FL, Heldt GP. Improved oxygenation during synchronized intermittent mandatory ventilation in neonates with respiratory distress syndrome: a randomized, crossover study. J Pediatr 1995; 126:407–411.
15. Tammela OK. Appropriate fluid regimens to prevent bronchopulmonary dysplasia. Eur J Pediatr 1995; 154:S15–S18.
16. Rush MG, Hazinski TA. Current therapy of bronchopulmonary dysplasia. Clin Perinatol 1992; 19:563–590.
17. Zimmerman JJ, Farrell PM. Advances and issues in bronchopulmonary dysplasia. Curr Probl Pediatr 1994; 24:159–170.
18. Abman SH, Groothius JR. Pathophysiology and treatment of bronchopulmonary dysplasia. Pediatr Clin North Am 1994; 41:277–315.
19. Barrington KJ, Finer NN. Treatment of bronchopulmonary dysplasia. Clin Perinatol 1998; 25:177–202.

20. Tuder RM, Flook BE, Voelkel NF. Increased gene expression for VEGF and the VEGF receptors KDR/Flk and Flt in lungs exposed to acute or to chronic hypoxia. Modulation of gene expression by nitric oxide. J Clin Invest 1995; 95:1798–1807.
21. Levy NS, Chung S, Furneaux H, Levy AP. Hypoxic stabilization of vascular endothelial growth factor mRNA by the RNA-binding protein HuR. J Biol Chem 1998; 273:6417–6423.
22. Karamsetty VS, Kane KA, Wadsworth RM. The effects of chronic hypoxia on the pharmacological responsiveness of the pulmonary artery. Pharmacol Ther 1995; 68:233–246.
23. Benatar A, Clarke J, Silverman M. Pulmonary hypertension in infants with chronic lung disease: non-invasive evaluation and short term effect of oxygen treatment. Arch Dis Child 1995; 72:F14–F19.
24. Berman W Jr, Katz R, Yabek SM, Dillon T, Fripp RR, Papile LA. Long-term follow-up of bronchopulmonary dysplasia. J Pediatr 1986; 109:45–50.
25. Groothius JR, Rosenberg AA. Home oxygen promotes weight gain in infants with bronchopulmonary dysplasia. Am J Dis Child 1987; 141:992–995.
26. Bernstein D, Bell JG, Kwong L Castillo RO. Alterations in postnatal intestinal function during chronic hypoxemia. Pediatr Res 1992; 31:234–238.
27. Poets CF, Southall DP. Noninvasive monitoring of oxygenation in infants and children: practical considerations and areas of concern. Pediatrics 1994; 93:737–746.
28. Walsh MC, Noble LM, Carlo WA, Martin RJ. Relationship of pulse oximetry to arterial oxygen tension in infants Crit Care Med 1987; 15:1102–1105.
29. Fan L, Voyles JB. Determination of inspired oxygen delivered by nasal cannula in infants with chronic lung disease. J Pediatr 1983; 103:923–925.
30. Moyle JT. Uses and abuses of pulse oximetry. Arch Dis Child 1996; 74:77–80.
31. Stoneham MD, Saville GM, Wilson IH. Knowledge about pulse oximetry among medical and nursing staff. Lancet 1994; 344:1339–1342.
32. Weber MW, Palmer A, Oparaugo A, Mulholland EK. Comparison of nasal prongs and nasopharyngeal catheter for the delivery of oxygen in children with hypoxemia because of a lower respiratory tract infection. J Pediatr 1995; 127:378–383.
33. Shann F, Gatchalian S, Hutchinson R. Nasopharyngeal oxygen in children. Lancet 1988; 2:1238–1240.
34. Chemrob S, Kaplan BS, Sherbotie JR, Aranda JV. Pharmacology of diuretics in the newborn Pediatr Clin North Am 1989; 36:1231–1250.
35. Tammela OK, Koivisto ME. Fluid restriction for preventing bronchopulmonary dysplasia? Reduced fluid intake during the first weeks of life improves the outcome of low-birth-weight infants. Acta Paediatr 1992; 81:207–212.
36. Engelhardt B, Elliott S, Hazinski TA. Short-and long-term effects of furosemide on lung function in infants with bronchopulmonary dysplasia. J Pediatr 1986; 109: 1034–1039.
37. Rush MG, Englehardt B, Parker RA, et al. Double-blind, placebo-controlled trial of alternate-day furosemide therapy in infants with chronic bronchopulmonary dysplasia. J Pediatr 1990; 117:112–118.
38. Kao LC, Warburton D, Cheng MH, et al. Effect of oral diuretics on pulmonary mechanics in infants with bronchopulmonary dysplasia: results of a double-blind crossover sequential trial 1984; 74:37–44.

39. Englehardt B, Blalock WA, Donlevy S, et al. Effect of spironolactone-hydrochlorothiazide on lung function in infants with chronic BPD. J Ped 1989; 114:619–624.
40. Albersheim SG, Solimano AJ, Sharma AK, et al. Randomized, double-blind, controlled trial of long-term diuretic therapy for bronchopulmonary dysplasia. J Pediatr 1989; 115:615–620.
41. Kao LC, Durand DJ, McCrea RC, Birch M, Powers RJ, Nickerson BG. Randomized trial of long-term diuretic therapy for infants with oxygen-dependent bronchopulmonary dysplasia. J Pediatr 1994; 124:772–781.
42. Segar JL, Robillard JE, Johnson KJ, Bell EF, Chemtob S. Addition of metolazone to overcome tolerance to furosemide in infants with bronchopulmonary dysplasia. J Pediatr 1992; 120:966–973.
43. Rastogi A, Luayon M, Ajayi OA, Pildes RS. Nebulized furosemide in infants with bronchopulmonary dysplasia. J Pediatr 1994; 125:976–979.
44. Adams ND, Rowe JC. Nephrocalcinosis. Clin Perinatol 1992; 19:179–195.
45. Karlowicz MG, Katz ME, Adelman RD, Solhaug MJ. Nephrocalcinosis in very low birth weight neonates: family history of kidney stones and ethnicity as independent risk factors. J Pediatr 1993; 122:635–638.
46. Alon US, Scagliotti D, Garola RE. Nephrocalcinosis and nephrolithiasis in infants with congestive heart failure treated with furosemide. J Pediatr 1994; 125:149–151.
47. Katz ME, Karlowicz MG, Adelman RD, Werner AL, Solhaug MJ. Nephrocalcinosis in very low birth weight neonates: sonographic patterns, histologic characteristics, and clinical risk factors. J Ultrasound Med 1994; 13:777–782.
48. Hoppe B, Hesse A, Neuhaus T, Fanconi S, Forster I, Blau N, Leumann E. Urinary saturation and nephrocalcinosis in preterm infants; effect of parenteral nutrition. Arch Dis Child 1993; 69:299–303.
49. Downing GJ, Egelhoff JC, Daily DK, Thomas MK, Alon U. Kidney function in very low birth weight infants with furosemide-related renal calcifications at ages 1 to 2 years. J Pediatr 1992; 120:599–604.
50. Stahlman MT, Orth DN, Grey ME. Immunocytochemical localization of epidermal growth factor in the developing human respiratory system and in acute and chronic lung disease in the neonate. Lab Invest 1989; 60:539–547.
51. De Boeck K, Smith J, Van Lierde S, Devlieger H. Response to bronchodilators in clinically stable 1-year-old patients with bronchopulmonary dysplasia. J Pediatr 1998; 157:75–79.
52. Nickerson BG, Taussig LM. Family history of asthma in infants with bronchopulmonary dysplasia. Pediatrics 1980; 65:1140–1144.
53. Hagen R, Minutillo C, French N, Reese A, Landau LI, LeSouëf PN. Neonatal chronic lung disease, oxygen dependency, and a family history of asthma. Pediatr Pulmonol 1996; 20:277–283.
54. Chambers HM, van Velzen D. Ventilator-related pathology in the extremely immature lung. Pathology 1989; 21(2):79–83.
55. Downing GJ, Kilbride HW. Evaluation of airway complications in high-risk preterm infants: application of flexible fiberoptic airway endoscopy. Pediatrics 1995; 95:567–572.

56. Zinman R. Tracheal stenting improves airway mechanics in infants with tracheobronchomalacia. Pediatr Pulmonol 1995; 19:275–281.
57. Panitch HB, Esteban N, Keklikian EN, Motley RA, Wolfson MR, Schidlow DV. Effect of altering smooth muscle tone on maximal expiratory flows in patients with tracheomalacia. Pediatr Pulmonol 1990; 9:170–176.
58. Davis GM, Nguyen HN, Faucher D. Respiratory responses to salbutamol and dexamethazone in BPD. Am J Respir Crit Care Med 1996; 153:A665.
59. Rubin BK, Albers GM. Use of anticholinergic bronchodilation in children. Am J Med 1996; 100:49S–53S.
60. Pierce MR, Bancalari E. The role of inflammation in the pathogenesis of bronchopulmonary dysplasia. Pediatr Pulmonol 1995; 19:371–378.
61. Nadel JA, Busse WW. Asthma. Am J Respir Crit Care Med 1998; 157:S130–S138.
62. Wagener JS, Kahn TZ, Copenhaver SC, Accurso FJ. Early inflammation and the development of pulmonary disease in cystic fibrosis. Pediatr Pulmonol Suppl 1997; 16:267–268.
63. Watterberg KL, Demers LM, Scott SM, Murphy S. Chorioamnionitis and early lung inflammation in infants in whom bronchopulmonary dysplasia develops. Pediatrics 1996; 97:210–215.
64. Yoon BH, Romero R, Jun JK, Park KH, Park JD, Ghezzi F, Kim BI. Amniotic fluid cytokines (interleukin-6, tumor necrosis factor-alpha, interleukin-1 beta, and interleukin-8) and the risk for the development of bronchopulmonary dysplasia. Am J Obstet Gynecol 1997; 177:825–830.
65. Groneck P, Gotze-Speer B, Oppermann M, Eiffert H, Speer CP. Association of pulmonary inflammation and increased microvascular permeability during the development of bronchopulmonary dysplasia; a sequential analysis of inflammatory mediators in respiratory fluids of high-risk preterm neonates. Pediatrics 1994; 93: 712–718.
66. Ozdemir A, Brown MA, Morgan WJ. Markers and mediators of inflammation in neonatal lung disease. Pediatr Pulmonol 1997; 23:292–306.
67. Munshi UK, Niu JO, Siddiq MM, Parton LA. Elevation of interleukin-8 and interleukin-6 precedes the influx of neutrolphils in tracheal aspirates from preterm infants who develop bronchopulmonary dysplasia. Pediatr Pulmonol 1997; 24:331–336.
68. Drazen JM. Pharmacology of leukotriene receptor antagonists and 5-lipoxygenase inhibitors in the management of asthma. Pharmacotherapy 1997; 17:22S–30S.
69. Watterberg KL, Murphy S. Failure of cromolyn sodium to reduce the incidence of bronchopulmonary dysplasia: a pilot study. Pediatrics 1993; 91:803–806.
70. Viscardi RM, Hasday JD, Gumpper KF, Taciak V, Campbell AB, Palmer TW. Cromolyn sodium prophylaxis inhibits pulmonary proinflammatory cytokines in infants at high risk for bronchopulmonary dysplasia. Am J Respir Crit Care Med 1997; 156:1523–1529.
71. Papile L, Stoll B, Donovan E, Tyson I, Bauer C, Wright L, Krause-Steinrauf H, Verter J. Dexamethasone therapy in infants at risk for chronic lung disease (CLD): a multi-center randomized, double-masked trial. Pediatr Res 1996; 39:236A.
72. Collaborative Dexamethasone Trial Group. Dexamethasone therapy in neonatal chronic lung disease: an international placebo-controlled trial. Pediatrics 1991; 88: 421–427.

73. Rastogi A, Akintorin SM, Bez ML, Morales P, Pildes RS. A controlled trial of dexamethasone to prevent bronchopulmonary dysplasia in surfactant-treated infants. Pediatrics 1996; 98:204–210.
74. Kari MA, Heinonen K, Ikonen RS, Koivisto M, Raivio KO. Dexamethasone treatment in preterm infants at risk for bronchopulmonary dysplasia. Arch Dis Child 1993; 68:566–569.
75. Watterberg KL, Scott SM. Evidence of early adrenal insufficiency in babies who develop bronchopulmonary dysplasia. Pediatrics 1995; 95:120–125.
76. Korte C, Styne D, Merritt TA, Mayes D, Wertz A, Helbock HJ. Adrenocortical function in the very low birth weight infant: improved testing sensitivity and association with neonatal outcome. J Pediatr 1996; 128:257–263.
77. Vijayakumar E, Soll RF, Bracken MB, Sinclair JC. Early postnatal corticosteroids for the prevention of chronic lung disease (CLD): meta-analysis of clinical trials. Pediatr Res 1995; 37:276A.
78. Watts CL, Bruce MC. Effect of dexamethasone therapy on fibronectin and albumin levels in lung secretions of infants with bronchopulmonary dysplasia. J Pediatr 1992; 121:597–607.
79. Kovacs LB, Davis M, Faucher DJ, Papageorgiou AN. Efficacy of early systemic and inhaled corticosteroid therapy in the prevention of chronic lung disease of prematurity. Pediatr Res 1996; 39:337A.
80. Cole CH, Bradish M, Frantz ID Jr. Utilization of aerosol therapy in neonates in USA NICU's. Pediatr Res 1996; 39:328A.
81. Cloutier MM. Nebulized steroid therapy in bronchopulmonary dysplasia. Pediatr Pulmonol 1993; 15:111–116.
82. Frank L. Antioxidants, nutrition, and bronchopulmonary dysplasia. Clin Perinatol 1992; 19:541–562.
83. Sosenko IR, Rodriguez-Pierce M, Bancalari E. Effect of early initiation of intravenous lipid administration on the incidence and severity of chronic lung disease in premature infants. J Pediatr 1993; 123:975–982.
84. Ehrenkranz RA, Ablow RC, Warshaw JB. Effect of vitamin E on the development of oxygen-induced lung injury in neonates. Ann NY Acad Sci 1982; 393:452–466.
85. Shenai JP, Kennedy KA, Chytil F. Clinical trial of vitamin A supplementation in infants susceptible to bronchopulmonary dysplasia. J Pediatr 1987; 111:269–277.
86. Tyson JE, Wright LL, Oh W, Kennedy KA, Mele L, Ehrenkranz RA, Stoll BJ, Lemons JA, Stevenson DK, Bauer CR, Korones SB, Fanaroff AA, Donovan EF, Carlo WA, Shankaran S, Stark AR, Papile L, Jobe A, Stacewicz-Sapuntzakis M, Verter J. A multi-center randomized trial of vitamin A supplementation for extremely low birth weight infants. 1998; in press.
87. Shenai JP, Rush MG, Parker RA, Chytil F. Sequential evaluation of plasma retinol-binding protein response to vitamin A administration in very-low-birth-weight neonates. Biochem Mol Med 1995; 54:67–74.
88. Boehm G, Bierback U, Moro G, Minoli I. Limited fat digestion in infants with bronchopulmonary dysplasia. J Pediatr Gastroenterol Nutr 1996; 22:161–166.
89. Pereira GR, Baumgart S, Bennett MJ, Stallings VA, Georgieff MK, Hamosh M,

Ellis L. Use of high-fat formula for premature infants with bronchopulmonary dysplasia: metabolic, pulmonary, and nutritional studies. J Pediatr 1994; 124:605–611.

90. Chessex P, Belanger S, Piedboeuf B, Pineault M. Influence of energy substrates on respiratory gas exchange during conventional mechanical ventilation of preterm infants. J Pediatr 1995; 126:619–624.
91. Yunis KA, Oh W. Effects of intravenous glucose loading on oxygen consumption, carbon dioxide production, and resting energy expenditure in infants with bronchopulmonary dysplasia. J Pediatr 1989; 115:127–132.
92. Billeaud C, Piedboeuf B, Chessex P. Energy expenditure and severity of respiratory disease in very low birth weight infants receiving long-term ventilatory support. J Pediatr 1992; 120:461–464.
93. Weinstein MR, Oh W. Oxygen consumption in infants with bronchopulmonary dysplasia. J Pediatr 1981; 99:958–961.
94. Orenstein SR. Gastroesophageal reflux disease. Semin Gastrointest Dis 1994; 5:2–14.
95. Anderson AH, Warady BA, Daily DK, Johnson JA, Thomas MK. Systemic hypertension in infants with severe bronchopulmonary dysplasia: associated clinical factors. Am J Perinatol 1993; 10:190–193.
96. Marciel JA, Rushing SF, Settles OL, Hazinski TA: Incidence of hypertension in oxygen-dependent infants with BPD. Pediatr Res 1997; 41:304A.
97. Tonini G, Pahor T, Colonna F, de Vonderweid U. Growth hormone does not prevent catabolic side effects of dexamethasone in extremely low birth weight preterm infants with bronchopulmonary dysplasia—a pilot study. J Pediatr Endocrinol Metab 1997; 10:291–294.
98. Furman L, Baley J, Borawski-Clark E, Aucott S, Hack M. Hospitalization as a measure of morbidity among very low birth weight infants with chronic lung disease. J Pediatr 1996; 128:447–452.
99. The Preventive Study Group. Reduction of respiratory syncytial virus hospitalization among premature infants and infants with bronchopulmonary dysplasia using respiratory syncytial virus immune globulin prophylaxis. Pediatrics 1997; 99:93–99.
100. The Impact-RSV Study Group. Palivizumab, a humanized respiratory syncytial virus monoclonal antibody, reduces hospitalization from respiratory syncytial virus infection in high-risk infants. Pediatrics 1998; 102:531–537.
101. Massaro GD, Massaro D. Postnatal treatment with retinoic acid increases the number of pulmonary alveoli in rats. Am J Physiol 1996; 270:L305–L310.
102. Massaro GD, Massaro D. Retinoic acid treatment abrogates elastase-induced pulmonary emphysema in rats. Nature Med 1997; 3:675–677.
103. Davis, JM, Rosenfeld WN, Richter DR, et al. Safety and pharmacokinetics of multiple doses of recombinant human CuZn superoxide dismutase administered intratracheally to premature neonates with respiratory distress syndrome. Pediatrics 1997; 100:24–30.
104. Coalson JJ, Winter V, deLemos RA. Decreased alveolarization in baboon survivors with bronchopulmonary dysplasia. Am J Respir Crit Care Med 1995; 152:640–646.

105. Hazinski TA, Cotton RB. Oxygen toxicity and oxidant stress in the developing lung. Semin Neonatol 1998; 3:103–111.
106. Cotton RB, Hazinski TA, Morrow JD, Roberts LJ, Steele S, Law AB. Effect of cimetidine on lipid peroxidation in the lungs of premature newborn infants. Pediatr Res 1996; 39:329A.
107. Cotton RB, Morrow JD, Hazinski TA, Roberts LJ, Law AB, Steele S. F_2-isoprostanes (F_2I) in tracheobronchial aspirate fluid (TBAF) indicate association between increased FIO_2 and lipid peroxidation in the lungs of premature infants. Pediatr Res 1996; 37:329A.
108. Banks BA, Ischiropoulos H, McClelland M, Ballard PL, Ballard RA. Plasma 3-nitrotyrosine is elevated in premature infants who develop bronchopulmonary dysplasia. Pediatrics 1998; 101:870–874.
109. Abman SH, Kinsella JP. Inhaled nitric oxide therapy for pulmonary disease in pediatrics. Curr Opin Pediatr 1998; 10:236–242.
110. Gutierrez HH, Nieves B, Chumley P, et al. NO regulation of superoxide-dependent lung injury: oxidant protective actions of endogenously produced and exogenously administered NO. Free Radic Biol Med 1996; 21:43–52.
111. Kinsella JP, et al. Effects of inhaled NO on pulmonary edema and neutrophil accumulation in severe experimental hyaline membrane disease. Pediatr Res 1997; 41: 457–463.
112. Cotton RB, Hazinski TA, Steele S, Capdevila JH, Zeldin DC. O_2 exposure is associated with the release of P450-derived arachidonic acid metabolities in the lung of premature infants at risk for bronchopulmonary dysplasia. Am J Respir Crit Care Med 1996; 153:665A.
113. Lentsch AB, Shanley TP, Sarma V, Ward PA. In vivo suppression of NF-kappa B and preservation of 1 kappa B alpha by interleukin-10 and interleukin-13. J Clin Invest 1997; 100:2443–2448.
114. Jones CA, Cayabyab RG, Kwong KY, Stotts C, Wong B, Hamdan H, Minoo P, deLemos RA. Undetectable interleukin (IL)-10 and persistent IL-8 expression early in hyaline membrane disease: a possible developmental basis for the predisposition to chronic lung inflammation in preterm newborns.
115. Tremblay L, Valenza F, Ribeiro SP, Li J, Slutsky AS. Injurious ventilatory strategies increase cytokines and c-*fos* m-RNA expression in an isolated rat lung model. J Clin Invest 1997; 99:944–952.

13

Nutritional Issues in Chronic Lung Disease of Premature Infants

ILENE R.S. SOSENKO

University of Miami School of Medicine
Miami, Florida

MICHAEL T. KINTER and ROBERT J. ROBERTS*

University of Virginia Health Science Center
Charlottesville, Virginia

I. Introduction

Nutrition is important to the processes that are involved in normal lung development and maturation. Discussions of the etiologies of chronic lung disease (CLD) in premature infants, such as oxidant injury, barotrauma, infectious agents, and aberrant intrinsic processes, require inclusion of nutritional influences (1–3). Several reports have appeared in the literature concerning the influence of nutritional status and specific nutrients, including lipid, protein, vitamins, and trace minerals, on lung function, development, and repair (4–7). Despite credible evidence on the ability of nutrition to influence normal lung development and function and to effect a major influence on the tolerance of the lung to adverse extrinsic challenges, particularly oxidant injury, little definitive information exists on the influence of nutrition in modulating the outcome of CLD in the human infant. The purpose of this chapter is to present evidence supporting the hypothesis that nutrition, including specific nutrients, can modulate the outcome of CLD in human infants through alteration in susceptibility to oxygen toxicity. The chapter also identifies a number of relevant current controversies.

---

*Deceased.

II. Negative Influence of General Undernutrition and Protein Malnutrition on Oxygen-Induced Lung Injury

Experimental manipulations that produce a decrease in general nutritional status increase the susceptibility of the whole animal, the lung, and lung cells in culture to hyperoxia-induced injury. One of the earliest studies of the influence of undernutrition on oxygen-induced toxicity reported that newborn mice with limited nutrition, produced by intermittent nursing, were more likely to die and had more microscopic evidence of lung pathology when exposed to hyperoxia, compared with control mice that were continuously nursed (8). Likewise, death from oxygen toxicity was accelerated in fasted newborn rats that were exposed to high concentrations of oxygen (9–11). Studies examining the effect of hyperoxic exposure plus total caloric deprivation showed that caloric deprivation produced an additive effect to the negative influence of hyperoxia on lung protein synthesis (12). Similarly, food deprivation accelerated lung injury, increased weight loss, and decreased DNA synthesis in lungs of mice that were rendered hyperoxic (13). The mechanism whereby undernutrition reduces survival in the presence of hyperoxia is unclear, and may be related to the combined inhibitory effects of oxygen and undernutrition on lung growth and DNA synthesis that are necessary for repair of oxygen-induced lung injury. This vulnerability does not appear to relate to an inability to mount a protective antioxidant enzyme (AOE) response to hyperoxia, as both normally fed and underfed rat pups responded to hyperoxic exposure with equivalent increases in lung AOEs (11,14,15).

When food intake of pregnant rats was limited to produce fetal growth retardation, the undernourished offspring had clearcut evidence of abnormal lung maturation, with reduced surfactant production. When exposed to hyperoxia, these undergrown newborn rats had a significant reduction in lung DNA, as well as a selected reduction in the glutathione arm of the antioxidant defense system (16). Other investigators have reported increased susceptibility of fasted mice to hyperoxic lung injury, associated with a significant reduction in lung glutathione content, but not with reduced amounts of AOEs in the lung. These findings prompted the authors to attribute to glutathione, but not to superoxide dismutase or catalase, a major role in the increased susceptibility of fasted animals to oxygen toxicity (17,18). Studies with a different species, the premature guinea pig, demonstrated that starvation increased mortality associated with hyperoxia and resulted in a decrease in both lung and liver glutathione content (19). The importance of glutathione reduction associated with undernutrition and its role in hyperoxic lung injury was reinforced by experiments showing that lung injury induced by oxygen and protein deprivation could be reversed by dietary manipulation designed to increase tissue levels of glutathione (20). Specifically, when protein nutritional deficiency was produced in rats by limiting protein intake for 6 days, these protein-deficient rats had increased mortality in hyperoxia compared with rats fed protein-sufficient diets. Furthermore, the increased susceptibility to oxygen produced by protein deprivation was prevented by dietary supplements of sulfur-containing amino acids (cysteine, cystine, or methionine), which yielded increased levels of glutathione in the lungs (20).

Studies of cells in culture also have demonstrated the influence of nutritional modification, in the form of medium replacement, on the toxic effects of oxygen exposure. Cultured hamster fibroblasts, provided either with medium replacement ever 24 hr or with medium replacement withheld for the study period, were exposed to hyperoxic conditions. Although lack of medium replacement may result in accumulation of toxic by-products associated with hyperoxic exposure, it is also likely that this experimental condition produces nutrient depletion (e.g., gluathione depletion). The cells provided with fresh medium every 24 hr and exposed to hyperoxia demonstrated decreased evidence of hyperoxic injury and increased resistance to the administration of the cytotoxic by-product of lipid peroxidation, 4-hydroxynonenal (4-HNE), compared with similarly exposed cells without medium replacement (21). Furthermore, this diffusible cytotoxin, 4-HNE, was detoxified by gluathione (22,23). These in vitro studies provide additional support for the role that cellular glutathione may play in protection against oxygen toxicity and also support the role of decreased glutathione levels associated with nutritional modification in the enhancement of oxidant injury.

III. Lipids and Oxygen-Induced Lung Injury: Helpful or Harmful?

Deficiency of essential fatty acids in the neonatal diet can have adverse effects on lipid membrane composition and general well-being, but it is unclear whether or not dietary lipids actually have a protective or a deleterious effect on oxidant lung injury in the neonatal lung. There is considerable experimental evidence suggesting that lipids, particularly those that are rich in polyunsaturated fatty acids (PUFA), are related to tolerance to hyperoxia in vivo. When pregnant rats were fed one of several diets that were high in PUFA, their newborn offspring had increased PUFA concentrations in their lungs, reflective of the diets themselves. For example, a diet that was high in the n-6 family of PUFA (safflower oil) generally produced high levels of the n-6 family of PUFA in lung lipids, and diets that were high in the n-3 family of PUFA (menhaden fish oil) produced high lung levels of the n-3 family of PUFA in lung (24,25). Likewise, in another report pregnant rats received a diet containing a lipid preparation (intralipid) that was high in the n-6 and n-3 families of PUFA, and the lungs of their offspring contained increased amounts of n-6 and n-3 PUFA (26). In yet another study, dietary supplementation of pregnant rats with palm oil, which contains low levels of PUFA, yielded offspring that showed decreased PUFA content in lung tissue

(24). In addition to these biochemical changes, the various high PUFA diets, including safflower oil-based, menhaden oil-based, and intralipid-based diets, produced superior survival and improved clinical and pathological status following prolonged hyperoxic exposure in the newborn rat offspring, whereas offspring of rats fed low PUFA (palm oil) diets were consistently the most susceptible to pulmonary oxygen toxicity and early death with hyperoxia. Postnatal dietary manipulation of PUFA also improved tolerance to hyperoxia in newborn rats, with similar degrees of oxygen tolerance associated with diets that contained high amounts of qualitatively different PUFA (24–26). These studies suggested that the high PUFA diets were not conferring protection against oxygen toxicity through effects on development of either the lung AOE system or the surfactant system, nor through enhanced induction of AOEs during hyperoxia (24–26). In contrast to these findings, additional studies that examined the influence of postnatal dietary modification on survival and lung injury of newborn rats and rabbits that were exposed to hyperoxia yielded more complex results. Mortality and lung injury associated with hyperoxia were greater with diets consisting of Ringer's lactate or lipid emulsion and less with a diet consisting of human milk alone (27). In the presence of protein deficiency, increased intake of PUFA produced an increase in lipid peroxidation in rats, a finding that was attributed to decreased antioxidant protection resulting from the protein deficiency (28).

The mechanism by which tolerance to hyperoxia is induced by high PUFA intake is unclear, but may relate to the increased pulmonary content of PUFA, which if located intracellularly, might function as an antioxidant, thereby conferring protection against oxygen toxicity (29). Studies of rabbit tracheal epithelial cells in culture showed that lipid supplementation of the culture medium led to increased PUFA content of the cells and decreased cytotoxicity from hyperoxia, with decreased lipid peroxidation (30).

Despite the aforementioned evidence of a protective effect of PUFA against oxidant injury, other in vitro studies have provided different and even opposite findings, consistent with the classic notion that unsaturated fatty acids are vulnerable to lipid peroxidation and oxidant damage. For instance, cultured hamster fibroblast cells that were grown in a medium that was enriched with PUFA had increased cell damage and death from hyperoxia. Specifically, fibroblasts exposed to 95% oxygen and supplemented with PUFA, either in the form of linoleic acid or eicosapentanoic acid, survived a shorter time than control cells did in hyperoxia (31). Other studies of porcine pulmonary artery endothelial cells in culture showed a protective effect of monounsaturation, as opposed to polyunsaturation, relative to oxidant-induced injury. Cultured endothelial cells that were supplemented with oleic acid (a monounsaturated fatty acid) before exposure to hydrogen peroxide had improved cell survival, as measured by lactate dehydrogenase (LDH) release (32,33).

How can these apparent inconsistencies concerning PUFA and oxidant damage be reconciled? Most of the evidence supporting increased oxidant damage associated with PUFA comes from in vitro studies, in which fatty acids were manipulated singly, whereas most of the evidence showing protection against oxidant damage by PUFA derives from in vivo studies, whereby multiple fatty acid changes were induced by using complex lipid oils consisting of various mixtures of different fatty acids. These complex dietary oils may have produced appreciable changes in a number of cellular fatty acids (rather than in one fatty acid, as in the in vitro studies), the combination of which may have yielded protection from injury. Differences between studies could relate to differences in the absolute quantity of individual fatty acids incorporated into cells, rather than the percentage changes in fatty acids, or they might relate to specific intracellular loci of changes in fatty acid composition. Another possible explanation for the harmful, rather than protective, effect of lipid on oxidant injury relates to triglyceride uptake by fetal rat lung, which is gestation-dependent (34). Thus, the premature lung, if its capacity to incorporate lipids is reduced, might accumulate exogenous lipids in cellular or extracellular sites, where the potential for peroxidation could have adverse effects on the lung.

These experimental findings could provide the basis for two apparently conflicting clinical hypotheses related to CLD of infants: (1) providing PUFA in the form of intralipid to premature infants might help protect them against oxidant lung injury and development of CLD; and (2) early initiation of intralipid might be harmful by increasing oxidant lung injury, thereby increasing the development of CLD. Which hypothesis has been substantiated by clinical trials or epidemiological evaluation?

Four prospective, controlled clinical trials have examined the effect of early delivery of intralipid to premature infants. The first, by Hammerman and coworkers (35), tested the hypothesis that "early intralipid" would have a harmful effect on pulmonary outcome. The investigators studied 20 infants who began receiving parenteral lipid infusion on postnatal day 3, compared with 22 control infants who did not receive lipid until 5 days later. The severity of CLD was greater in the infants who received intralipid early, but survival without CLD was not different between groups (35). A confounding variable that may have influenced the outcome of this study was that the early intralipid group had an average alveolar–arterial oxygen difference on day 1 that was 50% greater than that of controls. A subsequent study of Gilbertson et al. (36) focused on lipid tolerance and glucose homeostasis in low birth weight infants who received early intralipid administration beginning on postnatal day 1. Intralipid infusion had no detectable effect on respiratory morbidity, or on duration of oxygen therapy or ventilator therapy (36). Sosenko and co-workers (37) tested the hypothesis that "early" intralipid administration, given on the first postnatal day, would reduce the incidence of CLD. This study randomized 133 infants who were stratified according to two birth weight groups into "early" intralipid (initiated < 12 hr after birth) or controls (no intralipid until > 7 days after birth). There were no differences between the two groups in the number of infants who acquired CLD or who survived without CLD. This study did reveal, however, the unexpected findings of increased mortality and pulmonary hemorrhage in infants who weighed 600–800 g and who received early intralipid. In addition, more infants who received early intralipid continued to require supplemental oxygen 7 days after birth (37). In the fourth of these studies, Brownlee reported no differences in respiratory outcome of 129 infants who were randomly assigned to receive early (<36 hr old) versus late (postnatal day 6) intralipid administration (38).

In an epidemiological study of 659 infants who were 30 weeks or less gestation at birth, there was a significant association between the introduction of intravenous lipids early in life (first 21 days) and increased incidence or severity of CLD (39). A comparable retrospective survey of 799 premature infants with a birth weight less than 1500 g revealed that the administration of lipid was a significant predictor of the development of CLD (40).

Faced with the apparent discrepancies of the mostly favorable results with experimental animals, the mostly negative results with in vitro studies, and the lack of efficacy of early intralipid administration in premature infants, it is reasonable to speculate on why intralipid may have failed to protect against oxidant-related chronic lung damage in vulnerable preterm infants. One possibility is that PUFA protection from oxygen-related lung damage is species (rat)-specific. Another possible explanation is that toxic substances within the intralipid preparation itself, such as lipid peroxidation products (41,42), could directly damage lung cells or produce deleterious effects by causing an eicosanoid imbalance. Wispe et al. (43) reported evidence of increased lipid peroxidation in the form of expired ethane and pentane in infants who received intravenous lipid emulsion. A third possible explanation for lack of protection by early intralipid administration could relate to a relative overabundance of PUFA, particularly linoleic acid (50% of the intralipid preparation), which might have affected the quality and function of surfactant in the premature infants who were treated with intralipid. It is also possible that CLD of the low birth weight (LBW) infant may not be primarily related to oxygen toxicity. There is epidemiological support for this notion, as CLD often develops in premature infants who have little-or-no respiratory distress early in their course, and who require minimal or no supplemental oxygen over the first several days of life (44).

It is possible that early postnatal administration of lipid by the enteral route, perhaps because of better intestinal tolerance of the hydroperoxides and other products of lipid peroxidation, might enable the very premature infant to benefit from early PUFA-rich lipid. This is a testable hypothesis that merits further investigation. Development of an intravenous preparation that is free of lipid peroxidation products also warrants consideration. The potential role of dietary lipid in protecting the vulnerable premature infant from oxidant-mediated lung damage remains an important unresolved area of lung research.

IV. Influence of Additional Nutrients (Inositol, Selenium, and Vitamin A) on Oxygen-Induced Lung Injury

Inositol is a substance that is incorporated in cell membranes within the lung. There is evidence to suggest that dietary supplementation with inositol may help to inhibit development of CLD in preterm infants. Inositol is relatively abundant in breast milk, less so in premature formula, but virtually absent in parenteral nutrition solutions (45). Work with experimental animals indicated that administering inositol to immature rodents resulted in an increase in surfactant (46). From the preliminary observation that dietary inositol supplementation lessened CLD in infants who were born prematurely, Hallman and co-workers (47) carried out a double-blind, placebo-controlled randomized trial of inositol supplementation in 221 infants with respiratory distress whose gestation at birth was 24–32 weeks. Infants who received inositol supplementation had significantly greater survival without CLD than control infants had. It is noteworthy, however, that inositol supplementation afforded no discernible benefit among infants who also received surfactant treatment. The report suggested that inositol protects the developing lung by serving as a substrate for surfactant synthesis and secretion.

Selenium is a trace metal that serves as an essential cofactor in the antioxidant function of glutathione peroxidase. Selenium, similar to other trace metals, is acquired transplacentally during the last trimester of human gestation. Hence, human infants who are born prematurely are deficient in selenium (48). Several groups of investigators have demonstrated that selenium deficiency accentuates hyperoxic lung injury in experimental animals, presumably because of its vital role in glutathione peroxidase activity and in normal lung development (49–52). It is not known whether selenium deficiency contributes to CLD in preterm infants.

Vitamin A also is obtained by the human fetus mostly during the third trimester (48) and serves an important role in normal differentiation and maintenance of the integrity of epithelial cells in the conducting airways. Therefore, investigators have explored whether vitamin A may play an important role in protecting against CLD. Two studies examined the relation between plasma vitamin A concentration and development of CLD, and both reported lower levels of vitamin A during the first month in very LBW infants who subsequently acquired CLD (53,54). These findings provided the basis for the first randomized double-blind, controlled trial of vitamin A supplementation in preterm infants at risk for CLD (55). Infants who received supplemental vitamin A had consistently higher plasma concentrations of vitamin A and significantly less CLD than did infants who did not receive extra vitamin A (55). A subsequent study, however, failed to confirm these findings, perhaps because control infants had sufficient vitamin A in their plasma (56). The most recent study of the effect of vitamin A supplementation in protecting against CLD was conducted by the NICHD Neonatal Research Network, and included 405 vitamin A-treated infants (5000 IU three times per week for 28 days) and 402 control infants with birth weights of

Table 1 Potential Mechanisms for Nutritional Alteration of Oxygen-Induced Lung Injury

Mechanism	Altered outcome
1. Nutrients act as substrate for oxidant-induced reaction(s)	
Fatty acids → lipid peroxidation	
a. Production of toxic by-products	Increase injury
b. Loss of membrane integrity stability/function	Increase injury
c. Act as "sink" for energy of reactive molecules	Decrease injury
Amino acids/protein → degradation/adduct formation	
a. Production of toxic by-products	Increase injury
b. Loss of structural or enzymatic	Increase injury
c. Act as "sink" for energy of reactive molecules	Decrease injury
2. Nutrients influence the antioxidant protective systems	
Enzymatic process (SOD, catalase, glutathione system)	
a. Sufficient nutrition (protein, Se, Cu Zn)	Decrease injury
b. Undernutrition (protein, Se, Cu, Zn)	Increase injury
Nonenzymatic process (GSH, vit. E)	
a. Sufficient nutrition (GSH, vit. E)	Decreased injury
b. Undernutrition (GSH, vit. E)	Increased injury
3. Nutrients influence the cellular injury/repair processes (DNA)	
undernutrition, particularly protein deficiency	Increased injury and/or decrease repair

401–1000 g. This investigation found a small, but significant, reduction (55 vs. 62%) in the primary outcome variable, death or CLD, in vitamin A-supplemented versus control infants, respectively, and suggested that greater reductions in CLD might be detected if higher doses of vitamin A supplementation were given (57).

V. Conclusion

There is considerable experimental evidence that general undernutrition and, in particular, insufficient dietary protein, may increase the vulnerability of the preterm infant to oxidant lung injury and development of CLD. Dietary provision of lipid, in addition to preventing essential fatty acid deficiency, also may play a role in preventing or reducing the severity of CLD, although data are conflicting, and some studies suggest that early postnatal lipid administration may actually be harmful in terms of oxidant lung damage. Finally, additional nutrients, including those that may increase intracellular glutathione (such as sulfur-containing amino acids), inositol to serve as substrate for surfactant, selenium to function as an essential cofactor for the antioxidant enzyme glutathione peroxidase, and vitamin A for airway epithelial cell integrity, may provide the premature infant additional protection against the development of CLD. Table 1 summarizes the potential mechanisms for nutritional modification of oxygen-induced lung injury.

Given that optimal nutrition is recognized as an essential part of the management of premature infants, and that virtually every known nutrient is readily available for study, a concerted effort must be made to identify specific nutritional "therapy" that can provide both optimal growth and also serve to inhibit the development of chronic lung injury in LBW infants.

References

1. Roberts RJ. Implications of nutrition in oxygen-related pulmonary disease in the human premature infant. Adv Pharmacol Ther 1919; 8:53–64.
2. Sosenko IRS, Frank L. Nutritional influences on lung development and protection against lung disease. Semin Perinatol 1991; 15:462–468.
3. Frank L. Antioxidants, nutrition, and bronchopulmonary dysplasia. Clin Perinatol 1992; 19:541–567.
4. Curle DC, Adamson IYR. Retarded development of neonatal rat lung by maternal malnutrition. J Histochem Cytochem 1978; 26:401–408.
5. Kelly FJ, Fussell JC, Postle TD. Effect of acute food restriction on pulmonary growth and protein turnover in preterm guinea pigs. Am J Physiol 1992; 262:E240–E245.
6. Myers BA, Dubick MA, Gerreits J, Rucker RB, Jackson AC, Reiser KK Williams SK, Last JA. Protein deficiency: effects on lung mechanics and the accumulation of collagen and elastin in rat lung. J Nutr 1983; 113:2308–2315.

7. Deneke SM, Lynch BA, Fanburg BL. Effect of low protein diets or feed restriction on rat lung glutathione and oxygen toxicity. J Nutr 1985; 115:726–732.
8. Polgar G, Antagnoli W, Ferrigan LW, Martin EA, Gregg WP. The effect of chronic exposure to 100% oxygen in newborn mice. Am J Med Sci 1966; 580–587.
9. Bucher JR, Roberts RJ. alpha-Tocopherol (vitamin E) content of lung, liver and blood in the newborn rat and human infant: influence of hyperoxia. J Pediatr 1981; 98:806–811.
10. Roberts RJ, Rendak, Bucher JR. Lipid peroxidation in the newborn rat: influence of fasting and hyperoxia on ethane and pentane in expired air. Dev Pharmacol Ther 1983; 6:170–178.
11. Frank L, Groseclose E. Oxygen toxicity in newborn rats: the adverse effects of undernutrition. J Appl Physiol 1982; 53:1248–1255.
12. Massaro D. Hyperoxia: influence of food deprivation on protein synthesis by lung. Proc Soc Exp Biol Med 1973; 143:602–603.
13. Hackney JD, Evans MJ, Bils RF, Spier CE, Jones MP. Effects of oxygen at high concentrations and food deprivation on cell division in lung alveoli of mice. Exp Mol Pathol 1977; 26:350–358.
14. Bucher JR, Roberts RJ. The development of the newborn rat lung in hyperoxia: a dose–response study of lung growth, maturation and changes in antioxidant enzyme activities. Pediatr Res 1981; 15:999–1008.
15. Wispe JR, Knight M, Roberts RJ. Lipid peroxidation in newborn rabbits: effects on oxygen, lipid emulsion, and vitamin E. Pediar Res 1986; 20:505–510.
16. Frank L, Lewis PL, Garcia-Pons T. Intrauterine growth-retarded rat pups show increased susceptibility to pulmonary O_2 toxicity. Pediatr Res 1985; 19:281–286.
17. Smith LJ, Friedman K, Anderson J. Hyperoxic lung injury in mice: effect of neutrophil depletion and food deprivation. J Lab Clin Med 1988; 111:449–458.
18. Smith LJ, Anderson J, Shamsuddin K, Hsueh W. Effect of fasting on hyperoxic lung injury in mice. Am Rev Respir Dis 1990; 141:141–149.
19. Langley SC, Kelly FJ. Effect of food restriction on hyperoxia-induced lung injury in preterm guinea pigs. Am J Physiol 1992; 263:L357–L362.
20. Deneke SM, Gershoff SN, Fanburg BL. Potentiation of oxygen toxicity in rats by dietary protein or amino acid deficiency. J Appl Physiol 1983; 54:147–151.
21. Sullivan SJ, Roberts RJ, Spitz DR. Replacement of media in cell culture alters oxygen toxicity: possible role of lipid aldehydes and glutathione transferases in oxygen toxicity. J Cell Physiol 1991; 147:427–433.
22. Sullivan SJ, Oberley TD, Roberts RJ, Spitz, DR. A stable O_2-resistant cell line: role of lipid peroxidation by-products in O_2 mediated injury. Am J Physiol 1992; 262: L748–L756.
23. Spitz DR, Sullivan SJ, Malcolm RR, Roberts RJ. Glutathione dependent metabolism and detoxification of 4-hydroxy-2-nonenal. Free Radic Biol Med 1991; 11:415–423.
24. Sosenko IRS, Innis SK Frank L. Polyunsaturated fatty acids and protection of newborn rats from oxygen toxicity. J Pediatr 1988; 112:630–637.
25. Sosenko IRS, Innis SM, Frank L. Menhaden fish oil, n-3 polyunsaturated fatty acids and protection of newborn rats from oxygen toxicity. Pediatr Res 1989; 25:399–404.

26. Sosenko IRS, Innis SM, Frank L. Intralipid increases lung polyunsaturated fatty acids and protects newborn rats from oxygen toxicity. Pediatr Res 1991; 30:413–417.
27. Marshall TA, Roberts RL. In vitro and in vivo assessment of lipid peroxidation of infant nutrient preparations: effect of nutrition on oxygen toxicity. J Am Coll Nutr 1990; 9:190–199.
28. Huang CJ, Fwu ML. Protein insufficiency aggravates the enhanced lipid peroxidation and reduced activities of antioxidative enzymes in rats fed diets high in polyunsaturated fat. J Nutr 1992; 122:1182–1189.
29. Dormandy TL. Biological rancidification. Lancet 1969; 2:684–688.
30. Dennery PA, Kramer CM, Alpert SE. Effect of fatty acid profiles on the susceptibility of cultured rabbit tracheal epithelial cells to hyperoxic injury. Am J Respir Cell Mol Biol 1990; 3:137–144.
31. Spitz DR, Kinter MT, Kehrer JP, Roberts RJ. The effect of monosaturated and polyunsaturated fatty acids on oxygen toxicity in cultured cells. Pediatr Res 1992; 32: 366–372.
32. Hart CM, Tolson JK, Block ER. Supplemental fatty acids alter lipid peroxidation and oxidant injury in endothelial cells. Am J Physiol 1991; 260:L481–L488.
33. Hart CM Tolson JK, Block ER. Quantitative fatty acid analyses in cultured porcine pulmonary artery endothelial cells: the combined effects of fatty acid supplementation and oxidant exposure. J Cell Physiol 1992; 153:76–87.
34. Torday J, Hua J, Slavin R. Metabolism and fate of neutral lipids of fetal lung fibroblast origin. Biochim Biophys Acta 1995; 1254:198–206.
35. Hammerman C, Aramburo MJ. Decreased lipid intake reduces morbidity in sick premature neonates. J Pediatr 1988; 113:1083–1088.
36. Gilbertson N, Kovar IZ, Cox DJ, Crowe L, Palmer NT. Introduction of intravenous lipid administration on the first day of life in the very low birth weight neonate. J Pediatr 1991; 119:116–23.
37. Sosenko IRS, Rodriquez-Pierce K, Bancalari E. Effect of early initiation of intravenous lipid administration on the incidence and severity of chronic lung disease in premature infants. J Pediatr 1993; 123:975–982.
38. Brownlee KG, Kelly EJ, Ng PC, Kendall-Smith SC, Dear PRF. Early or late parenteral nutrition for the sick preterm infant? Arch Dis Child 1993; 69:281–283
39. Cooke RWI. Factors associated with chronic lung disease in preterm, infants. Arch Dis Child 1991; 66:776–779.
40. Wirtschafter DD, Jones M, Thomas JC. Intravenous lipid emulsion therapy confounds the assessment of respiratory distress syndrome interventions. Presented at Ross Laboratories Special Conference, 1991; Washington, DC: 321–328.
41. Pitkanen OM. Peroxidation of lipid emulsions: a hazard for the premature infant receiving parenteral nutrition? Free Radic Biol Med 1992; 13:239–245.
42. Helbock HJ, Motchnik PA, Ames BN. Toxic hydroperoxides in intravenous lipid emulsions used in preterm infants. Pediatrics 1993; 91:83–87.
43. Wispe JR, Bell EF, Roberts RJ. Assessment of lipid peroxidation in newborn infants and rabbits by measurements of expired ethane and pentane: influence of parenteral lipid infusion. Pediatr Res 1985; 19:374–379.
44. Rojas MA, Gonzalez A, Bancalari E, Claure N, Poole C, Silva-Neto G. Changing

trends in the epidemiology and pathogenesis of chronic lung disease. J Pediatr 1995; 126:605–610.

45. Pereira GR, Baker L, Egler J, Corcoran L, Chiavacci R. Serum *myo*inositol and concentrations in premature infants fed human milk, formula for infants, and parenteral nutrition. Am J Clin Nutr 1990; 51:589–593.
46. Hallman M, Saugstad OD, Porreco RP, Epstein BL, Gluck L. Role of *myo*-inositol in regulation of surfactant phospholipids in the newborn. Early Hum Dev 1985; 10: 245–254.
47. Hallman M, Bry K, Hoppu K, Lappi M, Pohjavouri M. Inositol supplementation in premature infants with respiratory distress. N Engl J Med 1992; 326:1233–1239.
48. Widdowson EM. Chemical composition and nutritional needs of the fetus at different stages of gestation. In: Aebi H, Whitehead R, eds. Maternal Nutrition During Pregnancy and Lactation. Berne: H Huber, 1980:39–48.
49. Cross CE, Hasegawa G, Reddy KA, Omaye ST. Enhanced lung toxicity of O_2 in selenium-deficient rats. Res Commun Chem Pathol Pharm 1977; 16:695–706.
50. Deneke SM, Gershoff SN, Fanburg BL. Changes in O_2 toxicity and glutathione peroxidase levels in selenium deficient rats. Chest 1983; 83:39S.
51. Forman HJ, Rotman EI, Fisher AB. Roles of selenium and sulfur-containing amino acids in protection against oxygen toxicity. Lab Invest 1983; 49:148–153.
52. Kim HY, Picciano MF, Wallig MA, Milner JA. The role of selenium nutrition in the development of neonatal rat lung. Pediatr Res 1991; 29:440–445.
53. Husted VA, Gutcher GR, Anderson SA, et al. Relationships of vitamin A (retinol) status and lung disease in the preterm infant. J Pediatr 1984; 105:610–615.
54. Shenai JP, Chytil F, Jhaveri A, et al. Plasma vitamin A and retinol-binding protein in premature and term neonates. J Pediatr 1981; 99:302–305.
55. Shenai JP, Kennedy KA, Chytil F, et al. Clinical trial of vitamin A supplementation in infants susceptible to bronchopulmonary dysplasia. J Pediatr 1987; 111:269–277.
56. Pearson E, Bose C, Snidow T, Ransom L, Young T, Bose G, Stiles A. Trial of vitamin A supplementation in very low birth weight infants at risk for bronchopulmonary dysplasia. J Pediatr 1992; 121:420–427.
57. Tyson JE, Ehrenkranz RA, Stoll BJ, et al. Vitamin A supplementation to increase survival without chronic lung disease in extremely low birth weight infants: a 14-center randomized trial [abstr]. Pediatr Res 1998; 43:199A.

14

Pulmonary Function in BPD and Its Aftermath

ERIC C. EICHENWALD

Harvard Medical School
Brigham and Women's Hospital
Boston, Massachusetts

ANN R. STARK

Harvard University Children's Hospital
Boston, Massachusetts

I. Introduction

Bronchopulmonary dysplasia (BPD) is the most common form of chronic lung disease affecting children. The spectrum of the disease has changed since Northway (1) first described the severe chronic lung disease that developed in premature infants with hyaline membrane disease (HMD) who required mechanical ventilation and high inspired oxygen concentrations. Advances in perinatal and neonatal care, including prenatal glucocorticoid therapy, exogenous surfactant, and newer modes of mechanical ventilation, have resulted in increased survival of smaller and more immature infants and a consequent increase in the incidence and absolute number of children in whom BPD is diagnosed (2). Although data are available on the short-term pulmonary outcome of infants with BPD, less is known about the effect of either extreme prematurity or of early lung injury on long-term pulmonary function. This chapter will review the clinical presentation and evaluation of infants and children with BPD after the newborn period, including advantages and limitations of techniques to assess pulmonary function, and provide an overview of what is known about their short- and long-term pulmonary outcome.

II. Clinical Evaluation of Infants and Children with BPD

Physical findings in infants and children with BPD reflect the severity of their pulmonary disease. During the first 24–36 months of life, however, dramatic changes in pulmonary function can occur secondary to somatic growth and lung repair (3). Thus, the clinical presentation of BPD depends on both the severity of the initial lung injury, as well as the infant's postnatal age and growth.

The clinical presentation of infants with BPD reflects the underlying pathology. In the acute and subacute stage of BPD, the major pathological features include focal hyperplastic changes at the level of the bronchi, terminal airways, and respiratory bronchioles (4). Bronchial lumens, particularly at the distal airway, may be completely occluded by hyperplastic squamous metaplasia and smooth-muscle hypertrophy. Emphysematous and fibrotic changes result in a diminished surface area for gas exchange. Perfusion to poorly ventilated areas may be preserved, resulting in ventilation–perfusion mismatch. As the lung begins to heal from its initial injury, glandular hyperplasia of the large airways, smooth-muscle proliferation and hyperplasia in the small airways, and areas of fibrosis interspersed with relatively normal lung are observed. Pulmonary vascular changes consistent with pulmonary hypertension may also be seen.

The major pulmonary signs and symptoms in infants and children with BPD reflect the pathological findings in the small airways. Infants are typically tachypneic, with chest wall retractions and intermittent or chronic wheezing. The increased respiratory rate helps preserve minute ventilation in the face of increased dead space ventilation and small tidal volumes. Chest retractions result from increased respiratory muscle activity on the compliant chest wall. This persistent deformation of the rib cage with respiratory muscle activity may be responsible for the ''flat chest'' (decreased anteroposterior diameter) often found in infants and older children with BPD (5). Reactive airway disease may appear as intermittent wheezing associated with exercise, cold-air challenge, and intercurrent lower airway infections. Persistent or chronic wheezing or a prolonged expiratory phase indicate more fixed lesions of the lower airways.

Inspiratory stridor, indicative of larger airway narrowing, also may be present. In one study, almost one-half of infants who required prolonged intubation and mechanical ventilation for BPD had abnormalities noted on bronchoscopy after extubation (6). These abnormalities included subglottic stenosis, vocal cord paresis, and laryngotracheobronchomalacia (6). Younger infants with severe BPD may suffer from acute airway obstruction during periods of agitation or crying, with resultant hypoxemia and hypercarbia (7). These so-called BPD spells result from collapse of abnormally compliant large airways, and they can be life-threatening.

Parenchymal abnormalities of the lung, most prominently alveolar septal fibrosis (8) and increased pulmonary vascular resistance contribute to abnormalities of gas exchange. Early in the course of BPD, infants typically have hypoxemia (oxygen saturation of hemoglobin less than 90%) during air breathing. Oxygen saturation usually improves even with minimal supplemental oxygen, indicating the contribution of ventilation–perfusion mismatch. Small increases of inspired oxygen concentration may reduce pulmonary vascular resistance, and thus increase pulmonary blood flow (9). Infants who do not require supplemental oxygen at rest may become hypoxemic when they are stressed, during feedings, or during sleep (10,11). Increased dead space ventilation secondary to ventilation–perfusion mismatch leads to a large arterial–alveolar difference in CO_2 tension, which contributes to hypercapnia. Marginal gas exchange and signs and symptoms of respiratory disease improve in most infants by early childhood, despite evidence for persistent pulmonary function abnormalities (12). Fewer than 10% of infants with BPD require supplemental oxygen therapy beyond 1 year of age, adjusted for prematurity.

Chest radiographic abnormalities in established BPD include interstitial infiltrates, general or focal hyperexpansion, and atelectasis (13,14). In most infants, major radiographic abnormalities gradually resolve over the first 4 years of life (14), although minor abnormalities may persist into childhood (15,16) and even adulthood (17).

III. Growth Failure in Infants with BPD

Most studies on growth of infants and children with BPD include only the first 2–3 years, and growth during late childhood is less well documented. Many infants, especially those who are severely affected, will have poor weight gain during the first 12–24 postnatal months (18). The abnormal growth pattern is directly related to the severity and duration of the pulmonary dysfunction, including the duration of supplemental oxygen and the frequency of recurrent lower respiratory infections (19). As pulmonary symptoms diminish after 2 years of age, linear and head growth usually accelerate followed more slowly by weight gain. As respiratory status improves, the growth pattern of infants with BPD does not differ significantly from that of premature infants without BPD. However, several short-term follow-up studies suggest that, although growth velocity improves with time, infants with BPD continue to be smaller than control infants of the same chronologic age, but without BPD (20–23). The greatest differences are observed in weight, with smaller differences in height and head circumference.

Northway's (17) follow-up study of adult survivors of BPD suggested that growth abnormalities observed in infants with BPD might persist into adulthood. In that study, 26 adults who were studied at a mean age of 18 years were significantly shorter and weighed less than a matched cohort of former premature infants without BPD. Studies of more recent survivors with BPD, who are of a lower gestational age and birth weight than were Northway's original subjects, indicate that patterns of growth may improve with age. Robertson (24) found no consistent differences in weight, length, and head circumference in 47 8-year-old children with a history of BPD, compared with age-matched premature and term infants. In the largest follow-up study to date of growth patterns in infants with BPD, Vrlenick (25) found significant decreases in weight and head circumference, but no difference in height at school age (8–10 years old) in 95 former premature infants with BPD compared with 311 infants without the disease. Differences in the growth indices were no longer apparent, however, when covariates that are known to affect growth (i.e., gestational age at birth, birth weight, race, maternal socioeconomic status) were taken into account. These results suggest that growth failure may be related more to extremely low birth weight and early gestational age, which are typical of the current population of infants with BPD, rather than to the disease itself.

The cause of the early growth failure in infants with BPD is likely multifactorial. Several studies have shown that resting oxygen consumption is increased (25–28). An elevated metabolic rate in the face of inadequate caloric intake may contribute to growth failure (26,27). The increased energy demands are only partly due to the increased work of breathing, in that improvement in respiratory status is not accompanied by a decrease in oxygen consumption (28). Repeated hypoxic episodes, common early in the course of BPD, also may affect growth. Treatment of the pulmonary disease with adequate home oxygen therapy (to maintain oxygen saturation above 92%) improves weight gain (29). Other possible mechanisms for the poor initial weight gain include inadequate caloric intake resulting from fluid restriction, in addition to behavioral and feeding difficulties, and the increased incidence of lower respiratory tract infections and rehospitalizations.

IV. Exacerbations with Intercurrent Illness

Respiratory exacerbations owing to recurrent lower respiratory tract infections occur frequently in infants with BPD and contribute to a higher rate of rehospitalization than in infants without BPD (19,30). In a recent follow-up study of infants enrolled in a randomized trial of high-frequency oscillatory ventilation, approximately 20% of the 432 study infants were readmitted to the hospital one or more times for respiratory infections (31). Respiratory syncytial virus (RSV) is a frequent cause of respiratory deterioration in infants with BPD during the winter months (32,33). Because these infants may have limited pulmonary reserve and marginal small airway caliber, they often deteriorate rapidly after the onset of even mild upper or lower respiratory tract infections. Recurrent respiratory infections may contribute to further damage to the lungs, and thus affect long-term pulmonary morbidity. The occurrence of a severe episode of RSV bronchiolitis during infancy has been associated with later development of reactive airway disease in normal-term infants (34). Thus, the more frequent occurrence of RSV bronchiolitis in infants with BPD may play a contributory role in the high incidence of reactive airway disease seen in these infants later in childhood. The role that intercurrent pulmonary infections play in the long-term outcome of infants with BPD has not been adequately studied. Recent data suggest that treatment with RSV immune globulin may help prevent severe RSV infections in infants with BPD (33). The effect that such therapy may have on long-term pulmonary outcome in these infants requires further study.

V. Techniques, Interpretation, and Limitations of Pulmonary Function Testing in Infants with BPD

A. Standard Measurements

Most of the techniques used to study pulmonary mechanics in adults require voluntary maneuvers that infants and young children are unable to perform. Thus, the study of short- and long-term pulmonary function in infants and children with BPD has been limited by the difficulties inherent in pulmonary function measurements in uncooperative subjects. Recently, however, innovative approaches developed to measure lung function in normal infants and children have been applied to infants with BPD. Self-contained computerized systems to study pulmonary function at the bedside have been developed as well, contributing to our understanding of lung function in infants with BPD. The excitement of the new technology, however, must be tempered with knowledge of its limitations and the implicit assumptions that may affect interpretation of results. This section will briefly review some of the techniques that have been used for the measurement of pulmonary function in infants and children with BPD, and outline their advantages and potential limitations.

Lung Volume Measurement

Accurate measurement of lung volume is important for standardizing measurements of lung mechanics in infants and children of different sizes. Functional residual capacity (FRC) is usually used as the standard lung volume. Between birth and approximately 1 year of age, infants use a breathing strategy to dynamically maintain an end-expiratory lung volume above the mechanically determined FRC (35,36). As a result of this breathing strategy, end-expiratory lung volume is more variable in infants than in older children and adults who breathe from a relaxed FRC. Despite this variability, two methods have been adapted for measurement of FRC in infants and children: gas equilibration and washout techniques, and body plethysmography.

The central assumptions of the gas dilution technique for the measurement of FRC are that complete equilibration and washout of the inhaled inert gas (helium or nitrogen) occurs within the short time period allowed for measurement, and the lung behaves in a homogeneous manner. These assumptions may not be correct in infants, especially those with lung disease (37). Trapped or poorly accessible gas within the lungs will not be measured by gas dilution techniques, but they are by plethysmography. Thus, measurements of FRC by gas dilution and washout techniques tend to underestimate lung volume (38). The amount of "trapped" gas in the lungs may be substantial in obstructive lung diseases, such as BPD, and thus FRC measured by this method can be variably underestimated by this method.

Body plethysmography for measurement of thoracic gas volume (TGV) has also been used in infants and children. Infants are placed in an air-tight body plethysmograph, and a face mask pneumotachograph apparatus outfitted with a shutter mechanism is applied. Airflow is occluded at end-expiration, and changes in pressure measured in the box and at the airway, allowing calculation of TGV. Infants and children usually require sedation for this technique.

Body plethysmographic measurements assume both a uniform distribution of pressure on the lung, and that mouth pressure accurately reflects mean alveolar pressure. These assumptions, however, may not always be valid in infants and children (39,40). For example, local variations of pleural pressure may occur in infants with paradoxical rib cage movement (41). Furthermore, in infants with reactive airway disease, lung volume measured by plethysmography was low despite clinical signs of air trapping while infants were wheezing (42), suggesting that mouth pressure may not accurately represent mean alveolar pressure in infants with airway obstruction.

Measurement of Lung Mechanics

Obtaining useful data on pulmonary mechanics requires measurement of airflow and airway and esophageal pressure. Flow is usually measured with a pneumotachograph with a differential pressure transducer attached to a face mask or nasal prongs; tidal volume is derived by integration of the flow signal. Volume changes also may be monitored in a plethysmograph. Airway (mouth) pressure is measured with a pressure transducer connected to a side port on the pneumotachograph. Transpleural pressure, needed to calculate dynamic lung compliance and respiratory resistance, is estimated by the difference between transesophageal pressure at the midthoracic esophagus and airway pressure. Esophageal pressure may be obtained using an esophageal balloon, or, more commonly utilized in infants, a fluid-filled catheter.

Most studies of pulmonary mechanics in infants and children with BPD have assessed changes in dynamic compliance and total pulmonary resistance over time. The compliance measurement is usually expressed as a function of body weight, length, or lung volume to compare infants of different ages and sizes. Airway, as opposed to total pulmonary resistance, can be measured using plethysmography, but this technique has not been widely reported in infants with BPD.

The accuracy of these techniques is based on the assumption that the pressure measured using the esophageal catheter represents average pleural pressure. Technical considerations, including positioning of the catheter within the esophagus and the frequency response of the system, may affect esophageal pressure measurements (43,44). Furthermore, esophageal catheters may sample only regional changes in pleural pressures (41,45). With paradoxical rib cage movement, which occurs in premature infants, in infants during rapid eye movement sleep, and in infants with obstructive lung disease, including BPD, different pleural pressure swings may occur at different catheter locations (45). In these situations, compliance and resistance measurements may not be accurate, for the esophageal pressure measurement does not represent an average across the lung.

Given the difficulty of measuring pulmonary mechanics in spontaneously breathing infants and children, investigators have modified the airway occlusion technique to assess the mechanical properties of the respiratory system. The occlusion technique takes advantage of the fact that infants and sedated children up to approximately 2 years of age have an active Hering-Breuer reflex that produces apnea when the airway is occluded at volumes above FRC (46,47). The passive mechanical properties of the respiratory system can be measured during the period of respiratory muscle relaxation (48). Compliance may be assessed by measurement of airway pressure and airflow/tidal volume during multiple airway occlusions at end-inspiration and at different points during expiration. Occlusions are maintained until airway pressure reaches a plateau, indicating relaxation of the respiratory muscles and equilibration between airway and alveolar pressure. From these measurements, a pressure–volume curve may be constructed; its slope represents passive compliance of the respiratory system.

An adaptation of the multiple occlusion technique can be used to measure both respiratory system compliance and resistance (48–50). In this technique, a single end-inspiratory occlusion is performed until an airway pressure plateau is reached, and flow and volume of the "passive" exhalation are displayed. From the linear portion of the flow–volume curve, the expiratory time constant, compliance, and resistance can be calculated.

These methods for measuring passive mechanics of the respiratory system also require several assumptions (44). First, the technique assumes that the occlusions result in complete relaxation of the respiratory muscles, which can be inferred only if an airway pressure plateau is reached. This may not occur in very small premature infants with weak Hering-Breuer reflexes or in infants with lung disease that is associated with increased respiratory drive and tachypnea. Second, the method assumes a constant resistance during expiration. Infants actively brake expiratory airflow with both postinspiratory diaphragmatic activity and laryngeal adduction (35). Laryngeal braking of expiratory airflow is not abolished by the Hering-Breuer reflex (44), so that the resistance to expiratory airflow may not be constant. In addition, these techniques assume a ''one-compartment'' lung model, where the time constant is uniform throughout the lung. This may not be true, especially in infants with significant lung disease, leading to a nonlinear flow–volume curve.

Maximal Forced Expiratory Flow

Assessment of airway function in infants with BPD has received considerable interest in recent years. Forced expiratory flows are determined by the dynamic mechanical properties of the intrathoracic airways, in contrast with resistance measurements, which are primarily influenced by the extrathoracic airways. Flow rates during the first half of expiration are limited by expiratory muscle effort and the resistance of the large airways. As lung volume decreases, forced expiratory flow also declines, a function of small airway resistance and decreased elastic recoil of the lung at lower lung volumes. Forced expiratory flow maneuvers can assess the severity of lower airways obstruction in individuals with lung disease. This technique also can be used to assess the reversible component of airway obstruction by comparing maximal expiratory flows before and after bronchodilator therapy.

Two techniques to measure maximal forced expiratory flows have been developed for infants and children. The first method uses rapid application of positive pressure to the chest and abdomen at end-inspiration for 3–5 sec by means of a ''squeeze'' jacket, inducing a forced expiration that is measured with a face mask and pneumotachograph (51,52). Because the forced expiratory volume usually proceeds below the spontaneous end-expiratory level with this maneuver, maximal expiratory flows are usually expressed as maximal expiratory flow at FRC (determined from the previous breaths or by direct measurement). The shape of the expiratory flow–volume curve also indicates the severity of airways obstruction. Forced expiratory maneuvers by this method in normal infants result in a convex flow-volume curve, while the resulting curve in infants with lower airways obstruction may be concave. In severe cases, the forced expiratory flow curve may be superimposed on the ''relaxed'' flow–volume tracing, indicative of expiratory flow limitation within the normal tidal breathing range (12).

Several methodological issues must be considered when evaluating results from forced expiratory flows measured by this technique (44). Sudden imposition of a large extrathoracic pressure may by itself produce airway compression, therefore, flow limitation. The level of positive pressure at which this occurs may be different among subjects, especially those with lung disease. This suggests that use of a single standard pressure to induce ''maximal'' expiratory flow may not be appropriate in all infants (53). In addition, representation of maximal expiratory flow at FRC assumes that end-expiratory lung volume in infants represents FRC, and it remains constant. However, as infants dynamically maintain their end-expiratory volume above FRC, this assumption is invalid, especially in younger infants (35). It is possible, therefore, that measured changes in flow at FRC represent changes in end-expiratory lung volume, not changes in airway dynamics.

The second method used to measure maximal expiratory flow is restricted to use in intubated and mechanically ventilated infants. In these infants, negative pressure is applied to the airway to induce a forced deflation (54). A constant lung volume history is set by three inflations to near total lung capacity before opening the airway to a 40-L negative-pressure reservoir. The advantage of this technique is that flows are measured from vital capacity to below FRC after a standardized volume history, similar to the technique used to measure maximal expiratory flows in adults. The obvious limitation of the technique is its restriction to use in intubated subjects. In addition, the presence of the endotracheal tube may artificially ''stiffen'' the trachea or change large airway resistance and alter expiratory flow characteristics if the trachea is a major site of flow limitation (55).

Most of the standard techniques just described were developed to study normal-term or preterm infants. Recognition of the limitations of the techniques in infants and children with lung disease is essential to the critical evaluation of data collected in this population. In these subjects, more variable or even erroneous results may be obtained, and significant intra- and interpatient variability is likely (56). In part, these limitations explain the relative paucity of data available on the short- and long-term pulmonary morbidity in infants and small children with BPD.

B. Indirect Measurement Techniques

Many of the methods to assess pulmonary mechanics in infants and children are somewhat invasive, requiring catheter placement or manipulation of the chest. Thus, successful completion of pulmonary function studies in infants beyond the newborn period often requires sedation, which may affect the measurements. Respiratory inductive plethysmography (RIP), a less invasive measurement technique to assess pulmonary function, has recently been used to study children with airway obstruction, including those with BPD (57,58). In this technique, elastic bands containing inductive coils are placed around the upper rib cage and the abdomen. Voltage changes in response to changes in band inductance are proportional to changes of the cross-sectional area of the measured compartment, allowing assessment of relative volume changes of the rib cage and abdomen.

Uncalibrated RIP has been used to quantitate relative timing, synchrony, and magnitude of the rib cage and abdominal motion by means of a Lissajous figure, a loop formed by the rib cage and abdominal signals displayed on an x–y plot. The phase angle measured from the Lissajous figure is an index of thoracoabdominal asynchrony, and the direction of the loop (clockwise or counterclockwise) indicates relative timing of the rib cage and abdomen during inspiration.

The degree of thoracoabdominal asynchrony is a reliable indicator of airflow obstruction and pulmonary mechanics in infants with and without BPD (57–59). It is especially useful in measurement of response to therapeutic interventions, such as bronchodilator treatment, when changes in the degree of thoracoabdominal asynchrony reflect changes in lung mechanics induced by the therapy (57). Advantages for this method of pulmonary function measurement are that it is noninvasive, well-tolerated, and may be used for prolonged periods without the need for sedation. Its use is limited, however, to younger infants and children whose rib cages are compliant enough to reflect changes in transpulmonary pressure swings. Similar correlations between the degree of thoracoabdominal asynchrony and pulmonary mechanical abnormalities are not seen with chronic obstructive lung disease in adults, who have stiffer rib cages than infants (60). This technique, although not used widely, is a potentially important adjunct for the assessment of pulmonary mechanics in infants and children with BPD.

VI. Pulmonary Function in BPD: Infancy and Beyond

Available pulmonary outcome data may not apply to today's intensive care unit graduate with BPD. The diagnosis of BPD is based on clinical history, radiographic changes, and the duration of oxygen therapy, not specific lung function abnormalities. Thus, the spectrum of pulmonary abnormalities and outcomes in infants with BPD is likely to be heterogeneous. In addition, the epidemiology of BPD is affected by changes in therapy. Infants who have BPD now have much lower birth weights and gestational ages than patients who have been evaluated previously in published pulmonary follow-up studies, especially studies of school-age children. Prematurity, birth weight, and treatment with mechanical ventilation also affect long-term pulmonary function in infants who do not acquire chronic lung disease (61,62). As BPD evolves into a disease primarily affecting the extremely premature infant, pulmonary outcome is likely to change. Nevertheless, review of available data on short- and long-term pulmonary outcomes of infants with BPD provides insight into the process of lung growth and repair in this population.

A. Infancy to 3 Years

Pulmonary function in infants with BPD is characterized by abnormalities in pulmonary mechanics, lung volume, energetics of breathing, and airflow dynamics. Gas-exchange abnormalities also exist early in the course of the disease. As infants grow, gas exchange becomes normal first, despite persistent and often severe abnormalities in other measures of lung function.

Pulmonary Mechanics

Lung compliance is significantly decreased in infants with BPD (3,63–64). In normal infants, lung compliance increases in close correlation with changes in body weight (3). This also appears to be true in infants with BPD (Fig. 1). Some studies suggest that lung compliance in infants with BPD may become normal by 6–12 months of age (63,65). Other studies indicate that, although improvements are seen with growth, dynamic compliance and specific compliance (the quotient of dynamic compliance and FRC) may remain below the normal range until close to 3 years of age (3,66). Decreased compliance in infants with BPD is likely secondary to morphological changes in the lung, including atelectasis, fibrosis, and interstitial edema. Lung compliance in infants with BPD may improve with bronchodilator therapy (67), suggesting that regional air trapping sec-

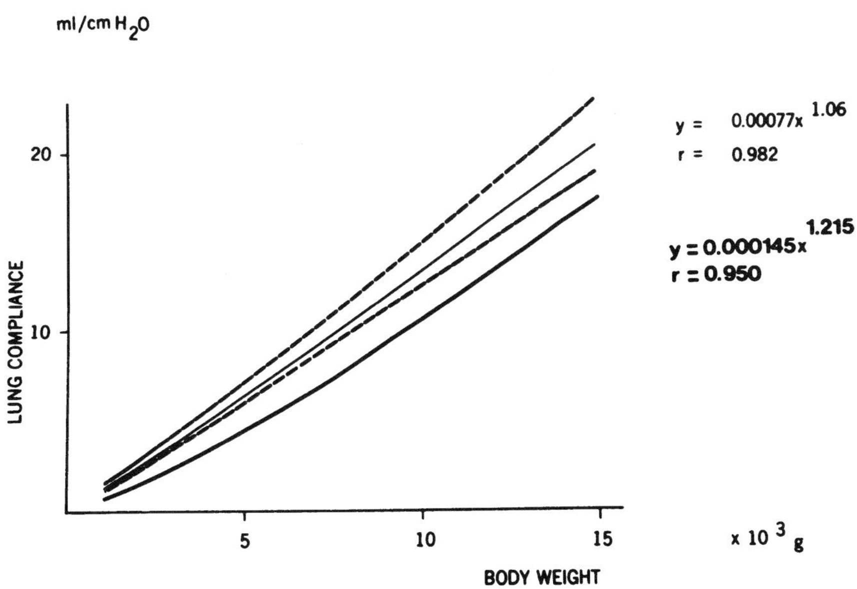

Figure 1 Relation of lung compliance to body weight in infants with BPD (heavy line) compared with normal infants (thin line; 95% confidence limits [dashed lines]). Lung compliance is decreased in infants with BPD, but improves with growth at a rate similar to normal infants. (From Ref. 3.)

ondary to increased airway resistance or obstruction also may contribute to abnormalities in compliance. The strong correlation between weight gain and improvements in compliance in infants with BPD suggests that it is related primarily to lung growth and formation of new alveoli (3).

Total pulmonary resistance is invariably elevated in infants with BPD (3,62,63,68,69). Early in the course of BPD, increased pulmonary resistance is likely related to airway narrowing caused by the pathological changes described earlier, including airway squamous metaplasia and proliferation of hypertrophied smooth muscle. These abnormalities persist despite adequate growth, although relative improvements occur when corrected for body weight. Resistance appears to change little over the first 6 postnatal months, but then gradually decreases between 6 and 36 months (3; Fig. 2). The lack of improvement in pulmonary resistance through early infancy may partly explain the susceptibility of infants with BPD to more severe lower respiratory tract infections during this period, because a minor change in small airway edema with infection may cause a marked reduction in airway resistance. Increases in pulmonary resistance in in-

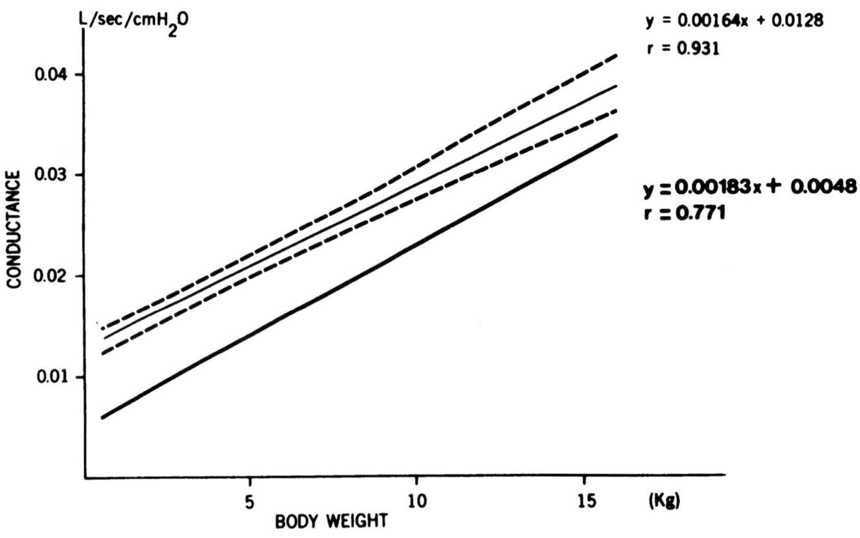

Figure 2 Relation of pulmonary conductance (reciprocal of resistance) to body weight in infants with BPD (heavy line) compared with normal infants (thin line; 95% confidence limits [dashed lines]). Pulmonary conductance is significantly less (i.e., higher resistance) in infants with BPD compared with normal infants. The relative difference between the pulmonary conductance in infants with BPD and normal infants decreases with growth, but remains significantly less. (From Ref. 3.)

fants with BPD also have a reversible component. Bronchodilator, methylxanthine, and diuretic therapy immediately, but transiently, decrease pulmonary resistance (67,70–72).

The decreased compliance and elevated resistance in infants with BPD is reflected in an increased work of breathing. Breath-to-breath esophageal pressure changes are larger in infants with BPD (31), indicative of increased respiratory muscle work. Despite the increased driving pressure, tidal volumes are significantly lower in infants with BPD compared with normal controls (64). Minute ventilation is higher, however, because respiratory rate is usually increased (3,31). The increased work of breathing and higher minute ventilation in infants with BPD is partly responsible for the observed increase in oxygen consumption and metabolic rate (27).

Lung Volumes

Some of the changes in pulmonary mechanics seen in infants with BPD over time have been attributed to changes in lung volume, particularly FRC. Earlier studies of lung volume in patients with BPD concluded that FRC was elevated secondary to air trapping (73). More recent studies, however, indicate that FRC, measured by gas dilution or washout techniques, probably is decreased early in the disease course (3,12). In these studies, FRC remained lower than normal until 6–10 months postnatal age, a finding that has been attributed to persistent atelectasis. Gerhardt (3) made serial determinations of pulmonary function in 39 infants with BPD from 1–36 months after birth. In that study, FRC returned to the normal range by about 12 months of age. After 12 months, the increase in FRC with growth was similar to that seen in normal infants, suggesting that infants with BPD had normal lung growth over this time period (Fig. 3). Studies comparing FRC to TGV measurements in infants with BPD have not been reported. FRC measurements by the gas dilution/washout techniques would tend to underestimate FRC when there is significant air trapping, whereas TGV measurements would include any "trapped" gas. In one study, TGV measurements in infants with BPD at 41 weeks postconceptional age were not significantly different from those in normal-term infants (67), consistent with the conclusion that air trapping is not a significant problem for most infants early in the course of BPD. Serial determinations of pulmonary mechanics in infants with BPD also support this conclusion. Lung compliance would be expected to decrease with air trapping because of associated alveolar overdistention. Contrary to this expectation, steady improvements in compliance with weight gain are seen in infants with BPD (3).

Airflow Mechanics and Reactive Airway Disease

Pulmonary resistance measurements primarily reflect the function of the larger airways and upper airway structures. The gradual decrease in pulmonary resis-

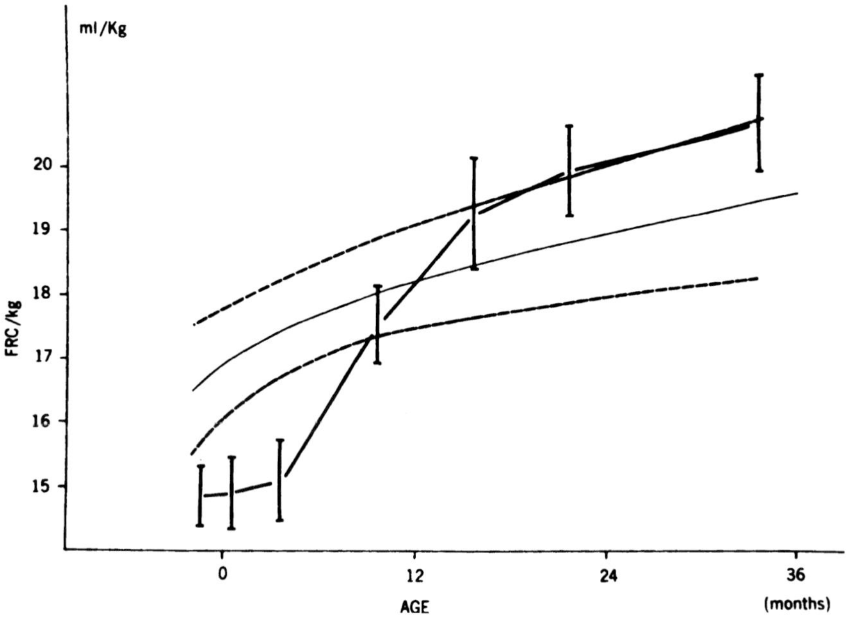

Figure 3 Functional residual capacity (FRC) per kilogram (kg) in infants with BPD from birth to 36 months (heavy line) compared with normal infants (thin line; 95% confidence limits [dashed lines]). FRC/kg is lower in infants with BPD in the first few postnatal months, but returns to the normal range by 12 months. After 12 months, the increase in FRC with growth is similar to that seen in normal infants. (From Ref. 3.)

tance with growth in infants with BPD results from large airway growth. Most of the pathological abnormalities in the airways of infants with BPD, however, are localized to the smaller peripheral airways. As might be expected from the pathology, assessment of small airway function by forced expiratory flow maneuvers in infants with BPD indicates that small airway obstruction persists throughout infancy, despite adequate growth (12,74). Tepper (12) measured partial maximal expiratory flow–volume curves using a "squeeze" jacket in 20 infants with BPD over the first postnatal year. The infants with BPD has significantly lower absolute and size-corrected expiratory flows as well as abnormally shaped flow–volume curves compared with a group of control infants who were matched for age and size (Fig. 4). Although maximal expiratory flow at FRC improved with growth, it did so at a significantly slower rate than in the normal infants, increasing the difference between the normal and affected infants. Mallory reported similar results in a small group of infants with severe BPD who required tracheos-

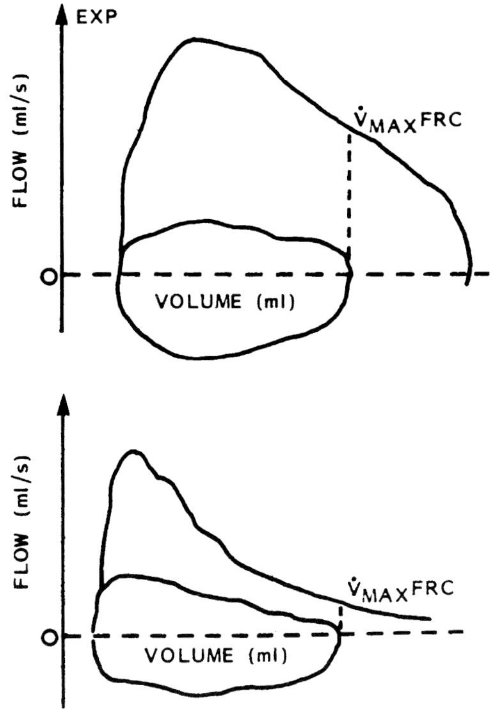

Figure 4 Partial expiratory flow–volume curves in a normal infant (top) and an infant with BPD (bottom). The smaller inner curve represents tidal breathing, and larger curve represents maximal expiratory flow generated by rapid compression technique. Note concave flow–volume curve in infant with BPD, demonstrating severe expiratory flow limitation. Maximal expiratory flow at FRC (V_{max} FRC) is significantly decreased in the infant with BPD compared with the normal infants, indicative of small airway obstruction. (From Ref. 12.)

tomy for prolonged mechanical ventilation, followed from 6 to 36 months of age (74). With a negative-pressure technique to measure forced vital capacity (FVC), all subjects at 6 months of age had decreased FVC and evidence for severe obstruction of the smaller intrathoracic airways. FVC progressively increased with age, indicating an increase in lung volume. FVC reached normal levels by 12 months of age in infants with less severe pulmonary disease (defined as shorter duration of mechanical ventilation). Maximal expiratory flow improved, but remained less than normal in this group of infants up to 36 months of age, indicative of persistent small airway obstruction. Despite small increases in FVC, no improvement in maximal expiratory flows was observed in the infants with the most severe disease.

The small airway obstruction seen in BPD is partly due to reversible small airway constriction. Evidence for airway reactivity in premature infants in whom BPD develops can be found as early as 12 days of age (54). In older infants with BPD, improvement in pulmonary mechanics, forced expiratory airflow, and thoracoabdominal asynchrony is consistently seen after bronchodilator therapy (12,58,71,74,75). Increased airway reactivity also can be demonstrated by cold air challenge (76). These findings are consistent with the histological appearance of hypertrophied smooth muscle in the airways of infants with BPD. Increased airway reactivity may be the consequence of oxygen toxicity or injury from high airway pressures or large tidal volumes. However, an increased incidence of airway hyperreactivity has been observed in the families of infants with BPD (77) and in women who deliver premature infants (78). A genetic predisposition to airway hyperreactivity may be a risk factor for the development of BPD. Other studies, however, have not confirmed this epidemiological association (79,80).

Summary

Changes in pulmonary function associated with growth of infants with BPD include normalization of pulmonary mechanics and lung volumes, but small airway obstruction and hyperreactivity persist. These observations suggest that the process of lung repair is different for the conductive airways than for the lung parenchyma. Formation and branching of the conductive airways is complete by the middle of the second trimester (81). In contrast, alveolar growth and multiplication is just beginning in the weeks before birth, and continues throughout early childhood. Although the pathological changes in BPD affect both airways and lung parenchyma, the number of branching airways is fixed at birth. With growth, damaged conductive airways can increase only in length and caliber, whereas alveoli increase in number, replacing areas of damaged parenchyma. Persistent small airway obstruction in infants with BPD suggests that abnormal functional development of existing damaged airways is a hallmark of the disease, despite improvement in other measures of pulmonary function.

B. Long-Term Pulmonary Outcome

Considerably less data are available on the longer-term pulmonary outcomes of infants with a history of BPD as they reach school age and adolescence. The few available studies, however, reveal that the airway obstruction and reactivity observed in younger children with BPD persist in school-age children. In contrast to findings reported during infancy, school-age children and adolescents with BPD have evidence for hyperinflation, as assessed by chest radiograph, and an increased ratio of residual volume to total lung capacity (17,80,82,83).

Children and adolescents are also more likely to have airway obstruction on pulmonary function tests (17,80,82–85). Reactive airway disease, a common feature in younger infants with a history of BPD, is also common in older survivors (17,80,82–86), despite a low incidence of clinically diagnosed asthma (80). Most studies have assessed airway reactivity by methacholine challenge. Exercise-induced bronchospasm in 10-year-old children with a history of BPD was associated with a decrease in oxygen saturation values (82), suggesting that functional limitations exist in these children. Such functional limitations may persist into adulthood. In Northway's (17) long-term follow-up of 26 adult survivors of a 1964–1973 BPD cohort, pulmonary dysfunction was rated to be either severe or responsible for respiratory symptoms in almost 25% of the patients.

Despite evidence for persistent pulmonary function abnormalities, improvements in function can occur late into childhood. Blayney (80) studied 32 patients with BPD at age 7 and 10 years. At the first examination, most children demonstrated airway obstruction, reactivity, and hyperinflation on pulmonary function testing. Children with the most significant degree of airway obstruction at age 7 showed improvement in function by age 10. Children with normal forced expiratory flows at age 7 continued to be normal at age 10, indicating continued lung growth and improvement in lung function during later childhood.

VII. Conclusions and Future Directions

Despite improvements in gas-exchange abnormalities, many children who have "recovered" from BPD continue to have airway obstruction, clinical as well as subclinical reactive airway disease, and exercise intolerance into late childhood and adolescence. These abnormalities suggest that the structural changes in the small airways seen in BPD persist into childhood and beyond, despite continued lung and somatic growth. Persistent abnormalities in pulmonary function may reflect fixed, irreversible structural changes within the lung from injury sustained in the neonatal period, as well as an alteration of subsequent growth of the lung as a consequence of the initial injury. Less severe lung growth and functional abnormalities also can be detected in later childhood in former premature infants who required mechanical ventilation without acquiring BPD, as well as in former premature infants without initial lung disease (68,78).

The more severe lung function abnormalities seen in children with BPD are likely to be superimposed on abnormal lung growth and development related to prematurity. Available pulmonary follow-up studies of children who acquired BPD in infancy have included a more mature population than the mostly extremely low birth weight infants currently diagnosed with BPD. The effects of recent changes in ventilatory management of extremely premature infants, including synchronized intermittent mandatory ventilation and high-frequency ventilation, on their short- and long-term pulmonary outcomes require extensive study. The effects of pharmacological agents used clinically or under investigation to treat or prevent BPD, including glucocorticoids, vitamin A, inositol, α_1-protease inhibitor, and superoxide dismutase, on long-term pulmonary growth and function remain unknown. Whether greater abnormalities in alveolar and capillary development will become evident as extremely premature infants born today reach adulthood remains to be seen, but emphasizes the need for continued follow-up studies. In addition to standard measurements of pulmonary function, it will be imperative to focus on the assessment of functional measurements that affect quality of life for these children. These might include sufficient respiratory reserve for an infant to feed without distress, for an older child to play, and for a teenager to participate fully in sports. Finally, in addition to outcome studies, future research efforts must focus on prevention of bronchopulmonary dysplasia and premature birth.

References

1. Northway WH, Rosan RC, Porter DY. Pulmonary disease following respiratory therapy of hyaline membrane disease. N Engl J Med 1967; 276:357–368.
2. Parker RA, Lindstrom DP, Cotton RB. Improved survival accounts for most, but not all, of the increase in bronchopulmonary dysplasia. Pediatrics 1992; 90:663–8.
3. Gerhardt T, Hehre D, Feller R, Reifenberg L, Bancalari E. Serial determination of pulmonary function in infants with chronic lung disease. J Pediatr 1987; 110:448–56.
4. Stahlman MT. Chronic lung disease in the newborn infant. In: Stern L, Vert P, eds. Neonatal Medicine. New York: Masson, 1987.
5. De Boeck K, Smith J, Van Lierde S, Van Gijsel D, Devlieger H. Flat chest in survivors of bronchopulmonary dysplasia. Pediatr Pulmonol 1994; 18:104–7.
6. Fan LL, Flynn JW, Pathak DR, Madden WA. Predictive value of stridor in detecting laryngeal injury in extubated neonates. Crit Care Med 1982; 10:453–5.
7. McCoy KS, Bagwell CE, Wagner M, Sallent J, O'Keefe M, Kosch PC. Spirometric and endoscopic evaluation of airway collapse in infants with bronchopulmonary dysplasia. Pediatr Pulmonol 1992; 14:23–7.
8. Stocker JT. Pathologic features of long-standing "healed" bronchopulmonary dysplasia. Hum Pathol 1986; 17:943–61.
9. Abman SH, Wolfe RR, Accurso FJ, Koops BL, Bowman CM, Wiggins JW Jr. Pulmonary vascular response to oxygen in infants with severe bronchopulmonary dysplasia. Pediatrics 1985; 75:80–4.
10. Garg M, Kurzner SI, Bautista DB, Keens TG. Clinically unsuspected hypoxia during sleep and feeding in infants with bronchopulmonary dysplasia. Pediatrics 1988; 81:635–42.
11. Singer L, Martin RJ, Hawkins SW, Benson-Szekely LJ, Yamashita TS, Carlo WA.

Oxygen desaturation complicates feeding in infants with bronchopulmonary dysplasia after discharge. Pediatrics 1992; 90:380–4.
12. Tepper RS, Morgan WJ, Cota K, Taussig LM. Expiratory flow limitation in infants with bronchopulmonary dysplasia. J Pediatr 1986; 109:1040–6.
13. Edwards D. Radiographic aspects of bronchopulmonary dysplasia. J Pediatr 1979; 823–9.
14. Mortensson W, Lindroth M. The course of bronchopulmonary dysplasia. Acta Radiol Diagn 1986; 27:19–22.
15. Griscom NT, Wheeler WB, Sweezey NB, Kim YC, Lindsey JC, Wohl MEB. Bronchopulmonary dysplasia: radiographic appearance in middle childhood. Radiology 1989; 171:811–14.
16. Oppenheim C, Mamou-Mani T, Sayegh N, deBlic J, Scheinmann P, Lallemand D. Bronchopulmonary dysplasia: value of CT in identifying pulmonary sequelae. Am J Roentgenol 1994; 163:169–72.
17. Northway WH Jr, Moss RB, Carlisle KB, Parker BR, Popp RL, Pitlick PT, Eichler I, Lamm RL, Brown BW Jr. Late pulmonary sequelae of bronchopulmonary dysplasia. N Engl J Med 1990; 323:1793–9.
18. Meisels SJ, Plunkett JW, Roloff DW, Pasick PL, Stiefel GS. Growth and development of preterm infants with respiratory distress syndrome and bronchopulmonary dysplasia. Pediatrics 1986; 77:345–52.
19. Cunningham CK, McMillan JA, Gross SJ. Rehospitalization for respiratory illness in infants of less than 32 weeks' gestation. Pediatrics 1991; 88:527–32.
20. Markestad T, Fitzhardinge PM. Growth and development in children recovering from bronchopulmonary dysplasia. J Pediatr 1981; 98:597–602.
21. Yu V, Orgill A, Lim SB, Bajuk B, Astbury J. Growth and development of very low birthweight infants recovering from bronchopulmonary dysplasia. Arch Dis Child 1983; 58:791–4.
22. Davidson S, Schrayer A, Wielunsky E, Krikler R, Lilos P, Reisner SH. Energy intake, growth and development in ventilated very low birthweight infants with and without bronchopulmonary dysplasia. Am J Dis Child 1990; 144:553–9.
23. Tammela OKT, Koivisto ME. A 1-year follow-up of low birth weight infants with and without bronchopulmonary dysplasia: health, growth, clinical lung disease, cardiovascular and neurological sequelae. Early Hum Dev 1992; 30:109–20.
24. Robertson CMT, Etches PC, Goldson E, Kyle JM. Eight-year school performance, neurodevelopmental, and growth outcome of neonates with bronchopulmonary dysplasia: a comparative study. Pediatrics 1992; 89:365–72.
25. Vrlenich LA, Bozynski MEA, Shyr Y, Schork M, Roloff DW, McCormick MC. The effect of bronchopulmonary dysplasia on growth at school age. Pediatrics 1995; 95: 855–9.
26. Weinstein MR, Oh W. Oxygen consumption in infants with bronchopulmonary dysplasia. J Pediatr 1981; 99:958–60.
27. Kurzner SI, Garg M, Bautista DB, Bader D, Merritt RJ, Warburton D, Keens TG. Growth failure in infants with bronchopulmonary dysplasia: nutrition and elevated resting metabolic expenditure. Pediatrics 1988; 81:379–84.
28. Kao L C, Durand DJ, Nickerson BG. Improving pulmonary function does not decrease oxygen consumption in infants with bronchopulmonary dysplasia. J Pediatr 1988; 112:616–21.

29. Groothuis JR, Rosenberg AA. Home oxygen promotes weight gain in infants with bronchopulmonary dysplasia. Am J Dis Child 1987; 141:992–5.
30. Kinney JS, Robertsen CM, Johnson KM, Gaddis M, Wheeler R, Jackson MA, Daily DK. Seasonal respiratory viral infections: impact on infants with chronic lung disease following discharge from the neonatal intensive care unit. Arch Pediatr Adolesc Med 1995; 149:81–5.
31. HiFi Study Group. High-frequency oscillatory ventilation compared with conventional mechanical ventilation in the treatment of respiratory failure in preterm infants: assessment of pulmonary function at 9 months of corrected age. J Pediatr 1990; 116: 933–41.
32. Groothuis JR, Gutierrez KM, Lauer BA. Respiratory syncytial virus infection in children with bronchopulmonary dysplasia. Pediatrics 1988; 82:199–203.
33. Groothuis JR, Simoes EA, Hemming VG. Respiratory syncytial virus (RSV) infection in preterm infants and the protective effects of RSV immune globulin (RSVIG). Respiratory Syncytial Virus Immune Globulin Study Group. Pediatrics 1995; 95: 463–7.
34. Sigurs N, Bjarnason R, Sigurbergsson F, Kjellman B, Bjorksten B. Asthma and immunoglobulin E antibodies after respiratory syncytial virus bronchiolitis: a prospective cohort study with matched controls. Pediatrics 1995; 95:500–5.
35. Kosch PC, Stark AR. Dynamic maintenance of end-expiratory lung volume in full-term infants. J Appl Physiol 1984; 57:1126–33.
36. Colin AA, Wohl MEB, Mead J, Ratjen FA, Glass G, Stark AR. Transition from dynamically maintained to relaxed end-expiratory volume in human infants. J Appl Physiol 1989; 67:2107–11.
37. Wall MA. Moment analysis of multibreath nitrogen washout in young children. J Appl Physiol 1985; 59:274–9.
38. Ronchetti R, Stocks J, Keith I, Godfrey S. An analysis of a rebreathing method for measuring lung volume in the premature infant. Pediatr Res 1975; 9:797–802.
39. Helms P. Problems with plethysmographic estimation of lung volume in infants and young children. J Appl Physiol 1982; 53:698–702.
40. Beardsmore CS, Stocks J. Silverman M. Problems in measurement of thoracic gas volume in infancy. J Appl Physiol 1982; 52:995–9.
41. Le Souef PN, Lopes JM, England SJ, Bryan MH. Bryan AC. Influence of chest wall distortion on esophageal pressure. J Appl Physiol 1983; 55:353–8.
42. Godfrey S, Beardsmore CS, Maayan C, Bar-Yishay E. Can thoracic gas volume be measured in infants with airways obstruction? Am Rev Respir Dis 1986; 133:245–51.
43. Beardsmore CS, Helms P, Stocks J, Hatch DJ, Silverman M. Improved esophageal balloon technique for use in infants. J Appl Physiol 1980; 49:735–42.
44. England SJ. Current techniques for assessing pulmonary function in the newborn and infant: advantages and limitations. Pediatr Pulmonol 1988; 4:48–53.
45. Heaf DP, Turner H, Stocks J, Helms P. The accuracy of esophageal pressure measurements in convalescent and sick intubated infants. Pediatr Pulmonol 1986; 2: 5–8.
46. Zin WA, Pengelly LD, Milk-Emili J. Single breath method for measurement of respiratory mechanics in anesthetized animals. J Appl Physiol 1982; 52:1266–71.

47. Shulman DL, Goodman A, Bar-Yishay E, Godfrey S. Comparison of single breath and volume recruitment techniques in the measurement of total respiratory compliance in anesthetized infants and children. Anesthesiology 1989; 70:921–7.
48. Mortola, JP, Fisher JT, Smith B, Fox G, Weeks S. Dynamics of breathing in infants. J Appl Physiol 1982; 52:1209–15.
49. Mortola JP, Saetta M. Measurements of respiratory mechanics in the newborn: a simple approach. Pediatr Pulmonol 1987; 3:123–30.
50. Le Souef PN, England SJ, Bryan AC. Passive respiratory mechanics in newborns and children. Am Rev Respir Dis 1984; 129:552–6.
51. Adler SM, Wohl MEB. Flow–volume relationship at low lung volumes in healthy term newborn infants. Pediatrics 1978; 61:636–40.
52. Taussig LM, Landau LI, Godfrey S, Arad I. Determinants of forced expiratory flows in newborn infants. J Appl Physiol 1982; 53:1220–7.
53. Le Souef PN, Hughes DM, Landau LI. Effect of compression pressure on forced expiratory flow in infants. J Appl Physiol 1986; 61:1639–46.
54. Motoyama EK, Fort MD, Klesh KW, Mutich RL, Guthrie RD. Early onset of airway reactivity in premature infants with bronchopulmonary dysplasia. Am Rev Respir Dis 1987; 136:50–7.
55. Jones JG, Frasier RB, Nadal JA. Effect of changing airway mechanics on maximum expiratory flow. J Appl Physiol 1975; 38:1012–21.
56. Nickerson BG, Durand DJ, Kao LC. Short-term variability of pulmonary function tests in infants with bronchopulmonary dysplasia. Pediatr Pulmonol 1989; 6:36–41.
57. Allen JL, Wolfson MR, McDowell K, Shaffer TH. Thoracoabdominal asynchrony in infants with airflow obstruction. Am Rev Respir Dis 1990; 141:337–42.
58. Allen JL, Greenspan JS, Deoras KS, Keklikian E, Wolfson MR, Shaffer TH. Interaction between chest wall motion and lung mechanics in normal infants and infants with bronchopulmonary dysplasia. Pediatr Pulmonol 1991; 11:37–43.
59. Wolfson MR, Greenspan JS, Deoras KS, Allen JL, Shaffer TH. Effect of position on the mechanical interaction between the rib cage and abdomen in preterm infants. Am Physiol Soc 1992; 1031–8.
60. Sackner MA, Gonzales H, Rodriguez M, Belsito A, Sackner DR, Grenvik S. Assessment of asynchronous and paradoxic motion between rib cage and abdomen in normal subjects and in patients with chronic obstructive pulmonary disease. Am Rev Respir Dis 1984; 130:588–93.
61. Greenspan JS, Abbasi S, Bhutani V. Sequential changes in pulmonary mechanics in the very low birth weight (< 1000 grams) infant. J Pediatr 1988; 113:732–7.
62. Abbasi S, Bhutani V, Spitzer AR, Fox WW. Pulmonary mechanics in preterm neonates with respiratory failure treated with high-frequency oscillatory ventilation compared with conventional mechanical ventilation. Pediatrics 1991; 87:487–93.
63. Morray JP, Fox WW, Kettrick RG, Downes JJ. Improvement in lung mechanics as a function of age in the infant with severe bronchopulmonary dysplasia. Pediatr Res 1982; 16:290–4.
64. Bhutani VK, Abbasi S. Long-term pulmonary consequences in survivors with bronchopulmonary dysplasia. Clin Perinatol 1992; 19:649–71.
65. Ahlstrom H. Pulmonary mechanics in infants surviving severe neonatal respiratory insufficiency. Acta Paediatr Scand 1975; 64:69–80.

66. Lindroth M, Mortensson W. Long-term follow-up of ventilator treated low birthweight infants. Acta Paediatr Scand 1986; 75:819–26.
67. Kao LC, Warburton D, Platzker ACG, Keens TG. Effect of isoproterenol inhalation on airway resistance in chronic bronchopulmonary dysplasia. Pediatrics 1984; 73: 509–14.
68. Moriette G, Gaudebout C, Clement A, Boule M, Bion B, Relier JP, Gaultier C. Pulmonary function at 1 year of age in survivors of neonatal respiratory distress: a multivariate analysis of factors associated with sequelae. Pediatr Pulmonol 1987; 3: 242–50.
69. Gerhardt T, Reifenberg L, Goldberg RN, Bancalari E. Pulmonary function in preterm infants whose lungs were ventilated conventionally or by high-frequency oscillation. J Pediatr 1989; 115:121–6.
70. Kao LC, Warburton D, Sargent CW, Platzker ACG, Keens TG. Furosemide acutely decreases airways resistance in chronic bronchopulmonary dysplasia. J Pediatr 1983; 103:624–9.
71. Kao LC, Durand DJ, Phillips BL, Nickerson BG. Oral theophylline and diuretics improve pulmonary mechanics in infants with bronchopulmonary dysplasia. J Pediatr 1987; 111:439–44.
72. Davis JM, Bhutani VK, Stefano JL, Fox WW, Spitzer AR. Changes in pulmonary mechanics following caffeine administration in infants with bronchopulmonary dysplasia. Pediatr Pulmonol 1989; 6:49–52.
73. Bryan MH, Hardie MJ, Reilly BJ, Swyer PR. Pulmonary function studies during the first year of life in infants recovering from the respiratory distress syndrome. Pediatrics 1973; 52:169–78.
74. Mallory GB Jr, Chaney H, Mutich RL, Motoyama EK. Longitudinal changes in lung function during the first three years of premature infants with moderate to severe bronchopulmonary dysplasia. Pediatr Pulmonol 1991; 11:8–14.
75. Logvinoff MM, Lemen RJ, Taussig LM, Lamont BA. Bronchodilators and diuretics in children with bronchopulmonary dysplasia. Pediatr Pulmonol 1985; 1:198–203.
76. Greenspan JS, DeGiulio PA, Bhutani V. Airway reactivity as determined by a cold air challenge in infants with bronchopulmonary dysplasia. J Pediatr 1989; 114: 452–4.
77. Nickerson BG, Taussig LM. Family history of asthma in infants with bronchopulmonary dysplasia. Pediatrics 1980; 65:1140–4.
78. Bertrand JM, Riley SP, Popkin J, Coates AL. The long-term pulmonary sequelae of prematurity: the role of familiar airway hyperreactivity and the respiratory distress syndrome. N Engl J Med 1985; 312:742–5.
79. Chan KN, Noble-Jamieson CM, Elliman A, Bryan EM, Aber VR, Silverman M. Airway responsiveness in low birthweight children and their mothers. Arch Dis Child 1988; 63:905–10.
80. Blayney M, Kerem E, Whyte H, O'Brodovich H. Bronchopulmonary dysplasia: improvement in lung function between 7 and 10 years of age. J Pediatr 1991; 118: 201–6.
81. Thurlbeck WM. Postnatal human lung growth. Thorax 1982; 37:564–71.
82. Bader D, Ramos AD, Lew CD, Platzker ACG, Stabile MW, Keens TG. Childhood

sequelae of infant lung disease: exercise and pulmonary function abnormalities after bronchopulmonary dysplasia. J Pediatr 1987; 110:693–9.

83. Hakulinen AL, Heinonen K, Länsimies E, Kiekara O. Pulmonary function and respiratory morbidity in school-age children born prematurely and ventilated for neonatal respiratory insufficiency. Pediatr Pulmonol 1990; 8:226–32.
84. Smyth JA, Tabachnik E, Duncan WJ, Reilly BJ, Levison H. Pulmonary function and bronchial hyperreactivity in long-term survivors of bronchopulmonary dysplasia. Pediatrics 1981; 68:336–40.
85. Andréasson, Lindroth M, Mortensson W, Svenningsen NW, Jonson B. Lung function eight years after neonatal ventilation. Arch Dis Child 1989; 64:108–13.
86. Duiverman EJ, den Boer JA, Roorda RJ, Rooyackers CMHM, Valstar M, Kerrebijn KF. Lung function and bronchial responsiveness measured by forced oscillometry after bronchopulmonary dysplasia. Arch Dis Child 1988; 63:727–32.

15

Cardiovascular Abnormalities in Bronchopulmonary Dysplasia

MICHAEL APKON, RODRIGO A. NEHGME, and GEORGE LISTER

Yale University School of Medicine
New Haven, Connecticut

I. Introduction

As documented by the other chapters in this monograph and numerous reviews, the consequences of bronchopulmonary dysplasia (BPD) and its treatment are protean, serious, and complex. The formerly premature infants who consume much of their energy merely to breathe have little left for growth or other activity. Although the primary focus of management traditionally has been to relieve respiratory insufficiency and pulmonary hypertension, the question frequently arises of whether there is merit in trying to manipulate the cardiac dysfunction that often results from these two disturbances. To put this question in perspective, it is our intent here to review what is known or can be reasonably deduced concerning cardiovascular function in infants with BPD. We will then discuss the rationale for various therapies that have been used to ''improve'' cardiovascular function in patients with BPD or analogous problems. Finally, the chapter provides an opportunity to delineate unresolved issues that are ripe for study and potentially important for understanding the pathogenesis and management of BPD.

For many aspects of cardiac function in BPD there are sufficient data to provide conclusions about mechanisms and consequences of this disorder. However, owing to the fragile state of many of the patients, their small size, their coexisting problems, and the difficulty of obtaining stable data, much of our understanding must be inferred from analogous conditions. The inference may not necessarily be valid. For instance, although infants with BPD and adults with chronic obstructive pulmonary disease (COPD) both have a high incidence of systemic hypertension, the cause is not known in either condition, and it is quite possible that the basis is different. Accordingly, we will try to highlight those assumptions that form the foundation for the analogy so that our rationale can be reexamined as new data arise. We recognize that most patients with BPD may have relatively mild compromise of cardiovascular function that may be undetected by routine clinical scrutiny and may have limited or no consequences. However, it is our intention here to focus on the more severe and clinically apparent disturbances in cardiovascular function. As a guide, Figure 1 indicates some of the cardiovascular consequences of severe BPD that are described in the following.

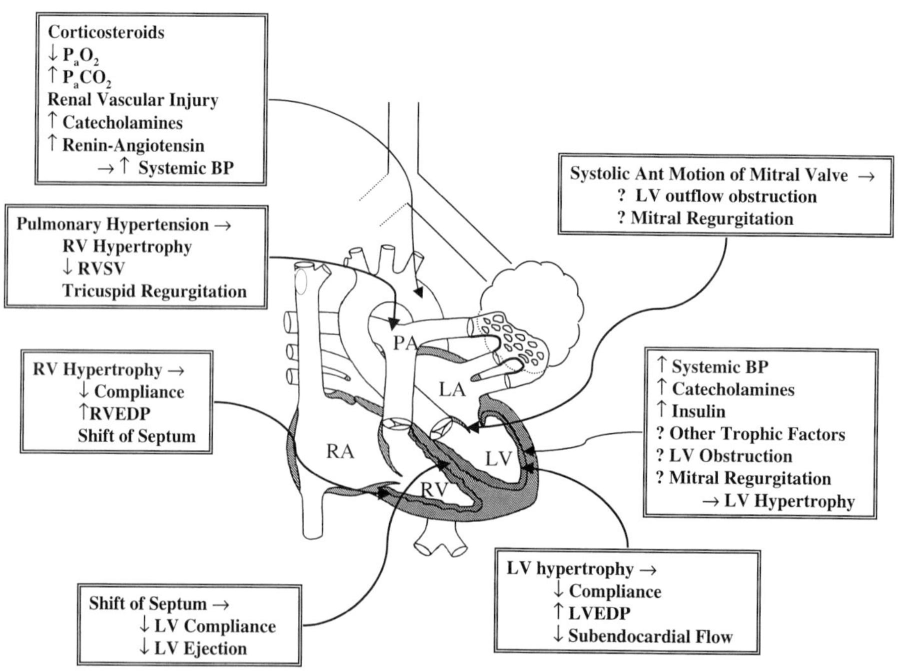

Figure 1 Schema showing hemodynamic changes and potential cardiocirculatory disturbances that occur with bronchopulmonary dysplasia. See text for discussion.

II. Disturbances in Cardiovascular Function

A. Cor Pulmonale

The presumption with BPD is that pulmonary hypertension, disturbances in blood gas tensions and acid–base homeostasis cause the cardiovascular dysfunction. Thus, it is common to describe the problem as *cor pulmonale*, which is defined as ''hypertrophy of the right ventricle resulting from diseases affecting the function and/or structure of the lungs, except when these pulmonary alterations are the result of diseases that primarily affect the left side of the heart, as in congenital heart disease'' (1). However, this definition is limited because it describes a structural change without reference to change in function, which is usually the signal for detecting problems in patients. Moreover, our ability to detect right ventricular hypertrophy in these patients is not very sensitive, because in early infancy, right ventricular forces are normally prominent, and echocardiography may be imprecise in a patient with hyperinflated lungs. The term cor pulmonale does not address or explain the left ventricular hypertrophy nor the systemic hypertension that often coexist in BPD (as well in adults with chronic lung disease; 2–7).

B. Effects on the Right Ventricle

Pathogenesis

It is well recognized that pulmonary hypertension is a common consequence of severe BPD (see Chap. 27), and the resultant elevation of right ventricular systolic pressure often leads to right ventricular hypertrophy. Pulmonary artery pressure is at systemic level during fetal life. With the onset of breathing at birth, pulmonary artery pressure decreases rapidly. The initial, rapid decrease occurs within hours to days (8), followed by a gradual decrease over ensuing weeks. The wall of the right ventricle is thick in utero and, shortly after birth, it develops a crescent shape with a concave septum and convex free wall. The right ventricle ejects its (pre)load at low peak pressure by shortening in the longitudinal direction (from tricuspid valve to the apex) as the free wall is compressed against the concave ventricular septum.

When there is a rapid increase in afterload resulting in tension on the ventricular wall during contraction, the right ventricle is unable to eject the normal stroke volume. This causes ventricular dilation, an increase in end-diastolic volume and pressure, and eventually, tricuspid regurgitation (9). In contrast, when afterload remains high from birth, the ventricle hypertrophies. Hypertrophy compensates for the increase in afterload [By the LaPlace relations, wall stress $= Pr/2h$, where P is pressure, r is the radius of curvature, and h is the wall thickness. This, however, is an oversimplification because the ventricle is not spherical. Therefore, meridional wall stress has been estimated as: $1.35\ Pd/[4h(1 + h/d)]$, where d is the ventricular minor axis.] This allows restoration of stroke volume, albeit at a higher pressure, while limiting the increase in wall stress (10). However, increases in wall thickness can decrease the diastolic compliance of the right ventricle, thereby altering ventricular-filling characteristics.

Systolic Function

Although the relation between pulmonary hypertension and respiratory insufficiency in BPD is not always predictable, reasonable inferences can be made for the consequences of elevated pulmonary vascular pressure. In response to the pulmonary hypertension, right ventricular stroke volume and ejection fraction may be diminished, as it is in adults with COPD (11,12). After using radionuclide assessment, Praud et al. (13) reported that right ventricular ejection fraction (RVEF) was decreased in five children, ages 1.5–5 years, who had a history of BPD. It is important to recognize, however, that changes in the commonly used indices of systolic function, such as stroke volume or ejection fraction, cannot necessarily be equated with a change in contractile function. Despite their simplicity, these and most other indices of ventricular function, such as rate of pressure change in the ventricle or rate of fiber shortening, depend on heart rate, preload and afterload, as well as contractility. Specifically, an increase in afterload may cause the ejection fraction to decrease without a change in contractility.

To develop a measure of contractility that is independent of preload or afterload, some investigators have assessed contractility by simultaneously measuring the change in pressure and volume of the ventricle in the intact circulation. These measurements are used to examine the end-systolic pressure–volume relation as preload or afterload changes. As the load changes, the different end-systolic pressure–volume points inscribe a line (or curve), for which the slope E_{max}, is a measure of contractility (Fig. 2). Although more complicated to obtain than other measures of systolic function, this approach, based on the work of Sagawa et al. (14,15), provides a measure of contractility that is relatively, but not entirely, independent of ventricular load. This approach was first applied to the left ventricle, and more recently, to the right ventricle (16). By using the end systolic pressure–volume point, MacNee et al. (17), and Burghuber and Bergmann (12) found that most stable adult patients with COPD have normal or supernormal right ventricular contractility, possibly from increased catecholamine stimulation. Similar data related to contractile function are not available for infants with BPD, but would be valuable. Thus, it is not known if decreases in RVEF in these infants result from diminished contractility or merely reflect changes in loading conditions.

Diastolic Function

To maintain stroke volume in the presence of diminished ejection fraction, right ventricular-filling volume must increase. In response to increased volume, end-

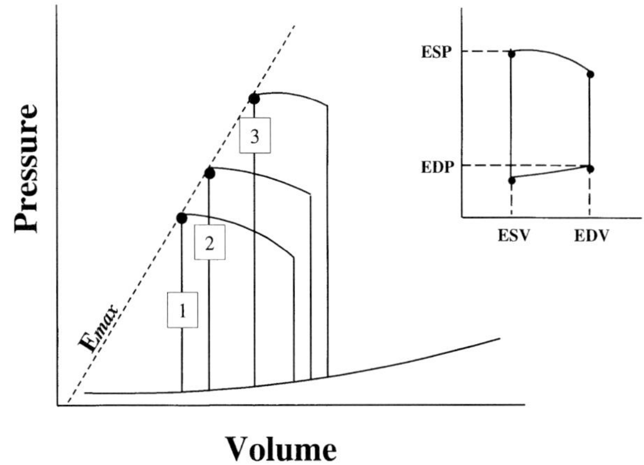

Figure 2 Relations between pressure and volume in a ventricle throughout the cardiac cycle as preload or afterload is varied (Inset) Changes from end-systolic (ESV) to end-diastolic (EDV) volume as ventricle fills during diastole along the curve that describes diastolic compliance; as the volume increases, the pressure also increases to end-diastolic pressure (EDP). During systole, pressure increases before ejection, and then volume decreases as the stroke volume (EDV − ESV) is ejected. At the end of systole, the ventricle attains the end-systolic pressure (ESP) just before relaxation. The figure demonstrates three pressure–volume curves, each with slightly different loading conditions. The end-systolic pressure–volume points lie on a single line with slope, E_{max}, or ventricular elastance, which represents a particular inotropic state. An increase in E_{max} is tantamount to an increase in inotropic function.

diastolic pressure, atrial pressure, and central venous pressure also will increase. Furthermore, the septum will become flattened, or can even become convex relative to the right ventricle. In this manner, a decrease in right ventricular compliance and an increase in filling pressure can change left ventricular filling characteristics and render it less compliant during diastole (Fig. 3; 18–25).

Increased filling pressure of the right ventricle, when transmitted to the systemic veins, can contribute to dysfunction of some organs. Protein-losing enteropathy has been well documented in patients with conditions that are associated with high systemic venous pressure, such as congestive heart failure and constrictive pericarditis (19,20). Protein-losing enteropathy was reported to occur in 7–10% of patients following an anastamosis between the vena cava and pulmonary artery (Fontan procedure; 21). Patients with severe chronic congestive heart failure commonly have elevation in bilirubin and hepatic enzymes, such as alanine aminotransferase (ALT) and aspartate aminotransferase (AST), but the relation of these abnormalities to right atrial pressure elevation or diminished cardiac

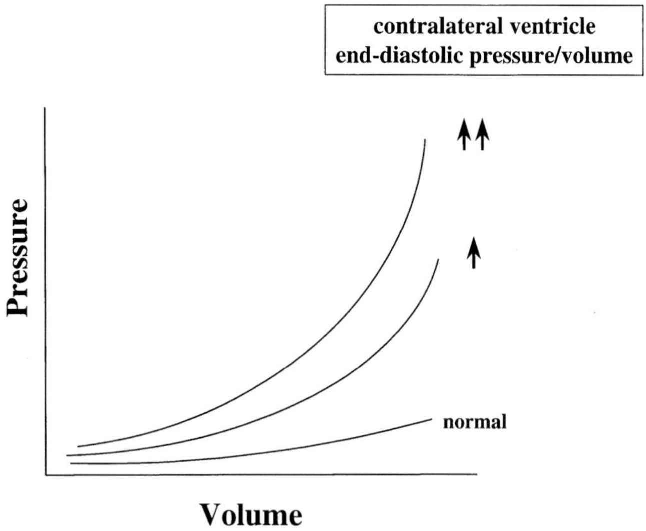

Figure 3 Effects on diastolic filling characteristics of a ventricle when end-diastolic pressure and volume of the contralateral ventricle are changed. A relatively compliant ventricle (normal curve) has relatively little increase in pressure as volume is increased. When the contralateral ventricle is filled, the compliance of a ventricle decreases, as shown by the upward or left shift in the pressure–volume relation. In this manner, elevated end-diastolic volume of the right ventricle can impede filling of the left ventricle, or conversely.

index is not strong. Data are not available on splanchnic function in children with BPD, but it is reasonable to presume that protein loss could contribute to the low serum protein concentration that often exists in infants with severe BPD.

If the right ventricle begins to fail, it may dilate and develop tricuspid regurgitation that aggravates systemic congestion and decreases right ventricular output. It may be difficult to distinguish these disturbances of organ function that are related to elevated venous pressure and reduced cardiac output from other common causes of organ dysfunction in an infant whose course has been complicated by premature birth and its aftermath.

Assessment of Function

The effects of BPD on the right ventricle can be evaluated by several noninvasive tests. The electrocardiogram of the premature infant often shows evidence of right ventricular hypertrophy early during the evolution of BPD. This is not a universal finding, however, and most infants with resolved BPD, and the majority of patients with persistent pulmonary disease, have normal electrocardiograms by 1 year after birth (26–29). Overall, right ventricular hypertrophy was noted in 35% of infants with well-established BPD and in only 16% of infants with either no lung disease or resolved BPD. Therefore, persistence of right ventricular hypertrophy should raise the possibility of persistent lung disease or the existence of undiagnosed cardiopulmonary abnormalities.

Cardiac ultrasonography has been an important tool, not only in the diagnosis of right ventricular hypertrophy, but also in the indirect assessment of pulmonary hypertension and in the diagnosis of associated cardiac anomalies in infants with BPD. Two-dimensional, M-mode, Doppler and color-Doppler echocardiography provide anatomical and functional diagnosis, and M-mode and Doppler studies can indirectly estimate the pulmonary artery pressures. The ratio of right ventricular preejection time to ejection time intervals (RVPET/RVET) has been used to assess the presence of pulmonary hypertension. The normal RVPET/RVET ratio in premature neonates older than 5 days is 0.28 ± 0.05 sec (30). A ratio higher than 0.3, measured by M-mode, has correlated well in some studies with the presence of pulmonary hypertension, severity of BPD, oxygen requirement, and decreased survival (30–34). Other investigators have not found right ventricular preejection and ejection intervals to be predictive of pulmonary artery pressure or pulmonary vascular resistance in patients with BPD who had cardiac catheterization, nor did these intervals change predictably when oxygen altered pulmonary hemodynamics (35).

In patients with tricuspid insufficiency, Doppler analysis of the regurgitant velocity can estimate the right ventricular systolic pressure by application of the Bernoulli equation (36). In most clinical circumstances the relation between right ventricular systolic pressure (P_{rv}), regurgitant velocity, and right ventricular end-diastolic pressure (estimated as central venous pressure; CVP) can be simplified as:

$$P_{rv}\text{, in mmHg} = 4 \times (\text{peak regurgitant velocity})^2 + \text{CVP, in mmHg}$$

The central venous pressure can be assumed normal at 2–4 mmHg, as it has little influence on the overall equation. The right ventricular systolic pressure is the same as the pulmonary artery pressure in the absence of obstruction to the outflow of the right ventricle. A similar analysis of a pulmonic insufficiency jet can be used to estimate the pulmonary artery diastolic pressure (P_{pad}):

$$P_{pad}\text{, in mmHg} = 4 \times (\text{peak regurgitant velocity})^2 + \text{CVP, in mmHg}$$

Although these estimates are useful, it is not uncommon to find difficulties in performing a good cardiac ultrasound examination in small infants with BPD, owing to limited transthoracic windows and lung hyperinflation.

An alternative imaging modality is radionuclide angiography, although it has not been used extensively in pediatric patients. This technique has been useful in the assessment of right ventricular size and function in adults and pediatric patients with chronic lung disease, and it also provides important information in the evaluation of immediate and long-term therapeutic interventions (37,38).

Lastly, cardiac catheterization should be reserved for those infants with suspected cardiac anomalies to further delineate the anatomy and hemodynamics and possibly to perform interventional procedure, such as closure of a patent ductus arteriosus (PDA).

Summary

Thus, it is likely, but not certain, that a stable infant with BPD will have relatively normal right ventricular contractile function in the presence of increased systolic and end-diastolic pressure. Until the right ventricle fails, the major consequences of the compensation for the high afterload and hypertrophy will be to cause systemic venous congestion or influence left ventricular function.

C. Effects on the Left Ventricle

Pathogenesis

Effects of BPD on the left ventricle can be subtler and less predictable than for the right ventricle. Several factors can alter left ventricular systolic and diastolic function, but the relative contribution of each factor is unknown, and the mechanisms for some of these abnormalities are uncertain, as they are in adult patients with COPD (22,23).

Diastolic Function

The cause for abnormal diastolic function can be attributed to at least two factors: changes in ventricular shape and changes in ventricular thickness. Leftward displacement of the interventricular septum decreases left ventricular compliance, which may induce even greater dysfunction of the right ventricle, as the left ventricular-filling pressure increases to preserve cardiac output. The high left ventricular-filling pressure causes left atrial and pulmonary venous hypertension which, in turn, will promote or aggravate pulmonary congestion, edema (24), increased airways resistance (25), impaired respiratory gas exchange, and pulmonary hypertension. A second cause of abnormal diastolic function is the left ventricular hypertrophy (39) (see following section), which is common in children with BPD.

Ventricular Hypertrophy

Left ventricular hypertrophy is often associated with right ventricular hypertrophy in infants with BPD (4,5), although the mechanism is not obvious. In a study by Stocker et al. (5), up to 70% of children who died with BPD had left ventricular hypertrophy. In adults with COPD, left ventricular hypertrophy and systolic dysfunction have been ascribed to an associated disease process, such as coronary artery disease or systemic hypertension (40–45). Because an association between left ventricular hypertrophy and late sudden death in infants with BPD has been suggested (46), it is worth considering some potential mechanisms of left ventricular hypertrophy in patients with BPD.

Anterior motion of the mitral valve during systole, which can partially obstruct left ventricular outflow, has been observed in some patients with BPD. In these patients, however, Doppler studies to detect mitral valve insufficiency or outflow obstruction were not performed (47). As the mitral valve moves anteriorly toward the ventricular septum in systole, mitral insufficiency can also develop which, in turn, elevates left atrial pressure and adversely affects patients with BPD and associated pulmonary hypertension. Left ventricular outflow obstruction and volume load from mitral regurgitation are independent stimuli for cardiac hypertrophy, and both should be considered when analyzing left ventricular function by echocardiography and Doppler measurements. The presence of systemic-to-pulmonary collateral circulation may contribute to the development of increased left ventricular hypertrophy by causing a volume overload in patients with BPD (48,49).

Systemic hypertension, which is a common finding in patients with BPD, may also contribute to the development of left ventricular hypertrophy. Trophic factors can promote left ventricular growth. Dexamethasone can induce a transient, but significant, increase in ventricular wall thickness, as well as a reduction in left ventricular end-diastolic dimension, without affecting the left ventricular ejection fraction (47). Although, it has been proposed that corticosteroids directly cause left ventricular hypertrophy in BPD (50), reports of left ventricular hypertrophy (4,51) preceded the widespread use of corticosteroids (52,53) for BPD.

Chronic adrenergic stimulation from ongoing stress and neurohumoral stimulation, exogenous administration of β-adrenergic agonists or phosphodiesterase inhibitors, and decreased lung clearance of norepinephrine, all have been implicated in the development of left heart hypertrophy in BPD (54,55). The mechanism responsible for the hypertrophy may relate to systolic hypertension from the catecholamine stimulation or from direct trophic effects of the catecholamines on the heart (56–58), similar to that which occurs with chronic administration of β-adrenergic agonists. The potential role of other growth factors, such as thyroid hormones and insulin in chronically ill infants, many of whom receive parenteral nutrition with high glucose concentration and insulin supplementation, has not been studied, but would be worth assessing. Experimental findings and specific clinical conditions, such as infants of diabetic mothers or nesidioblastosis, suggest that insulin per se may induce neonatal cardiac hypertrophy (59–62).

Systolic Function

Although many of the factors influencing diastolic function also might be expected to alter systolic function, there are very few data from which to derive conclusions about left ventricular contractile function in children with BPD. Leftward displacement of the ventricular septum, with associated diastolic dysfunction of the right ventricle, can also decrease left ventricular systolic function (63–66). Possible mechanisms for this impaired contractility include conformational changes in the ventricular chamber, causing outflow obstruction or impairment of coronary perfusion, hypoxemia, acidemia, changes in ventricular filling associated with negative pleural pressure, or ischemia.

Contractile function varies with left ventricular shape (67), and changes in shape can be readily produced by acute or chronic distension of the right ventricle (68,69). Distortion of the biconvex structure of the heart that contracts from apex to base can alter the ejection characteristics of the ventricle and give the appearance of decreased contractility. These effects have been demonstrated in dogs, in which progressive outflow obstruction of the right ventricle (raising end-diastolic pressure) caused a decrease in the ejection fraction of the left ventricle (18).

Studies with sheep have demonstrated that both hypoxemia and acidemia, especially in combination, can depress left ventricular contractile function (70–72), an effect that may be offset by a stress-related systemic catecholamine response. The independent effects of hypoxemia, hypercapnia, and acidemia on left ventricular function remain unclear in the absence of studies in which the response to a change of each variable is tested separately.

In patients with airflow obstruction caused by asthma, Permutt and others (73,74) have called attention to the marked increase in left ventricular afterload caused by the large decrease in pleural pressure at the end of inspiration (as low as $-30\ cmH_2O$). Given that the infant with BPD has both restrictive and obstructive lung disease, it is reasonable to assume that thc changes in pleural pressure might be as great as they are in asthmatic patients. Thus, the afterload imposed on the left ventricle could be substantial.

Whether there is any element of left ventricular ischemia that influences contractile function in BPD is uncertain. As discussed later, conditions associated with respiratory failure may lead to myocardial ischemia which, in turn, could worsen the balance between left ventricular demands and perfusion in BPD.

Summary

Thus, although there are limited studies to document the mechanisms for altering left ventricular function, it seems quite reasonable to assume that diastolic function is impaired by hypertrophy and distension of the right ventricle. Systolic function may be relatively well preserved except when pulmonary hypertension and right ventricular dilation are severe, or when there is a marked increase in afterload, possibly induced by a change in mechanical function of the respiratory system.

D. Systemic Hypertension

Systemic hypertension is another common cardiovascular complication of BPD. The reported incidence of hypertension varies between 13 and 43% in different studies of infants with BPD (6,7). These figures are clearly higher than those for the general neonatal population (0.7–3.0%) and higher than the one reported for neonatal intensive care graduates without BPD (1–9%; 75–78). In a retrospective study by Anderson et al. (7), the onset of hypertension occurred approximately 6 months after birth, with a range of 1–16 months. Systemic hypertension was associated with more severe lung disease and greater mortality rate than for infants without hypertension. Possible conditions that might contribute to the development of hypertension in these infants include thrombotic or embolic complications of umbilical artery catheterization; renal dysfunction and nephrocalcinosis; medications, such as theophylline, steroids, and furosemide; chronic volume depletion, with resultant release of renin and angiotensin; hypoxemia or hypercapnia during sleep; chronic adrenergic stimulation; and abnormal pulmonary catabolism of circulating norepinephrine. The etiology of systemic hypertension in BPD (6,7,54,55,78–81) remains unclear, however, and warrants further study to help provide some unifying theme for cardiovascular dysfunction.

E. Effects of Increased Metabolic Demands

Whereas many infants with BPD may have cardiovascular disturbances that are not apparent at rest, it is worth considering how stressful conditions that raise demands for blood flow may unmask dysfunction. The increase in metabolism that occurs with exercise serves as a useful paradigm for understanding the frequently appreciated signs of circulatory shock in marginally compensated infants with BPD when they become febrile or have other imposed metabolic stress.

The initial changes in the circulation when metabolism increases may be viewed by examining the relation between venous return and cardiac output as a function of atrial pressure during exercise (82; Fig. 4). In the healthy subject, sympathetic stimulation increases contractile function of the ventricle and causes arterioles and veins to constrict, except in working muscle. These circulatory responses cause a large increase in venous return and right ventricular output, with minimal change in right atrial pressure. The total increase in cardiac output is thereby nearly proportional to the increase in metabolic rate. The capacity of the pulmonary circulation to recruit nonperfused vessels, or further distend those vessels that are perfused, helps attenuate an exercise-related increase in pulmonary arterial pressure.

Infants with BPD, however, have a limited capacity to augment their car-

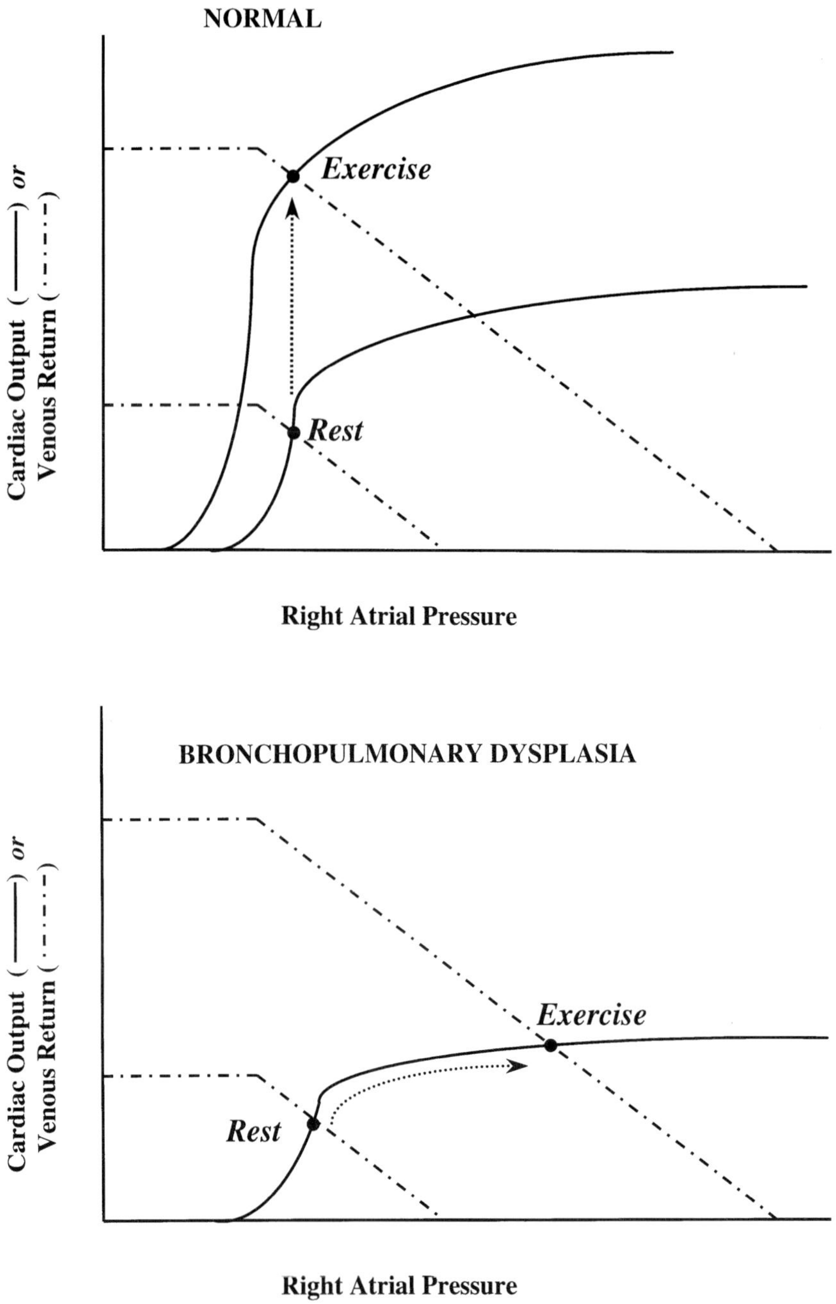
NORMAL
Exercise
Rest
Cardiac Output (———) or
Venous Return (· - · - · -)
Right Atrial Pressure
BRONCHOPULMONARY DYSPLASIA
Exercise
Rest
Cardiac Output (———) or
Venous Return (· - · - · -)
Right Atrial Pressure

diac output in response to an increase in metabolic demands. It is uncertain whether sympathetic stimulation in these infants leads to an increase in venous return. In some conditions that raise central venous pressure in infants, such as the Fontan procedure or positive end-expiratory pressure (PEEP), the ability to increase venous return is modest (83,84). If venous return does increase, an associated increase in right ventricular *afterload* and diminished ventricular *contractility* might limit the capacity of the right ventricle to pump more blood in response.

To consider afterload first, at least four factors can increase pulmonary vascular resistance or pressure. (1) As in the adult with COPD during exercise, increased pulmonary blood flow can lead to pulmonary hypertension because of limited pulmonary vascular recruitment or distension (85). (2) When metabolism increases, increased CO_2 production induces hyperpnea which, in turn, can worsen gas trapping, as it sometimes does in patients with COPD during exercise. Under these conditions, the increased alveolar pressure produced by trapped gas

---

Figure 4 Venous return and cardiac output curves in a normal subject and a subject with BPD at rest and during exercise: (Top) At *rest*, venous return (volume/time) from the periphery to the right atrium is shown; as right atrial pressure is altered. Venous return increases as right atrial pressure decreases until a plateau is reached, below which no further augmentation of venous return occurs because flow is no longer influenced by atrial pressure. Cardiac output from the ventricle increases at rest as right atrial pressure is increased, as described by the Starling relation. The intersection of the venous return and cardiac output curves, the equilibrium point, is the actual blood flow that is pumped by the right ventricle and right atrial pressure at this flow. During *exercise*, venous return increases owing to sympathetic constriction of vessels that diminishes capacitance and raises the driving pressure for blood flow from the periphery to the right atrium. Cardiac output increases because of the sympathetic stimulation that increases contractility and heart rate. The net result during exercise in the normal subject is a dramatic increase in right ventricular blood flow, with minimal increase in right atrial pressure. (Bottom) At *rest*, the output of the right ventricle is again determined by the intersection of the venous return and cardiac output curves in the patient with BPD. With *exercise*, or any stimulus that increases sympathetic drive, there is a decrease in venous capacitance; hence, there is a marked increase in venous return at any given right atrial pressure. We propose (see text), however, that unlike the normal subject, the cardiac function curve in the patient with BPD is very flat, with minimal increase in cardiac output as right atrial pressure rises. This occurs because of the increase in pulmonary artery pressure with any increase in blood flow (failure to recruit or dilate vessels), the hypoxemia and hypercarbia that depress contractile function, and possibly tricuspid regurgitation. The net result during stresses that increase metabolic demands may be a marked increase in right atrial pressure with little increase in cardiac output.

and lung overdistension increases pulmonary vascular resistance (86,87). (3) Polycythemia, resulting from prolonged hypoxemia in severe BPD, can also contribute to elevated pulmonary, as well as systemic, vascular resistance (88). (4) Pulmonary arterial hypoxemia also (see following discussion) can cause vasoconstriction in the lungs of infants BPD (89,90).

In addition to an increase in pulmonary arterial pressure, the potential for development of systemic hypoxemia, as demonstrated by the following argument, can worsen contractile function. Whenever metabolic demands and oxygen consumption increase, either cardiac output or arteriovenous oxygen content difference also must increase (91). If cardiac output does not increase in proportion to the increase in oxygen consumption, there must be an increase in peripheral oxygen extraction (i.e., widened arteriovenous oxygen content difference) and a decrease in mixed venous partial pressure of O_2. The resultant systemic venous desaturation will cause or exacerbate arterial hypoxemia (92) because the pulmonary venous blood from well-ventilated lung units will effectively be diluted with even more poorly oxygenated systemic venous blood. This will occur whether there is true intrapulmonary shunt or ventilation–perfusion (V/Q) mismatch producing arterial hypoxemia. In other words, for a given net intrapulmonary shunt fraction, any decrease in mixed systemic venous oxygen content or O_2 partial pressure will cause a decrease in arterial oxygen content or oxygen tension (93).

Hypoxemia can induce further systemic vasoconstrictive responses (94) and stimulate respiratory drive. The former will raise left ventricular afterload, and the latter will increase the high demands for blood flow to working respiratory muscle (92). It is also possible that a significantly elevated atrial pressure could reduce myocardial blood flow and, thereby, impair contractile function, because the right atrial pressure can be the relevant downstream pressure for coronary perfusion (95). This possibility has not been studied. Thus, the net response to increasing metabolic demands might be a minimal increase in cardiac output at an increased filling pressure (96), not a particularly productive response to stress.

The scenario just described may cause the infant with BPD to have hypoxemia, vasoconstriction, increased cardiac-filling pressures, and even worsening pulmonary edema, thereby yielding the appearance of circulatory shock in the presence of increased metabolic demands. In our experience, fever often abruptly produces these clinical signs, and the shock-like circulatory state is accentuated by the intense peripheral vasoconstriction that is essential for the increase in core temperature with a pyrogenic stimulus. These abnormal circulatory signs are often rapidly ameliorated by dissipation of the fever, even before the underlying problem is treated.

F. Myocardial Oxygen Supply and Demand

Although we know of no studies of myocardial oxygen supply and demand in BPD, the foregoing findings permit assessment of the important factors that

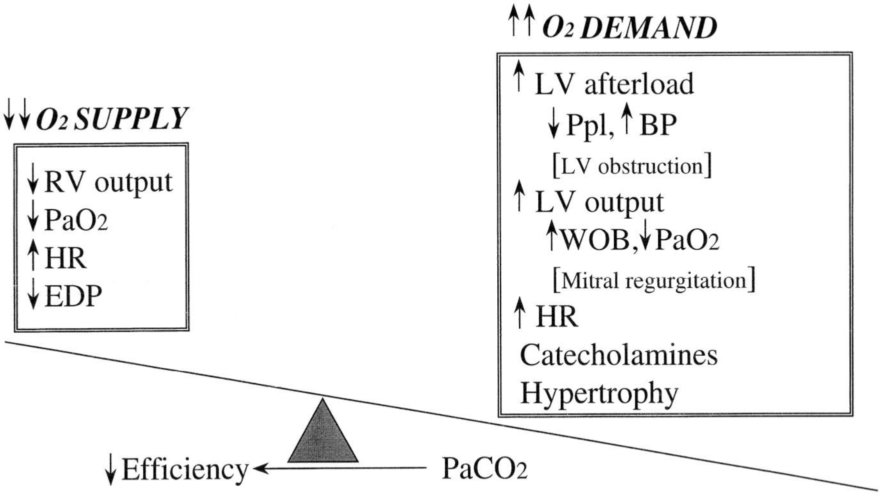

Figure 5 Myocardial oxygen supply and demand for the left ventricle in the presence of BPD: The figure identifies potential factors that can disrupt the balance between O_2 supply and demand in the left ventricle. Less important or less common factors are shown in [ ]. The factors that raise O_2 demands, as described in the text, include (1) increased left-ventricular (LV) afterload caused by decreased pleural pressure ($\downarrow P_{pl}$) and systemic hypertension ($\uparrow$ BP), and possibly LV outflow obstruction; (2) increased left ventricular output in response to the high work of breathing (WOB) and hypoxemia ($\downarrow$ Pao_2) and possibly from mitral regurgitation; (3) increased heart rate ($\uparrow$ HR); (4) increased catecholamines, which raise O_2 consumption related to external work and to excitation–contraction coupling; and (5) left ventricular hypertrophy. Factors that decrease O_2 supply include (1) decreased right ventricular (RV) output, (2) hypoxemia, (3) increased heart rate (shortening diastolic filling time), and (4) increased end-diastolic pressure ($\uparrow$ EDP). Finally, hypercapnic acidosis reduces efficiency and thereby, raises O_2 cost for any level of contractility.

would be expected to influence the relation between these two variables (Fig. 5). Myocardial oxygen demand will be increased by factors that increase left ventricular afterload and output. Decreased pleural pressure and systemic hypertension raise left ventricular afterload. To the extent that systolic anterior motion of the mitral valve obstructs left ventricular outflow, this too will increase left ventricular afterload. Increased work of breathing, hypoxemia, and catecholamine release raise the demands for systemic blood flow, as does mitral regurgitation, which raises both preload and afterload. Tachycardia and catecholamines raise demands for systemic flow and increase oxygen consumption related to both external work and excitation–contraction coupling. Finally, the increased muscle mass with left and right ventricular hypertrophy increases myocardial oxygen consumption.

Oxygen supply can be reduced by diminished right ventricular output which, in turn, will reduce left ventricular inflow, output, and coronary perfusion. An increase in end-diastolic pressure, could also limit coronary perfusion. Tachycardia, which shortens the fraction of time in diastole, and hypoxemia, which decreases the oxygen content of blood, will also decrease myocardial oxygen supply.

Finally, hypercapnic acidosis reduces efficiency of energy utilization and, thereby, raises the oxygen cost of myocardial contractility (97,98). It might be anticipated, therefore, that myocardial ischemia could be a consequence of BPD, although this important concern has yet to be studied. Moreover, we speculate that ischemia might contribute to what is often termed "BPD spells" in some of the less stable patients during episodes of respiratory distress that raise myocardial O_2 demand and limit supply.

III. Therapeutic Strategies

The cardiovascular pathology of chronic lung disease represents a formidable challenge to manage effectively. Therapeutic strategies, therefore, are often directed at minimizing the long-term cardiovascular consequences of lung disease, maximizing short-term cardiovascular performance, and counteracting the maladaptive consequences of homeostatic mechanisms that help preserve tissue perfusion at times of cardiocirculatory insufficiency. Because increased pulmonary vascular resistance is a dominant contributor to cardiocirculatory compromise in chronic lung disease, the administration of pulmonary vasodilators is the primary strategy aimed at optimizing hemodynamic function. In circulatory insufficiency, salt and water retention are typically induced as a homeostatic mechanism to improve effective tissue perfusion. When hypoxemia or hypercarbia activates these mechanisms in pulmonary disease, they can be maladaptive, leading to pulmonary and tissue edema. Thus, a second therapeutic strategy includes administration of diuretics.

Although these two general therapeutic strategies offer a wide range of pharmacological options, there is a remarkable paucity of data to support their application in the treatment of pediatric patients with chronic lung disease. Much of their consideration and application in such patients derives from experience in treating adult patients with chronic lung disease (primarily those with COPD).

Efficacy studies in adults and children are complicated by the lack of clear outcome-related experimental endpoints. Although short-term hemodynamic effects of therapy may be examined, there are no clear a priori relations between short-term hemodynamic responses and improvements in long-term mortality or morbidity. Investigation of efficacy in reducing morbidity and mortality for such a slowly progressing disease as cor pulmonale necessitates long prospective clinical studies. Studies in children with cardiac dysfunction as a consequence of

BPD are further complicated by the dynamic nature of the lung disease in this condition.

A. Pulmonary Vasodilation

The use of pulmonary vasodilation in cor pulmonale finds its theoretical underpinnings in the observation that patients with chronic lung disease who have elevated pulmonary arterial pressures have a higher mortality rate than patients with normal pulmonary hemodynamic variables (34,99,100). Furthermore, increased pulmonary vascular resistance can cause right ventricular dysfunction (11,101,102).

Assessing the effectiveness of various agents in causing vasodilation is complicated because it is often difficult to ascribe hemodynamic effects to specific reductions of pulmonary vascular tone (22,23). For example, pulmonary vascular resistance may decrease as a result of increases in cardiac output or increases in left atrial pressure, which may recruit or distend pulmonary blood vessels. This difficulty may be accentuated by the lack of specificity of most vasodilators for the pulmonary circulation. Hence, it may be difficult to attribute apparently beneficial effects on pulmonary vascular resistance to pulmonary vasodilation as opposed to systemic vasodilation or even noncardiovascular effects of these agents.

An additional difficulty with assessing efficacy arises because calculation of pulmonary vascular resistance requires invasive hemodynamic monitoring, so that such measurements are rarely made in young infants except in the cardiac catheterization laboratory. Noninvasive assessment of cardiovascular function by echocardiography, as in the measurement of the preejection period to ejection time, may unreliably estimate right ventricular afterload (103). Even estimates of pulmonary artery pressure from the velocity of retrograde flow across the pulmonic or tricuspid valve may be unreliable in assessing vascular tone because pulmonary arterial pressure may remain constant, even as pulmonary vascular resistance falls, provided there is an associated increase in cardiac output.

Finally, demonstration of beneficial short-term effects of vasodilators does not ensure sustained long-term hemodynamic responses or an improvement in morbidity or mortality. Moreover, lack of short-term effect does not preclude a potential beneficial long-term response. Despite these uncertainties, enthusiasm has persisted for the use of vasodilators because of apparent success in treating patients with primary pulmonary hypertension, as well as cor pulmonale, resulting from chronic obstructive pulmonary disease. With the exception of inhaled oxygen and nitric oxide, most vasodilating agents that have been studied are not selective for the pulmonary circulation.

Oxygen

Administration of oxygen in chronic lung disease is predicated on the assumption that chronic or intermittent hypoxemia is a significant contributor to pulmonary vasoconstriction and pulmonary vascular remodeling. Thus oxygen, perhaps more than other vasodilators, has the potential not only to reduce right ventricular afterload quickly, but also to arrest the progressive vasculopathy that results from chronic hypoxia.

Oxygen is a well-known pulmonary vasodilator. Maximal vasodilation occurs at a partial pressure of oxygen in the arterial blood (Pa_{O_2}) that is normally attained during air breathing. When Pa_{O_2} is less than normal, pulmonary vasoconstriction occurs (104–106). The ability to undergo hypoxic pulmonary vasoconstriction is a property of normal pulmonary arterial vascular smooth-muscle cells (107). Muscle contraction occurs because hypoxia suppresses the ionic current through voltage-activated potassium channels in the smooth-muscle cell that results in cell depolarization (108). Depolarization allows voltage-activated Ca^{2+} channels to open, thereby increasing the intracellular Ca^{2+} concentration and causing cell contraction (107,109). Pulmonary arterial smooth-muscle cells are influenced not only by the Pa_{O_2}, but also, and perhaps more importantly, by diffusion of gas from the alveolus to the precapillary arteries (110).

Initial Administration of Oxygen

The acute hemodynamic response to oxygen administration is variable in patients with BPD. Halliday et al. (32) measured by echocardiography, the ratio of RV preejection period to ejection time (RVPEP/RVET) in order to estimate RV afterload in ten preterm infants with BPD. These infants were all being treated with supplemental oxygen and were examined at a postconception age near term. In this group of infants, small decreases in inspired oxygen below that of the infants' typical O_2 environment (10% less than the prevailing F_{IO_2}) produced statistically significant increases in RVPEP/RVET. The RVPEP/RVET correlated with the Pa_{O_2}, suggesting that pulmonary vascular resistance was decreased in these subjects by raising the ambient F_{IO_2}.

Similar measurements were made by Berman and co-workers (35) in a group of older infants whose average age was 15 months, and who were treated with oxygen at home. Echocardiographic determinations of RVPEP/RVET were made in combination with invasive hemodynamic monitoring of pulmonary vascular resistance. These investigators failed to identify a significant effect of oxygen administration (F_{IO_2} 0.21, 0.40, and 0.88) on RVPEP/RVET, and they too found a poor correlation between changes in RVPEP/RVET and pulmonary vascular resistance. They did observe significant decreases in pulmonary vascular resistance in three of nine infants who were studied. The responders had higher baseline pulmonary vascular resistances and pulmonary arterial pressures, received more supplemental oxygen, and had lower Pa_{O_2} while breathing air.

A more uniform response to oxygen administration was observed by Abman and co-workers (111), who retrospectively reviewed cardiac catheterization data acquired in six patients with BPD who were studied while breathing room air or supplemental oxygen ($F_{IO_2} > 0.8$). These investigators found consistent decreases in mean pulmonary arterial pressure of at least 10 mmHg. These decreases correlated with increases in the arterial oxygen saturation. In three infants, oxygen was administered at different F_{IO_2} values, allowing mean pulmonary arterial pressure to be determined at three different arterial oxygen saturations. In these three infants, pulmonary arterial pressure decreased considerably when supplemental oxygen was administered to increase arterial oxygen saturation to 93%, but there was little or no change in vascular pressures when additional oxygen was given to raise the arterial oxygen saturation above 93%.

Differences in the responses to oxygen observed by different investigators may be related to differences among variables measured. It is perhaps even more likely that differences reflect differences in the patient populations who were studied. For example, it is possible that the responses observed in younger subjects by Halliday et al. (32) reflect the normally higher vascular responsiveness of younger subjects before physiological remodeling of the pulmonary circulation occurs. Alternatively, the lack of responsiveness in older subjects (35) may reflect progression of the pulmonary vascular disease to a stage at which irreversible vasculopathy has developed. Severity of disease also may influence the response to oxygen. The patients studied by Abman and co-workers (111) had higher mean pulmonary arterial pressures than those studied by Berman et al. (35), and patients in the latter study who did respond to oxygen were those patients with higher baseline pulmonary arterial pressures. It is important to consider other confounding variables that might cause some cohorts of patients to differ from others in their response to oxygen. For example, the patients included in the aforementioned studies (35,111) were all studied at altitudes well above sea level. Subjects reared at higher altitudes may have baseline muscular hypertrophy of pulmonary arteries (112) and an enhanced sensitivity to the pulmonary vascular effects of oxygen (113,114).

Long-Term Administration of Oxygen

There is little documentation to support the use of prolonged oxygen therapy in children with BPD. Nevertheless, enthusiasm derives from the belief that hypoxia contributes to pulmonary vascular remodeling and disease progression. The hope that long-term oxygen administration will be beneficial is reinforced by the finding that in adult patients with COPD, continuous oxygen therapy reduces mortality and progression of pulmonary hypertension.

Support for long-term oxygen administration is derived from two large randomized multicenter studies that have examined the beneficial effects of home oxygen therapy in adult patients with COPD (115–117). The British Medical Research Council randomized 87 patients to receive either oxygen therapy for at least 15 hr daily, or no oxygen therapy (116). Patients receiving oxygen therapy had significantly improved long-term survival, but had no significant improvement in either pulmonary arterial pressure or vascular resistance when compared with baseline values. Treated patients, however, had no significant increase in these variables over time. In contrast, patients who did not receive oxygen had progressive increases in pulmonary arterial pressure (~3 mmHg/year) and pulmonary vascular resistance (~100 dyne cm s^{-5}/year). This increase in right ventricular afterload was correlated with diminished survival.

A Nocturnal Oxygen Therapy Trial (NOTT) in North America compared the benefits of nocturnal oxygen administration with continuous oxygen administration (115). In this study, even though the mean daily duration of oxygen therapy differed by only 7 hr between groups, those patients who received continuous oxygen therapy had significantly better long-term survival (40.8 vs. 22.4% after 2 years). Cardiac catheterization during air breathing was performed before initiation of therapy and again after 6 months of oxygen therapy. Pulmonary arterial pressure and vascular resistance decreased significantly in those subjects who received continuous oxygen therapy at home, compared with patients who received only nocturnal oxygen therapy. The differences between treatment groups were even more apparent when the hemodynamic response to exercise was examined. Although both groups demonstrated expected decreases in pulmonary vascular resistance and increases in stroke volume index with exercise, these changes were considerably greater in those patients who received around-the-clock oxygen.

Thus, there is clear rationale for the administration of oxygen in the hypoxemic patient. The benefits of continuous oxygen delivery to infants with relatively normal arterial oxygen saturations is more difficult to determine, especially considering the toxicity of oxygen on the lungs. It is important to recognize, however, that a single estimate of arterial oxygen saturation at rest may be misleading, and it is likely that episodic decreases in arterial oxygen saturation contribute to the development of lung-related heart disease. Thus, the risk–benefit relation of continuous oxygen administration can be assessed only from carefully conducted, randomized clinical trials.

Nitric Oxide

Nitric oxide (NO) is an arterial vasodilator that is synthesized endogenously by vascular endothelium (118), as well as nonvascular cells (119). Although NO is a nonspecific vasodilator of systemic and pulmonary arterioles, its duration of biological activity is limited by rapid binding to hemoglobin. Because NO is a gas, it can be delivered preferentially to the lungs, where it can cause pulmonary vasodilation. The rapid binding to hemoglobin ensures that no biologically active NO passes from the pulmonary to the systemic circulation (120,121). This affords a high degree of specificity for the pulmonary circulation when NO is administered by inhalation (122).

The use of NO in hypoxic pulmonary hypertension is particularly interesting, for pulmonary vascular reactivity to changes in oxygen tension may be lost or attenuated in animals with hypoxia (123) and patients with COPD (124). Furthermore, inhaled NO reverses hypoxic pulmonary vasoconstriction in several species (122,125). When administered to adults with acute respiratory distress syndrome (ARDS), NO reversed the increase in pulmonary vascular resistance produced by hypercapnia (126). Pulmonary vascular resistance was also lowered in ten hypoxic children with ARDS (79).

Widespread enthusiasm for the use of inhaled NO in pulmonary vascular disease has been mitigated somewhat by the fact that NO cannot easily be administered continually or to ambulatory patients. Furthermore, long-term toxicity of NO therapy is unknown, and there is some concern that prolonged NO therapy could cause tissue injury by generation of reactive oxygen radicals and peroxynitrite (see Chap. 20). Short-term toxic effects of NO at doses that effectively decrease pulmonary vascular resistance appear to be minimal. Inhaled NO therapy has been used for more than 1 month in some patients without apparent side effects. Controlled trials are needed to study the effects of long-term NO inhalation on the outcome of patients with lung disease and associated pulmonary hypertension.

Administration of inhaled NO may also have a diagnostic role in evaluating the responsiveness of the pulmonary vasculature. By comparing the pulmonary vasomotor response to inhaled NO with the response to an endothelial-dependent vasodilator, such as acetylcholine, it may be possible to determine if the pulmonary arterioles have a capacity to dilate. This comparison may also help determine if the increased vascular tone in patients with pulmonary hypertension derives, at least in part, from endothelial cell dysfunction.

Prostacyclin

Besides producing and releasing NO, vascular endothelial cells also release prostacyclin, a vasodilator that derives from arachidonic acid. Similar to NO, prostacyclin has the capacity to dilate both pulmonary and systemic blood vessels, but is rapidly inactivated within the pulmonary circulation. Constitutive prostacyclin production may play a role in determining basal pulmonary vascular tone. In adult patients with either primary or secondary pulmonary hypertension, prostacyclin production is reduced, and the production of the vasoconstricting arachidonic acid metabolite thromboxane A_2 is increased (127); this imbalance does not exist in patients with chronic lung disease who do not have pulmonary hypertension.

The pulmonary vasodilatory effects of prostacyclin, combined with its rapid inactivation in the pulmonary circulation, led to the speculation that prostacyclin may act as a relatively specific pulmonary vasodilator when administered intravenously or by aerosol. In animal studies, prostacyclin decreases pulmonary vascular resistance when resistance has been increased by hypoxia (128,129) or by lung injury (130). Intravenous prostacyclin has been administered as a continuous infusion to adult patients with severe pulmonary hypertension. In these patients, prostacyclin decreased pulmonary vascular resistance and improved survival (131,132). One recent study suggests that long-term prostacyclin therapy results in a progressive decrease of pulmonary vascular resistance (133). Prostacyclin may also decrease pulmonary vascular resistance when administered as an aerosol in both adults (134) and children (135). To our knowledge, prostacyclin has not been widely used in infants with BPD, but its relatively selectivity for the pulmonary vascular bed and its potential for prolonged administration provide sufficient rationale to warrant further investigation.

Calcium Channel Blockers

The rationale for using Ca^{2+} channel blockers to treat hypoxia-related pulmonary hypertension derives from the pivotal role of Ca^{2+} influx through voltage-activated Ca^{2+} channels in regulating the tone of vascular smooth-muscle cells. Moreover, Ca^{2+} entry through voltage-activated channels is a key element in the development of hypoxic pulmonary vasoconstriction. Both verapamil and nifedipine blunt the pulmonary vasoconstriction that occurs in animals when they breathe a hypoxic gas mixture (136–139). This ability to blunt hypoxic pulmonary vasoconstriction is a direct effect on pulmonary blood vessels, for effects are observed in denervated, isolated, perfused lungs (136,139). In one model of chronic intermittent hypoxia, both verapamil and nifedipine inhibited the increase in pulmonary vascular resistance, the magnitude of right ventricular hypertrophy, and the hypertrophy of the pulmonary arterial smooth muscle, compared with hypoxic untreated controls (137).

Brief administration of nifedipine to patients with COPD decreases pulmonary vascular resistance without significant changes in pulmonary arterial pressure (140–143). Pulmonary arterial pressures remained elevated because nifedipine mediated decreases in systemic vascular resistance (independent of direct effects on pulmonary vascular resistance) and led to increases in cardiac output. In one of these studies (143), resting hemodynamic measurements were made before and after administration of a single dose of nifedipine and again after 2 months of repeated nifedipine therapy. Long-term therapy was associated with a slight decrease in resting pulmonary vascular resistance, but it was unclear from this report if the outcome reflected a difference in the state of the pulmonary vasculature or an effect of residual nifedipine. The immediate response to nifedipine administration was not predictive of the hemodynamic changes observed after long-term therapy. Long-term therapy was not associated with tachyphylaxis to nifedipine administration (143,144).

The acute hemodynamic effects of nifedipine have also been observed in children with BPD and pulmonary hypertension. Brownlee and co-workers (145) found that 0.5 mg/kg nifedipine, delivered enterally, decreased pulmonary arterial pressures and pulmonary vascular resistance. Cardiac output increased. In this study, nifedipine produced a greater reduction in pulmonary vascular resistance than did administration of 95% oxygen, and cardiac output increased only with nifedipine therapy. However, systemic oxygen transport increased equally with both therapies. Long-term studies of nifedipine administration to children with chronic lung disease are lacking.

Although other Ca^{2+} channel blockers blunt hypoxic pulmonary vasoconstriction in animals, no beneficial effects of diltiazem (146) or verapamil (147) were observed during investigations on subjects with COPD. Lack of effect of these agents may have resulted from inadequate dosing, a difference in the relative effects on pulmonary versus systemic blood vessels, or a greater negative inotropic effect compared with nifedipine.

B. Inotropic Agents

The finding that some patients with hypoxic pulmonary vascular disease have edema, right ventricular dilation, and decreased right ventricular ejection fraction suggests that inotropic agents that augment cardiac contraction in congestive heart failure also might have beneficial effects in these patients. The impetus for such therapy, however, is weakened when one considers that, despite these findings, the contractile function of the right ventricle appears to be well preserved in hypoxic pulmonary vascular disease. For example, the slope of the line relating right ventricular end-systolic pressure to end-systolic volume, often taken as an index of contractility, may be preserved in patients with COPD despite decreases in RV ejection fraction (102). In chronic lung disease, ejection fraction may decrease as a result of increased RV afterload, rather than decreased contractility per se.

Although it is possible that increasing the contractility of the heart to supranormal levels would increase ejection fraction, stroke volume, and cardiac output, there is concern that these increases will result in an increase in pulmonary artery pressure unless pulmonary vascular resistance is decreased simultaneously. Moreover, this increase in RV afterload will increase myocardial oxygen consumption, compounding the increase that results from the inotropic effects alone. This may be undesirable if hypoxia contributes directly to myocardial dysfunction. Thus, the potential benefit of inotropic agents may be self-limiting or even counterproductive in conditions associated with pulmonary hypertension.

There is little evidence to support the routine use of inotropic agents in heart disease associated with BPD or even in pulmonary heart disease in general. Historically, digoxin was often used to treat adult patients with pulmonary heart disease because of the similarity in symptoms between that syndrome and congestive heart failure (148). Two randomized, controlled studies in adult patients with COPD and right heart failure failed to demonstrate consistent benefit during digoxin therapy (149,150). In one of these studies (149), RV ejection fraction increased in some patients during digoxin therapy, but only in those patients who had reduced left ventricular ejection fractions, which digoxin corrected in these patients. Neither exercise performance nor general health improved in these patients (149). A study by Polic et al. (150) demonstrated some benefit of digoxin in patients with atrial fibrillation. Because atrial fibrillation is a common finding in adults with pulmonary heart disease, this suggests that some of the apparent benefit in patients with COPD may be related to the antiarrhythmic effects of digoxin.

The routine use of digoxin is made less appealing when one considers the low therapeutic index of this drug. Toxicity may be further compounded by the electrolyte disturbances that often exist in patients who are treated with diuretics for chronic lung disease. It is unclear which patients, if any, may benefit from digoxin therapy. The use of other inotropes is complicated by the need for parenteral delivery. Their use is often considered during acute exacerbations of lung disease that are complicated by diminished cardiac output. These agents may be most effective when left ventricular function is compromised.

C. Diuretic Therapy

Sodium and water retention may occur in pulmonary heart disease as a result of homeostatic mechanisms that serve to preserve cardiac output in the face of impaired ventricular function. These homeostatic mechanisms include release of renin, aldosterone, and vasopressin. Sodium and water retention may occur, however, as a result of gas-exchange abnormalities in chronic lung disease, even when cardiac function is normal. For example, hypoxia increases plasma renin activity in rats (151–153), dogs (154–156), and lambs (157). This effect of hypoxia appears to be magnified by simultaneous hypercapnia (151,154,156).

Manfredi and co-workers extended these observations in patients with COPD. In a series of studies, these investigators demonstrated elevated plasma renin activity in hypoxic nonedematous patients with COPD (158). Renin levels were particularly elevated in those patients with hypercapnia. Patients with carbon dioxide retention also had a decreased ability to excrete water and sodium loads (159–161). These investigators observed that impaired water excretion correlated closely with impaired salt excretion and suggested that an inability to excrete sodium was the primary excretory disturbance in hypercapnia. The mechanism of this disturbance remains unclear, but may be related to the increased net proximal tubular reabsorption of bicarbonate that is associated with hypercapnia, as originally suggested by Campbell and Short (162). Sodium would follow bicarbonate to maintain electroneutrality. This proximal reabsorption of sodium and bicarbonate could be accentuated further by the diminished renal plasma flow that occurs in patients with either hypercapnia (158) or diminished cardiac output.

Regardless of whether fluid retention occurs as a consequence of inadequate cardiocirculatory function or renal impairment secondary to blood gas abnormalities, diuretics may be useful in halting the cycle by which pulmonary dysfunction induces water retention that leads to pulmonary edema, further aggravating lung dysfunction. Therefore, many studies have focused on effects of diuretics on pulmonary function. Interpretation of these studies, however, is complicated somewhat by nonrenal effects of some of the diuretics studied.

Furosemide, a loop diuretic, caused decreases in pulmonary transvascular fluid filtration rate (163,164) and lung water (165) in experimental models of low-pressure pulmonary edema. These effects were observed in nephrectomized animals and so do not depend solely on enhanced salt and water excretion. Furosemide also decreases intrapulmonary shunting in anephric animals (165) and humans (166) with low-pressure pulmonary edema.

Furosemide improves pulmonary function in oxygen-dependent infants with chronic lung disease. In a placebo-controlled, double-blinded trial, McCann et al. (167) demonstrated improvements in pulmonary dynamic compliance after 1 week of twice-daily furosemide therapy. In another study of hypercapnic infants with BPD, Engelhardt et al. (168) demonstrated improvements in lung compliance, total pulmonary resistance, and arterial P_{CO_2} after a single dose of furosemide. Compared with a similar control period, these variables continued to improve during a 1-week therapeutic trial, except for the decrease in P_{CO_2}, which was not sustained. Similar beneficial effects were noted in a placebo-controlled trial of alternate-day furosemide (169). It is not known to what extent these beneficial effects of furosemide are related to decreases in interstitial water observed in infants with BPD (170) or to extrarenal effects of the diuretic. It is interesting, however, that lung compliance may increase, even when furosemide is delivered directly to the lungs by nebulization, even though no diuretic effect is observed with this route of administration (171).

Inasmuch as furosemide may improve pulmonary function by mechanisms other than diuresis and natriuresis, it is unclear whether other classes of diuretics will have similar benefit in infants with chronic lung disease. The combination of a thiazide diuretic and the aldosterone inhibitor spironolactone, for example, may produce a diuresis equivalent to that typically achieved with continued furosemide therapy. The beneficial effect of this diuretic combination on pulmonary mechanical function, however, has not been consistently demonstrated. Of three randomized, placebo-controlled studies examining the effects of long-term hydrochlorothiazide–spironolactone diuresis, two (172,173) demonstrated increases in total pulmonary compliance in the subjects who received diuretics. Both of these study protocols allowed furosemide to be administered at the discretion of the treating physician. The study by Albersheim and co-workers (172) also demonstrated an increased proportion of diuretic-treated subjects surviving to discharge, in comparison with the placebo-matched control subjects. Another study, however, failed to demonstrate any improvement in lung mechanics or oxygenation in subjects treated with the thiazide–spironolactone combination, despite significant increases in urine output (174).

IV. Summary

In this chapter our intent was to provide a framework for understanding the pathogenesis of cardiovascular abnormalities associated with BPD. Many of the findings follow logically from the response to the elevated pulmonary artery pressure at rest, or the presumed increase in pulmonary artery pressure during conditions that increase cardiac output. However, there remain important areas for study. Some issues relate to unresolved mechanisms and others to unproved therapy. It is clear that much of the focus of research should be directed at minimizing injury to the lungs and promoting their healthy postnatal growth. However, we believe that studies elucidating the mechanism(s) for left ventricular hypertrophy and systemic hypertension would be quite valuable, because these factors could contribute substantially to circulatory disturbances, even when pulmonary hypertension is not severe. The role of myocardial ischemia is uncertain, and it is plausible that this contributes to the apparent instability during episodes of increased respiratory distress. At the very least, conventional evaluation for ischemia, such as measurement of myocardial enzymes and assessment of ECG, would be useful. Estimates of the balance between myocardial oxygen supply and demand could also be obtained from measurement of arterial oxygen content and systemic and central venous pressure (95). There are currently few approaches to detect the near-failing right ventricle before cardiovascular collapse. In an era when heart and lung transplant might be considered (175), it would be essential to have better methods to predict ultimate failure of the right ventricle in infants and small children, and examination of function during changes in loading conditions would be quite useful. This might be accomplished in the ventilated patient by simply changing phase of respiration or transiently altering mean airway pressure to alter preload and afterload. Finally, although oxygen and other therapies have been used for short-term pulmonary vasodilation, it is unclear whether long-term use offers any benefit for survival or reduced morbidity. In a manner analogous to the nocturnal oxygen trials in adults with COPD, we think formal study, rather than anecdotal evidence or inference, should address these issues in therapy.

References

1. Report of an Expert Committee. Chronic cor pulmonale. Med Clin North Am 1963; 27:594–615.

2. Bishop JM. Cardiovascular complications of chronic bronchitis and emphysema. Med Clin North Am 1973; 57:771–780.
3. Fishman AP. State of the art: chronic cor pulmonale. Am Rev Respir Dis 1976; 114:775–794.
4. Malnick G, Pickoff AS, Ferrer PL, Peyser J, Bancalari E, Gelband H. Normal pulmonary vascular resistance and left ventricular hypertrophy in young infants with bronchopulmonary dysplasia: an echocardiographic and pathologic study. Pediatrics 1980; 66:589–596.
5. Stocker JT. Pathologic features of long-standing ''healed'' bronchopulmonary dysplasia: a study of 28 3- to 40-month-old infants. Hum Pathol 1986; 17:943–961.
6. Abman SH, Warady BA, Lum GM, Koops BL. Systemic hypertension in infants with bronchopulmonary dysplasia. J Pediatr 1984; 104:928–931.
7. Anderson AH, Warady BA, Daily DK, Johnson JA, Thomas MK. Systemic hypertension in infants with severe bronchopulmonary dysplasia: associated clinical factors. Am J Perinatol 1993; 10:190–193.
8. Reid LM. The pulmonary circulation: remodeling in growth and disease. Am Rev Respir Dis 1979; 119:531–546.
9. Vlahakes GJ, Turley K, Hoffman JI. The pathophysiology of failure in acute right ventricular hypertension: hemodynamic and biochemical correlations. Circulation 1981; 63:87–95.
10. Grossman W, Jones D, McLaurin LP. Wall stress and patterns of hypertrophy in the human left ventricle. J Clin Invest 1975; 56:56–64.
11. Brent BN, Berger HJ, Matthay RA, Mahler D, Pytlik L, Zaret BL. Physiologic correlates of right ventricular ejection fraction in chronic obstructive pulmonary disease; a combined radionuclide and hemodynamic study. Am J Cardiol 1982; 50: 255–262.
12. Burghuber OC, Bergmann H. Right-ventricular contractility in chronic obstructive pulmonary disease: a combined radionuclide and hemodynamic study. Respiration 1988; 53:1–12.
13. Praud JP, Cavailloles F, Boulhadour K, DeRecondo M, Guilleminault C, Gaultier C. Radionuclide evaluation of cardiac function during sleep in children with bronchopulmonary dysplasia. Chest 1991; 100:721–725.
14. Sagawa K. The end-systolic pressure–volume relation of the ventricle: definition, modifications and clinical use. Circulation 1981; 63:1223–1227.
15. Sagawa K, Suga H, Shoukas AA, Bakalar KM. End-systolic pressure/volume ratio: a new index of ventricular contractility. Am J Cardiol 1977; 40:748–753.
16. Maughan WL, Shoukas AA, Sagawa K, Weisfeldt ML. Instantaneous pressure–volume relationship of the canine right ventricle. Circ Res 1979; 44:309–315.
17. MacNee W, Hannan WJ, Flenley DC, Adie CJ, Muir AL. Assessment by radionuclide angiography of right and left ventricular function in chronic bronchitis and emphysema. Thorax 1983; 38:494–500.
18. Stool EW, Mullins CB, Leshin SJ, Mitchell JH. Dimensional changes of the left ventricle during acute pulmonary arterial hypertension in dogs. Am J Cardiol 1974; 33:868–875.
19. Davidson J, Goodman D, Waldmann T, Gordon R. Protein-losing enteropathy in congestive heart failure. Lancet 1961; 1:899–902.

20. Nelson DL, Blaese RM, Strober W, Bruce R, Waldmann TA. Constrictive pericarditis, intestinal lymphangiectasia, and reversible immunologic deficiency. J Pediatr 1975; 86:548–554.
21. Driscoll DJ, Offord KP, Feldt RH, Schaff HV, Puga FJ, Danielson GK. Five- to fifteen-year follow-up after Fontan operation. Circulation 1992; 85:469–496.
22. MacNee W. Pathophysiology of cor pulmonale in chronic obstructive pulmonary disease. Part II. Am J Respir Crit Care Med 1994; 150:1158–1168.
23. MacNee W. Pathophysiology of cor pulmonale in chronic obstructive pulmonary disease. Part I. Am J Respir Crit Care Med 1994; 150:833–852.
24. Staub NC. ''State of the art'' review. Pathogenesis of pulmonary edema. Am Rev Respir Dis 1974; 109:358–372.
25. Milic-Emili J, Ruff F. Effects of pulmonary congestion and edema on the small airways. Bull Physiopathol Respir 1971; 7:1181–1196.
26. Northway WJ, Rosan R. Radiographic features of pulmonary oxygen toxicity in the newborn: bronchopulmonary dysplasia. Radiology 1968; 91:49–58.
27. Northway WH Jr. Observations on bronchopulmonary dysplasia. J Pediatr 1979; 95:815–818.
28. Abman SH, Accurso FJ, Bowman CM. Unsuspected cardiopulmonary abnormalities complicating bronchopulmonary dysplasia. Arch Dis Child 1984; 59:966–970.
29. Walsh EP, Lang P, Ellison RC, Zierler S, Harned HS, Miettinen OS. Electrocardiogram of the premature infant at 1 year of age. Pediatrics 1986; 77:353–356.
30. Halliday H, Hirschfeld S, Riggs T, Liebman J, Fanaroff A, Bormuth C. Respiratory distress syndrome: echocardiographic assessment of cardiovascular function and pulmonary vascular resistance. Pediatrics 1977; 60:444–449.
31. Halliday H, Hirschfeld S, Riggs T, Liebman J, Fanaroff A. Echographic ventricular systolic time intervals in normal term and preterm neonates. Pediatrics 1978; 62: 317–321.
32. Halliday HL, Dumpit FM, Brady JP. Effects of inspired oxygen on echocardiographic assessment of pulmonary vascular resistance and myocardial contractility in bronchopulmonary dysplasia. Pediatrics 1980; 65:536–540.
33. Riggs T, Hirschfeld S, Borkat G, Knoke J, Liebman J. Assessment of the pulmonary vascular bed by echocardiographic right ventricular systolic time intervals. Circulation 1978; 57:939–947.
34. Fouron JC, Le Guennec JC, Villemant D, Perreault G, Davignon A. Value of echocardiography in assessing the outcome of bronchopulmonary dysplasia of the newborn. Pediatrics 1980; 65:529–535.
35. Berman W Jr, Yabek SM, Dillon T, Burstein R, Corlew S. Evaluation of infants with bronchopulmonary dysplasia using cardiac catheterization. Pediatrics 1982; 70:708–712.
36. Yock PG, Popp RL. Noninvasive estimation of right ventricular systolic pressure by Doppler ultrasound in patients with tricuspid regurgitation. Circulation 1984; 70:657–662.
37. Matthay RA, Berger HJ. Noninvasive assessment of right and left ventricular function in acute and chronic respiratory failure. Crit Care Med 1983; 11:329–338.
38. Alpert BE, Gainey MA, Schidlow DV, Capitanio MA. Effect of oxygen on right

ventricular performance evaluated by radionuclide angiography in two young patients with chronic lung disease. Pediatr Pulmonol 1987; 3:149–152.
39. Glantz SA, Parmley WW. Factors which affect the diastolic pressure–volume curve. Circ Res 1978; 42:171–180.
40. Williams JF Jr, Childress RH, Boyd DL, Higgs LM, Behnke RH. Left ventricular function in patients with chronic obstructive pulmonary disease. J Clin Invest 1968; 47:1143–1153.
41. Davies H, Overy HR. Left ventricular function in cor pulmonale. Chest 1970; 58: 8–14.
42. Fishman AP. The left ventricle in ''chronic bronchitis and emphysema.'' N Engl J Med 1971; 285:402–404.
43. Frank MJ, Weisse AB, Moschos CB, Levinson GE. Left ventricular function, metabolism, and blood flow in chronic cor pulmonale. Circulation 1973; 47:798–806.
44. Murphy ML, Adamson J, Hutcheson F. Left ventricular hypertrophy in patients with chronic bronchitis and emphysema. Ann Intern Med 1974; 81:307–313.
45. Steele P, Ellis JH, Van Dyke D, Sutton F, Creagh E, Davies H. Left ventricular ejection fraction in severe chronic obstructive airways disease. Am J Med 1975; 59:21–28.
46. Abman SH, Burchell MF, Schaffer MS, Rosenberg AA. Late sudden unexpected deaths in hospitalized infants with bronchopulmonary dysplasia. Am J Dis Child 1989; 143:815–819.
47. Werner JC, Sicard RE, Hansen TW, Solomon E, Cowett RM, Oh W. Hypertrophic cardiomyopathy associated with dexamethasone therapy for bronchopulmonary dysplasia. J Pediatr 1992; 120:286–291.
48. Ascher DP, Rosen P, Null DM, de Lemos RA, Wheller JJ. Systemic to pulmonary collaterals mimicking patent ductus arteriosus in neonates with prolonged ventilatory courses. J Pediatr 1985; 107:282–284.
49. Goodman G, Perkin RM, Anas NG, Sperling DR, Hicks DA, Rowen M. Pulmonary hypertension in infants with bronchopulmonary dysplasia. J Pediatr 1988; 112:67–72.
50. Brem AS, Bina RB, Klinger JR, King T, Werner JC. Glucocorticoid metabolism in the newborn rat heart. Proc Soc Exp Biol Med 1995; 209:146–151.
51. deSa DJ. Myocardial changes in immature infants requiring prolonged ventilation. Arch Dis Child 1977; 52:138–147.
52. Mammel MC, Green TP, Johnson DE, Thompson TR. Controlled trial of dexamethasone therapy in infants with bronchopulmonary dysplasia. Lancet 1983; 1:1356–1358.
53. Avery GB, Fletcher AB, Kaplan M, Brudno DS. Controlled trial of dexamethasone in respirator-dependent infants with bronchopulmonary dysplasia. Pediatrics 1985; 75:106–111.
54. Abman S, Schaffer M, Wiggins J, Washington R, Manco-Johnson M, Wolfe R. Pulmonary vascular extraction of circulating norepinephrine in infants with bronchopulmonary dysplasia. Pediatr Pulmonol 1987; 3:386–391.
55. Abman SH, Groothius JR. Pathophysiology and treatment of bronchopulmonary dysplasia. Current issues. Pediatr Clin North Am 1994; 41:277–315.
56. Simpson P, McGrath A, Savion S. Myocyte hypertrophy in neonatal rat heart cul-

tures and its regulation by serum and by catecholamines. Circ Res 1982; 51:787–801.

57. Simpson P, Bishopric N, Coughlin S, et al. Dual trophic effects of the alpha 1-adrenergic receptor in cultured neonatal rat heart muscle cells. J Mol Cell Cardiol 1986; 18:45–58.
58. Sheer D, Morkin E. Myosin isoenzyme expression in rat ventricle: effects of thyroid hormone analogs, catecholamines, glucocorticoids and high carbohydrate diet. J Pharmacol Exp Ther 1984; 229:872–879.
59. Stimmler L, Brazie J, O'Brien D. Plasma-insulin levels in the newborn infants of normal and diabetic mothers. Lancet 1964; 1:137–138.
60. Naeye RL. Infants of diabetic mothers: a quantitative morphologic study. Pediatrics 1965; 35:980–988.
61. Wolfe RR, Way GL. Cardiomyopathies in infants of diabetic mothers. Johns Hopkins Med J 1977; 140:177–180.
62. Gutgesell HP, Speer ME, Rosenberg HS. Characterization of the cardiomyopathy in infants of diabetic mothers. Circulation 1980; 61:441–450.
63. Elzinga G, Grondelle RV, Westerhof N, Bos GCVD. Ventricular interference. Am J Physiol 1974; 226:941–947.
64. Laver MB, Strauss HW, Pohost GM. Herbert Shubin Memorial Lecture. Right and left ventricular geometry: adjustments during acute respiratory failure. Crit Care Med 1979; 7:509–519.
65. Brinker JA, Weiss JL, Lappe DL, et al. Leftward septal displacement during right ventricular loading in man. Circulation 1980; 61:626–633.
66. Sibbald WJ, Driedger AA. Right ventricular function in acute disease states: pathophysiologic considerations. Crit Care Med 1983; 11:339–345.
67. Tischler MD, Niggel J, Borowski DT, LeWinter MM. Relation between left ventricular shape and exercise capacity in patients with left ventricular dysfunction. J Am Coll Cardiol 1993; 22:751–757.
68. Taylor RR, Covell JW, Sonnenblick EH, Ross J Jr. Dependence of ventricular distensibility on filling of the opposite ventricle. Am J Physiol 1967; 213:711–718.
69. Kelly DT, Spotnitz HM, Beiser GD, Pierce JE, Epstein SE. Effects of chronic right ventricular volume and pressure loading on left ventricular performance. Circulation 1971; 44:403–412.
70. Downing SE, Talner NS, Gardner TH. Influences of hypoxemia and acidemia on left ventricular function. Am J Physiol 1966; 210:1327–1334.
71. Fisher DJ. Comparative effects of metabolic acidemia and hypoxemia on cardiac output and regional blood flows in unanesthetized newborn lambs. Pediatr Res 1986; 20:756–760.
72. Fisher DJ. Acidaemia reduces cardiac output and left ventricular contractility in conscious lambs. J Dev Physiol 1986; 8:23–31.
73. Permutt S. Relation between pulmonary arterial pressure and pleural pressure during the acute asthmatic attack. Chest 1973; 63 (suppl):25S–28S.
74. Buda AJ, Pinsky MR, Ingels NB Jr, Daughters GTD, Stinson EB, Alderman EL. Effect of intrathoracic pressure on left ventricular performance. N Engl J Med 1979; 301:453–459.

75. Sheftel DN, Hustead V, Friedman A. Hypertension screening in the follow-up of premature infants. Pediatrics 1983; 71:763–766.
76. Friedman AL, Hustead VA. Hypertension in babies following discharge from a neonatal intensive care unit. A 3-year follow-up. Pediatr Nephrol 1987; 1:30–34.
77. Adelman RD. The hypertensive neonate. Clin Perinatol 1988; 15:567–585.
78. Johnson V. Systemic hypertension in infants with severe bronchopulmonary dysplasia. Am J Perinatol 1993; 10:260–261.
79. Abman SH, Griebel JL, Parker DK, Schmidt JM, Swanton D, Kinsella JP. Acute effects of inhaled nitric oxide in children with severe hypoxemic respiratory failure. J Pediatr 1994; 124:881–888.
80. Ng PC. The effectiveness and side effects of dexamethasone in preterm infants with bronchopulmonary dysplasia. Arch Dis Child 1993; 68:330–336.
81. Ezzedeen F, Adelman RD, Ahlfors CE. Renal calcification in preterm infants: pathophysiology and long-term sequelae. J Pediatr 1988; 113:532–539.
82. Guyton AC. Textbook of Medical Physiology. Philadelphia: WB Saunders, 1991: 1014.
83. Kelley JR, Mack GW, Fahey JT. Diminished venous vascular capacitance in patients with univentricular hearts after the Fontan operation. Am J Cardiol 1995; 76: 158–163.
84. Peters JK, Lister G, Nadel ER, Mack GW. Venous and arterial reflex responses to positive-pressure breathing and lower body negative pressure. J Appl Physiol 1997; 82:1889–1896.
85. Matthay RA, Niederman MS, Wiedemann HP. Cardiovascular–pulmonary interaction in chronic obstructive pulmonary disease with special reference to the pathogenesis and management of cor pulmonale. Med Clin North Am 1990; 74:571–618.
86. Wright JL, Lawson L, Pare PD, et al. The structure and function of the pulmonary vasculature in mild chronic obstructive pulmonary disease. The effect of oxygen and exercise. Am Rev Respir Dis 1983; 128:702–707.
87. Harris P, Segel N, Green I, Housley E. The influence of the airways resistance and alveolar pressure on the pulmonary vascular resistance in chronic bronchitis. Cardiovasc Res 1968; 2:84–92.
88. Lister G, Hellenbrand WE, Kleinman CS, Talner NS. Physiologic effects of increasing hemoglobin concentration in left-to-right shunting in infants with ventricular septal defects. N Engl J Med 1982; 306:502–506.
89. Bergofsky EH, Lehr DE, Fishman AP. Effect of changes in the hydrogen ion concentration on the pulmonary circulation. J Clin Invest 1962; 41:1492–1501.
90. Dawson CA. Role of pulmonary vasomotion in physiology of the lung. Physiol Rev 1984; 64:544–616.
91. Wasserman K, Whipp BJ. Exercise physiology in health and disease. Am Rev Respir Dis 1975; 112:219–249.
92. MacNee W, Morgan AD, Wathen CG, Muir AL, Flenley DC. Right ventricular performance during exercise in chronic obstructive pulmonary disease. The effects of oxygen. Respiration 1985; 48:206–215.
93. Lister G. Oxygen transport and consumption. In: Gluckman PD, Heymann MA, eds. Pediatrics and Perinatology. London: Arnold, 1996:778–790.

94. Sylvester JT, Scharf SM, Gilbert RD, Fitzgerald RS, Traystman RJ, Hypoxic and CO hypoxia in dogs: hemodynamics, carotid reflexes, and catecholamines. Am J Physiol 1979; 236:H22–H28.
95. Hoffman JI, Buckberg GD. The myocardial supply:demand ratio—a critical review. Am J Cardiol 1978; 41:327–332.
96. Sylvester JT, Goldberg HS, Permutt S. The role of the vasculature in the regulation of cardiac output. Clin Chest Med 1983; 4:111–126.
97. Hata K, Goto Y, Kawaguchi O, et al. Hypercapnic acidosis increases oxygen cost of contractility in the dog left ventricle. Am J Physiol 1994; 266:H730–H740.
98. Hata K, Takasago T, Saeki A, Nishioka T, Goto Y. Stunned myocardium after rapid correction of acidosis. Increased oxygen cost of contractility and the role of the $Na^{(+)}$–H^{+} exchange system. Circ Res 1994; 74:794–805.
99. Burrows B, Kettel LJ, Niden AH, Rabinowitz M, Diener CF. Patterns of cardiovascular dysfunction in chronic obstructive lung disease. N Engl J Med 1972; 286: 912–918.
100. Weitzenblum E, Hirth C, Ducolone A, Mirhom R, Rasaholinjanahary J, Ehrhart M. Prognostic value of pulmonary artery pressure in chronic obstructive pulmonary disease. Thorax 1981; 36:752–758.
101. Morrison D, Goldman S, Wright AL, et al. The effect of pulmonary hypertension on systolic function of the right ventricle. Chest 1983; 84:250–257.
102. Biernacki W, Flenley DC, Muir AL, MacNee W. Pulmonary hypertension and right ventricular function in patients with COPD. Chest 1988; 94:1169–1175.
103. Silverman N. Echo assessment of PVR. Circulation 1976; 54:525–526.
104. Viles PH, Shepherd JT. Relationship between pH, Po_2, and Pco_2 on the pulmonary vascular bed of the cat. Am J Physiol 1968; 215:1170–1176.
105. Barer GR, Howard P, Shaw JW. Sensitivity of pulmonary vessels to hypoxia and hypercapnia. J Physiol (Lond) 1970; 206:25P–26P.
106. Barer GR, Howard P, Shaw JW. Stimulus–response curves for the pulmonary vascular bed to hypoxia and hypercapnia. J Physiol (Lond) 1970; 211:139–155.
107. Madden JA, Vadula MS, Kurup VP. Effects of hypoxia and other vasoactive agents on pulmonary and cerebral artery smooth muscle cells. Am J Physiol 1992; 263: L384–L393.
108. Post JM, Hume JR, Archer SL, Weir EK. Direct role for potassium channel inhibition in hypoxic pulmonary vasoconstriction. Am J Physiol 1992; 262:C882–C890.
109. Salvaterra CG, Goldman WF. Acute hypoxia increases cytosolic calcium in cultured pulmonary arterial myocytes. Am J Physiol 1993; 264:L323–L328.
110. Jameson AG. Diffusion of gases from alveolus to precapillary artery. Science 1963; 139:826–828.
111. Abman SH, Wolfe RR, Accurso FJ, Koops BL, Bowman CM, Wiggins JW Jr. Pulmonary vascular response to oxygen in infants with severe bronchopulmonary dysplasia. Pediatrics 1985; 75:80–84.
112. Arias-Stella J, Saldana M. The muscular pulmonary arteries in people native to high altitude. Med Thorac 1962; 19:484–493.
113. Tucker A, Penney DG. Pulmonary vascular responsiveness in rats following neonatal exposure to high altitude or carbon monoxide. Exp Lung Res 1993; 19:699–713.

114. Grover RF, Johnson RL Jr, McCullough RG, et al. Pulmonary hypertension and pulmonary vascular reactivity in beagles at high altitude. J Appl Physiol 1988; 65: 2632–2640.
115. Nocturnal Oxygen Therapy Trial Group. Continuous or nocturnal oxygen therapy in hypoxemic chronic obstructive lung disease: a clinical trial. Ann Intern Med 1980; 93:391–398.
116. Stuart-Harris C, Bishop JM, Clark TJH, et al. Long term domiciliary oxygen therapy in chronic hypoxic cor pulmonale complicating chronic bronchitis and emphysema. Lancet 1981; 1:681–685.
117. Timms RM, Khaja FU, Williams GW, The Nocturnal Oxygen Therapy Trial G. Hemodynamic response to oxygen therapy in chronic obstructive pulmonary disease. Ann Intern Med 1985; 102:29–36.
118. Palmer RM, Ferrige AG, Moncada S. Nitric oxide release accounts for the biological activity of endothelium-derived relaxing factor. Nature 1987; 327:524–526.
119. Moncada S, Higgs A. The L-arginine–nitric oxide pathway. N Engl J Med 1993; 329:2002–2012.
120. Rimar S, Gillis CN. Selective pulmonary vasodilation by inhaled nitric oxide is due to hemoglobin inactivation. Circulation 1993; 88:2884–2887.
121. Stamler JS, Singel DJ, Loscalzo J. Biochemistry of nitric oxide and its redox-activated forms. Science 1992; 258:1898–1902.
122. Nelin LD, Moshin J, Thomas CJ, Sasidharan P, Dawson CA. The effect of inhaled nitric oxide on the pulmonary circulation of the neonatal pig. Pediatr Res 1994; 35:20–24.
123. Adnot S, Andrivet P, Chabrier PE, et al. Plasma levels of atrial natriuretic factor, renin activity, and aldosterone in patients with chronic obstructive pulmonary disease. Response to O_2 removal and to hyperoxia. Am Rev Respir Dis 1990; 141: 1178–1184.
124. Dinh-Xuan AT, Higenbottam TW, Clelland CA, et al. Impairment of endothelium-dependent pulmonary-artery relaxation in chronic obstructive lung disease. N Engl J Med 1991; 324:1539–1547.
125. Frostell C, Fratacci MD, Wain JC, Jones R, Zapol WM. Inhaled nitric oxide. A selective pulmonary vasodilator reversing hypoxic pulmonary vasoconstriction. Circulation 1991; 83:2038–2047.
126. Puybasset L, Stewart T, Rouby JJ, et al. Inhaled nitric oxide reverses the increase in pulmonary vascular resistance induced by permissive hypercapnia in patients with acute respiratory distress syndrome. Anesthesiology 1994; 80:1254–1267.
127. Christman BW, McPherson CD, Newman JH, et al. An imbalance between the excretion of thromboxane and prostacyclin metabolites in pulmonary hypertension. N Engl J Med 1992; 327:70–75.
128. Welte M, Zwissler B, Habazettl H, Messmer K. PGI_2 aerosol versus nitric oxide for selective pulmonary vasodilation in hypoxic pulmonary vasoconstriction. Eur Surg Res 1993; 25:329–340.
129. Zwissler B, Welte M, Messmer K. Effects of inhaled prostacyclin as compared with inhaled nitric oxide on right ventricular performance in hypoxic pulmonary vasoconstriction. J Cardiothorac Vasc Anesth 1995; 9:283–289.
130. Zobel G, Dacar D, Rodl S, Friehs I. Inhaled nitric oxide versus inhaled prostacyclin

and intravenous versus inhaled prostacyclin in acute respiratory failure with pulmonary hypertension in piglets. Pediatr Res 1995; 38:198–204.
131. Barst RJ, Rubin LJ, Long WA, et al. A comparison of continuous intravenous epoprostenol (prostacyclin) with conventional therapy for primary pulmonary hypertension. The Primary Pulmonary Hypertension Study Group. N Engl J Med 1996; 334:296–302.
132. Barst RJ, Rubin LJ, McGoon MD, Caldwell EJ, Long WA, Levy PS. Survival in primary pulmonary hypertension with long-term continuous intravenous prostacyclin. Ann Intern Med 1994; 121:409–415.
133. McLaughlin VV, Genthner DE, Panella MM, Rich S. Reduction in pulmonary vascular resistance with long-term epoprostenol (prostacyclin) therapy in primary pulmonary hypertension. N Engl J Med 1998; 338:273–277.
134. Olschewski H, Walmrath D, Schermuly R, Ghofrani A, Grimminger F, Seeger W. Aerosolized prostacyclin and iloprost in severe pulmonary hypertension. Ann Intern Med 1996; 124:820–824.
135. Santak B, Schreiber M, Kuen P, Lang D, Radermacher P. Prostacyclin aerosol in an infant with pulmonary hypertension. Eur J Pediatr 1995; 154:233–235.
136. McMurtry I, Davidson A, Reeves J, Grover RF. Inhibition of hypoxic pulmonary vasoconstriction by calcium antagonists in isolated rat lungs. Circ Res 1976; 38: 99–104.
137. Stanbrook HS, Morris KG, McMurtry IF. Prevention and reversal of hypoxic pulmonary hypertension by calcium antagonists. Am Rev Respir Dis 1984; 130:81–85.
138. Young TE, Lundquist LJ, Chesler E, Weir EK. Comparative effects of nifedipine, verapamil, and diltiazem on experimental pulmonary hypertension. Am J Cardiol 1983; 51:195–200.
139. Kennedy T, Summer W. Inhibition of hypoxic pulmonary vasoconstriction by nifedipine. Am J Cardiol 1982; 50:864–868.
140. Saadjian A, Philip-Joet F, Arnaud A. Hemodynamic and oxygen delivery responses to nifedipine in pulmonary hypertension secondary to chronic obstructive lung disease. Cardiology 1987; 74:196–204.
141. Singh H, Ebejer MJ, Higgins DA, Henderson AH, Campbell IA. Acute haemodynamic effects of nifedipine at rest and during maximal exercise in patients with chronic cor pulmonale. Thorax 1985; 40:910–914.
142. Muramoto A, Caldwell J, Albert RK, Lakshminarayan S, Butler J. Nifedipine dilates the pulmonary vasculature without producing symptomatic systemic hypotension in upright resting and exercising patients with pulmonary hypertension secondary to chronic obstructive pulmonary disease. Am Rev Respir Dis 1985; 132:963–966.
143. Sturani C, Bassein L, Schiavina M, Gunella G. Oral nifedipine in chronic cor pulmonale secondary to severe chronic obstructive pulmonary disease (COPD). Chest 1983; 84:135–142.
144. Saadjian AY, Philip-Joet FF, Vestri R, Arnaud AG. Long-term treatment of chronic obstructive lung disease by nifedipine: an 18-month haemodynamic study. Eur Respir J 1988; 1:716–720.
145. Brownlee JR, Beekman RH, Rosenthal A. Acute hemodynamic effects of nifedipine

in infants with bronchopulmonary dysplasia and pulmonary hypertension. Pediatr Res 1988; 24:186–190.

146. Clozel JP, Delorme N, Battistella P, Breda JL, Polu JM. Hemodynamic effects of intravenous diltiazem in hypoxic pulmonary hypertension. Chest 1987; 91:171–175.
147. Brown SE, Linden GS, King RR, Blair GP, Stansbury DW, Light RW. Effects of verapamil on pulmonary haemodynamics during hypoxaemia, at rest, and during exercise in patients with chronic obstructive pulmonary disease. Thorax 1983; 38: 840–844.
148. Doherty JE, Kane JJ, Phillips JR, Adamson JS. Digitalis in pulmonary heart disease (cor pulmonale). Drugs 1977; 13:142–151.
149. Mathur PN, Powles P, Pugsley SO, McEwan MP, Campbell EJ. Effect of digoxin on right ventricular function in severe chronic airflow obstruction. A controlled clinical trial. Ann Intern Med 1981; 95:283–288.
150. Polic S, Rumboldt Z, Dujic Z, Bagatin J, Deletis O, Rozga A. Role of digoxin in right ventricular failure due to chronic cor pulmonale. Int J Clin Pharmacol Res 1990; 10:153–162.
151. Raff H, Fagin KD. Measurement of hormones and blood gases during hypoxia in conscious cannulated rats. J Appl Physiol 1984; 56:1426–1430.
152. Martin IH, Baulan D, Basso N, Taquini AC. The renin–angiotensin–aldosterone system in rats of both sexes subjected to chronic hypobaric hypoxia. Arch Int Physiol Biochim 1982; 90:129–133.
153. Gould AB, Goodman SA. The effect of hypoxia on the renin–angiotensinogen system. Lab Invest 1970; 22:443–447.
154. Rose CE Jr, Kimmel DP, Godine RL Jr, Kaiser DL, Carey RM. Synergistic effects of acute hypoxemia and hypercapnic acidosis in conscious dogs. Renal dysfunction and activation of the renin–angiotensin system. Circ Res 1983; 53:202–213.
155. Liang CS, Gavras H. Renin–angiotensin system inhibition in conscious dogs during acute hypoxemia. Effects on systemic hemodynamics, regional blood flows, and tissue metabolism. J Clin Invest 1978; 62:961–970.
156. Raff H, Shinsako J, Dallman MF. Renin and ACTH responses to hypercapnia and hypoxia after chronic carotid chemodenervation. Am J Physiol 1984; 247:R412–R417.
157. Weismann DN, Williamson HE. Hypoxemia increases renin secretion rate in anesthetized newborn lambs. Life Sci 1981; 29:1887–1893.
158. Farber M, Kiblawi S, Strawbridge R, Robertson G, Weinberger M, Manfredi F. Studies on plasma vasopressin and the renin–angiotensin–aldosterone system in chronic obstructive lung disease. J Lab Clin Med 1977; 90:373–380.
159. Farber MO, Bright TP, Strawbridge RA, Robertson GL, Manfredi F. Impaired water handling in chronic obstructive lung disease. J Lab Clin Med 1975; 85:41–49.
160. Reihman DH, Farber MO, Weinberger MH, et al. Effect of hypoxemia on sodium and water excretion in chronic obstructive lung disease. Am J Med 1985; 78:87–94.
161. Farber MO, Roberts LR, Weinberger MH, Robertson GL, Fineberg NS, Manfredi F. Abnormalities of sodium and H_2O handling in chronic obstructive lung disease. Arch Intern Med 1982; 142:1326–1330.

162. Campbell E, Short D. The cause of oedema in "cor pulmonale." Lancet 1960; 1: 1184–1186.
163. Demling RH, Will JA. The effect of furosemide on the pulmonary transvascular fluid filtration rate. Crit Care Med 1978; 6:317–319.
164. Bland RD, McMillan DD, Bressack MA. Decreased pulmonary transvascular fluid filtration in awake newborn lambs after intravenous furosemide. J Clin Invest 1978: 601–609.
165. Ali J, Chiernicki W, Wood LDH. Effect of furosemide in canine low-pressure pulmonary edema. J Clin Invest 1979; 64:1494–1504.
166. Baltopoulos G, Zakynthinos S, Dimopoulos A, Roussos C. Effects of furosemide on pulmonary shunts. Chest 1989; 3:494–498.
167. McCann EM, Lewis K, Deming DD, Donovan MJ, Brady JP. Controlled trial of furosemide therapy in infants with chronic lung disease. J Pediatr 1985; 106:957–962.
168. Engelhardt B, Elliott S, Hazinski TA. Short- and long-term effects of furosemide on lung function in infants with bronchopulmonary dysplasia. J Pediatr 1986; 109: 1034–1039.
169. Rush MG, Engelhardt B, Parker RA, Hazinski TA. Double-blind, placebo-controlled trial of alternate-day furosemide therapy in infants with chronic bronchopulmonary dysplasia. J Pediatr 1990; 117:112–118.
170. O'Donovan BH, Bell EF. Effects of furosemide on body water compartments in infants with bronchopulmonary dysplasia. Pediatr Res 1989; 26:121–124.
171. Rastogi A, Luayon M, Ajayi OA, Pildes RS. Nebulized furosemide in infants with bronchopulmonary dysplasia. J Pediatr 1994; 125:976–979.
172. Albersheim SG, Solimano AJ, Sharma AK, et al. Randomized, double-blind, controlled trial of long-term diuretic therapy for bronchopulmonary dysplasia. J Pediatr 1989; 115:615–620.
173. Kao LC, Durand DJ, McCrea RC, Birch M, Powers RJ, Nickerson BG. Randomized trial of long-term diuretic therapy for infants with oxygen-dependent bronchopulmonary dysplasia. J Pediatr 1994; 124:772–781.
174. Engelhardt B, Blalock W, DonLevy S, Rush M, Hazinski T. Effect of spironolactone–hydrochlorothiazide on lung function in infants with chronic bronchopulmonary dysplasia. J Pediatr 1989; 114:619–624.
175. Rush MG, Hazinski TA. Current therapy of bronchopulmonary dysplasia. Clin Perinatol 1992; 19:563–590.

16

Long-Term Recovery from Bronchopulmonary Dysplasia

SOLOMON ALKRINAWI and VICTOR CHERNICK

University of Manitoba
Winnipeg, Manitoba, Canada

I. Introduction

The clinical, radiologic, and pulmonary function changes that occur with bronchopulmonary dysplasia (BPD) have not been extensively studied through infancy and childhood. Only a relatively few studies have attempted to look at pulmonary function years after suffering from BPD (Table 1). This is probably related to several factors. First, the disorder is relatively young, having been described only about 30 years ago (1,2). Second, the rapidly changing approach to the treatment of the preterm infant with hyaline membrane disease (HMD) has made follow-up studies difficult because the population of surviving infants keeps changing along with therapeutic modalities.

For example, in the 1970s, continuous positive-airway pressure (CPAP) and positive end-expiratory pressure (PEEP) were introduced and mortality from HMD abruptly decreased. In the late 1980s, surfactant replacement therapy again changed the population of surviving infants, and the influence of this therapy on the long-term prognosis for BPD has not been studied. No data are available on the effect of antenatal steroid treatment on BPD and long-term lung function. Similarly, the effect of high-frequency oscillating ventilation versus conventional ventilators on recovery from BPD has had only limited study (3). In this chapter

Table 1 Reported Pulmonary Function Tests in Children (≥6 years of age) with a History of BPD

Author (Ref.) yr	Number of BPD subjects (mean age: yr)	Number and type of control subjects	Results
Northway (7) 1992	26 (18.3)	26 preterm 53 term	68% mild airway obstruction; 24% fixed airway obstruction, hyperinflation, ↑ airway resistance, ↓ specific airway conductance; 52% AHR
Blayney (10) 1991	32 (serial study at 7 and 10 yr)	0	Mild airway obstruction, hyperinflation, 70% AHR, normal TLC, FRC
Kim (15)[a] 1988	9 (11)	9 RDS 10 preterm	Airway obstruction, AHR
Bader (8) 1987	10 (10.4)	8 term	Mild-to-moderate airway obstruction, hyperinflation; 50% EIB, on exercise: ↓ VE, ↑ $TcPco_2$, ↓ SaO_2
Andreasson (11) 1989	11 (8.6)	29 ventilated preterm	91% airway obstruction, in BPD vs. 31% in ventilated preterm infants
Smyth (16) 1981	9 (8.4)	nil	78% airway obstruction; 88% air trapping; 75% AHR, ↓ Po_2 ↑ Pco_2 (capillary)
Santuz (17) 1995	12 (8.1)	16 term	↓ FVC, ↓ FEV, on exercise: ↓ max Vo_2, ↓ V_E, ↓ Sao_2, ↓ anaerobic threshold, ↓ running time, 16% EIB
Mansell (13) 1987	8 (6.9)	26 preterm 10 RDS 18 term	No airway obstruction compared with preterm infants; low FEV_1 compared with full-term control
Hakulinen (12) 1990	10 (7.5)	19 ventilated preterm 13 preterm 30 term	↓ Specific airway conductance, ↑ RV/TLC, ↑ FRC compared with term
Wheeler (14)[a] 1984	11 (7.2)	15 RDS 14 preterm 11 term	Airway obstruction
Berman (23) 1986	10 (5.8)	nil	Difficult to interpret PFTs (5/10 BPD had moderate to severe developmental/motor delay)

Abbreviations: AHR, airway hyperreactivity; MCH, methacholine challenge test; EIB, exercise-induced bronchoconstriction; Sao_2, arterial oxygen saturation; V_E, minute ventilation; RDS, respiratory distress syndrome; $TePco_2$, transcutaneous Pco_2.
[a] Abstract only.

we will briefly review the few long-term studies related to physical examination, lung function, and radiographic study of the chest in subjects with BPD.

II. Physical Examination

A few studies have been done to relate BPD to changes in the chest wall, as assessed either by clinical or radiologic examination. Caliper measurements of the chest wall of 52 ventilated, preterm infants in the first year of life were done by de Boeck et al. (4). Of the 52 children 22 had BPD. Chest wall depth was significantly lower in children with BPD than in those without, but chest width and circumference did not differ between the two groups. The ratio of the transverse to anteroposterior chest diameter was significantly greater in infants with BPD than in those without. They speculated that this flattening of the chest wall was related to the disease process.

Edwards and Hilton (5) studied the chest radiographs of 18 children with BPD at a mean age of 444 days. The BPD groups was compared with 18 unaffected preterm patients and 110 normal patients. Width/thickness (W/T) ratio was higher in patients with BPD than in matched controls, again indicating a flattening of the chest wall in these patients. Thoracoabdominal asynchrony in subjects with BPD is related to the severity of the disorder (6), and in future studies, subsequent changes in the chest wall shape need to be related to an index of the severity of the disease process.

Northway et al. (7) found that adult subjects with BPD had significantly more pectus excavatum, overexpansion, and wheeze when compared with a normal-term control group, but there was no difference in physical examination between BPD subjects and a preterm nonventilated control group. However, the percentile height and weight in the subjects with BPD were significantly lower than normal controls or the matched preterm controls.

In contrast, Bader et al. (8) found that height and weight in BPD subjects were not different from a full-term control group. This is similar to the recent report by Vrlenick et al. (9), in which BPD subjects of school age did not have growth retardation. The more positive recent studies suggest that the current approach to nutritional support of preterm infants is preventing a long-term effect on body growth. Chest wall shape is clearly affected early, but carefully done long-term studies are needed to see whether or not the flattened chest improves with age.

III. Pulmonary Function

In 1990 Northway et al. (7) published the longest follow-up of patients with BPD to date. These adolescents and adults who were born preterm between 1964 and

1973, had undergone mechanical ventilation, required oxygen supplementation, and had chest radiographs at 4 weeks of age consistent with the diagnosis of BPD. Controls consisted of 26 subjects born during the same years, who were cared for in the neonatal intensive care unit, but did not require mechanical ventilation. A second control group of 53 subjects were age-matched, nonsmokers, who were not born prematurely (normal control group). The subjects performed standard pulmonary function and methacholine challenge tests. In addition, posteroanterior and lateral chest radiographs were obtained.

On average, mild expiratory airway obstruction was present in 68% (17/25) of subjects with BPD, and half had a significant response to isoproterenol or methacholine, suggesting the presence of reactive airways disease. Residual volume (RV)/total lung capacity (TLC) and functional residual capacity (FRC) were also increased compared with controls, indicating gas trapping and the presence of hyperinflation. These abnormalities correlated with the duration of postnatal ventilation and exposure to more than 80% O_2. The authors raised important concerns about the possibility of progressive obstructive pulmonary disease as these subjects get older and the potential adverse effects of cigarette smoke, which might be even more hazardous in individuals with a prior history of BPD. This study did not determine if the long-term pulmonary abnormalities were related to BPD, HMD, artificial ventilation, or a combination of events, for appropriate control groups were not studied.

Blayney et al. (10) studied 32 children with a history of BPD who showed significantly increased RV and RV/TLC at ages 7 and 10 years. Forty-two percent of the children with BPD had a normal 1-second forced expiratory volume (FEV_1) at age 7, and all remained normal at age 10. FEV_1 increased significantly with growth in the 58% of children who had a significantly low FEV_1 at age 7. In this group, FEV_1 changed from 65% of predicted to 72% of predicted, still lower than the normal predicted value. Specific airway conductance (SGaw) and FEV_1 in the BPD group were also no different from the preterm control group or the preterm group with a history of HMD, but without BPD. However, SGaw and FEV_1 were significantly less in the preterm children compared with the children born at full-term. TLC did not differ between groups. This study might be interpreted to indicate that preterm birth per se interferes with airway growth, but not with alveolar development.

Only three published studies have compared follow-up lung function of a preterm, ventilated control group with a preterm group with BPD (11–13). Andreasson et al. (11) studied children at about 9 years of age with a history of BPD compared with a ventilated preterm control group. There was evidence of airway obstruction in nearly all the children (10/11) with BPD. Interestingly, 9 of 27 (33%) preterm ventilated subjects without BPD also had evidence of airway obstruction. This study suggests that either artificial ventilation per se in preterm infants or neonatal lung disease is a risk factor for subsequent airway obstruction.

In contrast, Hakulinen et al. (12) found no difference in routine spirometry values at 6–9 years of age between BPD subjects and those ventilated for HMD, preterm infants without lung disease, and full-term subjects. However, specific airway conductance (SGaw) was significantly lower in the BPD group compared with full-term subjects, but was no different from the HMD and normal preterm groups.

In the report by Mansell at al. (14), children studied at ages 6–9 years who were born prematurely without lung disease had low SGaw and FEV_1 when compared with full-term infants. They found no difference in subsequent pulmonary function between those individuals with a history of HMD compared with those who had BPD or those who were born prematurely without lung disease. They concluded that preterm birth per se could lead to dysanaptic lung growth; that is, normal growth of lung volume, but not of airway size. A fourth study has not been published in full, and results are available only in abstract form (14,15; see Table 1). These data indicate that at age 7 years BPD subjects have airway obstruction (increased FRC and RV; decreased FEV_1) compared with infants who were born prematurely and had HMD without BPD; these abnormalities persisted at age 10 years.

In summary, the long-term effect of BPD on pulmonary function is difficult to ascertain from the current literature. It seems clear that BPD does not interfere with parenchymal growth. In the few studies where ventilated preterm infants without BPD are used as a control group, two found that BPD was associated with increased airway obstruction, whereas two studies found no differences between groups. Other confounding variables, such as type of ventilator, surfactant replacement therapy, use of steroids, and the changing clinical and radiologic definition of BPD render uncertain any conclusions about the effect of BPD itself on subsequent lung function. Long-term follow-up studies with appropriate control groups are needed.

IV. Airway Hyperreactivity

Northway et al. (7) concluded that of 25 subjects with BPD, 52% had evidence of airway hyperreactivity as assessed by response to inhaled isoproterenol (44%), or methacholine (8%). An additional 24% of patients with BPD had fixed airway obstruction and only 24% were considered normal. Interestingly, 31% of 16 individuals who were born prematurely without subsequent BPD also had positive methacholine challenge tests, as did 17% of subjects who were born at term. Blayney et al. (10) found approximately 70% of the 32 children with BPD had airway hyperreactivity at ages 7 and 10 years. Exercise-induced bronchoconstriction (EIB) was found in 50% (5/10) of children with BPD and none of the subjects born at term in the study by Bader et al. (8). Smyth et al. (16) found 67% (6/9) of BPD subjects had airway hyperreactivity on methacholine challenge testing, but they did not study a control group.

Andreasson et al. (11) using inhaled terbutaline, showed that there was a significant increase in FEV_1 in 5/11 (45%) 8-year-old children with a history of BPD and 4/29 (14%) children in a preterm ventilated control group. They did not have any children with EIB, in contrast with the study by Bader et al. (8). Santuz et al. (17) also found 2 of 12 BPD subjects had EIB. In a more recent study, this Finnish group reported that bronchial obstruction, bronchial lability, and increased bronchial responsiveness to histamine is common in prematurely born children of school age, independent of BPD (18).

In summary, only a relatively small number of former BPD patients have been tested for the presence of airway hyperreactivity by inhalation challenge, response to bronchodilator, or exercise challenge. Airway hyperreactivity is probably present in a substantial number of subjects with BPD. This is not surprising, in that BPD is associated with long-standing airway injury that may be slow to recover. Future studies of airway hyperreactivity in BPD subjects need to be done in a systematic manner and with appropriate control subjects. Indeed, as Riedel (19) suggests, artificial ventilation alone may be associated with increased airway hyperreactivity independent of BPD. Furthermore, if preterm birth itself leads to discordant growth of airway versus lung parenchyma, as indicated earlier in this chapter, future studies of airway hyperreactivity need to consider this factor.

V. Radiographic Study of the Chest

We are aware of only seven follow-up studies that have looked at the long-term effect of BPD on radiographic studies of the chest (Table 2). Five of these were published in the past decade, and in only three studies were the radiographs read in a blinded manner (7,12,20). In the study of Northway et al. (7), 26 adolescents and adults with BPD (mean age 18.3 years) had a radiographic score, composed of eight variables, which was significantly higher than the scores of matched preterm control subjects and normal-term subjects. The radiographic studies of the chest were assessed in a blinded manner by one observer. The abnormalities seen were generally subtle and included mild hyperexpansion, blebs, interstitial thickening, peribronchial cuffing, and pleural thickening.

Griscom et al. (20) studied 23 children with BPD in a blinded manner at a mean age of 8.7 years. The anteroposterior diameter was less than controls, and width/depth ratio was significantly greater than the controls. Of the children with a history of BPD, 52% had a flattened chest, 65% had radiographic evidence of fibrosis or deep pleural fissures and 18% had generalized thickening of interstitial tissue. Of the 23 children 6 had follow-up chest radiographs on average 2.7 years later, and their current radiographic findings showed no worsening or improvement.

Andreasson et al. (11) studied 40 children (11 BPD and 29 non-BPD) at

Table 2 Outcome of Chest Radiographic Studies of Children with a History of BPD

Author (Ref.) yr	Number of BPD subjects (mean age: yr)	Number and type of control subject	Results
Northway (7)[a] 1992	26 (18.3)	26 preterm 53 term	Hyperexpansion, blebs, interstitial thickening, peribronchial cuffing, pleural thickening
Griscom (20)[a] 1989	23 (8.7)	33 RDS 35 preterm	65% strands of fibrosis or pleural fissuring; 18% interstitial thickening 80% abnormal cxr: hyperinflation, interstitial fibrosis
Andreasson (11) 1989	11 (8.6)	29 ventilated preterm	89% abnormal cxr: hyperinflation, institial thickening, atelectasis and volume loss
Smyth (16) 1981	9 (8.4)	nil	40% had minor fibrotic changes
Hakulinen (12)[a] 1990	10 (7.5)	19 ventilated preterm 13 preterm 30 term	 62% coarse strands peribronchial thickening
Johnson (22) 1974	16 (5.7)	39 ventilated preterm	Interstitial infiltrate and hyperexpansion, one hyperexpansion without infiltrate
Harrold (21) 1974	15 (2.5)	7 ventilated preterm	

[a]Blinded study.

age 8–10 years who were ventilated in the neonatal period. Eight of ten children with severe BPD had an abnormal chest radiograph at an average of 8.6 years. The abnormal chest radiographs were found more frequently in the children who had abnormal radiographs just after they had been ventilated. The radiographic finding consisted of mild perihilar fibrosis or generalized hyperinflation. Four of eight children with hyperinflation also had focal areas of hyperinflation. The authors commented that the radiographic changes had improved in these children, who also had been studied 4 years earlier.

Smyth et al. (16) studied nine children with BPD at an average of 8.4 years, and in only one child was the chest radiograph considered normal. Four children had volume loss in the right upper lobe or the left lower lobe. Focal hyperinflation was found in eight of nine children. Suspected hypovascularity was found in four children and interstitial fibrosis in three children. The chest radiograph improved throughout childhood.

Hakulinen et al. (12) studied ten children with BPD compared with 19 ventilated children without a history of BPD, 13 preterm, and 30 full-term subjects at school age 6–9 years. All chest radiographic findings were markedly improved. Minor fibrotic changes were found in 4 children in the BPD group without signs of overinflation. Heart size and shape were normal. No pulmonary vascular abnormalities were seen.

Two reports from over 20 years ago showed that infants who survived mechanical ventilation and oxygen therapy for RDS, and who had subsequent BPD, had persistent chest radiographic abnormalities on follow-up (21,22).

In summary, studies of the outcome of chest radiographs in children with a history of BPD are fairly encouraging. Most reported chest radiographic abnormalities are minimal or mild-to-moderate over the long-term. Imaging studies using thin-section computed tomography (CT) scans would be of interest.

VI. Concluding Remarks

Long-term follow-up studies of this nature are difficult, but essential, if we are to monitor the effects of therapy on the preterm infant with lung disease. Since the advent of surfactant replacement therapy, more preterm infants born at a younger gestational age are surviving and the number of patients with BPD has actually increased. The effect of extreme prematurity on subsequent lung growth, independent of BPD, also deserves further study.

References

1. Northway WH Jr, Rosan RC, Porter DY. Pulmonary disease following respiratory therapy of hyaline membrane disease. N Engl J Med 1967; 276:357–368.

2. Pusey VA, MacPherson RI, Chernick V. Pulmonary fibroplasia following prolonged artificial ventilation of newborn infants. Can Med Assoc J 1969; 100:451–457.
3. HiFi Study Group. High frequency oscillatory ventilation compared with conventional mechanical ventilation in the treatment of respiratory failure in preterm infants: assessment of pulmonary function at nine months of corrected age. J Pediatr 1990; 116:933–941.
4. De Boeck K, Smith J, Van Lierde S, et al. Flat chest in survivors of bronchopulmonary dysplasia. Pediatr Pulmonol 1994; 18:104–107.
5. Edwards DK III, Hilton SW. Flat chest in chronic bronchopulmonary dysplasia. Am J Roentgenol 1987; 49:1213–1216.
6. Goldman MD, Pagani M, Trang HT, et al. Asynchronous chest movements during non-rapid eye movement and rapid eye movement sleep in children with bronchopulmonary dysplasia. Am Rev Respir Dis 1993; 147:1175–1184.
7. Northway WH Jr, Moss RB, Carlisle KB, et al. Late pulmonary sequelae of bronchopulmonary dysplasia. N Engl J Med 1990; 323:1793–1799.
8. Bader D, Ramos AD, Lew CD, et al. Childhood sequelae of infant lung disease: exercise and pulmonary function abnormalities after bronchopulmonary dysplasia. J Pediatr 1987; 110:693–699.
9. Vrlenich LA, Bozynski ME, Shyr Y, et al. The effect of bronchopulmonary dysplasia on growth at school age. Pediatrics 1995; 95:855–859.
10. Blayney M, Kerem E, Whyte H, et al. Bronchopulmonary dysplasia: improvement in lung function between seven and 10 years of age. J Pediatr 1991; 118:201–206.
11. Andreasson B, Lindroth M, Mortensson E, et al. Lung function eight years after neonatal ventilation. Arch Dis Child 1989; 64:108–113.
12. Hakulinen AL, Heinonen K, Lansimies E, et al. Pulmonary function and respiratory morbidity in school age children born prematurely and ventilated for neonatal respiratory insufficiency. Pediatr Pulmonol 1990; 8:226–232.
13. Mansel AL, Driscoll JM, James LS. Pulmonary follow-up of moderately low birth weight infants with and without respiratory distress syndrome. J Pediatr 1987; 110: 111–115.
14. Wheeler WB, Castile RG, Brown ER, et al. Pulmonary function in survivors of prematurity. Am Rev Respir Dis 1984; 129:A218.
15. Kim YC, Wheeler W, Longmate J. Longitudinal study of lung function in children following bronchopulmonary dysplasia. Am Rev Respir Dis 1988; 137:A18.
16. Smyth JA, Tabachnik E, Duncan WJ, et al. Pulmonary function and bronchial hyperreactivity in long-term survivors of bronchopulmonary dysplasia. Pediatrics 1981; 68:336–340.
17. Santuz P, Baraldi E, Zaramella P, et al. Factors limiting exercise performance in long-term survivors of bronchopulmonary dysplasia. Am J Respir Crit Care Med 1995; 152:1284–1289.
18. Pelkonen AS, Hakulinen AL, Turpeinen M. Bronchial lability and responsiveness in school children born very preterm. Am J Respir Crit Care Med 1997; 156:1178–1184.
19. Riedel F. Long-term effects of artificial ventilation in neonates. Acta Paediatr Scand 1987; 76:24–29.
20. Griscom NT, Wheeler WB, Sweezey NB, et al. Bronchopulmonary dysplasia: radiographic appearance in middle childhood. Radiology 1989; 171:811–814.

21. Harrod JR, L'Heureux P, Wangensteen OD, et al. Long-term follow-up of severe respiratory distress syndrome treated with IPPB. J Pediatr 1974; 84:277–286.
22. Johnson JD, Malachowski NC, Grobstein R, et al. Prognosis of children surviving with the aid of mechanical ventilation in the newborn period. J Pediatr 1974; 84: 272–276.
23. Berman W, Katz R, Yabek SM, et al. Long-term follow-up of bronchopulmonary dysplasia. J Pediatr 1986; 109:45–50.

17

The Goal
Prevention of BPD

MILDRED T. STAHLMAN

Vanderbilt University School of Medicine
Nashville, Tennessee

I. Introduction

Following severe injury, the lung can be repaired in a limited number of ways anatomically, of which functional repair eventually depends. Conducting airways undergoing necrotizing lesions that denude surfaces must be relined with stem cells arising largely from residual basal cells or from necks of tracheal and bronchial glands. These cells must migrate and differentiate into ciliated, goblet, and nonciliated secretory cells (Clara) if functional healing is to occur. However, if factors necessary for normal differentiation of these regenerating cells are absent, a squamous phenotype develops, resulting in functional impairment owing to loss of cilia, mucous secretion, secretions of Clara cells, water and chloride homeostasis, and impairment of neural functions of nerve endings and neuroendocrine cells present in normal conducting airway epithelium (1).

Terminal airways may also be widely denuded, requiring regeneration of lining stem cells, migration, and differentiation. In the absence of normal-healing factors, these airways reline with cells that are phenotypically type II cells, but may be quite dysplastic and of questionable functional integrity. Normal capillary invasion, a prerequisite for restoration of gas exchange, may not occur. The immature lung, which must continue to produce large numbers of terminal airway units with growth to maturity, is particularly vulnerable to the distortion of conducting airways during abnormal healing and to the failure of septation of terminal airways necessary for an adequate surface area for gas exchange (2).

Bronchopulmonary dysplasia (BPD) is the clinicopathological consequence of chronic or recurrent lung injury in the human preterm neonate. Its etiology is complex and involves interaction of many factors. Beginning with the original description in 1967 (3), BPD has been characterized as the end result of three major interacting factors: (1) pulmonary immaturity, especially of the surfactant system; (2) lung injury caused by oxygen therapy and mechanical ventilation; and (3) inadequate and inappropriate repair of the initial lung damage (3,4). BPD is characterized pathologically by widespread alveolar collapse with slit-like terminal airways relined with dysplastic type II cells and interstitial production of dense matrix collagens and elastic fibers (1). Those airways that are not collapsed are also lined with regenerating type II cells, but septation of alveoli may fail to occur, and regenerating capillaries fail to invade these terminal cuboidal-lined airspaces in a normal fashion, resulting in a limited air–blood interface for gas exchange. Conducting airways show areas of necrotizing tracheobronchitis and squamous metaplasia (2). These changes occur surprisingly rapidly. Other factors, including pulmonary edema (5), pulmonary air leak syndromes (6), and recurrent episodes of airway infection (7), also contribute to the development of the pathology of BPD. Before the mid-to-late 1970s, survival, or even intervention on behalf of infants born weighing less than 1000 g was rare except in some small-for-dates infants. Newer treatment strategies, such as surfactant replacement therapy and high-frequency ventilation, have been targeted primarily at prevention or minimization of acute lung injury. Hopes that these strategies would drastically reduce the incidence of BPD have not been realized, however. In fact, although recent treatment advances in the management of the very low birth weight (VLBW) infants have progressively lowered the thresholds of birth weight and gestational age survival, the incidence of chronic lung disease has increased as the survival of a susceptible population has increased (8). This increased survival of VLBW infants occurs in a population, many of whom have never had hyaline membrane disease (HMD), either because of prenatal maternal steroidal acceleration of lung maturation or because of maternal or fetal factors prematurely accelerating lung maturation (e.g., pregnancy associated hypertension, maternal smoking, or cocaine use). This survival has changed not only the incidence of BPD, but also its pathophysiology. Increasing numbers of surviving VLBW infants have milder and less protracted clinical courses, requiring only brief use of assisted ventilation and shortened exposure to high oxygen concentrations. The pathology of this type of chronic lung disease, if these patients die, may be more dominated by arrest in pulmonary development than by atelectasis, scarring, and distortion of terminal airways. Lack of progression of alveolar septation is prominent, and these large residual terminal airways often have incomplete or scanty capillary invasion of their cuboidal lining cells. The end result is a lung with far fewer terminal units than normal for the developmental period, and an attenuated air–blood interface for gas exchange.

II. Predisposing Factors

The myriad of predisposing factors that are related to the incidence of BPD have been documented and discussed in the preceding chapters. I will enumerate only those factors that I consider to be most important related to the incidence of BPD and discuss them briefly.

1. Preterm birth
2. Hyaline membrane disease
3. Birth asphyxia
4. Prolonged oxygen therapy
5. Prolonged assisted ventilation with barotrauma and air dissection
6. Secondary airway infection
   a. Bacterial
   b. Viral
7. Nutritional deprivation
   a. Protein and calorie deprivation
   b. Antioxidant vitamins
      1. Vitamin A
      2. Vitamin E
8. Persistent ductus arteriosus
9. Excessive fluid therapy especially with persistent ductus arteriosus
10. Family background of airway hyperactivity
11. Genetic background (e.g., SP-B deficiency)

The most important of these factors is preterm birth, which dictates the degree of lung immaturity. I will return to this essential later. As I have already indicated, there are now fewer cases of ''old'' BPD preceded by classic HMD than previously, partly owing to better obstetrical practices, especially with high-risk pregnancies, the avoidance of heavy sedation and perinatal asphyxia, the prenatal use of steroids to mature the lung, and the widespread use of surfactant replacement. However, ''new'' BPD is increasingly common, and most other predisposing factors are common to both. Prolonged oxygen therapy and assisted ventilation with the use of endotracheal tubes, the problems of barotrauma and air dissection, especially disseminated interstitial air (6), are considered particularly damaging to immature lungs, especially those already having underlying cell damage of HMD. Secondary airway infection of damaged lungs, with the release of inflammatory cytokines adds greatly to the complexity of the pathology. Most VLBW infants with respiratory distress, especially when intubated, are also nutritionally deprived, first of colostrum with its immune factors and, subsequently, of adequate calories. Despite the widespread use of total parenteral nutrition (TPN), including intralipid, adequate caloric intake is difficult to achieve early after birth. Antioxidant vitamins may also be inadequate in the amount delivered in TPN (9), and vitamin A has an important role in lung development and repair unrelated to its antioxidant properties (10–12). This increases its demand during the perinatal period, especially in the presence of lung injury (13).

The persistence of the patency of the ductus arteriosus is very common in VLBW infants in the presence of HMD, and often becomes symptomatic, especially with bouts of asphyxia or excessive fluid intake.

Although its influence is largely unknown in newborn lung disease, an allergic family background associated with airway hyperactivity may become an important component in symptomatic chronic lung disease in early childhood.

Finally, the effect of genetic mutations is just beginning to unfold, with the recognition of surfactant-associated protein-B deficiency of genetic origin, leading to fatal respiratory disease in term newborn infants (14). Other nonlethal mutations may be found in surfactant proteins, which could affect the incidence and severity of early chronic lung disease.

There is another set of factors that, although closely related to the predisposing factors, may minimize the incidence and severity of BPD. These include

1. Prevention of preterm birth by improving maternal health, prenatal care, and avoiding maternal and fetal stress, both physical and emotional
2. Prenatal acceleration of lung maturation with:
   a. Prenatal steroids
   b. Prenatal TRH
   c. Prenatal growth factors, such as EGF, in combination with differentiating factors, such as retinoids
3. Prevention and treatment of intrauterine, intrapartum, and neonatal asphyxia
4. Prophylactic surfactant instillation in high-risk groups of infants
5. Rescue surfactant instillation early in overt RDS
6. Minimize high oxygen inhalation therapy and barotrauma
   a. ? Liquid ventilation
7. Minimize barotrauma
   a. Early use of CPAP
   b. Selective use of high-frequency ventilation
   c. Careful regulation of airway pressure, especially when using surfactant or in the face of pulmonary edema or alveolar hemorrhage
8. Sterile techniques for suction, intravenous infusions, and blood sampling to avoid infection; nursery crowd control of infected visitors and personnel; and periodic bacteriological surveillance

9. Monitor infant vitamin levels, especially vitamin A, and maintain high intake throughout the first months of life
10. Early use of oral feeds, especially colostrum and breast milk, if possible, or early TPN and intralipid, if not
11. Prophylactic use of indomethacin in babies at high risk for symptomatic PDA
    a. Therapeutic use of CPAP, fluid restriction, indomethacin, or surgical ligation for symptomatic PDA
12. Judicious use of anti-inflammatory agents, such as steroids
13. Lung transplantation for SP-B gene deficiency and, possibly, for severe irreparable lung damage with chronic BPD, as a last resort

The prevention of preterm birth is the absolute prerequisite to the prevention of BPD. The importance of this in improving maternal health, good prenatal care, and the avoidance of maternal and fetal stress will be dealt with later.

The prenatal acceleration of lung maturation with steroids has been shown to be important in the prevention of HMD over the last 25 years (15). Despite the small percentage of pregnancies in which it is used appropriately in the United States, it ranks along with the postnatal use of surfactant replacement as the most seminal advancements improving the outcome of VLBW infants. The addition of TRH may prove additionally useful during the window of effective prenatal manipulation of lung maturation (16). Growth factors, such as epidermal growth factor (EGF), if combined with epithelial differentiating factors, such as retinoids, may also prove useful in the future as antepartum measures to promote lung maturation in the susceptible patient (17,18).

The prevention and treatment of intrauterine, intrapartum, and neonatal asphyxia by appropriate prenatal and neonatal care in the high-risk preterm neonate spares the lung from very low pulmonary blood flow associated with the redistribution of blood right-to-left through the ductus arteriosus associated with the "dive" reflex (19). If prolonged or repetitive, pulmonary hypertension and persistent fetal circulatory patterns can lead to secondary ischemic damage of lung lining epithelium. The neonatal use of nitric oxide inhalation is now under investigation in such circumstances (20,21).

Prophylactic surfactant instillation immediately after birth in very high-risk groups of infants undoubtedly prevents some infants from acquiring HMD and, thereby, lessens their chances for developing "old" BPD, with the disadvantage of one's not being able to evaluate the absolute need before treatment. The "rescue" instillation of surfactant early in the course of overt respiratory distress lessens the need for prolonged high concentration oxygen administration, and assisted ventilation (22), both important predisposing factors in the development of BPD. The minimization of high-concentration oxygen inhalation and barotrauma might both be promoted by the early use of liquid ventilation, and surfactant can be instilled in the perfluorocarbon liquid (23). Barotrauma may also be minimized by the early and judicious use of adequate constant distending airway pressure (CPAP), and by the selective use of high-frequency ventilation, especially in the face of disseminated interstitial air dissection (24).

The use of one or repeated doses of surfactant instilled into the trachea demands the careful regulation of airway pressure and inspired oxygen, as the rapidity of the surfactant's ability to change pulmonary mechanics and arterial oxygen levels may vary with type of surfactant used and the mode of its administration. Airway pressure regulation, always important, becomes crucial in the face of alveolar edema or hemorrhage, and air dissection becomes hazardous, even with the best of care.

It seems that, after more than 30 years of newborn intensive care, it would be unnecessary to mention the importance of sterile techniques for a very infection-susceptible and vulnerable population of patients, but the details of care are important. Repeated bouts of secondary infection, often with saprophytic organisms, in intubated or invasively instrumented infants are extremely common, and pulmonary infection is an important component leading to BPD's chronicity. Sterile techniques for airway suction, intravenous infusions, especially those containing protein, and blood sampling, especially through semipermanent lines, have importance in preventing such colonization that may, in the compromised host, lead to infection. Nursery crowd control of infected visitors and personnel may avert both bacterial and viral infections in patients, and periodic bacteriological surveillance is useful in monitoring pathogen source and spread. Hand-washing, a simple precaution, is still important. Monitoring infants' vitamin levels, especially that of vitamin A during periods of lung injury, repair, and accelerated growth, when requirements are increased, may promote lung healing as well as normal growth and development of the lung (13). The early use of oral feeds, especially with colostrum and breast milk, if possible, may provide the best substrate for gastrointestinal development and for tissue repair. The early use of TPN and intravenous fat is an alternative, but rarely meets early caloric needs and adds to the invasive hazards.

The prophylactic use of indomethacin in babies at high risk for symptomatic PDA may avoid the appearance of overt symptoms (25). The judicious use of CPAP and fluid restriction, combined with therapeutic indomethacin in the face of a symptomatic PDA may be helpful in avoiding the need for surgical ligation in a tiny, sick infant.

The short-term use of steroids during weaning from respirator care and extubation may prevent airway hyperreactivity and lessen tracheal edema. The prolonged use of steroids or other anti-inflammatory agents is becoming widespread, without adequate controlled clinical trials, including long-term anatomical and functional follow-up. The more prolonged use of steroids is thought to be useful in the prevention of fibrosis in severe BPD, but the long-term risks of prolonged steroid treatment on lung development, especially on the arrest of septation of alveoli, are not known in human infants and, therefore, should be used with caution (26–29).

Although lung transplantation for SP-B gene deficiency is being tried in selected cases (30), the scarcity of appropriate donors and the unknown long-term growth potential of the lung, especially in a chronically immunosuppressed recipient, make this approach difficult and potentially only palliative. Gene replacement would be the logical choice, but this may be some years away. The same problems, both ethical and medical, arise when considering lung or heart–lung transplantation for end-stage BPD and should be considered as an experimental treatment of last resort.

Most of the foregoing considerations of the predisposing factors of BPD and of those minimizing its incidence or its severity depend on meticulous attention to the details of management of pregnancy, labor, delivery, and neonatal care of the susceptible patient. As fewer experienced physicians in neonatal intensive care units have direct hands-on, minute-to-minute control over high-risk neonates, and as other types of personnel, such as nurses, respiratory therapists, pharmacists, x-ray and ultrasound technicians, and fluid therapists manipulate the infant at intermittent intervals, often without knowledge of the infant's immediate status or existing complications, more opportunities for deleterious events can occur. Continuity of care in decision making is important, especially at critical times, and the myriad of consultants, regardless of their expertise, may fragment a consolidated therapeutic approach. There is no substitute for careful acute care in preventing long-term sequelae, and BPD is a good example.

However, despite doing everything right and exercising all the proper precautions, many VLBW infants will end up with chronic lung disease, primarily because they are VLBW infants. The prevention of preterm birth is the only sure way to prevent BPD, since all its clinical, physiological, and pathological features are dependent, to one extent or another, on the immaturity of the lung and the necessity to increase its number of functional units from birth to maturity without distortion, severe scarring, chronic infection, or growth arrest. How does one prevent preterm birth? Maternal factors are dominant, with infection of extra-embryonic fetal tissue or uterine desidua being present in more than 25% of pregnancies complicating preterm labor. However, in many pregnancies, there is no clinical evidence of infection, and its importance in the initiation of preterm labor has recently been brought into question (31). At least 35–40% of pregnancies ending in preterm labor have no evidence of infection (32), and this suggests that preterm labor in this group is evoked by mechanisms different in some specific respects from those of normal parturition at term. Our ignorance about the onset of term or preterm labor should be a priority area for research. Fewer preterm labors are associated with other problems, such as premature rupture of membranes, pregnancy-induced hypertension, and abruption of the placenta). There has been no reduction in the incidence of preterm births in the United

States or Canada in recent years, notwithstanding the extensive use of tocolytic agents to halt preterm labor (33,34).

I believe we should look to the demographics of women who deliver preterm for some of the answers to its prevention. Prematurity has become largely a social, rather than a medical, disease in the United States, as our social structures have become more polarized toward the more well-off financially, better-educated segment of our population to whom access to medical care has always been available, versus the poor. This includes the working poor or those single women on welfare who tend to be poorly educated, have little or no job skills, and to whom access for medical care has been either nonexistent, physically difficult to reach, or beyond their financial means. It is little wonder that this group accounts for a high proportion of VLBW infants. This group of women live with stress from day to day for survival, and adequate prenatal care is realistically low on their priority list of necessities. Many of these mothers are children themselves, most commonly with no father figure involved in the pregnancy, and school drop-out is the rule. Many are second- and even third-generation welfare recipients, and poverty, poor health habits, poor nutritional patterns, and emotional turmoil is a way of life from infancy onward. Health care becomes a low priority in such a lifestyle. Drug use is also common in some segments of their society. Until our society ensures decent housing, good educational possibilities which lead to a job paying a living wage above the poverty line, reproductive education beginning at an early level, and priorities on family stability and responsibility, these social patterns will continue. Many women and girls who have VLBW infants are products of generations of poverty and a stressful lifestyle. The pattern of social deprivation that so often precedes VLBW births will not be easy to modify, for it will require great societal change before health, both mental and physical, of these mothers changes, beginning with their own intrauterine and birth experience and infancy. It may well take a full generation of healthy mothers to produce healthy babies.

Can BPD be prevented? Many of the medical factors discussed in the foregoing can be improved with better access to health care in general, and prenatal care in particular, good obstetrics, and meticulous attention to the details of perinatal care. The ultimate prevention of BPD, that of preventing preterm delivery of high-risk, VLBW infants, is, sadly, many years away.

References

1. Stahlman MT, Gray ME. Lung injury and repair in the neonate. In: Brigham and Stahlman, eds. Respiratory Distress Syndrome. Nashville: Vanderbilt University Press, 1990:3–11.
2. Stahlman MT, Gray ME. Remodeling of airways and epithelium. In: Brigham and

Stahlman, eds. Respiratory Distress Syndrome. Nashville: Vanderbilt University Press, 1990:188–197.
3. Northway WH Jr, Rosan RC, Porter DY. Pulmonary disease following respirator therapy of hyaline membrane disease: bronchopulmonary dysplasia. N Engl J Med 1967; 276:357–368.
4. Hazinski TA. Bronchopulmonary dysplasia. In: Chernick V, ed. Kendig's Disorders of the Respiratory Tract in Children. Philadelphia, WB Saunders, 1990:300–320.
5. O'Brodovich HM, Mellins RB. Bronchopulmonary dysplasia: unresolved neonatal acute lung injury. Am Rev Respir Dis 1985; 132:694–709.
6. Stahlman MT, Cheatham W, Gray ME. The role of air dissection in bronchopulmonary dysplasia. J Pediatr 1979; 95:878–882.
7. Stenmark KR, Voelkei NF. Potential role of inflammation and lipid mediators in the pathophysiology of bronchopulmonary dysplasia. In: Bancalari E, Stocker JT, eds. Bronchopulmonary Dysplasia. Washington: Hemisphere, 1988:58–77.
8. Parker RA, Lindstrom DP, Cotton RB. Improved survival accounts for most, but not all of the increase in bronchopulmonary dysplasia. Pediatrics 1992; 90:663–668.
9. Shenai JP, Stahlman MT, Chytil F. Vitamin A delivery from parenteral alimentation solution. J Pediatr 1981; 99:661–663.
10. Shenai JP, Chytil F. Vitamin A storage in lungs during perinatal development in the rat. Biol Neonate 1990; 57:126–132.
11. Popper H. Distribution of vitamin A in tissue as visualized by fluorescence microscopy. Physiol Rev 1944; 24:205–224.
12. Chytil F. The lungs and vitamin A. Am J Physiol 1992; 262:L517–L527.
13. Shenai JP, Kennedy KA, Chytil F, Stahlman MT. Clinical trial of vitamin A supplementation in infants susceptible to bronchopulmonary dysplasia. J Pediatr 1987; 111: 269–277.
14. Nogee LM, Garnier G, Dietz HC, et al. A mutation in the surfactant protein B gene responsible for fatal neonatal respiratory disease in multiple kindreds. J Clin Invest 1994; 93:1860–1863.
15. Liggins GC, Howie RN. A controlled trial of antepartum glucocorticoid treatment for prevention of the respiratory distress syndrome in premature infants. Pediatrics 1972; 50:515–525.
16. Ballard RA, Ballard PL, Creasy RK, et al. Respiratory disease in very-low-birth-weight infants after prenatal thyrotropin-releasing hormone and glucocorticoid. Lancet 1992; 339:510–515.
17. Sundell HW, Gray ME, Serenius FS, Escobedo MB, Stahlman MT. Effects of epidermal growth factor on lung maturation in fetal lambs. Am J Pathol 1980; 100:707–726.
18. Goetzman BW, Read LC, Plopper CG, et al. Prenatal exposure to epidermal growth factor attenuates respiratory distress syndrome in rhesus infants. Pediatr Res 1994; 35:30–36.
19. Grogaard J, Lindstrom DP, Stahlman MT, Marchal F, Sundell H. The cardiovascular response to laryngeal water administered in young lambs. J Dev Physiol 1982; 4: 353–370.
20. Roberts JD Jr, Polaner DM, Todres ID, Lang P, Zapol WM. Inhaled nitric oxygen

(NO): a selective pulmonary vasodilator for the treatment of persistent pulmonary hypertension of the newborn (PPHN). Circulation 1991; 84:A1279.
21. Abman SH, Kinsella JP, Shaffer MS, Wilkening RB. Inhaled nitric oxide in the management of a premature newborn with severe respiratory distress and pulmonary hypertension. Pediatrics 1993; 92:606–609.
22. The Vermont–Oxford Trials Network. Very low birth weight outcomes for 1990. Pediatrics 1993; 91:540–545.
23. Shaffer TH, Greenspan JS, Wolfson MR. Liquid ventilation. In: Boyton B, Carlo W, Jobe A, eds. New Therapies for Neonatal Respiratory Failure: A Physiologic Approach. Cambridge: Cambridge University Press, 1994.
24. Keszler M, Donn SM, Bucciarelli RL, et al. Multicenter controlled trial comparing high-frequency-jet-ventilation in newborn infants with pulmonary interstitial emphysema. J Pediatr 1991; 119:85–92.
25. Krueger E, Mellander M, Bratton D, Cotton R. Prevention of symptomatic patent ductus arteriosus with a single dose of indomethacin. J Pediatr 1987; 111:749–754.
26. Koizumi M, Frank L, Massaro D. Oxygen toxicity in rats: varied effect of dexamethasone treatment depending on duration of hyperoxia. Am Rev Respir Dis 1985; 131: 907–911.
27. Blanco LN, Frank L. The formation of alveoli in rat lung during the third and fourth postnatal weeks: effect of hyperoxia, dexamethasone, and deferoxamine. Pediatr Res 1993; 34:334–340.
28. Frank L. The use of dexamethasone in premature infants at risk for bronchopulmonary dysplasia or who already have developed chronic lung disease: a cautionary note [letter; comment]. Pediatrics 1991; 88:413–416.
29. Frank L. On dexamethasone in bronchopulmonary dysplasia [letter; comment]. Pediatr Pulmonol 1994; 17:205–206.
30. Hamvas A, Nogee LM, deMello DE, Cole FS. Pathophysiology and treatment of surfactant protein-B deficiency. Biol Neonate 1995; 67:18–31.
31. MacDonald PC, Cox SM, Casey ML. The accumulation of mediators of inflammation in amniotic fluid is a sequela of labor and not indicative that intrauterine infection initiates parturition preterm. 1995; submitted for publication.
32. Cunningham FG, MacDonald PC, Gant NF, Leveno KJ, Gilstrap LC. Williams Obstetrics. 19th ed. Norwalk, CT: Appleton & Lange, 1993.
33. Leveno KJ, Little BB, Cunningham FG. The national impact of ritodrine hydrochloride for inhibition of pre-term labor. Obstet Gynecol 1990; 76:12–15.
34. Canadian Preterm Labor Investigators Group. Treatment of preterm labor with the beta-adrenergic agonist ritodrine. N Engl J Med 1992; 327:308–312.

18

Unique Features of the Immature Lung That Make It Vulnerable to Injury

SCOTT H. RANDELL

University of North Carolina
Chapel Hill, North Carolina

STEPHEN L. YOUNG

Duke University Medical Center
Durham, North Carolina

I. Introduction

This chapter presents a ''snapshot'' of the human lung when it is developed to the point at which survival is just possible—about 25–27 weeks postconception. Our comments will focus on selected events of lung development that seem most likely to make the premature human lung vulnerable to injury during its precocious adaptation to the extrauterine environment. A prior review of this subject by Frank (1) and many of the discussions in other books (2) remain valuable. We will not address important nonlung components of respiration, including development of the thorax and abdomen, development of respiratory control centers, peripheral chemoreceptors, muscles of respiration and their innervation, and reflexes such as the diving and cough reflexes. We focus our review on information relevant to the late canalicular and early saccular stages of normal human lung development. Our comments are greatly amplified by other chapters in this volume and those authors also include important information about abnormal lung development after premature birth.

This chapter is roughly divided into a discussion of conducting airways and of the parenchyma.

II. The Airways

The lung bud forms as an outpocketing of the foregut endoderm at approximately 4 weeks postconception (pc; Fig. 1). As the primordial epithelium extends into the surrounding mesenchyme, a mutually instructive set of cell–cell and cell–matrix interactions controls the dichotomous branching of the forming airways (3–6) and by the end of the embryonic period, at about 8 weeks, all of the 19 bronchopulmonary segments are present (7). By the end of the pseudoglandular stage, at 16 weeks pc, all branches of the future conducting airway system have formed, including approximately 25,000 terminal bronchioles. The pulmonary acinus is ''born'' during the canalicular stage (17–27 weeks pc). At this stage, the acinus consists of a terminal bronchiole, prospective respiratory bronchioles, and a few generations of branched buds that will become the future distal airspaces (saccules). At the end of the canalicular stage, extrauterine viability is possible, but without benefit of the many maturational changes normally occurring during the saccular stage (28–36 weeks pc).

What is the developmental status of the premature conducting airway during the canalicular-to-saccular transition, and why is it predisposed to injury and maladaptation? Table 1 summarizes some of the potential factors and their possible clinical consequences. Events primarily affecting the distal lung parenchyma are addressed in the second half of this chapter.

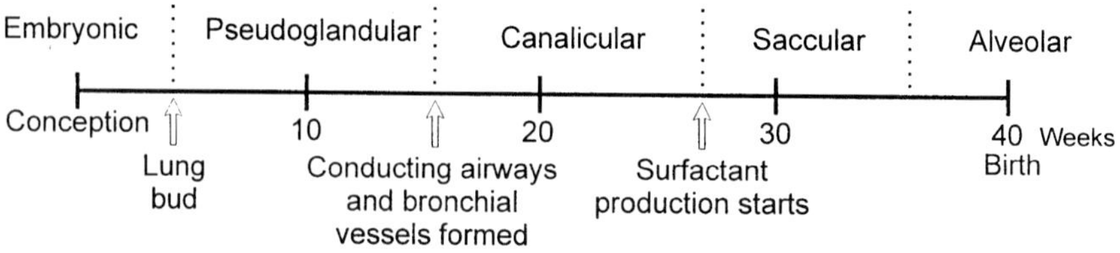

Figure 1 A highly schematic ''timeline'' of a few sentinel events in human lung development: The normal gestational period of about 40 weeks is shown, and five stages of lung development are given on the top of the line. The first outpocketing of the foregut endoderm occurs at about 4 weeks postconception and for the next 2½ months the advancing endoderm is producing the conducting airways by branching morphogenesis. The mesenchyme is developing capillaries and other differentiated structures as well as orchestrating many of the endodermal events. By about 25 weeks, the lung is still very immature, but airway and large vascular structures are in place. The later part of gestation is characterized by extensive expansion of the gas-exchange area and numerous crucial cellular events that prepare the lung for its role in gas exchange.

Table 1 Premature Airway Defects and Possible Clinical Outcome

Defect of premature airway	Possible clinical outcome
1. Poorly developed supporting structures (smooth muscle, cartilage) resulting in a high-compliance airway coupled to a low-compliance parenchyma	1. Overdistension of distal airway with disruption, interstitial emphysema and edema; chronic airway dysplasia
2. Incomplete neurogenic networks	2. Loss of neurotropic growth influence, hyperreactive airways
3. Neuroendocrine or neutral endopeptidase system immature	3. Loss of one mechanism for directing growth, hyperreactive airway response to neuropeptides
4. Airway epithelial cell populations immature, favoring increased mucous/serous cell ratio	4. Relative or absolute mucous hypersecretion with resultant obstruction
5. Inadequate intracellular or cell–cell adhesion	5. Epithelial sloughing
6. Decreased production of anitmicrobial and anti-inflammatory factors, underdeveloped immune accessory cell function	6. Loss of protective enzymes (e.g., lysozyme), susceptibility to lung infection, uncontrolled lung inflammatory reactions to stimuli
7. Immature cellular mechanisms for ion transport	7. Airway edema, inefficient airway clearance
8. Underdeveloped antioxidant protection	8. Heightened injury from inspired oxygen or other oxidants
9. Immature production or responses to cytokines, nitric oxide, prostaglandins, and poorly integrated physiological controls	9. Dysfunctional control over airway diameter; growth dysregulation
10. Incomplete development of bronchial circulation	10. Airway edema, bronchial airflow obstruction

A. Development of Airway Supporting Structures

The mesenchyme that surrounds the developing lung contributes cartilage, smooth muscle, and connective tissue components to airway structure (see Chap. 5). The functional status of these important airway structures in the preterm human lung at 25–28 weeks is partially understood, and it is generally accepted that underdeveloped airways are hypercompliant. Thus, they may be injured when high-inflation pressures are needed to expand the poorly compliant distal airspaces (8). Potential consequences include bronchiolar ectasia, with disruption and sloughing of the airway epithelium (9). Pathologically dilated terminal airways are a likely site for airway rupture and resultant air leaks that cause interstitial emphysema or pneumothorax. Smooth-muscle cells and tissue fibroblasts in the developing airway may be actively dividing and maturing at the time of premature birth, and they may be more susceptible to growth dysregulation resulting in airway smooth-muscle hyperplasia and fibrosis.

B. Innervation of the Airways

For detailed discussions of airway innervation, and neural and chemical regulation of bronchial caliber, the reader is referred to two volumes edited by Raeburn and Giembycz (10,11), as well as recent reviews (12,13). Noninnervated, bronchodilatory β-adrenergic receptors and bronchoconstrictive parasympathetic cholinergic nerves are important regulators of airway smooth muscle tone. Airways also contain bronchodilatory nonadrenergic, noncholinergic nerves as well as bronchoconstrictive C-fibers. The latter are thought to mediate neurogenic inflammation by neurokinin release. The airway epithelium itself is endowed with sensory and motor nerves that contain several neurotransmitters and neuropeptides. Complex interactions exist between the various neural components. Functional cholinergic responses are already present during the pseudoglandular stage of pig lung development and are hypothesized to play a role in normal growth (14).

There are wide gaps in our knowledge of the development of each of the airway neural systems, as well as the status of complex higher-order interactions, in the 25–28 week pc human fetus. Trophic influences and normal developmental patterning may be disrupted by the airway injury commonly accompanying premature birth. It is possible that the balance of regulatory forces in the preterm neonate favors airway hyperreactivity.

C. Neuroendocrine Epithelial Cells and Neutral Endopeptidase

Earlier than 8 weeks gestation, the primordial tracheobronchial airways are lined by undifferentiated columnar epithelial cells. Pulmonary neuroendocrine epithelial (PNE) cells, containing a wide variety of biogenic amines and peptides, may be the first developmentally differentiated airway epithelial cell type. In the human fetus, individual PNE cells and PNE clusters (neuroepithelial bodies) appear at approximately 8–10 weeks gestation (15,16), typically near nerve terminals and at airway branch points. Although the pattern of changes in PNE cell number and their content of secretory products (or mRNA) is complex, a generalized increase is observed during normal development, peaking during mid- or late gestation, and decreasing postnatally. There is a significant body of work on the biology of PNE cells, which was reviewed by Johnson (17) and in the Proceedings of a National Institutes of Health Workshop (18).

The PNE cells may modulate airway development, help regulate bronchial tone (and thus ventilation–perfusion matching), play a role in adaptation to chronic hypoxia and hypercarbia, and they are important in the genesis of certain pathological changes in the airways, including epithelial cancer. PNE cells appear to have a mitogenic paracrine effect on neighboring nonneuroendocrine epithelial cells (19), and recent studies demonstrate that PNE products stimulate airway epithelial mitosis, growth, and branching through specific receptor-mediated events (20–22).

The response of PNE cells to neonatal injury is dynamic, mirroring the evolution of respiratory distress syndrome (RDS) and bronchopulmonary dysplasia (BPD). Fewer PNE cells are present in areas of active epithelial necrosis, whereas there is PNE cell hyperplasia in repaired bronchioles (23,24). Greater numbers of PNE cells are also present in the Wilson–Mikity syndrome (23). It is unclear whether the increased number of PNE cells is of primary pathobiological significance, or if it is a secondary response to severe injury and alveolar gas abnormalities. PNE cell hyperplasia has also been reported in sudden infant death (SID) syndrome (25), in which the lungs are otherwise structurally normal. Although experimental animal data are highly suggestive, a causal relation between PNE cell products and airways hyperreactivity or structural modifications of the airway wall (fibrosis or smooth-muscle hypertrophy) in BPD has not yet been proved.

The bioactivity of peptides derived from PNE cells or airway nerves is modulated by endopeptidase enzymes (26). Neutral endopeptidase (NEP; the CD10 antigen also known as endopeptidase 24.11) is developmentally regulated in human lungs (27), and its inhibition enhances the growth-promoting effects of bombesin-like peptides (20,28). Airways exhibiting decreased levels of NEP owing to inflammation are hyperresponsive to bronchoconstrictors (29). NEP inactivates neuropeptide chemotaxins and mitogens for fibroblasts that are likely to be present in inflamed airways (30). Thus, NEP may modulate both short-term physiological responses and long-term structural remodeling. Other proteases, such as endopeptidase 24.15, which is localized to alveolar macrophages, airway nerves, and ciliated cells (31), can alter the activity of neuropeptides. The precise status of PNE cell products, neuropeptides, and their inhibitors in the 25–28 week gestation human fetus, and changes induced by precocious birth and its sequelae are not yet clear. One can speculate that the premature neonate is particularly sensitive to imbalance between the secretion and inactivation of these neuroendocrine peptides, which could contribute to the hyperreactivity and disordered growth characteristic of BPD. A focused research effort is needed to clarify these issues.

D. Cytodifferentiation of the Airway Epithelium

Although PNE cells are the first airway epithelial cell type to differentiate during development, they constitute only a small fraction of the total cell population. In the adult human, basal, ciliated, and non-PNE secretory (mucous, serous, and Clara) cells predominate, depending on airway generation and size (32). Airway epithelial cell differentiation has been reviewed elsewhere (15,16,33,34). Approximate developmental appearance times for each of the specific cell types in the human fetus are known, and detailed analysis of ciliogenesis and mucous cell development is available for the human trachea (35). However, quantitative ultrastructural studies that yield precise airway cell type ratios during development are available only for experimental animals. Humans differ from many of the small animal models used (rats, hamsters, ferrets), in which maturational changes occur very late in gestation or even postnatally. The timing of airway differentiation in the rhesus monkey (36) more closely approximates that of the human.

Ciliated cells first appear in the human trachea at 10 weeks pc and increase in number rapidly, so that by 24 weeks gestation they occupy approximately 80% of the epithial surface area (35). Because cytodifferentiation proceeds along a proximal to distal axis, it is surmised that ciliogenesis in the bronchi and bronchioles is delayed compared with that in the trachea, but the precise status of cytodifferentiation in the bronchi and bronchioles at 25–28 weeks remains unknown. Mucous secretory cells in the airways appear slightly later than do ciliated cells. In the trachea, mucous cell numbers peak by about 18 weeks gestation and decrease thereafter. Developmental changes in the number of mucous cells in the distal airways is less well defined than it is for the trachea. Although it is known that a relative decrease in mucous cells occurs during development, it is unknown whether this is complete by the time a viable birth is possible. An overabundance of mucous cells, or the fact that the epithelium is still in a transitional period may put the neonate at risk for mucous cell hypertrophy and hyperplasia which, in turn, may cause hypersecretion of mucus.

Identification of airway epithelial basal cells is hindered by an imprecise anatomical definition. Accurate estimates of human basal cell ontogeny are unknown. Structurally typical basal cells are visible by 16 to 18 weeks gestation in the central airways. Thus, basal cells develop relatively late compared with ciliated and secretory cells. Several studies performed with experimental animals suggest that basal cells are the precursors to other airway epithelial cell types in the mature respiratory tract (37). During development, however, secretory and ciliated cells are derived from an undifferentiated precursor, and there is a ciliated-to-secretory cell pathway. These observations suggest that the major cell lineages in airway epithelium may be different in the fetus and the adult. It remains unknown whether these differences predispose to disordered epithelial growth in the preterm neonate. It has been proposed that basal cells are specialized to facilitate attachment of overlying columnar cells (38). A decrease in structural integrity from fewer or more primitive basal cells may predispose to shedding of surface epithelial cells. Other factors that may contribute to epithelial integrity, such as desmosomes and tight junctions or integrin–extracellular matrix attachment sites, are probably developmentally regulated and require more study in the human.

In the adult respiratory tract, pseudostratified columnar airway epithelium changes to a cuboidal morphology, dominated by Clara and ciliated cells, in bronchioles of about 1-mm diameter (32). Clara cell differentiation in the human first occurs close to 15 weeks gestation. Thereafter, typical Clara cells with characteristic secretory granules increase in abundance, constituting about 11% of the bronchiolar surface epithelial cells in the 24 week gestation fetus (39). There are few studies of normal Clara cell development beyond 24 weeks, but it is known that terminal bronchiolar Clara cells are lost as a consequence of epithelial damage in RDS and BPD (39).

E. Submucosal Gland Development and the Production of Protective Factors

Submucosal glands form as evaginations of the surface epithelium in cartilaginous airways beginning at about 12 weeks gestation. Development proceeds along a proximal to distal axis and includes the formation and differentiation of mucous acini and tubules, serous acini, collecting ducts, and the ciliated ducts. For a detailed description of gland genesis the reader is referred to a prior review (16).

Mucous cells produce acidic mucin glycoproteins, and serous cells secrete (among other proteins) neutral glycoproteins, lactoferrin, lysozyme, and secretory leukoprotease inhibitor (SLPI) (40). Developmental changes during late gestation and childhood include a relative decrease in gland area and a shift from mostly mucous acini to a mixture of mucous and serous acini. Thus, there is a relative dominance of mucus-producing gland cells even following normal-term delivery. Extrapolation of this developmental pattern to the premature neonate would predict an even greater proportion of mucus-secreting cells. Jeffery et al. (16) proposed that gland hyperplasia in response to irritation might be more evident in the respiratory tract of young children than in adults. This might also be true for the premature neonate. Lysozyme and lactoferrin are antimicrobial proteins derived mainly from submucosal gland serous cells. Low lysozyme and lactoferrin levels in tracheal aspirates of RDS patients predict development of BPD (41), but a causal relation has not been proved. Well-developed submucosal glands, producing adequate protective factors, may be indicative of enhanced overall lung maturity and of a greater ability to face the challenges of premature birth and its necessary treatment.

F. Modulation of Immunity and Inflammation

The airway epithelium is an integral part of the secretory immune system of the lung (42,43). It is beyond the scope of this brief overview to discuss each of the many airway epithelial cells that likely participate in immune and inflammatory responses. It is important to recognize, however, that key immune cell functions, such as antigen processing by macrophages and by specialized epithelial cells (dendritic cells), regulation of leukocyte trafficking, and cytokine expression, may still be maturing during late gestation, and that immaturity may result in either an ineffective immune response or an unregulated inflammatory response. A relative inefficiency of the respiratory mucosal immune response has been attributed to immaturity of the neonatal T-cell system. Incomplete development of intraepithelial dendritic cells also may contribute to an immune deficiency (44). Regulation of dendritic cell activity may be influenced by granulocyte–macrophage colony-stimulating factor (GM–CSF) provided by alveolar epithelial cells (45). There is a need for research using animal and human models to characterize the developmental milestones for these complex interactions.

The secretory component (SC) of IgA is a secreted portion of the epithelial polymeric immunoglobulin receptor, the molecule that mediates transcytosis of IgA. Concentrations of secretory IgA in tracheal aspirate specimens from unborn infants were independent of gestational age, postnatal age, or respiratory status, and did not help predict subsequent development of BPD (46). Thus, although SC may be suitable as a reference protein in tracheal aspirate samples, its level is apparently not a useful predictor of progression to BPD. However, SC and IgA levels are not necessarily directly correlated, and IgA has not been quantified in lung secretions of premature neonates. Lower levels of secreted IgA in premature infants may be indicative of a less mature secretory immune system, which could predispose to infection.

Recent studies suggest that small antimicrobial peptides play a role in defense of airway surfaces (47,48). These peptides are classified based on nucleotide sequence and protein structure, and many share the common feature of cationic charge. Pathogens have evolved counterpeptide strategies that contribute to their virulence. A series of antimicrobial peptides with a conserved pattern of cystiene residues, termed defensins, have been isolated from human professional phagocytes (49). These are highly abundant in neutrophils and can be selectively induced in alveolar macrophages (50,51). Paneth cell defensins are thought to prevent bacterial invasion of intestinal crypts, and some defensins become strongly expressed only after birth (52–54). Bovine airways contain an abundant β-defensin named tracheal antimicrobial peptide, which is neonatally upregulated and is further induced by inflammatory stimuli (55,56). A novel series of anionic bactericidal peptides have been isolated from ovine pulmonary surfactant (57).

Two recently purified β-defensins, hBD-1 and -2, originally obtained from plasma and psoriatic skin flakes, respectively, are expressed in the human airway, and hBD-1 mRNA is upregulated neonatally (58–60). This rapidly unfolding evidence implicates defensin-like molecules as important, developmentally expressed and environmentally responsive components of airway mucosal innate immunity. Specific studies have not yet been performed to determine if a ''defensin-deficit'' contributes to increased susceptibility to infection of premature humans.

Tissue destruction caused by protease–protease inhibitor imbalance may be an important determinant of inflammatory airway injury (see Chaps. 32 and 35). SLPI is a major protective antiprotease that is derived from lung epithelium. SLPI, neutrophil numbers, and elastase activity were prospectively measured in tracheal lavage fluid from intubated infants (61). SLPI content increased over time, and whereas there were more neutrophils and greater elastase activity in the subgroup progressing to BPD, SLPI levels were equal in both groups. Thus, protease–protease inhibitor balance was unfavorable in those infants who went on to have BPD. It remains to be determined whether a more mature epithelium would respond to protease challenge by superinduction of SLPI, or if therapeutic augmentation of antiprotease levels will aid in prevention of the airway lesions of BPD.

G. Mucociliary Clearance

The postnatal development of the mucociliary clearance system has been studied in experimental animals, but few data are available from neonatal humans. The developmental status of mucous and goblet cells in late gestation is highly variable, depending on species. In studies performed with newborn sheep, the percentage of ciliated cells was high, as in humans, and cilia beat frequency was the same as that in adult sheep (62). However, there was an approximately threefold increase in the velocity of tracheal mucus during the first 8 weeks of postnatal life, and this was due to a decrease in mucous secretion, plus an elevated airway surface liquid absorption, which presumably enhance mucociliary coupling and thus clearance.

The conversion of the epithelium from predominantly Cl^- secretion to net sodium absorption at birth may be one of the major adaptations needed for air breathing, and is discussed in detail in Chapter 29. The study of sheep noted earlier suggests that airway surface liquid balance is ''fine tuned'' during neonatal adaptation to facilitate and improve mucociliary clearance. It is possible that similar changes occur in the neonatal human airway, and that the premature infant may be less capable of such adjustments and, therefore, prone to airflow obstruction.

H. Airway Epithelial Antioxidants

It is widely assumed that a significant fraction of cytotoxic neonatal lung injury is derived from reactive oxygen species, especially when high concentrations of supplemental oxygen are administered (protection against free radical injury is discussed at length in Chaps. 34 and 36). However, most investigations of antioxidant defenses have focused on whole-lung tissue, or on the alveolar epithelium. A study by Cohn et al. (63), indicates that the airway epithelium itself has an abundant capacity to scavenge the oxidant H_2O_2. Because epithelial necrosis is a prominent and early pathological feature predicting development of BPD, it is possible that antioxidant defenses in this specific compartment may be overwhelmed. Much still remains to be learned about the antioxidant status of the epithelium in premature human airways.

I. Dysregulated Epithelial Production of Mediators

The epithelium is a source of a wide variety of factors, including transforming growth factor-alpha (TGF-α), TGF-β, NO, endothelin, and arachidonate metabolites, some of which have well-known autocrine effects, as well as paracrine influences, on surrounding tissue cells. Fibroblasts in the lamina propria produce factors, such as keratinocyte growth factor, that serve as potent mitogens for the epithelium. This list is not comprehensive, and our purpose in mentioning the wide variety of mediators is simply to indicate that there is a complex and incompletely understood interplay of regulatory factors and their receptors that may be disrupted as a consequence of prematurity, which may then result in disordered growth or physiological control (4). These are potent mediators, the receptors of which are expressed in a highly regulated manner in developing animal lungs. Altered expression patterns have been noted in injury models. The field has the potential for yielding important new knowledge on the effectors of chronic lung injury in newborns, but we still lack data from humans, and cause-and-effect relations have not been proved.

J. The Bronchial Circulation

As noted in an early volume of this series (64), the ontogeny of the bronchial circulation in humans has not been studied in great detail. Bronchial artery sprouts apparently develop from the aorta at 8 weeks gestation. Growth parallels that of the bronchial tree, and by 26 weeks pc anastomoses between the bronchial and pulmonary circulations are present.

Maintenance of bronchial artery perfusion protected against extravascular lung water gain in one model of ischemia–reperfusion injury (65). Most studies of developmental changes in the bronchial circulation have been performed during the normal postnatal period in animals. Greater fluid transudation was present in the airways of young than in those of mature guinea pigs in response to histamine challenge (66). However, contrary data were obtained with tachykinins (67) and with a thromboxane-A_2 mimetic or leukotriene-D_4 (68), which argues against a simple interpretation of this data. When a sufficient number of studies are done to include prenatal time points, it should become possible to determine if the bronchial circulation in late gestation has greater susceptibility to fluid leakage and less ability to perform its purported protective functions.

III. The Parenchyma

Developmental immaturity and its possible clinical consequences for the distal, gas exchange, region of the lung are given in Table 2.

Table 2 Premature Parenchymal Defects and Possible Clinical Condition

Defect of premature parenchyma	Possible clinical condition
1. Poorly developed gas exchange surface	1. Insufficient area for gas exchange; poor lung compliance
2. Immature pulmonary vasculature	2. Insufficient area for gas exchange and hindered diffusion; high vascular resistance
3. Surfactant immaturity	3. Unstable alveoli; atelectasis, hypoxemia, high work of breathing and low compliance
4. Low tissue content of structural matrix (collagen and elastin)	4. Complications of mechanical ventilation; barotrauma, pulmonary vascular leaks
5. Immature development of nonstructural matrix	5. Lack of cellular differentiation, dysregulation of postnatal lung development
6. Underdeveloped antioxidant protection	6. Oxidant-induced alveolar damage
7. Immature cellular mechanisms for ion transport	7. Alveolar edema
8. Underdeveloped immune system	8. Susceptibilty to lung infection, uncontrolled lung inflammatory reactions to stress
9. Unfavorable protease-antiprotease balance	9. Inflammation; tissue destruction
10. Insufficient intermediary metabolism	10. Inadequate substrate utilization and production of key products such as fatty acids for surfactant secretion
11. Nutritional deficiencies	11. Inadequate protection from oxidants

A. Gas Exchange Surface

The current age limit of resuscitation of the premature infant is the time in gestation when the human lung is transitioning from the canalicular to the terminal sac stage of growth. At that early developmental point, there is only the beginning of a gas exchange surface, and true alveoli with their remarkably thin walls and rich capillary supply are absent (Fig. 2). The epithelium of immature lung saccules is mainly cuboidal, as contrasted with the attenuated mature alveolar epithelium. Compared with the mature alveolus, the capillaries in saccules are less numerous and more separated from the airspaces by interstitial tissue. Both conditions interfere with diffusion of gas from airspace to blood.

Growth of the gas exchange surface area within the lung is geometric, for the mechanism of increasing surface area is by dichotomous airway branching (Fig. 3; 69). Therefore, the surface area available for support of respiration by the premature infant is very sensitive to gestational age. It is seen in Figure 3 that small differences in gestational age during the later stages of intrauterine development correspond to substantial differences in the available gas exchange surface. Gas exchange demands of the newborn must be met at birth, and comparisons of animal and human data suggest that human infants have a relatively low ratio of available surface area to the rate of uptake of oxygen. This ratio can be calculated as even less favorable in the immature infant. Because premature birth imposes an immediate physiological demand on the lung to meet the infant's need for gas exchange, the present limits of clinical support are probably set by the physical immaturity of lung structure, and extrauterine survival of fetuses younger than about 24 weeks pc will likely require an extraordinary technology.

B. Pulmonary Vasculature

There are substantial data to assist an understanding of vascular dysfunction in the preterm lung (70). Development of the lung circulation has been reviewed (71), and vascular growth in the presence of chronic lung injury is presented in Chapters 25–27.

Pulmonary arteries and veins develop parallel to the development of the conducting airways, and they are in place by 16 to 19 weeks postconception. An extensive capillary network is delayed until the alveolar phase of maturation. The immature lung is susceptible to vascular dysfunction because its small poorly developed capillary bed has a small surface area and a longer tissue path length for gaseous diffusion. In addition to anatomical limitations, there are several

Figure 2 (a) Canalicular and (b) term human lung: Normal human lung at 23 weeks gestation and at term, respectively. (a, ×400; b, ×140).

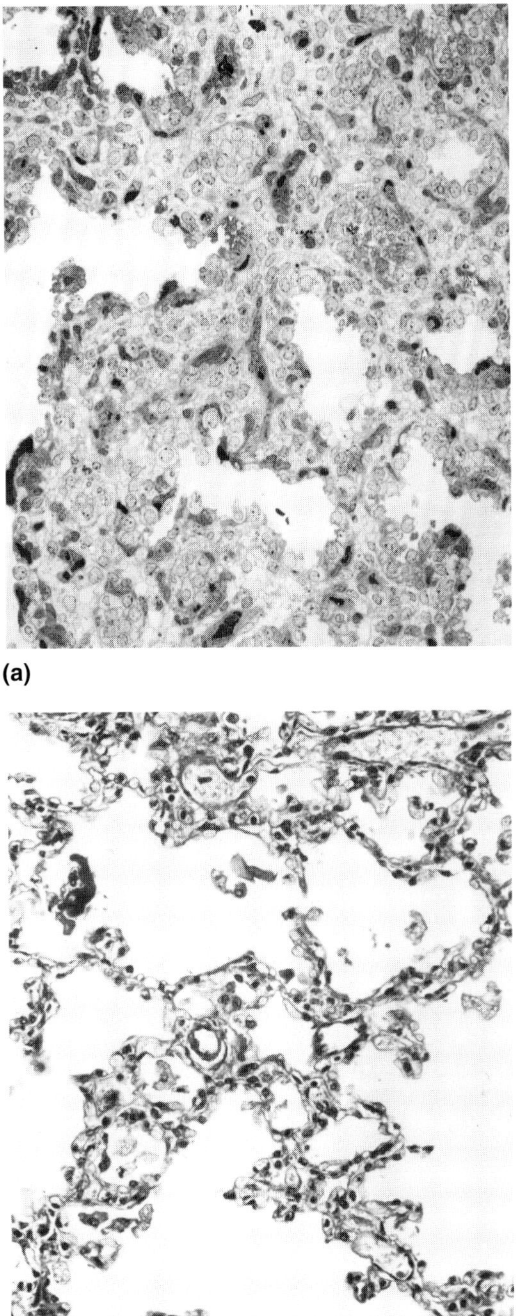

(a)

(b)

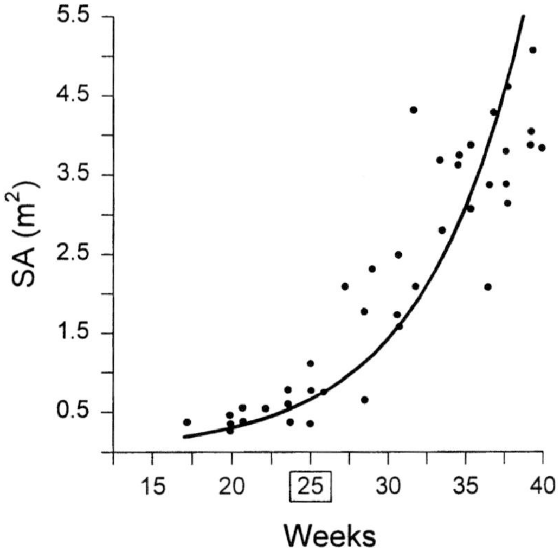

Figure 3 The results of a careful study showing the quantitative relation between gas exchange surface area (SA) and gestational age in humans. (From Ref. 69.)

physiological limitations of the immature vascular bed that predispose the premature lung to vascular injury.

There is smooth muscle in more peripheral branches of fetal lung blood vessels compared with limited distribution of smooth muscle in newborn lung at term. The tone of vascular smooth-muscle cells maintains the normally high pulmonary vascular resistance of the fetus and sustains the fetal circulatory shunt through the foramen ovale, but persistence of a high pulmonary vascular tone in the newborn is abnormal. Failure of the normal postnatal fall in pulmonary vascular resistance results in cyanosis and pulmonary hypertension, which may be fatal or produce lasting morphological injuries to the lung circulation.

Regulation of smooth-muscle tone by endothelial cell production of nitric oxide (NO), coupled with the potent effect of NO to relax vascular smooth muscle (70), is one important mechanism regulating pulmonary vascular resistance. Two developmentally regulated conditions may cause failure of this vasoregulatory system. Responsiveness of the immature vascular bed to the vasodilating effects of NO is delayed until the later stages of development; therefore, hyporesponsiveness to NO is present in the immature circulation. Second, there may be immaturity of the NO-producing enzyme system in the endothelial cells, which reduces NO availability.

A second physiological mechanism controlling lung vascular tone is the production and release of prostaglandins (PGs), especially prostacyclin (PGI_2).

The physiological role of PGI_2 to regulate lung blood flow after birth is clear enough, but its role in the pathophysiology of persistent pulmonary hypertension is not established (70).

The distensibility and structural integrity of blood vessel walls are partly determined by the extracellular matrix secreted by vascular cells. Fibroblast production of elastin is particularly interesting because it is highly upregulated late in lung development and accumulates during childhood, but de novo synthesis of elastin is nearly absent in the adult lung (72). We know that vessel wall elastin is abnormal in patients with BPD (73) and that abnormal elastolysis is part of the cause of vessel wall injury in some models of pulmonary vascular injury (74). Additionally, abnormal deposition of other supporting matrix molecules (e.g., collagen; 75) have been demonstrated in animal models. More work is required with the immature lung to understand its response to premature birth. The elegant primate model of BPD is attractive for its relevance to the premature infant (76).

C. Surfactant

A well-understood biochemical event that occurs at the limits of viability of the premature infant is the onset of surfactant production. Human lung tissue initiates surfactant lipid production early, compared with many other mammals, at about 60% of gestation or the beginning of the terminal sac stage (77). Certainly, the immature lung is vulnerable to injury owing to surfactant deficiencies (see Chap. 21). Air breathing creates demands on surfactant production that may exceed the immature epithelium's productive capacity. Diffuse alveolar collapse, hypoxemia, edema, and inflammation will result if surfactant is depleted, and these herald the onset of neonatal respiratory distress. The clinical success of replacement therapy for surfactant confirms that surfactant deficiency is a cause of respiratory distress in the premature infant, as proposed by Avery and Mead (78).

D. Extracellular Matrix

Structural Roles

The newborn lung has far less structural extracellular matrix (mainly collagens and elastin) than the adult lung has (79,80; see Chap. 28). The number of cells per unit lung weight in the adult human lung is only 30% of the number of cells in the 17-week fetal lung, but the adult has 11 times more collagen (81). Less structural matrix in the immature lung places it at risk of physical damage from stresses imposed by air breathing, especially the demands of mechanical ventilation. Interstitial emphysema, pneumothorax, and air emboli are the consequences of a lessened ability of the immature lung to resist mechanical stretch. Possibly a key region of injury in the very immature lung is the bronchoalveolar junction

(8), where the hypercompliant immature airways are joined to the noncompliant parenchyma.

Nonstructural Roles

Extracellular matrix has major nonmechanical roles, such as programming development, because of its effects on cellular processes. The cellular consequences of immaturity of the nonstructural matrix are difficult to report succinctly, but a few general effects should be considered.

Figure 4 schematically shows a few of the many known cell–matrix interactions. For example, the abundant extracellular matrix molecule fibronectin is capable of mediating migration, differentiation, and proliferation of epithelial cells when analyzed in cell culture systems. The critical importance to development of fibronectin was confirmed by genetic engineering of a mouse that lacks fibronectin. Animals with this defect fail to develop (82). The responses of cells in contact with fibronectin is mediated by a family of heteromeric cell surface receptors, the integrins (83).

Adding to the richness of matrix effects is the example that fibronectin–cell interactions are modulated by other matrix molecules. Tenascin is one example of an extracellular matrix molecule that is capable of modifying the actions of fibronectin on cells, possibly by physically covering critical domains of the fi-

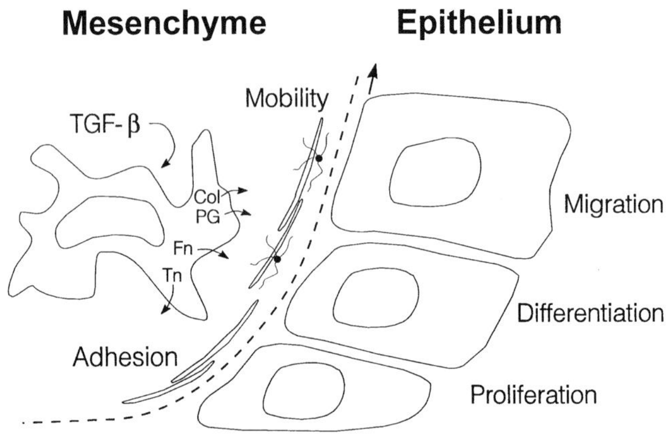

Figure 4 Schematic of a selected few of many reported interactions between extracellular matrix and the cells of developing tissues: in this scheme, which emphasizes the effects of TGF-β, epithelial cells are instructed by extracellular matrix proteins secreted by mesenchyme, and these interactions control cellular migration, differentiation, and proliferation.

bronectin dimer (84). Tenascin also interacts directly with cells by binding to integrins.

At all points in development, there are examples of highly coordinated events that govern the maturation of the animal or of a particular organ. The timing of expression of extracellular matrix molecules, their interactions with the cells by way of surface receptors, and the responses of the cells are all dependent on the conditions present at any particular moment in gestation. We know from animal experiments that the proper sequence of gestationally timed events is important to the outcome of development. We can predict that interference with this timing by premature birth, mechanical injury, environmental injury, drugs, infections, or other, will interfere with the development of a normal lung. Exploitation of new models and the use of drugs or gene manipulations to alter expression of extracellular matrix molecules should uncover useful information about cell–matrix interactions that might be important in the clinical care of the premature neonate.

E. Antioxidant Enzymes

The ability of the neonate to tolerate the extrauterine environment, which is hyperoxic relative to the intrauterine environment, is partly dependent on enzyme systems that can detoxify reactive products of oxygen metabolism (85–88). The developmental profile of rat lung antioxidant enzyme activity was reported by Tanswell and Freeman (87). The normal developmental profile of human whole-lung antioxidant enzyme activity is less understood than that of laboratory animals. Cell-specific data would be of use because there likely is a unique developmental profile for each different lung tissue compartment. Knowledge of the details of such cell-specific events may be crucial to assigning a hierarchy of importance to the acquisition of properties, such as antioxidant enzyme activities, and may benefit plans to target therapeutic supplementation to cell-specific locations.

Other antioxidant defenses include vitamins A, E, and C, ceruloplasm, and glutathione (86). Lung tissue levels of these antioxidants may be relatively low in the premature lung, and this may further weaken the tolerance to oxidant stress of the immature lung.

F. Host Defense

Macrophages

A main cellular defender of the lung, the macrophage, is present in low numbers at term and is even more severely reduced in the immature lung (see Chap. 33). Data from premature primate lungs illustrate some interesting correlations (89). Premature lungs of monkeys (*Macaca nemestrina*, about 85% gestation) had less than 25% as many lavageable alveolar macrophages as term animals had. Eighteen hours after birth there was normally a tenfold expansion of the alveolar macrophage population in both premature and term animals. Lavageable macrophages did not increase postnatally in premature monkeys that had hyaline membrane disease, but a causal relation between macrophage numbers and protection against lung injury was not established. Macrophages from rabbit neonates have a less well-developed oxidative postphagocytic metabolic response (90) than that of adult lung macrophages. Preterm rabbits exposed to an aerosol of group B streptococci had a sixfold greater proliferation of the microbes in their lungs than did term rabbit pups (91). More human experimentation of lung cellular defense is needed to confirm the predictions of the animal data.

Noncellular Defense

An exciting new research direction has developed with expanded knowledge of the non–surface-tension lowering properties of surfactant, although the therapeutic importance of the observations in this field remains to be determined.

Early work demonstrated that surfactant acted as an opsonin (92) and that it had bactericidal properties (93). Several reports suggest an effect on alveolar macrophage killing of organisms (94–96), although this property has not always been confirmed (97). The phospholipids of surfactant can downregulate the immune response, as reported by Ansfield and Benson (98,99). They noted inhibition of the proliferative response of lymphocytes to pokeweed mitogen when cells were incubated in the presence of surfactant lipids. This was true whether the lipids were extracted from natural sources or were synthetic. Recent in vitro experiments with surfactants that have been used for clinical support of premature infants (100) also showed effects of surfactant lipids. In these experiments, the release of inflammatory cytokines (IL-1, IL-6, and TNF-α) by human alveolar macrophages was inhibited by the lipid component(s) of the surfactants. Thus, the surfactant lipids may have anti-inflammatory actions in the alveolar space. One possible benefit to the lung of limiting the intrapulmonary inflammatory response would be to control or inhibit the leakage of serum into the interstitial and alveolar spaces, because such fluid accumulations would interfere with gas exchange.

Two of the surfactant-associated proteins may also play an immunoregulatory role in defense of the alveolar space against infectious agents. SP-A and SP-D are members of a family of proteins that bind carbohydrates (lectins) in a calcium-dependent manner and share structural features with other members of this C-lectin group, C1q and mannose-binding protein (MBP). Their immunomodulating properties are part of a non–cellular, non–antibody-mediated immune system termed the innate system. This primitive system may be designed for protection against environmental agents and has been proposed to play important roles in host defense, including opsonization of particles that enhances their phagocytosis, as well as enhanced killing of infectious organisms by macrophages. This subject has been reviewed (101).

SP-A binds specifically to macrophages (95) and will serve as an opsonin to several pathogenic organisms, including *Escherichia coli, Pseudomonas aeruginosa*, and *Staphylococcus aureus* (102). A surface glycoprotein of *Pneumocystis carinii* is a ligand for SP-A (103) and SP-A may serve as an opsonin to herpes simplex virus (104). SP-D binds *E. coli* and agglutinates the bacteria (105). These properties suggest a role for the lectin-type surfactant proteins in the lung's defense against several important pathogens. Because the development of surfactant protein metabolism is delayed into late gestation, these immunomodulatory properties of the proteins may be missing in the immature newborn.

Protease–Antiprotease

The balance of proteases and antiproteases in the lung has been established as a critical factor in the development of emphysema. When the major antiprotease, α_1-antitrypsin, is severely deficient in the serum, there is consequent damage to lung elastin over the early decades of life. Replacement of the missing antiprotease has logical support, but there are no convincing data to indicate benefit toward preventing the development of emphysema. A role for the balance of protease–antiprotease enzyme activities in the production or prevention of disease in the premature lung remains speculative.

The human fetus acquires nearly adult levels of serum α_1-antitrypsin at about 26 weeks gestation (106), but lung fluid measurements of this antiprotease in the normal fetus are unavailable. Measurements of α_1-antitrypsin in tracheal secretions of 26 intubated term and preterm infants was reported by Merritt and co-workers (91). Macrophages, neutrophils, and elastase activity increased, and antiprotease activity decreased in the tracheal aspirates of infants who subsequently had chronic lung disease. Evidence for elastolysis and the occurrence of emphysema-like lesions in BPD suggest that protease inhibitors might be applied as effective therapy of this condition (73,107,108). Secretory leukocyte protease inhibitor (SLPI; see foregoing) is another possibly important protector against structural damage to the lung during inflammation. In one study of low birth weight (less than 2000 g) infants (61), the tracheal aspirate concentration of SLPI increased postnatally in all patients, but in those with BPD, the neutrophil counts and elastase activity were higher. The authors concluded that a less favorable protease–antiprotease balance resulted. There is a need for a controlled therapeutic trial to determine the practical importance of the protective role of lung antiproteases in the development of BPD.

G. Cellular Pumps

One of the several functions attributed to the alveolar type II cell is that of fluid and electrolyte balance in the alveolar space. In the immature lung, epithelial transport of salt and water is probably important for normal growth, as well as for maintaining a dry airspace after birth (109; see Chap. 29). Because net lung fluid production during development is likely critical for lung growth (110), and net fluid absorption occurs after birth, there is a need for a developmentally regulated set of fluid and electrolyte pumps. Some of the complexities of these cellular pumps have been discovered in animal studies (111–115).

Sodium ion transport by at least two mechanisms (amiloride-sensitive channels and Na^+, K^+-ATPase) is important in fetal and adult lung, including adult human lung. Secretion of Cl^- into the lumen of the immature lung is also an important mechanism (113). Each of these transport mechanisms shows developmental dependency. Preparation for birth includes downregulation of the Cl^- channel(s) and upregulation of the Na^+ channel(s), which switches the lung from net fluid production to net fluid absorption. Premature birth leaves these "systems" in a potentially unfavorable condition that may promote formation of fetal lung liquid, whereas the poorly developed lung may lack normal Na^+ transport out of the airway lumen. The consequences could include pulmonary edema or obstructing airway secretions.

H. Metabolic Preparation for Birth

Lung lipid metabolism has been studied extensively (116) with the knowledge that surfactant is lipid-rich. The gestational acquisition of metabolic pathways for the production of saturated phospholipids and their secretion by the lung epithelium is well documented. It is clear that survival of the infant is correlated with the onset of surfactant lipid production.

Lung intermediary metabolism (the sum of all enzyme activities) is poorly studied, but in most ways, lung tissue metabolism appears similar to that of other tissues (117). Carbohydrate (mainly glucose) is the main energy source for the lung, and its metabolism by aerobic and anerobic pathways may be especially important to the maintenance of energy-demanding functions, such as maintenance of the membrane salt and water pumps.

References

1. Frank L. Preparation for birth. In: Hodson WA, ed. Development of the Lung. New York: Marcel Dekker, 1977:1141–1197.
2. Hodson WA, ed. Development of the Lung. New York: Marcel Dekker, 1977.
3. McGowan SE. Extracellular matrix and the regulation of lung development and repair [review]. FASEB J 1992; 6:2895–2904.

4. Minoo P, King RJ. Epithelial–mesenchymal interactions in lung development [review]. Annu Rev Physiol 1994; 56:13–45.
5. Taderera JV. Control of lung differentiation in vitro. Dev Biol 1967; 16:489–512.
6. Spooner BS, Wessells NK. Mammalian lung development: interactions in primordium formation and bronchial morphogenesis. J Exp Zool 1970; 175:445–454.
7. Boyden EA. Development and growth of the airways. In: Hodson WA, ed. Development of the Lung. New York: Marcel Dekker, 1977:3–35.
8. Frank L. Pathophysiology of lung injury and repair: special features of the immature lung. In: Polin RA, Fox WW, eds. Fetal and Neonatal Physiology. Philadelphia: WB Saunders, 1992:914–926.
9. Stocker JT. The respiratory tract. In: Stocker JT, Dehner LP, eds. Pediatric Pathology. Philadelphia: JB Lippincott, 1992:505–574.
10. Raeburn D, Giembycz MA, eds. Airways Smooth Muscle: Structure, Innervation and Neurotransmission. Basel: Birkhauser Verlag, 1994.
11. Raeburn D, Giembycz MA, eds. Airways smooth muscle: Development, and Regulation of contractility. Basel: Birkhauser Verlag, 1994.
12. Coleridge HM, Coleridge JC. Pulmonary reflexes: neural mechanisms of pulmonary defense [review]. Annu Rev Physiol 1994; 56:69–91.
13. Drazen JM, Gaston B, Shore SA. Chemical regulation of pulmonary airway tone [review]. Annu Rev Physiol 1995; 57:151–170.
14. Sparrow MP, Warwick SP, Everett AW. Innervation and function of the distal airways in the developing bronchial tree of the fetal pig. Am J Respir Cell Mol Biol 1995; 13:518–525.
15. Cutz E. Cytomorphology and differentiation of airway epithelium in developing human lung. In: McDowell EM, ed. Lung Carcinomas. New York: Churchill Livingstone, 1987:1–41.
16. Jeffery PK, Gaillard D, Moret S. Human airway secretory cells during development and in mature airway epithelium [review]. Eur Respir J 1992; 5:93–104.
17. Johnson DE. Pulmonary neuroendocrine cells. In: Farmer SG, Hay DWP, eds. The Airway Epithelium: Physiology, Pathophysiology, and Pharmacology. New York: Marcel Dekker, 1990:335–400.
18. Sorokin SP, Hoyt RF Jr. Workshop on pulmonary neuroendocrine cells in health and disease. Anat Rec 1993; 236:1–174.
19. Hoyt RF Jr, McNelly NA, McDowell EM, Sorokin SP. Neuroepithelial bodies stimulate proliferation of airway epithelium in fetal hamster lung. Am J Physiol 1991; 260:L234–L240.
20. Aguayo SM, Schuyler WE, Murtagh JJ Jr, Roman J. Regulation of lung branching morphogenesis by bombesin-like peptides and neutral endopeptidase. Am J Respir Cell Mol Biol 1994; 10:635–642.
21. Li K, Nagalla SR, Spindel ER. A rhesus monkey model to characterize the role of gastrin-releasing peptide (GRP) in lung development. Evidence for stimulation of airway growth. J Clin Invest 1994; 94:1605–1615.
22. King KA, Torday JS, Sunday ME. Bombesin and [Leu8]phyllolitorin promote fetal mouse lung branching morphogenesis via a receptor-mediated mechanism. Proc Natl Acad Sci USA 1995; 92:4357–4361.
23. Gillan JE, Cutz E. Abnormal pulmonary bombesin immunoreactive cells in Wil-

son–Mikity syndrome (pulmonary dysmaturity) and bronchopulmonary dysplasia. Pediatr Pathol 1993; 13:165–180.
24. Johnson DE, Anderson WR, Burke BA. Pulmonary neuroendocrine cells in pediatric lung disease: alterations in airway structure in infants with bronchopulmonary dysplasia. Anat Rec 1993; 236:115–119.
25. Perrin DG, McDonald TJ, Cutz E. Hyperplasia of bombesin-immunoreactive pulmonary neuroendocrine cells and neuroepithelial bodies in sudden infant death syndrome. Pediatr Pathol 1991; 11:431–447.
26. Nadel JA. Neurogenic inflammation in airways and its modulation by peptidases [review]. Ann NY Acad Sci 1992; 664:408–414.
27. Sunday ME, Hua J, Torday JS, Reyes B, Shipp MA. CD10/neutral endopeptidase 24.11 in developing human fetal lung. Patterns of expression and modulation of peptide-mediated proliferation. J Clin Invest 1992; 90:2517–2525.
28. King KA, Hua J, Torday JS, Drazen JM, Graham SA, Shipp MA, Sunday, ME. CD10/neutral endopeptidase 24.11 regulates fetal lung growth and maturation in utero by potentiating endogenous bombesin-like peptides [see comments]. J Clin Invest 1993; 91:1969–1973.
29. Lilly CM, Kobzik L, Hall AE, Drazen JM. Effects of chronic airway inflammation on the activity and enzymatic inactivation of neuropeptides in guinea pig lungs. J Clin Invest 1994; 93:2667–2674.
30. Harrison NK, Dawes KE, Kwon OJ, Barnes PJ, Laurent GJ, Chung KF. Effects of neuropeptides on human lung fibroblast proliferation and chemotaxis. Am J Physiol 1995; 268:L278–L283.
31. Choi HS, Lesser M, Cardozo C, Orlowski M. Immunohistochemical localization of endopeptidase 24.15 in rat trachea, lung tissue, and alveolar macrophages. Am J Respir Cell Mol Biol 1990; 3:619–624.
32. Mercer RR, Russell ML, Roggli VL, Crapo JD. Cell number and distribution in human and rat airways. Am J Respir Cell Mol Biol 1994; 10:613–624.
33. Jeffery PK, Reid LM. Ultrastructure of airway epithelium and submucosal gland during development. In: Hodson WA, ed. Development of the Lung. New York: Marcel Dekker, 1977:87–134.
34. Sturgess JM. Ontogeny of the bronchial mucosa. Am Rev Respir Dis 1985; 131: S4–7.
35. Gaillard DA, Lallement AV, Petit AF, Puchelle ES. In vivo ciliogenesis in human fetal tracheal epithelium. Am J Anat 1989; 185:415–428.
36. Plopper CG, Alley JL, Weir AJ. Differentiation of tracheal epithelium during fetal lung maturation in the rhesus monkey *Macaca mulatta*. Am J Anat 1986; 175:59–71.
37. Breuer R, Zajicek G, Christensen TG, Lucey EC, Snider GL. Cell kinetics of normal adult hamster bronchial epithelium in the steady state. Am J Respir Cell Mol Biol 1990; 2:51–58.
38. Evans MJ, Cox RA, Shami SG, Wilson B, Plopper CG. The role of basal cells in attachment of columnar cells to the basal lamina of the trachea. Am J Respir Cell Mol Biol 1989; 1:463–469.
39. Barth PJ, Wolf M, Ramaswamy A. Distribution and number of Clara cells in the normal and disturbed development of the human fetal lung. Pediatr Pathol 1994; 14:637–651.

40. Basbaum CB, Jany B, Finkbeiner WE. The serous cell [review]. Annu Rev Physiol 1990; 52:97–113.
41. Revenis ME, Kaliner MA. Lactoferrin and lysozyme deficiency in airway secretions: association with the development of bronchopulmonary dysplasia. J Pediatr 1992; 121:262–270.
42. Daniele RP. Immunoglobulin secretion in the airways [review]. Annu Rev Physiol 1990; 52:177–195.
43. Rankin JA. Pulmonary immunology. Clin Chest Med 1988; 9:387–393.
44. Nelson DJ, McMenamin C, McWilliam AS, Brenan M, Holt PG. Development of the airway intraepithelial dendritic cell network in the rat from class II major histocompatibility (Ia)-negative precursors: differential regulation of Ia expression at different levels of the respiratory tract. J Exp Med 1994; 179:203–212.
45. Christensen PJ, Armstrong LR, Fak JJ, Chen GH, McDonald RA, Toews GB, Paine RI. Regulation of rat pulmonary dendritic cell immunostimulatory activity by alveolar epithelial cell-derived granulocyte macrophage colony-stimulating factor. Am J Respir Cell Mol Biol 1995; 13:426–433.
46. Watts CL, Bruce MC. Comparison of secretory component for immunoglobulin A with albumin as reference proteins in tracheal aspirate from preterm infants. J Pediatr 1995; 127:113–122.
47. Smith JJ, Travis SM, Greenberg EP, Welsh MJ. Cystic fibrosis airway epithelia fail to kill bacteria because of abnormal airway surface fluid. Cell 1996; 85:1–20.
48. Goldman MJ, Anderson GM, Stolzenberg ED. Human beta-defensin-1 is a salt-sensitive antibiotic in lung that is inactivated in cystic fibrosis. Cell 1997; 88:553–560.
49. Ganz T, Leherer RI. Antimicrobial peptides of leukocytes. Curr Opin Hematol 1997; 4:53–58.
50. Ganz T, Selsted ME, Szklarek D, Harwig SS, Daher K, Bainton DF, Leherer RI. Defensins: natural peptide antibiotics of human neutrophils. J Clin Invest 1985; 76: 1427–1435.
51. Sherman MP, Ganz T. Host defense in pulmonary alveoli. Annu Rev Physiol 1992; 54:331–350.
52. Huttner KM, Ouellette AJ. A family of defensin-like genes codes for diverse cysteine-rich peptides in mouse paneth cells. Genome 1994; 24:99–109.
53. Jones DE, Bevins CL. Paneth cells of the human small intestine express an antimicrobial peptide gene. J Biol Chem 1992; 267:23216–23225.
54. Selsted ME, Miller SI, Henschen AH, Ouellette AJ. Enteric defensins: antibiotic peptide components of intestinal host defense. J Cell Biol 1992; 118:929–936.
55. Diamond G, Jones DE, Bevins CL. Airway epithelial cells are the site of expression of a mammalian antimicrobial peptide gene. Proc Natl Acad Sci USA 1993; 90: 4596–4600.
56. Diamond G, Zatuchni J, Eck H, Brattain DE, Maloy WL, Bevins CL. Tracheal antimicrobial peptide, a cysteine-rich peptide from mammalian tracheal mucosa: peptide isolation and cloning of a cDNA. Proc Natl Acad Sci USA 1991; 88:3952–3956.
57. Brogden KA, De Lucca AJ, Bland J, Elliott S. Isolation of an ovine pulmonary

surfactant-associated anionic peptide bactericidal for *Pasteurella haemolytica*. Proc Natl Acad Sci USA 1996; 93:412–416.
58. Bensch K, Raida M, Magert H-J, Schulz-Knappe P, Forssmann W-G. A novel b-defensin from human plasma. FEBS Lett 1995; 368:331–335.
59. Harder J, Bartels J, Christophers E, Schroder J-M. A peptide antibiotic from human skin. Nature 1997; 387:861.
60. McCray PB, Bentley L. Human airway epithelia express a beta-defensin. Am J Respir Cell Mol Biol 1997; 16:343–349.
61. Watterberg KL, Carmichael DF, Gerdes JS, Werner S, Backstrom C, Murphy S. Secretory leukocyte protease inhibitor and lung inflammation in developing bronchopulmonary dysplasia. J Pediatr 1994; 125:264–269.
62. Phipps RJ, Abraham WM, Mariassy AT, Torrealba PJ, Sielczak MW, Ahmed A, McCray M, Stevenson JS, Wanner A. Developmental changes in the tracheal mucociliary system in neonatal sheep. J Appl Physiol 1989; 67:824–832.
63. Cohn LA, Kinnula VL, Adler KB. Antioxidant properties of guinea pig tracheal epithelial cells in vitro. Am J Physiol 1994; 266:L397–L404.
64. Charan NB, Carvalho PG. Anatomy of the normal bronchial circulatory system in humans and animals. In: Butler J, ed. The Bronchial Circulation. New York: Marcel Dekker 1992:45–78.
65. Pearse DB, Wagner EM. Role of the bronchial circulation in ischemia–reperfusion lung injury. J Appl Physiol 1994; 76:259–265.
66. Arakawa H, Tokuyama K, Yokoyama T, Mochizuki H, Morikawa A, Kuroume T, Barnes PJ. Effect of maturation on histamine-induced airflow obstruction and airway microvascular leakage in guinea pig airways. Eur J Pharmacol 1992; 215:51–56.
67. Tokuyama K, Yokoyama T, Morikawa A, Mochizuki H, Kuroume T, Barnes PJ. Attenuation of tachykinin-induced airflow obstruction and microvascular leakage in immature airways. Br J Pharmacol 1993; 108:23–29.
68. Arakawa H, Lotvall J, Kawikova I, Tokuyama K, Lofdahl CG, Skoogh BE. Effect of maturation on airway plasma exudation induced by eicosanoids in guinea pig. Eur J Pharmacol 1994; 259:251–257.
69. Langston C, Kida K, Reed M, Thurlbeck WM. Human lung growth in late gestation and in the neonate. Am Rev Respir Dis 1984; 129:607–613.
70. Morin FC 3rd, Stenmark KR. Persistent pulmonary hypertension of the newborn [review]. Am J Respir Crit Care Med 1995; 151:2010–2032.
71. Hislop A, Reid LM. Formation of the pulmonary vasculature. In: Hodson WA, ed. Development of the Lung. New York: Marcel Dekker, 1977:37–86.
72. Bruce MC, Lo P-Y. A morphometric quantitation of developmental changes in elastic fibers in rat lung paryenchyma: variability with lung region and postnatal age. J Lab Clin Med 1991; 117:226–233.
73. Margraf LR, Tomashefski JF, Bruce MC, Dahms BB. Morphometric analysis of the lung in bronchopulmonary dysplasia. Am Rev Respir Dis 1991; 143:391–400.
74. Rabinovitch M. Investigational approaches to pulmonary hypertension [review]. Toxicol Pathol 1991; 19:458–469.
75. Tozzi CA, Christiansen DL, Poiani GJ, Riley DJ. Excess collagen in hypertensive

pulmonary arteries decreases vascular distensibility. Am J Respir Crit Care Med 1994; 149:1317–1326.
76. Coalson JJ, Winter V, deLemos RA. Decreased alveolarization in baboon survivors with bronchopulmonary dysplasia. Am J Respir Crit Care Med 1995; 152:640–646.
77. Clements JA, Tooley WH. Kinetics of surface-active material in the fetal lung. In: Hodson WA, ed. Development of the Lung. New York: Marcel Dekker, 1977:349–366.
78. Avery ME, Mead J. Surface properties in relation to atelectasis and hyaline membrane disease. Am J Dis Child 1959; 97:517–523.
79. Jackson JC, Clark JG, Standaert TA, Truog WE, Murphy JH, Juul SE, Chi EY, Hodson WA. Collagen synthesis during lung development and during hyaline membrane disease in the nonhuman primate. Am Rev Respir Dis 1990; 141:846–853.
80. Crystal RG. Lung collagen: definition, diversity, and development. Fed Proc 1974; 33:2248–2255.
81. Bradley K, McConnell-Breul S, Crystal RG. Collagen in the human lung quantitation of rates of synthesis and partial characterization and composition. J Clin Invest 1975; 55:543–550.
82. George EL, Georges-Labouesse EN, Patel-King RS, Rayburn H, Hynes RO. Defects in mesoderm, neural tube and vascular development in mouse embryos lacking fibronectin. Development 1993; 119:1079–1091.
83. Buck CA, Horwitz AF. Cell surface receptors for extracellular matrix molecules. Annu Rev Cell Biol 1987; 3:179–206.
84. Erickson HP, Bourdon MA. Tenascin: an extracellular matrix protein prominent in specialized embryonic tissues and tumors. Annu Rev Cell Biol 1989; 5:71–92.
85. Frank L, Bucher JR, Roberts RJ. Oxygen toxicity in neonatal and adult animals of various species. J Appl Physiol 1978; 45:699–704.
86. Freeman BA, Crapo JD. Free radicals and tissue injury. Lab Invest 1982; 47:412–426.
87. Tanswell AK, Freeman BA. Pulmonary antioxidant enzyme maturation in the fetal and neonatal rat I. Developmental profiles. Pediatr Res 1984; 18:584–587.
88. Tanswell AK, Freeman BA. Liposome-entrapped antioxidant enzymes prevent lethal O_2 toxicity in the newborn rat. J Appl Physiol 1987; 63:347–352.
89. Jacobs RF, Wilson CB, Palmer S, et al. Factors related to the appearance of alveolar macrophages in the developing lung. Am Rev Respir Dis 1985; 131:548–553.
90. Sherman MP, Lehrer RI. Oxidative metabolism of neonatal and adult rabbit lung macrophages stimulated with opsonized group B streptococci. Infect Immun 1985; 47:26–30.
91. Merritt TA, Cochrane CG, Holcomb K, Bohl B, Hallman M, Strayer DX, Edwards DK 3d, Gluck L. Elastase and $alpha_1$-proteinase inhibitor activity in tracheal aspirates during respiratory distress syndrome. Role of inflammation in the pathogenesis of bronchopulmonary dysplasia. J Clin Invest 1983; 72:656–666.
92. O'Neill SJ, Lesperance E, Klass DJ. Human lung lavage surfactant enhances staphylococcal phagocytosis by alveolar macrophages. Am Rev Respir Dis 1984; 130:1177–1179.

93. Coonrod JD, Lester RL, Hsu LC. Characterization of the extracellular bactericidal factors of rat alveolar lining material. J Clin Invest 1984; 74:1269–1279.
94. Juers JA, Rogers RM, McCurdy JB, Cook WW. Enhancement of bactericidal capacity of alveolar macrophages by human alveolar lining material [abstr]. J Clin Invest 1976; 58:271–275.
95. Pison U, Wright JR, Hawgood S. Specific binding of surfactant protein SP-A to rat alveolar macrophages. Am J Physiol 1992; 262:L412–L417.
96. O'Neill SJ, Lesperance E, Klass DJ. Rat lung lavage surfactant enhances bacterial phagocytosis and intracellular killing by alveolar macrophages. Am Rev Respir Dis 1984; 130:225–230.
97. Jonsson S, Musher DM, Goree A, Lawrence EC. Human alveolar lining material and antibacterial defenses. Am Rev Respir Dis [abstr]. 1986; 133:136–140.
98. Ansfield MJ, Benson BJ, Kaltreider HB. Immunosuppression by surface-active material: lack of species specificity [abstr]. Am Rev Respir Dis 1979; 120:949–952.
99. Benson BJ, Dobbs LG, Ansfield MJ. Immunopharmacology of lung surfactant. In: Newball HH, ed. Immunopharmacology of the Lung. New York: Marcel Dekker, 1985:209–241.
100. Thomassen MJ, Meeker DP, Antal JM, Connors MJ, Wiedemann HP. Synthetic surfactant (Exosurf) inhibits endotoxin-stimulated cytokine secretion by human alveolar macrophages. Am J Respir Cell Mol Biol 1992; 7:257–260.
101. Wright JR. Immunomodulatory functions of surfactant. Physiol Rev 1997; 77:931–962.
102. Manz-Keinke H, Plattner H, Schlepper-Schafer J. Lung surfactant protein A (SP-A) enhances serum-independent phagocytosis of bacteria by alveolar macrophages. Eur J Cell Biol 1992; 57:95–100.
103. Zimmerman PE, Voelker DR, McCormack FX, Paulsrud JR, Martin WJ. 120-kD surface glycoprotein of *Pneumocystis carinii* is a ligand for surfactant protein A. J Clin Invest 1992; 89:143–149.
104. Van Iwaarden JF, Van Strijp JAG, Ebskamp MJM, Welmers AC, Verhoef J, Van Golde LMG. Surfactant protein A is an opsonin in the phagocytosis of herpes simplex virus type 1 by rat alveolar macrophages. Am J Physiol 1993; 261:L204–L209.
105. Kuan S-F, Rust K, Crouch E. Interactions of surfactant protein D with bacterial lipopolysaccharides. J Clin Invest 1993; 90:97–106.
106. Gitlin D, Biasucci A. Development of gamma G, gamma A, gamma M, beta IC-beta IA, Cl esterase inhibitor, ceruloplasmin, transferrin, hemopexin, haptoglobin, fibrinogen, plasminogen, alpha$_1$-antitrypsin, orosomucoid, beta-lipoprotein, alpha$_2$-macroglobulin, and prealbumin in the human conceptus. J Clin Invest 1969; 48: 1433–1446.
107. Sanderson RJ, Gaddy L, Parra S, Takaro T. Alterations in stress distributions around interalveolar pores after exposure to papain in dogs. Am Rev Respir Dis 1981; 123: 327–332.
108. Poiani GJ, Greco M, Choe JK, Fox JD, Riley DJ. Liposome encapsulation improves the effect of antifibrotic agent in rat lung fibrosis. Am J Respir Crit Care Med 1994; 150:1623–1627.

109. Bland RD, Nielson DW. Developmental changes in lung epithelial ion transport and liquid movement. [review]. Annu Rev Physiol 1992; 54:373–394.
110. Wigglesworth JS. Pathology of the lung in the fetus and neonate, with particular reference to problems of growth and maturation. Histopathology 1987; 11:671–689.
111. Brown MJ, Olver RE, Ramsden CA, Strang LB, Walters DV. Effects of adrenaline and of spontaneous labour on the secretion and absorption of lung liquid in the fetal lamb. J Physiol 1983; 344:137–152.
112. O'Brodovich H, Canessa C, Ueda J, Rafii B, Rossier BC, Edelson J. Expression of the epithelial Na^+ channel in the developing rat lung. Am J Physiol 1993; 265: C491–C496.
113. Murray CB, Morales MM, Flotte TR, McGrath-Morrow SA, Guggino WB, Zeitlin PL. CIC-2: a developmentally dependent chloride channel expressed in the fetal lung and downregulated after birth. Am J Respir Cell Mol Biol 1995; 12:597–604.
114. Sakuma T, Okaniwa G, Nakada T, Nishimura T, Fujimura S, Matthay MA. Alveolar fluid clearance in the resected human lung [see comments]. Am J Respir Crit Care Med 1994; 150:305–310.
115. Tchepichev S, Ueda J, Canessa C, Rossier BC, O'Brodovich H. Lung epithelial Na channel subunits are differentially regulated during development and by steroids. Am J Physiol 1995; 269:C805–C812.
116. Rooney SA. The surfactant system and lung phospholipid biochemistry. Am Rev Respir Dis 1985; 131:439–460.
117. Tierney DF, Young SL. Glucose and intermediate metabolism of the lungs. In: Fishman AP, Fisher AB, eds. Handbook of Physiology—The Respiratory System. Bethesda, MD: American Physiology Society, 1985:255–275.

19

Hormonal Effects on Lung Maturation and Disease

PHILIP L. BALLARD and ROBERTA A. BALLARD

University of Pennsylvania School of Medicine
Children's Hospital of Philadelphia
Philadelphia, Pennsylvania

I. Introduction

The advances in neonatal intensive care over the past 20 years have greatly improved survival rates for all premature infants and, in particular, for infants of very low birth weight. A remaining problem, in part owing to our successes in lowering the age limits of viability, is the continuing occurrence of bronchopulmonary dysplasia (BPD) in premature infants. The incidence of BPD in infants less than 1500-g birth weight ranges from 25 to 40% in the United States, with a proportion of these infants acquiring a severe form of BPD that continues for many months or years and results in death or substantial disability associated with poor long-term neurodevelopmental outcome. A source of frustration for clinicians is the known contribution of hyperoxia and mechanical ventilation to the etiology of BPD, yet these supportive approaches are necessary for survival of infants with newborn lung disease.

There is accumulating evidence that the pathogenesis of BPD involves lung immaturity, iatrogenic damage to the lung, an inflammatory response producing additional lung injury, and a disorganized repair process (reviewed in 1). BPD is almost exclusively a disease of premature infants and is associated with occurrence of respiratory distress syndrome (RDS), emphasizing the importance of lung immaturity, which includes surfactant deficiency, inadequate structural development of alveoli and airways, and biochemical immaturity of systems, such as antioxidant and immune defenses. Support of these infants with supplemental oxygen and mechanical ventilation provides additional injury and induces an inflammatory process that involves both activation of macrophages and influx of neutrophils. Products of these cells, including proteases, phospholipases, and reactive oxygen and nitric oxide metabolites, further damage the lung by inactivating surfactant, altering lipids and proteins that affect various cell functions, and producing capillary leak that results in proteinaceous pulmonary edema. The consequences of this inflammatory process are abnormal cell proliferation, scarring and altered lung architecture, and in more severe cases, bronchoconstriction and pulmonary hypertension. Surviving infants often have marked disability, with an increased incidence of infection from respiratory syncytial virus (RSV), bronchiolitis, reactive airway disease, and long-term oxygen dependence, in addition to cardiac, renal, nutritional, and psychosocial problems.

As lung immaturity is a consistent feature of the occurrence and pathogenesis of BPD, some strategies for prevention of this disease have focused on approaches to accelerate lung development before premature delivery. This chapter reviews clinical and experimental results related to prenatal hormonal treatments, focusing on the recent studies of combined thyroid hormone and glucocorticoid therapy. Several possible mechanisms for the observed effects of combined treatment in experimental models are discussed.

II. Prenatal Corticosteroid Therapy and Newborn Lung Disease

Liggins was the first to observe accelerated pulmonary maturation after administration of glucocorticoids to fetal sheep (2). He was also the first to report a decreased incidence of RDS in infants after antenatal corticosteroid therapy (2,3). Since 1972, more than 25 randomized trials of antenatal corticosteroids have been performed and have established several statistically significant benefits for infant outcome, in particular decreased incidence of RDS, intraventricular hemorrhage and death, and better response to surfactant replacement (4). Corticosteroid therapy also may reduce the incidence of patent ductus arteriosus and necrotizing enterocolitis (5). These effects of glucocorticoid treatment are consistent with the concept that endogenous corticosteroids modulate differentiation of many fetal tissues and that increased levels of cortisol associated with fetal stress help to prepare the fetus for premature birth (reviewed in 6). The NIH Consensus Conference on the *Effect of Corticosteroids for Fetal Maturation on Perinatal Outcomes*, which was held in 1994, concluded that ''antenatal corticosteroid therapy is indicated for women at risk of premature delivery with few exceptions and will result in a substantial decrease in neonatal morbidity and mortality, as well as substantial savings in health care costs. The use of antenatal corticosteroids for fetal maturation is a rare example of a technology that yields substantial cost savings in addition to improving health'' (5).

The influence of this therapy on BPD is less certain. Doyle (7) first reported a decreased incidence of BPD after corticosteroid treatment (15 vs. 21% in the no-treatment group) in a cohort of consecutive very low birth weight infants; this difference was statistically significant by multivariate analysis for confounding factors. Van Marter et al. (8) analyzed the relation between prenatal glucocorticoid therapy and BPD in a group of low birth weight infants who were originally enrolled in a trial of neonatal phenobarbital for prophylaxis of intracranial hemorrhage. In this retrospective analysis of 223 infants, the incidence of BPD 28 days after birth was 35% for infants without prenatal glucocorticoid exposure, 46% for infants with longer than 24-h exposure to corticosteroid before delivery, and 25% for those born 1–7 days after a full course of prenatal dexamethasone or betamethasone. Stratification by gender and birth weight indicated benefit in all fully treated groups except male infants who weighed less than 1000 g. More recently, Kari et al. (9) in Finland carried out what will probably be the last trial of prenatal glucocorticoids to prevent RDS using a placebo-controlled population. This study enrolled women who were in premature labor at less than 32-weeks gestation and used prenatal dexamethasone combined with postnatal rescue surfactant for infants who required oxygen and mechanical ventilation at less than 24 hr of age. In the group of infants who were delivered 1–14 days after glucocorticoid therapy, there was a significant reduction in RDS, need for surfactant therapy, and intraventricular hemorrhage. Adverse outcome, defined as death or BPD, was less frequent in those infants whose mothers received dexamethasone, but the differences were not statistically significant. In a relatively small subpopulation of these infants ($\leq$ 30 weeks gestation), significantly more treated infants survived at 28 days without severe BPD (22/26) compared with the placebo group (9/19, $p = 0.02$). These findings underscore the benefits of prenatal corticosteroid therapy in reducing the incidence of RDS in the era of replacement surfactant and support the possibility of better long-term pulmonary outcome.

The relation between antenatal corticosteroid therapy and BPD has also been examined using clinical data from multicenter neonatal networks. In a recent retrospective analysis of five such observational data bases, each containing clinical information on more than 1000 preterm infants, the overall incidence of BPD ranged from 17 to 44% (10). The risk for BPD among all infants was significantly reduced by any prenatal glucocorticoid treatment in only one of the five data sets. Among 28-day survivors, the incidence of BPD was significantly less for corticosteroid-treated infants in three of the data sets (unadjusted odds ratios ranged from 0.59 to 0.79). In one data set, however, there was significantly increased risk for BPD. In a recent large clinical trial, in which all women received antenatal glucocorticoid treatment, the incidence of BPD among premature infants at 28 days after birth and at 36 weeks postmenstrual age was 42 and 29%, respectively (11). These incidence figures are comparable with those cited earlier in the 1990s when antenatal corticosteroids were not routinely used.

Thus, based on both observational data and results from a limited number of clinical trials, it is still unclear whether prenatal glucocorticoid therapy has any appreciable effect on development of BPD. The apparent lack of benefit from glucocorticoid suggests that the etiology of BPD is not closely linked with the incidence and severity of RDS, both of which are reduced by glucocorticoid treatment. In an attempt to develop more efficacious strategies for prevention of both RDS and BPD, other hormonal treatments have been investigated in both experimental and clinical studies.

III. Effects of Thyroid Hormones on Lung Maturation

Several studies have addressed effects of thyroid hormones and thyrotropin-releasing hormone (TRH) on lung maturation and incidence of newborn lung disease. Initially, Wu et al. (12) found that rabbit fetuses treated with thyroxine (T_4) had better air retention, more surface-active material in lung fluid, and enhanced morphological development than saline-treated litter mates. Administration of triiodothyronine (T_3) to fetal or pregnant rats stimulated the rate of choline incorporation into phosphatidylcholine (PC) in fetal lung without a change in endogenous corticosterone concentration (13). Both T_3 and T_4 stimulate the rate of precursor incorporation into PC and phosphatidylglycerol in organ cultures of fetal rat, rabbit, and human lung, establishing that fetal lung is a direct target tissue for thyroid hormones (reviewed in 14, 15). Thyroidectomy of fetal lambs delays the developmental increase in lecithin/sphingomyelin (L/S) ratio in tracheal fluid, supporting a physiological role for endogenous thyroid hormones in surfactant lipid production (16).

Thyroid function in the human fetus begins by 10 weeks of gestation as thyroid follicles appear and T_4 and thyrotropin (TSH) become detectable in the circulation. There is a progressive increase in serum T_4 and T_3, particularly during the third trimester, secondary to both increased TRH stimulation of TSH secretion and enhanced responsiveness of the thyroid (reviewed in 17). This temporal pattern is consistent with a role for endogenous thyroid hormones in human lung differentiation.

In initial clinical studies, Mashiach et al. (18) administered intra-amniotic T_4 to women before preterm delivery and found accelerated increases in the L/S ratio in amniotic fluid compared with the normal pattern. Subsequently, Schreyer et al. (19) and Romaguera et al. (20) both attempted to accelerate fetal lung maturation by injection of T_3 into the amniotic fluid. They observed an increase in the L/S ratio of amniotic fluid after 7 days and an apparent decreased occurrence of RDS among infants born to treated women. However, all of these studies were nonrandomized, and all of the treated women had complicated pregnancies whereas the control women had uncomplicated pregnancies. To date, there have been no controlled studies of intra-amniotic administration of T_4 or T_3, and the potential clinical usefulness of this therapy for RDS or BPD is uncertain.

IV. Combined Glucocorticoid and Thyroid Hormone Treatment

When thyroid hormone and dexamethasone treatment are combined, faster and supra-additive responses occur compared with corticosteroid or thyroid hormone treatment alone. Enhanced responses involve structural, biochemical and functional lung parameters, and these have been observed both in cultured lung tissue and in animal studies.

A. Surfactant Lipid

There is good agreement in the literature that in vivo treatment with TRH plus corticosteroid increases saturated PC content and lung stability. Some of the earliest studies were carried out by Liggins and colleagues, who treated fetal sheep with various hormonal combinations. Whereas TRH or cortisol treatment alone had only modest effects, combined treatment in utero for 6 days produced severalfold increases in maximal lung volume (V40), lung stability (V5), and content of phospholipids and saturated PC in lung lavage (21). In a companion set of experiments, these workers found that the combination of cortisol and T_3 increased lung distensibility and stability, as well as lavage fluid phospholipid content, more than treatment with either hormone alone. Addition of prolactin (PRL) to the treatment regimen further increased these functional parameters, but not alveolar phospholipids (22; Fig. 1). Similar effects of fetal TRH plus cortisol treatment on lung distensibility and stability in sheep have been reported by Campos et al. (23) and confirmed by Moraga et al. (24), who treated pregnant ewes with betamethasone and TRH in a regimen comparable with that used in women.

In similar experiments using slightly older fetuses, Warburton et al. (25) found additive or synergistic effects of combined TRH and cortisol treatment on lung mechanics and both tissue and lavage content of phospholipids. Based on studies of pulmonary β-adrenergic receptor-binding sites, these workers specu-

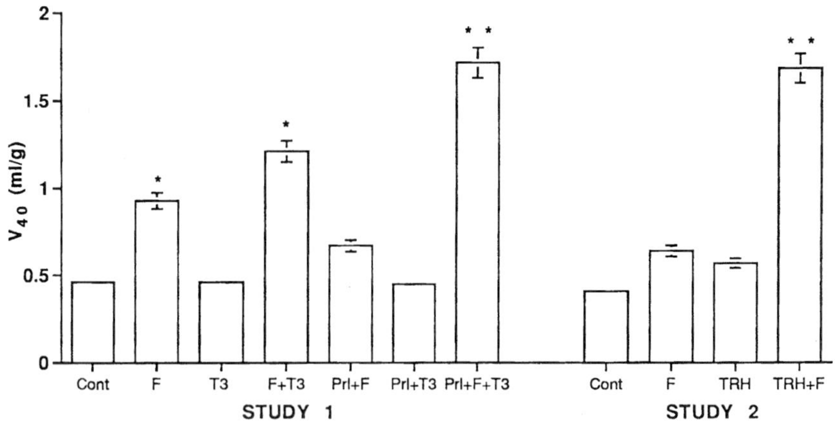

Figure 1 Lung volume at 40 cmH_2O in fetal lambs exposed to different hormone treatments: In study 1, fetuses were infused with cortisol (1 mg/hr), T_3 (25 μg/hr), ovine prolactin (30 μg/hr) or hormonal combinations for 4 days with delivery at 128 days gestation. In study 2, fetuses were infused with cortisol (1 mg/hr), TRH (25 μg/hr in 60-s pulses), or both hormones, and delivered on 128 days. Pressure volume studies were conducted on excised fetal lungs to determine lung volume. (From Refs. 22 and 21.)

lated that combined hormonal therapy may enhance adrenergic signal transduction, in addition to increasing phospholipid synthesis. Further evidence for involvement of the β-adrenergic system came from a subsequent study by Schellenburg et al. (26), who infused a β-adrenergic blocker along with TRH and cortisol, and, in so doing, prevented most of the improvement in lung mechanics and alveolar phospholipid produced by TRH plus cortisol treatment. These data support the concept that the synergistic response to combined hormonal treatment is dependent on the β-adrenergic system for maturation of lung mechanics and surfactant secretion, but not synthesis of surfactant.

These and other studies with sheep are of particular interest, because cortisol treatment of fetal sheep increases circulating levels of T_3 as a result of induction of a hepatic deiodinase, which increases conversion of T_4 to T_3, rather than reverse-T_3. Plasma concentrations of T_3 increase within 24 hr of cortisol infusion and are elevated tenfold after 3 days, reaching concentrations higher than those achieved with TRH infusion (21). This observation suggests that the response to in vivo combined treatment with cortisol plus TRH involves effects of hormones other than T_3. Given the studies of Schellenburg et al. (22), it is likely that stimulation of endogenous PRL in the fetal sheep contributes to the effect of combined therapy. Alternatively, the effects of TRH could be mediated through increases in T_4, decreased levels of reverse-T_3, or secondary to direct effects of TRH acting as a neurotransmitter.

Treatment with TRH has also been studied in rabbits, with observations generally similar to those obtained in sheep. In the first reported experiments with TRH, Rooney and colleagues (27) reported that TRH alone increased the content of saturated PC in lavage fluid, but not in lung tissue of fetal rabbits. Devaskar et al. (28,29) found that five injections of TRH to the pregnant rabbit improved fetal lung stability, but not distensibility. These experiments did not include a combined corticosteroid–TRH treatment protocol. Oulton et al. (30) examined the effects of cortisol and TRH treatment both alone and in combination, administering the steroid to the fetus and TRH intravenously to the doe. The intracellular pool of phospholipid increased to a similar extent with either hormone alone, and combined treatment produced an additive effect and also increased the percentage of PC. However, TRH treatment alone or in combination with cortisol did not significantly increase the extracellular phospholipid pool in these experiments. In studies with rats, combined treatment with TRH plus dexamethasone increased disaturated PC in fetal lung tissue more than did TRH alone (31).

The in vivo findings are supported by studies with cultured fetal lung. With either rat or human tissue (32,33), combined dexamethasone and T_3 treatment synergistically stimulates the rate of choline incorporation into PC, resulting in greater increases in choline incorporation at earlier times of exposure to hormone (Fig. 2). Furthermore, combined treatment is more effective than dexamethasone alone in stimulating type II cell cytodifferentiation, as judged by the number and size of lamellar bodies (33,34). Thus, there is a firm experimental basis for postulating effects of combined hormonal therapy on surfactant production in the human fetus.

Not all studies with prenatal TRH treatment in animals have found a positive interaction with corticosteroid treatment. For example, in studies with premature rabbit pups that were ventilated for 30 min after birth, compliance was increased with prenatal steroid therapy, but was not enhanced further by a variety of doses of TRH (35). Similar studies by the same group using sheep, found no significant effect of TRH alone or combined with corticosteroid on lung mechanics or phospholipid pools (36). These findings contrast with stimulatory effects observed by other investigators and could reflect different doses and administration regimens for TRH, or different exposures to mechanical ventilation after birth before measurements were performed. Another study in rabbits by Ikegami et al. (37) reported effects of TRH alone on compliance and ventilatory efficiency index in prematurely delivered pups, but there was no response to betamethasone alone or with TRH. The lack of steroid effect in this study may have resulted from the relatively late point in gestation (27 days) at which measurements were

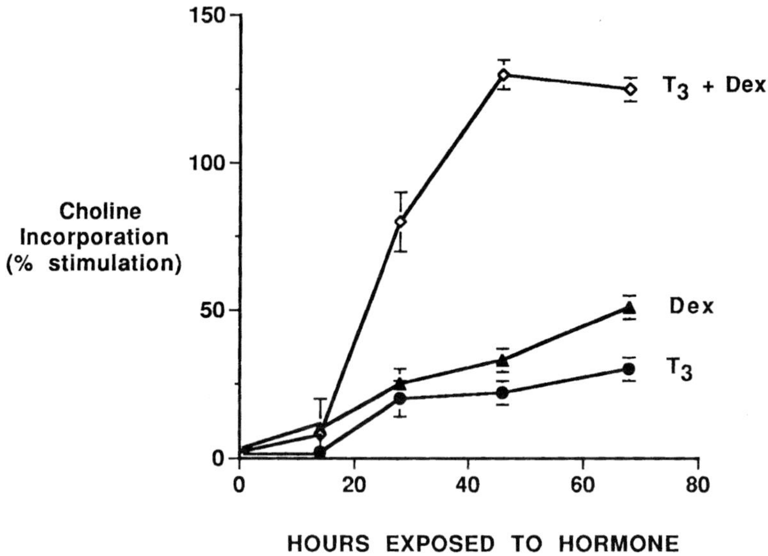

Figure 2 Interaction of dexamethasone and T_3 for stimulation of choline incorporation into PC of fetal rabbit lung: Explant of cultures from 23-day rabbit fetuses were assayed after various times exposure to T_3 (1 nM), dexamethasone (10 nM) or both hormones. A synergistic response is observed at earlier times of hormone treatment. Values are mean ± SE. (From Ref. 94.)

made. Gestational age also may be a factor accounting for the negative results reported by Seidner et al. (38), who failed to find effects of steroid or TRH on phospholipid synthesis in rabbit pups examined on fetal day 29. These negative results emphasize the importance of variables such as gestational age, hormone dose, treatment regimen, and perhaps, species, in the hormonal response.

The possible role of PRL in the response to TRH is not fully defined. Most in vivo studies have failed to demonstrate increased surfactant synthesis in response to PRL administration alone (reviewed in 14). Although one study using cultured explants of fetal rat lung showed that PRL increased PC synthesis (39), similar work using rabbit and human explants found no effect on choline incorporation or PC content (40,41). Studies of PRL binding in the lung have also provided inconsistent results (42–44). Thus, PRL may have a permissive role in the response to combined therapy, and increased levels appear to be required, at least in sheep.

The biochemical site of action of thyroid hormone in the biosynthesis of surfactant phospholipids is not established. In a study using two-dimensional gel electrophoresis and human fetal lung explants, T_3 treatment did not induce any of the approximately 800 lung proteins resolved (45). Thyroid hormone treatment of cultured tissue does not increase the activity of the enzyme fatty acid synthetase, a key enzyme in lipid production, which is induced by both glucocorticoids and cAMP (46). Cholinephosphate cytidylyltransferase is another rate-limiting enzyme that catalyzes formation of CDP-choline, which is used in the final step of PC synthesis. The activity of this enzyme in cultured lung tissue is increased by glucocorticoid and, to a lesser extent, by T_3. However, the increase in enzyme activity from combined T_3 plus dexamethasone treatment was no greater than that observed with dexamethasone alone (47). Thus, it is unlikely that this enzyme is the major biochemical site of T_3 action.

B. Surfactant Protein-A

There is one published observation that combined hormonal treatment has a synergistic effect on production of surfactant protein A (SP-A). In the aforementioned study by Ikegami et al. (36), lambs were examined at 128 days gestation after receiving fetal infusions of saline, cortisol, TRH, or both hormones. After 1.25 hr of ventilation, the lungs of the newborn lambs were lavaged and SP-A content was determined by radioimmunoassay. As shown in Figure 3, content of SP-A per kilogram body weight was similar in control, steroid, and TRH-treated

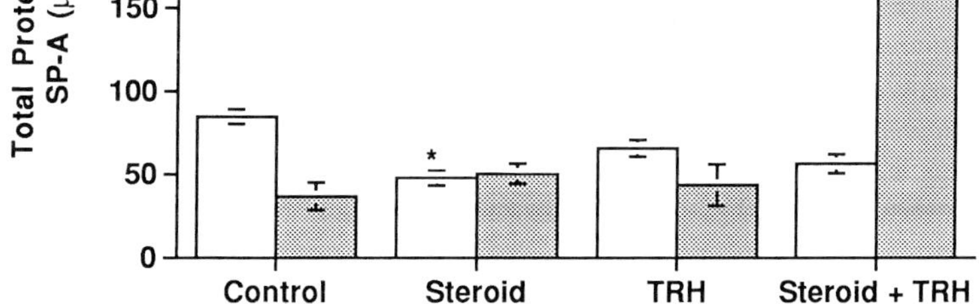

Figure 3 Effect of prenatal hormone therapy on alveolar-wash total protein and SP-A in fetal lambs. Fetuses were infused for 3 days with cortisol (~2.25 mg/hr), TRH (~30 μg/24 hr, given in intermittent boluses), or both hormones. Fetuses were delivered at 128 days gestation, ventilated for 1.25 hr and the amount of total protein and SP-A was determined in alveolar wash fluid. *$p < 0.05$ vs. control. (From data of Ref. 36.)

animals, but was increased about fivefold in lavage of animals exposed to steroid plus TRH. There was also a significant increase in SP-A with combined treatment when content was expressed relative to saturated PC.

SP-A has several properties that could contribute to enhanced lung function after hormonal treatment. SP-A is required for formation of tubular myelin, an alveolar form of surfactant that produces the surface active film at the air–aqueous interface, and in vitro, SP-A enhances the effect of the hydrophobic surfactant proteins on rate of film formation (48). Both in vitro and in vivo SP-A has overcome the inhibitory effects of plasma proteins such as albumin on the activity of surfactant (49). Mice that lack SP-A because of gene ablation have apparently normal respiratory function at birth and as adults. It is possible, however, that SP-A-deficient pups that are born prematurely would have impaired respiratory status compared with wild-type animals (50).

Surfactant protein-A is not produced by the human fetal lung until after 24-weeks gestation and does not appear in amniotic fluid until after 30 weeks, indicating that most premature infants are deficient in SP-A (15). Premature infants with RDS have much lower concentrations of SP-A in tracheal lavage fluid than do infants without RDS, and SP-A content increases in the first days after birth (51,52). Premature infants who died with RDS lacked both SP-A and tubular myelin in their lung tissue despite the presence of alveolar lamellar bodies (53,54).

At present there are no other data supporting the observation of Ikegami and colleagues that SP-A is induced by combined treatment with corticosteroid and TRH. In studies with cultured human fetal lung, lower doses and relatively short exposures to glucocorticoids increase production of SP-A, whereas synthesis is inhibited at higher hormone concentrations or with longer exposure (55,56). The physiological significance of this biphasic regulation of SP-A gene expression by corticosteroids is unclear. There is, however, evidence indicating a similar type of regulation in vivo (57). T_3 alone or in the presence of corticosteroid did not induce SP-A in cultured human lung or in rat fetuses (58,59); however, there have been no published reports of studies with glucocorticoid combined with both thyroid hormone and PRL or glucocorticoid plus TRH. There is also no effect of T_3 alone or of T_3 and corticosteroid on expression of SP-B and SP-C genes (Ballard, unpublished data).

C. Alveolar Structure

The maturational effects of corticosteroid treatment on lung structure, first described by Kikkawa et al. (60) in rabbits, are now well documented. Glucocorticoids accelerate developmental changes such as condensation of the interstitium, decrease in number of fibroblasts, apposition of capillaries and airspaces, and expansion of terminal airspaces. Treatment also decreases leak of plasma proteins into airspaces, which likely reflects a combination of factors, including perfusion pressure, endothelial cell tight junctions, tissue elasticity, and alveolar surface tension. As for other aspects of lung development, exposure to exogenous steroid appears to mimic the role of endogenous corticosteroids in modulating the rate of maturation. Recent experimental approaches demonstrating the role of endogenous corticosteroids in lung structural development are the knockout mouse models for corticotropin-releasing hormone (CRH) and glucocorticoid receptor. Homozygous pups for CRH deficiency, delivered of homozygous females, are deprived of both maternal and fetal sources of corticosterone in utero, and these pups die after birth with immature lungs (61). A similar delay in lung structural development was observed with glucocorticoid receptor-deficient animals (62).

Boshier et al. (63) performed morphometric analyses of alveolar structure in lungs of fetal lambs exposed to different hormonal treatments as described by Liggins (21). Compared with treatment with TRH or cortisol alone, combined treatment significantly decreased alveolar wall thickness and increased volume density of airspace. Jobe and co-workers, using direct fetal injection of hormones in fetal lambs, have found that administration of T_4 in combination with dexamethasone further augments the glucocorticoid effect on postnatal pulmonary function at 48 hr, but not at 24 hr (64,65). The effects occurred independently of observable effects on surfactant pool sizes, and thus likely reflect changes in lung structure. The accelerated structural development with hormonal therapy contrasts with the effects of hypophysectomy of the fetal lamb, which impairs the developmental changes in lung volume density and alveolar wall thickness (66). Supporting data for morphological effects of TRH come from the studies by Devaskar et al. (28,29,67), who described increased alveolar air expansion in fetal rabbit and mouse lungs after exposure to TRH in utero. In studies with mice, TRH treatment increased the ratio of airspace to parenchyma and the number of lamellar bodies per type II cell in the lung of the treated fetuses; however, combined therapy was not examined (67). Lung ultrastructural development also has been examined in a mouse line with a mutation in the TSH receptor, which produces hypothyroidism in homozygous animals. Hypothyroid newborn animals had delayed lung development, as indicated by thick alveolar septae and reduced airspace compared with control animals (68).

Information on possible biochemical events responsible for TRH-induced structural maturation comes from limited studies with glucocorticoid. Earlier studies noted increased content of both collagen and elastin in parenchyma of more distensible lungs resulting from various hormonal treatments. This change paralleled the developmental pattern of increasing content of both proteins (69,70). However, there has not yet been a detailed study of the synthesis, content, and distribution of lung matrix proteins during development and after hormone treatment. Recently, Pierce et al. (71) reported a developmental increase in tropoelastin gene expression in rat lung and a severalfold stimulation by dexamethasone treatment both in vivo and in cultured tissue. In the only reported study of TRH plus steroid effects on matrix proteins, Campos et al. (23) found a synergistic increase in tissue content of hydroxyproline and desmosine, reflecting collagen and elastin, respectively (Table 1). Because elastin is critical for development of terminal airspaces and normal elastic recoil, induction of this protein is likely an important component of glucocorticoid effects and a candidate target protein for responsiveness to combined treatment.

D. Lung Liquid

The synergistic effect of in vivo glucocorticoid and thyroid hormone treatment on lung maturity could partly relate to clearance of lung liquid. The strongest support for this hypothesis is the series of studies by Barker and colleagues (72,73) using a fetal lamb model. They showed that epinephrine-stimulated resorption of lung liquid occurs in late gestation, but not earlier. However, when thyroidectomized fetuses were treated with hydrocortisone and T_3, responsiveness to epinephrine was induced at an early stage in lung development, and reabsorption of lung water occurred (Fig. 4). Treatment with either hydrocortisone or T_3 alone had no effect, indicating a permissive or synergistic effect of the two hormones on absorption of lung liquid.

Both sodium and water channels, which are required for fluid flux, are present in the lungs of both fetal rats and humans (74,75). Levels of both channels are developmentally regulated in the rat fetus, and expression of epithelial sodium channel subunits is increased by treatment with dexamethasone. However, additive or synergistic responses to glucocorticoid plus thyroid hormone have not been described for either channel.

Other studies of combined hormonal therapy of fetal sheep have not noted decreased lung liquid in animals receiving both hormones, and Schellenberg et al. (26) reported statistically increased lung liquid in fetal sheep treated with TRH plus cortisol, compared with control fetuses. However, in these experiments the fetuses did not experience either labor or delivery and thus were not exposed to a surge of endogenous epinephrine. Moreover, Stein et al. (76) found that corticosteroid treatment, with or without TRH, reduced basal levels of both norepinephrine and epinephrine and markedly attenuated the postnatal increase in these hormones after delivery of preterm sheep. Although this change in catecholamine levels mimics the pattern that normally occurs in term fetuses, suppression of circulating epinephrine after hormonal treatment would not favor enhanced absorption of lung water.

E. Neurotransmitter TRH Effect

It has been proposed that TRH acts by its neurotransmitter function to augment the effects of corticosteroids on lung development, perhaps by increasing fetal

Table 1 Synergistic Effect of Combined Hormone Treatment on Connective Tissue Proteins of Fetal Lamb Lung

	Saline	TRH	Cortisol	TRH + cortisol
n	6	4	9	10
Hydroxyproline (μg/mg protein)	3.28 ± 0.9	3.53 ± 1.3 (+8%)	4.27 ± 0.8 (+30%)	10.1 ± 2.7 (+208%)
Desmosine (ng/mg protein)	31.5 ± 9.2	38.20 ± 8.3 (+21%)	41.0 ± 12.7 (+30%)	128.2 ± 38.2 (+307%)
V40 (mL/g)	0.4 ± 0.1	0.62 ± 0.07 (+55%)	0.66 ± 0.06 (+63%)	1.8 ± 0.11 (+350%)

Fetal lambs of 121 days received infusions of saline or TRH for 2.5 days and then cortisol or saline for an additional 2.5 days. Tissue hydroxyproline and desmosine content were analyzed by chromatography and reflect levels of collagen and elastin, respectively.
Source: Ref. 23.

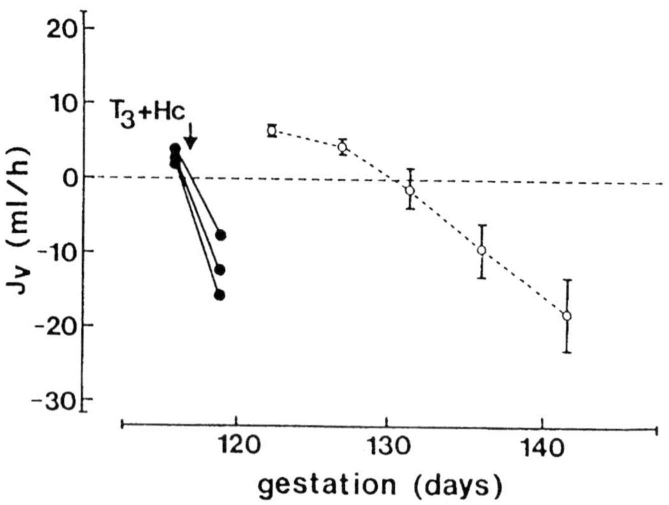

Figure 4 Assessment of lung liquid secretion and absorption rates in lamb fetuses receiving epinephrine infusion. Data are shown for control fetuses (open circle) and for three thyroidectomized fetal sheep before and after 3-days infusion of T_3 (60 μg/day) and hydrocortisone (10 mg/day). Hormone treatment induces sensitivity to epinephrine-mediated reabsorption of lung fluid comparable with that observed in older control animals. (From Ref. 73.)

breathing movements, which could enhance both synthesis and secretion of pulmonary surfactant and structural maturation by stretch-activated mechanisms. Administration of relatively high doses of TRH into the circulation, or lower doses into the lateral cerebral ventricles of fetal lambs, stimulates fetal-breathing movements, which become faster, deeper, and continuous (77,78). Although TRH effects on breathing in the human fetus have not been reported, treatment increases the frequency of fetal heart rate accelerations, which are closely associated with body and respiratory movements in the fetus (79,80). Furthermore, infants delivered after prenatal exposure to TRH plus betamethasone had shorter latencies in somatosensory-evoked potential compared with untreated preterm infants (81). By the end of the first week of life, the latency period had decreased in the untreated infants, possibly as a result of the postnatal thyroid hormone surge. These findings were interpreted to indicate neural maturation following prenatal betamethasone plus TRH treatment and to support the possibility of other neurotransmitter effects beneficial to lung development. Devaskar et al. (28) have tested the hypothesis that TRH-mediated lung maturation is through its neurotransmitter, rather than by neuroendocrine properties. They treated rabbits for 2 days before preterm delivery with either TRH or a TRH analogue designated DN1417. This compound functions as a neurotransmitter similar to TRH, but does not stimulate prolactin and has less than 3% of the TSH-releasing effect of TRH. Treatment with TRH and the analogue had comparable stimulatory effects on length of neonatal survival, lung stability, and alveolar air expansion. Additional studies are needed to confirm this finding and to examine responses in the presence of steroid treatment.

V. Clinical Trials of Antenatal Corticosteroid Plus TRH Therapy

The observations of additive effects of thyroid hormone and glucocorticoid on lung development in experimental models, described earlier, provided the basis for clinical trials to prevent RDS and BPD. Maternal administration of either T_3 or T_4 is not an effective approach to treat the fetus with thyroid hormone because binding by thyroid-binding globulin in the maternal circulation prevents these hormones from crossing the placenta to the fetus. In addition, the placenta expresses monodeiodinase activity, which inactivates maternally derived T_4 and T_3 (82). Thyrotropin-releasing hormone (TRH), however, is a tripeptide that crosses the placenta and stimulates the release of both thyroid hormone and prolactin (83–87).

In utero exposure to maternal treatment with TRH (400 μg) maximally increases both TSH and T_3 about twofold in fetal plasma (cord blood), compared with about a 50% increase in the corresponding maternal samples (87). Peak levels occur approximately 2 hr after TRH treatment, and T_3 concentrations return to control values 6–12 hr after treatment. The magnitude of the increases in fetal T_3 and free T_4 after in utero TRH can be considered physiological, in that they are comparable with those that normally occur immediately after birth. From findings with cultured tissue, the duration and levels of T_3 achieved in human fetuses after maternal TRH therapy should be sufficient to induce target proteins in the lung. A transient approximate twofold increase in plasma prolactin also occurs in infants of 26–30 weeks gestation who are exposed to TRH in utero (87). The effects of antenatal TRH on concentrations of thyroid hormones and prolactin in premature infants are summarized in Table 2.

Morales et al. (88) were the first to carry out a trial of combined TRH and betamethasone treatment of women in preterm labor. In this nonblinded study, RDS occurred in 28% of the TRH-treated infants versus 44% in infants of women receiving betamethasone alone (NS). In addition, there was a reported decrease in incidence of BPD from 24 to 8% ($p < 0.05$) with combined therapy.

Between 1986 and 1989, a multicenter, randomized double-blind clinical trial of TRH plus corticosteroid was conducted in the United States (89). In this

Table 2 Effect of Antenatal TRH on Plasma Concentrations of Thyroid Hormones and Prolactin in Premature Infants

	Control (n = 61)		TRH treatment 2–6 hr before delivery (n = 14)
	Birth	2 hr	Birth
TSH (mU/L)	9.7 ± 0.7	15.0 ± 1.2*	18.8 ± 2.5*
T_3 (nmol/L)	0.6 ± 0.04	1.6 ± 0.1*	1.2 ± 0.2*
Free T_4 (pmol/L)	14.5 ± 0.5	19.3 ± 0.9*	17.4 ± 1.8*
Prolactin (μg/L)	67.6 ± 5.3	85.7 ± 8.7	90.0 ± 25*

*$p < 0.05$ vs. control birth value.
Values are mean ± SE for infants 26–34 weeks gestation except for prolactin (26–30 weeks) who received antenatal corticosteroid plus either placebo (control) or TRH (400 μg).
Source: Ref. 87.

study, 404 women with threatened preterm delivery at 32 weeks or less gestation received betamethasone plus TRH (four doses of 400 μg at 8-hr intervals) or betamethasone plus placebo. Of the 103 infants who were fully treated (≥ 24 hr) and who weighed less than 1500 g at birth, there was a trend toward decreased occurrence of severe respiratory distress (12% in TRH and steroid vs. 25% in steroid alone, $p = 0.11$). Fewer TRH-treated infants required supplemental oxygen postnatally, and the incidence of chronic lung disease, defined as requirement for supplemental oxygen at 28 days of age, was 17.6 versus 43.9% in the control ($p < 0.01$). Both the need for supplemental oxygen and adverse outcome (defined as need for supplemental oxygen or death) were less at 36 weeks postmenstrual age in infants who were fully treated with TRH and corticosteroid versus those treated with corticosteroid alone (89).

Knight et al. (90), subsequently reported the results of a randomized placebo-controlled, double-blind trial of antenatal TRH in 378 New Zealand women less than 33 weeks gestation. Of the 405 liveborn infants delivered in the study, 175 were born between 24 hr and 10 days after the start of maternal treatment. Among these infants the incidence of RDS was 31 versus 52% (relative risk 0.61, 95% confidence interval 0.41–0.89) and the incidence of severe RDS was 20 versus 42% (RR 0.48; 95% Cl 0.29–0.78) for the TRH plus betamethasone group compared with betamethasone treatment alone, respectively. These investigators also found a significant decrease in adverse outcome with TRH therapy.

In 1994, Crowther and Alfirevic (91) reported results of a metanalysis of clinical trials of TRH plus betamethasone and found a significant decrease in both severe RDS and BPD in infants delivered 1–10 days after combined maternal therapy. In addition there was a strong trend toward a decrease in total RDS after just three doses of TRH (16 hr).

In 1995, however, a trial in Australia (Australian Collaborative Trial of Antenatal Thyrotropin-Releasing Hormone: ACTOBAT) reported no benefit of antenatal TRH on infant outcome. This study enrolled 1234 women between 24 and 32 weeks gestation into a randomized trial of TRH (four doses of 200 μg at a 12-hr interval) plus betamethasone versus corticosteroid alone (92). Some of the outcome data are shown in Table 3. There was no effect of TRH exposure on the incidence of either RDS or BPD among infants delivered within 10 days of maternal treatment. Moreover, among infants born more than 10 days after treatment, the incidence of RDS was slightly increased in the TRH-treated group (16%) compared with the placebo group (10%, $p = 0.01$). In this group, however, the incidence of severe RDS and the duration of mechanical ventilation were no different between the TRH and placebo infants. Thus, it is uncertain whether these observations of potential adverse effects of TRH are clinically important.

The North American TRH Trial enrolled 996 women in preterm labor at less than 30 week gestation at 13 centers between 1992 and 1996, randomizing to receive placebo or TRH (four doses of 400 μg at 8-hr intervals) in addition to corticosteroid (11). Outcome was evaluated for infants 32 weeks or less gestation (see Table 3), defined as the group at risk for lung disease, as well as infants born at 32 weeks or more. In both groups of infants, antenatal administration of TRH had no effect on incidence of either RDS or chronic lung disease evaluated at both 28 days of age and 36 weeks postmenstrual age. There was no indication that TRH treatment improved pulmonary outcome in any subgroup of infants as defined by gestation age or treatment interval before delivery. In addition, there was no evidence of either beneficial or adverse effects of TRH on the occurrence of other morbidities associated with prematurity, including intraventricular hem-

Table 3 Infant Outcome in Three Trials of Antenatal TRH (1995–1998)

	ACTOBAT	North American	Chile
Women enrolled	1231	996	370
Gestational age (wk)	24 < 32	24 < 30	24 < 33
Total number of infants studied	1369	1134	332
Infants delivered 1–10 days after treatment	506	333	207
RDS (%)–TRH/placebo	50/48	66/68	30/21
CLD or death day 28 (%)–TRH/placebo	41/42	43/41	29/24

None of the values for TRH versus placebo are significantly different.
Source: Refs. 11, 92, 93.

orrhage, patent ductus arteriosus, necrotizing entercolitis and retinopathy of prematurity. Similarly, no benefit of antenatal TRH was found in a recent trial carried out in Chile (93) that evaluated outcome in a smaller population of premature infants (see Table 3).

In comparison with the recent Australian, North American, and Chilean trials, the earlier trials that suggested efficacy involved fewer infants at risk of lung disease, and one study was unblinded (88). These limitations may have resulted in inaccurate conclusions. It is also possible that changes in management of premature infants in the past 5–10 years, which have improved survival of the smaller infants, influenced the response to TRH in the more recent studies. The recent trials involved more extremely premature infants (less than 26 weeks gestation) than the earlier studies. In these infants, immaturity of lung parenchymal structure may have a more dominant role in development of lung disease, whereas surfactant deficiency is likely of more importance in the older gestation infants. It seems unlikely, however, that age differences of infants between the initial and recent studies account for the observed difference in response to TRH treatment. It now appears that antenatal administration of TRH, at the dosing regimens that have been studied, provides no added benefit for infants compared with corticosteroid alone. This clinical finding was unexpected in view of the extensive data from experimental studies demonstrating additive effects of combined hormonal therapy on lung maturation.

VI. Summary

Although advances in intensive care have markedly improved survival for premature infants, occurrence of BPD and associated complications remain a major problem for these infants. It is well established that antenatal corticosteroid therapy accelerates fetal lung maturation and reduces mortality and the incidence of RDS and intraventricular hemorrhage in premature infants. This treatment may have some benefit for BPD, but this effect is not large nor firmly established. Various other agents have been investigated, both in the laboratory and in clinical studies, to determine effects on lung maturation. Much interest has focused on thyroid hormone and TRH. Combined treatment with glucocorticoid and T_3 or TRH has additive or synergistic effects on lung maturation, both in fetal animals and in cultured tissue. The mode of action of this combined hormonal treatment may involve (1) enhanced synthesis of surfactant phospholipids, (2) induction of SP-A, (3) accelerated lung structural maturation, and (4) faster clearance of lung liquid. The response to TRH in fetal sheep likely involves the action of both thyroid hormones and prolactin and may include direct effects of TRH acting as a neurotransmitter.

On the basis of experimental observations, clinical trials of betamethasone plus TRH for prevention of newborn lung disease have been carried out. Maternal treatment with 400 μg intravenous TRH produces a transient increase in cord blood thyroid hormones and PRL to peak levels approximating those achieved immediately after birth in the premature infant, indicating that this therapy mimics a physiological response. Initial clinical studies of maternal TRH plus betamethasone therapy found a significant decrease in both severe RDS and BPD in fully treated, premature infants who were born 1–10 days after therapy, compared with infants who were exposed to prenatal corticosteroid alone. Three more recent studies that had considerably larger numbers of premature infants found no reduction in the incidence of either RDS or BPD. The reasons for the discrepancy in clinical responses are unknown. The use of prenatal TRH therapy to enhance lung maturity is not now recommended.

References

1. Zimmerman JJ. Bronchoalveolar inflammatory pathophysiology of bronchopulmonary dysplasia. Clin Perinatol 1995; 22:429–456.
2. Liggins GC. Premature delivery of foetal lambs infused with glucocorticoids. J Endocrinol 1969; 45:515–523.
3. Liggins GC, Howie RN. A controlled trial of antepartum glucocorticoid treatment for prevention of the respiratory distress syndrome in premature infants. Pediatrics 1972; 50:515–520.
4. Crowley P. Antenatal corticosteroid therapy: a meta-analysis of the randomized trials, 1972 to 1994. Am J Obstet Gynecol 1995; 173:322–335.
5. NIH Consensus Development Panel. Effect of corticosteroids for fetal maturation on perinatal outcomes. JAMA 1995; 273:413–418.
6. Ballard PL, Ballard RA. Scientific basis and therapeutic regimens for use of antenatal glucocorticoids. Am J Obstet Gynecol 1995; 153:254–262.
7. Doyle LW, Kitchen WH, Ford GW, Rickards AL, Lissenden JV, Ryan MM. Effects of antenatal steroid therapy on mortality and morbidity in very low birth weight infants. J Pediatr 1986; 108:287–292.
8. Van Marter LJ, Leviton A, Kuban KCK, Pagano M, Allred EN. Maternal glucocorticoid therapy and reduced risk of bronchopulmonary dysplasia. Pediatrics 1990; 86: 331–336.
9. Kari MA, Hallman M, Eronen M, Teramo K, Virtanen M, Koivisto M, Iknen RS. Prenatal dexamethasone treatment in conjunction with human surfactant therapy—a randomized placebo-controlled multicenter study. Pediatrics 1994; 93:730–736.
10. Wright LL, Horbar JD, Gunkel H, Verter J, Younes N, Andrews EB, Long W. Evidence from multicenter networks on the current use and effectiveness of antenatal corticosteroids in low birth weight infants. Am J Obstet Gynecol 1995; 173:263–269.
11. Ballard RA, Ballard PL, Cnaan A, Pinto-Martin J, Davis DJ, Padbury JF, Phibbs RH, Parer JT, Hart MC, Mannino FL, Sawai SK. Antenatal thyrotropin-releasing hormone to prevent lung disease in preterm infants. N Engl J Med 1998; 338:493–498.

12. Wu B, Kikkawa Y, Orzalesi MM, Motoyama EK, Kaibara M, Zigas CJ, Cook CD. The effect of thyroxine on the maturation of fetal rabbit lungs. Biol Neonate 1973; 22:161–168.
13. Gross I, Dynia DW, Wilson CM, Ingleson LD, Gewolb IH, Rooney SA. Glucocorticoid–thyroid interactions in fetal rat lung. Pediatr Res 1984; 18:191–196.
14. Ballard PL. Hormones and lung maturation. In: Monographs on Endocrinology. Berlin: Springer-Verlag, 1986.
15. Ballard PL. Hormonal regulation of pulmonary surfactant. Endocr Rev 1989; 10: 165–181.
16. Erenberg A, Rhodes ML, Weinstein MM, Kennedy RK. The effect of fetal thyroidectomy on ovine fetal lung maturation. Pediatr Res 1979; 13:230–235.
17. Burrow GN, Fisher DA, Larsen PR. Maternal and fetal thyroid function. N Engl J Med 1994; 331:1072–1078.
18. Mashiach S, Barkai G, Sack J, Stem E, Brish M, Goldman B, Serr DM. The effect of intraamniotic thyroxine administration on fetal lung maturity in man. J Perinat Med 1979; 7:161–169.
19. Schreyer P, Caspi E, Letko Y, Ron-El R, Pinto N, Zeidman JL. Intraamniotic triiodothyronine instillation for prevention of respiratory distress syndrome in pregnancies complicated by hypertension. J Perinat Med 1982; 10:27–33.
20. Romaguera J, Zorrilla C, de la Vega A, Fromm R, Wallach RC, Rodriguez-Mariani A, Adamsons K. Responsiveness of L-S ratio of the amniotic fluid to intra-amniotic administration of thyroxine. Acta Obstet Gynecol Scand 1990; 69:119–122.
21. Liggins GC, Schellenberg JC, Manzai M, Kitterman JA, Lee CCH. Synergism of cortisol and thyrotropin releasing hormone on lung maturation in fetal sheep. J Appl Physiol 1988; 65:1880–1884.
22. Schellenberg J, Liggins GC, Manzai M, Kitterman JA, Lee CCH. Synergistic hormonal effects of lung maturation in fetal sheep. J Appl Physiol 1988; 65:94–100.
23. Campos, GA, Guerra FA, Brummer E, Munoz ML, Vega IA. Synergistic effect of cortisol and thyrotropin releasing hormone on lung maturation in the fetal sheep entails connective tissue maturation. Biol Res 1992; 25:95–100.
24. Moraga FA, Riquelme RA, López AA, Moya FR, Llanos AJ. Maternal administration of glucocorticoid and thyrotropin releasing hormone enhances fetal lung maturation in undisturbed preterm lambs. Am J Obstet Gynecol 1994; 171:729–734.
25. Warburton D, Parton L, Buckley S, Cosico L, Enns G, Saluna T. Combined effects of corticosteroid, thyroid hormones, and β-agonist on surfactant, pulmonary mechanics, and β-receptor binding in fetal lamb lung. Pediatr Res 1988; 24:166–170.
26. Schellenberg J, Liggins GC, Kitterman JA, Lee CCH. Sympathectomy and beta-adrenergic blockade during lung maturation stimulated by TRH and cortisol in fetal sheep. J Appl Physiol 1993; 75:141–147.
27. Rooney SA, Marino PA, Gobran LI, Gross I, Warshaw JB. Thyrotropin-releasing hormone increases the amount of surfactant in lung lavage from fetal rabbits. Pediatr Res 1979; 13:623–625.
28. Devaskar UP, deMello DE, Ackerman J. Effect of maternal administration of thyrotropin-releasing hormone or DN1417 on functional and morphologic fetal rabbit lung maturation and duration of survival after premature delivery. Biol Neonate 1991; 59:346–351.

29. Devaskar U, Nitta K, Szewczyk K, Sadiq F, deMello D. Transplacental stimulation of functional and morphologic fetal rabbit lung maturation: effect of thyrotropin-releasing hormone. Am J Obstet Gynecol 1987; 157:460–464.
30. Oulton M, Rasmusson MG, Yoon RY, Fraser CT. Gestation-dependent effects of the combined treatment of glucocorticoids and thyrotropin-releasing hormone on surfactant production by fetal rabbit lung. Am J Obstet Gynecol 1989; 160:961–967.
31. Rodriguez MP, Sozenko IRS, Antigua MC, Frank L. Prenatal hormone treatment with thyrotropin releasing hormone and with thyrotropin releasing hormone plus dexamethasone delays antioxidant enzyme maturation but does not inhibit a protective antioxidant enzyme response to hyperoxia in newborn rat lung. Pediatr Res 1991; 30:522–527.
32. Gross I, Wilson CM. Fetal lung in organ culture. IV. Supraadditive hormone interactions. J Appl Physiol Respir Environ Exerc Physiol 1982; 52:1420–1426.
33. Gonzales LW, Ballard PL, Ertsey R, Williams MC. Glucocorticoids and thyroid hormones stimulate biochemical and morphological differentiation of human fetal lung in organ culture. J Clin Endocrinol Metab 1986; 62:687–691.
34. Chinoy MR, Gonzales LW, Ballard PL, Fisher AB, Eckenhoff RG. Elemental composition of lamellar bodies from fetal and adult human lung. Am J Respir Cell Mol Biol 1995; 13:99–108.
35. Tabor BL, Ikegami M, Jobe A, Yamada T, Oetomo SB. Dose response of thyrotrophin-releasing hormone on pulmonary maturation in corticosteroid-treated preterm rabbits. Am J Obstet Gynecol 1990; 163:669–676.
36. Ikegami M, Polk D, Tabor B, Lewis J, Yamada T, Jobe A. Corticosteroids and thyrotrophin-releasing hormone effects on preterm sheep lung function. J Appl Physiol 1991; 70:2268–2278.
37. Ikegami M, Jobe AH, Pettenazzo A, Seidner SR, Berry DD, Ruffini L. Effects of maternal treatment with corticosteroids, T_3, TRH, and their combinations on lung function of ventilated preterm rabbits with and without surfactant treatments. Am Rev Respir Dis 1987; 136:892–898.
38. Seidner S, Rider E, Jobe A, Yamada T, Ikegami M. Effects of antenatal thyrotropin-releasing hormone, antenatal corticosteroids, and postnatal ventilation on surfactant mobilization in premature rabbits. Am J Obstet Gynecol 1992; 166:1551–1559.
39. Mullon DK, Smith YF, Richardson LL, Hamosh M, Hamosh P. Effect of prolactin on phospholipid synthesis in organ cultures of fetal rat lung. Biochim Biophys Acta 1983; 751:166–174.
40. Mendelson CR, Johnston JM, MacDonald PC, Snyder JM. Multihormonal regulation of surfactant synthesis by human fetal lung in vitro. J Clin Endocrinol Metab 1981; 53:307–317.
41. Cox MA, Torday JS. Pituitary oligopeptide regulation of phosphatidylcholine synthesis by fetal rabbit lung cells. Lack of effect with prolactin. Am Rev Respir Dis 1981; 123:181–184.
42. Josimovich JB, Merisko K, Boccella L, Tobon H. Binding of prolactin by fetal rhesus cell membrane fractions. Endocrinology 1977; 100:557–570.
43. Chan JSD, Robertson HA, Friesen HG. Distribution of binding sites for ovine placental lactogen in the sheep. Endocrinology 1978; 102:632–640.

44. Labbe A, Delcros B, Dechelotte P, Nouailles C, Grizard G. Comparative study of the binding of prolactin and growth hormone by rabbit and human lung cell membrane fractions. Biol Neonate 1992; 61:179–187.
45. Odom MW, Ertsey R, Ballard PL. Hormonally regulated proteins in cultured human fetal lung: analysis by two-dimensional polyacrylamide gel electrophoresis. Am J Physiol 1990; 259:L283–L293.
46. Gonzales L, Ballard PL, Gonzales J. Glucocorticoid and cAMP increase fatty acid synthetase mRNA in human fetal lung explants. Biochim Biophys Acta 1994; 1215: 49–58.
47. Sharma A, Gonzales LW, Ballard PL. Hormonal regulation of cholinephosphate cytidylyltransferase in cultured fetal lung. Biochim Biophys Acta 1993; 1170:237–244.
48. Hawgood S, Shiffer K. Structures and properties of the surfactant-associated proteins [review]. Annu Rev Physiol 1991; 53:375–394.
49. Yukitake K, Brown CL, Schulueter MA, Clements JA, Hawgood S. Surfactant apoprotein A modifies the inhibitory effect of plasma proteins on surfactant activity in vivo. Pediatr Res 1995; 37:21–25.
50. Korfhagen TR, Bruno MD, Ross GF, Huelsman KM. Ikegami M, Jobe AH, Wert SE, Stripp BR, Morris RE, Glasser SW, Bachurski CJ, Iwamoto HS, Whitsett JA. Altered surfactant function and structure in SP-A gene targeted mice. Proc Natl Acad Sci USA 1996; 93:9594–9599.
51. Gerdes J, Whitsett J, Long W. Elastase activity and surfactant protein concentration in tracheal aspirates from neonates receiving synthetic surfactant. J Pediatr 1992; 120:S34–S39.
52. Moya FR, Montes HF, Thomas VL, Mouzinho AM, Smith JF, Rosenfeld CR. Surfactant protein A and saturated phosphatidylcholine in respiratory distress syndrome. Am J Respir Crit Care Med 1994; 150:1672–1677.
53. deMello DE, Chi EY, Doo E, Lagunoff D. Absence of tubular myelin in lungs of infants dying with hyaline membrane disease. Am J Pathol 1987; 127:131–139.
54. deMello DE, Phelps DS, Patel G, Floros J, Lagunoff D. Expression of the 35 kDa and low molecular weight surfactant-associated proteins in the lungs of infants dying with respiratory distress syndrome. Am J Pathol 1989; 134:1285–1293.
55. Iannuzzi DM, Ertsey R, Ballard PL. Biphasic glucocorticoid regulation of pulmonary surfactant protein-A: characterization of the inhibitory process. Am J Physiol 1993; 264:L236–L244.
56. Odom MJ, Snyder JM, Boggaram V, Mendelson CR. Glucocorticoid regulation of the major surfactant associated protein (SP-A) and its messenger ribonucleic acid and of morphological development of human fetal lung in vitro. Endocrinology 1988; 123:1712–1720.
57. Schellhase DE, Shannon JM. Effect of maternal dexamethasone on expression of SP-A, SP-B, and SP-C in the fetal rat lung. Am J Respir Cell Mol Biol 1991; 4: 304–312.
58. Liley HG, Hawgood S, Wellenstein GA, Benson B, White RT, Ballard PL. Surfactant protein of molecular weight 28,000–36,000 in cultured human fetal lung: cellular localization and effect of dexamethasone. Mol Endocrinol 1987; 1:205–215.
59. Nichols KV, Floros J, Dynia DW, Veletza SV, Wilson CM, Gross I. Regulation of

surfactant protein A mRNA by hormones and butyrate in cultured fetal rat lung. Am J Physiol 1990; 259:L488–L495.

60. Kikkawa Y, Kaibara M, Motoyama EK, Orzalesi MM, Cook CD. Morphological development of fetal rabbit lung and its acceleration with cortisol. Am J Pathol 1971; 2:423–442.
61. Mugila L, Jacobson L, Dikkes P, Majzoub JA. Corticotropin-releasing hormone deficiency reveals major fetal but not adult glucocorticoid need. Nature 1995; 373: 427–432.
62. Cole TJ, Blendy JA, Monaghan AP, Krieglstein K, Schmidt W, Aguzzi A, Fantuzzi G, Hummler E, Unsiker K, Schutz G. Targeted disruption of the glucocorticoid receptor gene blocks adrenergic chromaffin cell development and severely retards lung maturation. Genes Dev 1995; 9:1608–1621.
63. Boshier CP, Holloway H, Liggins GC, Marshall RJ. Morphometric analyses of the effects of thyrotropin releasing hormone and cortisol on the lungs of fetal sheep. J Dev Physiol 1989; 12:49–54.
64. Jobe AH, Polk D, Ikegami M, Newnham J, Sly P, Kohen R, Kelly R. Lung responses to ultrasound-guided fetal treatments with corticosteroids in preterm lambs. J Appl Physiol 1993; 75:2099–2105.
65. Polk DH, Ikegami M, Jobe AH, Newnham J, Sly P, Kohen R, Kelly R. Postnatal lung function in preterm lambs: effects of a single exposure to betamethasone and thyroid hormones. Am J Obstet Gynecol 1995; 172:872–881.
66. Crone RK, Davies P, Liggins GC, Reid L. The effects of hypothesectomy, thyroidectomy, and postoperative infusion of cortisol or adrenocorticotropin on the structure of the ovine fetal lung. J Dev Physiol 1983; 5:281–288.
67. Devaskar U, Govindrajan R, Heyman S, Sosenko RS, deMello D. Fetal lung ultrastructural maturation is accelerated by maternal thyrotropin releasing hormone (TRH) treatment in a dose dependent manner [abstr]. Pediatr Res 1995; 37:329A.
68. deMello D, Heyman S, Govindarajan R, Sosenko IRS, Devaskar UP. Delayed ultrastructural lung maturation in the fetal and newborn hypothyroid (Hyt/Hyt) mouse. Pediatr Res 1994; 36:380–386.
69. Schellenberg JC, Liggins GC. Elastin and collagen in the fetal sheep lung. I. Ontogenesis. Pediatr Res 1987; 22:335–338.
70. Schellenberg JC, Liggins GC, Kitterman JA, Lee CCH. Elastin and collagen in the fetal sheep lung. II. Relationship to mechanical properties of the lung. Pediatr Res 1987; 22:339.
71. Pierce RA, Mariencheck WI, Sandefur S, Crouch EC, Parks WC. Glucocorticoids upregulate tropoelastin expression during late stages of fetal lung development. Am J Physiol 1995; 12:L491–L500.
72. Barker PM, Brown MJ, Ramsden CA, Strang LB, Walters DV. The effect of thyroidectomy in the fetal sheep on lung liquid reabsorption induced by adrenaline or cyclic AMP. J Physiol 1988; 407:373–383.
73. Barker PM, Markiewicz M, Parker KA, Walters DV, Strang LB. Synergistic action of triiodothyronine and hydrocortisone on epinephrine-induced reabsorption of fetal lung liquid. Pediatr Res 1990; 27:588–591.
74. O'Brodovich H, Canessa C, Ueda J, Rafii B, Rossier BC, Edelson J. Expression of the epithelial Na^+ channel in the developing rat lung. Am J Physiol 1993; 265:C491–C496.

75. McCray PB, Goodno S, Graeff RW, Acarregui MJ, McDonald FJ, Price MP, Welsh MJ. Ontogeny and regulation of expression of the amiloride-sensitive epithelial sodium channel (hENaC) subunits in human lung. Pediatr Res 1995; 37:342A.
76. Stein HM, Martinez A, Blount L, Oyama K, Padbury JF. The effects of corticosteroids and thyrotropin-releasing hormone on newborn adaptation and sympathoadrenal mechanisms in preterm sheep. Am J Obstet Gynecol 1994; 171:17–24.
77. Umans JG, Umans HR, Szeto HH. Effects of thyrotropin-releasing hormone in the fetal lamb. Am J Obstet Gynecol 1986; 155:1266–1271.
78. Bennet L, Gluckman PD, Johnston BM. The central effects of thyrotropin-releasing hormone on the breathing movements and electrocortical activity of the fetal sheep. Pediatr Res 1988; 23:72–75.
79. de Zegher F, Spitz B, Devlieger H. Prenatal treatment with thyrotrophin releasing hormone to prevent neonatal respiratory distress. Arch Dis Child 1992; 67:450–454.
80. Dawes GS, Visser GHA, Goodman JDS, Levine DC. Numerical analysis of the human fetal heart rate: modulation by breathing and movement. Am J Obstet Gynecol 1981; 140:535–544.
81. de Zegher F, de Vries L, Pierrat V, Daniels H, Spitz B, Casaer P, Devlieger H, Eggermont E. Effect of prenatal betamethasone/thyrotropin releasing hormone on somatosensory evoked potentials in preterm newborns. Pediatr Res 1992; 32:212–214.
82. Wu SY, Fisher DA, Polk DH. Maturation of thyroid hormone metabolism. In: Wu SY, ed. Thyroid Hormone Metabolism: Regulation and Clinical Implications. Boston: Blackwell Scientific, 1991; 293–320.
83. Roti E, Gnudi A, Braverman LE, Robuschi G, Emanuele R, Bandini P, Benassi L, Pagliani A, Emerson CH. Human cord blood concentrations of thyrotropin-releasing hormone. J Clin Endocrinol Metab 1976; 53:813–817.
84. Moya F, Mena P, Heusser F, Forafori A, Paiva E, Yazigi R, Michaud P, Gross I. Response of the maternal, fetal and neonatal pituitary–thyroid axis to thyrotropin-releasing hormone. Pediatr Res 1986; 20:982–986.
85. Moya F, Mena P, Foradori A, Becerra M, Inzunza A, Germain A. Effect of maternal administration of thyrotropin releasing hormone on the preterm fetal pituitary–thyroid axis. J Pediatr 1991; 119:966–971.
86. Jackson IM. Thyrotropin-releasing hormone. N Engl J Med 1982; 306:145–150.
87. Ballard PL, Ballard RA, Creasy RK, Padbury J, Polk DH, Bracken M, Moya FR, Gross I. Plasma thyroid hormones and prolactin in premature infants and their mothers after prenatal treatment with thyrotropin-releasing hormone. Pediatr Res 1992; 32:673–678.
88. Morales WJ, O'Brien WJ, Angel JF, Knuppel A, Sawai S. Fetal lung maturation: the combined use of corticosteroids and thyrotropin-releasing hormone. Obstet Gynecol 1989; 73:111–116.
89. Ballard RA, Ballard PL, Creasy RK, Padbury J, Polk DH, Bracken M, Moya FR, Gross I. Respiratory disease in very-low-birthweight infants after prenatal thyrotropin-releasing hormone and glucocorticoid. Lancet 1992; 339:510–515.
90. Knight DB, Liggins GC, Wealthall SR. A randomized controlled trial of antepartum thyrotropin-releasing hormone and betamethasone in the prevention of respiratory disease in preterm infants. Am J Obstet Gynecol 1994; 171:11–16.
91. Crowther CA, Alfirevic Z. Antenatal thyrotropin-releasing hormone (TRH) prior to

preterm delivery. In: Enkin MW, Keirse MJNC, Renfrew MJ, Neilson JP, eds. Pregnancy and Childbirth Module, 1994.

92. Crowther CA, Hiller JE, Haslam RR, Robinson JS, Group AS. Australian collaborative trial of antenatal thyrotropin-releasing hormone (ACTOBAT) for prevention of neonatal respiratory disease. Lancet 1995; 345:877–882.
93. Collaborative Santiago Surfactant Group. Collaborative trial of prenatal thyrotropin-releasing hormone and corticosteroids for prevention of respiratory distress syndrome. Am J Obstet Gynecol 1998; 178:33–39.
94. Ballard PL, Hovey ML, Gonzales LK. Thyroid hormone stimulation of phosphatidylcholine synthesis in cultured fetal rabbit lung. J Clin Invest 1984; 74:898–905.

20

Mechanisms and Physiological Sequelae of Reactive Species Injury to the Alveolar Epithelium

IMAD Y. HADDAD, SHA ZHU, SAMUEL J. TILDEN, and SADIS MATALON

University of Alabama at Birmingham
Birmingham, Alabama

I. Introduction and Purpose

Chronic lung disease of infancy (bronchopulmonary dysplasia; BPD) develops mainly in ventilated infants treated for hyaline membrane disease (HMD) with high concentrations of oxygen. The lungs of these infants are continuously exposed to both self-generated and exogenously derived oxidants. This oxidant stress is often mediated by reactive species, including $O_2^{\bullet -}$ (superoxide), H_2O_2 (hydrogen peroxide), and $^{\bullet}OH$ (hydroxyl radical). These species have been implicated as causal or contributory to lung injury by initiation of lipid peroxidation of biological membranes and oxidation of critical cellular proteins and nucleic acids.

Recently, another free radical with relatively high reactivity has been identified in the normal and diseased lung. Nitric oxide ($^{\bullet}NO$), produced by a variety of pulmonary cells, is a key signal transducing molecule with diverse physiological functions, including vasoregulation, neurotransmission, and immune host defense. However, the high level of $^{\bullet}NO$ production in disease states may contribute to respiratory epithelium cytopathology.

In addition, $^{\bullet}NO$ contains an unpaired electron and, therefore, can react with other free radicals such as $O_2^{\bullet -}$ to form peroxynitrite ($ONOO^-$), a potent oxidant. At physiological pH, $ONOO^-$ can be protonated to form peroxynitrous acid, which rapidly decomposes (~25% yield) to intermediates with the reactivity of $^{\bullet}OH$ and nitrogen dioxide ($^{\bullet}NO_2$; 3).

Following stimulation by proinflammatory cytokines and lipopolysaccharide, alveolar macrophages and epithelial cells produce large amounts of $^{\bullet}NO$ and $O_2^{\bullet -}$ for prolonged periods and can act as foci for the intense and localized production of $ONOO^-$ and its toxic intermediates, in close proximity to the pulmonary surfactant. These species may interact to form other potent oxidants that can injure the epithelium leading to clinically significant pathophysiological sequelae. The objectives of this chapter are (1) to summarize the evidence for the production of $^{\bullet}NO$ and $ONOO^-$ in the lung during inflammation and (2) to review in vitro and in vivo evidence indicating that $^{\bullet}NO$ may either enhance or sometimes diminish oxidant injury to the components of the alveolar epithelium. We will point out existing controversies and, whenever possible, attempt to reconcile existing differences.

II. Structure of the Newborn and Adult Alveolar Epithelium

The lining of the alveolar space consists of a continuous layer made of thin squamous type I epithelial cells interspersed with smaller, cuboidal, metabolically active type II epithelial cells. The tight junctions between epithelial cells are organized in such a manner that they provide a high-resistance barrier to fluid movement from the alveolar to the interstitial space. The alveolar epithelium is much less permeable to fluid than is the pulmonary vascular endothelium. Albumin and other proteins are restricted from entering the alveolar space, and the resulting osmotic pressure, along with the subatmospheric tissue pressure in the interstitial space, are important factors in limiting fluid flux from the extravascular to the airspaces (43).

In addition to the passive forces, active transepithelial ion transport plays a major role in regulating fluid transport. Results of studies with conscious animals, isolated perfused lungs, and cultured pneumonocytes indicate that alveolar type II cells contain amiloride-inhibitable sodium channels in their apical membranes, and ouabain-sensitive Na^+, K^+-ATPase in their basolateral membranes, and are capable of actively transporting sodium from the alveolar to the interstitial space (41,49). This important lung epithelial cell function helps explain the lack of significant amounts of alveolar edema in conditions associated with increased alveolar permeability to solute or with surfactant dysfunction.

The epithelial lining fluid (ELF) of normal lungs contains pulmonary surfactant that is synthesized by alveolar type II cells. This lipoprotein complex consists mainly of phospholipids and at least four different associated proteins, labeled surfactant proteins A, B, C, and D (SP-A, SP-B, SP-C, and SP-D). The main function of surfactant is to lower the surface tension of the air–liquid interface and to inhibit alveolar collapse at low lung volumes (79). This property decreases the work of breathing and prevents extravasation of fluid into the alveolar space. The hydrophobic surfactant proteins, SP-B and SP-C, enhance surfactant adsorption to the air–liquid interface and decrease the surface tension of the phospholipid lining the alveoli during lung deflation monolayer (65).

The most abundant surfactant protein, SP-A, causes lipid aggregation in the presence of calcium (27), which is necessary for the formation and stabilization of tubular myelin. SP-A also binds carbohydrates (19), and promotes adsorption of phospholipids to an air–fluid interface in the presence of SP-B (10).

SP-A can be structurally divided into four discrete domains. A short NH_2-terminal region, a collagen-like domain, a short (30- to 40-amino acid) domain, and a globular COOH-carbohydrate-binding terminal region. Recent work has examined the structure–function relation of SP-A (44), indicating that the globular COOH-terminal region of SP-A is required for lipid binding and aggregation.

SP-D binds to phosphatidylinositol and glucosylceramide and may act cooperatively with SP-A to induce lipid binding and moderate surfactant turnover (51). SP-D, as well as SP-A, can also interact specifically with a variety of microorganisms and alveolar macrophages (60), suggesting a role in pulmonary host defense.

III. Oxidant Stress in the Developing Lung

The importance of the influence of reactive oxygen or nitrogen species on the alveolar epithelium relative to chronic lung disease in premature infants requires consideration of certain maturational characteristics of the lung. At birth, the lung is not fully developed, and alveoli continue to increase in number and size postnatally. Therefore, lung injury and subsequent repair may interfere with the process of normal maturation, giving rise to unique diseases characteristic of the immature lung.

In the fetus, the potential alveolar spaces are filled with fluid. This fluid production ($\sim$3–5 mL hr^{-1} kg^{-1} of body weight) is driven by active chloride transport across the alveolar and airway epithelia (52). The presence of fluid is required for normal lung development in utero. Shortly before birth the alveolar epithelium starts to reabsorb sodium, a process that contributes significantly to the absorption of fetal lung liquid (9). Thus, the lungs of premature infants may be predisposed to alveolar edema if the normal physiological "switch" from secretory to absorptive epithelium is delayed.

Oxidative stress in the lung is a result of a delicate balance between the rate of oxidant production and the presence of antioxidants. The lung contains several potential enzymatic (superoxide dismutase, catalase, glutathione peroxidase) and nonezymatic antioxidants (vitamin E, vitamin C, glutathione). Depletion of antioxidant defenses contributes to the evolution of lung damage (25). Oxidant stress may induce lung antioxidant defenses, as in newborn rats exposed to hyperoxia, thereby facilitating oxygen tolerance in the developing lung (72).

IV. Biology of Reactive Oxygen and Nitrogen Species

A. Basic Review of Biochemistry

Under normal circumstances, most of the oxygen presented to mammalian cells (~98%) undergoes a four-electron catalytic reduction to form water by mitochondrial cytochrome *c*. The remaining oxygen (2%), may undergo sequential incomplete reduction to form reactive oxygen species (ROS), such as $O_2^{\bullet -}$ and H_2O_2. In the presence of iron, $O_2^{\bullet -}$ and H_2O_2 may combine to form $^{\bullet}OH$, an extremely toxic product of oxygen metabolism.

Under normal conditions, intracellular $O_2^{\bullet -}$ and H_2O_2 concentrations are kept at low levels (10 pM and 1–100 nM, respectively) by cytosolic and mitochondrial superoxide dismutases (SODs), cytosolic glutathione peroxidase, peroxisomal catalase, and several nonenzymatic antioxidants. This balance is disturbed by either a reduction in antioxidant defenses or an increase in the rate of reactive species formation. Several factors may exacerbate production of ROS in acute and chronic lung diseases. First, increased oxygen inhalation is often required to alleviate hypoxemia. Exposure of lung cells, subcellular organelles, and lung tissue to pure hyperoxia increases mitochondrial H_2O_2 production 10- to 15-fold (73). Second, in response to proinflammatory cytokines, activated neutrophils and macrophages migrate to the lungs and release ROS by the membrane-bound enzyme–complex NADPH oxireductase. Third, under conditions of ischemia, decreased perfusion, low oxygen tension, or trauma, xanthine dehydrogenase, the innocuous form of the enzyme, is converted to xanthine oxidase, which uses xanthine and molecular oxygen to produce partially reduced oxygen species. The results of several studies suggest that xanthine oxidase may be released from the intestine or liver into the circulation and bind to pulmonary endothelium, where it can stimulate production of ROS (77).

Although $O_2^{\bullet -}$ and H_2O_2 can be directly toxic to biological targets (16), their limited reactivity with many biological molecules has raised questions about their toxicity (70). Instead, it has been proposed that $O_2^{\bullet -}$ toxicity in vivo may derive from the conversion reduction of $O_2^{\bullet-}$ to the reactive $^{\bullet}OH$ by the iron-catalyzed Haber-Weiss reaction:

$$O_2^{\bullet-} + Fe^{3+} \rightarrow O_2 + Fe^{2+}$$

$$Fe^{2+} + H_2O_2 \rightarrow {}^{\bullet}OH + OH^- + Fe^{3+}$$

However, generation of $^{\bullet}OH$ by this reaction requires the interaction of three different species ($O_2^{\bullet-}$, H_2O_2, and Fe^{3+}), all of which are probably kept at very low concentrations in the ELF by the presence of catalase, SOD, and reduced glutathione (7). Most iron is chelated in a noncatalytic form by transferrin and ceruloplasmin in the ELF (55). In addition, ELF contains ascorbate in higher concentrations than $O_2^{\bullet-}$, and this also reduces Fe^{3+}, thereby preventing the formation of $^{\bullet}OH$.

Though the in vivo formation of the $^{\bullet}OH$ radical still may occur by the Haber-Weiss reaction, there is yet another pathway for the biological formation of activated species with the reactivity of the $^{\bullet}OH$, without the requirement for iron. Mammalian cells produce the stable free radical $^{\bullet}NO$ from the oxidative deamination of L-arginine by the low-output constitutive nitric oxide synthase (cNOS) and the high-output inducible nitric oxide synthase (iNOS). $^{\bullet}NO$ may combine with $O_2^{\bullet-}$ at near diffusion-limited rate (6.7×10^9 M^{-1} s^{-1}) to form $ONOO^-$ (57). With a p*K*a of 6.8, ~ 20% of $ONOO^-$ exists as peroxynitrous acid (ONOOH) at physiological pH, which rapidly decomposes to form potent oxidants with the reactivity of $^{\bullet}OH$ and $^{\bullet}NO_2$ without the need for metal catalysis (3).

$$^{\bullet}NO + O_2^{\bullet-} \rightarrow ONOO^- + H^+ \rightleftarrows ONOOH \rightarrow \text{“}^{\bullet}OH \ldots {}^{\bullet}NO_2\text{”}$$

B. Nitric Oxide in the Lung

$^{\bullet}NO$ detected in exhaled breath of normal individuals (36) plays an important physiological role in the lung. Basal low level production of $^{\bullet}NO$ by cNOS helps match ventilation and perfusion in the lungs and also influences pulmonary hypoxic vasoconstriction and airway reactivity (17). Because of its vasorelaxant properties and its rapid inactivation in the blood by its reaction with hemoglobin, $^{\bullet}NO$ inhalation has been advocated as a means of selectively reducing pulmonary hypertension and improving systemic oxygenation in a variety of clinical situations, including BPD (1), and the acute respiratory distress syndrome (ARDS; 67).

Besides basal $^{\bullet}NO$ production, alveolar macrophages (76), airway cells, and alveolar type II pneumocytes (63) release large amounts of $^{\bullet}NO$ in response to stimulation with tumor necrosis factor (TNF), interferon gamma (INF-γ), and lipopolysaccharide. In vitro exposure of these cells to these cytokines leads to abundant iNOS mRNA and associated production of nitrites and nitrates, the stable products of ˙NO, in the culture medium. iNOS, the enzyme responsible for ˙NO formation during inflammation has been immunolocalized to human lung tissue obtained from patients with pneumonia and sepsis (37). Furthermore, there have been reports of continuous expression of iNOS activity in bronchial and tracheal epithelial cells from normal humans (2).

Upregulation of ˙NO occurs in several animal models of lung injury and inflammation. Induction of immune complex and cytokine-induced alveolitis in rat lungs results in significant elevation of ˙NO decomposition products and albumin concentrations in the bronchoalveolar lavage (BAL) fluid (48). Exposure of rats to oxidant gases, such as ozone (58) or smoke (32), injured the alveolar epithelium, upregulated ˙NO production, and increased iNOS mRNA. Infecting hamster tracheal rings with *Bordetella pertussis* in vitro produced epithelial cytopathology, inhibited DNA synthesis, and induced ˙NO synthesis by the tracheal cells (28). In addition, intravenous injection of rats with bacterially derived lipopolysaccharide caused a time-dependent increase in iNOS mRNA expression in the lung (78).

A notable point of controversy is the capacity of human macrophages and neutrophils to produce ˙NO. In contrast to rodent macrophages, isolated human macrophages show relatively low production of nitrite (56). However, more recent evidence (8,15) is consistent with the production of reactive nitrogen species by human inflammatory cells, albeit in lower concentrations than those that have been measured in rodents.

The importance of this excess ˙NO production during inflammation remains unclear. Reactive nitric oxide has complex biological reactivity and its beneficial versus detrimental effects in the lungs may depend on the amount and duration of induction, on the nature of target molecule, and the copresence of other free radicals and oxidants. Excessive ˙NO, produced following a pathological event or an invading organism, may initially represent part of a host immune adaptive response against a variety of insults; however, sustained dysregulated levels may lead to toxic effects especially in the presence of $O_2^{\bullet -}$ anion leading to the formation of the potent oxidant, $ONOO^-$.

C. Beneficial ˙NO Effects

Several observations suggest that ˙NO can protect the lungs from oxidant stress. In buffer-perfused isolated rabbit lungs, inhaled ˙NO (24 ppm) ameliorated the increase in pulmonary vascular permeability produced by the intravascular generation of H_2O_2 (61), whereas inhibition of endogenous ˙NO exacerbated the oxidant-mediated increase in capillary filtration coefficient ($K_{f,c}$; 35). In patients with acute lung injury, inhaled ˙NO decreased permeability pulmonary edema (5) and suppressed proinflammatory cytokine production in the lung.

Potential mechanisms by which ˙NO may ameliorate tissue injury include (1) activation of guanylate cyclase, with resultant induction of cGMP-dependent effects, such as reducing adhesion of platelets and neutrophils to endothelium (39); (2) binding to the free coordination sites of heme-bound iron, thus indirectly acting as an iron chelator (34); (3) inhibiting oxidant-induced membrane and lipoprotein oxidation by annihilation of lipid radical species, thereby terminating radical chain propagation reactions (68); and (4) modulation of the inflammatory process by altering the production of soluble cytokines (14,59), and inhibiting the expression of adhesion molecules in endothelial cells (12).

D. Detrimental ˙NO Effects

Reactive nitric oxide participates in macrophage cytotoxicity against tumors (80) and host defense against pathogens, including bacteria (40) and viruses (11). However, these effects are nonspecific, and overproduction of ˙NO may be cytotoxic, not only for microbes, but also for the cells and tissues that produce it (28).

Several mechanisms for ˙NO cytotoxicity have been suggested. Exposure of cultured cells in vitro to activated macrophages or high concentrations of ˙NO depletes cells of their energy stores by interacting with iron–sulfur centers of essential enzymes such as mitochondrial aconitase, NADH–ubiquinone oxidoreductase (complex I), succinate–ubiquinone oxidoreductase (complex II) in the mitochondrial electron transport chain (71), and the important glycolytic enzyme glyceraldehyde-3-phosphate dehydrogenase (13). ˙NO also causes DNA strand breaks and the activation of the nuclear enzyme, poly-ADP-ribosyl transferase (81), with further consumption of ATP molecules.

E. The "Dark Side" of ˙NO: Reaction with $O_2^{\cdot-}$

Reactive nitric oxide is a weak oxidant, but it turns into a strong oxidant after its fast reaction with $O_2^{\cdot-}$ to form $ONOO^-$. Emerging evidence indicates that ˙NO-mediated *oxidant* reactions may be attributable to $ONOO^-$ or its decomposition products, and not ˙NO itself.

Although highly reactive, its modest rate of decomposition under physiological conditions allows $ONOO^-$ to diffuse for up to several cell diameters to critical cellular targets before becoming protonated and decomposing. $ONOO^-$ initiates iron-independent lipid peroxidation and oxidizes thiols, damages the mitochondria electron transport chain (64), and causes lipid peroxidation of human low-density lipoproteins. In addition, metal ions, such as Fe^{3+} EDTA and copper in the active site of SOD, catalyze the heterolytic cleavage of $ONOO^-$ to form a nitronium ion-like species (NO_2^+) that nitrates phenolics, including tyrosine in proteins (4).

Formation of $OONO^-$ is limited in normal tissue because the concentration of both $^{\bullet}NO$ (10–100 nM) and $O_2^{\bullet -}$ (10 pM) are much lower than SOD (~1 μM). Pathological conditions including inflammation can greatly increase the tissue concentrations of $^{\bullet}NO$ (1–5 μM) and $O_2^{\bullet -}$ to approach or exceed that of SOD. Under these conditions, the reaction rate constant of $^{\bullet}NO$ with $O_2^{\bullet -}$ is three times higher than the SOD-catalyzed dismutation of $O_2^{\bullet -}$ to H_2O ($2 \times 10^9\ M^{-1}\ s^{-1}$). Production of $OONO^-$ by human neutrophils (8), rat alveolar macrophages (33), and bovine aortic endothelial cells (38) has been demonstrated with luminol-dependent chemoluminescence. In the ELF, production of large amounts of $^{\bullet}NO$ and $O_2^{\bullet -}$ may create foci for the intense and localized production of $ONOO^-$, in close proximity to all components of the blood–gas barrier.

One way to demonstrate $ONOO^-$ formation in vivo is to detect the presence of stable by-products of its reaction with various biological compounds. 3-Nitrotyrosine, the product of the addition of a nitro group (NO_2) to the *ortho*-position of the hydroxyl group of tyrosine, is such a stable compound.

F. $ONOO^-$ Formation in ARDS

Acute respiratory distress syndrome, triggered by various pathological conditions, is a clinical syndrome that features severe lung inflammation with abnormal permeability of the alveolar epithelium. The edema is a result of injury to both endothelial and epithelial cells caused by reactive species and proteolytic enzymes released by activated neutrophils and alveolar macrophages. Despite the identification of many mediators that lead to neutrophil tissue infiltration and activation, overall mortality from ARDS remains at 50–70%. The lack of specific treatment for ARDS is due to the complex interplay between the different humoral mediators released by the initiating condition.

By using a polyclonal antibody that recognizes antigenic sites related to nitrotyrosine (22), we demonstrated increased immunostaining in the lung of pediatric patients who died with ARDS and in the lungs of rats exposed to sublethal hyperoxia (100% O_2 for 60 hr). Immunostaining was specific because it was blocked by the addition of an excess amount of antigen, and was absent when the nitrotyrosine antibody was replaced with nonspecific IgG (Figs. 1 and 2). Nitrotyrosine formation was detected only in rat lung sections incubated in vitro with $ONOO^-$, but not $^{\bullet}NO$ or reactive oxygen species (Fig. 3). The most likely candidate capable of nitrating tyrosine residues is $ONOO^-$. Thus, these data suggest that $ONOO^-$ is formed in the lungs of patients and animals with acute lung injury.

However, $ONOO^-$ may not be the only species capable of tyrosine nitration. $^{\bullet}NO_2$ can also nitrate tyrosine, although it is much less efficient than $ONOO^-$ because two molecules of $^{\bullet}NO_2$ are required to nitrate one tyrosine. Another pos-

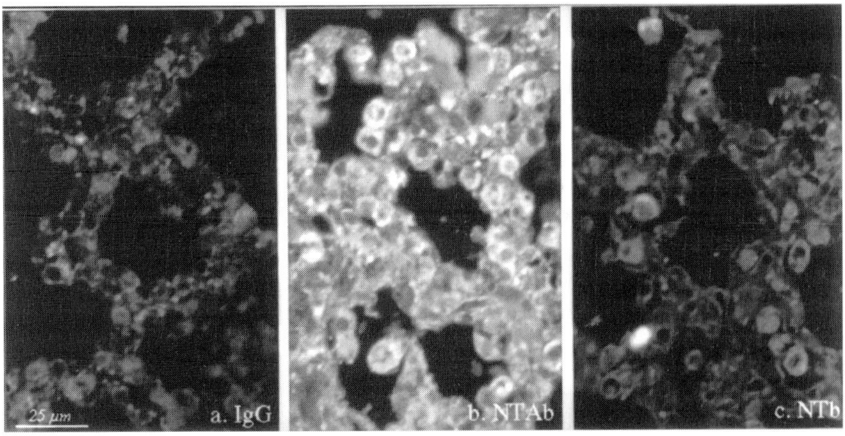

Figure 1 Epifluorescence images of paraffin-embedded, semithin (4–6 μm) lung sections from a patient with sepsis-induced ARDS, incubated with (a) nonspecific IgG; (b) the polyclonal antibody to nitrotyrosine (NTAb); or (c) the NTAb in the presence of 10 mM nitrotyrosine. All sections were then incubated with a secondary antibody, goat anti-rabbit IgG coupled to rhodamine. All pictures were obtained with identical camera and computer settings. Significantly higher specific immunostaining (white areas) was noted with lung sections incubated with the NTAb (mean pixel intensity = 155) compared with sections stained with nonspecific IgG (mean intensity = 90), or the NTAb in the presence of 10 mM nitrotyrosine (mean intensity = 96). Results were reproduced using either formalin-fixed or fresh-frozen sections from five patients with ARDS. (Reprinted from Ref. 21 with permission.)

sible nitration pathway is the reaction of ·NO-derived nitrite, with oxidants, such as H_2O_2 and hypochlorous acid, to form the nitrating species nitrosylchloride (74).

V. ·NO-Derived Effects on the Alveolar Epithelium

A. Oxidant-Mediated Injury to Surfactant

Prolonged continuous exposure of animals to high concentrations of oxygen (50), ozone (54), and $^{\cdot}NO_2$ (47) damages the pulmonary surfactant system, resulting in increased amounts of protein in the alveolar space, pulmonary atelectasis, arterial hypoxemia, and eventually death.

The mechanisms responsible for the development of surfactant deficiency

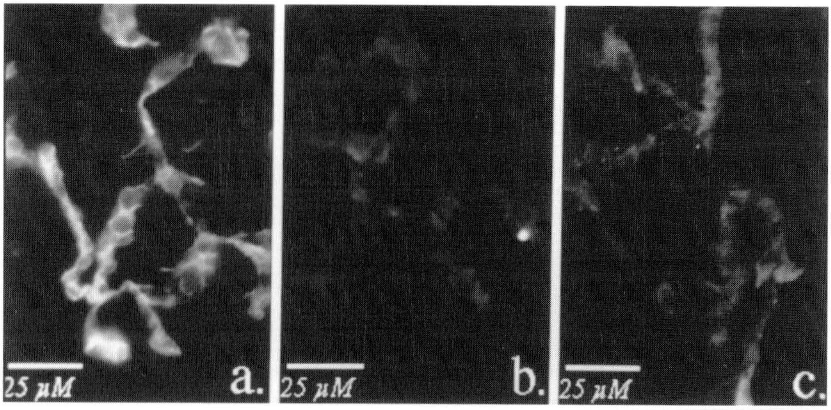

Figure 2 Frozen thin (6-μm) sections from lungs of rats that were exposed to (a, b) 100% oxygen for 60 hr or (c) room air: a and c were incubated with the polyclonal antibody against nitrotyrosine; b, with an equivalent amount of nonspecific IgG. All sections were then incubated with a secondary antibody coupled to rhodamine. All pictures were obtained with identical camera and computer settings. Notice the significantly higher level of fluorescence when an oxygen-exposed lung section was incubated with the nitrotyrosine antibody as compared with a room air control. (Reprinted from Ref. 21.)

after exposure to oxidants are complex. In vitro exposure of isolated alveolar type II cells to ROS resulted in decreased levels of surfactant synthesis and secretion (30). However, a decrease in the surfactant pool size may not necessarily lead to surfactant deficiency, because sufficient dipalmitoyl-phosphatidylcholine may be present to form a condensed surface film. Rabbits exposed to acute hyperoxia have normal lung compliance and total lung capacity in spite of a 40% reduction in lavaged phospholipids (31). The development of a surfactant-deficient state also may result from increased ELF concentrations of plasma proteins, cell membrane lipids, and hemoglobin following oxidant-induced increase of alveolar solute permeability. Plasma proteins compete with surfactant lipids for space in the air–fluid interface, thereby decreasing the surfactants' effectiveness (29). In vitro studies to measure surface tension of surfactant samples in a Wilhelmy balance or a pulsating bubble surfactometer indicated that both whole serum and albumin may inhibit surfactant adsorption in a dose-dependent manner. At low lung surfactant concentrations, protein inhibition of lung surfactant affects both the rate of adsorption and the minimum surface tension (surface tension at minimum bubble radius; T_{min}) achieved. At higher surfactant concentrations (> 0.125 mg/mL), the inhibition primarily affects adsorption rate, and the

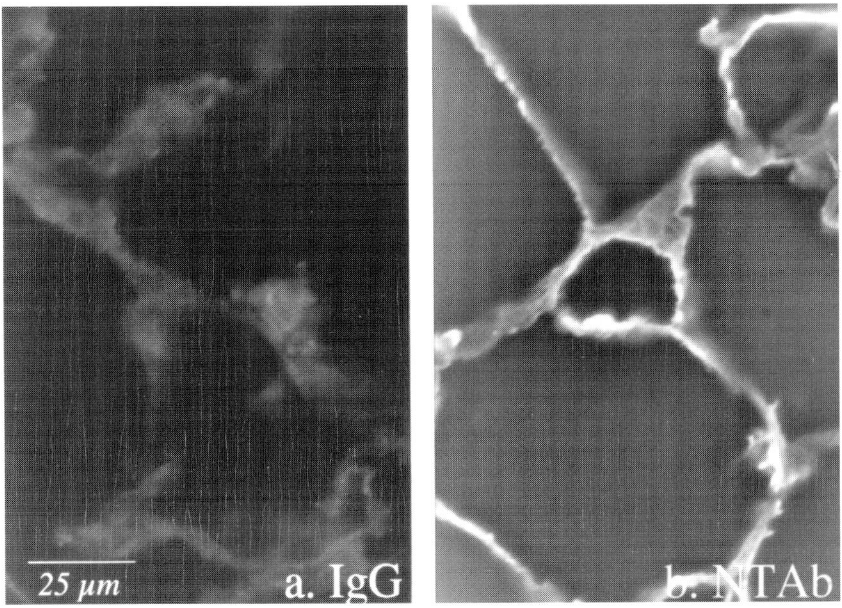

Figure 3 Epifluorescence images of semithin (4–6 μm), frozen rat lung sections. Sections were exposed to 1 mM ONOO for 15 min, by immersion in a 10-mM HEPES solution (pH 7.4) to which ONOO was added at time zero. They were then immunostained with either the polyclonal antibody to nitrotyrosine (NTAb; right panel), or an equivalent amount of nonspecific IgG (IgG; left panel), followed by the secondary antibody, goat antirabbit IgG conjugated to rhodamine. White areas contain higher fluorescence than background (black). Exposures were taken under identical conditions. (Reprinted from Ref. 21.)

T_{min} reached over time does not change. These data have led many investigators to reconsider the importance of this mechanism in causing a functional surfactant deficiency.

Probably the most important mechanism by which ROS cause surfactant dysfunction is by oxidizing unsaturated lipids and damaging surfactant proteins. In vitro exposure of purified natural lung surfactant to activated neutrophils and $FeCl_3$/ascorbate (69), or $FeCL_2/H_2O_2$ (18), which generates $^{\bullet}OH$ by the Fenton reaction, impaired the surfactant's ability to reach a T_{min} below 15 mN/m on dynamic compression in a pulsating bubble surfactometer. However, the concentrations of ROS generated by these agents were very large and may not be physiologically relevant. Polyacrylamide gel electrophoresis (SDS–PAGE) of pulmonary surfactant after exposure to neutrophils was consistent with SP-A fragmentation and cross-linking, which may impair the surfactant's function. SOD prevented the neutrophil-induced functional impairment of surfactant, but not the SP-A fragmentation, suggesting that $O_2^{\bullet -}$ also may have damaged the low molecular weight hydrophobic surfactant proteins SP-B and SP-C.

Evidence for oxidant-induced injury to SP-A was provided by in vitro exposure of SP-A to ozone and $^{\bullet}NO_2$, which resulted in partial loss of important physiological functions, including decreased ability to inhibit phosphatidylcholine secretion by alveolar type II cells, loss of mannose binding, and decreased enhancement of phagocytosis of herpes simplex virus by alveolar macrophages (46,53). Furthermore, in vitro exposure of SP-A to ozone resulted in a time-dependent oxidation of its methionine and tryptophan residues, and enhanced SP-A proteolysis by neutrophil elastase, suggesting a possible synergism between the action of proteases and ROS. Reactive species, present in oxidant gases or released by inflammatory cells in the ELF of patients with ARDS, may inactivate the α_1-protease inhibitor in vivo, which provides most of the protection against neutrophil elastase in the lower respiratory tract (62). Unopposed elastase may cause proteolytic inactivation of surfactant proteins, which may result in loss of important surfactant functions.

B. Role of $^{\bullet}NO$ in $O_2^{\bullet -}$-Mediated Injury to Pulmonary Surfactant

In addition to increased generation of ROSs, exposure of rats in vivo to ozone (58), endotoxin (78), or silica (6) also upregulated $^{\bullet}NO$ production and $ONOO^-$ generation. These reactive oxygen–nitrogen species secreted by epithelial cells and activated alveolar macrophages in the ELF may interact with the different components of the pulmonary surfactant system.

Chemical generators are often used to study the effects of reactive oxygen–nitrogen species in vitro. To relate these effects to biological systems, it is critical to measure the exact concentrations of reactive species released by these agents. The time course of $^{\bullet}NO$ production by spermine NONOate, *S*-nitrosopenicillamine (SNAP), and 3-morpholinosydnonimine (SIN-1), which simultaneously generates $^{\bullet}NO$ and $O_2^{\bullet -}$ to form $ONOO^-$ (20), is shown in Fig. 4. The production rate of $O_2^{\bullet -}$ by lumazine plus xanthine oxidase was measured as the SOD-inhibitable cytochrome *c* reduction at 550 nm (see Fig. 4A). $ONOO^-$ formation was quantified by the rate of rhodamine formation during the oxidation of dihydrorhodamine (DHR; Fig. 5). $ONOO^-$, but not $^{\bullet}NO$ or $O_2^{\bullet -}$ alone, oxidizes DHR to rhodamine (20).

To determine whether $^{\bullet}NO$ modifies $O_2^{\bullet -}$-mediated injury, we exposed a mixture containing phosphatidylcholine (PC) liposomes and SP-A (10% by weight) to increasing concentrations of $^{\bullet}NO$, generated by spermine NONOate, and constant $O_2^{\bullet -}$ levels, produced by the action of xanthine oxidase (5 mU/mL) on lumazine (100 μM) in the presence of Fe^{3+} (100 μM). The increase in the $^{\bullet}NO/O_2^{\bullet-}$ value resulted in suppression of $O_2^{\bullet-}$-induced lipid peroxidation, probably by scavenging lipid alkoxyl and peroxyl radicals (Fig. 6). However, the increase in $^{\bullet}NO/O_2^{\bullet-}$ ratio resulted in nitration of tyrosine residues of SP-A, and inhibited the ability of SP-A to enhance the aggregation of lipids and bind mannose in the presence of calcium, two important functional properties of SP-A. Similar nitration and inhibition of SP-A function was observed following exposure of SP-A to SIN-1 (20), chemically synthesized $ONOO^-$ (21), and tetranitromethane, a specific nitrating species at pH 8 (24). $^{\bullet}NO$ alone, generated by SNAP plus 100 μM L-cysteine, or spermine NONOate neither nitrated nor inhibited SP-A function. Taken as a whole, these data confirm that $^{\bullet}NO$ plays a dual role in the modification of oxidant-mediated injury. $^{\bullet}NO$ inhibited $O_2^{\bullet-}$-mediated lipid peroxidation, but enhanced $O_2^{\bullet-}$-induced injury to SP-A, by nitration of tyrosine residues of SP-A by $ONOO^-$, formed by the rapid reaction of $^{\bullet}NO$ and $O_2^{\bullet-}$.

The final translational product of human SP-A monomer contains eight tyrosine residues in the globular COOH-terminal region of the protein, the region responsible for the ability of SP-A to enhance the aggregation of lipids and to bind mannose. Nitration of tyrosine will decrease the pK_a of tyrosine from 10 to 7.5, rendering nitrotyrosine more hydrophilic, thus potentially inducing conformational change of the tertiary structure of the COOH-terminal region of SP-A secondary to alterations in the ionic charge.

Figure 4 (A) Time courses of release of $^{\bullet}NO$ by 200 μM spermine NONOate and generation of $O_2^{\bullet-}$ by lumazine (100 μM) plus xanthine oxidase (5 mU/mL): Steady-state concentration of $^{\bullet}NO$ was measured with ISO-NO meter in 10 mM HEPES buffer, pH 7.4 at 37°C. $O_2^{\bullet-}$ production rate was measured as SOD-inhibitable cytochrome *c* reduction at 550 nm in 10 mM HEPES buffer, pH 7.4, at 37°C. Results are of a typical experiment which was repeated three times (20). (B) Evolution of nitric oxide, measured with an ISO-NO meter, during a 2-hr period after addition of SIN-1 (1 mM), SNAP alone (1 mM), or 100 μM SNAP and 100 μM cysteine into a solution containing 10 mM HEPES. In the absence of a reductant, $^{\bullet}NO$ production by 1 mM SNAP reached a peak value of 1 μM within 5 min of its addition to the solution and decayed rapidly to zero. In contrast, when mixed with equimolar concentrations of L-cysteine, 100 μM SNAP generated a significantly higher amount of $^{\bullet}NO$. Under these conditions, the mean $^{\bullet}NO$ concentration during the 2-hr exposure period was about 1 μM. In the absence of SOD, no free $^{\bullet}NO$ could be detected by the decomposition of SIN-1. Addition of SOD (100 U/mL) to 1 mM SIN-1 in HEPES buffer led to the continuous and sustained release of $^{\bullet}NO$. Results are of a typical experiment which was reproduced at least three times. (From Ref. 20, with permission.)

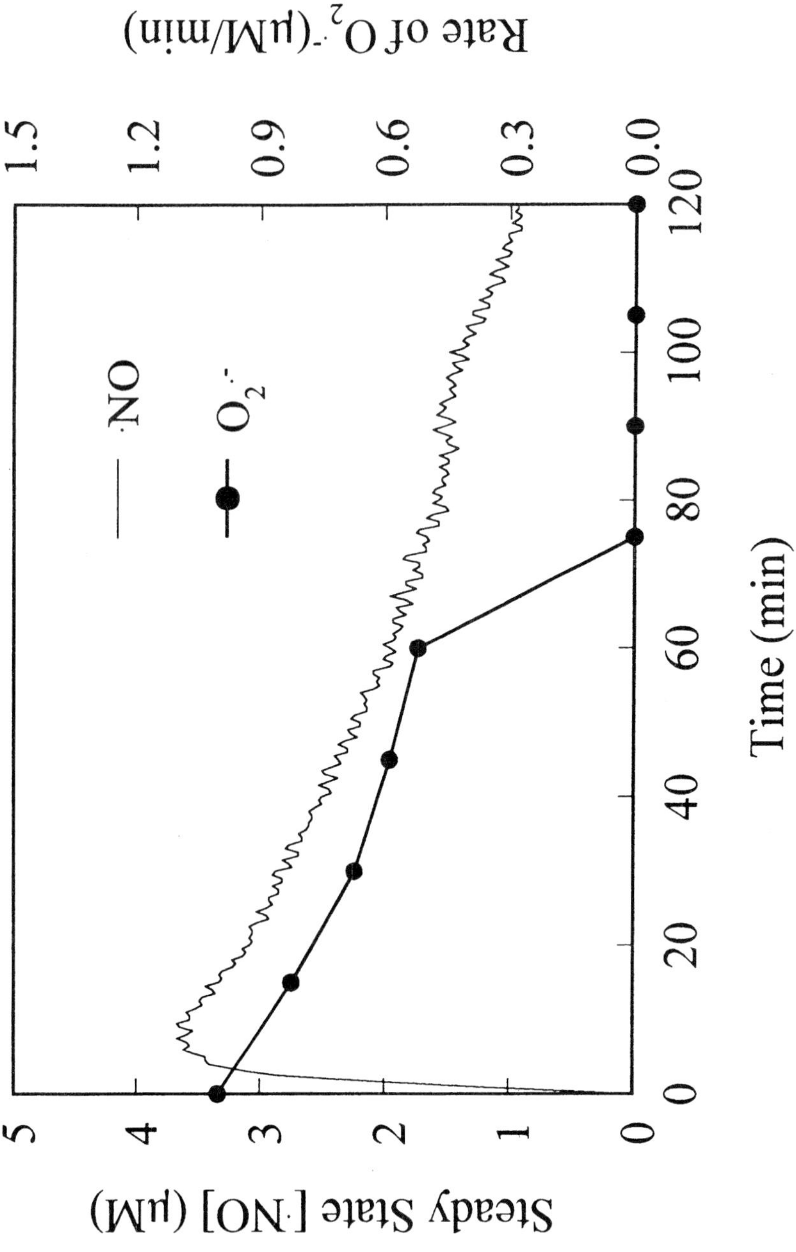
Steady State [·NO] (μM)
0
1
2
3
4
5
Rate of O$_2^{·-}$(μM/min)
0.0
0.3
0.6
0.9
1.2
1.5
·NO
O$_2^{·-}$
0
20
40
60
80
100
120
Time (min)

(A)

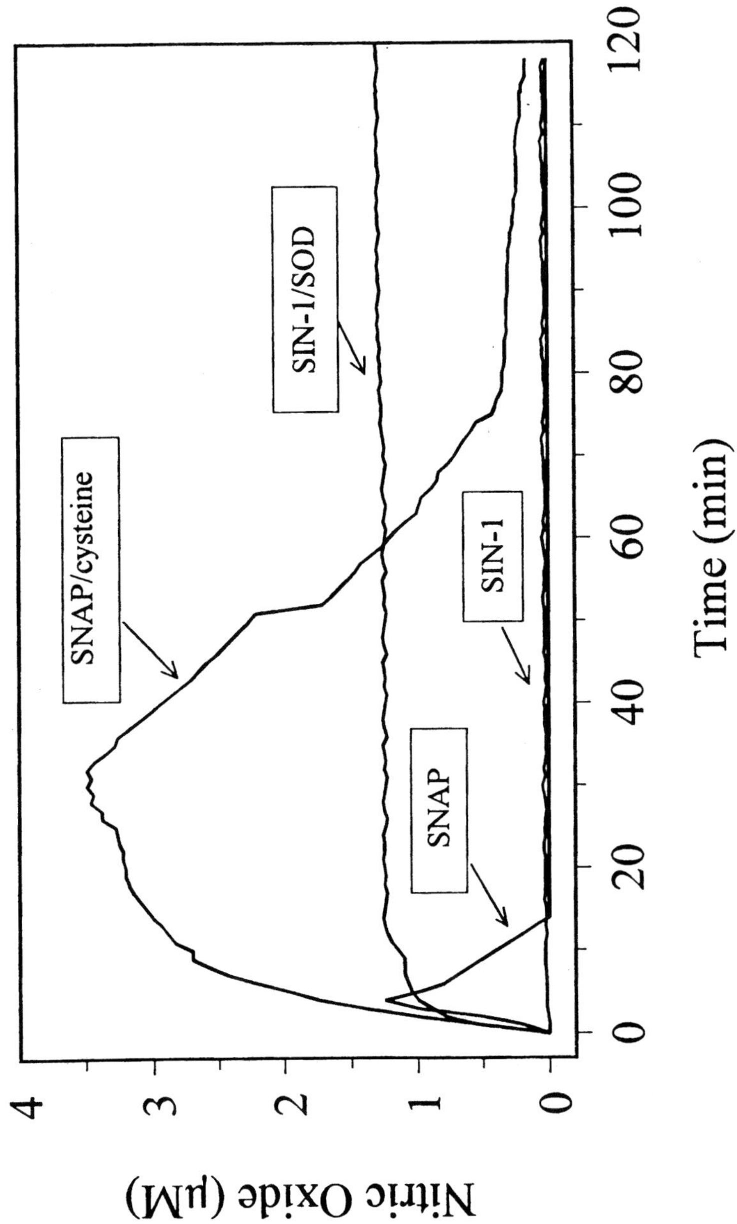
SNAP/cysteine
SIN-1/SOD
SIN-1
SNAP
Time (min)
Nitric Oxide (μM)
0
20
40
60
80
100
120
0
1
2
3
4

(B)

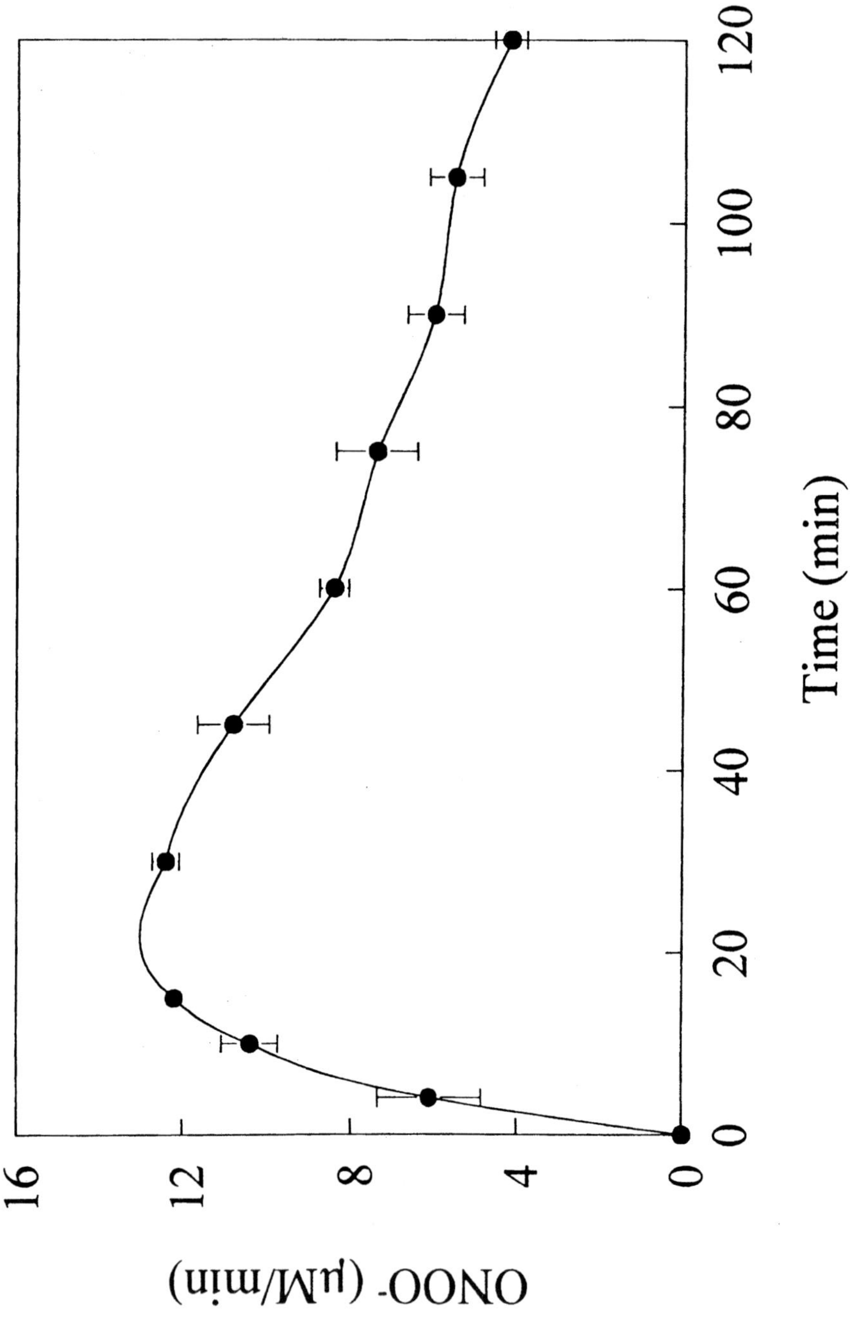
ONOO- (μM/min)
0
4
8
12
16
Time (min)
0
20
40
60
80
100
120

Several in vivo studies evaluated injury to surfactant following inhalation of nitric oxide gas (NO). Robbins et al. (66) demonstrated that exposure of newborn piglets to 100 ppm NO and 95% O_2 for 48 hr resulted in significant injury to pulmonary surfactant, manifested by inhibition of surface activity and worsened pulmonary inflammation. Injury to surfactant was attributed to the in vivo formation of $ONOO^-$. Matalon et al. exposed newborn lambs to various concentrations of NO for 6 hr and assessed various indices of surfactant function (42). T_{min} of surfactant samples isolated from the BAL fluid of newborn lambs breathing 80 or 200 ppm NO exhibited abnormal surface properties ($T_{min} > 8$ mN/m after 10 min of pulsation). In addition, SP-A, isolated from the lungs of lambs that breathed 200 ppm NO exhibited a small, but statistically significant, decrease in the ability to aggregate lipids (42). In contrast, Hallman et al. reported that NO gas (80 ppm) mitigated oxidant-induced inhibition of surface activity of natural surfactant in vitro (26). However, when hemoglobin was added to the surfactant, the same amount of NO promoted surfactant injury, presumably by the ·NO-induced conversion of hemoglobin to methemoglobin, which interferes with surfactant function in vitro and in vivo.

C. Regulation of Epithelial Metabolism by ·NO

Exposure of alveolar type II pneumocytes to 1–3 μM ·NO, generated by SNAP, or spermine NONOate resulted in an approximate 60% decrease in the rate of surfactant synthesis, as measured by the rate of incorporation of [methyl-^3H]choline into phosphatidylcholine, and 60–80% inhibition of cellular ATP levels (23). Incubation of freshly isolated alveolar type II pneumocytes with N-nitro-L-arginine methyl ester (L-NAME), an inhibitor of ·NO synthesis, increased surfactant synthesis, cell ATP content, and cellular oxygen consumption, suggesting that basal levels of ·NO regulated cell metabolism (45). Furthermore, exposure of human type II pneumocytes to the proinflammatory cytokine TNF-α decreased

---

Figure 5 Rate of $ONOO^-$ formation by SIN-1 measured by dihydrorhodamine (DHR) oxidation: Rhodamine formation, the oxidized product of DHR, was monitored for 2 min at 500 nm at 37°C ($\epsilon_{500nm} = 78{,}000\ M^{-1}\ cm^{-1}$) in cuvettes containing DHR (50 μM) and aliquots of the SIN-1 mixture obtained at the indicated times. ·NO alone, produced by spermine NONOate, or SNAP plus L-cysteine did not oxidize DHR (not shown). Values are means ± SE ($n = 3$). (Modified from Ref. 23.)

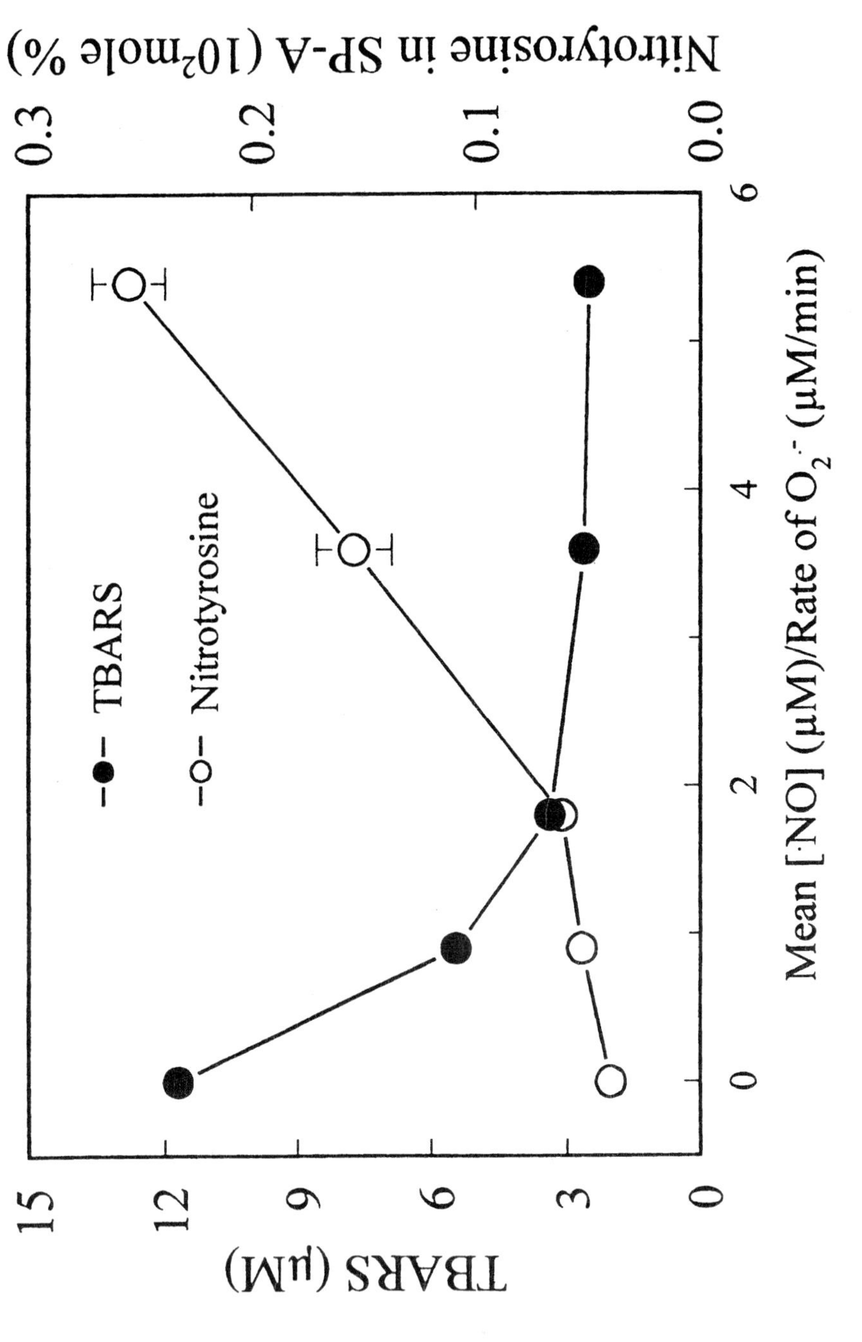
TBARS (μM)
15
12
9
6
3
0
Nitrotyrosine in SP-A (10²mole %)
0.3
0.2
0.1
0.0
TBARS
Nitrotyrosine
Mean [·NO] (μM)/Rate of O₂·⁻ (μM/min)
0
2
4
6

surfactant synthesis by a mechanism dependent, at least in part, on the induction of ·NO production by these cells (75).

VI. Lessons from Basic Research: Development of Rational Therapeutic Interventions to Limit Oxidant Injury

Instillation of SOD is currently undergoing clinical trials to determine its effectiveness in mitigating the onset and severity of BPD in infants with hyaline membrane disease. Antioxidant defense supplementation will be most effective when the location and nature of toxic species contributing to tissue injury are revealed and the antioxidants are site-directed in sufficient concentrations. Current techniques available to effectively deliver the antioxidants are suboptimal. Recently, vector-mediated gene therapy has shown promise in delivering therapeutic genes for both genetic and acquired diseases. Some antioxidant genes that have been cloned include manganese and copper–zinc SOD, catalase, and glutathione-related enzymes. With recombinant DNA technology, it is now possible to transfer these genes by intratracheal administration to cells subjected to oxidative stress. The effectiveness of this approach in humans is still unknown.

Reactive nitric oxide has both oxidant and nonoxidant reactions with diverse physiological and pathophysiological effects. Some reactions of ·NO promote oxidant injury, whereas other reactions may divert oxidants away from potentially harmful pathways. Clinical studies have demonstrated that inhaled NO can mitigate pulmonary hypertension and improve oxygenation in infants with chronic lung disease (1) by a cGMP-dependent mechanism. It is clear, however, that ·NO can undergo a variety of other effects in the lung, including reaction with other free radicals; inactivation of iron–sulfur centers of enzymes; interac-

---

Figure 6 Influence of variable $^{\cdot}NO/O_2^{\cdot -}$ ratio on lipid peroxidation and SP-A nitration: Mixtures of PC liposomes (5 mg/mL) and SP-A (0.5 mg/mL) were incubated with xanthine oxidase (5 mU/mL), 100 μM lumazine, 100 μM Fe^{3+}EDTA, and variable concentrations of ·NO released by spermine NONOate (0, 20, 40, 100, 200 μM) in 10 mM HEPES buffer, pH 7.4, at 37°C for 2 hr. The malondialdehyde (MDA) content of PC–SP-A mixture was determined by absorbance at 532 nm of the products formed after reaction of samples with 2-thiobarbituric acid. SP-A nitrotyrosine content was determined by a capture enzyme-linked immunosorbent assay (ELISA), using polyclonal antinitrotyrosine as primary antibody and nitrated bovine serum albumin as standard. Nitrotyrosine was expressed as percentage (%) of total moles of all amino acid residues. Values are means ± SE for $n = 4$.

tion with thiols or groups of proteins; and regulation of gene expression. These reactions of •NO need to be investigated to determine the role of endogenous and inhaled •NO in the diseased lung, especially during the critical period of lung development.

References

1. Abman SH, Griebel JL, Parker DK, Schmidt JM, Swanton D, Kinsella JP. Acute effects of inhaled nitric oxide in children with severe hypoxemic respiratory failure. J Pediatr 1994; 124:881–888.
2. Asano K, Chee CB, Gaston B, Lilly CM, Gerard C, Drazen JM, Stamler JS. Constitutive and inducible nitric oxide synthase gene expression, regulation, and activity in human lung epithelial cells. Proc Natl Acad Sci USA 1994; 91:10089–10093.
3. Beckman JS, Beckman TW, Chen J, Marshall PA, Freeman BA. Apparent hydroxyl radical production by peroxynitrite: implications for endothelial injury from nitric oxide and superoxide. Proc Natl Acad Sci USA 1990; 87:1620–1624.
4. Beckman JS, Ischiropoulos H, Zhu L, van der Woerd M, Smith C, Chen J, Harrison J, Martin JC, Tsai M. Kinetics of superoxide dismutase- and iron-catalyzed nitration of phenolics by peroxynitrite. Arch Biochem Biophys 1992; 298:438–445.
5. Benzing A, Brautigam P, Geiger K, Loop T, Beyer U, Moser E. Inhaled nitric oxide reduces pulmonary transvascular albumin flux in patients with acute lung injury. Anesthesiology 1995; 83:1153–1161.
6. Blackford JA Jr, Antonini JM, Castranova V, Dey RD. Intratracheal instillation of silica up-regulates inducible nitric oxide synthase gene expression and increase nitric oxide production in alveolar macrophages and neutrophils. Am J Respir Cell Mol Biol 1994; 11:426–431.
7. Cantin AM, North SL, Hubbard RC, Crystal RG. Normal alveolar epithelial lining fluid contains high levels of glutathione. J Appl Physiol 1987; 63:152–157.
8. Carreras MC, Pargament GA, Catz SD, Poderoso JJ, Boveris A. Kinetics of nitric oxide and hydrogen peroxide production and formation of peroxynitrite during the respiratory burst of human neutrophils. FEBS Lett 1994; 341:65–68.
9. Cassin S, Perks AM. Amiloride inhibits arginine vasopressin-induced decrease in fetal lung liquid secretion. J Appl Physiol 1993; 75:1925–1929.
10. Cockshutt AM, Weitz J, Possmayer F. Pulmonary surfactant-associated protein A enhances the surface activity of lipid extract surfactant and reverses inhibition by blood proteins in vitro. Biochemistry 1990; 29:8424–8429.
11. Croen KD. Evidence for an antiviral effect of nitric oxide: inhibition of herpes simplex virus type 1 replication. J Clin Invest 1993; 91:2446–2452.
12. De Caterina R, Libby P, Peng HB, Thannickal VJ, Rajavashisth TB, Gimbrone MA Jr, Shin WS, Liao JK. Nitric oxide decreases cytokine-induced endothelial activation. Nitric oxide selectively reduces endothelial expression of adhesion molecules and proinflammatory cytokines. J Clin Invest 1995; 96:60–68.

13. Dimmeler S, Lottspeich F, Brune B. Nitric oxide causes ADP-ribosylation and inhibition of glyceraldehyde-3-phosphate dehydrogenase. J Biol Chem 1992; 267: 16771–16774.
14. Eigler A, Moeller J, Endres S. Exogenous and endogenous nitric oxide attenuates tumor necrosis factor synthesis in the murine macrophage cell line RAW 264.7. J Immunol 1995; 154:4048–4054.
15. Evans TJ, Buttery LDK, Carpenter A, Springall DR, Polak JM, Cohen J. Cytokine-treated human neutrophils contain inducible nitric oxide synthase that produces nitration of ingested bacteria. Proc Natl Acad Sci USA 1996; 93:9553–9558.
16. Fridovich I. Biological effects of the superoxide radical. Arch Biochem Biophys 1986; 247:1–11.
17. Frostell CG, Blomqvist H, Hedenstierna G, Lundberg J, Zapol WM. Inhaled nitric oxide selectively reverses human hypoxic pulmonary vasoconstriction without causing systemic vasodilation. Anesthesiology 1993; 78:427–435.
18. Gilliard N, Heldt GP, Loredo J, Gasser H, Redl H, Merritt TA, Spragg RG. Exposure of the hydrophobic components of porcine lung surfactant to oxidant stress alters surface tension properties. J Clin Invest 1994; 93:2608–2615.
19. Haagsman HP, Hawgood S, Sargeant T, Buckley D, White RT, Drickamer K, Benson BJ. The major lung surfactant protein, SP 28-36, is a calcium-dependent, carbohydrate-binding protein. J Biol Chem 1987; 262:13877–13880.
20. Haddad IY, Crow JP, Hu P, Ye Y, Beckman J, Matalon S. Concurrent generation of nitric oxide and superoxide damages surfactant protein A. Am J Physiol 1994; 267:L242–L249.
21. Haddad IY, Ischiropoulos H, Holm BA, Beckman JS, Baker JR, Matalon S. Mechanisms of peroxynitrite-induced injury to pulmonary surfactants. Am J Physiol 1993; 265:L555–L564.
22. Haddad IY, Pataki G, Hu P, Galliani C, Beckman JS, Matalon S. Quantitation of nitrotyrosine levels in lung sections of patients and animals with acute lung injury. J Clin Invest 1994; 94:2407–2413.
23. Haddad IY, Zhu S, Crow J, Barefield E, Gadilhe T, Matalon S. Inhibition of alveolar type II cell ATP and surfactant synthesis by nitric oxide. Am J Physiol 1996; 270: L898–906.
24. Haddad IY, Zhu S, Ischiropoulos H, Matalon S. Nitration of surfactant protein A results in decreased ability to aggregate lipids. Am J Physiol 1996; 270:L281–L288.
25. Halliwell B, Hu ML, Louie S, Duvall TR, Tarkington BK, Motchnik P, Cross CE. Interaction of nitrogen dioxide with human plasma. Antioxidant depletion and oxidative damage. FEBS Lett 1992; 313:62–66.
26. Hallman M, Bry K, Lappalainen U. A mechanism of nitric oxide-induced surfactant dysfunction. J Appl Physiol 1996; 80:2035–2043.
27. Hawgood S, Clements JA. Pulmonary surfactant and its apoproteins. J Clin Invest 1990; 86:1–6.
28. Heiss LN, Lancaster JR Jr, Corbett JA, Goldman WE. Epithelial autotoxicity of nitric oxide: role in the respiratory cytopathology of pertussis. Proc Natl Acad Sci USA 1994; 91:267–270.

29. Holm BA, Enhorning G, Notter RH. A biophysical mechanism by which plasma proteins inhibit lung surfactant activity. Chem Phys Lipids 1988; 49:49–55.
30. Holm BA, Hudak BB, Keicher L, Cavanaugh C, Baker RR, Hu P, Matalon S. Mechanisms of H_2O_2-mediated injury to type II cell surfactant metabolism and protection with PEG-catalase. Am J Physiol 1991; 261:C751–C757.
31. Holm BA, Notter RH, Siegle J, Matalon S. Pulmonary physiological and surfactant changes during injury and recovery from hyperoxia. J Appl Physiol 1985; 59:1402–1409.
32. Ischiropoulos H, Mendiguren I, Fisher D, Fisher AB, Thom SR. Role of neutrophils and nitric oxide in lung alveolar injury from smoke inhalation. Am J Respir Crit Care Med 1994; 150:337–341.
33. Ischiropoulos H, Zhu L, Beckman JS. Peroxynitrite formation from macrophage-derived nitric oxide. Arch Biochem Biophys 1992; 298: 446–451.
34. Kanner J, Harel S, Granit R. Nitric oxide as an antioxidant. Arch Biochem Biophys 1991; 289:130–136.
35. Kavanagh BP, Mouchawar A, Goldsmith J, Pearl RG. Effects of inhaled NO and inhibition of endogenous NO synthesis in oxidant-induced acute lung injury. J Appl Physiol 1994; 76:1324–1329.
36. Kharitonov SA, Yates D, Barnes PJ. Increased nitric oxide in exhaled air of normal human subjects with upper respiratory tract infections. Eur Respir J 1995; 8:295–297.
37. Kobzik L, Bredt DS, Lowenstein CJ, Drazen J, Gaston B, Sugarbaker D, Stamler JS. Nitric oxide synthase in human and rat lung: immunocytochemical and histochemical localization. Am J Respir Cell Mol Biol 1993; 9:371–377.
38. Kooy NW, Royall JA. Agonist-induced peroxynitrite production from endothelial cells. Arch Biochem Biophys 1994; 310:352–359.
39. Kubes P, Suzuki M, Granger DN. Nitric oxide: an endogenous modulator of leukocyte adhesion. Proc Natl Acad Sci USA 1991; 88:4651–4655.
40. MacMicking JD, Nathan C, Hom G, Chartrain N, Fletcher DS, Trumbauer M, Stevens K, Xie QW, Sokol K, Hutchinson N. Altered responses to bacterial infection and endotoxic shock in mice lacking inducible nitric oxide synthase. Cell 1995; 81: 641–650.
41. Matalon S. Mechanisms and regulation of ion transport in adult mammalian alveolar type II pneumocytes. Am J Physiol 1991; 261:C727–C738.
42. Matalon S, DeMarco V, Haddad IY, Myles C, Skimming JW, Schurch S, Cheng S, Cassin S. Inhaled nitric oxide injures the pulmonary surfactant system of lambs in vivo. Am J Physiol Lung Cell Mol Physiol 1996; 270:L273–L280.
43. Matalon S, Egan EA. Interstitial fluid volumes and albumin spaces in pulmonary oxygen toxicity. J Appl Physiol 1984; 57:1767–1772.
44. McCormack FX, Calvert HM, Watson PA, Smith DL, Mason RJ, Voelker DR. The structure and function of surfactant protein A. Hydroxyproline- and carbohydrate-deficient mutant proteins. J Biol Chem 1994; 269:5833–5841.
45. Miles PR, Bowman L, Huffman L. Nitric oxide alters metabolism in isolated alveolar type II cells. Am J Physiol Lung Cell Mol Physiol 1996; 271:L23–L30.
46. Muller B, Barth P, von Wichert P. Structural and functional impairment of surfactant

protein A after exposure to nitrogen dioxide in rats. Am J Physiol 1992; 263:L177–L184.
47. Muller B, von Wichert P. Effect of nitrogen dioxide inhalation on surfactant phosphatidylcholine synthesis in rat alveolar type II cells. Biochim Biophys Acta 1993; 1170:38–43.
48. Mulligan MS, Hevel JM, Marletta MA, Ward PA. Tissue injury caused by deposition of immune complexes is L-arginine dependent. Proc Natl Acad Sci USA 1991; 88: 6338–6342.
49. Nici L, Dowin R, Gilmore-Hebert M, Jamieson JD, Ingbar DH. Upregulation of rat lung Na-K-ATPase during hyperoxic injury. Am J Physiol 1991; 261:L307–L314.
50. Novotny WE, Hudak BB, Matalon S, Holm BA. Hyperoxic lung injury reduces exogenous surfactant clearance in vivo. Am J Respir Crit Care Med 1995; 151:1843–1847.
51. Ogasawara Y, McCormack FX, Mason RJ, Voelker DR. Chimeras of surfactant proteins A and D identify the carbohydrate recognition domains as essential for phospholipid interaction. J Biol Chem 1994; 269:29785–29792.
52. Olver RE, Robinson EJ. Sodium and chloride transport by the tracheal epithelium of fetal, new-born and adult sheep. J Physiol (Lond) 1986; 375:377–390.
53. Oosting RS, van Greevenbroek MM, Verhoef J, van Golde LM, Haagsman HP. Structural and functional changes of surfactant protein A induced by ozone. Am J Physiol 1991; 261:L77–L83.
54. Oosting RS, Van Iwaarden JF, Van Bree L, Verhoef J, van Golde LM, Haagsman HP. Exposure of surfactant protein A to ozone in vitro and in vivo impairs its interactions with alveolar cells. Am J Physiol 1992; 262:L63–L68.
55. Pacht ER, Davis WB. Role of transferrin and ceruloplasmin in antioxidant activity of lung epithelial lining fluid. J Appl Physiol 1988; 64:2092–2099.
56. Padgett EL, Pruett SB. Rat, mouse and human neutrophils stimulated by a variety of activating agents produce much less nitrite than rodent macrophages. Immunology 1995; 84:135–141.
57. Padmaja S, Huie RE. The reaction of nitric oxide with organic peroxyl radicals. Biochem Biophys Res Commun 1993;195:539–544.
58. Pendino KJ, Laskin JD, Shuler RL, Punjabi CJ, Laskin DL. Enhanced production of nitric oxide by rat alveolar macrophages after inhalation of a pulmonary irritant is associated with increased expression of nitric oxide synthase. J Immunol 1993; 151:7196–7205.
59. Persson AH, Schornagel JK, Tilders HFF, Vente DJ, Berkenbosch F, Kraal G. Alveolar macrophages autoregulate IL-1 and IL-6 production by endogenous nitric oxide. Am J Respir Cell Mol Biol 1996; 14:272–278.
60. Pikaar JC, Voorhout WF, van Golde LM, Verhoef J, Van Strijp JA, Van Iwaarden JF. Opsonic activities of surfactant proteins A and D in phagocytosis of gram-negative bacteria by alveolar macrophages. J Infect Dis 1995; 172:481–489.
61. Poss WB, Timmons OD, Farrukh IS, Hoidal JR, Michael JR. Inhaled nitric oxide prevents the increase in pulmonary vascular permeability caused by hydrogen peroxide. J Appl Physiol 1995; 79:886–891.

62. Pryor WA, Stone K. Oxidants in cigarette smoke. Radicals, hydrogen peroxide, peroxynitrate, and peroxynitrite. Ann NY Acad Sci 1993; 686:12–27; see discussion 27–8.
63. Punjabi CJ, Laskin JD, Pendino KJ, Goller NL, Durham SK, Laskin DL. Production of nitric oxide by rat type II pneumocytes: increased expression of inducible nitric oxide synthase following inhalation of a pulmonary irritant. Am J Respir Cell Mol Biol 1994; 11:165–172.
64. Radi R, Rodriguez M, Castro L, Telleri R. Inhibition of mitochondrial electron transport by peroxynitrite. Arch Biochem Biophys 1994; 308:89–95.
65. Revak SD, Merritt TA, Hallman M, Cochrane CG. Reconstitution of surfactant activity using purified human apoprotein and phospholipids measured in vitro and in vivo. Am Rev Respir Dis 1986; 134:1258–1265.
66. Robbins CG, Davis JM, Merritt TA, Amirkhanian JD, Sahgal N, Morin FC 3rd, Horowitz S. Combined effects of nitric oxide and hyperoxia on surfactant function and pulmonary inflammation. Am J Physiol 1995; 269:L545–L550.
67. Rossaint R, Falke KJ, Lopez F, Slama K, Pison U, Zapol WM. Inhaled nitric oxide for the adult respiratory distress syndrome [see comments]. N Engl J Med 1993; 328:399–405.
68. Rubbo H, Radi R, Trujillo M, Telleri R, Kalyanaraman B, Barnes S, Kirk M, Freeman BA. Nitric oxide regulation of superoxide and peroxynitrite-dependent lipid peroxidation. Formation of novel nitrogen-containing oxidized lipid derivatives. J Biol Chem 1994; 269:26066–26075.
69. Ryan SF, Ghassibi Y, Liau DF. Effects of activated polymorphonuclear leukocytes upon pulmonary surfactant in vitro. Am J Respir Cell Mol Biol 1991; 4:33–41.
70. Sawyer DT, Valentine JS. How super is superoxide? Acct Chem Res 1981; 14:393–400.
71. Stuehr DJ, Nathan CF. Nitric oxide. A macrophage product responsible for cytostasis and respiratory inhibition in tumor target cells. J Exp Med 1989; 169:1543–1555.
72. Tanswell AK, Freeman BA. Pulmonary antioxidant enzyme maturation in the fetal and neonatal rat. I. Developmental profiles. Pediatr Res 1984; 18:584–587.
73. Turrens JF, Freeman BA, Crapo JD. Hyperoxia increases H_2O_2 release by lung mitochondria and microsomes. Arch Biochem Biophys 1982; 217:411–421.
74. van der Vliet A, Eiserich JP, O'Neill CA, Halliwell B, Cross CE. Tyrosine modification by reactive nitrogen species: a closer look. Arch Biochem Biophys 1995; 319: 341–349.
75. Vara E, Arias-Diaz J, Garcia C, Hernandez J, Balibrea JL. Both prostaglandin-E_2 and nitric oxide sequentially mediate the tumor necrosis factor alpha-induced inhibition of surfactant synthesis by human type II pneumocytes. Arch Surg 1995; 130: 1279–1285; see discussion 1286.
76. Warner RL, Paine R 3rd, Christensen PJ, Marletta MA, Richards MK, Wilcoxen SE, Ward PA. Lung sources and cytokine requirements for in vivo expression of inducible nitric oxide synthase. Am J Respir Cell Mol Biol 1995; 12:649–661.
77. Weinbroum A, Nielsen VG, Tan S, Gelman S, Matalon S, Skinner KA, Bradley E Jr, Parks DA. Liver ischemia–reperfusion increases pulmonary permeability in rat: role of circulating xanthine oxidase. Am J Physiol 1995; 268:G988–G996.

78. Wizemann TM, Gardner CR, Laskin JD, Quinones S, Durham SK, Goller NL, Ohnishi ST, Laskin DL. Production of nitric oxide and peroxynitrite in the lung during acute endotoxemia. J Leukoc Biol 1994; 56:759–768.
79. Wright JR, Wager RE, Hamilton RL, Huang M, Clements JA. Uptake of lung surfactant subfractions into lamellar bodies of adult rabbit lungs. J App Physiol 1986; 60: 817–825.
80. Xie K, Huang S, Dong Z, Juang SH, Gutman M, Xie QW, Nathan C, Fidler IJ. Transfection with the inducible nitric oxide synthase gene suppresses tumorigenicity and abrogates metastasis by K-1735 murine melanoma cells. J Exp Med 1995; 181: 1333–1343.
81. Zhang J, Dawson VL, Dawson TM, Snyder SH. Nitric oxide activation of poly(ADP-ribose) synthetase in neurotoxicity. Science 1994; 263:687–689.
82. Zhu S, Haddad IY, Matalon S. Modification of SP-A mamose-binding properties by reactive oxygen species. Arch Biochem Biophys 1996; 333:282–290.

21

Surfactant in Chronic Lung Injury

RICHARD J. KING

University of Texas Health Science Center
at San Antonio
San Antonio, Texas

SAMUEL HAWGOOD

University of California
San Francisco, California

I. Introduction

The last 30 years has been a time of significant advances in lung biology and medicine as related to pulmonary surfactant: the material has been isolated and analyzed, the genes of the proteins cloned, some progress achieved in understanding the complicated hormonal events involved in lung maturation and parturition, and substantial improvement has evolved in diagnosing and managing patients with acute and chronic lung injury, especially neonates with hyaline membrane disease (HMD). The legacy of this progress in saving increasingly smaller and more immature babies has been the emergence of a larger number of premature neonates with chronic lung disease (bronchopulmonary dysplasia; BPD) whose prolonged management to a successful outcome is still problematic. Likewise, since the first report on adult patients with chronic lung disease sharing the commonality of noncardiogenic pulmonary edema (1; adult respiratory distress syndrome; ARDS), there is now a substantially greater appreciation of the cellular processes involved in the evolution of this condition, although unfortunately, it has not yet resulted in substantial progress in treating this syndrome. This chapter concentrates on one rather limited aspect of these chronic lung injuries in the newborn and the adult—the potential involvement of pulmonary surfactant. Although the importance of pulmonary surfactant is clear and favorably exploited in the treatment of HMD, its role in BPD is far less certain. Patients with ARDS sometimes manifest changes in the properties and composition of pulmonary surfactant that are evident and readily linked to the pathophysiology. In other patients, the correlations are less sure. This chapter will attempt to summarize current information on surfactant in chronic lung injury in both the adult and neonate, for there is increasing evidence that many of the cellular events in both age groups are similar, although they may occur with different time courses and severities (2). Similar to most disease processes, the pathophysiological outcome is a result of several intervening factors, of which surfactant is but one, and this is apparent by the many topics covered in this volume. We will not attempt to provide comprehensive coverage of all aspects of the injury processes. The experiments and clinical cases that are included herein were chosen because of their intended design or emphasis on questions of surfactant, possibly to the exclusion of other factors that also may be affecting etiology and outcome in patients or experimental animals.

II. Composition and Functions of Pulmonary Surfactant

Given the complex cellular response of the alveolar epithelium to injury, it is reasonable to suppose that the composition and function of surfactant, one of the important secretions of the alveolar epithelium, might be affected during the evolution of chronic lung injury. A brief overview of the structure and function of normal surfactant components is presented here to provide a background for our following discussion of the limited experimental and clinical studies of surfactant in chronic lung disease (CLD).

Surfactant is composed of several different phospholipid-rich lipoproteins, including the contents of the lamellar inclusions in pulmonary type II epithelial cells, an extracellular form called tubular myelin, the surface film itself, and other vesicular structures of various sizes and shapes (3,4). These lipoproteins constitute a metabolic cycle that maintains a stable intra-alveolar pool of surfactant, despite wide fluctuations in breathing rates and patterns. For the most part, regulation of the metabolic cycle is poorly understood and will not be reviewed here. Phospholipids make up most of the mass of surfactant (5), but similar to other lipoprotein systems, the structure and activity of the various surfactant fractions are determined by specific apoproteins. Abnormalities in the relative abundance of various surfactant forms, most commonly an accumulation of protein-poor vesicular structures, are commonly reported in lung injury.

A. Lipid Composition and Function

Phospholipids of several types are the major components in all forms of surfactant. Although particular phospholipids, notably dipalmitoylphosphatidylcholine

(DPPC) and phosphatidylglycerol (PG), are markedly enriched in surfactant relative to those found in other mammalian membranes, there are no phospholipids in surfactant which are specific to it. This is important to the interpretation of bronchoalveolar lavage studies of the surfactant system in chronic lung disease, when cell and bacterial debris may contaminate the surfactant preparations. Suspensions of many phospholipid mixtures will spontaneously form a surface film if an air–fluid interface is present. This process is termed adsorption and refers to the formation of an insoluble film at the fluid surface. By excluding water molecules from the surface layer, phospholipids effectively lower the surface tension of water from 70 mN m^{-1} to values of approximately 25 mN m^{-1} (6). This value (25 mN m^{-1}) is the approximate equilibrium surface tension of a film formed by most naturally occurring phospholipids (7). Compression of the surface film caused by a reduction in area of the film results in a further fall in surface tension. The molecular mechanisms underlying phospholipid adsorption to an air–fluid interface are not well understood, but are important in the physiology of pulmonary surfactant, as adsorption is presumably the mechanism by which the alveolar surface film is formed from the surfactant that is secreted in the fluid layer lining the alveoli.

Experimentally, the kinetics of the process depend on many factors, including the type of phospholipid, the extent of lipid aggregation, and the presence of other components, particularly proteins. Although some proteins enhance adsorption, an excess of nonsurfactant protein in the fluid phase markedly inhibits adsorption, an observation that is often cited to explain surfactant dysfunction in lung injury, wherein the amount of surfactant present frequently appears normal (8). The stability of compressed phospholipid films (area reduced to less than the area at which the surface tension is 25 mN m^{-1}) varies markedly with the composition of the film. Films of DPPC, the single most abundant phospholipid in pulmonary surfactant (9), can be compressed to surface tensions as low as 1 mN m^{-1} or less and show remarkable metastability at such low nonequilibrium surface tensions (10). Most models of alveolar function assume the surface film is highly enriched in DPPC. Pulmonary surfactant secreted into the fluid of the alveolus contains several components, both lipid and protein, in addition to DPPC, which appear to facilitate the rapid formation of DPPC-rich surface films (11).

Unsaturated phosphatidylcholines make up about 25% of the phospholipids in surfactant. The unsaturated phospholipids contribute to the very broad temperature range for the gel-to-liquid crystalline transitions of surfactant, perhaps favoring the adsorption process. A relatively high content of PG is found in the pulmonary surfactant of most, but not all, species (12). PG is found in very low concentrations in most mammalian membranes, but is quite enriched in surfactant, constituting 5–15% of the phospholipids. PG facilitates adsorption of phospholipid mixtures in vitro (13). It is possible that electrostatic interactions between the anionic phosphatidylglycerol head group and either calcium or cationic regions on the surfactant apoproteins may be important in regulating surfactant structure and activity (14). Other phospholipid classes, including phosphatidylethanolamine and phosphatidylserine, have been consistently found in low amounts in isolated surfactant preparations.

Neutral lipids cholesterol, and triglycerides make up about 10% of the surfactant mass (11). Although these lipids modify the behavior of mixed phospholipid films in vitro, a clear role for them in surfactant function has not been established. Finally, several glycolipids have also been purified from surfactant preparations (15), but again, there is insufficient information available to assign them any definite functional role. It is possible that some of these minor components are contaminants, rather than specific surfactant components. Improved methods of surfactant purification and fractionation will be required to resolve this uncertainty. Ensuring the purity of surfactant preparations is particularly troublesome in the setting of lung injury.

B. Protein Structure and Function

The protein content of surfactant preparations varies considerably, depending on the isolation procedures used. Variable amounts of presumably nonspecifically associated proteins, predominantly serum proteins, can contaminate these preparations (11). This problem initially led to considerable confusion over the importance of proteins in surfactant function. Currently four proteins, SP-A, SP-B, SP-C, and SP-D, are generally accepted as surfactant apolipoproteins.

Two homologous collagen-like lectins (collectins), SP-A and SP-D, are secreted by the type II cell into the alveolar lumen. SP-A is almost all lipid-bound and makes up about 3–4% of the total mass of isolated surfactant. SP-D is less abundant and is found predominantly in the lipid-depleted supernatant of lavage fluid (16). The genes for human SP-A (17) and SP-D (18) are both located on chromosome 10. Both proteins are expressed in type II pulmonary epithelial cells and nonciliated cells of the airways (19–21). For the purposes of general description, four clearly distinct structural domains can be recognized in all collectins. A short NH_2-terminal region, containing one or more interchain disulfide bridges, is followed by a variable number of glycine–hydroxyproline-rich triplets, the collagen-like domain. The next domain forms a short helical coiled–coil (22) that links the collagen chains to a calcium-dependent carbohydrate recognition domain (21,23,24). Both SP-A and SP-D are oligomerized into structurally complex multimers of 18 and 12 monomers, respectively.

Both collectins bind certain phospholipids, although the mechanism of binding appears different. SP-D binds and aggregates glycolipids in a calcium-dependent fashion, using the carbohydrate recognition domain (25). Phosphatidylinositol (PI), a ligand for SP-D, is found in surfactant and is often increased during lung injury. The relevance of the interaction between SP-D and PI to surfactant function is uncertain. Despite the sequence homology between the two collectins, the interaction between SP-A and phospholipids does not depend on calcium or carbohydrates (26,27). SP-A binds reversibly to DPPC and DPPC–PG mixtures (28). In the presence of calcium, SP-A–phospholipid mixtures form large heterogeneous aggregates of lipid and protein (27,29). This ability to aggregate surfactant lipids appears to be critical to the proposed role of SP-A in adsorption and film spreading. Calcium binds directly to SP-A, regulating several of the protein's putative functions, including roles in the conversion of lamellar bodies to tubular myelin, the adsorption process, and the interaction of SP-A with alveolar cells.

Two smaller proteins have also been isolated from surfactant. These proteins, SP-B and SP-C, have unusual solution properties because of their remarkable hydrophobicity. Both preferentially partition into most organic solvents from aqueous suspensions of surfactant. SP-B and SP-C are present in surfactant in roughly equal abundance and together make up 2–5% of the surfactant mass. The human SP-B gene is localized to chromosome 2 (30). SP-B is expressed in the lung by both type II cells and nonciliated bronchiolar cells (19). SP-B is translated as a 381-amino acid preproprotein (31–33). Extensive processing of the proprotein in multivesicular bodies, involving the removal of glycosylated NH_2- and COOH-terminal flanking sequences, is required to generate the mature 79-amino acid form of SP-B (34,35). Mature SP-B has a high content of cysteines (9%), positively charged residues (7%), and hydrophobic residues (45%). SP-B appears to have a role in the organization of lamellar bodies (36) and tubular myelin (14,37,38), and in the adsorption process (31,39). Several families that carry a mutation in codon 121 of the SP-B gene have been identified (40). The fatal respiratory distress suffered by infants homozygous for this mutation underscores the importance of SP-B in surfactant function (41).

SP-C also is translated as a larger proprotein (42), which is processed to a smaller, very hydrophobic mature form of the protein. The human SP-C gene is found on chromosome 8 (43). The proprotein (197 residues) is processed to a mature form of only 35 amino acids (44). SP-C, similar to the other surfactant components, is found in lamellar bodies. The mature SP-C sequence is remarkable for a very hydrophobic stretch of 24 amino acids at the COOH-terminal end of the protein. This region forms an α-helix and is presumably in contact with the hydrophobic interior of surfactant membranes (45). SP-C is made even more hydrophobic by covalently attached palmitic acid close to the NH_2-terminus (46). In vitro SP-C markedly increases the rate of phospholipid adsorption (39,42,47), but the mechanisms involved are unknown.

The cumulative experimental data suggest that one important role of the apoproteins is their ability to facilitate the formation of a DPPC-rich surface film. There is evidence for complementary interaction between apoproteins in this function, but the precise mechanisms are not understood (31). SP-A may be particularly important when the surfactant concentration is low or when interfering proteins are present (48,49). Both situations pertain in acute and chronic lung injury. Other roles for the apoproteins have been proposed and extensively discussed in recent reviews (50). SP-B may have a critical role in the assembly of lamellar bodies (36), a hypothesis that is strongly supported by findings of SP-B deficiency in a mouse model (51). Based on in vitro experiments, SP-A may regulate the alveolar surfactant pool size by controlling rates of surfactant exocytosis and endocytosis in type II cells (52). SP-A and SP-D may have additional roles in maintaining the alveolar space and small airways free of pathogenic organisms (53).

III. Experimental Studies on Surfactant in Chronic Lung Injury

A. Adult Animals

Exudative (Inflammatory) Phase

Several animal homologues of ARDS have been used, but most of the work on surfactant has been derived from experiments on animals breathing oxidant gases. Additional studies have been published using chemical carcinogens or the antineoplastic agent bleomycin. Rodents or rabbits have been the choice for most studies, as would be anticipated because of their cost, availability, and experimental convenience, but these species exhibit limited longevity breathing 100% oxygen continuously, and all generally die within 3–4 days, with extensive alveolar edema. Deterioration from sustained hyperoxia is very rapid. After 48 hr of exposure to 100% oxygen, the damage is minimal, with only the beginning of the formation of alveolar edema, reflecting a largely intact capillary endothelium. By 72 hr, however, there is extensive edema, diffusing capacity has dropped to 25% of normal, and death is common (54). Protocols have been devised to extend the duration of the injury (55,56), but a comprehensive pathological assessment of the injury that ensues is often not described. Thus, it is sometimes difficult to know the stage of injury at the time of death. There is, however, enough consistency in the data to allow some generalizations concerning the status of the surfactant system during the acute (inflammatory) aspects of the injury, as compared with the later fibroproliferative phase.

The results show that the metabolism of surfactant phosphatidylcholines is reduced in the time period between 48 and 72 hr of continuous oxidative stress, and this deficit in metabolic capacity results in significant reductions in the amounts of phospholipid that can be harvested from the bronchoalveolar lavage (57). The chemical *composition* of the lavage pool of phosphatidylcholines, however, is largely unchanged. There are substantial alterations in other characteristics of the lavage surfactant; most notably, phosphatidylglycerol is substantially reduced, whereas SP-A and SP-B are increased by severalfold. Cellular distribution is nonuniform, however, and the changes in SP-A and SP-B may result primarily from the effects of injury to Clara cells. A few individual studies on the effects of high oxygen concentrations on surfactant phospholipids in rodents and rabbits, selected because their results are generally consistent with other findings in a relatively large database, may be useful to the reader interested in the primary literature (58–63).

In contrast with the *decreased* phosphatidylcholine pools measured in whole lung and in isolated type II cells of rodents after they breathe 100% oxygen for 60 hr, SP-A subtractive cloning indicates an analagous *increase* in the expression of SP-A mRNA (64), a finding that was verified by Minoo et al. (56). Neither the mechanism nor the significance of this apparent difference in PC and SP-A regulation during the early stages of oxidative stress have been explained, but several studies indicate that tissue SP-A exceeds lamellar body SP-A by several fold (65,66), suggesting that SP-A exists in several pools. The increase in total lung SP-A may partly reflect changes in SP-A content in small-airway cells (64). It is noteworthy, however, that Allred et al. (67) reported a decrease in SP-A mRNA in rats that breathed 100% oxygen for 60 hr. Thus, like other aspects of oxidative injury in the lung, the early effects on SP-A are still not completely clear.

We know of only three studies on the effects of oxidative stress on the other surfactant proteins in adult rodents. Wikenheiser et al. (68) exposed mice to 100% oxygen for up to 5 days and measured steady-state mRNA levels of SP-B in lung tissue. These observations were correlated with in situ hybridization and immunocytochemistry studies showing the cellular distribution of the mRNA and protein. Lung tissue mRNA was increased tenfold after 3 days of hyperoxia and was maintained throughout the subsequent period of oxygen exposure. The distribution of the increased mRNA was nonuniform. SP-B message was markedly increased in the cells of the bronchial epithelium, whereas it was decreased in the alveolar epithelium, and the distribution of mRNA and protein correlated well.

Minoo and co-workers (56) used hamsters that were exposed to 100% oxygen, interrupted by daily 20-min periods of air breathing, to develop an oxidatively-induced lesion that extends over 8 days, a time period more typical of that found in primates with chronic respiratory failure. Survival was high through 8 days, but by day 8 the animals were in extreme distress and died quickly when they were placed in room air. Histological changes were undetectable before day 4; from day 4 through day 8 there was increasing peribronchial and alveolar wall cellularity, edema, and an alveolitis associated with increased numbers of polymorphonuclear lymphocytes (PMNs) and alveolar macrophages (AMs), characteristic of a lesion of mixed exudative–reparative diffuse alveolar damage.

Phospholipid content in lavage increased by twofold at day 4 and by fourfold at day 6; the composition, however, also changed with a 25% increase in DSPC and a 40% decrease in PG. Surface tension–surface area properties indicated a more concentrated surface packing, consistent with the higher amount of DSPC, but surface adsorption rate was substantially reduced. SP-A mRNA doubled at day 4, consistent with the change in phospholipids, but then decreased to about 25% of controls by day 8. In contrast, SP-B and SP-C mRNAs declined continuously with time in oxygen, without the initial increase observed with SP-A. Surfactant proteins were not quantified, but sodium dodecylsulfate–polyacrylamide gel electrophoresis (SDS–PAGE) suggested significant losses of all surfactant proteins in the lavage surfactant by day 6. Allred's study (65) also found decreased expression of SP-B and SP-C.

Nonhuman primates have been used in some of the earliest experiments on oxidative stress (69), but the primary emphasis in these experiments was on the morphological changes and the distribution of cell types. There are, to our knowledge, only two sets of studies on the effects of 100% oxygen on surfactant in the nonhuman primate. Coalson and co-workers (70,71) exposed baboons to 100% oxygen for 5–6 days, followed by ventilation with 50% oxygen for varying periods to study primarily changes in surfactant during stages of the injury in which reparative processes were dominant. These findings are described in the following section. In these experiments, however, bronchoscopic lavage samples for lipid analysis were taken on day 4 of mechanical ventilation, although morphological correlation was not possible. DSPC, quantified as a fraction of total phospholipids, decreased to about 85% that of nonventilated controls, and the ratio of PG to PI decreased to less than 30% of control, nonventilated animals. Lavage and cellular surfactant pools were not quantified.

In a series of studies reported from the laboratories of Young and Crapo (72,73), baboons were mechanically ventilated with 100% oxygen for 4 days to explore the effects of surfactant replacement on the progression of acute lung injury. The injury at 96 hr included diffuse epithelial and endothelial cell injury, interstitial widening, and neutrophil accumulation. The number densities of type I alveolar epithelial cells and endothelial cells decreased, whereas those of type II cells and interstitial cells were unchanged. The average volume of type II cells more than doubled, but there was no change in the lamellar body density. There was denuding of the basement membrane and severe lung edema. Total levels of PC and DSPC in lung lavage of oxygen treated baboons were decreased by about 50%, but the composition of the PC pools was unchanged. PG, however, decreased significantly. In contrast, lamellar body DSPC increased in an amount almost identical with the decrease in the lavage pool, suggesting that the primary target of the oxidative stress may have been secretory pathways. SP-A content in lavage was not changed with oxygen exposure, whereas lamellar body content of SP-A was doubled.

Fibroproliferative Phase

Generalizations about surfactant function and composition during the latter stages of the injury, when fibroblasts and type II-like cells are dividing more rapidly, and epithelial and mesenchymal hyperplasia are evident, are more difficult to establish. Animal homologues are not easy to maintain for the required times, morphological and physiological correlations are sometimes sketchy, and the results are not always consistent. The data do show, however, that surfactant obtained from animals in the hyperplastic phase of the injury is abnormal in either composition or amount, or both.

The antineoplastic agent bleomycin has been used to induce fibrosis in rats (74) and baboons (75). As used in these studies, the agent induced severe edema, followed by a diffuse interstitial mononuclear cell infiltrate, typical of the inflammatory response described in other modes of injury. Type II cell hyperplasia followed within 1–2 weeks after transtracheal administration of bleomycin in rats, and there was increased synthesis of collagen (76) and detectable collagen deposition in interstitial and alveolar sites as early as 1 week after bleomycin was given (77). Fibrotic lesions were prominent. Static lung compliance was decreased at 3, 7, and 14 days after bleomycin, but returned to normal values by 30 days. The reduced lung compliance was attributed to changes in surfactant properties at 3 and 7 days; reduced lung compliance at 14 days was attributed to changes in tissue elasticity (77). Total PC and DPPC pools were doubled by 14 days (77,78), but the amount of PG was unchanged, resulting in a decrease in the percentage of PG. PG is characteristically found in relatively high amount in surfactant compared with phospholipid constituents in other tissues, but its physiological role is unknown (79). The changes in PG reported by Thrall et al. (77) and Low et al. (78) are, in themselves, unlikely to result in functional defects, but they do indicate that regulatory pathways are sensitive to the evolving fibroproliferative changes. Of the surfactant proteins, only SP-A was measured. SP-A content was unchanged, and the SP-A/PC ratio was reduced (80).

N-Nitroso-*N*-methylurethane injected subcutaneously in dogs results in a lesion that evolves over a 20-day period, and it shares some of the pathological features of ARDS (81). Liau and co-workers observed an acute inflammatory-type injury that was apparent by day 4 and peaked at day 7. Recovery began at day 10 and was recognized by a prominent regeneration of the epithelium associated with type II cells that were abnormally laden with lamellar bodies. At the peak of the injury all lipid components in the recoverable lavage were reduced by about 50%, but lipid composition was unchanged (81). Surfactant proteins were not quantified, but the results of SDS-PAGE suggested a reduction in SP-A content, peaking at day 7, that partially reversed with recovery. The physical properties of the surfactants changed with the progression. The principal forms of normal canine surfactant have isopycnic densities of 1.05 and 1.09 g/mL. At peak injury, this decreased to 1.02 g/mL (characteristic of the lipid mixture) and reversed at day 15–20. Surface tension of the lavage surfactant was elevated at days 2–8, but recovered by day 15–20. The shift in buoyant densities may partly reflect, an increase of activity in a surface cycling-dependent enzyme described by Gross and Narine (82). Higuichi et al. (83) studied the in vitro conversion of lavage surfactants obtained from normal rabbits and from rabbits that were injected with *N*-nitroso-*N*-methylurethane. Conversion to the lighter subtypes was greater in the lavage from the injured animals. SP-A supplemented in concentrations greater that 4.5% stimulated the conversion.

Young (84) and Nogee (85) and co-workers studied rats exposed continuously to 85% oxygen for up to 9 days. Under these conditions rats lost weight for 3–5 days, as their food intake decreased. Appetite and activity returned at 5 days, and by day 7 the animals acquired tolerance to 100% oxygen. Type II cells were increased in size and doubled in number, lamellar bodies were prominent, and lamellar body and lavage DSPC were both increased by four- to fivefold. DSPC production, as measured by the turnover of the lavage pool, was four- to sixfold greater than it was in air-breathing controls, but lamellar body phospholipid composition, and presumably, lavage composition, were unchanged. SP-A content was increased 20-fold in lavage and 10-fold in tissue, with similar increases in steady-state mRNA. The results indicate that the adaptation to 85% oxygen results in substantial increases in the surfactant pools, with unchanged composition, at least as measured by SP-A and phospholipids. These changes may be consistent with those observed by Holm et al. (86), who exposed rabbits to 60% oxygen for up to 21 days. Physiological changes in this study were modest—a 10-mmHg decrease in $Pa\text{O}_2$ and a 30% increase in wet-to-dry weight—yet total lavage phosphatidylcholine doubled, as did the rate of incorporation of choline into PC and DSPC in isolated type II cells.

There is limited information on the effects of chronic lung injury on surfactant in nonhuman primates. Huang (72) and Fracia (73) and co-workers exposed baboons to 100% oxygen for up to 4 days (72,73); their findings are summarized in the preceding section. Coalson et al. (70) and King et al. (71), in parallel studies, examined the effects of longer exposures to oxygen and bacterial infection. Adult baboons were subjected to three protocols to develop conditions commonly found in patients: (1) Intravenous injection with oleic acid to induce an inflammatory-like initial lesion, and then ventilation continuously with 100% oxygen for 5–7 days. $F\text{IO}_2$ was then reduced to 0.5 and ventilation continued for up to 14 more days until the animals were killed. (2) Continuous ventilation with 100% oxygen for 4–5 days, followed by 6 days with 50% oxygen. (3) Continuous ventilation with 80% oxygen for 6 days. On day 6, 10^8 *Pseudomonas aeruginosa* were innoculated in each lung, and ventilation was continued for 5 days with 50% oxygen.

The pathological assessment indicated severe lesions in the three injury groups, with greater than fivefold increases in type II cells, twofold increases in interstitial cells, and decreases in endothelial and type I epithelial cells. Type II cell volume density was increased tenfold, whereas lamellar bodies were small and atypical. Lung compliance, diffusing capacity, and Pa_{O_2} were severely decreased in animals in all protocols. Phospholipid composition of lavage surfactant was perturbed in the three injury modes, but the most significant changes were induced in the oleic acid–100% oxygen protocol, wherein the most extensive postinjury repair occurred. Surfactant proteins and mRNAs were not quantified, but qualitative assessment by SDS–PAGE suggested decreases in SP-A content. Surface tension–area curves were abnormal.

Summary

It is evident that the regulation of the surfactant system in conditions of protracted injury can be expressed variably, depending on the mode of injury, its duration, and species. Although the acute phase appears to be associated with decreases in surfactant phosphatidylcholines and an increase in SP-A, there is very limited information on the other surfactant proteins, and that which is available is not consistent. Thus, in the study by Wikenheiser et al. (68), SP-B mRNA and protein were markedly increased, whereas Minoo (56) and Allred (67) and co-workers found decreases in SP-B and SP-C mRNA protein. In more protracted injuries induced in primates (71), DPPC was substantially reduced. In hamsters, however, DPPC was increased by over fourfold, whereas all surfactant proteins were decreased (56). The effects of reductions in the amounts of disaturated phosphatidylcholines, and in their relative abundance among the other constituents of surfactant, are relatively easy to evaluate—it is clear that DPPC needs to be present in adequate amounts to cover the alveolar surface with a relatively stable film. Changes in the amounts of the surfactant proteins, however, are less predictable. The functions of SP-C are unknown. SP-B is essential for life (41) and is required for surface adsorption or film stability (31). SP-A participates in a variety of functions (see previous section), but the extent to which decreases in SP-A might complicate chronic lung injury is still speculative. Mice with deletion of the SP-A gene appear to have normal physiological function in spite of reduced amounts of tubular myelin (87). However, in response to intratracheal instillation with group B streptococci, they display a greater sensitivity as evaluated by the number of bacteria in lung and spleen, and the amount of pulmonary infiltration (88). It is noteworthy, however, that BPD and ARDS are usually associated with extensive alveolar edema fluid that may contain substances that can bind to surfactant and interfere with its physical properties or otherwise inhibit surfactant activity (89). These conditions may not be identical with those that prevail when mice breathe 100% oxygen continuously. Several recent studies have shown that interference with surfactant function may be related to the content of surfactant proteins, at least as evaluated by in vitro experiments (90,91). Thus, it is possible that a compromise in SP-A abundance could exacerbate the pathophysiology of oxygen-induced lung injury, simply based on the importance of SP-A in forming tubular myelin or resisting inhibitor interaction.

B. Newborn Animals

Although data on the status of surfactant in patients with BPD are still fragmentary (relevant studies are summarized in the next section), and abnormalities in surfactant may have importance in the etiology of this disease, there are almost no controlled studies on surfactant in animal homologues of BPD, probably because of the technical demands in duplicating this condition in experimental animals. Fetal animals delivered at sufficiently early gestational ages are very difficult to maintain for the times required to develop a BPD-like lesion, although such efforts are now underway and are promising (92). Alternatively, premature baboons delivered at about 75% of term and then ventilated with 100% oxygen acquire a condition that mimics many of the features of BPD (93,94), and the physiological and pathological changes that accompany this animal homologue of BPD are now well described (95). The only other animal model of BPD uses prematurely delivered sheep (96,97), but there are no published studies on surfactant in this preparation. Animal preparations suitable for the study of BPD have been reviewed previously (95) and are discussed elsewhere in this volume.

Coalson (98) and King (99) and co-workers have analyzed changes in parenchymal cell populations and surfactant components in the 100% oxygen-ventilated baboon homologue of BPD. Animals were delivered by cesarean section at 140 $\pm$ 2 days gestational age (term = 183 days) and ventilated continuously with 100% oxygen for 11 days. On day 11, oxygen concentrations were reduced to maintain a Pao_2 of about 40 mmHg for 5 additional days of ventilation. These animals were considered the "BPD" group. In a separate set of animals, 10^8 *Escherichia coli* were instilled intratracheally on day 11, concomitant with the reduced FiO_2, and these animals constituted the "BPD-infected" group. Three control groups were studied: nonventilated fetal animals of 140 days-gestation; nonventilated fetal animals of 156 days gestation; and 140-day–premature animals ventilated for the 16-day experimental period with oxygen concentrations sufficient to maintain a Pao_2 of more than 60 mmHg. The two injury groups were similar in their responses to oxidative stress and infection. All animals showed saccular wall fibrosis and alternating areas of overinflation and atelectasis. Hyperplastic type II cells were evident, with few type I cells. The appearance of the type II cells varied widely, with substantial heterogeneity of cell volume, glycogen content, and lamellar body size and number. Numerical densities of the type II cells in the two injury groups were increased compared with the ventilated controls, whereas type I cells were decreased, leading to a fivefold increase in the ratio of type II cells to type I cells. The percentage of interstitial cells, however, did not change. Alveolar macrophages were prominent in the alveolar spaces. The small airways at the respiratory bronchiolar level showed either residual hyaline membranes or thin, regenerating epithelium. Animals in the BPD-infected group showed a superimposed organizing pneumonia and more extensive airway changes.

Immunostaining and in situ hybridization indicated various patterns of SP-A mRNA and protein localization compared with ventilated controls. SP-A mRNA was markedly decreased in bronchiolar epithelial and type II epithelial cells, whereas SP-A protein localization was more variable. SP-A was abundant in the hyperplastic cells in peribronchial sites, but there was minimal staining in grossly fibrotic sites in the distal lung. Steady-state SP-A mRNA in whole-lung tissue of both BPD and BPD-infected animals was about 50% of steady-state SP-A mRNA that was present in lungs of ventilated controls. Tissue SP-A protein content was unchanged in the BPD group, but was reduced by 50% in the BPD-infected animals. SP-A content in lavage surfactant was about 35% of that in the ventilated control animals and was comparable in amount with that of the 156-day–nonventilated control. Tissue mRNAs of SP-B and SP-C were unchanged from those of the ventilated control animals, but immunostaining of the proteins indicated considerable variability among the different cell types. Areas with remodeled and fibrobrotic walls showed strong staining in type II and small airway cells, whereas there was minimal or no staining in areas of atelectasis. The composition and amount of phospholipid in surfactant recovered from lavage was unchanged. Surface properties of the lavage surfactant displayed abnormally high surface tension.

The results indicate that in the nonhuman primate with chronic lung injury, surfactant proteins are significantly altered, either in amounts or in cellular localization, with the most striking changes being in the content of SP-A mRNA and protein. Although the best studied attribute of SP-A is its ability to team with other surfactant proteins and induce functional rearrangements in the organization of surfactant phospholipids (31), it contributes to other aspects of lung cell function, as discussed previously. The indications of work to date are that the changes in surfactant composition found in this model of premature lung injury are less extensive that those seen in adult animals (70,71), but that the neonatal injury is still associated with significant changes in lung compliance, atelectasis, and surface tension–area properties, and some of these changes may be related to alterations in surfactant proteins. The importance of these changes of surfactant in BPD, in relation to the other pathophysiological events that occur in parallel, is still incompletely understood.

IV. Involvement of Surfactant in Patients with Chronic Lung Injury

There is a paucity of data about surfactant in human infants with established chronic lung disease. The limited data that are available come from studies of tracheobronchial aspirates and a few postmortem immunohistochemical studies.

A. Tracheobronchial Aspirates

Surfactant, measured as phosphatidylcholine concentration in tracheobronchial aspirates, rises from day 4 to day 7 after premature birth, coincident with resolution of HMD (100). Likewise, the concentration of surfactant proteins in tracheobronchial aspirates rises to normal or supernormal levels within days of birth in premature infants with HMD (101). Very few studies have examined the subsequent changes in tracheobronchial concentrations of surfactant during the evolution of chronic lung disease. Kari and colleagues measured concentrations of surfactant components in tracheobronchial lavage specimens in 2-week-old infants with signs of evolving chronic lung disease (102). This report did not include values for healthy age-matched infants, but control data were published by some of the same group of investigators in an earlier study (100), indicating that SP-A and phosphatidylcholine concentrations are reduced in chronic lung disease. The particularly marked reduction in the SP-A/PC ratio in infants chronic lung disease may be of functional significance, for SP-A has been reported to protect surfactant against protein inhibition (48). Predictably, Kari et al. (102) reported a marked elevation of total protein concentrations in tracheobronchial lavage specimens in infants with chronic lung disease, and the surfactant obtained from these infants was functionally inhibited in vitro (100). This functional inhibition may be more important physiologically than are abnormalities of surfactant composition or concentration.

There are serious methodological problems in assuming that tracheobronchial concentrations of surfactant constituents reflect concentrations within the alveolus, and it is difficult to interpret the tracheobronchial data in the face of immunohistochemical studies that have indicated that the number of type II cells and the cell content of surfactant proteins is increased in chronic lung disease. Nevertheless, the available data suggest that chronic lung disease may be a disease that is associated with surfactant dysfunction. Only one study, to our knowledge, has directly tested this hypothesis by treating infants with early chronic lung disease with replacement surfactant. In this uncontrolled study, ten infants with early chronic lung disease who were treated with surfactant had a significant, although transient, reduction in supplemental oxygen requirements after treatment (103).

B. Postmortem Studies

Margraf et al. studied the distribution of SP-A in lungs of infants who died with chronic lung disease (104). They found that hypertrophied type II cells formed a continuous alveolar epithelial lining in lungs with chronic lung disease, and that these cells stained intensely with an anti SP-A antibody. Secretions in the airspaces also stained for SP-A. Stahlman and colleagues reported similar findings for SP-B (105). In their study of 18 infants who died with chronic lung disease between 12 days and 7 months after birth, these investigators found abundant SP-B in type II cells lining expanded areas of the lung and in secretions within the airspaces. These lining cells contained small, abnormal-appearing lamellar bodies, and led the authors to consider the possibility that the lamellar body lipid content might be abnormal in chronic lung disease and during reparative stages of lung injury. There are no human lung data that support or refute this speculation. In contrast with the findings in the expanded areas, the collapsed areas of the lungs in Stahlman's study did not stain with the SP-B antibody or have SP-B in the potential airspaces. These two studies did not examine the function of the surfactant that was present in apparent abundance in the expanded airspaces, but the results do indicate that lining type II cells in chronic lung disease do synthesize and secrete surfactant apoproteins.

These immunohistochemical results are in apparent conflict with the results from studies that examined tracheobronchial aspirates. The differences may reflect differences in the stage of the disease sampled, for all tracheobronchial data are from relatively early disease, whereas most autopsy immunohistochemical data are from well-established disease, often complicated by repeated infections and chronic oxygen exposure. Sampling error and difficulty in quantifying results are problematic from both types of study. It is fair to conclude, however, that there is a paucity of data on the synthesis, secretion, and function of pulmonary surfactant at all stages of chronic lung disease in human infants.

V. Conclusions

In spite of considerable recent efforts to investigate the status of the surfactant system in chronic lung injury, there remain more questions than answers. Most important: Is surfactant altered in chronic lung injury? The work with experimental homologues of BPD indicate the potential for perturbations, either through interactions with extraneous components altering the physicochemical properties of surfactant, or through damage and changing phenotype of type II cells. Reports in the clinical literature, unfortunately infrequent and with less than optimal controls, also suggest that some of these changes in surfactant may occur in humans with chronic injury, particularly in adults. Assessing the extent of these changes is difficult. Even when conditions are relatively well defined, as in animal models with experimentally induced injury, the alterations in surfactant that are found in the reparative–fibroproliferative phase are very inconsistent. The most abundant information relates to SP-A and DPPC. These data, both experimental and clinical, suggest that the component of surfactant most sensitive to injury is SP-A. It is unclear, however, how the change occurs, as both increases and decreases have been reported, depending on the extent or the progression of the injury. An understanding of the effects of diminished amounts of SP-A on the pathogenesis of injury will require additional data.

Acknowledgments

Supported in part by HL43704, HL52648, and HL24075 awarded by the National Heart, Lung, and Blood Institute.

References

1. Ashbaugh DG, Bigelow DB, Petty TL, Levine BE. Acute respiratory distress in adults. Lancet 1967; 2:319–323.
2. Coalson JJ, Kuehl TJ, Prihoda TJ, deLemos RA. Diffuse alveolar damage in the evolution of bronchopulmonary dysplasia in the baboon. Pediatr Res 1988; 24:357–366.
3. Manabe T. Freeze-fracture study of alveolar lining layer in adult rat lungs. J Ultrastruct Res 1979; 69:86–97.
4. Magoon MW, Wright JR, Baritussio A, Williams MC, Goerke J, Benson BJ, Hamilton RL, Clements JA. Subfractionation of lung surfactant. Implications for metabolism and surface activity. Biochim Biophys Acta 1983; 750:18–31.
5. Wright JR, Benson BJ, Williams MC, Goerke J, Clements JA. Protein composition of rabbit alveolar surfactant subfractions. Biochim Biophys Acta 1984; 791:320–332.
6. Davies JT, Rideal EK. Interfacial Phenomena. New York: Academic Press, 1963: 217–277.
7. Goerke J, Clements JA. Alveolar surface tension and lung surfactant. In: Macklem PT, Mead J, eds. Handbook of Physiology. Vol. 3. Washington, DC: American Physiological Society, 1986:247–261.
8. Seeger W, Stohrg G, Wolf HR, Neuhof H. Alternation of surfactant function due to protein leakage: special interaction with fibrin monomer. J Appl Physiol 1985; 58:326–338.
9. Brown ES. Isolation and assay of dipalmityl lecithin in lung extracts. Am J Physiol 1963; 207:402–406.
10. Goerke J, Gonzales J. Temperature dependence of dipalmitoyl phosphatidylcholine monolayer stability. J Appl Physiol Respir Environ Exerc Physiol 1981; 51:1108–1114.
11. King RJ, Clements JA. Surface active materials from dog lung. II. Composition and physiological correlations. Am J Physiol 1972; 223:715–726.
12. Hallman M, Gluck L. Phosphatidylglycerol in lung surfactant. III. Possible modifier of surfactant function. J Lipid Res 1976; 17:257–262.
13. Bangham AD, Morley CJ, Phillips MC. The physical properties of an effective lung surfactant. Biochim Biophys Acta 1979; 573:552–556.
14. Suzuki Y, Fujita Y, Kogishi K. Reconstitution of tubular myelin from synthetic lipids and proteins associated with pig pulmonary surfactant. Am Rev Respir Dis 1989; 140:75–81.
15. Slomiany A, Smith FB, Slomiany BL. Isolation and characterization of a sulfated glyceroglucolipid from alveolar lavage of rabbit. Eur J Biochem 1979; 98:47–51.

16. Kuroki Y, Shiratori M, Ogasawara Y, Tsuzuki A, Akino T. Characterization of pulmonary surfactant protein D: its copurification with lipids. Biochim Biophys Acta 1991; 1086:185–190.
17. Bruns G, Stroh H, Veldman GM, Latt SA, Floros J. The 35 kd pulmonary surfactant-associated protein is encoded on chromosome 10. Hum Genet 1987;76:58–62.
18. Crouch E, Rust K, Veile R, Donis-Keller H, Grosso L. Genomic organization of human surfactant protein D (SP-D). SP-D is encoded on chromosome 10q22.2-23.1. J Biol Chem 1993; 268:2976–2983.
19. Phelps DS, Floros J. Localization of surfactant protein synthesis in human lung by in situ hybridization. Am Rev Respir Dis 1988; 137:939–942.
20. Walker SR, Williams MC, Benson B. Immunocytochemical localization of the major surfactant apoproteins in type II cells, Clara cells, and alveolar macrophages of rat lungs. J Histochem Cytochem 1986; 34:1137–1148.
21. Crouch E, Parghi D, Kuan S-F, Persson A. Surfactant protein D: subcellular localization in nonciliated bronchiolar epithelial cells. Am J Physiol 1992; 263:L60–L66.
22. Hoppe HJ, Barlow PN, Reid KB. A parallel three stranded alpha-helical bundle at the nucleation site of collagen triple-helix formation. FEBS Lett 1994; 344:191–195.
23. Haagsman HP, Hawgood S, Sargeant T, Buckley D, White RT, Drickamer K, Benson BJ. The major lung surfactant protein, SP 28–36, is a calcium-dependent, carbohydrate-binding protein. J Biol Chem 1987; 262:13877–13880.
24. Haagsman HP, White RT, Schilling J, Lau K, Benson BJ, Golden J, Hawgood S, Clements JA. Studies of the structure of lung surfactant protein SP-A. Am J Physiol 1989; 257:L421–L429.
25. Persson AV, Gibbons BJ, Shoemaker JD, Moxley MA, Longmore WJ. The major glycolipid recognized by SP-D in surfactant is phosphatidylinositol. J Biol Chem 1992; 267:19846–19853.
26. King RJ, Klass DJ, Gikas EG, Clements JA. Isolation of apoproteins from canine surface active material. Am J Physiol 1973; 224:L788–L795.
27. King RJ, Carmichael MC, Horowitz PM. Reassembly of lipid–protein complexes of pulmonary surfactant. Proposed mechanism of interaction. J Biol Chem 1983; 258:10672–10680.
28. King RJ, Phillips MC, Horowitz MC, Dang S-C. Interaction between the 35 kDa apolipoprotein of pulmonary surfactant and saturated phosphatidylcholines. Effects of temperature. Biochim Biophys Acta 1986;879:1–13.
29. Hawgood S, Benson BJ, Hamilton RL Jr. Effects of a surfactant-associated protein and calcium ions on the structure and surface activity of lung surfactant lipids. Biochemistry 1985; 24:184–190.
30. Pilot-Matias TJ, Kister SE, Fox JL, Kropp K, Glasser SW, Whitsett JA. Structure and organization of the gene encoding human pulmonary surfactant proteolipid SP-B. DNA 1989; 8:75–86.
31. Hawgood S, Benson BJ, Schilling J, Damm D, Clements JA, White RT. Nucleotide and amino acid sequences of pulmonary surfactant protein SP 18 and evidence for cooperation between SP 18 and SP 28–36 in surfactant lipid adsorption. Proc Natl Acad Sci USA 1987; 84:66–70.

32. Jacobs KA, Phelps DS, Steinbrink R, Fisch J, Kriz R, Mitsock L, Dougherty JP, Taeusch HW, Floros J. Isolation of a cDNA clone encoding a high molecular weight precursor to a 6-kDa pulmonary surfactant-associated protein. J Biol Chem 1987; 262:9808–9811.
33. Glasser SW, Korfhagen TR, Weaver T, Pilot-Matias T, Fox JL, Whitsett JA. cDNA and deduced amino acid sequence of human pulmonary surfactant-associated proteolipid SPL(Phe). Proc Natl Acad Sci USA 1987; 84:4007–4011.
34. Weaver TE, Lin S, Bogucki B, Dey C. Processing of surfactant protein B proprotein by a cathepsin D-like protase. Am J Physiol 1992;263:L95–L103.
35. Voorhout WF, Veenendaal T, Haagsman HP, Weaver TE, Whitsett JA, van Golde LM, Geuze HJ. Intracellular processing of pulmonary surfactant protein B in an endosomal/lysosomal compartment. Am J Physiol 1992; 263:L479–L486.
36. Hawgood S, Latham D, Borchelt J, Damm D, White T, Benson B, Wright JR. Cell-specific posttranslational processing of the surfactant-associated protein SP-B. Am J Physiol 1993; 264:L290–L299.
37. Poulain FR, Allen L, Williams MC, Hamilton RL, Hawgood S. Effects of surfactant apolipoproteins on liposome structure: implications for tubular myelin formation. Am J Physiol 1992; 262:L730–L739.
38. Williams MC, Hawgood S, Hamilton RL. Changes in lipid structure produced by surfactant proteins SP-A, SP-B, and SP-C. Am J Respir Cell Mol Biol 1991; 5: 41–50.
39. Curstedt T, Jörnvall H, Robertson B, Bergman T, Berggren P. Two hydrophobic low-molecular-mass protein fractions of pulmonary surfactant. Characterization and biophysical activity. Eur J Biochem 1987; 168:255–262.
40. Nogee LM, Garnier G, Dietz HC, Singer L, Murphy AM, deMello DE, Colten HR. A mutation in the surfactant protein B gene responsible for fatal neonatal respiratory disease in multiple kindreds. J Clin Invest 1994; 93:1860–1863.
41. Nogee ML, DeMello DE, Dehner LP, Colten HR. Brief report: deficiency of pulmonary surfactant protein B in congenital alveolar proteinosis. N Engl J Med 1993; 328:406–410.
42. Warr RG, Hawgood S, Buckley DI, Crisp TM, Schilling J, Benson BJ, Ballard PL, Clements JA, White RT. Low molecular weight human pulmonary surfactant protein (SP5): isolation, characterization, and cDNA and amino acid sequences. Proc Natl Acad Sci USA 1987; 84:7915–7919.
43. Glasser SW, Korfhagen TR, Perme CM, Pilot-Matias TJ, Kister SE, Whitsett JA. Two SP-C genes encoding human pulmonary surfactant proteolipid. J Biol Chem 1988; 263:10326–10331.
44. Johansson J, Curstedt T, Robertson B, Jörnvall H. Size and structure of the hydrophobic low molecular weight surfactant-associated polypeptide. Biochemistry 1988; 27:3544–3547.
45. Johansson J, Szyperski T, Curstedt T, Wüthrich K. The NMR structure of the pulmonary surfactant-associated polypeptide SP-C in an apolar solvent contains a valyl-rich alpha-helix. Biochemistry 1994; 33:6015–6023.
46. Curstedt T, Johansson J, Persson P, Eklund A, Robertson B, Lowenadler B, Jornvall H. Hydrophobic surfactant-associated polypeptides; SP-C is a lipopeptide with two

palmitoylated cysteine residues whereas SP-B lacks covalently linked fatty acyl groups. Proc Natl Acad Sci USA 1990; 87:2985–2989.

47. Takahashi A, Fujiwara T. Proteolipid in bovine lung surfactant: its role in surfactant function. Biochem Biophys Res Commun 1986; 135:527–532.
48. Cockshutt AM, Weitz J, Possmayer F. Pulmonary surfactant-associated protein A enhances the surface activity of lipid extract surfactant and reverses inhibition by blood proteins in vitro. Biochemistry 1990; 29:8425–8429.
49. Schürch S, Possmayer F, Cheng S, Cockshutt AM. Pulmonary SP-A enhances adsorption and appears to induce surface sorting of lipid extract surfactant. Am J Physiol 1992; 263:L210–L218.
50. Johansson J, Curstedt T, Robertson B. The proteins of the surfactant system. Eur Respir J 1994; 7:372–391.
51. Clark JC, Wert SE, Bachurski CJ, Stahlman MT, Stripp BR, Weaver TE, Whitsett JA. Targeted disruption of the surfactant protein B gene disrupts surfactant homeostasis, causing respiratory failure in newborn mice. Proc Natl Acad Sci USA 1995; 92:7794–7798.
52. Dobbs LG, Wright JR, Hawgood S, Gonzalez R, Venstrom K, Nellenbogen J. Pulmonary surfactant and its components inhibit secretion of phosphatidylcholine from cultured rat alveolar type II cells. Proc Natl Acad Sci USA 1987; 84:1010–1014.
53. Crouch EC, White MR, Eggleton P, Tauber AI, Chang D, Sastry K. Evidence for a protective role of pulmonary surfactant protein D (SP-D) against influenza A viruses. J Clin Invest 1994; 94:311–319.
54. Frank L, Bucher JR, Roberts RJ. Oxygen toxicity in neonatal and adult animals of various species. J Appl Physiol 1978; 45:699–704.
55. Frank L, Iqbal J, Hass M, Massaro D. New ''rest period'' protocol for inducing tolerance to high O_2 exposure in adult rats. Am J Physiol 1989; 257:L226–L231.
56. Minoo P, King RJ, Coalson JJ. Surfactant proteins and lipids are regulated independently during hyperoxia. Am J Physiol 1992; 263:L291–L298.
57. Putman E, van Golde MG, Haagsman HP. Toxic oxidant species and their impact on the pulmonary surfactant system. Lung 1997; 175:75–103.
58. Holm BA, Notter RH, Siegle J, Matalon S. Pulmonary physiological and surfactant changes during injury and recovery from hyperoxia. J Appl Physiol 1985; 59:1402–1409.
59. Holm BA, Matalon S, Finkelstein JN, Notter RH. Type II pneumocyte changes during hyperoxic lung injury and recovery. J Appl Physiol 1988; 65:2672–2678.
60. Gross NJ, Smith DM. Impaired surfactant phospholipid metabolism in hyperoxic mouse lungs. J Appl Physiol 1981; 51:1198–1203.
61. Välimäki M, Pelliniemi TT, Niinikoski J. Oxygen-induced changes in pulmonary phospholipids in the rat. J Appl Physiol 1975; 39:780–787.
62. Crim C, Simon RH. Effects of oxygen metabolites on rat alveolar type II cell viability and surfactant metabolism. Lab Invest 1988; 58:428–437.
63. Haagsman HP, van Golde LMG. Lung surfactant and pulmonary toxicology. Lung 1985; 163:275–303.
64. Veness-Meehan KA, Cheng ER, Mercier CE, Blixt SL, Johnston CJ, Watkins RH, Horowitz S. Cell-specific alterations in expression of hyperoxia-induced mRNAs of lung. Am J Respir Cell Mol Biol 1991; 5:516–521.

65. Randell SH, Silbajoris R, Young SL. Ontogeny of rat lung type II cells correlated with surfactant lipid and surfactant apoprotein expression. Am J Physiol 1991; 260: L562–L570.
66. Young SL, Ho YS, Silbajoris RA. Surfactant apoprotein in adult rat lung compartments is increased by dexamethasone. Am J Physiol 1991; 260:L161–L167.
67. Allred TF, Thomas RF, Autin RL. Surfactant apoprotein A, B, and C mRNA are suppressed after brief exposures to 95% oxygen in rats. Am J Respir Crit Care Med 1992; 149:A99.
68. Wikenheiser KA, Clark JC, Linnoila RI, Stahlman MT, Whitsett JA. Distinct effects of oxygen on surfactant protein B expression in bronchiolar and alveolar epithelium. Am J Physiol 1992; 262:L32–L39.
69. Kapanci Y, Weibel ER, Kaplan HP, Robinson FR. Pathogenesis and reversibility of the pulmonary lesions of oxygen toxicity in monkeys. II. Ultrastructural and morphometric studies. Lab Invest 1969; 20:101–118.
70. Coalson JJ, King RJ, Winter VT, Prihoda TJ, Anzueto AR, Peters JI, Johanson WG Jr. O_2- and pneumonia-induced lung injury. I. Pathological and morphometric studies. J Appl Physiol 1989; 67:346–356.
71. King RJ, Coalson JJ, Seidenfeld JJ, Anzueto AR, Smith DB, Peters JI. O_2- and pneumonia-induced lung injury. II. Properties of pulmonary surfactant. J Appl Physiol 1989; 67:357–365.
72. Huang Y-CT, Caminiti SP, Fawcett TA, Moon RE, Fracica PJ, Miller FJ, Young SL, Piantadosi CA. Natural surfactant and hyperoxic lung injury in primates. I. Physiology and biochemistry. J Appl Physiol 1994; 76:991–1001.
73. Fracica PJ, Caminiti SP, Piantadosi CA, Duhaylongsod FG, Crapo JD, Young SL. Natural surfactant and hyperoxic lung injury in primates. II. Morphometric analyses. J Appl Physiol 1994; 76:1002–1010.
74. Snider GL, Celli BR, Goldstein RH, O'Brien JJ, Lucey EC. Chronic interstitial pulmonary fibrosis produced in hamsters by endotracheal bleomycin. Lung volumes, volume–pressure relations, carbon monoxide uptake, and arterial blood gas studies. Am Rev Respir Dis 1978; 117:289–297.
75. McCullough B, Collins JR, Johanson WG Jr, Grover FL. Bleomycin-induced diffuse interstitial pulmonary fibrosis in baboons. J Clin Invest 1979; 61:79–88.
76. Phan SH, Thrall RS, Ward PA. Bleomycin-induced pulmonary fibrosis in rats:biochemical demonstration of increased rate of collagen synthesis. Am Rev Respir Dis 1980; 121:501–506.
77. Thrall RS, Swendsen CL, Shannon TH, Kennedy CA, Frederick DS, Grunze MF, Sulavik SB. Correlation of changes in pulmonary surfactant phospholipids with compliance in bleomycin-induced pulmonary fibrosis in the rat. Am Rev Respir Dis 1987; 136:113–118.
78. Low RB, Adler KB, Woodcock-Mitchell J, Giancola MS, Vacek PM. Bronchoalveolar lavage lipids during development of bleomycin-induced fibrosis in rats. Am Rev Respir Dis 1988; 138:709–713.
79. Beppu OS, Clements JA, Goerke J. Phosphatidylglycerol-deficient lung surfactant has normal properties. J Appl Physiol 1983; 55:496–502.
80. Horiuchi T, Mason RJ, Kuroki Y, Cherniack RM. Surface and tissue forces, surfactant protein A, and the phospholipid components of pulmonary surfactant in bleo-

mycin-induced pulmonary fibrosis in the rat. Am Rev Respir Dis 1990; 141:1006–1013.
81. Liau DF, Barrett CR, Bell AL, Ryan SF. Functional abnormalities of lung surfactant in experimental acute alveolar injury in the dog. Am Rev Respir Dis 1987; 136: 395–401.
82. Gross NJ, Narine KR. Surfactant subtypes of mice: metabolic relationships and conversion in vitro. J Appl Physiol 1989; 67:414–421.
83. Higuchi R, Lewis J, Ikegami M. In vitro conversion of surfactant subtypes is altered in alveolar surfactant isolated from injured lungs. Am Rev Respir Dis 1992; 145: 1416–1420.
84. Young SL, Crapo JD, Kremers SA, Brumley GW. Pulmonary surfactant lipid production in oxygen-exposed rat lungs. Lab Invest 1982; 46:570–576.
85. Nogee LM, Wispe JR, Clark JC, Whitsett JA. Increased synthesis and mRNA of surfactant protein A in oxygen-exposed rats. Am J Respir Cell Mol Biol 1989; 1: 119–125.
86. Holm BA, Notter RH, Leary JF, Matalon S. Alveolar epithelial changes in rabbits after a 21-day exposure to 60% O_2. J Appl Physiol 1987; 62:2230–2236.
87. Korfhagen TR, Bruno MD, Ross GF, Huelsman KM, Ikegami M, Jobe AH, Wert SE, Stripp BR, Morris RE, Glasser SW, Bachurski CJ, Iwamoto HS, Whitsett JA. Proc Natl Acad Sci USA 1996; 93:9594–9599.
88. LeVine AM, Bruno HD, Huelsman KM, Ross GF, Whitsett JA, Korfhagen TR. Surfactant protein-A deficient mice are susceptible to group B streptococcal infection. J Immunol 1997; 158:4336–4340.
89. Jobe A, Ikegami M. Surfactant for the treatment of respiratory distress syndrome. Am Rev Respir Dis 1987; 136:1256–1275.
90. Seeger W, Gunther A, Thede C. Differential sensitivity to fibrinogen inhibition of SP-C- vs. SP-B-based surfactants. Am J Physiol 1992; 261:L286–L291.
91. Holm BA, Waring AJ. Designer surfactants. The next generation in surfactant replacement. Clin Perinatol 1993; 20:813–829.
92. Seidner SR, McCurnin D, Coalson J, Correll D, Castro R. A new model of chronic lung injury in surfactant-treated preterm baboons delivered at very early gestations. Pediatr Res 1993; 33:344A.
93. Escobedo MB, Hilliard JL, Smith F, Meredith K, Walsh W, Johnson D, Coalson JJ, Kuehl TJ, Null DM Jr, Robotham JL. A baboon model of bronchopulmonary dysplasia. I. Clinical features. Exp Mol Pathol 1982; 37:323–334.
94. Coalson JJ, Kuehl TJ, Escobedo MB, Hilliard JL, Smith F, Meredith K, Null DM Jr, Walsh W, Johnson D, Robotham JL. A baboon model of bronchopulmonary dysplasia. II. Pathologic features. Exp Mol Pathol 1982; 37:335–350.
95. deLemos RA, Coalson JJ. The contribution of experimental models to our understanding of the pathogenesis and treatment of bronchopulmonary dysplasia. Clin Perinatol 1992; 19:521–539.
96. Bland R, Cho S, Carlton D, Albertine K, Davis P. Chronic lung injury in mechanically ventilated preterm lambs. FASEB J 1995; 9:A275.
97. Albertine KH, Carlton DP, Cho S, Davis PL, Bland RD. Histopathology of chronic lung injury in preterm lambs. FASEB J 1995; 9:A275.
98. Coalson JJ, King RJ, Yang F, Winter V, Whitsett JA, deLemos RA, Seidner SR.

SP-A deficiency in primate model of bronchopulmonary dysplasia with infection. In situ mRNA and immunostains. Am J Respir Crit Care Med 1995; 151:854–866.

99. King RJ, Coalson JJ, deLemos RA, Gerstmann DR, Seidner SR. SP-A deficiency in a primate model of BPD. Am J Respir Crit Care Med 1995; 151:1989–1997.

100. Hallman M, Merritt A, Akino T, Bry K. Surfactant protein A, phosphatidylcholine, and surfactant inhibitors in epithelial lining fluid. Am Rev Respir Dis 1991; 144: 1376–1384.

101. Chida S, Phelps DS, Cordle C, Soll R, Floros J, Taeusch HW. Surfactant-associated proteins in tracheal aspirates of infants with respiratory distress syndrome after surfactant therapy. Am Rev Respir Dis 1988; 137:943–947.

102. Kari MA, Raivio KO, Venge P, Hallman M. Dexamethasone treatment of infants at risk for chronic lung disease: surfactant components and inflammatory parameters in airway specimens. Pediatr Res 1994; 36:387–393.

103. Pandit PB, Dunn MS, Kelly EN, Perlman M. Surfactant replacement in neonates with early chronic lung disease. Pediatrics 1995; 95:851–854.

104. Margraf LR, Paciga JE, Balis JU. Surfactant-associated glycoproteins accumulate in alveolar cells and secretions during reparative stage of hyaline membrane disease. Hum Pathol 1990; 21:392–396.

105. Stahlman MT, Gray ME, Whitsett JA. The ontogeny and distribution of surfactant protein B in human fetuses and newborns. J Histochem Cytochem 1992; 40:1471–1480.

22

The Regulation of the Formation of Pulmonary Alveoli

DONALD J. MASSARO and GLORIA D. MASSARO

Georgetown University School of Medicine
Washington, D.C.

I. Introduction

This chapter will consider architectural, cellular, and regulatory aspects of the formation of alveoli and hence of the dimensions of the lung gas-exchange surface area (Sa). We shall focus on four topics we think are especially relevant to neonatologists: the effect on the developing lung of hyperoxia, hypoxia, corticosteroids, and retinoic acid.

The lung may be usefully divided into two components: the conducting airways and the gas-exchange region. In all species studied, the conducting airways are formed in utero; therefore, their formation is somewhat protected from environmental challenges (e.g., high altitude, inadequate availability of food by maternal adaptations). In contrast to the conducting airways, the timing of the development of the gas-exchange region varies in a manner that seems to correspond to the activity ''lifestyle'' of the species to which the newborn belongs. At birth members of so-called precocial species, such as guinea pigs and some range animals, have fur, sight, and within hours of birth considerable locomotor activity. In these species, the formation of alveoli occurs in utero, and the lung at birth is, except for size, architecturally mature (1–6). Members of altricial species, such as rat, mouse, rabbit, and human, are rather helpless and have poor locomotor ability at birth; in these species the formation of alveoli is a postnatal event, or as in humans occurs during late gestation and the first few postnatal years (7–15).

In a very important and pioneering paper, Tenney and Remmers demonstrated that across species the size of the gas-exchange surface area (Sa) scales directly and linearly with the organisms' total oxygen consumption ($\dot{V}O_2$), alveolar size varies inversely with the species body mass-specific $\dot{V}O_2$, and lung volume is an almost constant fraction of body volume (16). Thus, when a large Sa per body mass is needed, it is achieved by greater partitioning of the lung's internal surface (i.e., formation of smaller and relatively more alveoli), rather than generation of a larger lung volume per body mass. These observations on balancing Sa to mass-specific metabolic rate, aside from their intrinsic interest to the biology of the lung, have important implications for potential therapies to generate more Sa in individuals with an insufficient number of alveoli for their metabolic needs (see later Sec. III. E).

II. Architectural Maturation of the Lung's Gas-Exchange Region: From Saccules to Alveoli

The gas-exchange region of the architecturally immature lung is composed of large structures, referred to as *saccules* (9). The smaller, more numerous structures that compose the gas-exchange region of the architecturally mature lung are designated *alveoli*. The latter are formed, in part, by subdivision (*septation*) of the saccules (9). We shall maintain this nomenclature. However, in situations where septation of saccules has not occurred, the resulting structures, although still larger and unseptated (or incompletely septated) will, nevertheless, be referred to as alveoli.

In all species in which it has been studied in detail, the architectural events that convert the gas-exchange region from immature to mature are quite similar, although the timing of the events varies widely among species (3,4,7,9–13,15,17). The process entails the outgrowth of septa from the walls of the saccules that form the gas-exchange regions of the immature lung (9). Septation is advantageous because it allows an increase in Sa, without a proportional increase of lung volume (i.e., alveoli have a larger surface/volume ratio than saccules) (9).

Concomitant with septation, the alveolar wall becomes thinner and its cellular composition changes (9,18). In the rat, in which septation of the gas-exchange saccules occurs mainly from postnatal days 4 to 14 (9), the thickness of the alveolar wall decreases about 20% and the air–gas barrier (the distance between alveolar gas and capillary blood) diminishes about 25% (18). The volume density (volume fraction) of alveolar type I cells increases about 45%, consistent with the large increase in Sa, whereas the volume density of interstitial fibroblasts decreases 22% (18). Most of this latter change is due to a fall in volume density of fibroblasts that have intracellular lipid granules, hereafter referred to as *lipid-interstitial fibroblasts* (LIF) (18). The volume density of the matrix and of the capillary lumen in the gas-exchange region do not change during septation (18). We suggest that the cellular changes are accompanied by differentiation of some of the cell types that ends their ability to promote septation. As septation of the gas-exchange saccules present at birth is ending, important remodeling of the microvasculature of the gas-exchange wall begins. The capillaries, which form double capillary layers in the immature gas-exchange region, are remodeled to form a single capillary layer. This process is completed in the rat by about the third postnatal week (19).

Three additional observations should be mentioned concerning the timing of septation and its consequences:

1. The available information indicates the serum concentration of the species' major glucocorticosteroid hormone is low during the time septation occurs and increases as septation ends and remodeling of the alveolar microvasculature begins (20). These observations have been experimentally exploited and are relevant to the development of the lung in humans with bronchopulmonary dysplasia (BPD; see later Sec. III. D).
2. Septation takes place mainly before (i.e., guinea pigs and some range animals) or after (rat, mouse, rabbit) the late gestational maturation of the lungs surfactant system (21) and rise of activity of some lung antioxidant enzymes (22). These interspecies differences in timing of septation, in relation to late gestational events, seem programmed to spread out the energy requirement of the offspring–maternal unit, but still meet the newborn's need for motor activity at birth.
3. Septation occurs under vastly different oxygen tensions in different species and, in humans, within species. Thus, septation takes place in utero in guinea pigs at a Po_2 of approximately 25 torr, postnatally in rats at an alveolar Po_2 of about 100 torr, and in humans it occurs in utero at a Po_2 of about 25 torr and continues after birth at an alveolar Po_2 of about 100 torr. Yet, allowing rats to be born and raised in 13% O_2 by dams acclimatized to 13% O_2 impairs septation in a seemingly irrevocable manner (23,24).

III. Formation of Alveoli

A. Quantitation of Septation and "Other" Methods of Forming Alveoli

Burri et al., in two very important papers, provided morphological and morphometric evidence that the large saccules that compose the gas-exchange region of the architecturally immature lung undergo septation to form smaller and more numerous gas-exchange structures (alveoli) of architecturally mature lungs (9,25). Subsequent work extended these reports by the use of serial lung sections, which enable alveoli to be distinguished from alveolar ducts, and by the use of stereological procedures that allow the selection of alveoli for analysis by unbiased methods (i.e., selection not influenced by alveolar size, shape, or distribution; (24,26). In this manner, Randell et al. (32) reported for rats a sixfold decrease in volume of an average gas-exchange saccule as it was septated to form alveoli. More importantly, their data indicate that over the period studied (birth to age 7 days), septation could account for only about one-third of the alveoli formed. This finding in rats was confirmed and the time studied was extended over the entire period of septation; during this period, septation of gas-exchange saccules present at birth accounted for only 26% of alveoli present at age 14 days (24). Therefore, about three-quarters of alveoli made in rats during the period of "septation" are formed by "other" means. These reports (24,26) confirm the previously expressed notion that alveoli are formed during the period of septation by two methods: septation of the gas-exchange saccules present at birth (27) and by other, as yet unidentified mechanisms. Furthermore, using serial sections to distinguish alveoli from alveolar ducts and unbiased methods for the selection and quantitation of alveoli, we showed that alveoli continue to form after septation of the original gas-exchange saccules has been completed (28); however, alveoli are formed more rapidly during the period of septation (24). Evidence supports the thesis that following septation of the gas-exchange saccules present at birth additional alveoli are formed mainly at the periphery of the lung (29). The mechanism by which alveoli are formed after completed septation of saccules that are present at birth is unknown.

B. Hyperoxia and the Formation of Alveoli

Hyperoxia impairs the formation of alveoli. Exposure of neonatal animals to a high Po_2 diminishes septation, the development of alveolar capillaries, and the developmental increase of Sa (26,30–33). In an especially important paper, Randell et al. used serial lung sections to identify alveoli and unbiased methods to measure them; they found that exposure of rats to a high Po_2 from birth to age 7 days prevented septation and the normal increase in the number of alveoli (26). Calculations based on the number of alveoli formed and the number expected to have been formed by septation indicate hyperoxia diminished the number of alveoli formed by septation and by other means. Randell et al. (26) also reported on recovery after exposure of rats to hyperoxia from birth to age 7 days. At age 40 days, Sa, alveolar number, and the size of alveoli were equal in rats previously exposed to a high Po_2 compared with rats that were never exposed to hyperoxia. It is noteworthy that the size distribution of alveoli differed at age 40 days; rats previously exposed to hyperoxia had significantly more very small and very large alveoli than rats that were not previously exposed to hyperoxia. We suggest that the large alveoli represent saccules that failed to septate during exposure to hyperoxia, the cells of which experienced accelerated differentiation during that period that permanently impaired their ability to foster septation. We propose that the presence of very small alveoli represents an effort to match the size of Sa to the organism's metabolic rate ($\dot{V}O_2$).

C. Hypoxia and the Formation of Alveoli

Biomedical interest and studies on the effect of a low inspired PO_2 on the lung have been fostered mainly because of the large thorax and large lung volume of individuals native to high altitudes (34). We shall refer to these natives of high altitude who remain at high altitudes as highlanders; individuals of the same race who are born and live at sea level are referred to as lowlanders.

Highlanders have a 38% higher residual lung volume than lowlanders (34) and are reported to have larger and more numerous alveoli than lowlanders (35,36). Highlanders have a lower maximum expiratory flow rate and a lower upstream conductance than lowlanders (37). These characteristics have suggested that gestation and postnatal growth of highlanders at high altitudes cause dysanaptic lung growth (disproportionate growth among different parts of an organ; 14). It has been suggested that the lung's gas-exchange region, which in humans septates in part postnatally, does so under the presumed stimulatory effect of a low PO_2 and thereby becomes too large for the cross-sectional area of the conducting airway; the latter, which achieve architectural maturity in utero, would not experience during their development the presumed stimulation of the low PO_2 of high altitude because of maternal adaptive response (e.g., greater placental surface area and high concentrations of hemoglobin).

The available evidence indicates that in the rat, a species that septates postnatally (9), birth into and maintenance in 13–14% O_2 during the period that septation normally occurs markedly impairs septation, and the septation of the saccules present at birth does not occur even after the rats are placed in a normoxic environment (23,24). By contrast, members of species that septate in utero, but have lived at high altitudes for generations, do not have abnormal dimensions of their gas-exchange structures (38). This supports the notion that structures that develop in utero are protected from the effects of a low PO_2, presumably by maternal adaptations. The study showing that exposure of rats to a low PO_2 during the period they normally septate blocks septation and diminishes the developmental increase in Sa (23,24), taken with the demonstration that exposure of rats to a PO_2 after the period of septation increases Sa (23,30,31), indicates the developmentally dependent sensitivity of alveolus formation.

The hypoxia-induced impairment of septation in rats results in fewer alveolar attachments to small conducting airways and to small conducting blood vessels (23). This raises the possibility that, much as occurs in emphysema, during which alveolar septa have been destroyed and there are fewer attachments to conducting airways (39), diminished alveolar attachments to conducting airways in low-O_2 rats might result in premature closure of conducting airways and consequent air-trapping. This possibility is supported by the higher lung volume in low-O_2 rats than in rats raised in 20.9% O_2, even though the former are smaller because of their diminished somatic growth from hypoxia (23,24). If the large gas-exchange units reported in highlanders (36) do represent impaired septation, the putative fewer septal attachments to small conducting airways could be responsible for the high residual lung volume, low volume-specific maximum expiratory flow rate, and low upstream conductance in highlanders (34,37).

D. Corticosteroid Effects on Alveolar Formation

Eruption and elongation of structures such as alveolar septa are brought about by folding epithelium into ridges, a process that requires cell division. Because glucocorticosteroid hormones inhibit cell division in several tissues (40), including the lung (41), it was suspected that they might inhibit the formation of septa, their elongation, or both processes (27). Furthermore, an analysis of the serum concentration of the predominant glucocorticosteroid hormone in rats (42) and guinea pigs (43) revealed the serum concentration of the glucocorticosteroid is low during the period in which septation normally occurs, and the glucorticosteroid's concentration begins to increase as septation ends and alveolar wall thinning accelerates (18). These considerations led to an attempt to maintain a high serum concentration of a glucocorticosteroid hormone in rats during the period in which their lungs normally septated (27). Treatment of rats with dexamethasone from postnatal day 3 or 4 to postnatal day 13, the period of lung septation in rats, was associated with impaired septation and reduced numbers of alveoli (27,28). Furthermore, and of great importance, the impairment of septation persisted after dexamethasone was discontinued at age 13 days up to age 60 days—the time the rats were killed (27,28)—and, in another study, to the time the rats were killed at age 99 days (44).

Blanco and Frank reported that treatment of rats with dexamethasone for 10 days, beginning at age 18 days, does not affect Sa, alveolar number, or alveolar volume (45). However, these authors did not report if dexamethasone, in the dose they used, had any effect on the rats (e.g., on body weight). This latter information is necessary to interpret their results because between ages 4 and 14 days there is a clear relation between the dose of dexamethasone and its effect on body weight and on the dimensions of the terminal gas-exchange units and Sa (27). Removal of the adrenal glands in adult rats increases lung weight, without a change in the lung's wet/dry weight ratio (46), and adrenalectomy results in enlargement of the Sa (47). We therefore believe that without information to show that the dose of dexamethasone used by Blanco and Frank (45) had some biological effect, a conclusion cannot be drawn that dexamethasone does not influence Sa or alveolar number after the early postnatal period.

The cellular and molecular basis for the inhibition of septation by dexamethasone is unknown, but there are some clues. Thinning and diminished cellularity of the gas-exchange wall is a key component of the architectural maturation of the lung's gas-exchange region; these events are markedly accelerated by treatment with dexamethasone. By 48 hr after the first of two treatments, rats that received dexamethasone beginning at age 4 days had almost as much alveolar wall thinning as normally takes place in diluent-treated rats during the entire period of septation—postnatal days 4–14 (18). This rapid wall thinning is at least partly due to an equally rapid 30–40% fall in the volume fraction of the fibroblasts in the gas-exchange wall (18). This may reflect corticosteroid-induced apoptosis. In the LIFs of the interstitium of the alveolar wall the volume fraction of lipid granules, which are lung storage sites for vitamin A (48), also falls (18).

The molecular basis by which dexamethasone inhibits septation is unknown, but there are several molecular changes that may play a role. Three proteins, the actions of which in other systems indicate that they influence developmental events, have a peak of expression in rat lung during the time septation normally takes place. These proteins are a 14-kDa β-galactoside-binding protein (49,50; galectin-1, by current terminology), cellular retinol-binding protein (51), and cellular retinoic acid-binding protein (51). Treatment of neonatal rats with dexamethasone diminishes the peak of expression of galectin-1 (52), and treatment of adult rats with dexamethasone decreases the expression of lung cellular retinol-binding proteins within 3 hr (52). The lung has receptors for retinoic acid, a metabolite of vitamin A that affects developmental events in other systems (53). Of particular interest, retinoic acid increases elastin synthesis by lung LIFs (54), a process that is considered important for septation, and one that increases markedly in rat lung during septation. Retinoids and glucocorticosteroid hormones exhibit some mutually antagonistic actions (52,55,56). Infants with bronchopulmonary dysplasia (BPD) are commonly treated with glucocorticosteroid hormones. Many prematurely born babies with BPD have a lower plasma concentration of retinol than premature infants without BPD (57,58) and lung septation is impaired in babies with BPD (59,60).

E. Retinoic Acid and the Postnatal Formation of Alveoli

The observations recorded in the preceding paragraph led to the notion that treatment of neonatal rats with retinoic acid might prevent the inhibition of septation by dexamethasone and, in otherwise untreated rats, might increase septation. Treatment of rats with retinoic acid, begun at age 3 days and continued during treatment with dexamethasone from age 4 through 13 days, largely prevented the inhibition of septation by dexamethasone (Fig. 1), (61). Retinoic acid treatment also prevented the low body mass-specific Sa caused by dexamethasone. Of equal

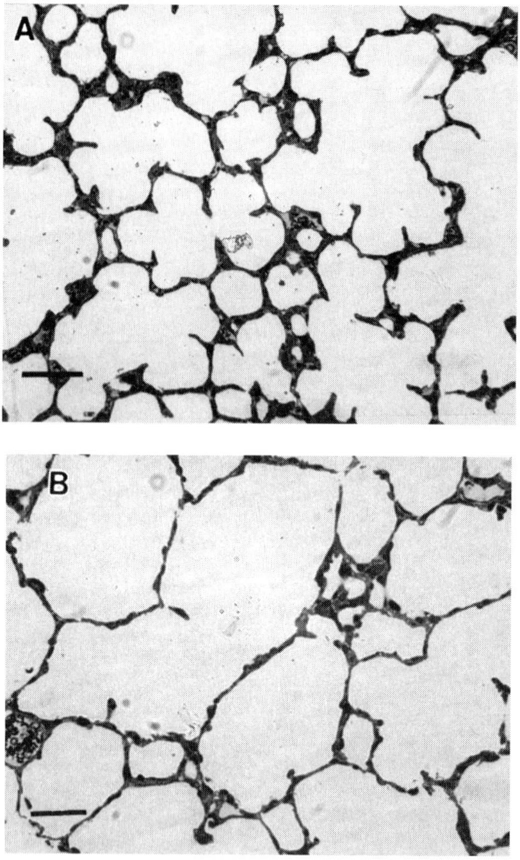

Figure 1 Histological sections of lung: Rats were injected with (A) Dil or (C) RA (500 μg/kg) daily from age 3 days through age 13 days; Dex treatment (0.25 μg/day) was started at age 4 days and (B) given alone or (D) with RA daily through age 13 days. All rats were killed at age 14 days. Scale markers, 50 μm. (From Ref. 61.)

importance, the administration of retinoic acid from age 3 to 13 days, to otherwise untreated rats, increases the number of alveoli formed: in these studies, it induced the formation of smaller alveoli than were present in diluent-treated pups and thereby did not increase Sa (61).

The basis for the lack of increase of Sa in the presence of more, but smaller, alveoli in rats treated with retinoic acid is unclear. We propose that it is due to the presence of a control mechanism that inhibits the growth of alveoli, and hence of Sa, in the absence of a need for additional Sa. This notion has led us to envision

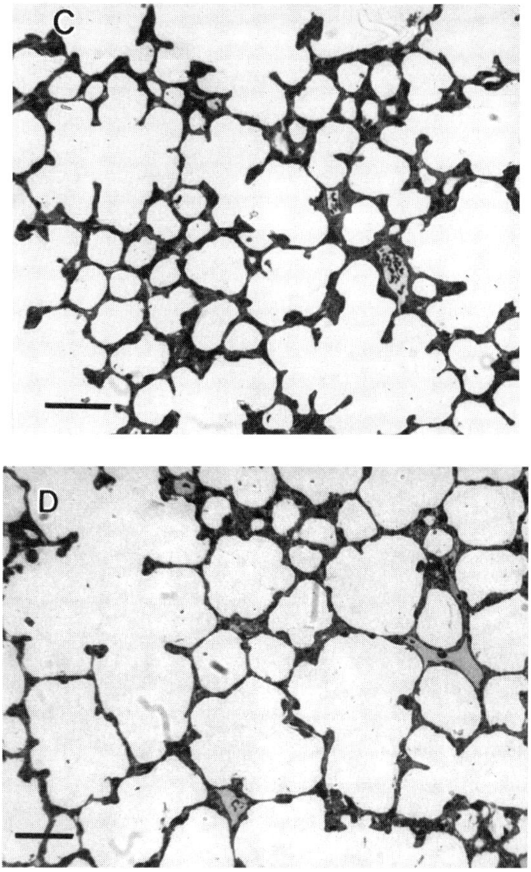

Figure 1 Continued

two distinct processes in the formation of alveoli: eruption of a septum, and its subsequent elongation. We further propose that eruption and elongation are under different regulatory control: retinoic acid, for example, induces eruption of a septum, whereas other agents or conditions may regulate septal length. If there are excess eruptions, as there are in rats treated with retinoic acid, without a need for extra Sa owing to increased O_2 consumption, septum length is curtailed. Such a control mechanism would prevent the use of energy to support the formation and maintenance of unneeded gas-exchange tissue. In the presence of disease states that result in too few alveoli for normal gas exchange, we believe this mechanism would allow septa to lengthen to increase Sa.

In considering potential clinical applications of treatment with retinoic acid in lung disorders, it is important to remember that the bony thorax limits the increase in Sa that can be achieved by forming larger than normal alveoli, and that lung volume is an almost constant fraction of body mass among all species tested (16). In particular, species with a high body-mass specific $\dot{V}O_2$ do not have a greater lung volume/body mass ratio than species with a low body mass-specific $\dot{V}O_2$ (16). Rather, in species with a high mass-specific $\dot{V}O_2$, a large mass-specific Sa is achieved by greater partitioning of the lung's internal surface (i.e., by the formation of smaller, but more numerous, alveoli; 16). These considerations indicate this pharmacological attempt to increase Sa in individuals with inadequate Sa for their VO_2 would have to achieve it mainly by the induction of more numerous, but smaller alveoli. The induction by retinoic acid of more but smaller alveoli meets this requirement. However, it remains to be seen if in diseased conditions (e.g., experimentally induced emphysema), treatment with retinoic acid causes an increase in alveolar number and, if so, if sufficient alveoli are formed to return Sa toward or to normal values.

Possibly clinical application of retinoic acid to induce the formation of alveoli include its use in prematurely born infants and in adults with emphysema. Retinoic acid treatment might be relevant to prematurely born infants for three reasons: First, even in the absence of treatment with glucocorticosteroids, some infants with BPD fail to septate (60). This failure, in the absence of treatment with glucocorticosteroids, may be due to treatment with high concentrations of oxygen (26,30–33). The ability of retinoic acid to induce the formation of alveoli in otherwise untreated neonatal rats may presage successful use in premature infants not treated with glucocorticosteroids. Second, the prevention of the inhibition of septation by dexamethasone in rats raises the possibility that retinoic acid would have the same effect in prematurely born infants treated with glucocorticosteroids. Finally, the ability of retinoic acid to induce the formation of alveoli in otherwise untreated rats by treatment with retinoic acid provides hope for specific remedial therapy of other chronic lung diseases. These diseases—pulmonary emphysema and pulmonary fibrosis—are characterized by having too few alveoli to provide sufficient Sa for adequate gas exchange and for which lung transplantation is the only available remedial therapy.

IV. Relation of Experimental Work to the Lung and Its Development in Prematurely Born Infants with Bronchopulmonary Dysplasia

Prematurely born infants who have inadequate gas-exchange are often treated with a high concentration of O_2 and glucocorticosteroid hormones, but because of obstruction of conducting airways with mucus they also may have local areas of alveolar hypoxia. Furthermore, prematurely born organisms, including humans, may have inadequately developed antioxidant enzyme expression (22,62), making even 20.9% O_2 "hyperoxia" (63). All these conditions—hyperoxia, hypoxia, and treatment with glucocorticosteroid hormones—impair septation in animals. Thus, the impairment of septation and the large alveoli and low Sa in prematurely born infants with BPD probably have multiple causes. It is important to know if retinoic acid, which increases alveolar number in rats and prevents the dexamethasone-induced decrease in septation (61), has the same effect in prematurely born humans.

Acknowledgments

Supported in part by NIH grants HL-20366 and HL-37666. D. Massaro is Cohen Professor of Pulmonary Research.

References

1. Alcorn DG, Adamson TM, Maloney JE, Robinson PM. A morphologic and morphometric analysis of fetal lung development in the sheep. Anat Rec 1981; 201:655–667
2. Castleman WL, Lay JC. Morphometric and ultrastructural study of postnatal lung growth and development in calves. Am J Vet Res 1990; 51:789–795.
3. Collins MH, Kleinerman J, Moessinger AC, Collins AH, James LS, Blanc WA. Morphometric analysis of the growth of the normal fetal guinea pig lung. Anat Rec 1986; 216:381–391.
4. Lechner AJ, Banchero N. Advanced pulmonary development in newborn guinea pigs (*Cavia porcellus*). Am J Anat 1982; 163:235–246.
5. Winkler GC, Cheville NF. Morphometry of postnatal development in the porcine lung. Anat Rec 1984; 211:427–433.
6. Winkler GC, Cheville NF. The neonatal porcine lung: ultrastructural morphology and postnatal development of the terminal airways and alveolar region. Anat Rec 1984; 210:303–313.
7. Amy RW, Bowes D, Burri PH, Haines J, Thurlbeck WM. Postnatal growth of the mouse lung. J Anat 1977; 124:131–151.
8. Boyden EA, Tompsett DH. The postnatal growth of the lung in the dog. Acta Anat 1961; 47:185–215.
9. Burri PH. The postnatal growth of the rat lung. III. Morphology. Anat Rec 1974; 180:77–98.
10. Dingler EC. Wachstrum der Lung nach der Geburt. Acta Anat 1986; 32 (suppl 30): 1–86.
11. Dubruil G, Lacoste A, Raymond R. Observations sur le development du poumon humain. Bull Histol Appl Physiol Pathol Tech Microsc 1936; 13:135–145.

12. Engle S. The structure of the respiratory tissue in the newly born. Acta Anat 1953; 19:353–365.
13. Langston C, Kida K, Reed M, Thurlbeck WM. Human lung growth in late gestation and in the neonate. Am Rev Respir Dis 1984; 129:607–613.
14. Reid L. The embryology of the lung. In: de Reuck, AVS ed. Development of the Lung. London: Churchill Livingston, 1967:109–130.
15. Zeltner TB, Burri PH. The postnatal development and growth of the human lung. II. Morphology. Respir Physiol 1987; 67:269–282.
16. Tenney SM, Remmers JE. Comparative quantitative morphology of the mammalian lung diffusing area. Nature 1963; 197:54–56.
17. Boyden EA, Tompsett DH. The changing patterns of the developing lungs of infants. Acta Anat 1965; 61:164–192.
18. Massaro D, Massaro GD. Dexamethasone accelerates postnatal alveolar wall thinning and alters wall composition. Am J Physiol 1986; 251:R218–R224.
19. Burri PH. Development and growth of the human lung. In: Fishman AP, Fisher AB, eds. Handbook of Physiology. The Respiratory System. Bethesda, MD: American Physiology Society, 1985; 1:1–46, 572.
20. Massaro GD, Massaro, D. Formation of pulmonary alveoli and gas-exchange surface area: quantitation and regulation. Annu Rev Physiol 1996; 58:73–92.
21. Kitterman JA, Liggins GC, Campos GA, Clements JA, Forster CS, Lee CH, Creas RK. Post-partum maturation of the lung: relation to cortisol. J Appl Physiol 1981; 51:384–390.
22. Sosenko IRS, Frank L. Prenatal development of lung antioxidant enzymes in four species. J Pediatr 1987; 110:106–110.
23. Massaro GD, Olivier J, Dzikowski C, Massaro D. Postnatal development of lung alveoli: suppression by 13% O_2 and a critical period. Am J Physiol 1990; 258: L321–L327.
24. Blanco LN, Massaro D, Massaro GD. Alveolar size, number and surface area: developmentally dependent response to 13% O_2. Am J Physiol 1991; 261: L370–L377.
25. Burri PH, Dbaly J, Weibel ER. The postnatal growth of the rat lung. I. Morphometry. Anat Rec 1974; 178:711–730.
26. Randell SH, Mercer RR, Young SL. Postnatal growth of pulmonary acini and alveoli in normal and oxygen-exposed rats studied by serial section reconstructions. Am J Anat 1989; 186:55–68.
27. Massaro D, Teich N, Maxwell S, Massaro GD, Whitney P. Postnatal development of alveoli: regulation and evidence for a critical period in rats. J Clin Invest 1985; 76:I297–I305.
28. Blanco LN, Massaro GD, Massaro D. Alveolar dimensions and number: developmental and hormonal regulation. Am J Physiol 1989; 257:L240–L247.
29. Massaro GD, Massaro D. Postnatal lung growth: evidence that the gas-exchange region grows fastest at the periphery. Am J Physiol 1993; 265:L319–L322.
30. Bartlett D Jr. Postnatal growth of the mammalian lung: influence of low and high oxygen tensions. Respir Physiol 1970; 9:58–64.
31. Burri PH, Weibel ER. Morphometric estimation of pulmonary diffusion capacity II. Effect of Po_2 on the growing lung. Adaptation of the growing rat lung to hypoxia and hyperoxia. Respir Physiol 1971; 11:247–264.

32. Randell S, Mercer RR, Young SL. Neonatal hyperoxia alters the pulmonary alveolar and capillary structure of 40-day old rats. Am J Pathol 1990; 136:1259–1266.
33. Bucher JR, Roberts RJ. The development of the newborn rat lung in hyperoxia: a dose response study of lung growth, maturation, and changes in antioxidant enzyme activity. Pediatr Res 1981; 15:999–1008.
34. Hurtado H. Animals in high altitudes: resident man. In: Bill DB, Adolph EF, eds. Handbook of Physiology Adaptation to the Environment. Washington, DC: American Physiology Society, 1964:Sec 4 843–860.
35. Campos Rey De Castro J, Iglesias B. Mechanisms of natural acclimatization: preliminary report on anatomic studies at high altitudes. US Air Force School of Aviation Medicine, San Antonio, Texas. 1956; Report 33–97.
36. Saldana M, Garcia-Oyola E. Morphometry of the high altitude lung. Lab Invest 1970; 22:509.
37. Brody JS, Lahiri S, Simpser M, Motoyama EK, Velasquez T. Lung elasticity and airways dynamics in Peruvian natives to high altitude. J Appl Physiol 1977; 42:245–251.
38. Tenney SM, Remmers JE. Alveolar dimensions in the lungs of animals raised at high altitude. J Appl Physiol 1966; 21:1328.
39. Saetta M, Ghezzo H, Kim WD, King M, Angus GE, Wang N, Cosio MG. Loss of alveolar attachments in smokers. A morphometric correlate of lung function impairment. Am Rev Respir Dis. 1985; 132:894–900.
40. Loch JN. Corticosteroids and growth. N Engl J Med 1976; 295:547–552.
41. Morishige WK, Jouns NS. Influence of glucocorticosteroids on postnatal lung development in the rat: possible modulation by thyroid hormones. Endocrinology 1982; 11:1587–1594.
42. Henning SJ. Plasma concentration of total and free corticosterone during development in the rat. Am J Physiol 1978; 235:E452–E456.
43. Jones CT. Corticosteroid concentration in the plasma of fetal and maternal guinea pigs during gestation. Endocrinology 1974; 95:1129–1133.
44. Sahebjami H, Domino M. Effects of postnatal dexamethasone treatment on development of alveoli in adult rats. Exp Lung Res 1989:961–973.
45. Blanco LN, Frank L. The formation of alveoli in rat lung during the third and fourth postnatal weeks: effect of hyperoxia, dexamethasone, and deferoxamine. Pediatr Res 1993:334–340.
46. Liebowitz D, Massaro GD, Massaro D. Adrenalectomy and surfacant in adult rats. J Appl Physiol Respir Environ Exerc Physiol 1984; 56:564–567.
47. Adkisson VT, Callas G. Morphometric changes in the lungs of rats following adrenalectomy supplemented by desiccated thyroid. Anat Rec 1982; 203:147–156.
48. Okabe T, Yorifuji H, Yamada E. Exp Cell Res 1984; 154:125–135.
49. Powell JT, Whitney PL. Postnatal development of rat lung: changes in lung lectin, elastin, acetylcholinesterase and other enzymes. Biochemistry 1980; 188:1–8.
50. Clerch LB, Whitney P, Massaro D. Rat lung lectin gene expression is regulated developmentally and by dexamethasone. Am J Physiol 1989; 256:C501–C505.
51. Ong D, Chytil F. Changes in levels of cellular retinol- and retinoic-acid-binding proteins of liver and lung during perinatal development of rat. Proc Natl Acad Sci USA 1976; 73:3976–3978.

52. Rush MG, Riaz-Ul-Haq, Chytil F. Opposing effects of retinoic acid and dexamethasone on cellular retinol-binding protein ribonucleic acid levels in the rat. Endocrinology 1991; 129:705–709.
53. Gudas LJ. Retinoids and vertebrate development. J Biol Chem 1994; 269:15399–15402.
54. Liu R, Harvey CS, McGowan SE. Retinoic acid increases elastin in neonatal rat lung fibroblast cultures. Am J Physiol 1993; 265:L430–L43.
55. Franckhauser J, Antras-Ferry J, Robin P. Robin D, Forest C. Glucocorticoids antagonize retinoic acid stimulation of *pepck* gene transcription in 3T3-F442A adipocytes. Cell Mol Biol 1994; 40:723–729.
56. Goradeski GI, Eckert RL, Utian WH, Sheean L, Rorke EA. Retinoids, sex steroids and glucocorticoids regulate ecotcervical cell envelope formation but not the level of the envelope precursor, involucrin. Differentiation 1989; 42:75–80.
57. Hustead VA, Gutcher GR, Anderson SA, Zachman RD. Relationship of vitamin A (retinol) status to lung disease in the preterm infant. J Pediatr 1984; 105:610–615.
58. Shenai JP, Chytil F, Stahlman MT. Vitamin A status of neonates with bronchopulmonary dysplasia. Pediatr Res 1985; 19:185–189.
59. Sobonya RE, Logrinoff MM, Taussig LM, Theriault A. Morphometric analysis of the lung in prolonged bronchopulmonary dysplasia. Pediatr Res 1982; 16:969–972.
60. Margraf LR, Tomashefski JR Jr, Bruch MC, Dahms BB. Morphometric analysis of the lung in bronchopulmonary dysplasia. Am Rev Respir Dis 1991; 143:391–400.
61. Massaro GD, Massaro D. Postnatal treatment with retinoic acid increases the number of pulmonary alveoli in rats. Am J Physiol 1996; 270:L305–L310.
62. Autor AP, Frank L, Roberts RJ. Developmental characteristics of pulmonary superoxide dismutase: relationship to idiopathic respiratory distress syndrome. Pediatr Res 1976; 10:154–158.
63. Clerch LB, Neithardt G, Spencer U, Melendez JA, Massaro GD, Massaro D. Pertussis toxin treatment alters manganese superoxide dismutase activity in lung: evidence for lung oxygen toxicity in air-breathing rats. J Clin Invest 1994; 93: 2482–2489.

23

Factors Mediating Cell Growth in Lung Injury

A. KEITH TANSWELL, SHILPA BUCH, MINGYAO LIU, and MARTIN POST

University of Toronto
The Hospital for Sick Children
Toronto, Ontario, Canada

I. Introduction

The term bronchopulmonary dysplasia (BPD) was coined by Northway et al. (1) to reflect the involvement of all lung tissue elements. The described features included airway mucosal metaplasia, airway and vascular smooth-muscle hyperplasia, saccular emphysema, and atelectasis. The same group of investigators subsequently emphasized the additional feature of widespread interstitial fibrosis (2). An intriguing feature of BPD, as seen in the current era, has been a reduced frequency of airway injury (3,4). This may simply reflect a change in population characteristics, in that there has been a proportional increase in the representation of very low birth weight infants among those who survive and go on to acquire BPD. Alternatively, there may have been some unattributed change in management that has resulted in a decrease in the degree of airway injury. There are likely to be multiple factors that result in the histological changes seen with the development of BPD, but the three major candidates are pulmonary oxygen toxicity, barotrauma, and cellular immaturity. Unlike injury to the adult lung, in which lung cell proliferation is superimposed on an essentially growth-arrested organ, BPD occurs in an organ that is normally in a state of active cell division. In the most severely affected infants BPD is characterized by a long-term global reduction in alveolar number and surface area (5). However, this long-term failure of lung growth is preceded, in the early stages of injury, by reparative pneumonocyte hyperplasia and later, in those who develop fibrosis, patchy areas of fibroblast hyperplasia. These specific cellular hyperplasia are superimposed on an overall pattern of development in which formation of new alveoli is retarded. Whether these changes reflect an altered pattern of secretion of those polypeptide growth factors that control normal lung growth, or the appearance of different factors, is unknown. There is very little direct information available about the role of polypeptide growth factors, either in normal human lung development or in BPD. In part, this has been due to limited availability of human tissue in the early stages of disease development and, until relatively recently, uncertainty over the identity of likely mediators of cell growth. Although the factors that influence cell growth in BPD remain unknown, there has been considerable recent information obtained from several in vitro and in vivo models of growth, repair, and injury that suggest that immaturity, oxygen concentration, and barotrauma, all may influence the expression of growth factors in the developing lung.

II. Regulation of Cell Division

Smith and Stiles (6) have suggested that growth factors fall into two categories. Those that act on genes controlling early cell cycle events (G_0 and early G_1) are known as competence factors, whereas those that act later in the cell cycle (late G_1) are known as progression factors. Cells require exposures to both a competence and a progression factor for completion of cell division. As the known growth factors fall into one or other category, division of any one cell type during normal growth or repair would appear to require the presence of at least two growth factors. The competence and progression model of sequential growth factor effects was developed through the study of fibroblast-derived cell lines in vitro. Concerns have been aired about the validity of this model for epithelial cells, or even fibroblasts in primary cell culture as, under serum-free conditions, they may appear to respond to a single growth factor. It now seems likely that the model is valid, and the response to a single exogenous growth factor can be explained by the autocrine release of the necessary second growth factor into the culture medium. Primary cultures of premature lung fibroblasts and pneumonocytes synthesize both autocrine and paracrine factors (7). From the information available at that time, some of our early in vitro studies suggested that the positive effectors of lung cell growth following lung injury could be lung-specific autocrine and paracrine growth factors (8,9). Subsequent recognition of a wide variety of growth factor homologues, and of growth factor-binding proteins with varying molecular sizes and isoelectric points (10), makes it likely that these partially characterized factors were members of the major growth factor families.

There are several ways in which growth factors may reach a responsive cell. They may be synthesized elsewhere and be blood-borne in an endocrine fashion. Alternatively, they may be synthesized locally by one cell type and then passively diffuse to act on a different cell type in a paracrine fashion, or target the originating cell in an autocrine loop. More recently recognized modes of growth factor transfer are two juxtacrine mechanisms. Direct transfer can occur through gap junctions at cell-to-cell contacts, which are under oncogene control (11) and may be hormonally activated (12). The second juxtacrine mechanism involves the presentation of a membrane-bound proform of a growth factor on one cell to an appropriate receptor on an adjacent cell (13).

There are four major signal transduction pathways by which growth factor binding to cells influences DNA synthesis and cell division. In the first pathway, growth factors binding to plasma membrane receptors act through G proteins to cause a phospholipase C-mediated generation of diacylglycerol (DG) and inositol triphosphate (IP_3). Together, DG and IP_3 activate protein kinase C (PKC), which can then phosphorylate various cellular proteins responsible for cell cycle control (14). Second, growth factors, such as platelet-derived growth factor (PDGF) and fibroblast growth factors (FGFs) may bind to their membrane protein tyrosine kinase receptor to activate a PKC, which is an integral part of the receptor complex (15). The third pathway involves a growth factor-mediated increase in intracellular cyclic AMP (cAMP), which may either stimulate or inhibit DNA synthesis through effects on various protein kinases or by cAMP-responsive elements in the promoters of various genes (16). Last, certain cytokines can bind to their receptors with a resultant direct phosphorylation of three ''Stat'' proteins, which then aggregate to act as a transcription complex (17). To exert their effect, protein kinases that exert cell cycle control bind to members of the cyclin family. Separate cyclin–protein kinase complexes act independently to control transition from G_1 to S and from G_2 to M (18).

From the foregoing description, it is clear that there are multiple sites at which control of the altered cell proliferation seen in BPD may be exerted. The response of any given lung cell to growth factors in its environment is subject to a complex array of intrinsic and extrinsic regulators. The development of BPD is associated, as are many lung injuries, with a requirement for greater inspired O_2 concentrations, yet increased O_2 concentrations can slow repair from lung injury (19). Weiss and Kavanau (20) first suggested a negative-feedback model of organ growth, requiring both positive and negative regulators. Lung cell hyperplasia following injury may be due to an increase in positive regulators, a reduction in negative regulators, or a combination of the two. Putative homeostatic negative regulators, or chalones, have been extracted from mouse lung tissue (21), whereas bronchoalveolar lavage of healthy rats contains inhibitors of both fibroblast and pneumonocyte growth that disappear following injury with ozone (22,23). Several novel growth inhibitors have been characterized in other organs (24) but, with the exception of the transforming growth factor-β (TGF-β) family, little information is available for the lung. A 3.5- to 12.5-kDa inhibitor of lung fibroblast growth, that is released only at specific stages of lung development, has recently been detected in the conditioned medium of pneumonocytes isolated from premature rat lung (25). It should be remembered, particularly under conditions of injury, that cell death is a potent regulator of specific cell populations. This may be through a direct unprogrammed cytotoxic effect of the agent responsible for injury, or through activation of genes leading to programmed cell death, or apoptosis (26). An important function of certain growth factors in adaptation to lung injury may be to inhibit apoptosis (27).

Chronic lung injury is associated with changes in extracellular matrix composition. A detailed description of these changes falls outside our mandate for this chapter, but are provided in various recent reviews (28–31), as well as elsewhere in this volume. Such changes, however, may play a significant role in the responsivity of lung cells to growth factors in their microenvironment. Pneumonocytes (32), fibroblasts (33), and endothelial cells (34) from immature lung, all show variable responses to growth stimuli in vitro, depending on the composition of their substratum. Some extracellular matrix proteins have growth factor-like domains with direct growth-promoting activity (35), whereas others modify cell shape, which indirectly influences sensitivity to growth factors (36). Extracellular matrix proteins can function as a reservoir for growth factors that are inert until released by proteases (37), can hold growth factors in an active form while protecting them from inactivation (38), or can bind growth factors to inhibit their binding to cell surface receptors (39). Alternatively, extracellular matrix components may facilitate delivery of growth factors to a cell through receptor-dependent (40) or receptor-independent (41) pathways. As assessed by immunohistochemistry, expression of growth factor receptors, following lung injury, may be transient compared with expression of the ligand (42,43). Such considerations complicate the interpretation of altered growth factor expression in lung injury. Any temporal relations between increased growth factor expression and cell proliferation, while suggestive, can only be considered a correlation until intervention studies can confirm a cause-and-effect relation.

Having said this, interventional studies, with certain exceptions (44), await better definition of which growth factors have increased expression following lung injury. What growth factors might one expect to mediate changes in cell proliferation in a neonatal lung injury, such as BPD? Are they likely to emulate the changes observed in the normally quiescent adult lung following injury, or will they represent altered expression of those growth factors that control normal prenatal and postnatal lung growth? The concept that at least some component of the proliferative changes observed in the injured adult lung is likely to represent a reactivation of normal fetal and neonatal growth controls is attractive. As shown in Figure 1, pneumonocytes, or prepneumonocytes, isolated from fetal, neonatal, and adult lung differ in their sensitivity to growth factors, and it would not be surprising if the same were true for lung fibroblasts. The stage of lung development at the time of birth, O_2-exposure, and forces generated during positive-pressure ventilation, are all likely to be contributory factors to the abnormal lung cell growth pattern seen during the development of BPD.

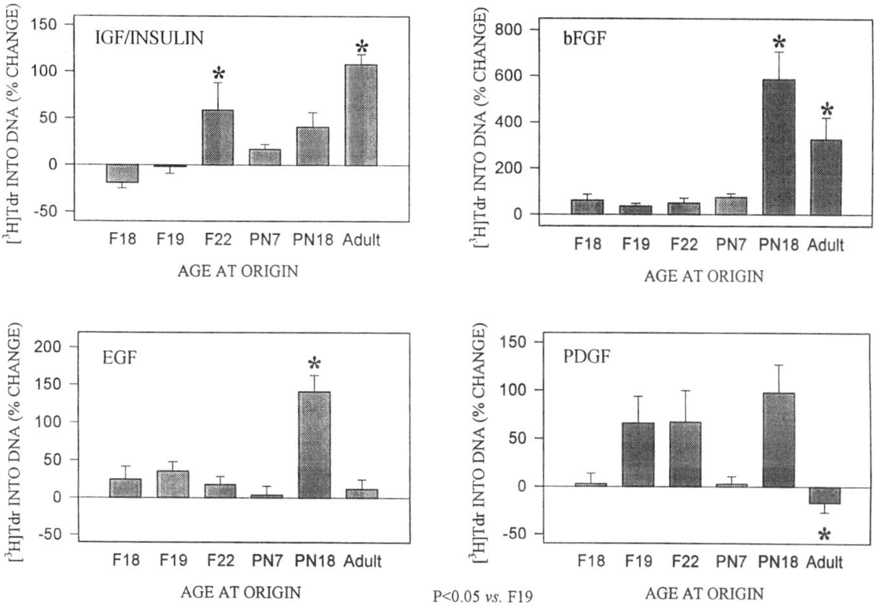

Figure 1 The response of distal lung epithelial cells to growth factors is dependent on the age of the donor at the time of cell purification. Cells were purified from fetal rats at 18, 19, or 22 days gestation; from postnatal rats at 7 or 18 days of age; or from adult rats. They were cultured at the same cell density in serum-free medium on a poly-D-lysine substratum, and the response to various growth factors was assessed by the uptake of [^{3}H]thymidine ([^{3}H]Tdr) into DNA. The responses to IGF-I (20 ng/mL) with insulin (50 μg/mL), bFGF (20 ng/mL), EGF (50 ng/mL), and PDGF-BB (20 ng/mL) are shown as M ± SEM for four- to seven-cell preparations * = $p < 0.05$ vs. F19. At F19, the lungs are at the canalicular stage of lung development, which is the stage of development at delivery of those human infants most susceptible to the development of BPD.

III. Regulation of Normal Lung Growth by Growth Factors

That premature infants are more susceptible to the development of chronic lung disease than their full-term counterparts could reflect a fundamental difference in the ability of the developing lung to undergo an efficient and controlled repair process. Ideally, the repair processes that follow lung injury would mimic ontogeny. This would make economic sense, in that the use of processes for repair different from those used in morphogenesis would require a greater repertoire of genetic regulatory programs. It, therefore, seems likely that if we are to understand the repair processes within the lung of the premature infant, we first need to understand the physiology of normal lung growth.

The mammalian lung originates from an endodermal tube derived from an invagination of the primitive foregut, entering the surrounding mesoderm. This embryonic stage is followed by the pseudoglandular stage of sequential tubular bifurcations. In the subsequent canalicular stage there is vascularization of the developing lung, which is followed by the saccular stage of acinar development and then alveolarization. Fetal lung morphogenesis involves major structural changes that are associated with cell proliferation (reviewed in Ref. 45). Lung cell proliferation is mainly confined to morphogenetically active regions that shift from central to peripheral tubules during development. The rate of proliferation of both epithelial and mesenchymal cells decreases during development, but the decline is unequal. The proportion of dividing epithelial cells increases initially during fetal development, but declines dramatically near term (46–48). Studies with isolated fetal lung epithelial cells have confirmed this growth pattern (49). The decline in epithelial mitotic activity is associated with an increase in cellular differentiation (reviewed in Ref. 50). The proportion of dividing cells of mesenchymal origin (endothelial cells and fibroblasts) decreases in the initial stages of lung development, but increases sharply at the canalicular phase of development, owing to capillary growth. Growth of fibroblasts progressively declines during late fetal life (25). Capillary formation continues at a rapid rate during late fetal life and, consequently, mesenchymal cells are the major dividing cell type near term (46–48). These developmental differences in proliferation rates between epithelial and mesenchymal cells are also reflected in the ratio of the total numbers of epithelial cells to mesenchymal cells. The ratio increases from 1:4 at the pseudoglandular stage of development to 1:1 at the late canalicular stage, before decreasing again at term (47). The period of alveolarization is accompanied by a phase of rapid cellular proliferation in both epithelial and mesenchymal cell populations. Interstitial fibroblasts actively proliferate early in this phase, but then slow down, whereas endothelial cell growth is brisk throughout. The dividing endothelial and interstitial cells are primarily located in septal crests. Epithelial cell division in this period occurs on septal buds and walls. Both alveolar epithelial cell populations, type I and type II cells, increase during this growth period.

However, only alveolar epithelial type II cells proliferate (45,46), indicating that the alveolar type I cell population arises from type II cells.

The mechanism(s) controlling this ontogenic pattern of lung cell proliferation remains to be elucidated. However, embryonic lung morphogenesis (branching and budding) is guided by instructive interactions between lung endoderm and mesoderm (51). Therefore, it seems logical to hypothesize that similar interactions are involved in regulation of cell proliferation during development. Several studies have shown that increasing quantities of bronchial mesenchyme stimulate bronchial epithelial growth (52,53). In addition, recombinations between bronchial mesenchyme and tracheal epithelium have resulted in the induction of supernumerary buds in the normally unbranched tracheal epithelium (54–56). The latter suggests that bronchial mesoderm influences the mitotic rate of the tracheal endoderm which, in turn, leads to budding. A recent autoradiographic study (55) revealed elevated proliferation rates of epithelium in supernumerary tracheal buds induced by combining tracheal epithelium and bronchial mesenchyme. It appears that bronchial mesenchyme has the ability to maintain most or all of the epithelial cells in the cell cycle, which seems to be required for further mesenchymal–epithelial interactions leading to branching morphogenesis (57). These findings suggest that lung mesodermal cells can stimulate endodermal multiplication and that lung mesoderm may even induce endodermal growth at precise sites by keeping the endodermal cells at those sites in the cell cycle. Mesenchymal–epithelial interactions in the lung at late fetal gestation also control epithelial cell growth. Fibroblasts obtained at the pseudoglandular stage of lung development stimulate epithelial cell growth, whereas fibroblasts at the saccular stage promote epithelial cell differentiation, but not proliferation (58). Regulation of epithelial cell growth by mesoderm has also been reported for other tissues, and this suggests qualitative differences in mesenchymes from different organs (59,60). Even postnatal epithelial growth is stimulated by fetal mesenchyme. Implantation of fetal mammary mesenchyme in the adult mammary fat pad results in an invasion of the mesenchyme by the host's gland epithelium, which is then stimulated in its proliferation (61). The canalicular and saccular stages of lung development are marked by thinning of mesenchymal tissue. This regression of mesenchymal tissue appears to be controlled by mesenchymal–epithelial tissue interactions. Although the exact nature of the factors involved in mesenchymal–epithelial tissue interactions during fetal lung development is unknown, several growth factors have been implicated in lung morphogenesis.

Both transforming growth factor-alpha (TGF-α) and epidermal growth factor (EGF) are expressed in the fetal lung (62,63). Both are mitogenic through binding to the EGF receptor (EGF-R), although they may have different potencies owing to different ligand–receptor processing (64). It has been suggested that TGF-α may play an EGF-like role in the fetus that, after birth, is taken over by EGF (65), in a fashion somewhat analogous to insulin-like growth factors-II and

I (IGF-II, IGF-I). In the preterm rodent lung EGF and TGF-α mRNA are found mainly in mesenchyme (66,67), whereas immunoreactive TGF-α and EGF are localized to airway and saccular epithelial cells (68). The receptor is localized to both epithelial and mesenchymal cells (66,68). These data suggest that EGF and TGF-α play an autocrine and paracrine role in lung cell growth. The autocrine role for TGF-α had previously been suggested by in vitro studies with type II pneumonocytes (69). EGF-R has been reported to be found in airway, but not saccular, epithelial cells of ovine fetal and human fetal and neonatal lung (70–72). However, others have reported the presence of EGF-R in the airway and alveolar epithelium of adult human lung (73). Whether these discrepancies reflect true species or maturational differences, or are simply due to antibody sensitivity, awaits further study. Both EGF and TGF-α influence growth and branching morphogenesis in vitro (68,74). However, genetic studies have suggested that EGF receptor signaling is not essential for lung branching (75–77). Administration of EGF to fetal rabbit (78), lamb (79), and rhesus monkey (80) also accelerates the morphological and physiological maturation of the lung. The mechanism by which EGF may act to stimulate lung maturation is unknown. EGF does not directly affect surfactant phosphatidylcholine formation by fetal type II cells (81), but it may stimulate fetal lung fibroblasts to produce a differentiation factor for epithelial cells (81,82), fibroblast–pneumonocyte factor (FPF).

As discussed herein, and reviewed by Stiles and D'Ercole (83), there is considerable indirect evidence to support a role for IGF-I and -II in normal lung growth. IGF-I and -II have been immunolocalized to the respiratory epithelium (84,85). Gene expression for IGF-I occurs in the mesenchyme of the lung (85,86), whereas IGF-II mRNA expression is predominantly localized to airway epithelium (86). The type 1 IGF receptor is expressed in virtually all cells in the developing lung (86). In contrast, the transcripts for type 2 IGF receptor are mainly found in the mesenchyme (86). Expression of both receptors changes little during development (86). IGF-I mRNA is less abundant than IGF-II mRNA in fetal lung, implying that IGF-II is the somatomedin important for fetal lung growth (87). Mice carrying null mutations of the IGF-I type 1 IGF receptor die at birth from respiratory failure, but no histopathological defects of lung development were observed (88). Transgenic mice with a disrupted IGF-II gene are small, but no abnormal lung morphology is noted (89). Thus, the precise role of IGFs in fetal lung growth remains uncertain.

Acidic and basic fibroblast growth factors (aFGF, bFGF) have been immunolocalized in fetal (90,91), postnatal, and adult (92) rat lungs. In normal adult rat lung aFGF (FGF-1) colocalizes with EGF to airway and alveolar epithelium, to interstitial cells, and to smooth-muscle cells (92). In contrast, bFGF (FGF-2) was primarily confined to alveolar and vascular basement membranes, and to the external laminae of smooth muscle (92). In fetal lung, bFGF appears to be sequestered by the extracellular matrix (ECM), and its role in lung branching remains to be elucidated (90). Two FGF receptors (FGF-R1 and FGF-R2) have been localized to embryonic lung epithelium (90,93). The ligand for a FGF-R2 splice variant (FGFR2-IIIB) is keratinocyte growth factor (KGF/FGF-7). KGF mRNA expression is localized to embryonic lung mesenchyme (94). At late fetal gestation, lung fibroblasts secrete KGF into their medium, which stimulates adult type II cell proliferation (95). A targeted expression of a dominant–negative FGF-R2 in transgenic mice inhibits secondary bronchial branching (96), whereas antisense oligonucleotides or antibodies to KGF and FGF-R2 inhibit branching in embryonic rat lung explants (97).

Transforming growth factor-β, which may modulate extracellular matrix composition, also appears to play a role in lung-branching morphogenesis (98,99). High concentrations of TGF-β_1 inhibit lung-branching morphogenesis in vitro (99). However, inactivation of the mouse TGF-β_1 gene does not affect lung branching (100). TGF-β_2 null mice exhibit perinatal mortality and a wide range of developmental defects (101). Prenatal lung morphology of the mutant mice was, however, normal. Mice lacking TGF-β_3 exhibit an arrest in lung development at the late pseudoglandular stage (102). These genetic analyses suggest that none of the TGF-β isoforms play a major biological role in early lung development. However, it is plausible that redundancy or leakage of maternal TGF-βs across the placenta rescues the early developmental events in these transgenic mice. At later stages of fetal lung development, minute quantities of TGF-β stimulate fetal type II cell proliferation, whereas high concentrations inhibit lung maturation (25,103). During an earlier developmental epoch, fetal lung fibroblasts release an inhibitor of type II cell maturation, the programmed loss of which, as lung development proceeds, could set the stage for FPF to trigger the maturational process. The inhibitor appears to be a TGF-β homologue (104). Interestingly, Müllerian-inhibiting substance (MIS), which has a high homology with TGF-β and is responsible for Müllerian duct regression in the male, has been proposed to delay male lung maturation (105,106).

Platelet-derived growth factor is also implicated in fetal lung development. In the embryonic lung and other organs, both PDGF isoforms, AA and BB, are synthesized in the epithelium, whereas the PDGF receptors, α and β, are expressed in the mesenchyme (107–114). Translational arrest of endogenous PDGF-BB, using an antisense oligodeoxynucleotide strategy, results in significant smaller lungs (109). The degree of branching is unaffected. Also, mice deficient for PDGF-B (110) and β-receptor (111) show no abnormal lung branching. The AA isoform of PDGF (112), and the PDGF α-receptor (114) seem to play a critical role in early lung-branching morphogenesis. A PDGF-A knockout is lethal at two restriction points, one in early embryonic development, and one after birth (115). The lung phenotype of dying mutant embryos was not further investigated and, thus, it is not clear whether PDGF-A is involved in the early formation of the lung. The observation that PDGF-A-deficient mice surviving beyond birth have normal fetal lung development argues against PDGF-A being involved in early-branching morphogenesis. Alternatively, PDGF-A's role may be replaced by other non-PDGF factors, or maternal leakage of PDGF may rescue the early developmental events in the knockout mice. PDGF-A-deficient mice that survive the embryonic bottleneck develop postnatal lung emphysema, secondary to a failure of alveologenesis, attributed to a lack of alveolar myofibroblast differentiation (115). Mice carrying a targeted disruption in the PDGF α-receptor gene die during embryonic development and exhibit severe developmental defects (116). However, early lung development proceeds normally in the α-receptor null mutants. PDGF expression increases at the early canalicular stage of lung development, but then declines before type II pneumonocyte cytodifferentiation (117). PDGF-BB stimulates fetal type II cells' proliferation, but does not affect their maturation (25).

Other factors affecting prenatal lung growth include physical factors, which is discussed separately, as well as hormonal factors. It is widely recognized that hormones, such as glucocorticoids, androgen, thyroid hormone, and insulin, affect lung differentiation. Their physiological role in lung growth remains to be established. Several studies have suggested that glucocorticoids affect lung growth. Maternal administration of glucocorticoids inhibits fetal lung growth (118–120). Morphologically, the proportion of epithelial type II cells in the population diminishes after glucocorticoid treatment, whereas that of type I cells increases (121,122). Consistent with these findings are the observations that exposure of fetal lung cells to glucocorticoids also results in reduced DNA synthesis (123). Recent studies suggest that two IGF-binding proteins, IGFBP-1 and IGFBP-2, may be involved in mediating the marked growth retardation secondary to glucocorticoid excess (124). As exogenous glucocorticoids decrease lung growth, it is plausible that endogenous glucocorticoids also reduce the rate of cell proliferation. However, ablation experiments, such as fetal hypophysectomy, do not support this idea. Fetal hypophysectomy retards lung growth, but the lung weights are normal when corrected for body weight (125). Human anencephaly may represent another model of lung development in a reduced hormonal environment. Anencephalics frequently demonstrate hypoplastic lungs that are less mature. Although lack of hormonal influences cannot be totally excluded, recent evidence indicates that lung hypoplasia in anencephalics is primarily due to thoracic abnormalities (126). Although thyroid hormones have been reported to influence circulating concentrations of IGF-I and IGFBPs (127), IGF receptor expression (128), as well as EGF (129) and EGF-R (130) mRNAs, thyroid hormone appears to stimulate lung maturation, but not lung growth (131). Thyroidectomy slows lung growth (132) but, again, lung weights are normal when corrected for body weight. Female lungs contain more cuboidal epithelial cells than male lungs before epithelial differentiation (133), implying a variability in lung growth. Indeed, the rate of lung growth of females at this stage of development is greater than that of males (47). Moreover, the proportion of dividing epithelial cells is greater in females than males. At this period of development, interstitial cells are the predominant multiplying cell type in males. With advancing gestation, the rate of lung growth in males increases and catches up with females (47). At term, size differences between male and female lungs are eliminated. Substantial evidence suggests that androgens cause this sexual dimorphism in lung development. Infants of diabetic mothers (IDMs) have elevated circulating levels of insulin (134). The higher insulin levels are probably responsible for the macrosomia seen in some IDMs (135), and it has been argued that insulin may play a significant role in normal fetal growth (136).

IV. The Influence of Physical Factors on Lung Cell Growth

A variety of physical factors influence normal fetal lung growth (137,138). These include the volumes of amniotic and lung fluid (139–143), available space for the lung in the thorax (144–148), and fetal respiration (139–151). The importance of lung fluid volume in fetal lung growth has been clearly demonstrated. Distention of the lung by tracheal ligation stimulates lung growth (139,140). Conversely, tracheal drainage inhibits lung growth (139), probably by diminishing the distending fluid pressure. Obstruction of the trachea and bronchus in the human fetus has been associated with lung hyperplasia (141). The precise role of amniotic fluid in normal fetal lung growth is unknown. The rate of lung fluid production also influences the amount of amniotic fluid volume. Experimental introduction of oligohydramnios by amniotic drainage (152–154), nephrectomy (155), or obstructive uropathy (156) of fetal animals reduces lung growth. Restoring normal amniotic fluid volume, after drainage, reverses changes in lung weight (153). Tracheal ligation reverses the pulmonary hypoplasias associated with fetal nephrectomy (155). Clinically, lack of amniotic fluid (oligohydramnios) has been associated with lung hypoplasia (143,156). In humans, lung hypoplasia has also been associated with decreased pulmonary arterial flow (157). Other studies have indicated that pulmonary arterial ligation decreases lung growth by reducing lung fluid production (158,159).

Although experiments of nature and whole-animal experiments demonstrate a relation between lung fluid and normal fetal lung growth, its direct influence on embryonic lung growth was recently demonstrated in studies with cultured lung explants (160). Restriction of lung liquid secretion by blockage of transepithelial [Cl^-] transport resulted in smaller lungs, but did not affect branching. Amniotic fluid deficits may also cause a sufficient uterine constraint to reduce the thoracic space. Decreased thoracic space may diminish the distending force in the lungs, thereby reducing lung growth. Indeed, lesions such as diaphragmatic hernia (146,148) and thoracic abnormalities (126,145) that limit the available space for lung growth, have been associated with lung hypoplasia. Experimental compression of the lung in animals also diminishes fetal lung growth (144,147). Pulmonary hypoplasia caused by reduced thoracic space has also been observed in newborns with congenital adenomatoid malformation (161). Interestingly, tracheal ligation accelerates lung growth and reverses the effect of pulmonary hypoplasia in congenital diaphragmatic hernias (162). Uterine and thoracic constraints may also restrict fetal respiration. The reduced distention of the lung caused by diminished fetal respiration may then lead to hypoplasia. Several lines of evidence support the concept that normal lung growth is affected by intermittent stretch caused by fetal breathing movements. Disruption of the intermittent distension of the lung by spinal cord section (149,151) or phrenectomy (139,163) results in diminished lung growth. Inhibition of fetal-breathing movements with curare has a similar effect (150). In contrast, increases in fetal respiration caused by maternal CO_2 inhalation results in accelerated lung development (164). A reduction in the amplitude of pressure changes during fetal respiration also results in hypoplasia (165). Fetal-breathing movements do not appear to stimulate fetal lung growth through changes in pulmonary blood flow (166), but rather affect lung growth by causing regional changes in lung fluid volume, which transiently increase or decrease distending pressures during fetal respiration (167,168). In many nonpulmonary tissues and cell types, physical force functions as a regulator of cell proliferation and differentiation (169). How physical factors specifically affect lung cell growth remains to be defined, but available evidence strongly supports the concept that stretch can stimulate the expression of such growth factors as PDGF (170–174), IGF-I (175,176), and TGF-β (170). Conversely, physical force may decrease DNA synthesis by altering the shape of fetal lung cells (177).

To simulate fetal breathing movements in vitro, several cell strain systems have been recently developed and applied (171,178–180). Mechanical strain induces growth of premature rat lung cells maintained in a three-dimensional culture system (171,172). That this effect is mediated by an increased synthesis of endogenous growth factors is suggested by the growth-stimulatory activity of conditioned medium from strained cells, but not from control cells (181). The mitogenic activity of conditioned medium from an embryonic lung fibroblast cell line has also been reported to be increased after mechanical strain (178). Mechanical strain of premature lung cells increased their content of PDGF-B and its β-receptor (PDGF-βR) mRNA within 5 min of the onset of strain. Increased PDGF-BB and PDGF-βR proteins were detected following a 24-hr exposure to intermittent strain. The strain-induced stimulatory effect on premature lung cell proliferation could be blocked by antisense PDGF-B oligodeoxynucleotides (ODN), neutralizing PDGF-BB antibody, a PDGF receptor-associated tyrosine kinase inhibitor (tyrphostin 9), and by antisense PDGF-βR ODN (173). These in vitro findings are consistent with recent in vivo observations by Harding et al.

(167), who found that abolition of fetal-breathing movements by spinal cord transection led to a reduction in both DNA synthesis and IGF-II gene expression. Changes in lung volume, from tracheal obstruction or lung liquid drainage, also altered IGF-II expression in fetal sheep (175).

Adult type II pneumonocytes stretched in vitro, have increased mobilization of intracellular calcium, which mediates release of surfactant (182). In premature lung cells, both intra- and extracellular calcium modulate strain-induced proliferative activity. The rapid entry of calcium (<1 min) through a gadolinium-sensitive pathway, presumably an activated ion channel, contributed to strain-induced PKC activation and proliferative activity (183). Intracellular concentrations of both IP_3 and DAG were dramatically increased after a short period of strain associated with the activation of phospholipase C-γ (183). The specific activity of PKC increased five to sevenfold shortly after strain, remained elevated throughout a 48-hr period of intermittent strain. PKC inhibitors blocked strain-induced DNA synthesis (184). Activation of protein tyrosine kinases seems to be an upstream event of the PKC-phospholipase C-γ pathway (185). Stretch-induced prostacyclin (186) and cAMP (179,186) synthesis increased in cells from premature rat lung exposed to a relatively high amplitude strain. Such secondary changes could influence growth factor gene expression in lung cells. Resnick et al. (173) have recently identified a *cis*-acting fluid shear–stress-responsive element (SSRE) on the PDGF-B chain promoter. This putative transcription factor-binding site is also present in the promoters of TGF-β_1, tissue plasminogen activator, intercellular adhesion molecule 1, c-*fos*, c-*jun*, and monocyte chemotactic protein 1, which are all present in endothelial cells and have been demonstrated to be shear responsive. By directly injecting DNA into beating hearts, Aoyagi and Izumo (187) mapped the promoter element of the protooncogene c-*fos* in myocardium subjected to left ventricular pressure overload in vivo. Deletion and point mutations of the serum response element (SRE) of the c-*fos* promoter, resulted in a loss of pressure-induced reporter gene expression, indicating that the pressure response element (PRE) coincides with the SRE. Mechanical strain-induced intracellular signaling may regulate gene expression through these and other similar response elements.

After birth, physical forces still play an important role in regulation of lung growth, function, structure, and metabolism (188,189). Ferrets exposed to a continuous positive airway pressure of 6 cmH_2O for 2 weeks have accelerated lung growth (190). Barotrauma is an important and potentially lethal complication of mechanical ventilation. In addition to the most widely recognized form, the presence of extra-alveolar air, diffuse lung injury has also been attributed to barotrauma (191). Overdistention of the lung appears to be the fundamental mechanism underlying ventilator-associated lung injury (192–194). Ventilation with high tidal volumes can increase vascular filtration pressures, produce stress fractures of capillary endothelium, epithelium, and basement membrane, and cause lung rupture (195), as well as stimulate the release of proinflammatory cytokines (196). The structural immaturity and low tensile strength of premature lung tissue may contribute to ventilator-induced microvascular permeability (197). Of both clinical and experimental relevance is the observation that particulate water in the gas mixture used for ventilation can independently affect lung structure (198).

The risk of ventilator-induced lung injury may be minimized by preventing overdistention of functional lung units during therapeutic ventilation. Pohlandt et al. (199) reported that preterm infants ventilated at 60 cycles/min with a short inspiratory time (0.33 sec) had a significantly reduced incidence of extra-alveolar air leakage or death before air leak, when compared with infants ventilated at 30 cycles/min with a longer inspiratory time (1 sec). Patients less than 2 years of age with thermal lung injury treated with ventilators that employ a high-frequency progressive accumulation of subtidal volumes in a pressure-limited format have decreased pulmonary barotrauma (200). The effects of various ventilation strategies on growth factor gene expression awaits future experimentation.

V. The Influence of Oxygen on Lung Cell Growth

Exposure of lung tissue to increased concentrations of oxygen leads to an increase in the formation of reactive oxygen species (ROS). The formation of ROS, their cytotoxicity, and the importance of endogenous and exogenous antioxidant defenses in limiting lung injury are discussed elsewhere in this volume. We will limit our discussion to a summary of the known effects of ROS on cell growth. There is increasing evidence to support the hypothesis, put forward by Saran and Bors (201), that ROS may play important physiological roles as intra- and intercellular messengers modulating the growth and differentiation status of target cells. This has been the subject of a recent comprehensive review by Burdon (202). Low concentrations of superoxide and hydrogen peroxide stimulate the growth of multiple cell types in vitro, whereas growth is inhibited at higher concentrations (202). Conversely, addition of the antioxidant enzymes, catalase and superoxide dismutase, can inhibit the growth of some cell types (202), suggesting an autocrine growth-stimulating effect of cell-derived ROS.

Newborn rats exposed to more than 95% O_2 for 1 week have complete arrest of lung growth with essentially undetectable lung cell DNA synthesis, as assessed by [^{3}H]thymidine autoradiography. If such animals are then allowed to recover in air, they have considerable catch-up lung growth with ultimately only a modest reduction in alveolar number and an increase in the variability of alveolar size measurements (203). The initial growth arrest by O_2 concentrations higher than 95% may be a protective response mediated by a cellular oxygen sensor. There are a considerable number of redox-sensitive cellular sites where such a sensor may be located (202), and the sensor may vary with different cell types. In pulmonary neuroepithelial cells, one O_2 sensor appears to be NADPH associated with a potassium channel (204). For growth-arrested lung cells a more likely candidate may be a hemoprotein such as aconitase. In *Escherichia coli*, aconitase, a critical tricarboxylic acid (TCA) cycle enzyme, is a sensitive target for the superoxide radical (205). It is also rapidly inactivated in whole lung by exposure to 100% O_2 (206). The advantage of aconitase, an enzyme vital for the interconversion of citrate and isocitrate, being sensitive to oxidative attack by superoxide is that the enzyme can act as a "circuit breaker" which, by its sensitivity to ROS, can shut down mitochondrial respiration and limit the production of ROS by mitochondria. This may spare DNA and other critical cell components from a potentially suicidal oxidative injury (207). Decreased growth rate, caused by TCA cycle impairment, decreases the lethality of radiation (208) and paraquat (209) to *E. coli*. Hassan and Fridovich (210) have demonstrated a requirement for a reducing substrate for paraquat lethality. Horowitz and his colleagues (211–214) have demonstrated that neonatal and adult rabbits, as well as adult mice, exposed to O_2 concentrations sufficient to produce growth arrest ($> 95\%$) have cell-specific increases in mRNAs for surfactant apoprotein, tissue inhibitor of metalloprotease (TIMP-I), and metallothioneins (MT-I and MT-II), all of which may serve protective functions.

Adult rats exposed to 100% O_2 for 48 hr, then allowed to recover in air for 48 hr, have reparative pneumonocyte proliferation (215). Bui et al. (216), using this model, have recently reported an increase in A- and D-type cyclins and of $p34^{cdc2}$ histone H1 kinase in pneumonocytes during the proliferative recovery phase. In contrast to the lung growth arrest generally seen with breathing more than 95% O_2, lower O_2 concentrations may directly stimulate lung cell growth, without the need for a recovery period. An example of this situation is the adult rat exposed to 85% O_2 for 2 weeks, in which there is a marked increase in the number of lung fibroblasts and type II pneumonocytes (217). A different profile of gene induction to that seen with greater than 95% O_2 concentration would be expected, although the similarity of gene expression to the recovery model has not yet been explored. In the 85% O_2 model we have observed an O_2-mediated increase in the expression of various growth factor genes, as described later. How oxygen toxicity brings about an increase in mammalian growth factor gene expression is presently unknown. It may be by a direct action of ROS on DNA, as observed in prokaryotes, or the effect may be mediated by some change in signal transduction molecules that then results in altered growth factor gene expression. Some bacteria adapt to lethal effects of oxidants by induced expression of protective stress genes under the control of the *oxy*R and *sox*R regulons. The *oxy*R gene product is a regulatory protein OxyR that undergoes a conformational change, and is activated, when exposed to hydrogen peroxide (218,219). Several of the proteins regulated by *oxy*R have been identified and include catalase, encoded by *kat*G; glutathione reductase, encoded by *gor*A; and an alkyl hydroperoxide reductase, encoded by *ahp*FC (220,221). Strains carrying deletions of *oxy*R are unable to induce these proteins and show an increased sensitive to hydrogen peroxide and other oxidants (220). The *sox*RS gene product is a transcriptional activator protein SoxR that specifically senses changes in superoxide concentration using a redox-active iron–sulfur center (222). The *sox*RS regulon mediates the transcription of several genes, including manganese-containing superoxide dismutase, *sod*A (223). As yet there is no direct evidence for specific mammalian homologues of the bacterial *oxy*R and *sox*R genes, but the recent identification of two oxygen-responsive elements in the 5′-flanking region of the human glutathione peroxidase gene (224) suggests that the same, or similar, mechanisms will be uncovered in mammalian cells. In contrast to O_2-mediated increases in glutathione peroxidase activity, resulting from increased transcription (224), O_2-mediated increases in catalase activity are not due to an increase in transcription, but rather, to an increased mRNA stability (225). This mechanism may also occur with growth factor mRNAs.

In vitro studies of premature lung cells exposed to high concentrations of O_2 have shown that they have a marked increase in prostaglandin synthesis (226,227), and *cis*-unsaturated fatty acids, including arachidonic acid, can directly stimulate PKC in some cell types (228). Activation of PKC may also occur in response to a change in the ratio of oxidized to reduced glutathione (229), and hyperoxic premature lung cells in vitro become rapidly depleted of reduced intracellular nonprotein thiols (230). Not only may oxidative stress influence growth factor transduction pathways by alterations of protein tyrosine phosphorylation through protein tyrosine kinase but also through altered protein tyrosine phosphatase activity (231). Protein kinases can also be activated by a rise in intracellular calcium which, in some cell types, occurs in response to an increase in certain prostaglandins (232). In addition to effects on protein kinases and protein phosphatases, ROS can affect another group of molecules critical for the regulation of gene expression: the nuclear transcription factors. Exposure to low concentrations of ROS can stimulate the expression of the early growth-related genes c-*fos* and c-*jun* in a variety of cell types (202). In turn, the binding of the Fos–Jun heterodimer to the AP-1 promoter site is dependent on the redox state of a cysteine residue in the DNA-binding domain of the proteins (233). This same mechanism mediates the stimulation of the DNA-binding of the Fos–Jun heterodimer by the nuclear protein Ref-1 (234,235), as well as of other transcription factors (201). Redox-dependent activation of the transcription factor NF-κB is by a different mechanism involving release from an inactive cytoplasmic complex (236), which may also be regulated by the degree of glutathione oxidation (237). Exposure of pneumonocytes from premature rat lung to 95% O_2 results in DNA breaks (230), a phenomenon that has been linked to modulation of c-*fos* expression (238). Activation of c-*fos*, as well as ROS-mediated activation of the *erg*1 transcription factor gene, requires modification of the serum response factor (239,240).

A wide awareness of the potential for O_2-mediated lung cell cytotoxicity encourages a desire to wean infants with BPD from supplemental O_2 as quickly as possible. This often means maintaining basal arterial O_2 concentrations at the low end of the normal range, which may be associated with episodic hypoxemia. This could contribute to the development of pulmonary hypertension (241). Pulmonary endothelial cells subjected to a hypoxic stimulus secrete factors that are mitogenic for pulmonary smooth muscle (242).

Both O_2 and pressure share common pathways by which they may influence cell growth. Early studies suggested that increased airway pressure could enhance the lethal effects of lambs breathing 100% O_2 (243), and additive effects on growth factor expression have yet to be explored in the laboratory. Such experiments will not be simple. As assessed by depletion experiments, a role for neutrophils in pulmonary oxygen toxicity has yet to be firmly established (244–249). However, studies by Kawano et al. (250) demonstrated that barotrauma-mediated changes in airway pathology are phagocyte-mediated when the ventilated lung is surfactant-insufficient, suggesting that ex vivo or surfactant-sufficient preparations may have limitations as experimental models for barotrauma sustained shortly after preterm delivery. The introduction of routine surfactant replacement therapy may have played some part in the changing pattern of lung pathology in BPD.

VI. Epithelial–Mesenchymal Interactions in Lung Injury

Mesenchymal–epithelial interactions are recognized as an essential part of normal lung development. Several groups have suggested that epithelial cell-derived factors may play a critical role in the fibroblast hyperplasia of lung injury (215,251,252). As will be described in the following, several recent studies have confirmed lung epithelium as a source of growth factors that can stimulate fibroblast growth. Alveolar macrophages are also a rich source of growth factors in injured lung (253). Both cell types are susceptible to pharmacological manipulation of the airway, which is why the discussion in the next section focuses heavily on the cellular origins and destinations of individual growth factors. Lung injury studies have demonstrated that fibroblast growth is promoted in the absence of epithelium (252,254,255). Restoration of the epithelium suppresses this enhanced fibroblast proliferation. Studies with cultured fetal lung cells (25,256) demonstrated that epithelial cells release a potent inhibitor of fetal lung fibroblast proliferation.

VII. Specific Growth Factors in Lung Injury

A. IGFs

Insulin-like growth factors have been implicated in compensatory growth of liver (257), kidney (258), and lung (83). IGF-I has also been implicated in experimental pulmonary hypertension induced by continuous air embolization (259). This observation is consistent with our own observations that IGF-I and type I IGF receptor mRNAs and proteins are increased in the lung parenchyma of adult rats exposed to 85% O_2, and that the increase in the IGF receptor was localized to perivascular and peribronchial smooth muscle and endothelial cells (260). We have also used a neonatal rat model, in which a 2-week exposure to 60% O_2 results in patchy areas of tissue thickening and active cell growth interspersed with emphysematous areas of arrested cell growth (261). Areas of absent cell growth had a reduction in immunoreactive IGF-I and type I IGF receptor, compared with air-exposed lungs, whereas thickened areas of active DNA synthesis had an increase in immunoreactive IGF-I and its receptor (261). Exposure of newborn rats to 80–90% O_2 for 4–6 weeks results in a markedly increased expression of both IGF-I and IGF-II (262). Given that both surface forces and oxygen regulate IGF gene expression in experimental models, it is very likely that IGFs will be found to play a role in BPD.

B. EGF and TGF-α

Studies with transgenic mice, in which respiratory epithelial cells overexpressed TGF-α, support a paracrine pathway for epithelial cell-derived TGF-α leading to pulmonary fibroblast hyperplasia (263). Type II pneumonocytes from O_2-exposed rabbits produce increased amounts of TGF-α (264), but following oxidant injury, hamster lung fibroblasts also synthesize TGF-α (265), suggesting that cell interactions in the injured lung may differ from those in normal lung. The two studies of which we are aware that looked at tissue from infants with BPD had conflicting results. Stahlman et al. (266) described the presence of bronchiolar EGF in infants with BPD, which was not seen in unaffected infants. Strandjord et al. (267) detected EGF and its receptor in all lung epithelium and TGF-α in airway epithelium of normal children, whereas children with BPD had increased EGF, EGF receptor, and TGF-α in alveolar macrophages.

C. PDGF

Human patients with idiopathic pulmonary fibrosis have mRNA for PDGF-B in both alveolar macrophages (AMs) and alveolar epithelial cells (268–270), with similar findings observed in experimental asbestosis (271). Under these conditions, it seems that the major source of the peptide is the AM, to which PDGF-BB can be localized by immunohistochemistry. PDGF-B mRNA and PDGF-BB peptide, as well as the PDGF-β-receptor mRNA and protein, have also been found by several groups (42,272,273) to be increased in adult rats subjected to hyperoxia. Under these conditions, Western blot analysis suggested that the PDGF-BB extracted from O_2-exposed lungs was not primarily of AM origin (42). This is supported by immunohistochemistry, in which some PDGF-BB can be localized to AMs, but a great excess of cells immunoreactive for PDGF-BB were not AMs. These findings are consistent with the observed increase in PDGF production by type II pneumonocytes isolated from adult rats subjected to hyperoxia (264), and the in vitro upregulation of PDGF genes in premature rat lung cells by increased O_2 (274), suggesting an O_2-mediated paracrine mode of transmission that results in perisaccular fibroblast hyperplasia. PDGF has been implicated in the obliterative bronchiolitis, sometimes seen after lung transplantation (275), and has been localized to the airways of adult rats exposed to 85% O_2. In the 60% O_2 neonatal rat model used for the study of IGFs, we have also seen a marked upregulation of the PDGF-β-receptor following O_2 exposure (unpublished observations). In combination, these data make it likely that PDGF isoforms will be found to play some role in the cellular changes seen in BPD, but immunohistochemical and in situ hybridization analyses of human tissue are awaited.

D. FGFs

The FGFs are a superfamily of growth factors, of which several may play a role in normal and abnormal lung growth. Exposure to 85% O_2 for 6 days results in increased bFGF mRNA and protein, along with a change in bFGF distribution from the matrix to alveolar epithelial cells in the adult rat (43). In common with various other growth factors, bFGF can apparently be stored in matrix, from which it can be released to exert a mitogenic effect (276). In adult rats exposed to 85% O_2, there is also a transient appearance of bFGF receptor at a time of active pneumonocyte proliferation (43), although bFGF uptake by cells may be by receptor-mediated or receptor-independent pathways (277), and the lack of detectible receptor does not exclude bFGF from exerting a mitogenic effect. In human patients dying 10–28 days after an acute lung injury, much of the observed intra-alveolar bFGF appears to be contributed by macrophages (278). Both aFGF and bFGF are mitogenic for type II pneumonocytes (279). This property is shared by members of the FGF family, keratinocyte growth factor (KGF), and hepatocyte growth factor (HGF), which has considerable homology with KGF (97,280). KGF and KGF receptor mRNAs are constitutively expressed in lung tissue (97). Type II pneumonocytes have the HGF receptor (280) but HGF mRNA in normal lung is localized to macrophages (281). An intriguing observation has been that lung endothelial cell-derived HGF may serve an endocrine function following unilateral nephrectomy or partial hepatectomy (281).

E. TGF-βs

The TGF-βs are a superfamily of multifunctional peptide growth factors of which one or other isoform is expressed in virtually all cells, although most cells will possess functional membrane-bound receptors for members of this family (282). Increased expression of TGF-β_1 has been reported in the lungs of animals subjected to experimental silicosis (283), bleomycin-induced pulmonary fibrosis (284), asbestosis (285), hypersensitivity pneumonitis (286), and pulmonary oxygen toxicity (287). The intracellular form has been localized to airway epithelium and to alveolar macrophages and epithelium, whereas the extracellular form has been localized to matrix in human idiopathic pulmonary fibrosis (288). The origin of TGF-βs in the injured lung may be from a variety of cell types at differing time points following the onset of the injury process. In bleomycin-mediated injury, for example, the initial source is epithelium, followed by macrophages and then interstitial cells (289). Intervention studies, using antibodies to three TGF-β isoforms, have limited collagen deposition in experimental bleomycin-induced pulmonary fibrosis (44). Such an intervention might also be expected to limit changes in the synthesis of other collagens (290), elastin (291), and proteoglycans (292). Although the role of TGF-βs in the matrix deposition of lung injury has been confirmed by intervention studies, they may also be influencing cell proliferation. There is a temporal relation between TGF-β expression and cell proliferation in bleomycin-induced pulmonary fibrosis (293). Proliferation of fibroblasts in response to TGF-β may be mediated through an autocrine release of PDGF (294), or restoration of PDGF receptors (295). Inhibition of airway epithelial cell proliferation may be by an effect on EGF receptor phosphorylation (296). Although TGF-β may play a role in matrix remodeling in neonatal lung injury, we have been unable to show a significant effect of TGF-β_1 on immature lung fibroblast DNA synthesis (58), even though, very low concentrations do stimulate DNA synthesis by immature pneumonocytes (25). One other effect of TGF-β that may be of relevance in BPD is a capacity, shared with FGFs, to regulate nitric oxide synthase activity (297,298).

F. Other Growth Factors

Exposure to 100% oxygen impairs the synthesis of VEGF by epithelial cells, which may contribute to impaired postnatal microvascular development (299). This chapter has focused on the classic group of polypeptide growth factors. Other cytokines may also serve a direct or indirect role as growth factors. Interleukin-6 has been reported to be an autocrine mitogen for murine lung fibroblast subsets (300), but it is unclear whether this is a direct effect or is an example of cytokine induction of a polypeptide growth factor (301). Neuroendocrine cells containing gastrin-releasing peptide increase in the airways of infants with BPD, and there is good evidence that gastrin-releasing peptide is a growth factor for airway epithelium (302). A role for 5-hydroxytryptamine as a fibroblast mitogen is suggested by studies of experimental radiation-induced pulmonary fibrosis (303). Adult cryptogenic fibrosing alveolitis is associated with an increased expression of endothelin-1 in airway and alveolar epithelial cells, particularly at sites adjacent to granulation tissue, as well as in endothelial cells (304). Endothelin-1 is a known mitogen for vascular smooth-muscle cells (305) and may play a role in the pulmonary hypertension seen in BPD. Thrombin, which has also been reported to be mitogenic for smooth muscle, appears to exert this effect through bFGF (306).

VIII. Problems of Interpretation

As growth factor expression in lung injury becomes better characterized, especially in BPD, it is likely that a very complex picture of interactions will appear. These include potential interactions between O_2, mechanical forces, and gestational age (Table 1), as well as interactions between individual growth factors. TGF-β_1, for example, has been reported to enhance the TGF-α- or EGF-mediated upregulation of the EGF-R (130,307). PDGF and TGF-β have each been reported to downregulate the other's receptor (308). IGF-II expression and IGF-I receptor abundance may be affected by exposure to bFGF (309). PDGF and EGF can increase IGF-I receptor (310), whereas EGF can increase IGF-I synthesis (311).

Table 1 Exposure to Elevated O_2 Concentrations, to High Surface Pressures Through Mechanical Ventilation and of Delivery Are All believed to Contribute to the Development of BPD[a]

Growth factor	Induced by oxygen	Induced by mechanical forces	Gest
aFGF	?	?	
bFGF	+	?	
EGF	?	?	
IGF-I	+	+	
IGF-II	?	?	
PDGF-AA	+/−	+	
PDGF-BB	+	+	
TGF-α	+	?	
TGF-β	+	+	

[a]Individually, each of these putative contributors has been shown to modify the expression of several growth factors in the lung.
+, increased expression; +/−, variably reported to increase expression or have no effect; ?, effect unknown.

HGF may be induced by PDGF, EGF, or bFGF in some cells (312). An understanding of such interactions in lung injury will be critical for interpretation of intervention studies. Superimposed on these difficulties is the problem of different subpopulations of fibroblasts being nonhomogeneous in their response to, or secretion of, growth factors (300,313). Alveolar macrophages may change from synthesis of stimulatory growth factors to synthesis of growth inhibitors, or vice versa, over the course of an injury process (314,315).

Growth factors may serve numerous functions other than inducing cell division. Of particular relevance to BPD is the induction or derepression of genes that regulate synthesis of matrix components, such as type I collagen (316) and elastin (317), whereas other growth factors may repress the expression of the same genes (318,319). It is probable that most, if not all, of the polypeptide growth factors will serve duel functions, either simultaneously or sequentially.

A potential confounding variable for the study of tissue from infants with BPD is the widespread use of steroid therapy to reduce O_2 and ventilator requirements. Glucocorticoids inhibit the expression of many growth factor genes (320,321), and their repeated or sustained use could, theoretically, compound the inhibition of lung growth that is the consequence of severe BPD. Paradoxically, dexamethasone has been reported to increase alveolar macrophage PDGF mRNA (322).

IX. Foci for Future Research

As is obvious from the foregoing discussion, there are many outstanding questions, and few answers, for the role of growth factors in BPD. Listed in the following are four areas that we believe deserve special attention in future studies.

1. The growth factors that mediate the relatively slow changes of evolving BPD, and the timing of their expression, cannot be accurately predicted from brief studies of lung injury in adult animals. Of the currently available animal models, the immature baboon is the most likely to follow a pattern of disease progression comparable with premature human infants. We believe a high priority should be placed on investigating growth factor expression in this model. Data would need to be compared with results from a bank of human tissue, fixed appropriately for in situ hybridization and immunohistochemistry, for confirmation.

2. A thorough understanding of the signal transduction pathways for O_2- and pressure-mediated gene regulation, and their ontogeny of response, will allow the relative contributions of the different putative etiologic agents to be defined through highly specific interventions. It seems probable that specific pathways will be shared by contributing factors, which may then become appropriate targets for therapeutic intervention.

3. In situ hybridization and immunohistochemistry for growth factors and growth factor receptors will allow testable hypotheses to be developed for the sources and targets of individual growth factors. In some instances, this may be facilitated by Western blot analyses of tissue samples, to allow quantitation of growth factors—derived from specific cell types—which may differ in molecular weight. The role of the epithelium and of alveolar macrophages, as sources of factors mitogenic for fibroblasts and smooth-muscle cells, needs to be clearly defined, for both are easily accessible for therapeutic intervention from the airway.

4. Development of pharmacological approaches consistent with interventions that may need to be effective over several weeks. Antibodies against specific growth factors or growth factor receptors, or antisense oligodeoxynucleotides against their mRNAs, have been used successfully in the laboratory, but are likely to have significant limitations in clinical practice. Gene therapy, using transient expression systems, offers a tantalizing promise for the future.

References

1. Northway WH, Rosan RC, Porter DY. Pulmonary disease following respirator therapy of hyaline membrane disease: bronchopulmonary dysplasia. N Engl J Med 1967; 276:357–368.
2. Bonikos DS, Bensch KG, Northway WH, Edwards DK. Bronchopulmonary dysplasia: the pulmonary pathological sequel of necrotizing bronchiolitis and pulmonary fibrosis. Hum Pathol 1976; 7:643–666.
3. Chambers HM, van Velzen D. Ventilator-related pathology in the extremely immature lung. Pathology 1989; 21:79–83.
4. Van Lierde S, Cornelis A, Devlieger H, Moerman P, Lauweryns J, Eggermont E. Different patterns of pulmonary sequelae after hyaline membrane disease: heterogeneity of bronchopulmonary dysplasia? Biol Neonate 1991; 60:152–163.
5. Margraf LR, Tomashefski JF, Bruce MC, Dahms BB. Morphometric analysis of the lung in bronchopulmonary dysplasia. Am Rev Respir Dis 1991; 143:391–400.
6. Smith JC, Stiles CD. Cytoplasmic transfer of the mitogenic response to platelet-derived growth factor. Proc Natl Acad Sci USA 1981; 78:4363–4367.
7. Stiles AD, Smith BT, Post M. Reciprocal autocrine and paracrine regulation of growth of mesenchymal and alveolar epithelial cells. Exp Lung Res 1986; 11:165–177.
8. Tanswell AK. Cellular interactions in pulmonary oxygen toxicity in vitro: I. Hyperoxic induction of fibroblast factors which alter growth and lipid metabolism of pulmonary epithelial cells. Exp Lung Res 1983; 5:23–36.
9. Tzaki MG, Byrne PJ, Tanswell AK. Cellular interactions in pulmonary oxygen toxicity in vitro. II. Hyperoxia causes adult rat lung fibroblast cultures to produce apparently autocrine growth factors. Exp Lung Res 1988; 14:403–419.

10. Sara VR, Hall K. Insulin-like growth factors and their binding proteins. Physiol Rev 1990; 70:591–614.
11. Loewenstein WR. Cell-to-cell communication and the control of growth. Am Rev Respir Dis 1990; 142 (suppl):48–53.
12. Munari-Silem Y, Audebet C, Rousset B. Hormonal control of cell to cell communication: regulation by thyrotropin of the gap-junction mediated dye transfer between thyroid cells. Endocrinology 1991; 128:3299–3309.
13. Massagué J. Transforming growth factor-α. A model for membrane-anchored growth factors. J Biol Chem 1990; 265:21393–21396.
14. Farago A, Nishizuka Y. Protein kinase C in transmembrane signalling. FEBS Lett 1990; 268:350–354.
15. Yarden Y, Ullrich A. Growth factor receptor protein kinases. Annu Rev Biochem 1988; 57:443–478.
16. Dumont JE, Jauniaux JC, Roger PP. The cyclic AMP-mediated stimulation of cell proliferation. Trends Biochem Sci 1989; 14:67–71.
17. Ihle JN, Wirtthuhn BA, Quelle FW, Yamamoto K, Thierfelder WE, Kreider B, Silvennoinen O. Signalling by the cytokine receptor superfamily: JAKs and STATs. Trends Biochem Sci 1994; 19:222–227.
18. Pines J. Cyclins and cyclin-dependent kinases: take your partners. Trends Biochem Sci 1993; 18:95–99.
19. Hackney JD, Evans MJ, Spier CE, Anzar UT, Clark KW. Effect of high concentrations of oxygen on reparative regeneration of damaged alveolar epithelium in mice. Exp Mol Pathol 1981; 34:338–344.
20. Weiss P, Kavanau JL. A model of growth and growth control in mathematical terms. J Gen Physiol 1957; 41:1–47.
21. Simnett J, Fisher JM, Heppelston AG. Tissue-specific inhibition of lung alveolar cell mitosis in organ culture. Nature 1969; 223:944–946.
22. Tanswell AK, Fraher LJ, Grose EC. Circulating factors that modify lung cell DNA synthesis following exposure to inhaled oxidants. I. Effect of serum and lavage on lung fibroblasts following exposure of adult rats to 1 ppm ozone. J Toxicol Environ Health 1989; 27:239–254.
23. Tanswell AK, Fraher LJ, Grose EC. Circulating factors that modify lung cell DNA synthesis following exposure to inhaled oxidants. II. Effect of serum and lavage on lung pneumocytes following exposure of adult rats to 1 ppm ozone. J Toxicol Environ Health 1990; 29:131–144.
24. Miyazaki K, Horio T. Growth inhibitors: molecular diversity and roles in cell proliferation. In Vitro Cell Dev Biol 1989; 25:866–872.
25. Caniggia I, Tseu I, Rolland G, Edelson J, Tanswell AK, Post M. Inhibition of fibroblast growth by epithelial cells in fetal rat lung. Am J Respir Mol Cell Biol 1995; 13:91–98.
26. Ueda N, Shah SV. Apoptosis. J Lab Clin Med 1994; 124:169–177.
27. Harrington EA, Bennett MR, Fanidi A, Evan GI. c-*myc*-induced apoptosis in fibroblasts is inhibited by specific cytokines. EMBO J 1994; 13:3286–3296.
28. Raghu G, Striker LJ, Hudson LD, Striker GE. Extracellular matrix in normal and fibrotic human lungs. Am Rev Respir Dis 1985; 131:281–289.
29. Dunnill MS. Pulmonary fibrosis. Histopathology 1990; 16:321–329.

30. Crouch E. Pathobiology of pulmonary fibrosis. Am J Physiol 1990; 259:L159–L184.
31. McGowan SE. Extracellular matrix and the regulation of lung development and repair. FASEB J 1992; 6:2895–2904.
32. Jassal D, Han RNN, Caniggia I, Post M, Tanswell AK. Growth of distal fetal rat lung epithelial cells in a defined serum-free medium. In Vitro Cell Dev Biol 1991; 27:625–632.
33. Tanswell K, Rolland G, Jassal D, Buch S, Post M. The fibroblast hyperplasia observed in pulmonary O_2 toxicity may depend on both a local increase in growth factors and a change in subcellular matrix composition [abstr]. Am Rev Respir Dis 1992; 145:828.
34. Tanswell AK, Han RNN, Jassal D, Fraher LJ, Post M. The response of small vessel endothelial cells from fetal rat lung to growth factors. J Dev Physiol 1991; 15:199–209.
35. Engel J. EGF-like domains in extracellular matrix proteins: localized signals for growth and differentiation? FEBS Lett 1989; 251:1–7.
36. Ingber D. Extracellular matrix and cell shape: potential control points for inhibition of angiogenesis. J Cell Biochem 1991; 47:236–241.
37. Vlodavsky I, Fuks Z, Ishai-Michaeli R, Bashkin P, Levi E, Korner G, Bar-Shavit R, Klagsbrun M. Extracellular matrix-resident basic fibroblast growth factor: implications for the control of angiogenesis. J Cell Biochem 1991; 45:167–176.
38. Murphy-Ullrich JE, Schultz-Cherry S, Höök M. Transforming growth factor-β complexes with thrombospondin. Mol Biol Cell 1992; 3:181–188.
39. Raines EW, Lane TF, Iruela-Arispe ML, Ross R, Sage EH. The extracellular glycoprotein SPARC interacts with platelet-derived growth factor (PDGF)-AB and -BB and inhibits the binding of PDGF to its receptors. Proc Natl Acad Sci USA 1992; 89:1281–1285.
40. Gitay-Goren H, Soker S, Vlodavsky I, Neufeld G. The binding of vascular endothelial growth factor to its receptors is dependent on cell surface-associated heparin-like molecules. J Biol Chem 1992; 267:6093–6098.
41. Roghani M, Moscatelli D. Basic fibroblast growth factor is internalized through both receptor-mediated and heparan sulfate-mediated mechanisms. J Biol Chem 1992; 267:22156–22162.
42. Han RNN, Buch S, Freeman BA, Post M, Tanswell AK. Platelet-derived growth factor and growth-related genes in rat lung II. Effect of exposure to 85% O_2. Am J Physiol 1992; 262:L140–L146.
43. Buch S, Han RNN, Liu J, Moore A, Edelson JD, Freeman BA, Post M, Tanswell AK. Basic fibroblast growth factor and growth factor receptor gene expression in 85% O_2-exposed rat lung. Am J Physiol 1995; 268:L455–L464.
44. Giri SN, Hyde DM, Hollinger MA. Effect of antibody to transforming growth factor β on bleomycin induced accumulation of lung collagen in mice. Thorax 1993; 48: 959–966.
45. Kauffmann SL. Cell proliferation in the mammalian lung. Int Rev Exp Pathol 1980; 22:131–191.
46. Adamson IYR, Bowden DH. Derivation of type 1 epithelium from type 2 cells in the developing rat lung. Lab Invest 1975; 32:736–745.

47. Adamson IYR, King, GM. Sex differences in development of fetal rat lung. I. Autoradiographic and biochemical studies. Lab Invest 1984; 50:456–460.
48. O'Hare KH, Townes PL. Morphogenesis of albino rat lung: an autoradiographic analysis of the embryological origin of the type I and II pulmonary epithelial cells. J Morphol 1970; 132:69–82.
49. Buch S, Jassal D, Han R, Liu J, Caniggia I, Edelson J, Tanswell K, Post M. Ontogeny and regulation of platelet-derived growth factor gene expression in distal fetal rat lung epithelial cells. Am J Respir Cell Mol Biol 1994; 11:251–261.
50. Post M, Smith BT. Hormonal control of surfactant metabolism. In: Robertson B, Van Golde LMG, Batenburg JJ, eds. Pulmonary Surfactant: From Molecular Biology to Clinical Practice. New York: Elsevier, 1992:379–424.
51. Post M. Tissue interactions. In: Crystal RG, West J, eds. The Lung: Scientific Foundations. New York: Raven Press, 1997:1003–1011.
52. Alescio T, Colombo Piperno E. A quantitative assessment of mesenchymal contribution to epithelial growth rate in mouse embryonic lung developing in vitro. J Embryol Exp Morphol 1967; 17:213–227.
53. Alescio T, DiMichelle M. Relationship of epithelial growth to mitotic rate in mouse embryonic lung developing in vitro. J Embryol Exp Morphol 1968; 19:227–237.
54. Alescio T, Cassini A. Induction in vitro of tracheal buds by pulmonary mesenchyme grafted on tracheal epithelium. J Exp Zool 1962; 150:83–94.
55. Goldin GV, Wessels NK. Mammalian lung development: the possible role of cell proliferation in the formation of supernumerary tracheal buds and in branching morphogenesis. J Exp Zool 1979; 208:337–346.
56. Shannon JM. Induction of alveolar type II cell differentiation in fetal tracheal epithelium by grafted distal lung mesenchyme. Dev Biol 1994; 166:600–614.
57. Lawson KA. Stage specificity in the mesenchyme requirement of rodent lung epithelium in vitro: a matter of growth control? J Embryol Exp Morphol 1983; 74: 183–206.
58. Caniggia I, Tseu I, Han RNN, Smith BT, Tanswell K, Post M. Spatial and temporal differences in fibroblast behaviour in fetal rat lung. Am J Physiol 1991; 261:L424–L433.
59. Lawson KA. The role of mesenchyme in the morphogenesis and functional differentiation of rat salivary epithelium. J Embryol Exp Morphol 1972; 27:497–513.
60. Kratochwil K. Organ specificity in mesenchymal induction demonstrated in the embryonic development of the mammary gland of the mouse. Dev Biol 1969; 20: 46–71.
61. Sakakura T, Sakagami S, Niskizyka Y. Persistence of responsiveness of adult mouse mammary gland to induction by embryonic mesenchyme. Dev Biol 1979; 72:201–210.
62. Snead ML, Luo W, Olizer P, Don-Wheeler G, Bessem C, Bell GI, Rall LB, Slavkin HC. Localization of epidermal growth factor precursors in tooth and lung during embryonic mouse development. Dev Biol 1989; 134:420–429.
63. Partanen A-M. Epidermal growth factor and transforming growth factor-α in the development of epithelium–mesenchymal organs of the mouse. Curr Top Dev Biol 1990; 24:31–55.
64. Ebner R, Derynck R. Epidermal growth factor and transforming growth factor-α:

differential routing and processing of ligand-receptor complexes. Cell Regul 1991; 2:599–612.
65. Freemark M, Comer M. Epidermal growth factor (EGF)-like transforming growth factor (TGF) activity and EGF receptors in ovine fetal tissues: possible role for TGF in ovine fetal development. Pediatr Res 1987; 22:609–615.
66. Standjord TP, Clark JG, Madtes DK. Expression of TGF-α, EGF, and EGF receptor in fetal rat lung. Am J Physiol 1994; 267:L384–L389.
67. Snead ML, Luo W, Olizer P, Don-Wheeler G, Bessem C, Bell GI, Rall LB, Slavkin HC. Localization of epidermal growth factor precursors in tooth and lung during embryonic mouse development. Dev Biol 1989; 134:420–429.
68. Warburton D, Seth R, Shum L, Horcher PG, Hall FL, Werb Z, Slavkin HC. Epigenetic role of epidermal growth factor expression and signalling in embryonic mouse lung morphogenesis. Dev Biol 1992; 149:123–133.
69. Raaberg L, Nexø E, Buckley S, Luo W, Snead ML, Warburton D. Epidermal growth factor transcription, translation and signal transduction by rat type II pneumocytes in culture. Am J Respir Cell Mol Biol 1992; 6:44–49.
70. Johnson MD, Gray ME, Carpenter G, Pepinsky RB, Sundell H, Stahlman MT. Ontogeny of epidermal growth factor receptor/kinase and of lipocortin-1 in the ovine lung. Pediatr Res 1989; 25:535–541.
71. Johnson MD, Gray ME, Carpenter G, Pepinsky RB, Stahlman MT. Ontogeny of epidermal growth factor receptor and lipocortin-1 in fetal and neonatal human lungs. Hum Pathol 1990; 21:182–191.
72. Ruocco S, Lallemand A, Tournier JM, Gaillard D. Expression and localization of epidermal growth factor-α, and localization of their common receptor in fetal human lung development. Pediatr Res 1996; 39:448–455.
73. Aida S, Tamai S, Sekiguchi S, Shimizu N. Distribution of epidermal growth factor and epidermal growth factor receptor in human lung: immunohistochemical and immunoelectron-microscopic studies. Respiration 1994; 61:161–166.
74. Ganser GL, Stricklin GP, Matrisian LM. EGF and TGFα influence in vitro lung development by the induction of matrix-degrading metalloproteinases. Int J Dev Biol 1991; 35:453–461.
75. Threadgill DW, Dlugosz AA, Hansen LA, Tennenbaum T, Lichti U, Yee D, LaMantia C, Mourton T, Herrup K, Harris RC, Barnard JA, Yuspa SH, Coffey RJ, Mjagnuson T. Targeted disruption of mouse EGF receptor: effect of genetic background on mutant phenotype. Science 1995; 269:230–234.
76. Hardie WD, Kerlakian CB, Bruno MD, Huelsman KM, Wert SE, Glasser SW, Whitsett JA, Korfhagen TR. Reversal of lung lesions in transgenic transforming growth factor α mice by expression of mutant epidermal growth factor receptor. Am J Respir Cell Mol Biol 1996; 15:499–508.
77. Miettinen PJ, Berger JE, Meneses J, Phung Y, Pederson RA, Werb Z, Derynck R. Epithelial immaturity and multiorgan failure in mice lacking epidermal growth factor receptor. Nature 1995; 376:337–341.
78. Catteron WZ, Escobedo MB, Sexson, WR, Gray E, Sundell HW, Stahlman MT. Effects of epidermal growth factor on lung maturation in fetal lambs. Pediatr Res 1979; 13:104–108.
79. Sundell HW, Gray ME, Serenius FS, Escobedo MB, Stahlman MT. Effects of epi-

dermal growth factor on lung maturation in fetal lambs. Am J Pathol 1980; 100: 707–726.

80. Plopper CG, St George JA, Read LC, Nishio SJ. Weir AJ, Edwards L, Tarabtal AF, Pinkerton KE, Merritt TA, Whitsett JA. Acceleration of alveolar type II cell differentiation in fetal rhesus monkey lung by administration of EGF. Am J Physiol 1992; 262:L313–L321.
81. Sen N, Cake MH. Enhancement of desaturated phosphatidylcholine synthesis by epidermal growth factor in cultured fetal lung cells involves a fibroblast–epithelial cell interaction. Am J Respir Cell Mol Biol 1991; 5:337–343.
82. Nielsen HC. Epidermal growth factor influences the developmental clock regulating maturation of the fetal lung fibroblasts. Biochim Biophys Acta 1989; 1012:201–206.
83. Stiles AD, D'Ercole AJ. The insulin-like growth factors and the lung. Am J Respir Cell Mol Biol 1990; 3:93–100.
84. Han VKM, Hill DJ, Strain A, Towle AC, Lauder JM, Underwood LE, D'Ercole AJ. Identification of somatomedin/insulin-like growth factor immunoreactive cells in the human fetus. Pediatr Res 1987; 22:245–249.
85. Klempt M, Hutchins A-M, Gluckman PD, Skinner SJM. IGF binding protein-2 gene expression and location of IGF-I and IGF-II in fetal rat lung. Development 1992; 115:765–772.
86. Retsch-Bogart GZ, Moats-Staats BM, Howard K, D'Ercole AJ, Stiles AD. Cellular localization of messenger RNAs for insulin-like growth factors (IGFs), their receptors and binding proteins during fetal rat lung development. Am J Respir Cell Mol Biol 1996; 14:61–69.
87. Wallen LD, Han VKM. Spatial and temporal distribution of insulin-like growth factors I and II during development of rat lung. Am J Physiol 1994; 267:L531–L542.
88. Liu JP, Baker J, Perkins AS, Robertson EJ, Efstratiadis A. Mice carrying null mutations of the genes encoding insulin-like growth factor I (IGF-1) and type 1 IGF receptor (IGFlr). Cell 1993; 75:59–72.
89. DeChiara TM, Efstratiadas A, Robertson EJ. A growth-deficiency phenotype in heterozygous mice carrying an insulin-growth factor II gene disrupted by targeting. Nature 1990; 345:78–80.
90. Han RNN, Liu J, Tanswell AK, Post M. Expression of basic fibroblast growth factor and receptor. Immunolocalization studies in developing rat fetal lung. Pediatr Res 1992; 31:435–440.
91. Fu Y, Spirito P, Yu Z-X, Biro S, Sasse J, Lei J, Ferrans VJ, Epstein SE, Casscells W. Acidic fibroblast growth factor in the developing rat embryo. J Cell Biol 1991; 114:1261–1273.
92. Sannes PL, Burch KK, Khosla J. Immunohistochemical localization of epidermal growth factor and acidic and basic fibroblast growth factors in postnatal developing and adult rat lungs. Am J Respir Cell Mol Biol 1992; 7:230–237, 1992.
93. Orr-Utreger A, Givol D, Yayon A, Yarden Y, Lonai P. Developmental expression of two murine fibroblast growth factor receptors, flg and bek. Development 1991; 113:1419–1434.
94. Mason JJ, Fuller-Pace F, Smith R, Dickson C. FGF-7 (keratinocyte growth factor)

expression during mouse development suggests roles in myogenesis, forebrain regionalisation and epithelial–mesenchymal interactions. Mech Dev 1994; 45:15–30.
95. Panos RJ, Rubin JS, Csaky KG, Aaronson SA, Mason RJ. Keratinocyte growth factor and hepatocyte growth factor/scatter factor are heparin-binding growth factors for alveolar type II cells in fibroblast-conditioned medium. J Clin Invest 1993; 92:969–977.
96. Peters K, Werner S, Liao X, Wert S, Whitsett JA, Williams LT. Targeted expression of a dominant negative FGF receptor blocks branching morphogenesis and epithelial differentiation of the mouse lung. EMBO J 1994; 13:3296–3301.
97. Post M, Souza P, Liu J, Tseu I, Wang J, Kuliszewski M, Tanswell AK. Keratinocyte growth factor and its receptor are involved in regulating early lung branching. Development 1996; 122:3107–3115.
98. Heine UI, Munoz EF, Flanders KC, Roberts AB, Sporn MB. Colocalization of TGF-beta 1 and collagen I and III, fibronectin and glycosaminoglycans during lung branching morphogenesis. Development 1990; 109:29–36.
99. Sera R, Pelton RW, Moses HL. TGFβ_1 inhibits branching morphogenesis and *N-myc* expression in lung bud organ cultures. Development 1994; 120:2153–2161.
100. Kulkarni AB, Huh C-G, Becker D, Geiser A, Light M, Flanders KC, Roberts AB, Sporn MB, Ward JM, Karlsson S. Transforming growth factor-β_1 null mutation in mice causes excessive inflammatory response and early death. Proc Natl Acad Sci USA 1993; 90:770–774.
101. Sanford LP, Ormsby I, Gittenberg-de Groot AC, Sariola H, Friedman R, Biovin GP, Cardell EL, Doetschman T. TGFβ_2 knockout mice have multiple developmental defects that are nonoverlapping with other TGFβ knockout phenotypes. Development 1997; 124:2659–2670.
102. Kaartinen V, Voncken JW, Shuler C, Warburton D, Bui D, Heisterkamp N, Groffen J. Abnormal lung development and cleft palate in mice lacking TGF-β_3 indicates defects of epithelial-mesenchymal interaction. Nature Genet 1995; 11:415–421.
103. Whitsett JA, Weaver TE, Lieberman MA, Clark JC, Daugerty C. Differential effects of epidermal growth factor and transforming growth factor-β on synthesis of *M*R = 35,000 surfactant-associated protein in fetal lung. J Biol Chem 1987; 262: 7908–7913.
104. Torday JS, Kourembanas S. Fetal rat lung fibroblasts produce a TGFβ homolog that blocks alveolar type II cell maturation. Dev Biol 1990; 139:35–41.
105. Catlin EA, Manganaro TF, Donahoe PK. Müllerian inhibiting substance depresses accumulation in vitro of disaturated phosphatidylcholine in fetal rat lung. Am J Obstet Gynecol 1988; 159:1299–1303.
106. Catlin EA, Powell SM, Manganaro TF, Hudson PL, Ragin C, Epstein J, Donahoe PK. Sex-specific fetal lung development and müllerian inhibiting substance. Am Rev Respir Dis 1990; 141:466–470.
107. Han RNN, Mawdsley C, Souza P, Tanswell AK, Post M. Platelet-derived growth factors and growth-related genes in rat lung III. Immunolocalization during fetal development. Pediatr Res 1992; 31:323–329.
108. Han RNN, Liu J, Tanswell AK, Post M. Ontogeny of platelet-derived growth factor receptor (PDGFR) in fetal rat lung. Microsc Res Tech 1993; 26:381–388.

109. Souza P, Sedlackova L, Kuliszewski M, Wang J, Liu J, Tseu I, Tanswell K, Post M. Antisense oligonucleotides targeting PDGF-B mRNA inhibit cell proliferation during embryonic rat lung development. Development 1994; 120:2163–2173.
110. Levéen P, Pekny M, Gebre-Medhin S, Swolin B, Larsson E, Betsholtz C. Mice deficient for PDGFB show renal, cardiovascular, and hematological abnormalities. Genes Dev 1994; 8:1875–1887.
111. Soriano P. Abnormal kidney development and hematological disorders in PDGF β-receptor mutant mice. Genes Dev 1994; 8:1888–1896.
112. Souza P, Kuliszewski M, Wang J, Tseu I, Tanswell AK, Post M. PDGF-AA and its receptor influence early lung branching morphogenesis via an epithelial–mesenchymal interaction. Development 1995; 121:2559–2567.
113. Orr-Utreger A, Lonai P. Platelet-derived growth factor-A and its receptor are expressed in separate, but adjacent cell layers of the mouse embryo. Development 1992; 115:1045–1058.
114. Souza P, Tanswell AK, Post M. Different roles for PDGF-α and -β receptors in embryonic lung development. Am J Respir Cell Mol Biol 1996; 15:551–562.
115. Boström H, Willetts K, Pekny M, Leveen P, Lindahl P, Hedstrand H, Pekna M, Hellstrom M, Gebre-Medhin S, Schalling M, Nilsson M, Kurland S, Törnell J, Heath JK, Betsholtz C. PDGF-A signaling is a critical event in lung alveolar myofibroblast development and alveogenesis. Cell 1996; 85:863–873.
116. Soriano P. The PDGFα receptor is required for neural crest cell development and for normal patterning of the somites. Development 1997; 124:2691–2700.
117. Buch S, Jones C, Sweezey N, Tanswell AK, Post M. Platelet-derived growth factor and growth related genes in rat fetal lung: I. Developmental expression. Am J Respir Cell Mol Biol 1991; 5:371–376.
118. Carson SH, Taeusch HW, Avery ME. Inhibition of lung cell division after hydrocortisone injection in fetal rabbits. J Appl Physiol 1973; 34:660–664.
119. Kotas RV, Avery ME. Accelerated appearance of pulmonary surfactant in the fetal lung. J Appl Physiol 1971; 30:358–361.
120. Kotas RV, Mims L, Hart L. Reversible inhibition of lung cell numbers after glucocorticoid injection. Pediatrics 1974; 53:358–361.
121. Kikkawa Y, Kaibaira M, Motoyama EK, Orzalesi MM, Cook CD. Morphologic development of fetal rabbit lung and its acceleration with cortisol. Am J Pathol 1971; 64:423–433.
122. Motoyama E, Orzalesi M, Kikkawa Y, Kaibaira M, Wu B, Zigas C, Cook CD. Effect of cortisol on the maturation of fetal rabbit lungs. Pediatrics 1971; 48:547–555.
123. Franco G, Stiles AD, Carlson KS, Post M. Endogenous and exogenous growth potential of fetal lung cells [abstr]. Pediatr Res 1986; 20:187.
124. Price WA, Stiles AD, Moats-Staats BM, D'Ercole AJ. Gene expression of insulin-like growth factors (IGFs), the type I IGF receptor, and IGF-binding proteins in dexamethasone-induced fetal growth retardation. Endocrinology 1992; 130:1424–1432.
125. Liggins GC. Growth of fetal lung. J Dev Physiol 1984; 6:237–248.
126. Cooney TP, Thurlbeck WM. Lung growth and development in anencephaly and hydrancephaly. Am Rev Respir Dis 1985; 132:596–601.

127. Latimer AM, Hausman GJ, McCusker RH, Buonomo FC. The effects of thyroxine on serum and tissue concentrations of insulin-like growth factors (IGF-I and -II) and IGF-binding proteins in the fetal pig. Endocrinology 1993; 133:1312–1319.
128. Pfeifle B, Ditschuneit H. Regulation of receptors for insulin-like growth factors in cultured arterial smooth muscle cells by thyroid hormone. Endocrinology 1983; 98: 373–379.
129. Walker P. Thyroxine increases neonatal mouse submandibular gland mRNA-directed synthesis of epidermal growth factor. Biochem Cell Biol 1986; 64:290–296.
130. Fernandez-Pol JA, Klos DJ, Hamilton PD. Modulation of transforming growth factor alpha-dependent expression of epidermal growth factor receptor gene by transforming growth factor beta, triiodothyronine, and retinoic acid. J Cell Biochem 1989; 41:159–170.
131. Bartlett D. Postnatal growth of the mammalian lung: influence of exercise and thyroid activity. Respir Physiol 1970; 9:50–57.
132. Erenberg A, Rhodes RL, Weinstein MM, Kennedy RL. The effect of thyroidectomy on ovine fetal lung maturation. Pediatr Res 1969; 13:230–235.
133. Adamson IYR, King GM. Sex-related differences in cellular composition and surfactant synthesis of developing fetal rat lungs. Am Rev Respir Dis 1984; 129:130–134.
134. Robert MF, Neff RK, Hubell JF, Taeusch HW, Avery ME. Association between maternal diabetes and the respiratory-distress syndrome in the newborn. N Engl J Med 1976; 294:357–360.
135. Horger EO, Miller MC, Conner ED. Relation of large birthweights to maternal diabetes mellitus. Obstet Gynecol 1975; 45:150–159.
136. Gluckman PD. The role of pituitary hormones, growth factors and insulin in the regulation of fetal growth. Oxford Rev Reprod Biol 1986; 8:1–60.
137. Harding R, Hooper SB. Regulation of lung expansion and lung growth before birth. J Appl Physiol 1996; 81:209–224.
138. Kitterman JA. The effects of mechanical forces on fetal lung growth. Clin Perinatol 1996; 23:727–740.
139. Alcorn D, Adamson TM, Lambert TE, Maloney JE, Ritchie BC, Robinson PM. Morphological effects of chronic ligation and drainage in the fetal lamb lung. J Anat 1977; 130:683–695.
140. Carmal JA, Friedman F, Adamson FH. Fetal tracheal ligation and lung development. Am J Dis Child 1965; 109:450–456.
141. Griscom NT, Harris GBS, Wohl ME, Vawter GF, Eraklis AJ. Fluid filled lung during airway obstruction in the newborn. Pediatrics 1969; 48:383–390.
142. Perelman M, Levin M. Fetal pulmonary hypoplasia, anuria and oligohydramnios: clinicopathologic observations and review of the literature. Am J Obstet Gynecol 1974; 118:1119–1123.
143. Thomas IT, Smith DW. Oligohydramnios, cause of non-renal features of Potter's syndrome, including pulmonary hypoplasia. J Pediatr 1974; 84:811–814.
144. deLorimier AA, Tierney DF, Parker HR. Hypoplastic lungs in fetal lambs with surgically produced congenital diaphragmatic hernia. Surgery 1967; 62:12–17.
145. Finegold MJ, Katzew H, Genieser NB, Becker MH. Lung structure in thoracic dystrophy. Am J Dis Child 1971; 122:153–159.

146. George DK, Cooney TP, Chiu BK, Thurlbeck WM. Hypoplasia and immaturity of the terminal lung unit (acinus) in congenital diaphragmatic hernia. Am Rev Respir Dis 1987; 136:947–950.
147. Harrison MR, Bressack MA, Chung AM, deLorimier AA. Correction of congenital diaphragmatic hernia in utero. Stimulated correction permits fetal lung growth with survival at birth. Surgery 1980; 88:260–268.
148. Reale FR, Esterly JR. Pulmonary hypoplasia: a morphometric study of the lungs of infants with diaphragmatic hernia, anencephaly, and renal malformations. Pediatrics 1973; 51:91–96.
149. Liggins GC, Campos GA, Kitterman JA, Lee CH. The effect of spinal cord transection on lung development in fetal sheep. J Dev Physiol 1981; 3:267–274.
150. Moessinger AC, Marone P, James LS, Blanc WA. Fetal akinesia and lung growth [abstr]. Lab Invest 1980; 42:175.
151. Wigglesworth JS, Desai R. Effects on fetal lung growth of cervical cord section in the rabbit fetus. Early Hum Dev 1979; 3:51–65.
152. Moessinger AC, Collins MH, Blanc WA, Rey HR, James LS. Oligohydramnios-induced lung hypoplasia: the influence of timing and duration in gestation. Pediatr Res 1986; 20:951–954.
153. Nakayama DK, Glick PL, Harrison MR, Villar RL, Noall R. Experimental hypoplasia due to oligohydramnios and its reversal by relieving thoracic compression. J Pediatr Surg 1983; 18:347–353.
154. Higuchi M, Kato T, Yoshino H, Matsuda K, Gotoch K, Hirano H, Koyama K, Maki M. The influence of experimentally produced oligohydramnios on lung growth and pulmonary surfactant content in fetal rabbits. J Dev Physiol 1991; 16:223–227.
155. Wilson JM, DiFiori JW, Peters CA. Experimental fetal tracheal ligation prevents the pulmonary hypoplasia associated with fetal nephrectomy: possible application for congenital diaphragmatic hernia. J Pediatr Surg 1993; 28:1433–1439.
156. Peters CA, Reid LM, Docimo S, Lutetic T, Carr M, Retik AB, Mandell J. The role of the kidney in lung growth and maturation in the setting of obstructive uropathy and oligohydramnios. J Urol 1991; 146:597–600.
157. Hislop A, Sanderson M, Reid L. Unilateral congenital dysplasia of lung associated with vascular anomalies. Thorax 1973; 28:435–441.
158. Wallen LD, Perry SF, Alson JT, Maloney JE. Fetal lung growth; influence of pulmonary arterial flow and surgery in sheep. Am J Respir Crit Care Med 1994; 149: 1005–1011.
159. Wallen LD, Kulisz E, Maloney JE. Main pulmonary artery ligation reduces lung fluid production in fetal sheep. J Dev Physiol 1991; 16:173–179.
160. Souza P, O'Brodovich H, Post M. Lung fluid restriction affects growth but not airway branching of embryonic rat lung. Int J Dev Biol 1995; 39:629–635.
161. Neilson IR, Russo P, Laberge JM, Filiatrault D, Nguyen LT, Collin PP, Guttman FM. Congenital adenomatoid malformation of the lung: current management and prognosis. J Pediatr Surg 1991; 26:975–980.
162. DiFiori JW, Fauza DO, Slavin R, Peters CA, Fackler JC, Wilson JM. Experimental fetal tracheal ligation reverses the structural and physiological effects of pulmonary hypoplasia in congenital diaphragmatic hernia. J Pediatr Surg 1994; 29:248–256.

163. Fewell JE, Lee C, Kitterman JA. Effects of phrenic nerve section on the respiratory system of fetal lambs. J Appl Physiol 1981; 51:293–297.
164. Nagai A, Thurlbeck WM, DeBoeck C, Ioffe S, Chernick V. The effect of maternal CO_2 breathing on lung development of fetuses in the rabbit. Am Rev Respir Dis 1987; 135:130–136.
165. Liggins GC, Vilos GA, Campos GA, Kitterman JA, Lee CH. The effect of bilateral thoracoplasty on lung development in fetal sheep. J Dev Physiol 1981; 3:275–282.
166. Savich RD, Guerra FA, Lee CC, Kitterman JA. The effect of fetal breathing movements on pulmonary blood flow in fetal sheep. Pediatr Res 1994; 35:484–489.
167. Harding R, Hooper SB, Han VKM. Abolition of fetal breathing movements by spinal cord transection leads to reductions in fetal lung liquid volume, lung growth, and IGF-II gene expression. Pediatr Res 1993; 34:148–153.
168. Murai D, Lee C, Kitterman JA. Breathing movements transiently increase lung volume [abstr]. Pediatr Res 1983; 17:385.
169. Frangos JA. Physical Forces and the Mammalian Cell. San Diego: Academic Press, 1993.
170. Liu M, Liu J, Buch S, Tanswell AK, Post M. Antisense oligonucleotides against PDGF-B and its receptor inhibit mechanical strain-induced fetal lung cell growth. Am J Physiol 1995; 269:L178–L184.
171. Liu M, Skinner SJM, Xu J, Han RNN, Tanswell AK, Post M. Stimulation of fetal rat lung cell proliferation in vitro by mechanical stretch. Am J Physiol 1992; 263: L376–L383.
172. Liu M, Xu J, Souza P, Tanswell B, Tanswell AK, Post M. The effect of mechanical strain on fetal rat lung cell proliferation: comparison of two- and three-dimensional culture systems. In Vitro Cell Dev Biol 1995; 31:858–866.
173. Resnick N, Collins T, Atkinson W, Bonthron DT, Dweey CF Jr, Gimbrone MA Jr. Platelet-derived growth factor B chain promoter contains a *cis*-acting fluid shear–stress-responsive element. Proc Natl Acad Sci USA 1993; 90:4591–4595.
174. Hsieh H-J, Li N-Q, Frangos JA. Shear-induced platelet-derived growth factor gene expression in human endothelial cells is mediated by protein kinase C. J Cell Physiol 1992; 150:552–558.
175. Hooper SB, Han VKM, Harding R. Changes in lung expansion alter pulmonary DNA synthesis and IGF-II gene expression in fetal sheep. Am J Physiol 1993; 265: L403–L409.
176. Perrone CE, Fenwick-Smith D, Vandenburgh A. Collagen and stretch modulate autocrine secretion of insulin-like growth factor-1 and insulin-like growth factor binding proteins from differentiated skeletal muscle cells. J Biol Chem 1995; 270: 2099–2106.
177. Singhvi R, Kumar A, Lopez GP, Stephanopoulos GN, Wand DIC, Whitesides GM, Ingber DE. Engineering cell shape and function. Science 1994; 264:696–698.
178. Bishop JE, Mitchell JJ, Absher PM, Baldor L, Geller HA, Woodcock-Mitchell J, Hamblin MJ, Vacek P, Low RB. Cyclic mechanical deformation stimulates human lung fibroblast proliferation and autocrine growth factor activity. Am J Respir Cell Mol Biol 1993; 9:126–133.
179. Scott JE, Yang S-Y, Stanik E, Anderson JE. Influence of strain on [^{3}H]thymidine

incorporation, surfactant phospholipid synthesis, and cAMP levels in fetal type II alveolar cells. Am J Respir Cell Mol Biol 1993; 8:258–265.
180. Skinner SJM. Fetal breathing movements: a mechanical stimulus for fetal lung cell growth and differentiation. In: Johnston BM, Gluckman PD, eds. Research in Perinatal Medicine (VIII), Advances in Fetal Physiology. Ithaca, NY: Perinatology Press, 1989:133–141.
181. Liu M, Xu J, Tanswell AK, Post M. Stretch-induced growth-promoting activities stimulate fetal rat lung epithelial cell proliferation. Exp Lung Res 1993; 19:505–517.
182. Wirtz HRW, Dobbs LG. Calcium mobilization and exocytosis after one mechanical stretch of lung epithelial cells. Science 1990; 250:1266–1269.
183. Liu M, Xu J, Tanswell AK, Post M. Inhibition of mechanical strain-induced fetal rat lung cell proliferation by gadolinium, a stretch-activated channel blocker. J Cell Physiol 1994; 161:501–507.
184. Liu M, Xu J, Liu J, Kraw ME, Tanswell AK, Post M. Mechanical strain-enhanced fetal lung cell proliferation is mediated by phospholipases C and D and protein kinase C. Am J Physiol 1995; 268:L729–L738.
185. Liu M, Qin Y, Liu J, Tanswell AK, Post M. Mechanical strain induces pp60src activation and translocation to cytoskeleton in fetal rat lung cells. J Biol Chem 1996; 271:6625–6630.
186. Skinner SJM, Somervell CE, Olson DM. The effects of mechanical stretching on fetal rat lung cell prostacyclin production. Prostaglandins 1992; 43:413–433.
187. Aoyagi T, Izumo S. Mapping of the pressure response element of the c-*fos*gene by direct DNA injection into beating hearts. J Biol Chem 1993; 268:27176–27179.
188. Riley DJ, Rannels DE, Low RB, Jensen L, Jacobs TP. Effect of physical forces on lung structure, function, and metabolism. Am Rev Respir Dis 1990; 142:910–914.
189. Thurlbeck WM. Postnatal growth and development of the lung. Am Rev Respir Dis 1975; 111:803–844.
190. Zhang S, Garbutt V, McBride JT. Strain-induced growth of the immature lung. J Appl Physiol 1996; 81:1471–1476.
191. Marcy TW. Barotrauma: detection, recognition, and management. Chest 1993; 104: 578–584.
192. Dreyfuss D, Soler P, Basset G, Saumon G. High inflation pressure pulmonary edema. Am Rev Respir Dis 1988; 137:1159–1164.
193. Carlton DP, Cummings JJ, Scheerer RG, Poulain FR, Bland RD. Lung overexpansion increases pulmonary microvascular protein permeability in young lambs. J Appl Physiol 1990; 69:577–583.
194. Manning HL. Peak airway pressure: why the fuss? Chest 1994; 105:242–247.
195. Parker JC, Hernandez LA, Peevy KJ. Mechanisms of ventilator-induced lung injury. Crit Care Med 1993; 21:131–143.
196. Tremblay L, Valenza F, Ribeiro S, Li J, Slutsky AS. Injurious ventilation strategies increase cytokines and c-*fos* mRNA expression in an isolated rat lung model. J Clin Invest 1997; 99:944–952.
197. Adkins WK, Hernandez LA, Coker PJ, Buchanan B, Parker JC. Age affects susceptibility to pulmonary barotrauma in rabbits. Crit Care Med 1991; 19:390–393.

198. Todd DA, John E. Lung injury and repair in rabbits from ventilation with moist air. Br J Exp Pathol 1989; 70:637–645.
199. Pohlandt F, Saule H, Schroder H, Leonhardt A, Hornchen H, Wolff C, Bernsau U, Oppermann H-C, Obladen M, Feilen K-D, and the study group. Decreased incidence of extra-alveolar air leakage or death prior to air leakage in high versus low rate positive pressure ventilation: results of a randomised seven-centre trial in preterm infants. Eur J Pediatr 1992; 151:904–909.
200. Rodeberg DA, Maschinot NE, Housinger TA, Warden GD. Decreased pulmonary barotrauma with the use of volumetric diffusive respiration in paediatric patients with burns. J Burn Care Rehabil 1992; 13:506–511.
201. Saran M, Bors W. Oxygen radicals acting as chemical messengers: a hypothesis. Free Radic Res Commun 1989; 7:3–6.
202. Burdon RH. Superoxide and hydrogen peroxide in relation to mammalian cell proliferation. Free Radic Biol Med 1995; 18:775–794.
203. Randell SH, Mercer RR, Young SL. Postnatal growth of pulmonary acini and alveoli in normal and oxygen exposed rats studied by serial section reconstruction. Am J Anat 1989; 186:55–68.
204. Youngson C, Nurse C, Yeger H, Cutz E. Oxygen sensing in airway chemoreceptors. Nature 1993; 365:153–155.
205. Gardner PR, Fridovich I. Effect of glutathione on aconitase in *Escherichia coli*. Arch Biochem Biophys 1993; 301:98–102.
206. Gardner PR, Nguyen D-DH, White CW. Aconitase is a sensitive and critical target of oxygen poisoning in cultured mammalian cells and in rat lungs. Proc Natl Acad Sci USA 1994; 91:12248–12252.
207. Halliwell B, Gutteridge JMC. Oxygen toxicity, oxygen radicals, transition metals and disease. Biochem J 1984; 219:1–14.
208. Gillies NE, Alper T. Reduction in the lethal effects of radiations on *Escherichia coli* β by treatment with chloramphenicol. Nature 1959; 183:237–238.
209. Minakami H, Fridovich I. Relationship between growth of *Escherichia coli* and susceptibility to the lethal effect of paraquat. FASEB J 1990; 4:3239–3244.
210. Hassan HM, Fridovich I. Regulation of the synthesis of superoxide dismutase in *Escherichia coli*. J Biol Chem 1977; 252:7667–7672.
211. Horowitz S, Dafni N, Shapiro D, Holm BA, Notter RH, Quible DJ. Hyperoxic exposure alters gene expression in the lung: induction of the tissue inhibitor of metalloproteinase mRNA and other mRNAs. J Biol Chem 1989; 264:7092–7095.
212. Horowitz S, Shapiro DL, Finkelstein JN, Notter RH, Johnston CJ, Quible DJ. Changes in gene expression in hyperoxia-induced lung injury. Am J Physiol 1990; 258:L107–L111.
213. Veness-Meehan KA, Cheng ERY, Mercier CE, Blixt SL, Johnston CJ, Watkins RH, Horowitz S. Cell-specific alterations in expression of hyperoxia-induced mRNAs of lung. Am J Respir Cell Mol Biol 1991; 5:516–521.
214. Piedboeuf B, Johnston CJ, Watkins RH, Hudak BB, Lazo JS, Cherian MG, Horowitz S. Increased expression of tissue inhibitor of metalloproteinases (TIMP-I) and metallothionein in murine lungs after hyperoxic exposure. Am J Respir Cell Mol Biol 1994; 10:123–132.

215. Adamson IYR, Hedgecock C, Bowden DH. Epithelial cell-fibroblast interactions in lung injury and repair. Am J Pathol 1990; 137:385–392.
216. Bui KC, Buckley S, Wu F, Uhal B, Joshi I, Liu J, Hussain M, Makhoul I, Warburton D. Induction of A- and D-type cyclins and cdc2 kinase activity during recovery from short-term hyperoxic lung injury. Am J Physiol 1995; 268:L625–L635.
217. Crapo JD, Barry BE, Foscue HA, Shelburne J. Structural and biochemical changes in rat lungs occurring during exposures to lethal and adaptive doses of oxygen. Am Rev Respir Dis 1980; 122:123–143.
218. Stortz G, Tartaglia LA, Ames B. Transcriptional regulator of oxidative stress inducible genes: direct activation by oxidation. Science 1990; 248:189–194.
219. Stortz G, Tartaglia LA. OxyR: a regulator of antioxidant genes. J Nutr 1990; 122: 627–630.
220. Christman MF, Morgan RW, Jacobson FS, Ames BN. Positive control of a regulon for defences against oxidative stress and some heat shock proteins in *Salmonella typhimurium*. Cell 1985; 41:753–762.
221. Morgan RW, Christman MF, Jacobson FS, Storz G, Ames BN. Hydrogen peroxide-inducible proteins in *Salmonella typhimurium*: overlap with heat shock and other proteins. Proc Natl Acad Sci USA 1986; 83:8059–8063.
222. Hidalgo E, Demple B. An iron–sulphur centre essential for transcriptional activation by redox sensing SoxR protein. EMBO J 1994; 13:138–146.
223. Storz G, Tartaglia LA, Farr SB, Ames BN. Bacterial defences against oxidative stress. Trends Genet 1990; 6:1–6.
224. Cowan DB, Weisel RD, Williams WG, Mickle DAG. Identification of oxygen responsive elements in the 5′-flanking region of the human glutathione peroxidase gene. J Biol Chem 1993; 36:26904–26910.
225. Clerch LB, Massaro D. Rat lung antioxidant enzymes: differences in perinatal gene expression and regulation. Am J Physiol 1992; 263:L466–L470.
226. Tanswell AK, Olson DM, Freeman BA. Response of fetal rat lung fibroblasts to elevated oxygen concentrations after liposome-mediated augmentation of antioxidant enzymes. Biochim Biophys Acta 1990; 1044:269–274.
227. Tanswell AK, Olson DM, Freeman BA. Liposome-mediated augmentation of antioxidant defences in fetal rat pneumocytes. Am J Physiol 1990; 258:L165–L172.
228. Dell KR, Severson DI. Effects of *cis*-unsaturated fatty acids on aortic protein kinase C. Biochem J 1989; 258:171–175.
229. Kass GEN, Duddy SK, Orrenius S. Activation of protein kinase C by redox-cycling quinones. Biochem J 1989; 260:499–507.
230. Christie NA, Slutsky AS, Freeman BA, Tanswell AK. A critical role for thiol, but not ATP, depletion in 95% O_2-mediated injury in preterm pneumocytes. Arch Biochem Biophys 1994; 313:131–138.
231. Keyse SM, Emslie EA. Oxidative stress and heat shock induce a human gene encoding a protein tyrosine phosphatase. Nature 1992; 359:644–647.
232. Suzuki A, Kozawa O, Saito H, Oiso Y. Effects of prostaglandin $F_{2\alpha}$ on Ca^{2+} influx in osteoblast-like cells: function of tyrosine kinase. J Cell Biochem 1994; 54:487–493.

233. Abate C, Patel L, Rauscher FJ, Curran T. Redox regulation of Fos and Jun DNA-binding in vitro. Science 1990; 249:1157–1161.
234. Xanthoudakis S, Curran T. Identification and characterization of Ref-1, a nuclear protein that facilitates AP-1 DNA-binding activity. EMBO J 1992; 11:653–665.
235. Xanthoudakis S, Miao G, Wang F, Pan Y-CE, Curran T. Redox activation of Fos–Jun DNA binding activity is mediated by a DNA repair enzyme. EMBO J 1992; 11:3323–3335.
236. Schreck R, Rieber P, Baeuerle PA. Reactive oxygen intermediates as apparently widely used messengers in the activation of the NF-κB transcription factor and HIV-1. EMBO J 1991; 10:2247–2258.
237. Galter D, Mihm S, Dröge W. Distinct effects of glutathione disulphide on the nuclear transcription factors κB and the activator protein-1. Eur J Biochem 1994; 221: 639–648.
238. Amstad PA, Krupitza G, Cerutti P. Mechanism of c-*fos* induction by active oxygen. Cancer Res 1992; 52:3952–3960.
239. Datta R, Taneja N, Sukhatme VP, Qreshi SA, Weichselbaum R, Kufe DW. Reactive oxygen intermediates target $CC(A/T)_6GG$ sequence to mediate activation of early growth response 1 transcription factor gene by ionising radiation. Proc Natl Acad Sci USA 1993; 90:2419–2422.
240. Treisman RH. Identification of a protein binding site that mediates transcriptional response of the c-*fos* gene to serum factors. Cell 1986; 46:567–574.
241. Abman SH, Wolfe RR, Accurso FJ, Koops BL, Bowman CM, Wiggins JWJ. Pulmonary vascular response to oxygen in infants with severe bronchopulmonary dysplasia. Pediatrics 1985; 75:80–84.
242. Vender RL, Clemmons DR, Kwock L, Friedman M. Reduced oxygen tension induces pulmonary endothelium to release a pulmonary smooth muscle mitogen(s). Am Rev Respir Dis 1987; 135:622–627.
243. Liland AE, Zapol WM, Qvist J, Nash G, Skoskiewicz M, Pontopoppidan H, Lowenstein E, Laver MB. Positive airway pressure in lambs spontaneously breathing air and oxygen. J Surg Res 1976; 20:85–92.
244. Raj JU, Bland RD. Neutrophil depletion does not prevent oxygen-induced lung injury in rabbits. Chest 1983; 83(suppl):20–21.
245. Kreiger BP, Loomis WH, Spragg RG. Granulocytes and hyperoxia act synergistically in causing acute lung injury. Exp Lung Res 1984; 7:77–83.
246. Raj JU, Hazinski TA, Bland RD. Oxygen-induced lung microvascular injury in neutropenic rabbits and lambs. J Appl Physiol 1985; 58:921–927.
247. Boyce NW, Campbell D, Holdsworth SR. Granulocyte independence of pulmonary oxygen toxicity in the rat. Exp Lung Res 1989; 15:491–498.
248. Wegner CD, Wolyniec WW, LaPlante AM, Marschman K, Lubbe K, Haynes N, Rothlein R, Letts LG. Intercellular adhesion molecule-1 contributes to pulmonary oxygen toxicity in mice: role of leukocytes revised. Lung 1992; 267–279.
249. Kubo K, King LS, Kobayashi T, Newman JH. Differing effects of nitrogen mustard and hydroxyurea on lung O_2 toxicity in adult sheep. Am Rev Respir Dis 1992; 145: 13–18.
250. Kawano T, Mori S, Cybulsky M, Burger A, Ballin A, Cutz E, Bryan AC. Effect

of granulocyte depletion in a ventilated surfactant-depleted lung. J Appl Physiol 1987:27–33.

251. Haschek WM, Witschi H. Pulmonary fibrosis—a possible mechanism. Toxicol Appl Pharmacol 1979; 51:475–487.

252. Witschi HP, Haschek WM, Klein-Sjanto AJP, Hakkinen PJ. Potentiation of diffuse lung damage by oxygen: determining variables. Am Rev Respir Dis 1981; 123: 98–103.

253. Pierce GF. Macrophages: important physiologic and pathologic sources of polypeptide growth factors. Am J Respir Cell Mol Biol 1990; 2:233–234.

254. Terzaghi M, Nettesheim P, Williams ML. Repopulation of denuded tracheal grafts with normal, preneoplastic and neoplastic epithelial cell populations. Cancer Res 1979; 38:4546–4553.

255. Adamson IYR, Young L, Bowden DH. Relationship of alveolar epithelial injury and repair to the induction of pulmonary fibrosis. Am J Pathol 1988; 130:377–383.

256. Adamson IYR, Young L, King GM. Reciprocal epithelial: fibroblast interactions in the control of fetal and adult rat lung cells in culture. Exp Lung Res 1991; 17: 821–835.

257. Scott CD, Ballesteros M, Baxter RC. Increased expression of insulin-like growth factor-II/mannose-6-phosphate receptor in regenerating rat liver. Endocrinology 1990; 127:2210–2216.

258. Stiles AD, Sosenko IRS, D'Ercole AJ, Smith BT. Relation of kidney tissue somatomedin-C/insulin-like growth factor I to postnephrectomy renal growth in the rat. Endocrinology 1985; 117:2397–2401.

259. Perkett EA, Badesch DB, Roessler MK, Stenmark KR, Meyrick B. Insulin-like growth factor I and pulmonary hypertension induced by continuous air embolization in sheep. Am J Respir Cell Mol Biol 1992; 6:82–87.

260. Han RNN, Han VKM, Buch S, Freeman BA, Post M, Tanswell AK. Insulin-like growth factor-I and type I insulin-like growth factor receptor in 85% O_2-exposed rat lung. Am J Physiol 1996; 271:L139–L149.

261. Han RNN, Buch S, Tseu I, Young J, Christie NA, Frndova H, Lye SJ, Post M, Tanswell AK. Changes in structure, mechanics, and insulin-like growth factor-related gene expression in the lungs of newborn rats exposed to 60% oxygen. Pediatr Res 1996; 39:921–929.

262. Veness-Meehan KA, Moats-Staats BM, Price WA, Stiles AD. Re-emergence of a fetal pattern of insulin-like growth factor expression during hyperoxic rat lung injury. Am J Respir Cell Mol Biol 1997; 16:538–548.

263. Korfhagen TR, Swanz RJ, Wert SE, McCarty JM, Kerlakian CB, Glasser SW, Whitsett JA. Respiratory epithelial cell expression of human transforming growth factor-α induces lung fibrosis in transgenic mice. J Clin Invest 1994; 93:1691–1699.

264. Finkelstein JN, Kramer CM. Alveolar epithelial proliferation and production of growth factors and cytokines in pulmonary fibrosis [abstr]. Am Rev Respir Dis 1993; 147:153.

265. Vivekananda J, Lin A, Coalson JJ, King RJ. Acute inflammatory injury in the lung precipitated by oxidant stress induces fibroblasts to synthesize and release transforming growth factor-α. J Biol Chem 1994; 269:25057–25061.

266. Stahlman MT, Orth DN, Gray ME. Immunocytochemical localization of epidermal growth factor in the developing human respiratory system and in acute and chronic lung disease in the neonate. Lab Invest 1989; 60:539–547, 1989.
267. Strandjord TP, Clark JG, Guralnick DE, Madtes DK. Immunolocalization of transforming growth factor-α, epidermal growth factor (EGF), and EGF-receptor in normal and injured developing human lung. Pediatr Res 1995; 38:851–856.
268. Antoniades HN, Bravo MA, Avila RE, Galanopoulos T, Neville-Golden J, Maxwell M, Selman M. Platelet-derived growth factor in idiopathic pulmonary fibrosis. J Clin Invest 1990; 86:1055–1064.
269. Vignaud JM, Allam M, Martinet N, Pech M, Plenat F, Martinet Y. Presence of platelet-derived growth factor in normal and fibrotic lung is specifically associated with interstitial macrophages, while both interstitial macrophages and alveolar epithelial cells express the c-*cis* proto-oncogene. Am J Respir Cell Mol Biol 1991; 5: 531–538.
270. Marinelli WA, Polunovsky VA, Harmon KR, Bitterman PB. Role of platelet-derived growth factor in pulmonary fibrosis. Am J Respir Cell Mol Biol 1991; 5: 503–504.
271. Brody AR. Control of lung fibroblast proliferation by macrophage-derived platelet-derived growth factor. Ann NY Acad Sci 1994; 725:193–199.
272. Fabisiak JP, Evans JN, Kelley J. Increased expression of PDGF-B (c-*cis*) mRNA in rat lung precedes DNA synthesis and tissue repair during chronic hyperoxia. Am J Respir Cell Mol Biol 1989; 1:181–189.
273. Powell PP, Chung Wang C, Jones R. Differential regulation of the genes encoding platelet-derived growth factor receptor and its ligand in rat lung during microvascular and alveolar wall remodelling in hyperoxia. Am J Respir Cell Mol Biol 1992; 7:278–285, 1992.
274. Buch S, Moore A, Post M, Tanswell AK. In vitro expression of the genes for platelet-derived growth factor and its receptors in fetal lung cells exposed to hyperoxia [abstr]. Pediatr Res 1992; 31:303.
275. Hertz MI, Henke CA, Nakleh RE, Harmon KR, Marinelli WA, Fox JMK, Kubo SH, Shumway SJ, Bolman RM, Bitterman PB. Obliterative bronchiolitis after lung transplantation: a fibroproliferative disorder associated with platelet-derived growth factor. Proc Natl Acad Sci USA 1992; 89:10385–10389.
276. Moscatelli D, Flaumenhaft R, Saksela O. Interaction of basic fibroblast growth factor with extracellular matrix and receptors. Ann NY Acad Sci 1991; 638:177–181.
277. Roghani M, Moscatelli D. Basic fibroblast growth factor is internalized through both receptor-mediated and heparan sulfate-mediated mechanisms. J Biol Chem 1992; 267:22156–22162.
278. Henke C, Marinelli W, Jessurun J, Fox J, Harms D, Peterson M, Chiang L, Doran P. Macrophage production of basic fibroblast growth factor in the fibroproliferative disorder of alveolar fibrosis after lung injury. Am J Pathol 1993; 134:1189–1199.
279. Leslie CC, McCormick-Shannon K, Mason RJ. Heparin-binding growth factors stimulate DNA synthesis in rat alveolar type II cells. Am J Respir Cell Mol Biol 1990; 2:99–106.
280. Mason RJ, Leslie CC, McCormick-Shannon K, Deterding RR, Nakamura T, Rubin

JS, Shannon JM. Hepatocyte growth factor is a growth factor for rat alveolar type II cells. Am J Respir Cell Mol Biol 1994; 11:561–567.

281. Yanagita K, Nagaike M, Ishibashi H, Niho Y, Matsumoto K, Nakamura T. Lung may have an endocrine function producing hepatocyte growth factor in response to injury of distal organs. Biochem Biophys Res Commun 1992; 182:802–809.
282. Sporn MB, Roberts AB. The transforming growth factor-betas: past, present, and future. Ann NY Acad Sci 1990; 593:1–9.
283. Williams AO, Flanders KC, Saffiotti U. Immunohistochemical localization of transforming growth factor-β_1 in rats with experimental silicosis, alveolar type II hyperplasia, and lung cancer. Am J Pathol 1993; 142:1831–1840.
284. Khalil N, O'Connor RN, Flanders KC, Shing W, Whitman CI. Regulation of type II alveolar cell proliferation by TGF-β during bleomycin-induced lung injury in rats. Am J Physiol 1994; 11:498–507.
285. Perdue TD, Brody AR. Distribution of transforming growth factor-β_1, fibronectin, and smooth muscle actin in asbestos-induced pulmonary fibrosis in rats. J Histochem Cytochem 1994; 42:1061–1070.
286. Denis M, Ghadirian E. Transforming growth factor-β is generated in the course of hypersensitivity pneumonitis: contribution to collagen synthesis. Am J Respir Cell Mol Biol 1992; 7:156–160.
287. Moore AM, Buch S, Han RNN, Freeman BA, Post M, Tanswell AK. Altered expression of type I collagen, TGF-β_1, and related genes in rat lung exposed to 85% O_2. Am J Physiol 1995; 268:L78–L84.
288. Khalil N, O'Connor R, Unruh H, Warren P, Kemp A, Greenberg A. Enhanced expression and immunohistochemical distribution of transforming growth factor-β in idiopathic pulmonary fibrosis. Chest 1991; 99 (suppl):65–66.
289. Khalil N, Bereznay O, Sporn M, Greenberg AH. Macrophage production of transforming growth factor-β and fibroblast collagen synthesis in chronic pulmonary inflammation. J Exp Med 1989; 170:727–737.
290. Grande J, Melder D, Zinsmeister A, Killen P. Transforming growth factor-β_1 induces collagen IV gene expression in NIH-3T3 cells. Lab Invest 1993; 69:387–395.
291. Katchman SD, Hsu-Wong S, Ledo I, Wu M, Uitto J. Transforming growth factor-β up-regulates human elastin promoter activity in transgenic mice. Biochem Biophys Res Commun 1994; 203:485–490.
292. Maniscalco WM, Campbell MH. Transforming growth factor-β induces a chondroitin sulfate/dermatan sulfate proteoglycan in alveolar type II cells. Am J Physiol 1994; 266:672–680.
293. Raghow R, Irish P, Kang AH. Coordinate regulation of transforming growth factor-β gene expression and cell proliferation in hamster lungs undergoing bleomycin-induced pulmonary fibrosis. J Clin Invest 1989; 84:1836–1842.
294. Moses HL, Coffey RJ, Leof EB, Lyons RM, Keski-Oja J. Transfroming growth factor-β regulation of cell proliferation. J Cell Physiol 1987; 5 (suppl):1–7.
295. Psarras S, Kletsas D, Stathakos D. Restoration of down-regulated PDGF receptors by TGF-β in human embryonic fibroblasts. FEBS Lett 1994; 339:84–88.
296. Chess PR, Ryan RM, Finkelstein JN. Tyrosine kinase activity is necessary for

growth factor-stimulated rabbit type II pneumocyte proliferation. Pediatr Res 1994; 36:481–486.

297. Perrella MA, Yoshizumi M, Fen Z, Tsai J-C, Hsieh C-M, Kourembanas S, Lee M. Transforming growth factor-β_1, but not dexamethasone, down regulates nitric-oxide synthase mRNA after its induction by interleukin-1β in rat smooth muscle cells. J Biol Chem 1994; 269:14595–14600.
298. Goureau O, Lepoivre M, Becquet F, Courtois Y. Differential regulation of inducible nitric oxide synthase by fibroblast growth factors and transfroming growth factor-β in bovine retinal pigmented epithelial cells: inverse correlation with cellular proliferation. Proc Natl Acad Sci USA 1993; 90:4276–4280.
299. Maniscalco WM, Watkins RH, D'Angio CT, Ryan RM. Hyperoxic injury decreases alveolar epithelial cell expression of vascular endothelial growth factor (VEGF) in neonatal rabbit lung. Am J Respir Cell Mol Biol 1997; 16:557–567.
300. Fries KM, Felch ME, Phipps RP. Interleukin-6 is an autocrine growth factor for murine lung fibroblast subsets. Am J Respir Cell Mol Biol 1994; 11:552–560.
301. Kovacs EJ, Kelley J. Lymphokine regulation of macrophage-derived growth factor secretion following pulmonary injury. Am J Pathol 1985; 121:261–268.
302. Sunday ME, Kaplan LM, Motoyama E, Chin WW, Soindel ER. Gastrin-releasing peptide (mammalian bombesin) gene expression in health and disease. Lab Invest 1988; 59:5–24.
303. Aldenborg F, Nilsson K, Jarlshammer B, Bjermer L, Enerbäck L. Mast cells and biogenic amines in radiation-induced pulmonary fibrosis. Am J Respir Cell Mol Biol 1993; 8:112–117.
304. Gaid A, Michel RP, Stewart DJ, Sheppard M, Corrin B, Hamid Q. Expression of endothelin-1 in the lungs of patients with cryptogenic fibrosing alveolitis. Lancet 1993; 341:1550–1554.
305. Komoro I, Kurihara H, Sagiyama T, Takaku F, Yazaki Y. Endothelin stimulates c-*fos* and c-*myc* expression and proliferation of vascular smooth muscle cells. FEBS Lett 1988; 238:249–252.
306. Weiss RH, Maduri M. The mitogenic effect of thrombin in vascular smooth muscle cells is largely due to basic fibroblast growth factor. J Biol Chem 1993; 268:5724–5727.
307. Fernandez-Pol JA, Hamilton PD, Klos DJ. Transcriptional regulation of proto-oncogene expression by epidermal growth factor, transfroming growth factor-β_1 and triiodothyronine in MDA-468 cells. J Biol Chem 1989; 264:4151–4156.
308. Leholta L, Nistér M, Höltä E, Westermark B, Alitalo K. Down-regulation of cellular platelet-derived growth factor receptors induced by an activated *neu* receptor tyrosine kinase. Cell Regulation 1991; 2:651–661.
309. Rosenthal SM, Brown EJ, Brunetti A, Goldfine ID. Fibroblast growth factor inhibits insulin-like growth factor-II (IGF-II) gene expression and increases IGF-I receptor abundance in BC3H-1 muscle cells. Mol Endocrinol 1991; 5:678–684.
310. Yoshinouchi M, Baserga R. The role of the IGF-I receptor in the stimulation of cells by short pulses of growth factors. Cell Prolif 1993; 26:139–146.
311. Barreca A, Voci A, Minuto F, deMarchis M, Cecchelli E, Fugassa E, Giordano G, Gallo G. Effect of epidermal growth factor and insulin-like growth factor-I (IGF-

I) and IGF-binding protein synthesis by adult rat hepatocytes. Mol Cell Endocrinol 1992; 84:119–126.

312. Gohda E, Matsunaga T, Kataoka H, Takebe T, Yamamoto I. Induction of hepatocyte growth factor in human skin fibroblasts by epidermal growth factor, platelet-derived growth factor and fibroblast growth factor. Cytokine 1994; 6:633–640.
313. Silviera MR, Sempowski GD, Phipps RP. Expression of TGFβ isoforms in THY-1^+ and Thy-1^- pulmonary fibroblast subsets: evidence for TGFβ as a regulator of IL-1-dependent stimulation of IL-6. Lymphokine Cytokine Res 1994; 13:277–285.
314. Lugano EM, Dauber JH, Elias JA, Bashey RI, Jiminez SA, Daniele RP. The regulation of lung fibroblast proliferation by alveolar macrophages in experimental silicosis. Am Rev Respir Dis 1984; 129:767–771.
315. Lemaire I, Beaudoin H, Dubois C. Cytokine regulation of lung fibroblast proliferation: pulmonary and systemic changes in asbestos-induced pulmonary fibrosis. Am Rev Respir Dis 1986; 134:653–658.
316. Goldstein RH. Control of type I collagen formation in the lung. Am J Physiol 1991; 261:L29–L40.
317. Noguchi A, Nelson T. IGF-I stimulates tropoelastin synthesis in neonatal rat pulmonary fibroblasts. Pediatr Res 1991; 30:248–251.
318. Brettell LM, McGowan SE. Basic fibroblast growth factor decreases elastin production by neonatal rat lung fibroblasts. Am J Respir Cell Mol Biol 1994; 10:306–315.
319. Tan EML, Rouda S, Greenbaum SS, Moore JH, Fox JW, Solberg S. Acidic and basic fibroblast growth factors down-regulate collagen gene expression in keloid fibroblasts. Am J Pathol 1993; 142:463–470.
320. Beck F, Samani NJ, Senior P, Byrne S, Morgan K, Gebhard R, Brammer WJ. Control of IGF-II mRNA levels by glucocorticoids in the neonatal rat. J Mol Endocrinol 1988; 1:5–8.
321. Matsumoto K, Tajima H, Okazaki H, Nakamura T. Negative regulation of hepatocyte growth factor gene expression in human lung fibroblasts and leukemic cells by transforming growth factor-β_1 and glucocorticoids. J Biol Chem 1992; 267:24917–24920.
322. Haynes AR, Shaw RJ. Dexamethasone-induced increase in platelet-derived growth factor (B) mRNA in human alveolar macrophages and myelomonocytic HL60 macrophage-like cells. Am J Respir Cell Mol Biol 1992; 7:198–206.

24

Developmental Airway Structure and Function in Health and Chronic Lung Injury

HOWARD B. PANITCH

University of Pennsylvania School of Medicine
Children's Hospital of Philadelphia
Philadelphia, Pennsylvania

THOMAS H. SHAFFER

Temple University School of Medicine
Philadelphia, Pennsylvania

I. Introduction

Airway injury with subsequent dysfunction is a hallmark of bronchopulmonary dysplasia (BPD). Although the conducting airways are formed well in advance of fetal viability, they must still undergo significant maturational changes in late gestation. Until they attain characteristics of more mature airways, they are more susceptible to damage. Controversy continues to exist concerning the pathogenesis of BPD in the neonate; however, prolonged mechanical ventilation and oxygen toxicity appear to be major factors. Serial assessments of pulmonary function during the first year of life in infants with BPD have indicated that the duration and pressures of mechanical ventilation, rather than increased inspired oxygen tensions, damage the airways and interfere with their growth (1,2). Within this context, greater assisted ventilatory requirements of the very premature infant relative to the older infant yield an age-related predisposition for airway damage. The present chapter will summarize morphology and functional characteristics of the developing airways and the effect of mechanical ventilation on airway function. In addition, clinical assessment of airway function will be reviewed.

II. Developmental Morphology

A. Airway Formation and Growth

Airway formation is one of the earliest events of lung development. The trachea and main bronchi form during the fourth gestational week, lobar bronchi can be identified in a 5-week fetus, and segmental bronchi are seen by the sixth week of gestation (3,4). By the 16th week, the branching pattern of the conducting airways is complete (3,4; Table 1). The second half of gestation, however, is marked by continuing maturation and remodeling of the airways. The airways not only increase in length and diameter, but also become less collapsible and distensible.

Growth and maturation of the conducting airways do not proceed uniformly throughout the tracheobronchial tree. Tracheal growth follows a pattern different from that of other preacinar airways. Furthermore, differentiation of endoderm and mesenchyme into epithelium, cartilage, muscle, and glands occurs centrifugally, so that at any given gestational age, central airways are at an advanced developmental stage compared with more peripheral airways. The trachea in the neonate is a funnel-shaped structure that becomes more cylindrical in the older child (5). The trachea also undergoes three distinct phases of growth: in the last 12 weeks of gestation, the midtracheal internal perimeter enlarges by 2.6 mm/10-cm increase in crown–rump length; prepubertal growth velocity doubles to 5 mm/10-cm increase in crown–rump length; and postpubertal growth slows to 2.6 mm/10-cm increase in crown–rump length (5). In contrast, the mean luminal

Table 1 Landmarks of Airway Development

Gestational age (wk)	Structural formation	Cellular events
4	Trachea and main bronchi	
6	Segmental bronchi	
7	Tracheal cartilage	
8		Pulmonary neuroendocrine cells identifiable
10	Main bronchial cartilage	Differentiation of epithelial cells Cilia appear
12	Segmental bronchial cartilage	Mucosal glands appear
13		Submucosal glands appear
16	Branching pattern of conducting airways complete	Goblet cells appear
25		Cartilage deposition complete

diameter of more peripheral airways increases linearly from late gestation to at least the first 8 months of postnatal life (6). Hislop et al. (7) also noted that from main bronchi to terminal bronchioles, the length and diameter of preacinar airways grow proportionally from birth to adulthood. They suggested that the preacinar airways of the newborn are a miniature version of the mature airways, and that growth in this region remains proportional throughout postnatal life (6,7).

The major components that contribute to the mechanical properties of the conducting airway walls include cartilage, connective tissue, and muscle. The observation that airways become stiffer with maturation (8,9) may be explained by constitutional changes in these tissues, thickening of the airway wall in relation to its diameter, relative changes in the amounts of either cartilage or muscle in the airway wall, or changes in the geometric configuration of these basic elements of wall composition.

B. Cartilage

Cartilage rings and plates develop in zones of precartilage, a relatively hypercellular substance with little or no extracellular matrix (3). With advancing gestational age, a ground substance devoid of collagen surrounds the cells. It slowly increases in amount and undergoes changes in mucoprotein composition. Cartilage formation lags behind the actual formation of the airways. Tracheal cartilage is first identified at 7 weeks and main bronchial cartilage at 10 weeks of gestation, but cartilage does not reach the level of the segmental bronchi until about 12 weeks (3). Cartilage continues to grow after bronchial branching is complete, with new cartilage steadily appearing until the 25th week of gestation (3). Because of this lag in cartilage maturation, distal conducting airways at term contain plates in the immature or precartilage form (3,10).

Cartilage does not attain its final properties for 15–20 weeks (3). Maturational changes in the compositional characteristics of airway cartilage include an increase in the amount of glycosaminoglycans (3,11); an alteration in the type of proteoglycan, as determined by the appearance of proteoglycans resistant to digestion by testicular hyaluronidase (11); and an increase in collagen content. Proteoglycans confer rigidity to cartilage (12,13), thereby allowing it to withstand compressive and some distensive forces. Their experimental depletion by enzymatic digestion renders the trachea more susceptible to collapse with exposure to compressive forces (14). Tracheal cartilage becomes stiffer with maturation (15), a change that parallels these biochemical alterations.

C. Muscle

There is also a maturational increase in the stiffness of airway smooth muscle, reflected in the amount of stress (force per cross-sectional area) generated in response to stretch (16). In isolated muscle strips or tracheal rings, passive force at the length at which active tension generation is maximal (L_0) increases throughout the fetal period and into adulthood (16–19). When passive force is normalized, however, it appears that any increase in passive stress of tracheal smooth muscle is largely a postnatal event. We have noted (17) that the passive stress of sheep tracheal smooth muscle remained constant over the last third of gestation, but increased threefold from preterm to adult. Over the same period of gestation, however, tracheal-specific compliance decreased by 53% (20). The postnatal change in passive stress could not be accounted for by a change in the relative proportions of muscle to connective tissue within the muscle bundle, for these remained constant (Fig. 1). We speculated that either constitutional changes within the connective tissue ground substance, or increases in the concentration of contractile proteins or in the number of cross-bridges within the myocyte, could account for the observed increase in passive stress. Nevertheless, although changes in the passive properties of airway smooth muscle may contribute to the observed decrease in airway compliance, it is unlikely that such changes are a major determinant of airway stiffness.

D. Epithelium

Epithelial cell differentiation begins at 10 weeks gestation centrally, and proceeds peripherally so that differentiated cells can be seen in the peripheral airways by 13 weeks (21). In the trachea, cilia can be identified at 10 weeks, and by 12 weeks mucosal glands appear (22). Initially, bronchial epithelium is lined by nonciliated columnar cells that become cuboidal and ciliated (22). The first cell type to undergo differentiation in any airway is the pulmonary neuroendocrine cell (PNEC; 23,24). These cells have been identified with significant cytoplasmic differentiation as early as 8 weeks (23). They are found initially in the midst of largely undifferentiated cells, and in significantly greater numbers in the fetal and immediate newborn period compared with adulthood (23–25). These observations have led to the speculation that PNECs play an important role in lung development and in the transition from intrauterine to extrauterine life.

Submucosal glands arise from epithelial cells that migrate into the submucosa. Differentiation of these cells into mucous glands is first recognized by 13

Figure 1 Histological sections of tracheal muscle strips from (a) preterm, (b) newborn, and (c) adult sheep. Computerized densitometric analysis was performed within each box to distinguish muscle fibers from intervening connective tissue, and repeated along the entire length of the muscle. The ratios of muscle to connective tissue for the pictured samples were preterm, 76.2%; newborn, 67.8%; and adult, 73.3% (original magnification 40×). (From Ref. 17.)

a)

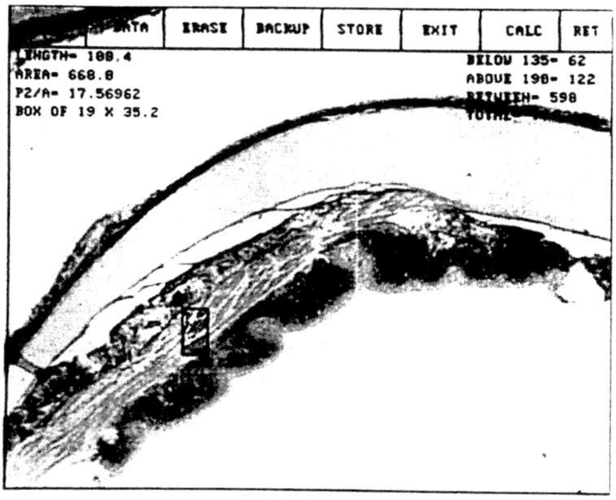

PRETERM

b)

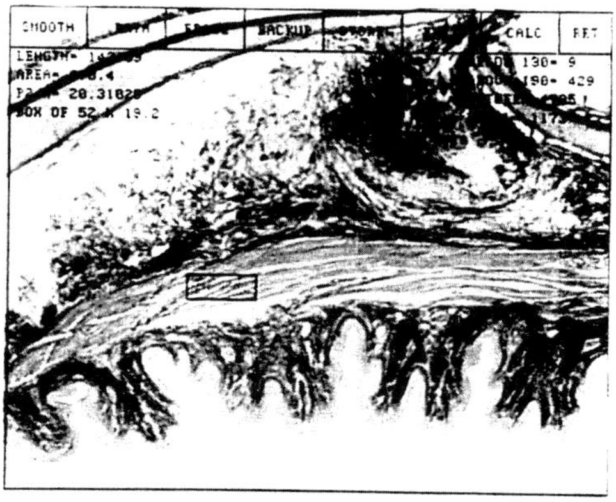

NEWBORN

c)

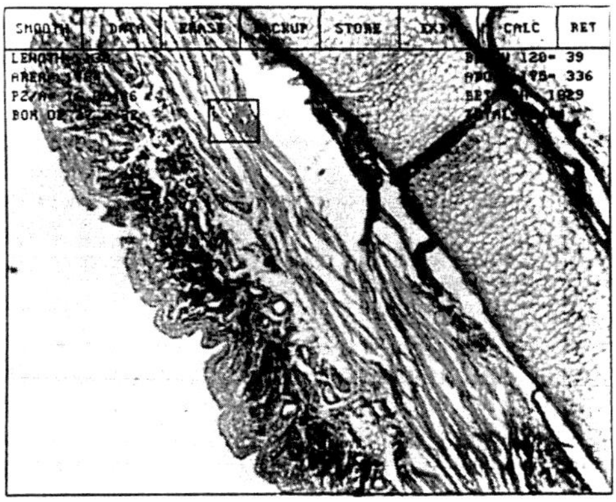

ADULT

weeks (22). Earlier studies suggested that the area of glands composing the airway wall in major bronchi was greater in children than in adults (26). More recent data, however, suggested that the relative gland area of the airway wall increased linearly throughout gestation up to 8 months of age, and that there was a further increase in relative gland area in the hilar and large bronchi into adulthood (6). There was also a maturational change in the composition of mucus produced, with increasing amounts of neutral glycoprotein being produced during late fetal life and infancy (6). Goblet cells, which appeared centrally and extended peripherally with development, also markedly increased in number within the first 4 weeks after birth. These cells also demonstrated a postnatal transition from production of a sulfated glycoprotein to a less viscid sialomucin during the first 12 weeks of postnatal life (6).

By the end of the second trimester, when fetal viability is possible, the human lung contains its full complement of conducting airways. Although these developing airways resemble mature airways structurally, there are important differences in the composition, biochemistry, mechanical characteristics, and geometry of the immature airways that render them particularly vulnerable to pressure-induced trauma.

E. The Morphological Basis for Developmental Changes in Airway Compliance

Although both cartilage and muscle undergo maturational changes in their inherent mechanical characteristics, both also increase in amount with airway growth. Possible mechanisms that would account for the observed maturational increase in airway stiffness include an increase in wall thickness relative to luminal size, or an increase in the amount of cartilage relative to muscle in the airway wall. Within the trachea, however, the relations between cartilage or muscle thickness and airway radius remain constant throughout prenatal development (11). Furthermore, any increase in tracheal perimeter is achieved by a proportional lengthening of cartilage and muscle, so that the ratio of cartilage to muscle length or amount remains constant throughout pre- and postnatal development (27–29). Thus, it appears that changes within each component of the airway, rather than a change in the relative proportions, are responsible for developmental stiffening of the airway.

Patterns of bronchial growth are less clear. Matsuba and Thurlbeck (26) demonstrated that the cartilage and muscle content of the major bronchi remained constant from birth through adulthood. There was always a greater proportion of smooth muscle in small airways (< 2 mm nonalveolated airways) compared with the major bronchi at any age, but the amount of smooth muscle in small airways in children was significantly less than that found in the small airways of adults. More recently, Sward-Comunelli et al. (30) also found that bronchial and bronchiolar muscle mass remained constant relative to airway size from 25 weeks gestation to term, and was proportionally greater in airways smaller than 1 mm compared with larger airways. Hislop and Haworth, however, showed that between 22 weeks gestation and 8 months of postnatal life, there was a linear increase in the amount of cartilage relative to airway perimeter in the main bronchus, although the proportion of cartilage to airway perimeter remained constant in other airways (6). Furthermore, they demonstrated that bronchial smooth muscle increased linearly in relation to airway perimeter as a function of postconceptional age. They noted a dramatic increase in the amount of bronchial smooth muscle immediately after birth. By using α-smooth-muscle antibody stains, airway smooth muscle has been identified in the smallest preterminal bronchioles from infants 23 weeks gestation to term (30).

Deoras and co-workers have suggested that a difference in structural geometry within the posterior wall of the trachea exists, which contributes to the greater compliance and susceptibility to deformation of the preterm airway (11,28). Shortening of the mature trachealis muscle pulls the free ends of the cartilage together to form a nearly complete cartilaginous ring (31). The trachealis muscle of the lamb spans the gap between the free ends of the cartilage ring and inserts on the inner aspect of the perichondrium, in a manner similar to that of the human. In the preterm lamb trachea, the free ends of the cartilage beyond the muscle–cartilage junction overlap each other in a random, deformed way (11,28). In the term trachea, however, the free ends abut each other with minimal overlap. Such an arrangement would favor formation of a complete cartilage ring with even a small amount of muscle shortening, and thereby, strengthen the airway wall. Thus, there is decreased structural support of the posterior tracheal wall in the preterm airway. Altogether, it appears that a change in the mechanical characteristics of components of the airway wall, as well as a change in the geometry of those tissues, contribute to observed developmental changes in airway compliance.

F. Effects of Chronic Exposure to Positive-Pressure Ventilation on Airway Structure

The effects of protracted positive-pressure ventilation (PPV) on airway structure have been elucidated by postmortem studies of infants who required prolonged courses of PPV in the newborn period and who died either as a result of respiratory insufficiency or by causes independent of their lung disease, and by animal studies of the effects of PPV on neonatal airways. In most of these studies, the relative contributions of pressure volume trauma, oxygen toxicity, and alterations of temperature and humidity of the inspired gas to airway damage cannot be separated. Furthermore, when PPV is administered through an artificial airway, additional airway damage can result from mechanical trauma of endotracheal or tracheostomy tubes and suction catheters.

Damage from PPV

Several investigators have described a progression of injuries in those infants exposed to PPV and high levels of oxygen, with a direct relation between the degree of injury and length of exposure to PPV or high concentrations of supplemental oxygen. The most common central airway lesions reported in acute and long-standing BPD include focal or diffuse epithelial damage (27,32–39), submucosal gland hyperplasia (6,34,35), and smooth-muscle hyperplasia (6,24,30,34,35). The increase in the amount of bronchial smooth muscle has been attributed to an increase in muscle cell number, rather than to an increase in cell size (24). Pulmonary neuroendocrine cells are also seen in increased numbers in the airways of infants with BPD, but their role in smooth-muscle hyperplasia or epithelial regeneration is unclear (24).

Bonikos et al. compared both the length of therapy and the degree of supplemental oxygen exposure with the type of injuries sustained in 21 infants who acquired BPD before death (32). There was great variability in the severity of damage seen in infants who died before 4 weeks of age, consisting of marked structural alterations in airways, as well as fibroproliferative activity. Histopathological changes in those infants who survived for more than 4 weeks were more uniform and were graded as severe to very severe. There was focal loss of cilia, as well as metaplasia and necrosis of bronchial and bronchiolar epithelium, often accompanied by an acute and chronic inflammatory reaction involving the underlying wall of the airway and adjacent stroma. Airway lumina were often filled with a mixture of inflammatory cells, epithelial cell debris, and mucinous secretions. Lesions became more pronounced with longer exposures to high concentrations of supplemental oxygen.

Anderson and Engel studied 73 infants who died after more than 2 days of mechanical ventilator therapy (33). They grouped subjects by length of survival, and found three patterns of lung damage: an exudative early reparative stage in infants of shortest survival that was replaced by a subacute fibroproliferative stage, and ultimately a chronic fibroproliferative stage associated with widespread interstitial fibrosis. In the early stage, small bronchi and bronchioles occasionally contained eosinophilic debris, and occasional focal bronchial wall necrosis was present. Changes seen in both the early and middle stages included nodular foci of fibrosis, and development of obliterative bronchiolitis in association with organization of the intrabronchiolar exudate. Furthermore, cystic bronchiolectasis was present in several subjects in this group. In the chronic fibroproliferative stage, obliterative bronchiolitis and cystic bronchiolectasis were absent, whereas interstitial fibrosis was prominent. In contrast, Erickson et al. studied a group of infants of similar age, but found a different progression of damage (40). These investigators found evidence of interstitial fibrosis in the youngest group, normal conducting bronchi with marked distal airspace enlargement in the oldest, and a mixture of the two in the intermediate group. An alternative scheme was described by Van Lierde and co-workers (41). They found two different patterns of injury in their review of 37 infants who died after hyaline membrane disease. One group had marked interstitial fibrosis without airway lesions, whereas the second group had marked airway lesions consisting of epithelial erosions, squamous metaplasia, and bronchiolitis obliterans, along with alveolar and interstitial emphysema. In comparison with the first group, the second group had more severe clinical disease and a requirement for more intensive ventilator and supplemental oxygen support even during the first few days of life. Because some infants in the series demonstrated both types of histopathological changes, the authors reasoned that the two presentations represent extremes along the spectrum of chronic lung injury after hyaline membrane disease. In contrast, Chambers and van Velzen described yet another pattern of lung injury in infants who were born prematurely between 23 and 30 weeks gestation, were supported for more than 10 days by positive-pressure ventilation and high concentrations of supplemental oxygen, and died within 156 days (42). In this group, central airway lesions were much less prominent, whereas simplification of alveolar architecture and interstitial changes in lung parenchyma distal to the terminal bronchiole predominated. These authors speculated that the reduction in central airway pathology was the result of improved respiratory care. In an animal model of BPD, Coalson et al. also noted that central airway lesions were significantly less severe than those reported in earlier studies, perhaps because of newer techniques of respiratory management (43). In summary, central airway lesions are present in some, but not all, infants who undergo positive-pressure ventilation in the newborn period. It is possible that these lesions are markers for more severe parenchymal disease when higher pressures and oxygen concentrations are required to maintain adequate ventilation and oxygenation. In addition, those infants who require extended courses of mechanical ventilatory support would be more likely to sustain central airway damage.

Investigations that have quantified airway wall components of those infants who required prolonged courses of mechanical ventilation have demonstrated abnormalities in the conducting airways. Hislop and Haworth compared the airway architecture of (1) four infants who were born prematurely and who did not require mechanical ventilation, (2) seven infants who were born between 25 and 42 weeks gestation and who required from 6 days to 5 weeks of mechanical ventilation, and (3) normal infants of varying gestational and postnatal ages (6). They noted that the proportion of cartilage within the airway wall did not differ from normal in the infants who were born prematurely, whether or not they required mechanical ventilation. In contrast, there was a significant increase in the amount of smooth muscle found in the main, large, and small bronchi of infants exposed to PPV when compared with normals. Those infants born prematurely who did not receive PPV demonstrated quantities of smooth muscle similar to those of normal infants of the same postnatal age. Prematurity per se was associated with an increase in the proportion of goblet cells for a given postconceptional age, whereas exposure to PPV was also associated with an increase in the proportion of goblet cells as a function of postnatal age. Ventilated infants also showed a significant increase in submucosal gland area in the large bronchi.

These findings were confirmed by Margraf and co-workers, who examined the lung development of eight infants with BPD who had required mechanical ventilation for 2–12 months (34). When compared with six normal infants and young children, there was a proportionate increase in the volume of submucosal glands present in the central bronchi of infants with BPD. The amount of smooth muscle was also relatively increased in the central airways of patients with BPD, although the amount of cartilage and connective tissue was no different from that of controls. Focal areas of squamous metaplasia were present within the bronchial mucosa, and mild to moderate submucosal fibrosis was found in six of the infants with BPD. Mucosal squamous metaplasia, epithelial dysplasia, smooth-muscle hyperplasia, and chronic inflammation were also seen in small airways ($<$ 2 mm diameter) of these patients. No evidence of obliterative bronchiolitis was found.

In an autopsy study of long-term survivors of BPD, Stocker (35) examined the lungs of 28 infants who required mechanical ventilatory support for a minimum of 3 weeks and who survived for 3–40 months. The most common tracheal lesion was squamous metaplasia of varying degrees. Focal and diffuse epithelial necrosis, submucosal fibrosis and inflammation, and glandular hyperplasia were frequently also seen. There was diffuse or focal stenosis of the tracheal lumen in 9 infants, and pseudopolyp formation was noted in 3 infants. Bronchial changes were fewer and less severe than those seen in the trachea, with ''normal''-appearing structures in almost one-half of the subjects. Abnormalities in the remainder consisted of primarily mild squamous metaplasia, submucosal fibrosis, muscular and glandular hyperplasia, and submucosal inflammation.

It is difficult to compare findings of these various studies directly, because of differences in gestational and postconceptional ages, and in the medical and ventilatory management of the subjects. The findings must be interpreted carefully, for there are no published series of findings from lung biopsies of human infants with less severe disease. As several authors have noted, the pulmonary histopathology of infants with BPD, who died of respiratory failure, probably represents an extreme, so that extrapolation to survivors of neonatal respiratory insufficiency must be made with caution.

Epithelial lesions, similar to those described in the human neonate, have also been described in animal models of BPD, even when high distending pressures were avoided (27,36,37,39). Preterm rabbits that were supported by high-frequency oscillations (mean airway pressures 6–8 cmH_2O) without surfactant replacement acquired necrosis and desquamation of bronchiolar epithelium (39).

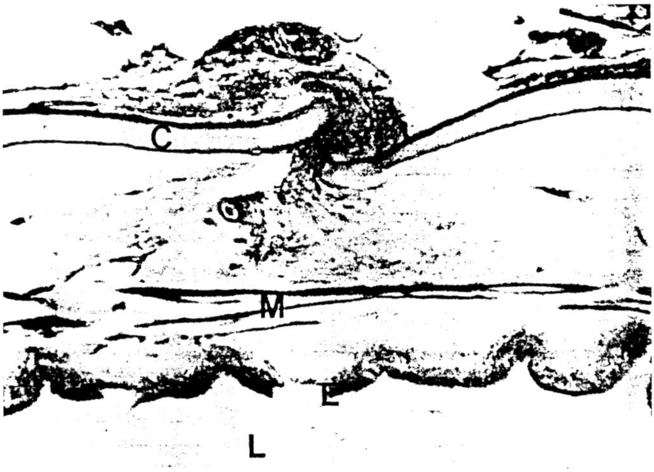

Figure 2 Transverse section of a preterm lamb trachea exposed to mechanical ventilation. There are focal abrasions of the epithelium present after only 2–3 hr of ventilation. (C, cartilage; M, muscle; L, lumen; E, epithelium; magnification 60×). (From Ref. 27.)

The authors speculated that shear forces developed and caused epithelial damage in the lungs of preterm lambs in which expansion was nonuniform. Deoras et al. showed that after only 2–3 hr of PPV at mean airway pressures of 5–12 cmH_2O, the tracheal epithelial layer was flattened and focally abraded (27; Fig. 2). Additionally, the anteroposterior diameter of ventilated airways, along with the length of the trachealis muscle, was significantly greater compared with unventilated controls. There was also a thinning of the tracheal cartilage and trachealis muscle, and decreased overlap of the posterior free ends of the tracheal cartilage. Bhutani et al. (44) also demonstrated dramatic increases in tracheal diameter, volume, and length in immature airways following brief periods of PPV or application of continuous positive airway pressure (CPAP). Furthermore, in the most immature group, the magnitude of these structural alterations increased with longer durations of PPV for up to 2 hr (45). McFawn and Mitchell found that inflation of immature pig bronchi to 20 cmH_2O resulted in significant thinning of the bronchial wall, although no such thinning was detected in adult bronchi (46). They reasoned that the reduction in wall area occurred because of compression of the submucosa. Such findings demonstrate structural changes in the airways of preterm animals and characterize alterations in the geometric arrangement of the muscle and cartilage following PPV.

Damage from Artificial Airways

Endotracheal tubes have been associated with injury to supraglottic, glottic, subglottic, and tracheal tissues in newborns, even after brief periods of tracheal intubation (47–52). Two prospective studies of infants who required intubation in the newborn period found the incidence of moderate to severe subglottic stenosis to be 9.8 and 12.8% (53,54). Typical lesions include focal or extensive necrosis of epithelium, mucosa, and submucosa (48,49). In infants intubated for as few as 6 days, superficial ulcerations with subsequent granulation formation and collagen deposition have been noted (55). Such superficial lesions seen at the time of extubation often resolve without sequelae (51–53), but some infants go on to acquire significant subglottic scarring and obstruction for reasons that are not well understood.

Factors postulated to be important in the genesis of acquired subglottic stenosis include gestational age, birth weight, endotracheal tube size relative to the size of the patient, number of intubations, duration of intubation, route of intubation (naso- vs. orotracheal), frequency of tube changes, trauma of intubation, and presence of infection or hypotension with poor perfusion. Evidence to support each of these factors, however, is conflicting. Several investigators found no differences in gestational age or birth weight between those infants who acquired subglottic stenosis and those who did not (50,53,54). Although Jones did not find a relation between duration of mechanical ventilation and subglottic stenosis (50), others showed that duration of intubation or mechanical ventilation and number of tube insertions both were significant risk factors for acquiring subglottic stenosis (53,54).

Use of inappropriately large endotracheal tubes is an important risk factor for the development of subglottic stenosis (47,53,54). Endotracheal tube size, standardized for gestational age, but not for birth weight or length, correlated significantly with development of subglottic stenosis in a group of 49 infants (53). A ratio of tube size to gestational age (in weeks) of greater than 0.1 was associated with acquired airway obstruction. These criteria were subsequently applied to a separate population of 44 infants who were significantly more premature than those in the previous study (56). When "appropriately" sized tubes were used, the incidence of acquired subglottic stenosis was decreased: only 1 of 36 infants acquired significant subglottic stenosis compared with 9 of 49 in the previous study and 3 of 8 who were intubated with a larger-than-recommended endotracheal tube. In addition, no patient who received less than 25 days of mechanical ventilation had subglottic stenosis.

Central airway obstruction from tracheal and bronchial stenosis and granuloma formation has been described in infants with BPD who were between the ages of 3 weeks and 17 months. Bronchoscopic evaluation disclosed airway narrowing or occlusion by thickened respiratory mucosa or circumferential nodular or polypoid granulations in the distal trachea, often extending into main bronchi (57–60). Histologically, the masses of granulation tissue were accompanied by squamous metaplasia, ulceration of the overlying epithelium, and fibrosis in the mucosa and submucosa (57,60). Several investigators have speculated that stenosis and granulation formation are not complications of BPD, but of extended endotracheal intubation, because lobar emphysema resolved following removal of granulation tissue (57,58,60,61). Repeated mucosal abrasion from suction catheters or from the tip of the endotracheal tube has been implicated as the likely cause of such injury, for those lesions most commonly occur in the distal trachea and right-sided bronchi, where suction catheters and displaced endotracheal tubes are most likely to migrate (57–63.)

Several studies have demonstrated acute mucosal injury to the carina and main bronchi from unrestricted or ''deep'' suctioning (64,65). Bailey and coworkers used light and electron microscopy to assess the effects of deep or shallow suctioning techniques in young rabbits (64). Airways from the group receiving deep suctioning consistently showed more mucosal inflammation and necrosis than did airways that had been treated with shallow suctioning. Necrosis in the deep suction group ranged from 40 to 100% of the airway circumference, and there was almost total loss of cilia and markedly increased mucus in the epithelium of the tracheal bifurcation.

In another study, the airways of two groups of infants who weighed less than 1250 g at birth and who died after prolonged intubation were examined microscopically for signs of damage (65). One group had received deep suctioning routinely, whereas the second group was treated with shallow suctioning. Mucosal changes were found in 25 of 51 autopsy specimens. Severe changes were equally distributed between the two groups, but damage was more severe in the group that was treated routinely with deep suctioning. Although the patients from the shallow suction group were younger and received a longer course of mechanical ventilation, 16% fewer infants among those who were autopsied had moderate or severe tracheal injury.

III. Functional Characteristics of the Immature Airway

Neonatal airways are more compliant than are adult airways. As shown in Figure 3, early studies in necropsied human tracheobronchial segments indicated that airway pressure–volume relations were altered with maturity (8,9). Reduction in airway compliance with maturity results in decreased collapsibility and increased resistance to deformation during positive-pressure ventilation. Therefore, the immature airway is more likely to sustain deformational changes resulting from barotrauma and volutrauma compared with the less compliant airway of the older infant or adult.

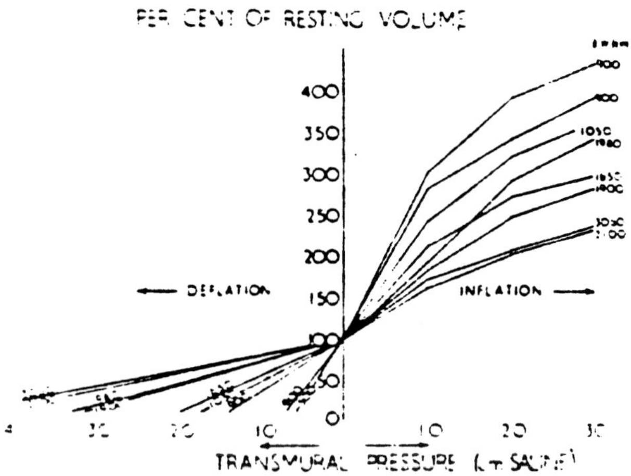

Figure 3 Comparison of pressure–volume relations of airways (tracheae and main bronchi) from infants of different gestational ages. There is an inverse relation between maturity and compliance. *Deflation pressure* was defined as that pressure necessary to collapse the segment to 10% of its resting volume. (From Ref. 8.)

A. Physiology of the Developing Airway

Animal tracheae have been used extensively as a model to study mechanisms that determine maturational changes in airway function. Studies of rabbit tracheal segments have shown that there is an age-related decrease in compliance (66) that parallels changes observed in human neonates (8). Similar developmental changes in airway compliance and an age-related decrease in the relaxation time constant of the trachea have been noted in vivo in sheep (20). Measurements of in vivo specific tracheal compliance were less than in vitro measurements. Such differences may reflect the influence of surrounding connective tissue, or of neural–humoral effects on airway smooth-muscle tone and the elastic properties of the developing airway. The decrease in relaxation time constant with maturation implies that there may be age-related differences in active smooth-muscle tone in vivo. Differences in the magnitude of smooth-muscle contraction modulate mechanical properties and pressure–flow relations of the trachea in both preterm and term newborn lambs (67–69). In general, tracheae stimulated with acetylcholine become stiffer and less compressible, as indicated by lower resistance to airflow when subjected to compressive forces (69–71). The effect of pharmacological stimulation on airway mechanics is age-dependent, and airway smooth muscle of the preterm trachea may be less able to decrease airway compliance and increase flow than can smooth muscle from more mature airways (69). The

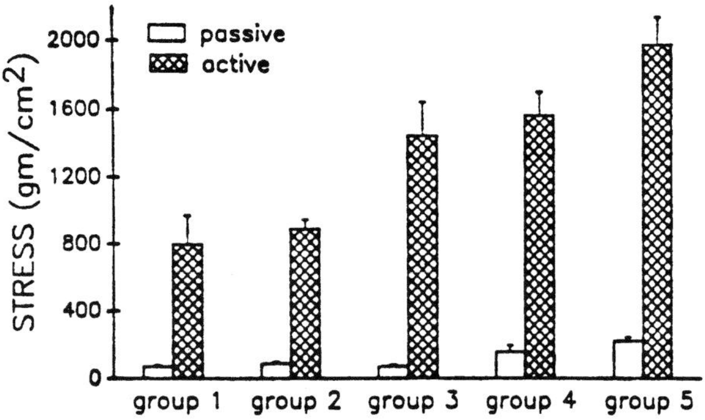

Figure 4 Active and passive stress of isolated trachealis muscle strips from preterm, newborn, and adult sheep, normalized for cross-sectional area and for percentage of muscle fibers within the strip. Group 1, < 110 days gestation ($n = 8$); group 2, 110–124 days gestation ($n = 25$); group 3, 125–140 days gestation ($n = 5$); group 4, newborns ($n = 10$); group 5, adults ($n = 16$). There was a significant increase in both active and passive stress as a function of age ($p < 0.001$). Post hoc analysis disclosed significant differences in active stress between group 1 and groups 3, 4, and 5, and between group 2 and groups 4 and 5. Similarly, passive stress increased between groups 1–3 and group 5. Values are mean ± SEM. Term is 147 ± 3 days. (From Ref. 17.)

reduced capacity of smooth muscle in immature airways to generate as much force as the smooth muscle in adult airways probably contributes to this limitation.

The effect of postnatal aging on the maximal force generated by airway smooth muscle and sensitivity to various agonists remains controversial (72). Some studies show that contractility and sensitivity increase with age (17,73,74), whereas others suggest that contractility and sensitivity reach their peak early in postnatal life, and thereafter decline (18,75). When the extremes of the developmental spectrum are compared, however, a clear pattern emerges. Several investigators have shown that maximal contractility of airway smooth muscle increases between two- and fourfold from preterm or term newborn to adult stages of development (16–18,72). Furthermore, maximum contractility increases significantly during late gestation in both lambs (17; Fig. 4) and pigs (19). This change was not the result of an increase in smooth-muscle mass. In a recent study, Driska (76) identified age-related differences in morphometry in airway smooth-muscle cells isolated from preterm and adult sheep (Fig. 5). Isolated airway smooth muscle cells from preterm airways were about half as long and thick as those of adult cells, but shortening velocities were similar.

Airway epithelium plays an important role in the modulation of smooth-muscle function. In adult airways, airway epithelium generates relaxant and con-

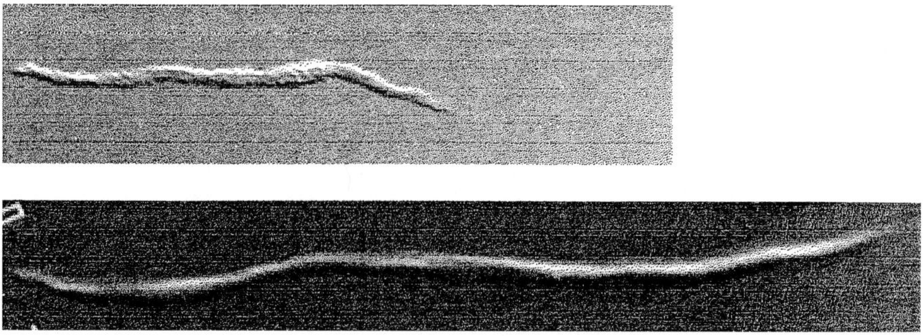

Figure 5 Tracheal smooth muscle cells isolated from adult and preterm sheep: Both images were obtained with 40× differential interference contrast (Nomarski) optics using an Olympus IMT-2 inverted microscope. Top panel: Smooth-muscle cell from a preterm trachea; cell length is 121 μm. Bottom panel: Smooth-muscle cell from an adult trachea; cell length is 249 μm. (Courtesy of Dr. Steven Driska, Department of Physiology, Temple University School of Medicine.)

tractile factors that modulate the tone of the underlying smooth muscle (77–81). Moreover, epithelial damage has been associated with bronchial hyperreactivity (82). In a study of de-epithelialized preterm lamb trachea, force generation in response to acetylcholine stimulation was increased compared with the intact tracheal smooth-muscle strip (83; Fig. 6). These data demonstrate that preterm airway epithelium can modulate the responsiveness of smooth muscle. Furthermore, the magnitude of the effect did not change with maturation from premature newborn to adult. Thus, even during late gestation, epithelial integrity may be an important determinant of smooth-muscle function, bronchial hyperreactivity, and bronchodilator responsiveness. It is not completely understood whether regional differences in airway epithelium exert differential contractile–relaxant influences on airway smooth muscle in the developing airway.

The structural arrangement of muscle and cartilage in the adult trachea is different from that in the bronchi, and suggests that the functional effects of muscle contraction may also be different in these tissues (84). Studies of the adult trachea suggest that the elasticity of the passive trachealis muscle and connective tissue is greater than that of the bronchial wall (85). Moreover, tracheal smooth muscle is capable of generating larger circumferential tensions than bronchial muscle, in all likelihood because of the circumferential alignment and relatively greater proportion of smooth-muscle cells in the trachealis muscle than in the helical orientation and fewer smooth-muscle cells in the bronchial wall.

Regional differences in force generation have also been noted in the airway of premature sheep (86). Passive, active, and total stress development decreased

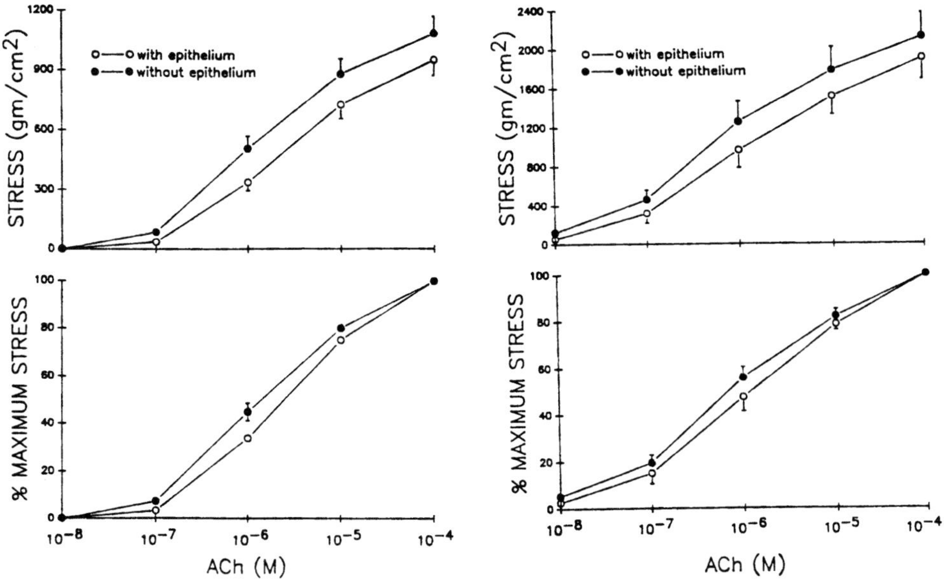

Figure 6 Effect of epithelium removal on concentration–effect curves from preterm (left panels) and adult (right panels) trachealis muscle stimulated with acetylcholine (ACh). Top: forces normalized for cross-sectional area. Bottom: values expressed as percentage of active maximum stress. Epithelium removal resulted in a significant increase in maximum stress in preterm but not in adult strips. In both preterm and adult strips, however, there was a significant decrease in the half-maximal response to ACh resulting from epithelium removal, indicating an increase in sensitivity to the agonist. Values are mean ± SEM. Preterm, $n = 14$; adult, $n = 9$. (Adapted from Ref. 83.)

significantly as a function of airway generation, from trachea (generation 0) to the subsegmental bronchi (generation 4). The receptor-mediated response to acetylcholine was significantly less in generations 0, 1, and 2 than in generations 3 and 4. In addition, the ratio of internal radius to wall thickness (r/t) decreased from trachea to fourth generation airway. The law of LaPlace predicts that because of this decline in r/t, the trachea would be exposed to the greatest degree of wall stress during PPV (86). Taken together these data help explain the structural changes and physiological alterations in airway reactivity that can occur in the premature infant after mechanical ventilation.

Although the intact trachea is suitable for studying the mechanical function of the muscle and cartilage, it is important to consider the individual differences in airway smooth-muscle function and the contribution of cartilage. Several authors have suggested that airway cartilage plays an important role in determining airway compressibility and inflatibility (14,15,84). Moreno et al. (14) softened rabbit tracheas with papain and demonstrated alterations in unstressed tracheal volume and compliance. In a related study using papain-treated rabbits, McCormack et al. (87) observed changes in pulmonary function indicative of increased airway collapsibility when the cartilage was softened. Penn et al. (15) showed that tracheal cartilage of preterm lambs is extremely compliant relative to that of the adult sheep. McFawn and Mitchell (46) noted that premature pig bronchi, which do not generate spontaneous active tone, also are more compliant than bronchi from 1-week-old or adult pigs. Thus, maturational changes in cartilage stiffness also contribute to airway function. Other investigators suggested that these age-related changes in cartilage paralleled developmental differences in tracheal smooth muscle and tracheal mechanics (16,17,66). Therefore, age-related differences in airway mechanical function may reflect an increase in stiffness of both airway muscle and cartilage.

B. Effects of Mechanical Ventilation on Airway Function

Mechanical ventilation has little effect on size and proportions of adult airways (44), but it does affect the dimensions (27,44,88) and mechanical properties of preterm and newborn airways (45,89). The extent of ventilation-induced deformation appears to be directly related to the compliance of the airway and inversely related to age (Fig. 7). We have observed an increase in tracheal diameter, thinning of cartilage and muscle, disruption of the muscle–cartilage junction, and focal abrasions of the epithelium following several hours of mechanical ventilation of preterm lambs (27). In comparison with unventilated trachea, decreased inflation and increased collapsing compliance of the trachea following ventilation yield a structure analogous to a firehose, which is collapsible but difficult to expand (89). In addition, ventilated tracheae showed greater resistance to airflow than did unventilated tracheae of similar-aged preterm animals. The clinical implications of these studies include increased dead space, flow limitation, increased airway resistance and work of breathing, and gas trapping (90).

The mechanisms that are responsible for the alterations in mechanical properties of the ventilated trachea are unclear and have not been studied. We speculate that disruption of the muscle–cartilage junction may reduce the ability of the trachea to resist compressive forces during exhalation, such as excessive positive intrapleural pressures produced by infants with airflow obstruction. In addition, pressure-induced alterations in the orientation of airway smooth-muscle fibers may affect the force-generating capabilities or affect the ability of smooth-muscle contraction to stiffen the airway and resist deformation. Finally, it is also possible that pressure-induced alterations in the alignment of cartilage components (i.e.,

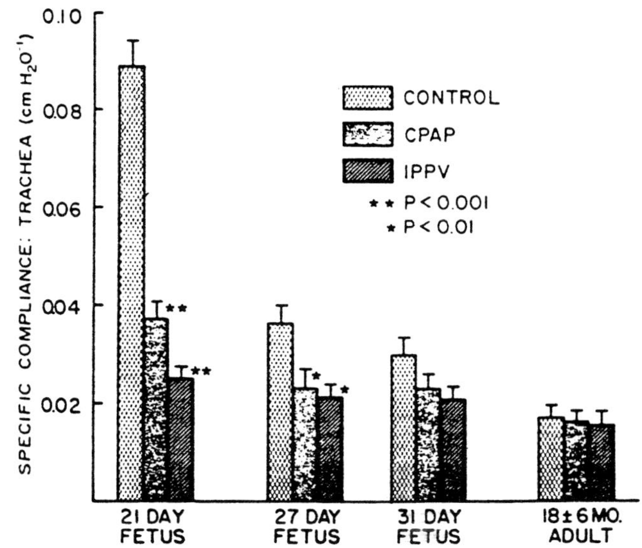

Figure 7 Changes in specific tracheal compliance (change in volume normalized to resting volume/pressure) following CPAP or intermittent PPV (IPPV) in isolated rabbit tracheal segments: 21 days, 67% gestation; 27 days, 87% gestation; 31 days, term. (From Ref. 44.)

proteoglycan–collagen configuration) may attenuate the contribution of cartilage as a structural support for the trachea. Histological studies of ventilated neonatal human and animal lungs describe widening of both the trachea and the peripheral airways after positive-pressure ventilation (91,92). Apart from the qualitative assessment of dimensions, the effect of ventilation on the peripheral airways is unclear and has not been extensively studied. Presumably, age, as well as regional differences in amount of cartilage and smooth muscle, orientation of muscle fibers, force-generating capabilities, and receptor sensitivity of airway smooth muscle, all may influence the effect of ventilation on the relatively more compliant distal compared with the proximal airways. These effects would be potentiated further by a ventilatory pattern in which inspiration is prolonged. Long inspiratory times favor equilibration of pressures throughout the tracheobronchial tree, thereby increasing the length of time that the highly compliant distal airways are subjected to pressure-induced stretch. However, high-frequency jet ventilation (HFJV), evaluated in preterm rabbits, showed significant dimensional and mechanical deformation of tracheal segments and an increased propensity toward collapse following HFJV (93). Therefore, ventilation techniques that attempt to minimize pulmonary barotrauma may still have adverse effects on immature proximal airways. It is difficult to determine which mechanical ventilation strategies are associated with a reduction in airway injury because of the paucity of well-controlled prospective studies designed to evaluate them (94).

Structural alterations of the conducting airways can accentuate luminal narrowing following airway smooth-muscle (ASM) contraction (95–97). In general, factors that enhance airway narrowing for a given amount of ASM shortening include (1) an increase in the amount of smooth muscle in the airway wall; (2) secretions that obstruct the lumen; (3) an increase in the wall thickness relative to lumen diameter; (4) high chest wall compliance; and (5) low elastic recoil pressure (97). These alterations often are present in mechanically ventilated infants. Airways of infants exposed to PPV contain a greater proportion of smooth muscle and submucosal glands then do the airways of normal age-matched infants (6,30,34,35). In addition, acute and chronic submucosal inflammation (32,34,35) serve to increase wall thickness. These changes in airway wall architecture may also be accompanied by a smaller afterload, against which ASM must contract and shorten. Forces that oppose ASM shortening include elastic properties of the airway wall and lung parenchyma. A stiff chest wall contributes to lung parenchymal recoil forces. The chest wall, however, is more compliant in healthy infants and children younger than 2 years of age (98), although chest wall compliance in infants with BPD has not been quantified. Because permanent chest wall distortion can occur in these infants (99), extrapolation from normative data may not be accurate. Similarly, whether elastic recoil pressure is increased or decreased in infants with BPD, compared with normal infants, is also not well established. Quasistatic methods of measuring respiratory system compliance have demonstrated that alterations in the elastic properties of the lung contribute significantly to the observed decrease in compliance (100). Morphological data, however, demonstrate a striking reduction in the number of alveoli and, therefore, in the number of alveolar wall attachments to the airways in infants exposed to chronic PPV (34,40,101,102) or baboon survivors with BPD (43). Alveolar septal attachments are the bridges by which recoil forces exert their effects on the airways and help maintain luminal patency. The balance between the reduced number of wall attachments (decreasing elastic recoil pressure) and the degree of alveolar septal fibrosis (increasing elastic recoil forces) will determine the magnitude of force that ASM must overcome to shorten and to reduce the airway lumen. Taken together, these factors may contribute to excessive airway narrowing following smooth-muscle stimulation, and help account for the high incidence of airway hyperreactivity and bronchodilator responsiveness described in infants with BPD (103–110). In addition to these factors, epithelial damage that is commonly found in the conducting airways of infants exposed to PPV (27,32–39) results in a loss of smooth-muscle modulation (83), which can contribute to the accentuated bronchoconstrictor response to inhaled agonists frequently observed in infants with pulmonary dysfunction resulting from chronic lung disease (111).

Airway smooth-muscle tone also plays an important role in modulating the dimensions and conductance of the adult tracheobronchial tree (112). Increased muscle tone can increase the rigidity of the trachea in the full-term newborn lamb (68). Because a stiffer airway resists pressure-induced deformation better than a more compliant one, this finding provides evidence of a mechanism by which ventilation-induced alterations of the airway can be ameliorated. If the ability of ASM to increase tone in response to pharmacological stimulation is age- and or regionally dependent, then smooth muscle stimulation with a bronchoconstrictor, such as bethanechol, before ventilation might have differential effects on proximal versus peripheral airways of the developing animal.

IV. Clinical Assessment of Airway Function

Several modalities exist to assess airway function clinically in infants. These include measurements of lung function during tidal breathing or forced exhalation, radiography and fluoroscopy, and airway endoscopy. These tests can be used to identify and quantify the predicted functional abnormalities found in preterm airways exposed to PPV, including elevated resistance, decreased forced expiratory flows, airway hyperreactivity, and excessive central airway collapsibility. These tests have provided important insight into the effects of early injury on future airway growth and function, and they can be used to test the effectiveness of new therapies. They are especially useful and should be considered in an infant whose course is not one of gradual improvement or is marked by frequent severe pulmonary exacerbations, and in infants who demonstrate stridor, chronic wheezing, or focal areas of chronic atelectasis or hyperinflation.

A. Measurements of Lung Mechanics During Tidal Breathing and Forced Expiration

Values of dynamic pulmonary compliance, as measured by the esophageal balloon technique, are significantly less in infants who go on to acquire CLD compared with those of normal infants or of infants who recover uneventfully from neonatal respiratory distress (113–115). Dynamic pulmonary compliance improves over time and approaches normal values by 2 years of age (114,115). Resistance measurements, including airway resistance, as determined by plethysmography, pulmonary resistance measured by the esophageal balloon technique, or respiratory system resistance determined by the airway occlusion technique, are significantly elevated in infants with BPD (108,109,114–116). When measurements of resistance or its reciprocal, conductance, have been made serially, values have approached normal over the first 2–3 years of life (114,115). Size-corrected values of resistance or conductance (i.e., *specific conductance*, defined as the conductance divided by lung volume at FRC), however, rose only minimally and remained below normal at the end of the study period, suggesting that airway growth is impaired over the first 3 years of life (114). Arad and co-workers found that specific conductance rose from 57 ± 7% of predicted in infancy to 90 ± 8% of predicted by 5–7 years of age, although the children who required mechanical ventilation in infancy demonstrated air trapping and small airway obstruction in childhood (117).

Forced expiratory flows, produced by either the rapid thoracic compression technique (116,118,119) or the rapid deflation technique (110,120) have been measured in infants with BPD to obtain information more reflective of small airways, and to compare data obtained in infancy more easily with spirometric measurements routinely performed later in childhood. Such studies also demonstrate significant airway obstruction in infancy, with evidence of incomplete recovery with growth. Maximum expiratory flow–volume (MEFV) curves, generated by the rapid-deflation technique, in a group of intubated preterm infants during the acute phase of BPD showed severe small-airway obstruction, as determined by a marked reduction in $\dot{V}max_{25}$, and an MEFV curve shape concave to the volume axis (110). When patients with moderate BPD, who were weaned from mechanical ventilation before 5 months of age, were studied longitudinally with the same technique, there was a gradual increase in $\dot{V}max_{25}$ to approximately 40% of predicted by 3 years of age (120). In contrast, those patients who required extended periods of mechanical ventilation ($\geq$ 10 months) showed no increase in $\dot{V}max_{25}$ over the same time period.

Similar evidence of airway obstruction in young infants with BPD has been demonstrated using the rapid compression technique to produce partial expiratory flow–volume (PEFV) curves over the tidal range of breathing, during which flow is quantified by measuring maximal flow at FRC ($\dot{V}$maxFRC; 116,118). In infants with BPD, forced expiratory flows, corrected for body size, were only half that of normal control values, and did not increase by 14–22 months of age (118). Furthermore, the slope of the regression equation for $\dot{V}$maxFRC versus age was lower in the BPD group compared with normal infants (Fig. 8). These data suggest that early exposure to PPV and high concentrations of oxygen not only caused early airway damage, but also interfered with subsequent normal airway growth. In addition, the separation between tidal and forced flow curves, interpreted as a measure of expiratory flow reserve (118), showed that in infants with BPD there was a smaller expiratory flow reserve compared with normals.

Values of $\dot{V}$maxFRC are usually considered as representative of small-airway function. However, central airway collapsibility (i.e., tracheomalacia or bronchomalacia) can cause a marked reduction in values of $\dot{V}$maxFRC and appear graphically similar to small-airway obstruction (Fig. 9; 119,121). Panitch and co-

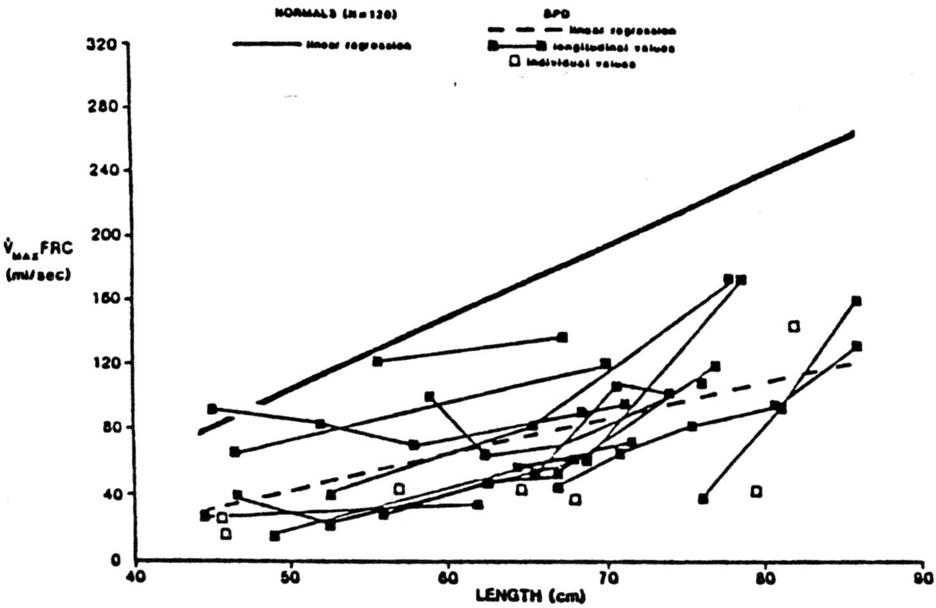

Figure 8 Individual and longitudinal values of $\dot{V}$maxFRC versus body length in infants with BPD. The slope of the regression equation for the group (r = 0.62; dashed line) is significantly lower than that of normal controls (r = 0.48; bold line), suggesting persistent airway dysfunction. (From Ref. 118.)

workers studied five infants with BPD who, by the rapid compression technique had bronchoscopic evidence of tracheobronchomalacia (119). When CPAP was applied to the airway opening, there was an incremental increase in $\dot{V}$maxFRC. Additionally, in several subjects there was a change in the shape of the PEFV curve from concave to convex, suggesting that CPAP acted as an intra-airway stent to prevent collapse (Fig. 10). Furthermore, the ratio of forced-to-tidal flows at midexpiration, a reflection of expiratory flow reserve, increased with application of CPAP. Thus, it is possible that reductions in $\dot{V}$maxFRC, which were previously ascribed to small-airway damage in infants with BPD, may partly reflect central airway injury.

The raised volume rapid thoracic compression technique is a new method of measuring forced expiratory flows in infants (122–124). By inflating the lungs of infants above tidal volumes, airflow obstruction can be identified with greater sensitivity and less variability than with PEFV curve analysis (124). Simultaneous measurement of FRC allows fractioning of lung volumes in the same way conventional pulmonary functions in older children are analyzed, thus facilitating

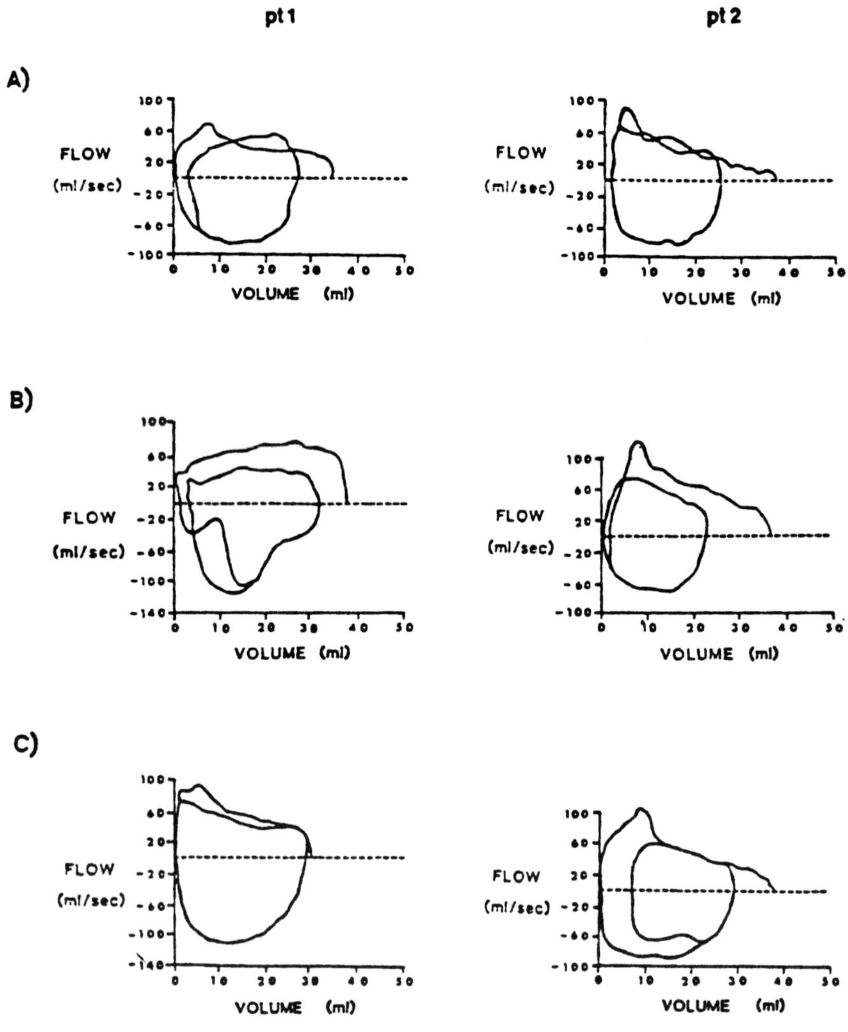

Figure 9 Series of PEFV curves from two infants with bronchoscopically proved tracheomalacia: (A) baseline PEFV curve; (B) following inhalation of methacholine; (C) following inhalation of albuterol. Baseline curves demonstrate flow limitation during tidal breathing, with $\dot{V}$maxFRC values below tidal flow values. With an increase in smooth-muscle tone following methacholine administration, the trachea becomes less collapsible and $\dot{V}$maxFRC increases. Expiratory flow reserve is also present. Following relaxation of airway smooth muscle with albuterol, forced flows fall back to baseline. These curves demonstrate that central airway obstruction can influence values of $\dot{V}$maxFRC and appear graphically similar to small airway obstruction. (Adapted from Ref. 121.)

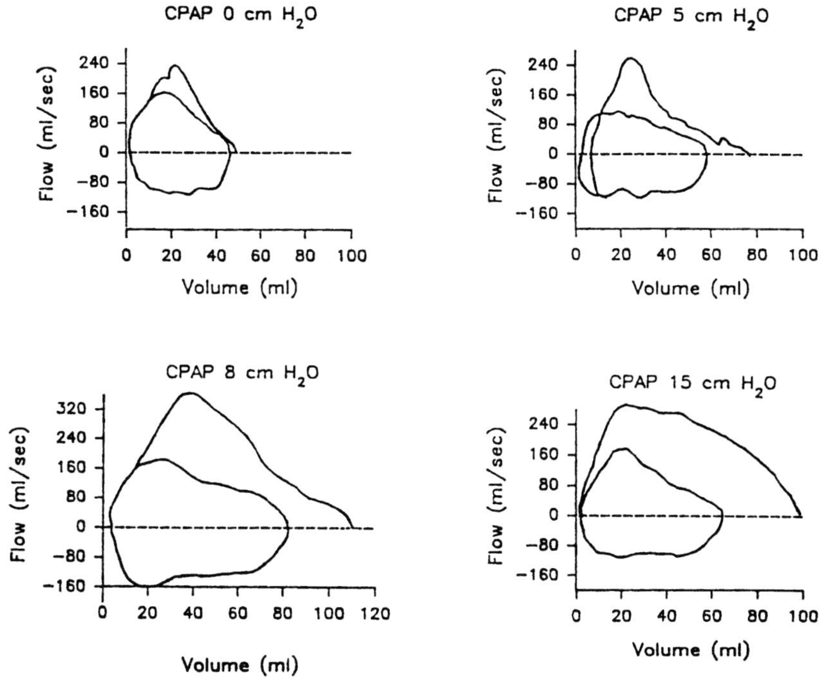

Figure 10 Series of PEFV curves from an infant with BPD and bronchoscopically documented tracheobronchomalacia, showing the effect of increasing levels of CPAP. Off CPAP, the curve shape is concave to the volume axis. As CPAP is increased to 8 cmH_2O, the curve becomes straight, and at higher levels of CPAP it becomes convex. At each level of CPAP, expiratory flow reserve increases as well. Values of $\dot{V}$maxFRC at each level of CPAP are (mL/sec) 26 (0 cmH_2O), 53 (5 cmH_2O), 120 (8 cmH_2O), and 204 (15 cmH_2O). (From Ref. 119.)

comparisons of flows and volumes in longitudinal studies. This method has not yet been applied to infants and young children with BPD.

B. Radiographic Determinations of Central Airway Injury

Bhutani et al. (88) described roentgenographic evidence of acquired tracheomegaly in preterm neonates weighing less than 1000 g at birth who had received mechanical ventilatory support. Increases in tracheal width at the level of the thoracic inlet and carina were present when compared with weight-matched, non-ventilated control infants. The authors speculated that the persistent airway dimensional deformation seen in these infants resulted in increased anatomical dead space and contributed to carbon dioxide retention following extubation.

Acquired tracheomalacia has been evaluated fluoroscopically and by computed tomography (CT). Sotomayor et al. (125) used fluoroscopy in anteroposterior, oblique, or lateral views to document central airway collapse in five infants with BPD who required mechanical ventilation for periods of 3 weeks to 4 months. The authors also employed fluoroscopy to determine the amount of distending pressure required to maintain airway patency in these infants. The range of applied pressures varied between 8 and 20 cmH_2O. McCubbin and co-workers used a cine-CT technique to study central airway collapse in ten infants with BPD (126). The age of the subjects ranged from 3.3 to 20.5 months. A group of seven children of similar age with glottic or supraglottic obstruction, but no evidence of lower airway disease, served as controls. The median percentage decrease in airway cross-sectional area during exhalation in the BPD group was 63.5% (range, 23–100%), whereas that of the control group was only 9% (range, 5–13%). This significant difference in collapsibility was present in a short segment of airway in six and was diffuse in the other four patients. Because narrowing was not always diffuse, these authors speculated that the underlying cause must include local sites of injury, as well as transmural pressure changes.

C. Endoscopic Evaluation of Central Airway Injury

Airway endoscopy permits both diagnosis and treatment of anatomical lesions of supraglottic, glottic, and subglottic regions, as well as of the trachea and bronchi extending to the segmental level (51,53,54,56,58,62,127). The incidence of fixed anatomical lesions other than subglottic stenosis in the population with BPD is unknown. Endoscopy was not used routinely in populations in other series; rather, it was employed when infants presented with acquired lobar emphysema, persistent lobar atelectasis, or unexplained medical failure (57–60,62,128). When lobar emphysema occurred, the right lower lobe and right middle lobes were more commonly affected (57–63).

Direct visualization of the airways during spontaneous breathing is the most accurate method of identifying central airway collapse. Although both open tube (''rigid'') and flexible fiberoptic bronchoscopy are available for the study of pediatric airways, general anesthesia is required for rigid bronchoscopy, usually requiring assisted ventilation during the procedure. Consequently, the patient's effort of breathing is decreased and exhalation may be completely passive. Thus, many cases of central airway collapse can be missed using this method.

In contrast, flexible bronchoscopy is usually performed using conscious sedation. The patient breathes spontaneously, but must breathe around the bronchoscope as well. Variations in expiratory effort can influence the degree of intrathoracic airway collapse noted. McCoy and co-workers (129) observed tracheal collapse bronchoscopically, and cessation of airflow spirometrically in eight infants with BPD following a toe pinch maneuver. When the infants were quieted, however, tracheal caliber and airflow returned to normal baseline conditions. Because of these technical considerations and lack of universally agreed-on criteria, the frequency of diagnosis of central airway collapse varies from center to center. To circumvent these inconsistencies, some authors have based the diagnosis on percentage of airway narrowing during exhalation (119,127,130). Mair and Parsons (130) recommended a grading system based on percentage of airway narrowing present at end-expiration during spontaneous respiration together with an increase in the membrane/cartilage ratio. Others have defined tracheobronchomalacia as collapse resulting in more than 50% (119,131) or 75% (125) obstruction during spontaneous breathing, with no mention of changes in the proportion of membrane to cartilage. Acquired extrathoracic tracheomalacia has also been described in patients with BPD (54).

V. Summary

Over the last several decades, considerable progress has been made in characterizing developmental (preterm, newborn, and adult) differences in the physiology of the conducting airways relative to pressure–volume and pressure–flow relations, the effects of mechanical ventilation, and of pharmacological stimulation. These studies have used in vivo, in vitro and muscle bath preparations to lend valuable insight into how the very premature infant may differ from the later preterm and full-term neonate relative to airway function. Nevertheless, little is known about how positive-pressure ventilation alters the cellular, biochemical, and molecular constituents of the components of the immature airway, and why severe airway dysfunction develops in some mechanically ventilated premature infants and not in others. Ultrastructure studies that assess structural damage with greater sensitivity, and biochemical analyses that can detect alterations in collagen, muscle, and connective tissue composition, would improve our understanding of the pathogenesis of pressure/stretch-related injury. These data, together with carefully controlled mechanical ventilation protocols in premature infants and experimental animal models of BPD, can help establish schemes to reduce the likelihood of airway injury. Finally, longitudinal clinical evaluation of airway function of infants with BPD will lend insight into the effects of early injury on subsequent airway growth and function, as well as repair processes. Such studies will also permit objective evaluation of mechanical or pharmacological interventions, such as prolonged use of CPAP, bronchodilators, or anti-inflammatory agents, on airway growth and repair.

References

1. Stocks J, Godfrey S. The role of artificial ventilation, oxygen, and CPAP in the pathogenesis of lung damage in neonates: assessment by serial measurements of lung function. Pediatrics 1976; 57:352–362.
2. Stocks J, Godfrey S, Reynolds EOR. Airway resistance in infants after various treatments for hyaline membrane disease: special emphasis on prolonged high levels of inspired oxygen. Pediatrics 1978; 61:178–183.
3. Bucher U, Reid L. Development of the intrasegmental bronchial tree: the pattern of branching and development of cartilage at various stages of intrauterine life. Thorax 1961; 16:207–218.
4. Reid L. The lung: its growth and remodeling in health and disease. Am J Roentgenol 1977; 129:777–788.
5. Wailoo M, Emery JL. Structure of the membranous trachea in children. Acta Anat 1980; 106:254–261.
6. Hislop AA, Haworth SG. Airway size and structure in the normal fetal and infant lung, and the effect of premature delivery and artificial ventilation. Am Rev Respir Dis 1989; 140:1717–1726.
7. Hislop A, Muir DCF, Jacobsen M, Simon G, Reid L. Postnatal growth and function of the pre-acinar airways. Thorax 1972; 27:265–274.
8. Burnard ED, Grattan-Smith P, Picton-Warlow CG, Grauaug A. Pulmonary insufficiency in prematurity. Aust Paediat J 1965; 1:12–38.
9. Croteau JR, Cook CD. Volume–pressure and length–tension measurements in human tracheal and bronchial segments. J Appl Physiol 1961; 16:170–172.
10. Itoh K, Itoh H. A study of cartilage development in pulmonary hypoplasia. Pediatr Pathol 1988; 8:65–81.
11. Deoras KS, Wolfson MR, Searls RL, Hilfer SR, Shaffer TH. Developmental changes in tracheal structure. Pediatr Res 1991; 30:170–175.
12. Kempson GE, Muir H, Swanson SAV, Freeman MAP. Correlations between stiffness and the chemical constituents of cartilage on the human femoral head. Biochim Biophys Acta 1970; 215:70–77.
13. Hassell JR, Kimura JH, Hascall VC. Proteoglycan core protein families. Annu Rev Biochem 1986; 55:539–567.
14. Moreno RH, McCormack GS, Mullen JBM, Hogg JC, Bert J, Pare PD. Effect of intravenous papain on tracheal pressure–volume curves in rabbits. J Appl Physiol 1986; 60:247–252.
15. Penn RB, Wolfson MR, Shaffer TH. Developmental differences in tracheal cartilage mechanics. Pediatr Res 1989; 26:429–433.
16. Panitch HB, Allen JL, Ryan JP, Wolfson MR, Shaffer TH. A comparison of preterm and adult airway smooth muscle mechanics. J Appl Physiol 1989; 66:1760–1765.
17. Panitch HB, Deoras KS, Wolfson MR, Shaffer TH. Maturational changes in airway smooth muscle structure–function relationships. Pediatr Res 1992; 31:151–156.
18. Sparrow MP, Mitchell HW. Contraction of smooth muscle of pig airway tissues from before birth to maturity. J Appl Physiol 1990; 68:468–477.

19. Booth RJ, Sparrow MP, Mitchell HW. Early maturation of force production in pig tracheal smooth muscle during fetal development. Am J Respir Cell Mol Biol 1992; 7:590–597.
20. Shaffer TH, Bhutani VK, Wolfson MR, Penn RB, Tran NN. In vivo mechanical properties of the developing airway. Pediatr Res 1989; 25:143–146.
21. Thurlbeck WM. Prematurity and the developing lung. Clin Perinatol 1992; 19:497–519.
22. Crelin ES. Development of the lower respiratory system. Clinical Symposia. Vol. 27 (4). Summit, NJ: CIBA Pharmaceutical, 1975.
23. Cutz E, Gillan JE, Bryan AC. Neuroendocrine cells in the developing human lung: Morphologic and functional considerations. Pediatr Pulmonol 1985; 1:S21–S29.
24. Johnson DE, Anderson WR, Burke BA. Pulmonary neuroendocrine cells in pediatric lung disease: alterations in airway structure in infants with bronchopulmonary dysplasia. Anat Rec 1993; 236:115–119.
25. Johnson DE, Georgieff MK. Pulmonary neuroendocrine cells: their secretory products and their potential roles in health and chronic lung disease in infancy. Am Rev Respir Dis 1989; 140:1807–1812.
26. Matsuba K, Thurlbeck WM. A morphometric study of bronchial and bronchiolar walls in children. Am Rev Respir Dis 1972; 105:908–913.
27. Deoras KS, Wolfson MR, Bhutani VK, Shaffer TH. Structural changes in the tracheae of preterm lambs induced by ventilation. Pediatr Res 1989; 26:434–437.
28. Deoras KS, Wolfson MR, Searls RL, Hilfer SR, Sheffield JB, Shaffer TH. Use of a touch sensitive screen and computer assisted image analysis for quantitation of developmental changes in pulmonary structure. Pediatr Pulmonol 1990; 9:109–118.
29. Wailoo MP, Emery JL. Normal growth and development of the trachea. Thorax 1982; 37:584–587.
30. Sward-Comunelli SL, Mabry SM, Truog WE, Thibeault DW. Airway muscle in preterm infants: changes during development. J Pediatr 1997; 130:570–576.
31. James AL, Pare PD, Moreno RH, Hogg JC. Quantitative measurement of smooth muscle shortening in isolated pig trachea. J Appl Physiol 1987; 63:1360–1365.
32. Bonikos DS, Bensch KG, Northway WH Jr, Edwards DK. Bronchopulmonary dysplasia: the pulmonary pathologic sequel of necrotizing bronchiolitis and pulmonary fibrosis. Hum Pathol 1976; 7:643–666.
33. Anderson WR, Engel RR. Cardiopulmonary sequelae of reparative stages of bronchopulmonary dysplasia. Arch Pathol Lab Med 1983; 107:603–608.
34. Margraf LR, Tomashefski JF Jr, Bruce MC, Dahms BB. Morphometric analysis of the lung in bronchopulmonary dysplasia. Am Rev Respir Dis 1991; 143:391–400.
35. Stocker JT. Pathologic features of long-standing ''healed'' bronchopulmonary dysplasia: A study of 28 3- to 40-month-old infants. Hum Pathol 1986; 17:943–961.
36. Coalson JJ, Kuehl TJ, Escobedo MB, et al. A baboon model of bronchopulmonary dysplasia: II. Pathologic features. Exp Mol Pathol 1982; 37:335–350.
37. Coalson JJ, Winter VT, Gerstmann DR, Idell S, King RJ, deLemos RA. Pathophysiologic, morphometric, and biochemical studies of the premature baboon with bronchopulmonary dysplasia. Am Rev Respir Dis 1992; 145:872–881.

38. Lee RMKW, O'Brodovich H. Airway epithelial damage in premature infants with respiratory failure. Am Rev Respir Dis 1988; 137:450–457.
39. Nilsson R, Berggren P, Curstedt T, Grossmann G, Renheim G, Robertson B. Surfactant treatment and ventilation by high frequency oscillation in premature newborn rabbits: effect on survival, lung aeration, and bronchiolar epithelial lesions. Pediatr Res 1985; 19:143–147.
40. Erickson AM, de la Monte SM, Moore GW, Hutchins GM. The progression of morphologic changes in bronchopulmonary dysplasia. Am J Pathol 1987; 127:474–484.
41. Van Lierde S, Cornelis A, Devlieger H, Moerman P, Lauweryns J, Eggermont E. Different patterns of pulmonary sequelae after hyaline membrane disease: heterogeneity of bronchopulmonary dysplasia? Biol Neonate 1991; 60:152–162.
42. Chambers HM, van Velzen D. Ventilator-related pathology in the extremely immature lung. Pathology 1989; 21:79–83.
43. Coalson JJ, Winter V, deLemos RA. Decreased alveolarization in baboon survivors with bronchopulmonary dysplasia. Am J Respir Crit Care Med 1995; 152:640–646.
44. Bhutani VK, Rubenstein D, Shaffer TH. Pressure-induced deformation in immature airways. Pediatr Res 1981; 15:829–832.
45. Bhutani VK, Shaffer TH. Time-dependent tracheal deformation in fetal, neonatal, and adult rabbits. Pediatr Res 1982; 16:830–833.
46. McFawn PK, Mitchell HW. Bronchial compliance and wall structure during development of the immature human and pig lung. Eur Respir J 1997; 10:27–34.
47. Strong RM, Passy V. Endotracheal intubation: complications in neonates. Arch Otolaryngol 1977; 103:329–335.
48. Rasche RH, Kuhns LR. Histopathologic changes in airway mucosa of infants after endotracheal intubation. Pediatrics 1972; 50:632–637.
49. Joshi VV, Mandavia SG,Stern L, Wiglesworth FW. Acute lesions induced by endotracheal intubation: occurrence in the upper respiratory tract of newborn infants with respiratory distress syndrome. Am J Dis Child 1972; 124:646–649.
50. Jones R, Bodnar A, Roan Y, Johnson D. Subglottic stenosis in newborn intensive care unit graduates. Am J Dis Child 1981; 135:367–368.
51. Fan LL, Flynn JW, Pathak DR, Madden WA. Predictive value of stridor in detecting laryngeal injury in extubated neonates. Crit Care Med 1982; 10:453–455.
52. Fan LL, Flynn JW, Pathak DR. Risk factors predicting laryngeal injury in intubated neonates. Crit Care Med 1983; 11:431–433.
53. Sherman JM, Lowitt S, Stephenson C, Ironson G. Factors influencing acquired subglottic stenosis in infants. J Pediatr 1986; 109:322–327.
54. Downing GJ, Kilbride HW. Evaluation of airway complications in high-risk preterm infants: application of flexible fiberoptic airway endoscopy. Pediatrics 1995; 95:567–572.
55. Hawkins DB. Hyaline membrane disease of the neonate: prolonged intubation in management. Effects on the larynx. Laryngoscope 1978; 88:201–224.
56. Sherman JM, Nelson H. Decreased incidence of subglottic stenosis using an "appropriate-sized" endotracheal tube in neonates. Pediatr Pulmonol 1989; 6:183–185.
57. Nagaraj HS, Shott R, Fellows R, Yacoub U. Recurrent lobar atelectasis due to acquired bronchial stenosis in neonates. J Pediatr Surg 1980; 15:411–415.

58. Miller RW, Woo P, Kellman RK, Slagle TS. Tracheobronchial abnormalities in infants with bronchopulmonary dysplasia. J Pediatr 1987; 111:779–782.
59. Grylack LJ, Anderson KD. Diagnosis and treatment of traumatic granuloma in tracheobronchial tree of newborn with history of chronic intubation. J Pediatr Surg 1984; 19:200–201.
60. Miller KE, Edwards DK, Hilton S, Collins D, Lynch F, Williams R. Acquired lobar emphysema in premature infants with bronchopulmonary dysplasia: an iatrogenic disease? Radiology 1981; 138:589–592.
61. Cooney DR, Menke JA, Allen JE. ''Acquired'' lobar emphysema: a complication of respiratory distress in premature infants. J Pediatr Surg 1977; 12:897–904.
62. Greenholz SK, Hall RJ, Lilly JR, Shikes RH. Surgical implications of bronchopulmonary dysplasia. J Pediatr Surg 1987; 22:1132–1136.
63. Moylan FMB, Shannon DC. Preferential distribution of lobar emphysema and atelectasis in bronchopulmonary dysplasia. Pediatrics 1979; 63:130–134.
64. Bailey C, Kattwinkel J, Teja K, Buckley T. Shallow versus deep endotracheal suctioning in young rabbits: pathologic effects on the tracheobronchial wall. Pediatrics 1988; 82:746–751.
65. Brodsky L, Reidy M, Stanievich JF. The effects of suctioning techniques on the distal tracheal mucosa in intubated low birth weight infants. Int J Pediatr Otorhinolaryngol 1987; 14:1–14.
66. Bhutani VK, Rubenstein SD, Shaffer TH. Pressure–volume relationships of tracheae in fetal newborn and adult rabbits. Respir Physiol 1981; 43:221–231.
67. Bhutani VK, Koslo RJ, Shaffer TH. The effect of tracheal smooth muscle tone on neonatal airway collapsibility. Pediatr Res 1986; 20:492–495.
68. Koslo RJ, Bhutani VK, Shaffer TH. The role of tracheal smooth muscle contraction on neonatal tracheal mechanics. Pediatr Res 1986; 20:1216–1220.
69. Penn RB, Wolfson MR, Shaffer TH. Effect of tracheal smooth muscle tone on collapsibility of immature airways. J Appl Physiol 1988; 65:863–869.
70. Cobum RF, Thorton D, Arts R. Effect of trachealis muscle contraction on tracheal resistance to airflow. J Appl Physiol 1972; 16:170–172.
71. Knudson RJ, Knudson DE. Effect of muscle constriction on flow-limiting collapse of isolated canine trachea. J Appl Physiol 1975; 38:125–131.
72. Fisher JT. Airway smooth muscle contraction at birth: in vivo versus in vitro comparisons to the adult. Can J Physiol Pharmacol 1992; 70:590–596.
73. Rodriguez RJ, Dreshaj IA, Kumar G, Miller MJ, Martin RJ. Maturation of the cholinergic response of tracheal smooth muscle in the piglet. Pediatr Pulmonol 1994; 18:28–33.
74. Haxhiu-Poskurica B, Emsberger P, Haxhiu MA, Miller MJ, Cattarossi L, Martin RJ. Development of cholinergic innervation and muscarinic receptor subtypes in piglet trachea. Am J Physiol 1993; 264:L606–L614.
75. Murphy TM, Mitchell RW, Blake JS, et al. Expression of airway contractile properties and acetylcholinesterase activity in swine. J Appl Physiol 1989; 67:174–180.
76. Driska SP, Laudadio RE, Wolfson MR, Shaffer TH. A method for isolating adult and neonatal airway smooth muscle cells and measuring shortening velocity. J Appl Physiol 1999; 86:427–435.

77. Cuss FM, Barnes PJ. Epithelial mediators. Am Rev Respir Dis 1987; 136:S32–S35.
78. Aizawa H, Miyazaki N, Shigematsu N, Tomooka M. A possible role of airway epithelium in modulating hyperresponsiveness. Br J Pharmacol 1988; 93:139–145.
79. Barnes PJ, Cuss FM, Palmer JB. The effect of airway epithelium on smooth muscle contractility in bovine trachea. Br J Pharmacol 1985; 86:685–691.
80. Flavahan NA, Aarhus LL, Rimele TJ, VanHoutte PM. Respiratory epithelium inhibits bronchial smooth muscle tone. J Appl Physiol 1985; 58:834–838.
81. Stuart-Smith K, VanHoutte PM. Airway epithelium modulates the responsiveness of porcine bronchial smooth muscle. J Appl Physiol 1988; 65:721–727.
82. Laitinen LA, Heino M, Laitinen A, Kava T, Haahtela T. Damage of the airway epithelium and bronchial reactivity in patients with asthma. Am Rev Respir Dis 1985; 131:599–606.
83. Panitch HB, Wolfson MR, Shaffer TH. Epithelial modulation of preterm airway smooth muscle contraction. J Appl Physiol 1993; 74:1437–1443.
84. Gunst SJ, Lai-Fook SJ. Effect of inflation on trachealis muscle tone in canine tracheal segments in vitro. J Appl Physiol 1983; 54:906–913.
85. Olsen CR, Stevens AE, McIlroy MB. Rigidity of tracheae and bronchi during muscular constriction. J Appl Physiol 1967; 23:27–34.
86. Gauthier SP, Wolfson MR, Deoras KS, Shaffer TH. Structure–function of airway generations 0 to 4 in the preterm lamb. Pediatr Res 1992; 31:157–162.
87. McCormack GS, Moreno RH, Hogg JC, Pare PD. Lung mechanics in papain-treated rabbits. J Appl Physiol 1986; 60:242–246.
88. Bhutani VK, Ritchie WG, Shaffer TH. Acquired tracheomegaly in very preterm neonates. Am J Dis Child 1986; 140:449–452.
89. Penn RB, Wolfson MR, Shaffer TH. Effect of ventilation on mechanical properties and pressure–flow relationships of immature airways. Pediatr Res 1988; 23:519–524.
90. Wolfson MR, Bhutani VK, Shaffer TH, Bowen FW. Mechanics and energetics of breathing helium in infants with bronchopulmonary dysplasia. J Pediatr 1984; 104: 752–757.
91. Reynolds EOR, Roberton NRC, Wigglesworth JS. Hyaline membrane disease, respiratory distress, and surfactant deficiency. Pediatrics 1968; 42:758–768.
92. Ackerman NB Jr, Coalson JJ, Kuehl TJ, et al. Pulmonary interstitial emphysema in the premature baboon with hyaline membrane disease. Crit Care Med 1984; 12: 512–516.
93. Bhutani VK, Shaffer TH, Abbasi S, Spitzer AR, Fox WW. Effect of high-frequency jet ventilation on preterm and rabbit tracheal mechanics. Pediatr Pulmonol 1986; 2:327–331.
94. Truog WE, Jackson JC. Alternative modes of ventilation in the prevention and treatment of bronchopulmonary dysplasia. Clin Perinatol 1992; 19:621–647.
95. James AL, Pare PD, Hogg JC. The mechanics of airway narrowing in asthma, Am Rev Respir Dis 1989; 139:242–246.
96. Sterk PJ, Bel EH. Bronchial hyperresponsiveness: the need for a distinction between hypersensitivity and excessive airway narrowing. Eur Respir J 1989; 2:267–274.

97. Panitch HB. Maturational aspects of human airway smooth muscle function. Monaldi Arch Chest Dis 1996; 51:413–418.
98. Papastamelos C, Panitch HB, England SE, Allen JL. Developmental changes in chest wall compliance in infancy and early childhood. J Appl Physiol 1995; 78: 179–184.
99. Breysem L, Smet MH, Lierde SV, deVlieger H, Boeck KD, Marchal G. Bronchopulmonary dysplasia: correlation of radiographic and clinical findings. Pediatr Radiol 1997; 27:642–646.
100. Tepper RS, Pagtakhan RD, Taussig LM. Noninvasive determination of total respiratory system compliance in infants by the weighted-spirometer method. Am Rev Respir Dis 1984; 130:461–466.
101. Sobonya RE, Logvinoff MM, Taussig LM, Theriault A. Morphometric analysis of the lung in prolonged bronchopulmonary dysplasia. Pediatr Res 1982; 16:969–972.
102. Hislop AA, Wigglesworth JS, Desai R, Aber V. The effects of preterm delivery and mechanical ventilation on human lung growth. Early Hum Dev 1987; 15:147–164.
103. Denjean A, Guimaraes H, Migdal M, Miramand JL, Dehan M, Gaultier C. Dose-related bronchodilator response to aerosolized salbutamol (albuterol) in ventilator-dependent premature infants. J Pediatr 1992; 120:974–979.
104. Cabal LA, Larrazabal C, Ramanathan R, et al. Effects of metaproterenol on pulmonary mechanics, oxygenation, and ventilation in infants with chronic lung disease. J Pediatr 1987; 110:116–119.
105. Gomez-Del Rio M, Gerhardt T, Hehre D, Feller R, Bancalari E. Effect of a beta-agonist nebulization on lung function in neonates with increased pulmonary resistance. Pediatr Pulmonol 1986; 2:287–291.
106. Kao LC, Warburtion D, Platzker AC, Keens TG. Effect of isoproterenol inhalation on airway resistance in chronic bronchopulmonary dysplasia. Pediatrics 1984; 73: 509–514.
107. Sosulski R, Abbasi S, Bhutani VK, Fox WW. Physiologic effects of terbutaline on pulmonary function of infants with bronchopulmonary dysplasia. Pediatr Pulmonol 1986; 2:269–273.
108. Kao LC, Durand DJ, Nickerson BG. Effects of inhaled metaproterenol and atropine on the pulmonary mechanics of infants with bronchopulmonary dysplasia. Pediatr Pulmonol 1989; 6:74–80.
109. Wilkie RA, Bryan MH. Effect of bronchodilators on airway resistance in ventilator-dependent neonates with chronic lung disease. J Pediatr 1987; 111:278–282.
110. Motoyama EK, Fort MD, Klesh KW, Mutich RL, Guthrie RD. Early onset of airway reactivity in premature infants with bronchopulmonary dysplasia. Am Rev Respir Dis 1987; 136:50–57.
111. Mirmanesh SJ, Abbasi S, Bhutani VK. alpha-Adrenergic bronchoprovocation in neonates with bronchopulmonary dysplasia. J Pediatr 1992; 121:622–625.
112. Buckley CJ. The role of bronchial musculature. Lancet 1989; 2:836–837.
113. Bryan MH, Hardie MJ, Reilly BJ, Swyer PR. Pulmonary function studies during the first year of life in infants recovering from the respiratory distress syndrome. Pediatrics 1973; 52:169–178.

114. Gerhardt T, Hehre D, Feller R, Reifenberg L, Bancalari E. Serial determination of pulmonary function in infants with chronic lung disease. J Pediatr 1987; 110:448–456.
115. Morray JP, Fox WW, Kettrick RG, Downes JJ. Improvement in lung mechanics as a function of age in the infant with severe bronchopulmonary dysplasia. Pediatr Res 1982; 16:290–294.
116. Kao LC, Durand DJ, Phillips BL, Nickerson BG. Oral theophylline and diuretics improve pulmonary mechanics in infants with bronchopulmonary dysplasia. J Pediatr 1987; 111:439–444.
117. Arad I, Bar-Yishay E, Eyal F, Gross S, Godfrey S. Lung function in infancy and childhood following neonatal intensive care. Pediatr Pulmonol 1987; 3:29–33.
118. Tepper RS, Morgan WJ, Cota K, Taussig LM. Expiratory flow limitation in infants with bronchopulmonary dysplasia. J Pediatr 1986; 109:1040–1046.
119. Panitch HB, Allen JL, Alpert BE, Schidlow DV. Effects of CPAP on lung mechanics in infants with acquired tracheobronchomalacia. Am J Respir Crit Care Med 1994; 150:1341–1346.
120. Mallory GB Jr, Chaney H, Mutich RL, Motoyama EK. Longitudinal changes in lung function during the first three years of premature infants with moderate to severe bronchopulmonary dysplasia. Pediatr Pulmonol 1991; 11:8–14.
121. Panitch HB, Keklikian EN, Motley RA, Wolfson MR, Schidlow DV. Effect of altering smooth muscle tone on maximal expiratory flows in patients with tracheomalacia. Pediatr Pulmonol 1990; 9:170–176.
122. Turner DJ, Stick SM, Lesouef KL, Sly PD, Lesouef PN. A new technique to generate and assess forced expiration from raised lung volume in infants. Am J Respir Crit Care Med 1995; 151:1441–1450.
123. Feher A, Castile R, Kisling J, et al. Flow limitation in normal infants: a new method for forced expiratory maneuvers from raised lung volumes. J Appl Physiol 1996; 80:2019–2025.
124. Turner DJ, Lanteri CJ, LeSouef PN, Sly PD. Improved detection of abnormal respiratory function using forced expiration from raised lung volume in infants with cystic fibrosis. Eur Respir J 1994; 7:1995–1999.
125. Sotomayor JL, Godinez RI, Borden S, Wilmott RW. Large-airway collapse due to acquired tracheobronchomalacia in infancy. Am J Dis Child 1986; 140:367–371.
126. McCubbin M, Frey EE, Wagener JS, Tribby R, Smith WL. Large airway collapse in bronchopulmonary dysplasia. J Pediatr 1989; 114:304–307.
127. Duncan S, Eid N. Tracheomalacia and bronchopulmonary dysplasia. Ann Otol Rhinol Laryngol 1991; 100:856–858.
128. Hauft SM, Perlman JM, Siegel MJ, Muntz HR. Tracheal stenosis in the sick premature infant. Am J Dis Child 1988; 142:206–209.
129. McCoy KS, Bagwell CE, Wagner M, Sallent J, O'Keefe M, Kosch PC. Spirometric and endoscopic evaluation of airway collapse in infants with bronchopulmonary dysplasia. Pediatr Pulmonol 1992; 14:23–27.
130. Mair EA, Parsons DS. Pediatric tracheobronchomalacia and major airway collapse. Ann Otol Rhinol Laryngol 1992; 101:300–309.
131. Couvreur J, Grimfield A, Tournier G. La dyskinesia tracheale (tracheomalacie) chez l'enfant. Reflexions a propos de 127 cas reconnus par endoscopie. Ann Pediatr (Paris) 1980; 27:561–570.

25

Lung Development and the Effects of Chronic Hypoxia

SHEILA G. HAWORTH

Institute of Child Health
London, England

I. Introduction

Chronic hypoxia in the perinatal period leads to a persistently elevated pulmonary vascular resistance, irrespective of its etiology. The immediate morbidity and mortality is high, and after the insult has been removed, permanent damage can result. The normal processes of adaptation to extrauterine life and subsequent ordered growth are disturbed in both the airways and vasculature, and development proceeds along the wrong track. The aim is to identify the most important factors instigating abnormal development, to control them, to reverse abnormal structural and functional changes and to reestablish the normal pattern of growth and development.

This chapter describes normal development and then discusses the effect of chronic hypoxia. In the course of this presentation, some of the most important lines of research for further investigation become self-evident.

II. Normal Development of the Human Lung

The lungs start to develop about 22 days after fertilization, when a ventricular diverticulum, lined by epithelium of endodermal origin, protrudes from the foregut. The bud divides during the fourth week of gestation to form the lung primordia, and the trachea becomes separated from the esophagus by the rostral extension of a septum formed by fusion of epithelial ridges at the root of the lung buds. Incomplete fusion results in a tracheobronchial fistula. Splanchnic mesoderm invests the growing lung and later condenses and differentiates to form the cartilage and the smooth muscle developing around the bronchial tree. A plexus of capillaries and angioblasts lying below the foregut gives rise to the pulmonary and bronchial circulations within the lung. It was once thought that the bronchial arteries arose from the aorta at about 12 weeks gestation, but it now seems probable that all intrapulmonary vessels have the same origin (1). At about 37 days gestation the pulmonary plexus becomes connected to the aortic sac by the pulmonary arteries. These vessels were thought to originate from the sixth branchial arches, but recent experimental studies indicate that the pulmonary artery is the most cranial vessel of a system of ventral splanchnic vessels connecting the pulmonary plexus with the dorsal aorta and the only vessel to persist, all others being transient (2,3). Initially, the lung primordia are drained by systemic veins, until the extrapulmonary veins connect with the left atrium at 4–5 weeks gestation. Following this period of embryogenesis, four overlapping phases of fetal lung development are recognized:

1. Pseudoglandular: 5–17 weeks gestation, when the preacinar (nonrespiratory) airway and arterial-branching pattern is established.
2. Canalicular: 16–26 weeks, when the respiratory region begins to develop as the vascularization of the peripheral mesenchyme accelerates and capillaries form beneath the thinning epithelium of terminal lung buds.
3. Saccular: 24–36 weeks, when additional airways and the future respiratory units (acini) are laid down.
4. Alveolar: 36 weeks gestation to 3 years of postnatal life.

The pattern of lung development is determined by the airway-branching pattern. The airways extend by rapid cell proliferation of the epithelial bronchial buds and branching is dependent on epithelial–mesenchyme interaction (4,5). Remodeling is determined by interactions between cell–cell and cell–substrate adhesion molecules and extracellular matrix proteins; growth factors that stimulate epithelial cell multiplication, such as insulin-like growth factor and epidermal growth factor, and those that inhibit multiplication, such as transforming growth factor-β (6). One of the fibroblast growth factor receptor genes, *FGFR2* is expressed in embryonic lung epithelium, and the targeted expression of a dominant negative FGF receptor blocked airway branching and epithelial cell differentiation in the transgenic mouse lung (7).

The pulmonary arteries accompany the airways and branch with them. Approximately 70% of the preacinar airways and arteries are formed between the

10th and 14th week of gestation, airway branching being complete by 16 weeks and arterial branching by 20 weeks (8,9). The airway lumen diameter, from bronchi to terminal bronchioli, increases in a linear fashion from 22 weeks gestation until growth is complete after birth. Cartilage appears in the trachea during the 4th week and in the main and segmental bronchi by the 10th and 12th weeks, respectively. Cartilage plates continue to form peripherally until the second month of postnatal life, and then each cartilage mass increases in size. The sympathetic and parasympathetic systems are defined by 6 weeks, and by 10 weeks the second-generation bronchi, large arteries, and veins are innervated (10). At birth, the distribution of both sympathetic and parasympathetic nerves to the airways is similar to that in the adult, and nerves extend to the alveolar ducts. The development of receptors is poorly understood. β-Adrenoreceptors and receptors for vasoactive intestinal peptide are present after 14 weeks gestation and increase thereafter, whereas α_1-adrenoreceptors and muscarinic receptors have not been detected before 23 weeks gestation (11,12).

After the preacinar airways are formed, peripheral branching continues. As it does so, the epithelium becomes thinner and the lumen enlarges to make saccules by 25 weeks gestation (13). The amount of interstitial tissue between the saccules decreases between 19 and 30 weeks. Alveoli are recognizable at about 28 weeks, as cup-shaped depressions in the saccule wall delineated by the crests of elastin and collagen that appear to support them (Figs. 1 and 2). The blood–gas barrier becomes as thin as it is in postnatal life, 0.2 μm, by 34–35 weeks gestation. Babies of only 23 weeks gestation have survived, and 50% of those born at 26 weeks gestation survive. The total alveolar number increases from approximately 30 million at 29 weeks to 150 million at term, about one-third to one-half of the adult complement, with a total surface area of 1/20 that of the adult (13–15). The peripheral pulmonary arteries and veins form as the peripheral airways develop; they also continue to form after birth. Thus, alveolar and intra-acinar pulmonary arterial and venous multiplication is extremely vulnerable to fetal, perinatal, and neonatal insults, such as chronic hypoxia.

A. Development of the Airway Wall

All epithelial cells—ciliated, mucus-secreting (goblet), indeterminate, basal, and Clara cells–originate from primitive endodermal cells. Differentiation proceeds in a centrifugal manner from proximal to peripheral airways (16). The epithelium becomes ciliated at 11–16 weeks gestation, as cartilage and bronchial smooth muscle develop. In vitro studies suggest that waves of ciliogenesis pass along the airway until the adult complement of 200–300 cilia per cell is achieved (17). Mature basal cells are recognizable during the canalicular and saccular stages of development. They are thought to be the main epithelial progenitor cell. Clara cells form during the second half of gestation and by 36 weeks are producing

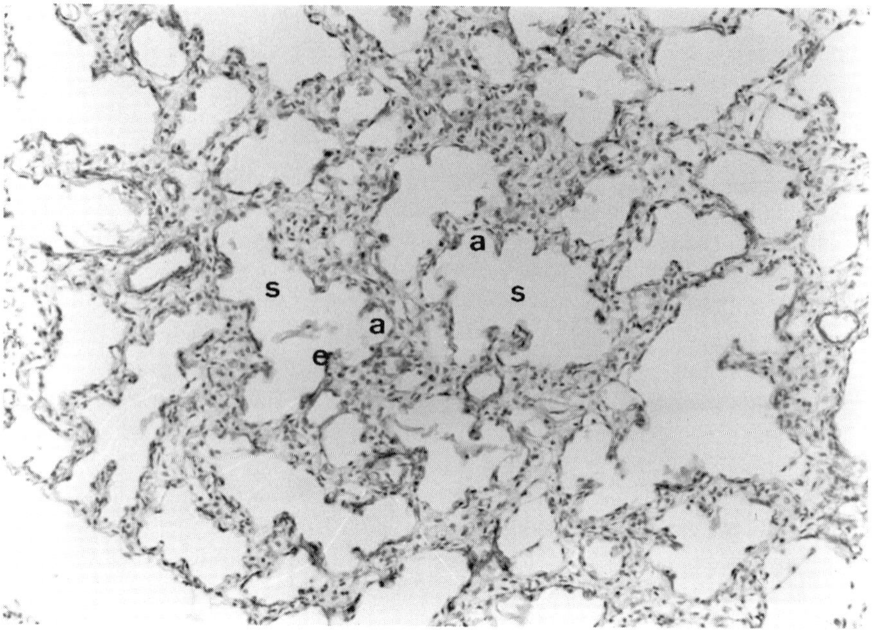

Figure 1 Photomicrograph of human lung tissue at 29 weeks: Saccules (s), many with shallow thick-walled alveoli (a), are separated by relatively thick connective tissue septa. e, elastin (elastic van Gieson stain counterstained with hematoxylin; magnification × 187).

antileukoprotease, thought to be a protective antiprotease (18). Mucous cells are first seen at 13 weeks gestation (19,20). By 22 weeks they are present at the distal end of the large bronchi and by term are found in the bronchioles. After birth the proportion of goblet to ciliated cells increases rapidly during the first 4 weeks of life. This also occurs in preterm babies who, therefore, have an increased number of goblet cells for their postconceptional age and airway size (21). Submucosal glands are present by 10 weeks gestation (22). They also form in a centrifugal manner, extending from the trachea to the bronchi by 16 weeks. Few new glands are formed after 23 weeks gestation. Gland complexity increases during childhood, and in early life the proportion of the airway wall occupied by submucosal glands is greater than in the adult. Neuroendocrine or dense-core granulated cells are thought to be the first mature cell type to differentiate in the primitive airway epithelium and are identifiable at 8 weeks gestation (23). Initially, they contain serotonin and neuron-specific enolase. Bombesin is present 2 weeks later in the late fetal and neonatal period and then declines. The function

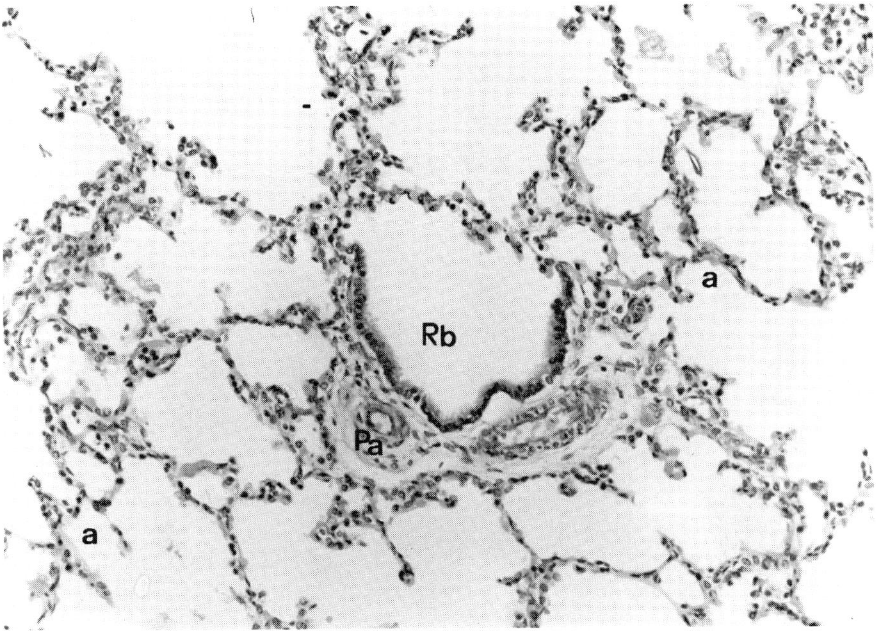

Figure 2 Photomicrograph of human lung tissue at term: Alveoli (a) are mature and thin-walled; Rb, respiratory bronchioli; Pa, pulmonary artery (hematoxylin and eosin stain; magnification × 187).

of these cells is uncertain, but they may influence growth and differentiation, and they change in an hypoxic environment. Their numbers are increased in babies recovering from hyaline membrane disease and in those with bronchopulmonary dysplasia (BPD), and they undergo intracellular changes in young hypoxic rats (24,25).

The airway epithelium modulates airway smooth-muscle contraction, and epithelial damage is associated with airway hyperreactivity (26). Removal of the epithelium from the isolated trachealis smooth muscle of the preterm fetal sheep increased both the maximal contractile response and the sensitivity to acetylcholine. The mechanism by which the epithelium alters smooth-muscle responsiveness is unknown, but possible explanations include release of a relaxing factor (27) and protection from various agonists. In addition, the epithelium contains more β-adrenoreceptors than do smooth-muscle cells, and so loss of epithelial cells deprives the airway wall of the potential to relax to isoproterenol (28).

Airway smooth-muscle cells appear in the tracheal wall at 6–8 weeks gestation and develop sequentially along the airways. In vitro studies show that first-trimester airway smooth-muscle cells contract spontaneously, strongly enough to move intraluminal fluid and distend the distal ends of epithelial tubes (29). This may be an important determinant of early lung development. As in the adult, fetal smooth-muscle cells contract in response to acetylcholine and carbachol, contractions inhibited by calcium channel blockers, and relax in response to isoproterenol and the KATP channel agonist levcromakalim (29). Muscle appears in the walls of small bronchi at between 22 and 24 weeks and in the more peripheral airways, destined to become terminal and respiratory bronchioli, by 26 weeks gestation. The amount of bronchial smooth muscle increases immediately after birth, probably owing to the onset of air breathing (21). Therefore, preterm babies have more muscle than is appropriate for either their postconceptional age or airway size. Bronchial smooth muscle is mature at birth, as judged by its contractile protein and cytoskeletal composition, at which time it is innervated and contractile (30,31). Physiological airway studies indicate that there is a reduction in muscarinic receptor function and an increase in β-adrenoreceptor activity during the first year of extrauterine life (32). Reactivity appears to be greater in young infants than in older children.

Experimental studies have not yet clarified the relation between structural and functional maturation of airway smooth muscle. In porcine smooth muscle, the proportion of the mature myosin heavy chain (200-kDa) isoform 2 increases after birth (33). This change occurs at the same time that the maximum shortening velocity during the early phase of contraction increases, itself suggesting that the ATPase activity of the rapidly cycling cross-bridges increases with maturation (34). Contractile force generation in response to vagal stimulation appears to decrease between 2 and 10 weeks of postnatal life in porcine tracheal muscle, probably owing to the increased functional expression of acetylcholinesterase (35). However, electrical vagal stimulation of tracheal smooth muscle gave only a weak contraction during the first week of life, in comparison with the response at 2–3 and 10 weeks of age (36). This was thought to be due to absent G protein coupling to muscarinic receptors. The total density of muscarinic receptors and of the M_1 and M_3 subtypes did not change during this time interval. Most experimental studies carried out on airway smooth muscle use the trachealis muscle, but airway reactivity shows regional heterogeneity (37); therefore, such studies may not affect bronchial or bronchiolar reactivity.

B. Development of Pulmonary Vessel Walls

By the 19th week of gestation the preacinar arterial pathway down to the seventh generation has an elastic wall structure, as in the adult lung; beyond the seventh generation it is muscular (8). In the smaller arteries, wall structure is related to arterial diameter, the muscle gradually giving way to a nonmuscular structure at the same diameter in the fetus as in the adult lung, but obviously at a more

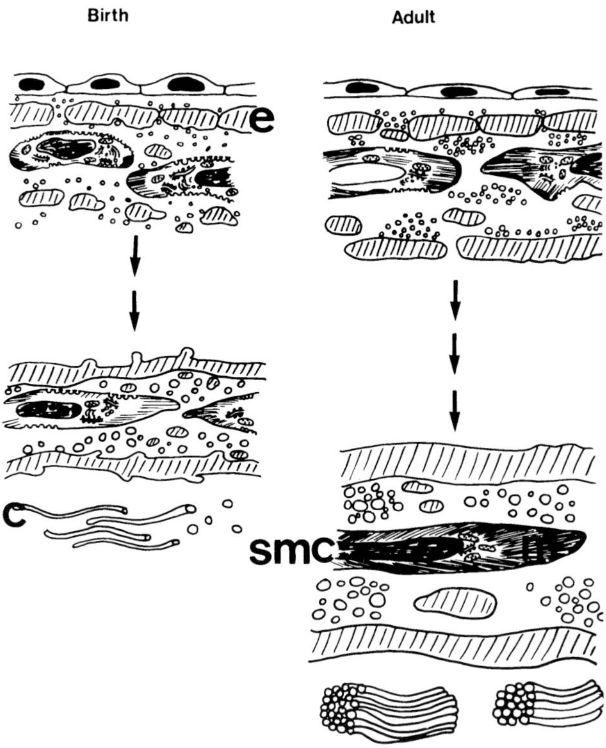

Figure 3 Diagram of wall of an intrapulmonary artery, at birth and in the adult: Each lamellar unit increases in thickness, elastin profiles (e) become thicker and longer, collagen type I fibrils (c) increase in number, and fibrils in the outer media and adventitia become thicker. Smooth muscle cell (smc) myofilament volume density (m) increases in all cells with age, but the concentration is always greater in cells in the outer part of the media.

proximal level along the arterial pathway. At birth, therefore, relatively few intra-acinar arteries contain muscle. Muscle cells gradually differentiate in progressively more peripheral arteries as the vessels grow (Fig. 3). Thus, as gestation advances, the number of muscularized arteries increases, thereby increasing the amount of smooth muscle per unit area of lung tissue. Premature infants are born with arteries that are slightly smaller than normal; consequently, they have less muscle than is normal at term.

Innervation appears to follow muscularization and, therefore, as the intra-acinar arteries increase in size and acquire a muscle coat, so the nerves appear

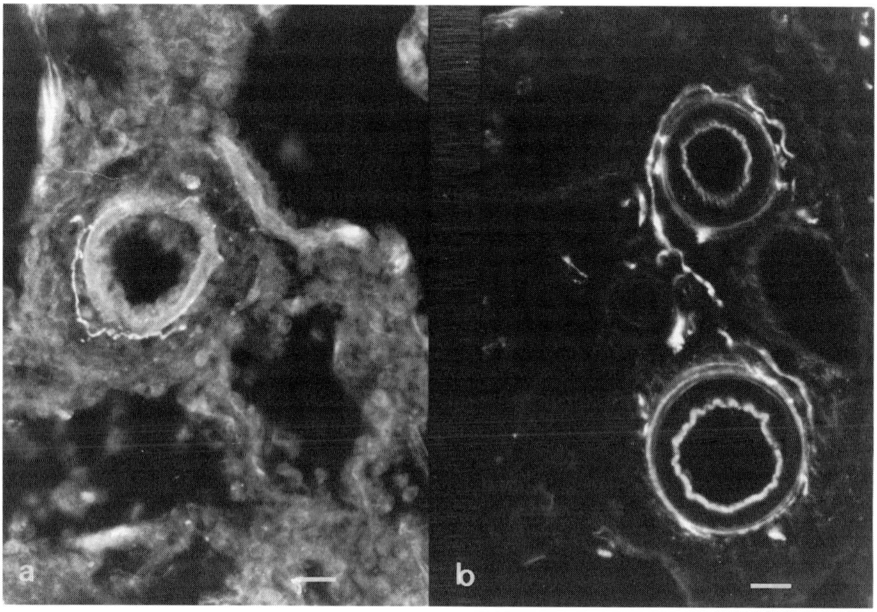

Figure 4 Tyrosine hydroxylase immunoreactive perivascular nerve fibers at the adventitial–medial border of an alveolar duct artery: (a) in the normal lung of a child aged 2 months and (b) in pulmonary hypertension, at 2 years. Scale bar = 50 μm.

(38; Fig. 4). The vasoactive peptides in these nerves are predominantly vasoconstrictor. Pulmonary arterial media is thick during fetal life and thins rapidly immediately after birth. By contrast, the vein wall is thin throughout fetal and postnatal life, and muscle cells are rarely found before 28 weeks of gestation.

At birth, ultrastructural studies show that all of the pulmonary arterial smooth-muscle cells, from the hilum to the capillary bed, are immature. Synthetic, rather than contractile, organelles predominate (30,39,40; see Fig. 3). Contractile myofilament concentration increases rapidly during the first 6 months after birth, but maturation is not well advanced until 2 years of age. At birth the deposition of connective tissue, rather than contractility, appears to have priority. At all ages, the smooth-muscle cells of the media of large arteries form a phenotypically heterogeneous, highly organized cell population. The cells between the elastic laminae close to the adventitia contain a greater concentration of myofilaments, immunoreactive for vinculin, calponin, and desmin, than do those closer to the intima; therefore, these cells might be considered more highly differentiated. The greater concentration of contractile myofilaments in the outer media may relate to their close proximity to sympathetic vasoconstrictor nerves that

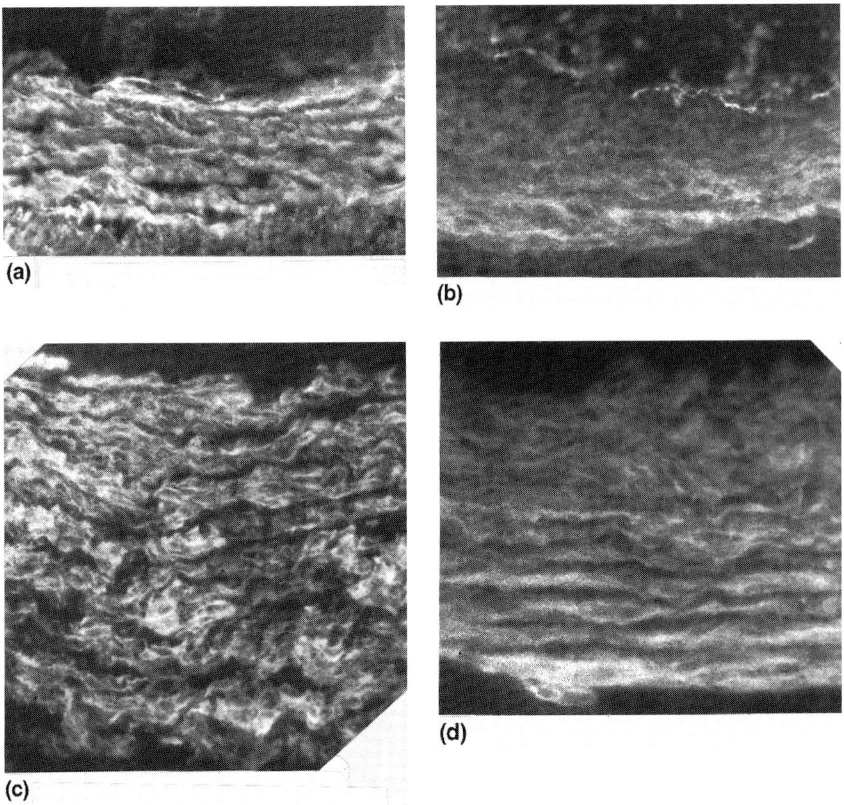

Figure 5 Cryosections of small elastic porcine intrapulmonary arteries stained with an antibody for smooth-muscle-specific 204-kDa myosin heavy-chain isoform SM_1 in(a) normal at birth; (b) normal at 3 days shows transient loss of SM_1 from inner cell layers; (c) normal, at 14 days, showing staining of all cell layers; (d) chronically hypoxic pulmonary hypertensive animals at 3 days showing retention of staining of inner cell layers (magnification: a and c, × 950; b and d, × 1875).

accelerate smooth-muscle cell differentiation in vitro. In the porcine lung at birth all the cells of the large intrapulmonary elastic arteries contain smooth muscle, with specific isoforms of both myosin and actin, and the associated actin-binding and regulatory proteins vinculin and calponin (Fig. 5). Caldesmon, another actomyosin-regulating process, is absent during the first week of life. Desmin, generally considered to be a marker of cell differentiation, is present in a few cells scattered throughout the media. In both bovine and porcine pulmonary arteries, clusters of metavinculin-staining cells are found in the outer part of the media.

Cells in the smaller muscular vessels contain less of the lighter myosin heavy-chain isoform (200 kDa), but contain caldesmon and not calponin. It is becoming increasingly difficult to define smooth-muscle cell phenotypes. At least during development, the term maturation has little meaning. Each cell is appropriately differentiated for the function it must perform at a given type and size of extra- or intrapulmonary artery at that particular stage of development.

The structure of the pulmonary trunk reflects the high pulmonary vascular resistance of fetal life. Before birth the pulmonary trunk, which continues as the ductus arteriosus into the descending thoracic aorta, has a wall structure similar to that of the aorta, with concentric, compact, parallel elastic fibers of uniform thickness.

C. Adaptation to Extrauterine Life

Pulmonary vascular resistance falls rapidly at birth. It decreases in the ovine lung from 1.6 to 0.3 mmHg mL^{-1} min^{-1} kg^{-1}, and blood flow increases from 31 to 145 mL kg^{-1} min^{-1} (41). The main determinant of pulmonary flow is the pulmonary vascular resistance, but bidirectional shunting can occur as long as the ductus arteriosus remains open, depending on the relative resistances of the pulmonary and systemic circulations. This is the unstable transitional circulation.

The wall thickness of the peripheral pulmonary arteries decreases during the initial weeks after birth. Adaptation involves the entire arterial pathway, the elastic and large muscular conducting arteries, in addition to the resistance arteries. The earliest and most dramatic changes, however, are seen in precapillary arteries (42). These vessels consist of only endothelial cells surrounded by pericytes. The endothelial cells at birth are squat and have a narrow base on the subendothelium, a low surface/volume ratio, and many surface projections. Within the first 5 min after birth, the endothelial cells have become thinner and gradually show less cell–cell overlap. Quantitative studies on the porcine lung show that the surface/volume ratio increases, and few if any surface projections remain. The vessel walls become thinner, and lumen diameter increases. Similar structural changes are evident in small muscular arteries immediately after birth. The cells become thinner and spread within the vessel wall, without there being any reduction in the amount of pulmonary vascular smooth muscle. These changes may be facilitated by the lack of fixed interstitial connective tissue in the walls of the peripheral pulmonary arteries at birth. Correlation between structure and function is impossible to study in the normal human infant, but the structural remodeling that takes place during the first two postnatal weeks in the porcine lung helps reduce the mean pulmonary arterial pressure from 55 to 14 mmHg, reduces the pulmonary/systemic resistance ratio from 0.7 to 0.18, and halves the power output of the right ventricle from 10.4 to 5.4 mW kg^{-1}.

The mechanisms responsible for the postnatal fall in pulmonary vascular resistance include mechanical ventilation, oxygen, the preterm reduction in vasoconstrictor leukotrienes, the increase in prostacyclin associated with the onset of breathing, and endothelial-derived relaxing factor(s). Nitric oxide helps moderate the pulmonary arterial pressure in the intact ovine fetus and contributes to the postnatal fall in pressure (43). Immediately after birth, however, endothelium-dependent relaxation of isolated intrapulmonary arteries to a variety of agonists, such as acetylcholine, bradykinin, and the calcium ionophore calcimycin (A23187), is absent or poor, depending on the species, as compared with the response seen a few days after birth. Poor endothelium-dependent relaxation is not due to a lack of nitric oxide synthase. Endothelial cells produce nitric oxide synthase near the end of the first trimester (43 days) in the ovine fetus (44). In the porcine lung there appears to be more nitric oxide synthase in the pulmonary arterial endothelial cells at birth than subsequently, peaking at 2–3 days after birth (45). Within pulmonary arterial smooth-muscle cells, the sensitivity to exogenous nitric oxide and phosphodiesterase inhibitors is less at birth than subsequently, increasing rapidly during the first 10 days of postnatal life. Despite the smaller response to nitric oxide, the basal generation of cyclic guanosine monophosphate (cGMP) is particularly high at birth (46). Potassium channel activation is an alternative relaxation pathway, and KATP channel activation is almost as effective at birth as subsequently, in both conduit and resistance porcine pulmonary arteries (47). Newborn porcine pulmonary arteries contract in response to KCI and $PGF_{2\alpha}$, but the tension developed during the first weeks of life is less than that seen in adult vessels (48).

Receptors link vascular structure and function, and the receptors to many agonists change in density and distribution after birth. The muscarinic receptor subtype M_3 is thought to be responsible for endothelium-dependent relaxation in the adult lung, possibly also with the involvement of the M_1 subtype (49). The density of muscarinic receptors increases rapidly after birth. Expression of mRNA by the M_1 and M_3 subtypes changes with age, changes that are reflected in the pharmacological response to muscarinic stimulation and the influence of specific muscarinic antagonists, which indicate a transient role for the M_1 receptor subtype in the relaxant response soon after birth. Other receptors that change in density and distribution in the neonatal period include the ET_A and ET_B receptors to endothelin and receptors to vasoactive intestinal peptide and calcitonin gene-related peptide (50).

III. Effect of Chronic Hypoxia on Lung Development

Newborn babies who are continuously hypoxic are usually suffering from parenchymal lung disease or, less commonly, pulmonary hypoplasia. The picture is complex.

A. Airway Development

Chronic hypoxia leads to an increase in lung volume and gas exchange surface area, both in humans who are native to high altitude and in experimental animals. On the first day of extrauterine life, ventilatory oxygen extraction is greater in babies who are born at high altitude than in those who are born at low altitude (51), and at 4–6 years of age their pulmonary-diffusing capacity is greater by at least 25% (52). In rat fetuses that were exposed to maternal hypoxia, the lung weight, protein, and DNA content was reduced (53,54), and alveolar septation was diminished. Such enlargement of the air spaces would contribute to the higher respiratory compliance seen in high-altitude infants and possibly to their higher pulmonary diffusing capacity. In newborn rats who were first exposed to hypoxia 4 h after birth, oxygen consumption decreased initially, and then became normal (55), as in high altitude babies (51), and dry lung weight increased. In other rats made hypoxic for 6 hr to 7 days, an initial increase in lung weight was followed by an increase in DNA synthesis and cell proliferation (56). Lung distension followed, arguing against the hypothesis that it is the distension associated with chronic hypoxia that causes an increase in protein synthesis. Thus, the response of the lung to a reduced oxygen tension is age-dependent and, after birth, may lead to enhanced lung growth. Enlarged air spaces and an increase in lung volume should not, however, be confused with growth.

The lungs of babies dying with BPD show patchy areas of over distended airspaces, but in this condition the initial hypoxic insult has been followed by the traumatic effects of mechanical ventilation, hyperoxia, and possibly infection. The dominant finding is a reduction in alveolar number, even in the mild, relatively nonfibrotic forms of BPD.

Airway and Alveolar Development in BPD

Newborn infants who remain oxygen-dependent for 4 weeks can be said to have chronic lung disease, (CLD) and the more severely compromised will have BPD. The histological appearance of the lungs reflects the degree of immaturity and the structural remodeling that occurs in response to long-term ventilatory support. Traditionally, BPD consists of three evolving phases: a reparative phase in the first 2 weeks, followed by a subacute fibroproliferative phase during the third and fourth weeks, and a subsequent chronic fibroproliferative phase (57,58). Twenty years ago the lungs of babies dying with BPD showed extensive bronchial wall thickening, with epithelial hyperplasia, metaplasia and exudate, bronchial smooth-muscle cell hypertrophy, and areas of interstitial thickening and fibrosis, alternating with grossly dilated air spaces (59). Improved ventilation procedures, particularly the use of lower inflation pressures, has reduced the severity of the changes in the bronchi and bronchioli, but the alveolar abnormalities remain. In a 1989 study of premature, very low birth weight infants with gestational ages of

23.5–30 weeks, the terminal respiratory units were oversimplified (60), denoting failure of alveolarization. The radial alveolar counts were low. In another group of babies of similar gestational age, reported in 1991, Van Lierde et al. (61) described two pathological variants of BPD: bronchiolar and interstitial. Those with the bronchiolar pattern had notable airway lesions and alveolar emphysema. These infants required prolonged ventilatory support and had a higher mortality than did those infants with the interstitial pattern, whose lungs showed predominantly interstitial fibrosis, without severe airways disease. Babies who survived the initial respiratory illness and died later appeared to have fewer alveoli than normal on quantitative morphometric examination. Although the alveolar number appeared to have increased in a group of babies who died after age 3 months, the increase was not sufficient to compensate for the early developmental failure. Radial alveolar counts were reduced in a group of 15 babies with a gestational age of 25–31 weeks, who died at between 13 days and 42 months of age. Margraf and colleagues also found a decrease in total alveolar number in 8 babies of 24–30 weeks gestation who died at 2–28 months of age (62). Lung internal surface was reduced and the mean linear intercept was increased.

It has become increasingly difficult to accept that it is only the most severely affected children, those who die, in whom alveolar development is severely compromised. Surviving adults who were treated for BPD in the 1970s had more respiratory tract infections and wheezing episodes than did age-matched controls, whether they were born prematurely or at term (63). These patients, who were studied by Northway et al. and presented in a 1990 report (63) had a reduction of 25–50% in the mean values of a range of lung function tests, and more than 50% of patients appeared to have airway obstruction. Some of these functional abnormalities no doubt reflect the bronchial and bronchiolar damage sustained by these patients treated so long ago. In an attempt to discover the outcome of BPD when the injury was less severe, baboons were delivered prematurely and treated with hyperoxic ventilation for 21 days and then sacrificed 33 weeks later (64). The lungs showed reduced alveolarization, with enlarged, ''unclassifiable'' air spaces. In the human lung, most alveoli are formed during late fetal life and during the first 2 years of postnatal life, and the lungs of babies who have survived and have been relatively well at a time when the potential for rapid alveolar development is at its highest, still have too few alveoli (65). There is a discrepancy between airway and alveolar development, because airway diameter is generally normal for postconceptional age.

It is difficult to distinguish the effect of treatment from the effect of the primary disease process. The lungs invariably show areas of overexpanded and grossly underexpanded saccular or incompletely alveolarized air spaces. This appearance might be explained by an initial, irregular loss of normal epithelial and endothelial function, leading to greater impairment of surfactant activity in one region than another. Well-ventilated areas of lung would then be exposed to the effects of mechanical ventilation and hyperoxia, whereas nonventilated areas would be hypoxic. Hypoxia is associated with an increase in fibroblast and pulmonary arterial smooth-muscle expression of mRNAs for proelastin and procollagens, and increased net synthesis and deposition of connective tissue (66).

Effects of Mechanical Ventilation on Lung Development

Mechanical ventilation appears to have a profound effect on lung development. When examined at autopsy by quantitative morphometric techniques, the lungs of mechanically ventilated premature infants have fewer alveoli and a lower surface area than expected for their lung volume and airway diameter (21). Prematurity, itself, does not seem to disturb lung development. In the absence of neonatal respiratory distress, airway and alveolar development progress normally (67). Respiratory function, FEV_1, and airway reactivity were normal in healthy children who had been born prematurely and studied at 7–12 years of age (68). Moreover, a group of infants who had developed the respiratory distress syndrome, but had not been mechanically ventilated, had normal respiratory function tests at 4–10 months of age (69). But morphological studies have shown that premature infants have, for their postconceptional age, an increase in the amount of bronchial smooth muscle and goblet cells, and that these changes are significantly greater in those who have been ventilated, whether or not they had hyaline membrane disease (21). In adults with chronic obstructive lung disease, elevated airway resistance correlates well with bronchial smooth-muscle volume (70), but not with increased reactivity. In infants who have been mechanically ventilated, airway obstruction and bronchial hyperactivity have been described up to 10 months after birth (69).

Mechanical Ventilation with Superimposed Infection

Many ventilated babies also become infected, further compromising lung development. After birth, all babies have an increase in bronchial smooth muscle, while submucosal gland area and goblet cell numbers increase and the mucus becomes more viscous. All these factors increase the likelihood of acquiring respiratory tract infections, particularly in premature infants with small airways. Ventilated infants have a higher risk of acquiring more frequent and more severe infections than do nonventilated infants (71). When young rats were infected with a parainfluenza type I virus, the infection had a more marked effect on 5-day-old rats in the proliferative stage of lung growth than it did in 25-day-old rats (72,73). Growth of secondary septa into the alveoli was impaired, alveoli were enlarged, and alveolar surface density was reduced. The alveolar growth pattern followed the pattern of viral replication and induced inflammation and was predominantly centriacinar. Airway development was also affected, and terminal bronchiolar diameter was reduced. On recovery, lung growth continued, but did not compensate for the early abnormalities in alveolar and bronchiolar growth, which were associated with increasing respiratory resistance and decreased lung compliance (72,73).

Mechanical Ventilation with Superimposed Hyperoxia

While receiving ventilatory support, the ventilated areas of lung are exposed to relatively high oxygen tensions. Hyperoxia permanently reduces alveolar septation in newborn rats (74,75). Hyperoxia also causes airway hyperresponsiveness in 21-day-old rats (76). Pulmonary diffusion capacity, determined morphometrically, is reduced, airspaces are enlarged, and the alveoli and alveolar ducts are unevenly dilated. Thibeault and co-workers (74) found an increase in gas-exchanging airspace, resting lung volume, and decreased elastic recoil in the midvolume range in rats exposed to hyperoxia from 6 days of age. Dexamethasone has similar effects, and the same group found that the effects of dexamethasone and hyperoxia were additive (74). A high oxygen tension can suppress DNA synthesis and selectively reduce type II cell proliferation, thereby influencing cellular repair (75,77).

The difficulty of disentangling the direct effects of chronic hypoxia from those of treatment, and the complexity of the cellular responses emphasizes the crucial need for continued experimental study.

B. Pulmonary Vascular Development

The syndrome of persistent pulmonary hypertension has a mortality rate of 20–50%; the most common cause of persistent pulmonary hypertension is hypoxia (78). In babies who die soon after birth of persistent pulmonary hypertension precipitated by severe intrauterine or intrapartum hypoxia, without significant parenchymal lung damage, postmortem examination shows thick-walled, undilated respiratory unit arteries. Such vessels are seen in the normal porcine lung during the first 12 hr of life and not later. They are not seen in the lungs of babies dying a noncardiopulmonary death. Their continued presence in babies with persistent pulmonary hypertension suggests that the failure of small precapillary arteries to dilate after birth may be important in the pathogenesis of persistent pulmonary hypertension. In a group of seven apparently healthy fetuses born at term following an obstetric emergency such as accidental hemorrhage, the mean percentage arterial medial thickness [$(2 \times$ medial thickness $\div$ external diameter$) \times 100\%$] between 10 and 32 hr after birth was similar to that seen in normal fetuses (79). In babies who survive for a few days, the medial smooth muscle cells differentiate into a more contractile phenotype than normal, and connective tissue deposition, predominantly elastin and collagen type I, is excessive. The vessels appear to have become fixed in an incompletely dilated state. The pericytes and intermediate cells in the walls of arteries accompanying respiratory bronchioli and alveolar ducts and lying within the alveolar walls differentiate into smooth-muscle cells, and muscle is then said to show abnormal extension along the arterial pathway. The vessel wall is innervated by sympathetic-like vasoconstrictor nerves (38; see Fig. 4). Changes are uniform throughout the lung. Similar changes are present when pulmonary hypertension results from hypoxic lung disease, caused by aspiration of meconium, amniotic fluid and blood, pulmonary infection, pulmonary hemorrhage, and hyaline membrane disease. The entire pulmonary arterial bed is abnormal, but the changes are most severe in the regions of lung showing the greatest parenchymal damage.

Chronic intrauterine ''hypoxia'' in animals produces pulmonary vascular abnormalities similar to those seen in newborn babies who die of persistent pulmonary hypertension. In the offspring of pregnant rats exposed to hypoxia and in lambs undergoing chronic umbilical cord compression, the peripheral pulmonary arteries show medial hypertrophy (80). After birth, the timing of the hypoxic insult determines the structural response, the most marked abnormalities occurring in animals exposed to hypoxia from birth. When newborn pigs were exposed to chronic hypobaric hypoxia (380 torr) from the moment of birth, the endothelial and smooth-muscle cells in the peripheral pulmonary arteries retained their fetal appearance after 3 days (81; Fig. 6). The cells failed to ''spread'' and had a low surface/volume ratio. In animals that were first allowed to adapt normally to extrauterine life in room air and then exposed to hypoxia, the pulmonary arteries did not revert to a fetal appearance (81). However, ultrastructural studies showed that the smooth muscle cells of all animals exposed to hypoxia for 3 days during the first week of life have an increase in contractile myofilament concentration and excessive connective tissue deposition, predominantly collagen type 1. In animals exposed to hypoxia from birth, the connective tissue appeared to fix the arteries in an incompletely dilated state. In animals first exposed to hypoxia from postnatal age of 14 days smooth-muscle cell myofilament concentration did not increase significantly. A longer period of hypoxia is required in older animals to elicit the same response.

In piglets exposed to chronic hypoxia from birth, the initial failure of the smooth-muscle cells to adapt to extrauterine life involves abnormal cytoskeletal remodeling, which appears to mimic the fetal pulmonary hypertensive state (81). In elastic arteries, the transient cytoskeletal disassembly normally seen after birth failed to occur, the cells contained an excessive amount of γ-actin and myosin heavy-chain isoform SM_1 and the total amount of actin, assessed biochemically, did not decrease immediately after birth, as it does in normal animals (see Fig. 5). Immunohistochemical studies revealed accelerated cell differentiation, with an increase in the number of desmin-containing cells and the premature appearance of cells with caldesmon-containing filaments.

In babies, persistent ventilation can harm the pulmonary vasculature as well as the airways. Hyperoxia causes pulmonary vascular remodeling (82,83). In

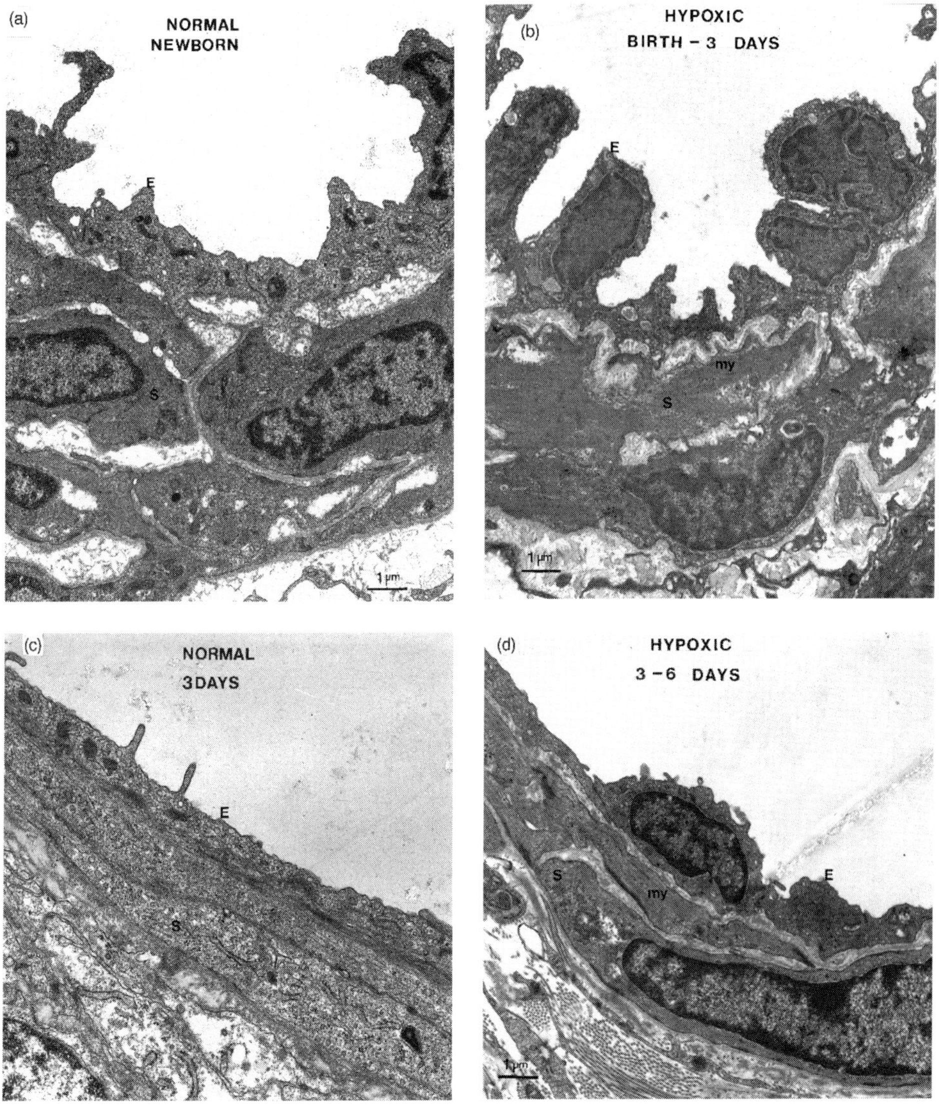

Figure 6 Electronmicrographs of transverse sections of terminal bronchiolar arteries from pigs showing (a) normal at birth, (b) 3-day-old exposed to hypoxia from birth, (c) normal at 3 days, and (d) 6-day-old exposed to hypoxia from 3 days. Note similarity between (a) and (b) and excessive smooth muscle cell myofilaments (my) in (b) and (d); E, endothelium; S, smooth muscle cell.

young rats prolonged hypoxia gives rise to pulmonary hypertension within 7 days, and by 8 days leads to chronic intra-acinar pulmonary arterial medial hypertrophy and a reduction in peripheral arterial number (82,83). On recovery, gas exchange surface area is reduced, but alveolar capillary density increases. In pulmonary hypertension, the development of a thick muscle coat in small precapillary arteries is thought to be due to the differentiation and growth of preexisting pericytes and intermediate cells. In experimental hyperoxia, however, periadventitial fibroblasts migrate into the vessel wall and act as or become, smooth-muscle cells (83).

Premature babies who recover from a neonatal respiratory illness, but then fail to thrive and later die, may have significant structural abnormalities in the pulmonary vasculature, whether or not they have the clinical or pathological features of cor pulmonale. In a recent study, some children died in the first 3 months without recovering from the initial illness, and the morphological findings suggested the presence of persistent pulmonary hypertension (65). Others died at 4–15 months and had a marked increase in pulmonary arterial medial thickness, with extension of muscle into more peripheral arteries than normal. Others died at 6 months with pulmonary hypertension and the clinical features of cor pulmonale (Fig. 7). They had a greater increase in pulmonary arterial muscularity than did those dying at a younger age. Few babies ever have the severe fibrotic pulmonary dysplasia described by Northway et al. (59). In the aforementioned study, however, the amount of bronchial smooth muscle and connective tissue was increased, the alveoli varied in shape and size, and the number of alveoli was reduced (65). Because the ratio of alveoli to arteries was normal, there were fewer than the normal number of peripheral arteries in these children, some of whom had developed cor pulmonale. There seemed to be no difference in the severity of the initial illness between those who later acquired cor pulmonale and those who did not. The later clinical course also varied considerably, although the children with end-stage cor pulmonale had usually survived longer.

In chronic hypoxia with persistent pulmonary hypertension, the pulmonary arteries appear thick-walled and incompletely dilated, and fail to relax normally when exposed to vasodilators. Endothelium-dependent and independent relaxation is impaired in the isolated vessels of chronically hypoxic newborn piglets (46). Exposure to chronic hypobaric hypoxia from birth prevented the normal postnatal establishment of both the receptor-mediated relaxant response to acetylcholine and the nonreceptor-dependent response to the calcium ionophore, calcimycin (A23187) in isolated porcine pulmonary arteries (46). Chronic hypoxia inhibited the established response in animals first exposed to it from either 3 or 14 days of age. Endothelium-dependent relaxation was impaired, despite the presence of abundant endothelial nitric oxide synthase. The explanation is not clear, but an excess of reactive oxygen species might be responsible for inactivat-

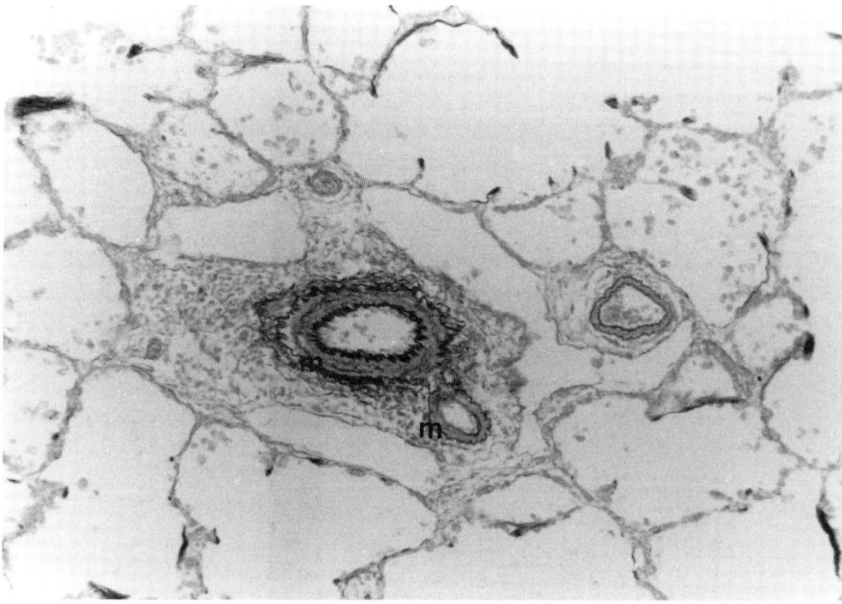

Figure 7 Photomicrograph of lung tissue from a 7-month-old child who died of cor pulmonale, showing a pulmonary artery with thick media (m) and perivascular collagen, and large, but thin-walled alveoli.

ing any nitric oxide released (84). Nitric oxide synthase activates soluble guanylate cyclase (85). Relaxation of chronically hypoxic newborn pulmonary arteries to atrial natriuretic peptide, which activates particulate guanylate cyclase, was not impaired. Studying endothelium-independent relaxation, the relaxant response of the smooth-muscle cells to exogenous nitric oxide and phosphodiesterase inhibitors was attenuated, despite an appropriate increase in cGMP generation. This suggests a block in the relaxation pathway distal to cGMP generation. Basal generation of cGMP, normally higher at birth than subsequently, was not attenuated by exposure to chronic hypoxia in newborn pigs, nor is it attenuated in chronically hypoxic adult rats. The relaxant response to the KATP channel agonist levcromakalim was not impaired, and the sensitivity to levcromakalim was increased in resistance arteries (47). Thus, chronic hypoxia selectively impairs certain relaxation pathways while sparing others. In the adult rat lung, smooth-muscle cells of different phenotypes show a predominance of different potassium channels (86). Within the vessel wall, radioligand-binding studies show that not all smooth-muscle cells have the same receptors. The relation between the effect

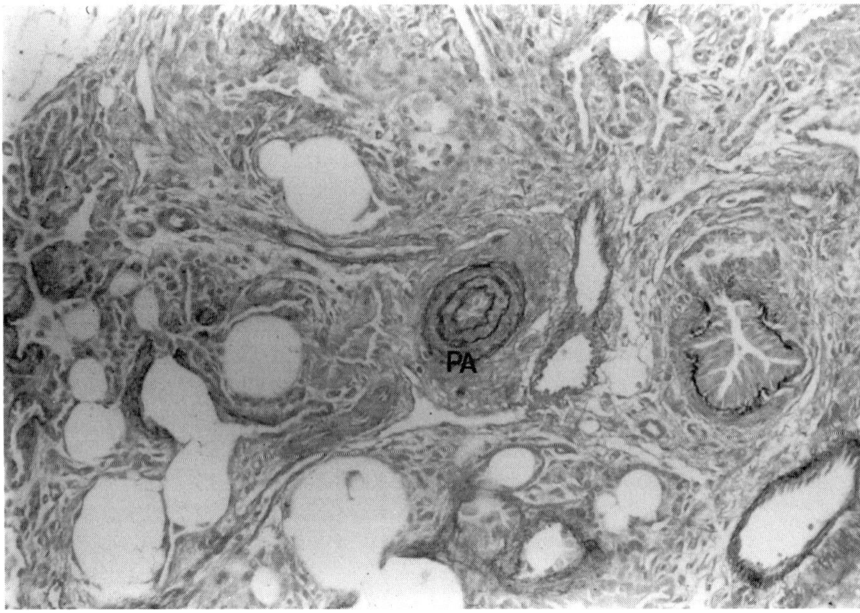

Figure 8 Photomicrograph of lung tissue taken at 6 weeks of age from a term baby showing pulmonary dysplasia and evidence of severe pulmonary hypertension after 6 weeks of NO therapy. Pulmonary artery (PA) shows severe medial hypertrophy (magnification × 200).

of chronic hypoxia on the different pulmonary arterial smooth-muscle cell phenotypes of the newborn lung and the reactivity of each of these phenotypes is yet to be established.

In clinical practice, the management of babies with persistent pulmonary hypertension has been revolutionized by nitric oxide. Failure to respond is usually due to extensive parenchymal lung disease. Failure to sustain an initial response to nitric oxide can be due to pulmonary hypoplasia and dysplasia (87; Fig. 8). Failure of normal alveolarization is seen on lung biopsies and at autopsy. Thick interstitial walls separate saccules, rather than alveoli, ''alveolar'' counts are reduced, and tall columnar epithelium is seen, inappropriately lining distal airways. Babies who do respond satisfactorily to NO may be difficult to wean from NO, and this can be associated with failure to sustain adequate generation of cGMP (88).

On recovery, the structural and functional abnormalities return to normal more slowly in animals exposed to hypoxia from birth than in those that are first allowed to adapt normally to extrauterine life (89). In piglets recovering from chronic hypoxia, after 6 days the pulmonary arterial muscularity had decreased significantly in all animals, but was still greater than normal in those exposed from birth. Endothelium-dependent and independent relaxation returned to normal more slowly in the youngest animals, but was normal by 6 days, although the peripheral pulmonary arteries were still abnormally thick-walled. The contractile response to $PGF_{2\alpha}$ and KCl in normal newborn isolated intrapulmonary arteries is less than it is in adults, and chronic hypoxic remodeling did not increase contractility. The contractile response did, however, increase during recovery, irrespective of the age of the animal.

Exposure to chronic hypoxia probably alters the density and distribution of many vasoactive receptors and changes their signal transduction pathways, modifying the changes that normally take place after birth. For example, the density of ETA receptors on the pulmonary arterial smooth-muscle cells of chronically hypoxic newborn pigs increases and on recovery remains high for some time on the muscular pulmonary arteries of animals exposed to hypoxia from birth, decreasing more rapidly in older animals (90; Fig. 9). The ETB receptors, which appear transiently at postnatal day 3 in the normal lung (exogenous endothelin vasodilates the newborn porcine isolated perfused lung; 91), fail to appear in the hypoxic lung, nor do they appear on recovery (90). Their absence during hypoxic exposure might contribute to impaired endothelium-dependent relaxation by the nitric oxide pathway.

IV. The Future: Where Do We Go from Here?

In both the airways and pulmonary vasculature, our understanding of normal adaptation to extrauterine life and early postnatal development is so deficient that it is difficult to identify the early crucial factors that are altered by chronic hypoxia and that instigate the cascade of abnormal structural and functional changes. These changes become increasingly difficult to reverse with the passage of time. During the acute illness, the effects of chronic hypoxia must be distinguished from the effects of treatment. We need to understand how chronic hypoxia alters the contractile and cytoskeletal apparatus of both bronchial and pulmonary vascular smooth muscle, and how these and other abnormalities of structural remodeling translate into functional disturbances. The interaction between epithelium and bronchial smooth muscle, between endothelium and vascular smooth muscle cells, and the crosstalk that must occur between airway and vasculature during postnatal lung development needs close scrutiny. Decreased lung compliance and increased airways resistance is a feature of pulmonary hypertension in older children. Understanding the potential for structural and functional recovery will determine what we could hope to achieve in practice. Enhancing alveolar and peripheral arterial multiplication and extending the phase of rapid postnatal

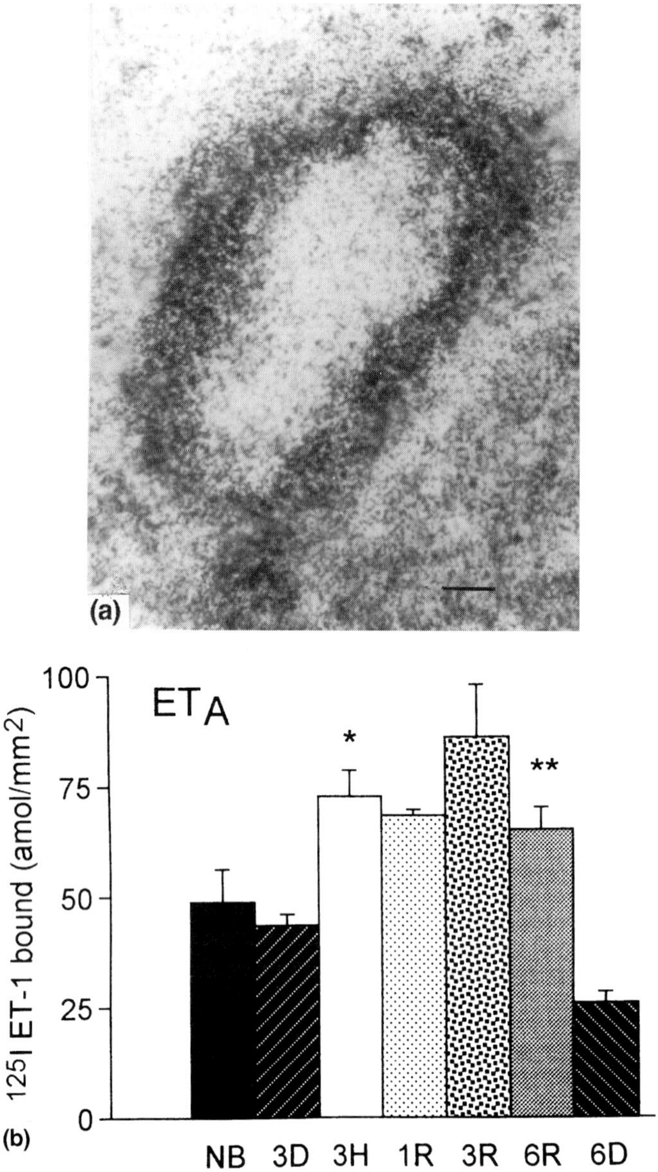

Figure 9 Endothelin receptors in newborn porcine pulmonary arteries: (a) Photomicrograph of muscular pulmonary artery from normal newborn after incubation with ^{125}I ET-1 and exposure to photographic emulsion, showing silver grains only over media; bar, 67 μm. (b) Mean density of ^{125}I ET-1 binding in the presence of the ETB agonist sarafatoxin 6c, demonstrating density of ETA receptors.

development would improve long-term outcome, and is feasible. Transplantation of an immature lung into a healthy adult animal will make the native, recipient mature lung form new arteries and alveoli (92). We need to understand the signaling mechanisms that determine lung growth to promote these changes at will.

References

1. Boyden EA. The time lag in the development of bronchial arteries. Anat Rec 1970; 166:611–614.
2. Congdon ED. Transformation of the aortic-arch system during the development of the human embryo. Contrib Embryol 1922; 14:47–110.
3. De Ruiter MC, Gittenberger-De-Groot AC, Rammos S, Poelmann RE. The special status of the pulmonary arch artery in the branchial arch system of the rat. Anat Embryol 1989; 179:319–325.
4. Masters JRW. Epithelial-mesenchymal interaction during lung development: The effect of mesenchymal mass. Dev Biol 1976; 51:98.
5. McGowan SE. Extracellular matrix and the regulation of lung development and repair. FASEB J 1992; 6:2895–2904.
6. Jetten AM. Growth and differentiation factors in tracheobronchial epithelium. Am J Physiol 1991; 260:L361–L373.
7. Peters K, Werner S, Lao Z, Wert S, Whitsett J, Williams L. Targeted expression of a dominant negative FGF receptor blocks branching morphogenesis and epithelial differentiation of the mouse lung. EMBO J 1994; 13:3296–3301.
8. Hislop A, Reid L. Intrapulmonary arterial development during fetal life—branching pattern and structure. J Anat 1972; 113:35–48.
9. Bucher U, Reid L. Development of the intrasegmental bronchial tree: the pattern of branching and development of cartilage at various stages of intra-uterine life. Thorax 1961; 16:207–218.
10. Loosli CG, Hung KS. Development of pulmonary innervation. In: Hodson WA, ed. Development of the Lung. New York: Marcel Dekker, 1977:269.
11. Sharma RK, Jeffery PK. Adrenoreceptors and muscarinic receptors in developing and adult lung [abstr]. Eur Respir J 1989; 281S.
12. Sharma RK, Jeffery PK. Autoradiographic localization of VIP receptors in developing and adult human lung [abstr]. Eur Respir J 1989; 281S.
13. Hislop A, Wigglesworth JS, Desai R. Alveolar development in the human fetus and infant. Early Hum Dev 1986; 13:1–11.
14. Zeltner TB, Caduff JH, Gehr P, Pfenninger J, Burri PH. The postnatal development and growth of the human lung. I. Morphometry. Respir Physiol 1986; 67:247–267.
15. Langston C, Thurlbeck WM. Lung growth and development in late gestation and early postnatal life. In: Rosenberg SG, Bernstein J, ed. Perspectives in Pediatric Pathology. New York: Masson, 1982:203–235.
16. Jeffery PK, Reid L. The ultrastructure of the airway lining and its development. In: Hodson A, ed. The Development of the Lung. New York: Marcel Dekker, 1977: 87–134.

17. Fawcett DW. The Cell. Philadelphia: WB Saunders, 1981.
18. Willems LNA, Kramps JA, Jeffery PK, Dijkman JH. Detection of antileukoprotease in the developing fetal lung. Thorax 1988; 43:784–786.
19. Bucher U, Reid L. Development of the mucus-secreting elements in human lung. Thorax 1961; 16:219–225.
20. De Haller R. Development of mucus-secreting elements. In: Emery J, ed. Anatomy of the Developing Lung. Oxford: Heinemann, 1969:94.
21. Hislop AA, Haworth SG. Airway size and structure in the normal fetal and infant lung and the effect of premature delivery and artificial ventilation. Am Rev Respir Dis 1989; 140:1717–1726.
22. Tos M. Development of the mucous glands in the human main bronchus. Anat Anz 1968; 376–389.
23. Cutz E, Gillan JE, Track MS. Pulmonary endocrine cells in developing human lung and during neonatal adaptation. In: Becker KL, Gazdar AF, ed. Endocrine Lung in Health and Disease. Philadelphia: WB Saunders, 1984:210.
24. Stahlman MT, Castleburg AG, Orth DN, Gray NM. Ontogeny of neuroendocrine cells in human fetal lung. An immunohistochemical study. Lab Invest 1985; 52:52–60.
25. Lauweryns JM, Cokelaere M. Hypoxia-sensitive neuro-epithelial bodies: intrapulmonary secretory neuro-receptors modulated by the CNS. Z Microsk Anat Forsch 1973; 145:521–540.
26. Panitch HB, Wolfson MR, Shaffer TH. Epithelial modulation of preterm airway smooth muscle contraction. J Appl Physiol 1993; 74:1437–1443.
27. Vanhoutte PM. Airway epithelium and bronchial reactivity. Can J Physiol Pharmacol 1987; 65:448–450.
28. Zue QF, Maurer R, Engel G. Selective distribution of beta- and $alpha_1$-adrenoreceptors in rat lung visualized by autoradiography. Arch Int Pharmacodyn Ther 1983; 266:308–314.
29. McCray PBJ. Spontaneous contractility of human fetal airway smooth muscle. Am J Respir Cell Mol Biol 1993; 8:573–580.
30. Allen K, Haworth SG. Cytoskeletal features of immature pulmonary vascular smooth muscle cells and the influence of pulmonary hypertension on normal human development. J Pathol 1989; 158:311–317.
31. Hislop A, Wharton J, Allen K, Polak J, Haworth S. Immunohistochemical localisation of peptide-containing nerves in the airways of normal young children. Am J Respir Cell Mol Biol 1990; 3:191–198.
32. Tepper RS. Airway reactivity in infants: a positive response to metacholine and metaproterenol. J Appl Physiol 1987; 62:1155–1159.
33. Murphy TM, Mitchell RW, Halayko A, et al. Effect of maturational changes in myosin content and morphometry on airway smooth muscle contraction. Am J Physiol 1991; 260:L471–L480.
34. Ikeda K, Mitchell RW, Guest KA, et al. Ontogeny of shortening velocity in porcine trachealis. Am J Physiol 1992; 262:L280–L285.
35. Murphy TM, Mitchell RW, Blake JS, et al. Expression of airway contractile properties and acetylcholinesterase activity in swine. J Appl Physiol 1989; 67:174–180.
36. Haxhiu-Poskurica B, Ernsberger P, Haxhiu MA, Miller MJ, Cattarossi L, Martin RJ.

Development of cholinergic innervation and muscarinic receptor subtypes in piglet trachea. Am J Physiol 1993; 8:L606–L614.
37. Murphy TM, Roy L, Phillips IJ, Mithcell RW, Kelly EA, Munoz NM, et al. Effect of maturation on topographic distribution of bronchoconstrictor responses in large diameter airways of young swine. Am Rev Respir Dis 1991; 143:126–131.
38. Allen KM, Wharton J, Polak JM, Haworth SG. A study of nerves containing peptides in the pulmonary vasculature of healthy infants and children and of those with pulmonary hypertension. Br Heart J 1989; 62:353–360.
39. Hall S, Haworth SG. Conducting pulmonary arteries: structural adaptation to extra-uterine life in the pig. Cardiovasc Res 1986; 21:208–216.
40. Allen K, Haworth SG. Human postnatal pulmonary arterial remodelling: ultrastructural studies of smooth muscle cell and connective tissue maturation. Lab Invest 1988; 59:702–709.
41. Teitel D, Iwamoto H, Rudolph A. Effects of birth-related events on central blood flow patterns. Pediatr Res 1987; 22:557–566.
42. Hall SM, Haworth SG. Normal adaptation of pulmonary arterial intima to extrauterine life in the pig: ultrastructural studies. J Pathol 1986; 149:55–66.
43. Abman SH, Chatfield BA, Hall SL, McMurtry IF. Role of endothelium-derived relaxing factor during transition of pulmonary circulation at birth. Am J Physiol 1990; 259:H1921–H1927.
44. Halbower AC, Tuder RM, Franklin WA, Pollock JS, Forstermann U, Abman SH. Maturation-related changes in endothelial nitric oxide synthase immunolocalization in developing ovine lung. Am J Physiol Lung Cell Mol Physiol 1994; L585–L591.
45. Hislop AA, Springall DR, Buttery LDK, Pollock JS, Haworth SG. Abundance of endothelial nitric oxide synthase in newborn intrapulmonary arteries. Arch Dis Child 1995; 12:F17–F21.
46. Tulloh RMR, Hislop AA, Boels PJ, Deutsch J, Haworth SG. Chronic hypoxia inhibits postnatal maturation of porcine intrapulmonary artery relaxation. Am J Physiol 1997; 272:H2436–H2445.
47. Boels PJ, Gao B, Deutsch J, Haworth SG. K^+(ATP)-channel activation in isolated normal and hypertensive newborn and adult porcine pulmonary vessels. Pediatr Res 1997; 42:1–10.
48. Levy M, Tulloh R, Komai H, Stuart-Smith K, Haworth SG. Maturation of the contractile response and its endothelial modulation in newborn porcine intrapulmonary arteries. Pediatr Res 1995; 38:25–29.
49. Rubanyi GM, McKinney M, Vanhoutte PM. Biphasic release of endothelium-derived releasing factor(s) by acetylcholine from perfused canine femoral arteries. Characterisation of muscarinic receptors. J Pharmacol Exp Ther 1987; 240:802–808.
50. Hislop AA, Zhao YD, Springall DR, Polak JM, Haworth SG. Postnatal changes in endothelin-1 binding in porcine pulmonary vessels and airways. Am J Respir Cell Mol Biol 1995; 12:557–566.
51. Mortola JP, Frappell PB, Frappel DE, Villena-Cabrera N, Villena-Cabrera M, Pena F. Ventilation and gaseous metabolism in infants born at high altitude, and their responses to hyperoxia. Am Rev Respir Dis 1992; 146:1206–1212.
52. Vargas E, Beard J, Haas J, Cudkowicz L. Pulmonary diffusing capacity in young Andean highland children. Respiration 1982; 43:330–335.

53. Faridy E, Sanii MR, Thilveris JA. Fetal lung growth: influence of maternal hypoxia and hyperoxia in rats. Respir Physiol 1988; 73:225–242.
54. Larson JE, Thurlbeck WM. The effect of experimental maternal hypoxia on fetal lung growth. Pediatr Res 1988; 24:156–159.
55. Piazza T, Lauzon AM, Mortola JP. Time course of adaptation to hypoxia in newborn rats. Can J Physiol Pharmacol 1988; 66:152–158.
56. Faridy EE, Yang WZ. Role of hyperventilation and hypoxia on lung growth in rats. Respir Physiol 1989; 76:179–190.
57. Anderson WR, Engle RR. Cardiopulmonary sequelae of reparative stages of bronchopulmonary dysplasia. Arch Pathol Lab Med 1983; 107:603–608.
58. Askin F. Respiratory tract disorders in the fetus and neonates. In: Wigglesworth J, Singer DB, eds. Textbook of Fetal and Perinatal Pathology. Oxford: Blackwell Scientific, 1991:643–688.
59. Northway WH, Rosan RC, Porter DY. Pulmonary disease following respiratory therapy of hyaline membrane disease: bronchopulmonary dysplasia. N Engl J Med 1967; 276:357–368.
60. Chambers HM, van Velzen D. Ventilatory related pathology in the extremely immature lung. Pathology 1989; 21:79–83.
61. van Leirde S, Cornelis A, Devlieger H. Different patterns of pulmonary sequelae after hyaline membrane disease: heterogeneity of bronchopulmonary dysplasia. Biol Neonate 1991; 60:152–162.
62. Margraf LR, Tomashefski JFJ, Bruce MC, Dhams BB. Morphometric analysis of the lung in bronchopulmonary dysplasia. Am Rev Respir Dis 1991; 141:391–400.
63. Northway WH, Moss RB, Carlisle KB, et al. Late pulmonary sequelae of bronchopulmonary dysplasia. N Engl J Med 1990; 323:1793–1799.
64. Coalson JJ, Winter V, Delemos RA. Decreased alveolarization in baboon survivors with bronchopulmonary dysplasia. Am J Respir Crit Care Med 1995; 152:640–646.
65. Hislop A, Haworth S. Pulmonary vascular damage in the development of cor pulmonale following hyaline membrane disease. Pediatr Pulmonol 1990; 9:152–161.
66. Stenmark KR, Aldashev AA, Orton EC, et al. Cellular adaptation during chronic neonatal hypoxic pulmonary hypertension. Am J Physiol 1991; 261:97–104.
67. Hislop A, Wigglesworth JS, Desai R, Aber V. The effects of preterm delivery and mechanical ventilation on human lung growth. Early Hum Dev 1987; 15:147–164.
68. Bertrand JM, Riley SP, Popkin J, Coates AL. The longterm pulmonary sequelae of prematurity: the role of familial airway reactivity and the respiratory distress syndrome. N Engl J Med 1986; 312:742–745.
69. Stocks J, Godfrey S, Reynolds EOR. Airway resistance in infants after various treatments for hyaline membrane disease: special emphasis on prolonged high levels of inspired oxygen. Pediatrics 1978; 61:178–183.
70. Dalquen P, Oberholzer M, Wyss H, Specht H, Rohr HP, Herzog H. Bronchus morphometry: correlations between morphometric data and lung function parameters in obstructive airway disease. Respiration 1977; 34:121–130.
71. Myers MG, McGuinness GA, Lachenbruch PA, Koontz FP, Hollingshead R, Olson DB. Respiratory illnesses in survivors of infant respiratory distress syndrome. Am Rev Respir Dis 1986; 133:1011–1018.

72. Castleman WL, Sorkness RL, Lemanske RF, Grassee G, Suyemoto MM. Neonatal viral bronchiolitis and pneumonia induces bronchiolar hypoplasia and alveolar dysplasia in rats. Lab Invest 1988; 59:387–396.
73. Castleman WL, Brundage-Anguish LJ, Kreitzer L, Neuenschwander SB. Pathogenesis of bronchiolitis and pneumonia induced in neonatal and weanling rats by parainfluenza (Sendai) virus. Am J Pathol 1987; 129:277–286.
74. Thibeault DW, Heimes B, Rezaiekhaligh M, Mabry S. Chronic modifications of lung and heart development in glucocorticoid-treated newborn rats exposed to hyperoxia or room air. Pediatr Pulmonol 1993; 16:81–88.
75. Massaro D, Teich N, Maxwell S, Massaro GD, Whitney P. Postnatal development of alveoli: regulation and evidence for a critical period in rats. J Clin Invest 1985; 1297–1305.
76. Hershenson MB, Aghili S, Punjabi N, et al. Hyperoxia-induced airway hyperresponsiveness and remodelling in immature rats. Am J Physiol 1992; 6:L236–L269.
77. Blanco LN, Massaro GD, Massaro D. Alveolar dimensions and number: developmental and hormonal regulation. Am J Physiol 1989; 257:L240–L247.
78. Fox WW, Duara S. Persistent pulmonary hypertension in the neonate: diagnosis and management. J Pediatr 1983; 103:505–514.
79. Haworth SG, Godman MJ, Marquis RM, ed. Pulmonary vascular structure in persistent fetal circulation. In: Paediatric Cardiology. Heart Disease in the Newborn. Edinburgh: Churchill Livingstone, 1979:67–78.
80. Soifer SJ, Kaslow D, Roman C, Heymann MA. Umbilical cord compression produces pulmonary hypertension in newborn lambs: a model to study the pathophysiology of persistent pulmonary hypertension in the newborn. J Dev Physiol 1987; 9: 239–252.
81. Allen KM, Haworth SG. Impaired adaptation of pulmonary circulation to extrauterine life in newborn pigs exposed to hypoxia: an ultrastructural study. J Pathol 1986; 150:205–212.
82. Jones R, Zapol WM, Reid L. Pulmonary artery remodeling and pulmonary hypertension after exposure to hyperoxia for 7 days. A morphometric and hemodynamic study. Am J Pathol 1984; 117:273–285.
83. Jones R. Ultrastructural analysis of contractile cell development in lung microvessels in hyperoxic pulmonary hypertension. Am J Pathol 1992; 141:1491–1505.
84. Vanhoutte PM, Rubanyi GM, Miller VM, Houston DS. Modulation of vascular smooth muscle contraction by the endothelium. Annu Rev Physiol 1986; 48:307–320.
85. Ignarro LJ, Byrns RE, Wood KS. Endothelium-dependent modulation of cGMP levels and intrinsic smooth muscle tone in isolated bovine intrapulmonary artery and vein. Circ Res 1987; 60:82–92.
86. Archer SL, Hampl V, Reeve HL, Huang JMC, Tolarova S, Michelakis E, et al. Regional diversity of vascular myocyte K channel types between conduit and resistance arteries explains vascular reactivity to hypoxia and nitric oxide. Circulation 1995; 92:I635 Abstract.
87. Goldman AP, Tasker RC, Haworth SG, Sigston RE, Macrae DJ. Four patterns of response to inhaled nitric oxide for primary pulmonary hypertension of the newborn. Pediatrics 1996; 98(4 pt 1): 706–713

88. Goldman AP, Haworth SG, Macrae DJ. Does inhaled nitric oxide suppress endogenous nitric oxide production? Cardiovasc Thorac Surg 1996; 12:541–542.
89. Tulloh RMR, Hislop AA, Haworth SG. Increased pulmonary vascular reactivity on recovery from neonatal pulmonary hypertension. Am J Respir Crit Care Med 1995; 151:A517.
90. Noguchi Y, Hislop AA, Haworth SG. Influence of hypoxia on endothelin-1 binding sites in neonatal porcine pulmonary vasculature. Am J Physiol 1997; 272:H669–H678.
91. Perreault T, De Marte J. Endothelin-1 has a dilator effect on neonatal pig pulmonary vasculature. J Cardiovasc Pharmacol 1991; 18:43–50.
92. Hislop AA, Rinaldi M, Lee R, McGregor CGA, Haworth SG. Growth of the immature lung transplanted into an adult recipient. Am J Physiol 1993; 264(1 pt 1): L60–L65.

26

Altered Development of the Pulmonary Circulation in Chronic Lung Injury

MARLENE RABINOVITCH

University of Toronto
The Hospital for Sick Children
Toronto, Ontario, Canada

I. Introduction

It is not possible to step twice into the same river
Heraclitus, circa 540–480 BC

The ancient Greek philosophers appreciated the difficulties inherent in trying to unravel dynamic processes in nature. In developmental biology, the dynamics are equally complex, with a host of cell–cell, cell–matrix interactions all occurring at the same time. The superimposition of disease further complicates the process. Despite this, there have been many recent advances in uncovering the mechanisms that underlie perturbations in lung vascular development in association with chronic lung injury (CLI). Clinical and experimental studies have related morphological abnormalities in vascular growth and maturation to a host of etiologic factors that include infection, hypoxia, hyperoxia (oxygen toxicity), airway pressure-induced trauma, and high blood flow and pressure. Recent studies have identified common cellular and molecular features that provide new therapeutic targets.

II. Structural Changes in Pulmonary Arteries

Regardless of etiology, the structural changes that occur in the pulmonary arteries are similar and represent disease superimposed on abnormal development. When vessels are landmarked according to the airway they accompany, those in the acinus in the newborn (i.e., associated with respiratory bronchioli) are partially muscular, and arteries accompanying alveolar ducts and alveolar walls are normally nonmuscular (1). Vessels become more muscular as they increase in external diameter, but normally those associated with the alveoli remain nonmuscular or only partially muscular, even in adulthood. In response to chronic lung injury there is abnormal extension of muscle into peripheral arteries that are normally nonmuscular, so that vessels accompanying the alveolar ducts and alveoli, even as small as 15-μm–external diameter, are often muscularized. This inappropriate muscularization results from abnormal differentiation of precursor cells (pericytes and intermediate cells) into mature smooth-muscle cells (2; Fig. 1), and there also appears to be recruitment of fibroblasts, which differentiate into smooth-muscle cells (3,4).

Under normal conditions, muscular arteries dilate very early in the postnatal period; thus, beginning with the smallest vessels (< 250 μm) at 4 days and extending to those at the hilum by 4 months, the wall thickness, as a percentage of the external diameter, is at adult level. This is in keeping with the regression of right ventricular dominance by 4 months. There may be some loss of muscle cells, but the reduction of vessel diameter is largely a function of dilation and reorganization of the cells and connective tissue compartments (5; Fig. 2). With chronic lung injury, there is not only failure of the normal process of medial thinning, but also there is medial hypertrophy of normally muscular arteries. This feature may be in response to the hemodynamic effects of vasoconstriction, or the increased resistance produced by a muscularized peripheral pulmonary vascular bed. Medial hypertrophy usually reflects an increase in the size and number of vascular smooth-muscle cells and an increase in the intercellular connective tissue components (e.g., elastin, collagen, glycosaminoglycans; 2). In addition, there is frequently a reduction in the number of small peripheral arteries, which may be the result of failure of these vessels to grow normally, or loss of vessels from either resorption, or from destruction of lung parenchyma.

III. Acute and Chronic Infection

Various clinical studies have related pre- and postnatal infections to the development of chronic lung disease (6). In experimental studies, these pathogens directly and indirectly induce changes in pulmonary vascular endothelium, smooth-muscle cells, and fibroblasts, and impede the normal process of growth and devel-

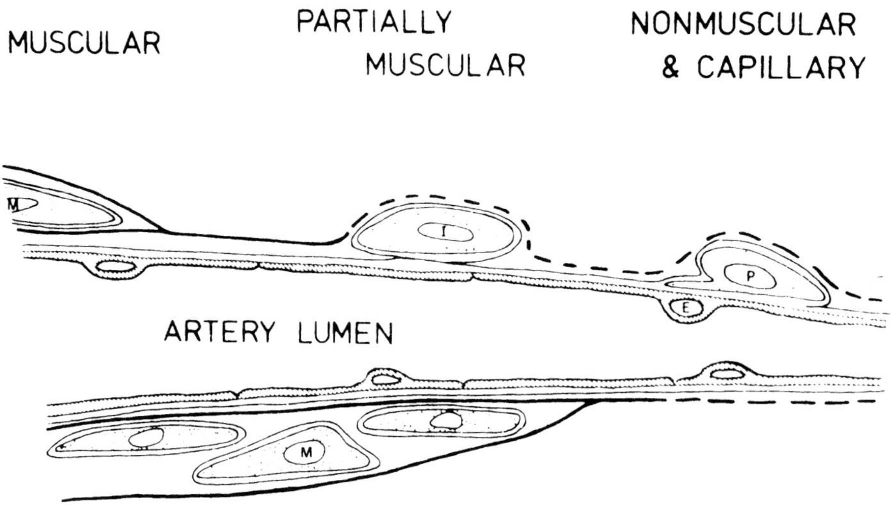

Figure 1 Diagrammatic representation of the cells in the wall of the distal part of a rat pulmonary artery: The smooth-muscle cells (M) of the medial muscular coat are surrounded by a discrete basement membrane and are situated between both an internal and external elastic lamina (thick black lines). In the nonmuscular regions of the partially muscular artery, the "intermediate" cell (I) is seen. This cell is surrounded by a basement membrane that fuses, in some regions, with that of the endothelial cell-(E) and is situated internal to the single fragmented internal elastic lamina (broken line). Thus, it has an intimal position. The pericyte (P) is in the wall of the nonmuscular artery and alveolar capillary. This cell is ensheathed by a basement membrane that is continuous with that of the endothelial cell. Similar to the "intermediate" cell, it is situated internal to the single elastic lamina. With exposure to hypoxia, it is the pericyte and intermediate cell that hypertrophy and divide to form "new" muscle. (From Ref. 62.)

opment of the peripheral lung vasculature. This, coupled with recent work in systemic vascular pathobiology implicating inflammatory cells and the induction of cell surface adhesion molecules, strengthens the potential detrimental influence of infections on the structure of the pulmonary circulation.

Infections may induce alterations in pulmonary vascular reactivity and structural changes in pulmonary arteries that contribute to persistent and progressive elevation in pulmonary vascular resistance. For example, β-streptococcal infection increases pulmonary vascular reactivity in newborn animals (7), as do inflammatory cytokines, such as tumor necrosis factor-alpha (TNF-α; 8,9). The induction of pulmonary hypertensive changes results from repeated injections of

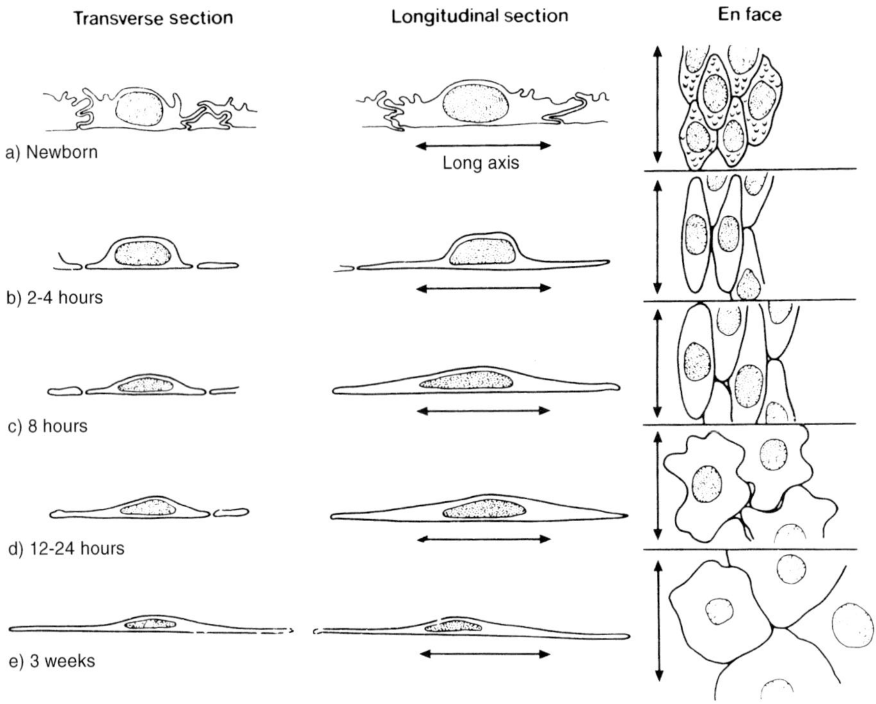

Figure 2 Diagram illustrating en force shape changes in the endothelial cells of non- and partially muscular arteries during the first 3 weeks of life. Two phases of change are illustrated; (a–c) stretching during inflation; (d–e) spreading during dilatation. (From Ref. 5.)

endotoxin in rats (10). These studies have shown extension of muscle into peripheral, normally nonmuscular arteries, medial hypertrophy of muscular arteries, and reduced arterial numbers relative to alveolar number. The direct effects of infectious agents and their by-products are compounded by the secondary changes that result from damage to the lung parenchyma, hypoxia, and parenchymal loss, and by therapeutic regimens that frequently involve ventilator-induced stretch and high oxygen tension.

Infectious agents and the by-products of inflammation may cause an increase in pulmonary artery pressure and resistance, owing to the liberation of vasoactive mediators. On the other hand, there are direct effects on cell function resulting from immune and inflammatory processes that can cause pulmonary vascular remodeling. This is certainly suggested by the development of pulmonary vascular disease in autoimmune disorders, such as scleroderma (11), and experimentally in association with toxins and cytokines (12). We have developed a model in which an immune–inflammatory mechanism stimulates remodeling in coronary arteries, and it is likely that a similar pathophysiology could contribute to remodeling in the pulmonary circulation (13–17). The induction of endothelial injury and the influx of inflammatory cells results in the upregulation of cell surface adhesion molecules (17). These and other endothelial cell surface molecules assure that the inflammatory cells will ''roll'' and adhere to the endothelium and migrate into the subendothelium (18). There is also evidence that influx of inflammatory cells into the adventitia may contribute to invasion of the vessel wall. The inflammatory cells release cytokines, and we have shown that reciprocal coinduction of TNF-α and interleukin-1β (IL-1β) upregulate production of fibronectin, which stimulates both transendothelial migration of T cells (19) and vascular smooth-muscle cell migration (20) into the subendothelium. Serine elastase(s) produced by inflammatory cells and vascular smooth-muscle cells (21) can induce medial hypertrophy by liberating potent smooth-muscle cell mitogens, such as basic fibroblast growth factor (22), that are normally stored in the extracellular matrix in an inactive form attached to proteoglycans. Serine elastases, acting through elastin peptides, can also upregulate production of fibronectin which, in turn, contributes to neointimal formation (23). How inflammation may induce smooth-muscle cell differentiation, which is necessary for the abnormal extension of muscle into peripheral arteries that normally are nonmuscular, is less well understood; although this too may involve protease-mediated liberation of growth factors that are also differentiation factors. In addition, the degradation of matrix and subsequent liberation of matrix peptides (e.g., elastin and fibronectin peptides) may provide highly chemotactic stimuli (24) that could induce migration of fibroblasts and associated differentiation of muscle in peripheral arteries. The mechanism whereby loss of the number of peripheral arteries can be induced by inflammatory stimuli is purely speculative, but conceivably could be related to T-cell-induced apoptosis (25).

The toxin produced by an infectious agent also may have similarities to toxins that induce vascular disease by direct injury to the endothelium. Monocrotaline, which has been studied as a toxin, has been injected experimentally in rats and appears to induce pulmonary vascular changes in neonatal, infant, and adult animals by initiating an endothelial injury (26; Fig. 3). The subsequent cascade of changes in the pulmonary arteries include extension of muscle, medial hypertrophy, and loss of small, peripheral arteries. The working hypothesis is that secondary to endothelial injury, there is loss of the barrier function of the endothelium and, as a direct result of a serum-factor leak or release of endothelial-derived factors from damaged cells, there is induction of elastase activity in vascular smooth muscle cells (27). This has been shown in vitro and appears to involve an intracellular-signaling pathway that involves tyrosine kinase activity, gene transcription, and translation. The elastase then liberates mitogens and in-

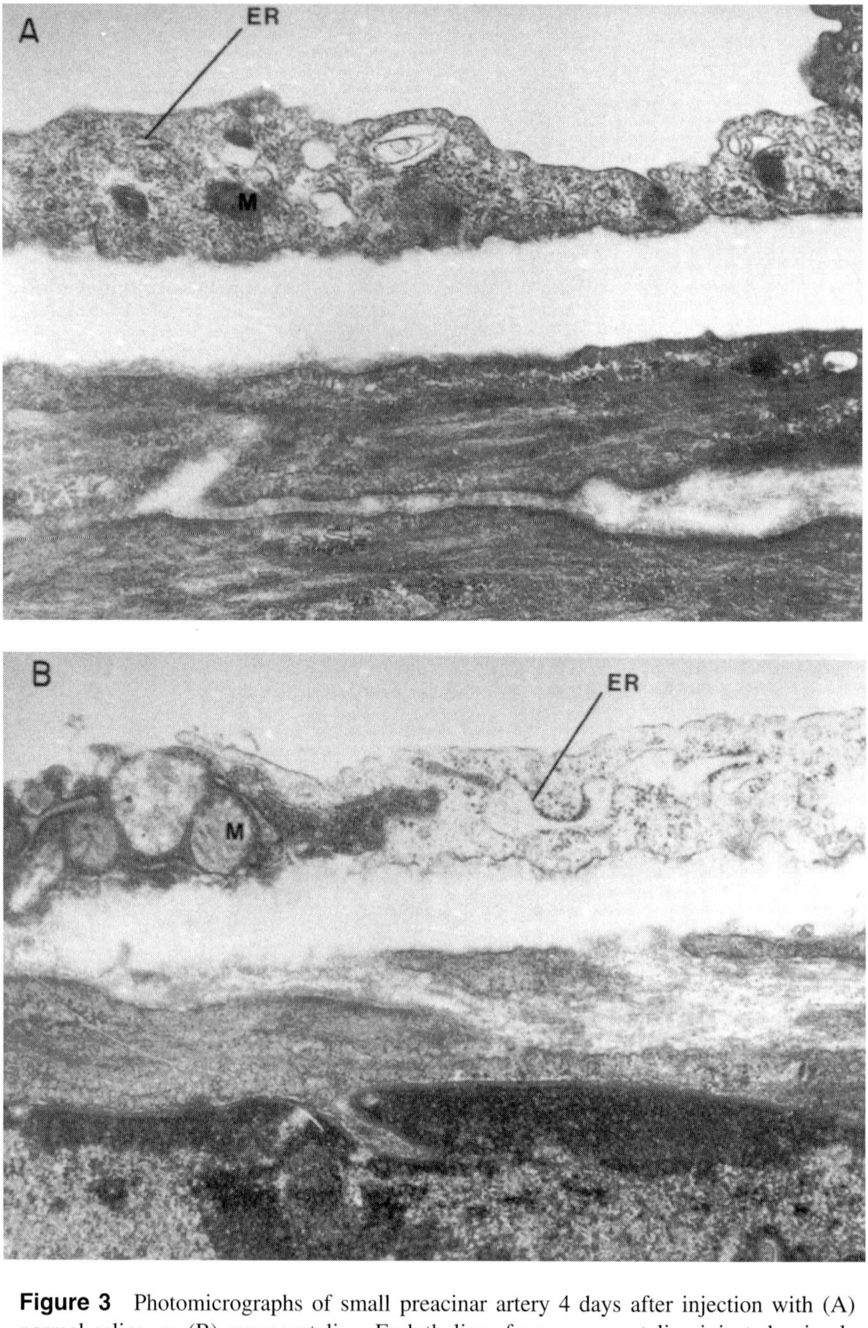

Figure 3 Photomicrographs of small preacinar artery 4 days after injection with (A) normal saline, or (B) monocrotaline. Endothelium from monocrotaline-injected animals appears swollen and less dense. Note swollen mitochondria (M) and dilated endoplasmic reticulum (ER). (From Ref. 26.)

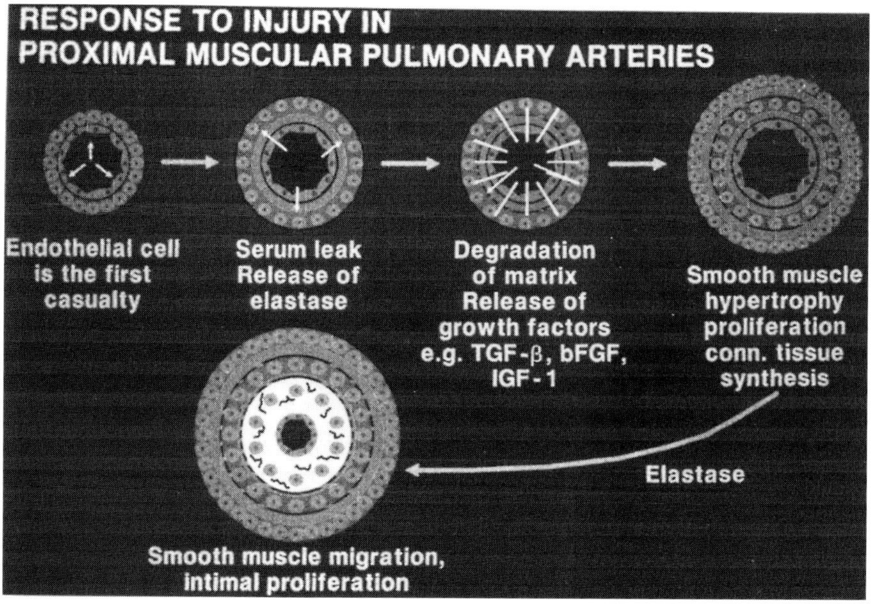

Figure 4 Schema for elastase in the pathogenesis of pulmonary vascular disease: The hypothesis described in the text is related to structural features associated with progressive elevation in pulmonary artery pressure and resistance. (From Ref. 63.)

duces smooth-muscle cell changes that have been previously described (Fig. 4). The imbalance between elastases and elastase inhibitors is most apparent when the toxin is given to neonatal rats, since there is emphysema, perhaps as a result of elastolytic activity in a rapidly developing lung. Infant rats that receive the toxin show lack of progression of their vascular disease when compared with adult rats in which the injury is malignant, causing right ventricular hypertrophy and heart failure (28). This age-related difference may be due to a more persistent increased activity of the adipsin-related serine elastase in the adult rat (29).

Hypoxia-induced pulmonary hypertension, which is nonprogressive and potentially reversible, is also associated with an early increase in elastase activity before vascular changes develop, but there is no persistent increase in elastase activity once medial hypertrophy has occurred (30; Fig. 5). Moreover, inhibition of the early increase in elastase activity prevents later development of pulmonary vascular abnormalities. Administration of elastase inhibitors to monocrotaline-injected adult rats following the development of medial hypertrophy prevents the

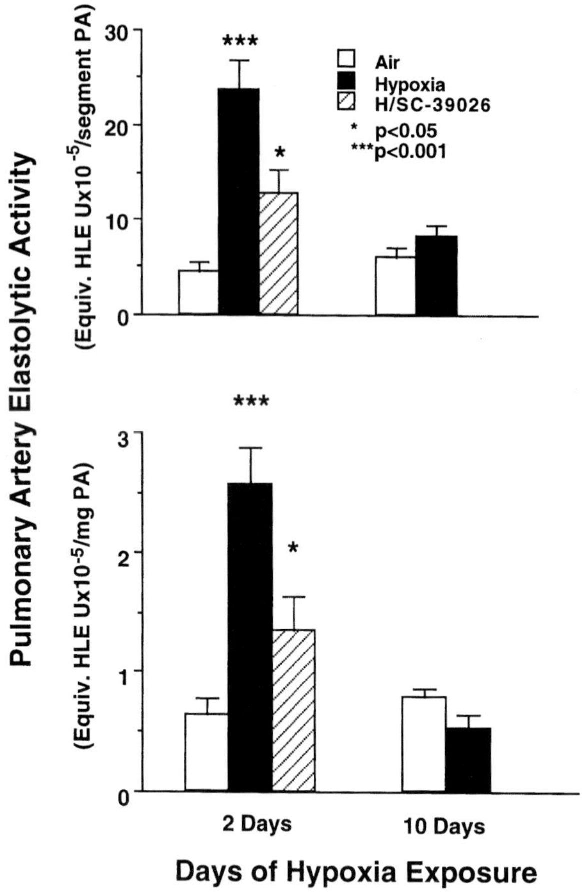

Figure 5 Elastolytic activity in central pulmonary arteries after hypoxia exposure. Elastolytic activity expressed per pulmonary artery segment (seg/PA) as units (U) of human neutrophil (leukocyte) elastase (HLE) standard. Values from vessels of rats that were kept in room air are denoted by open bars and values from vessels of hypoxic rats by solid bars. Triplicate assessments were made from eight pooled pulmonary arteries at each time point, and assays were repeated three times at the 2-day and twice at the 10-day time points. Bars are means ± SE from nine values at 2 days and from six values at 10 days. There were three values obtained from pooled arteries from eight elastose inhibitor SC-39026 (SC-1)-treated hypoxic rats (hatched bar). Significantly higher elastolytic activity is evident in vessels from rats after 2 days of hypoxia when compared with normoxia control animals (***$p < 0.001$), but values are significantly reduced in hypoxia SC-1 rats (*$p < 0.05$). Values from hypoxia and normoxia rats at 10 days are similar to 2-day controls. (From Ref. 30.)

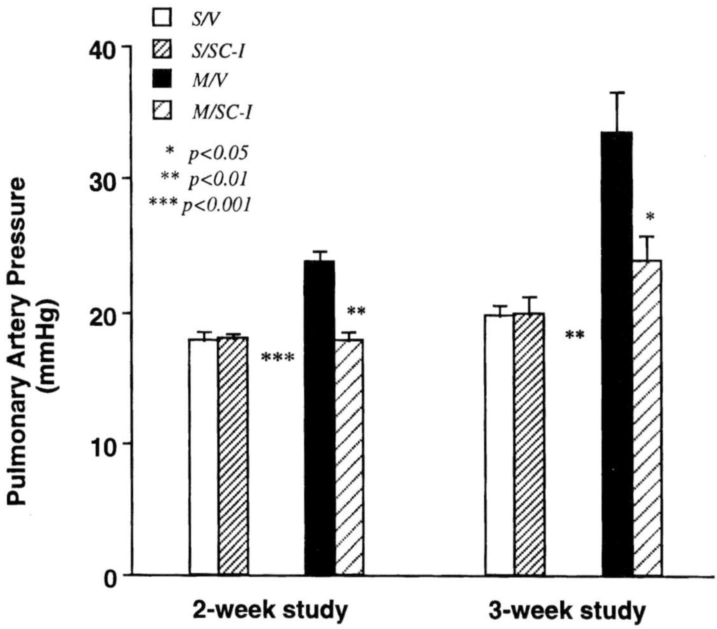

Figure 6 Mean pulmonary artery pressures: S, saline; V, vehicle; SC-1 (elastase inhibitor), SC-37698 (2 mg/day in 2-week study and 3 mg/day in 3-week study); M, monocrotaline. Two-week study: S/V ($n = 6$), M/V ($n = 7$), M/SC-1 ($n = 6$). Three-week study: S/V ($n = 3$), S/SC-1 ($n = 3$), M/V ($n = 6$), M/SC-1 ($n = 6$). Values are means ± SE. (From Ref. 31.)

associated increase of elastase activity and, thereby, retards the progression of vascular changes (31; Fig. 6).

The increase in elastase activity observed with progressive disease may also be a function of inactivation or a lack of a naturally occurring inhibitor. The naturally occurring inhibitor of the endogenous vascular elastase may be elafin. Elafin is a highly specific serine elastase inhibitor that is naturally found in bronchial secretions and in the skin (32). We have shown that elafin is expressed in the developing vasculature and lung and is prevalent throughout neonatal and adult life in the experimental animal (unpublished observations).

Recent studies have also implicated induction of the extracellular matrix glycoprotein, tenascin, in the pathophysiology of (33), pulmonary vascular changes in patients with congenital heart defects in experimental rats with monocrotaline-induced pulmonary hypertension (34). Tenascin expression colocalizes

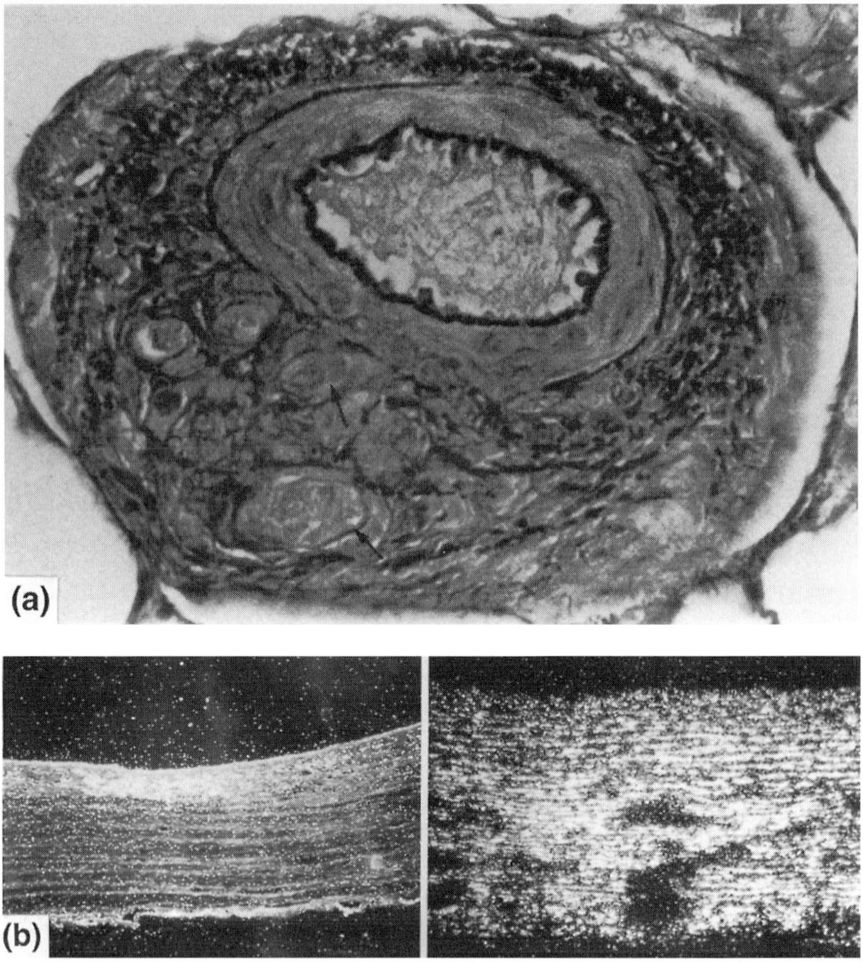

Figure 7 (a) An artery from the lung of a 2-week-old calf raised from birth at a simulated altitude of 4300 m. Pulmonary artery systolic pressure was 100 mgHg. There is marked medial hypertrophy (m) and adventitial thickening with neovascularization (arrow; elastic tissue stain, × 400). (Courtesy of K. Stenmark.) (b) In situ hybridization localization of tropoelastin mRNA in control and hypertensive vessels from neonatal calves. White staining over areas indicates tropoelastin mRNA labeling. In normotensive vessels (left), labeled cells (^{35}S-labeled T66-T7) were confined to the inner media. Minimal signal is noted in the outer vessel wall. In vessels from hypertensive animals (day 14 of hypoxia; right), intense autoradiographic signal was observed throughout the media, albeit in a patchy distribution. (From Ref. 39.)

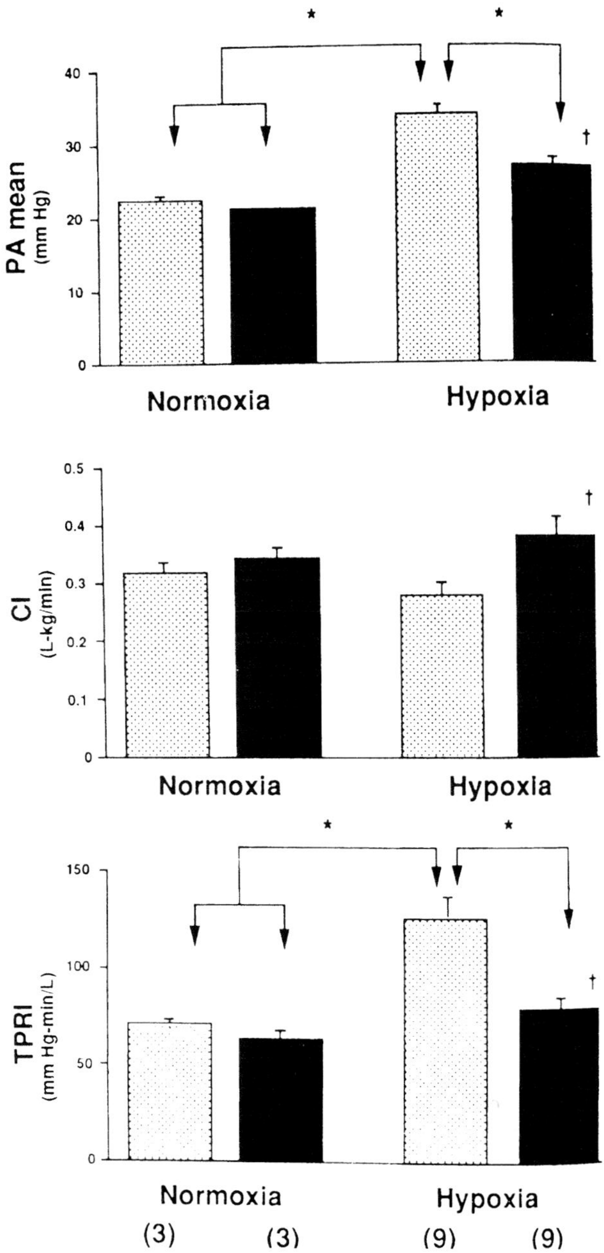

Figure 8 Hemodynamic assessment: Comparisons of pulmonary artery (PA) mean pressure, cardiac index (CI), and total pulmonary resistance index (TPRI) were made in both normoxic and hypoxic rats treated with either saline (stippled bars) or BQ 123 (solid bars) for 2 weeks; $p < 0.05$ from groups as shown † p is not significant from normoxic rats with and without BQ 123 endothelin receptor blocker. (From Ref. 43.)

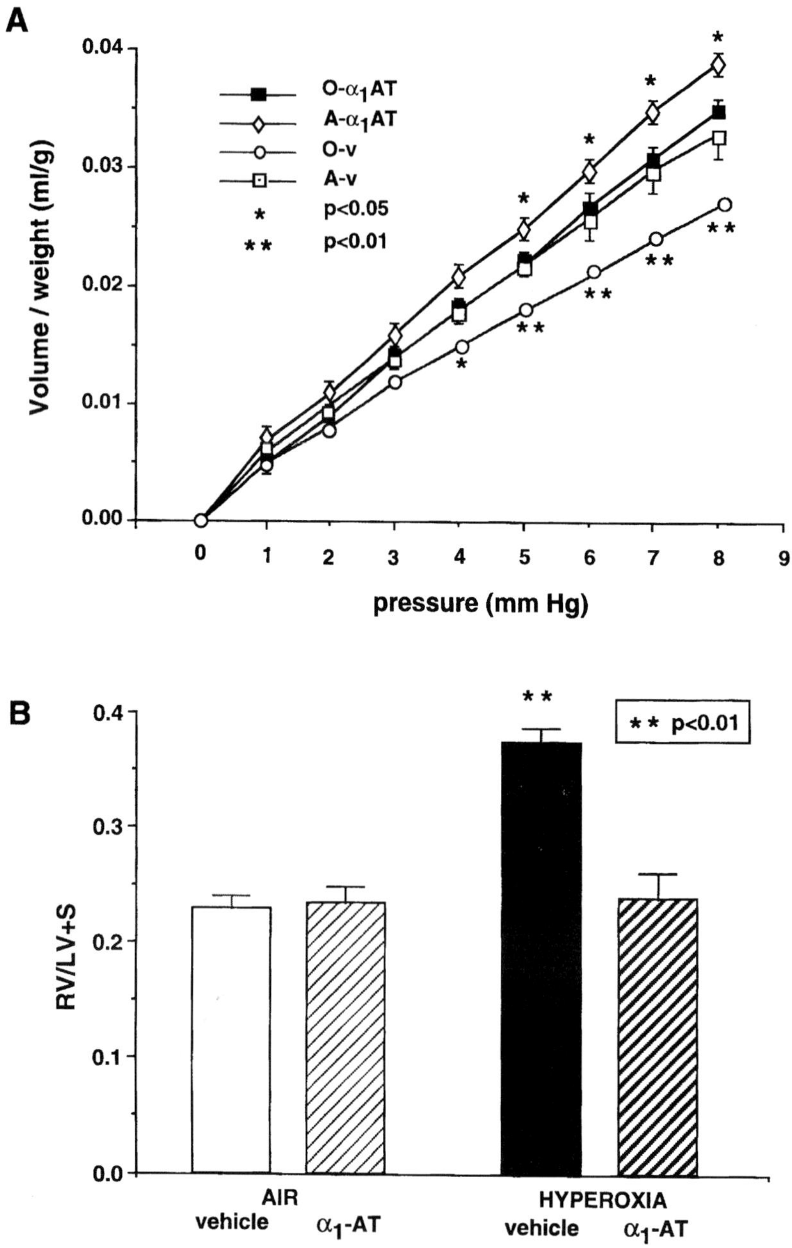
A
0.04
0.03
0.02
0.01
0.00
O-α1AT
A-α1AT
O-v
A-v
* p<0.05
** p<0.01
Volume / weight (ml/g)
0 1 2 3 4 5 6 7 8 9
pressure (mm Hg)
B
0.4
0.3
0.2
0.1
0.0
** p<0.01
RV/LV+S
AIR
vehicle α1-AT
HYPEROXIA
vehicle α1-AT

with proliferating smooth-muscle cells and in cultured cells alters cell shape, permitting rapid phosphorylation of the receptor for epidermal growth factor (EGF) (35). The relative ''suppression'' of tenascin in the infant rat may provide a clue as to why vascular disease in the infant may not progress, and perhaps why regression of vascular smooth muscle may occur during early development (unpublished data).

IV. Hypoxia

Hypoxia can induce structural changes in pulmonary arteries that likely derive from a direct effect of the vasoconstricting influence. That is, in experiments in which animals are subjected to chronic hypoxia, but in which the pulmonary artery is banded to prevent the increase in pressure, hypoxia-induced structural changes of medial hypertrophy and extension of muscle do not occur (36). Alternatively, infusion of angiotensin during hypoxia, in doses that will stimulate prostacyclin production, also prevents vascular disease (37). Recent studies, however, suggest that the efficacy of inhibitors of angiotensin-converting enzyme in reducing vascular disease may result from a cellular, rather than a hemodynamic, effect of angiotensin that is present in chronic hypoxia (38). Chronic hypoxia is also associated with the production of a pulmonary artery elastase, and hypoxia-induced pulmonary vascular disease is inhibited by serine elastase inhibitors (30).

Tropoelastin synthesis is maintained in the pulmonary artery of neonatal calves subjected to chronic hypoxia (39,40; Fig. 7), but how hypoxia or mechanical forces regulate the production of tropoelastin remains to be determined. In addition, these studies have shown that there is heterogeneity in the response of vascular smooth muscle cells, for all cells do not respond synchronously with

Figure 9 (A) Graph of lung compliance assessed as pressure–volume curves corrected for body weight: O, hyperoxia; A, room air; v, vehicle. The data show a decrease in lung compliance in the hyperoxia/vehicle relative to the room air/α_1-antitrypsin (α_1-AT) group at pressures as low as 4 mmHg ($p < 0.05$), and a decrease compared with all other groups at pressures higher than 5 mmHg ($p < 0.01$). An increase in compliance in the room air/α_1-AT compared with the other groups is observed at pressures of 5 mmHg and higher ($p < 0.05$). Values are mean ± SEM. $n = 5$ rats per group. (B) Graph of right ventricular weight (RV) compared with that of left ventricle and septum (LV + S). There is a significant increase in this measurement (an index of right ventricular hypertrophy) in the hyperoxia–vehicle group compared with the other three groups, room air–vehicle group compared with the other three groups, room air–vehicle, room air–α_1-AT, and hyperoxia–α_1-AT ($p < 0.05$). Values are mean ± SEM; $n = 5$ rats per group. (From Ref. 46.)

increased expression of tropoelastin. Frid et al. (41) have described metavinculin as a marker for a smooth-muscle cell subtype that has a different growth potential within the pulmonary artery. Growth potential can be stimulated by insulin-like growth factor and is associated with the activation of protein kinase C (42). At least one report has provided evidence that vasoconstriction and vascular remodeling associated with sustained hypoxia may be related to increased production of endothelin (43; Fig. 8). Previous experimental studies by our group have shown that when a young animal is exposed to hypoxia throughout the period of lung development, recovery and regression of vascular changes on return to room air may be impaired when compared with the adult animal (44).

V. Oxygen Toxicity and Barotrauma

The chronic injurious effects of oxygen toxicity on the developing vasculature have been studied in a variety of experimental models. Infant and neonatal rats, on exposure to high oxygen concentrations, show features of muscular extension into peripheral arteries, medial hypertrophy of muscular arteries, and loss of small arteries, with associated development of right ventricular hypertrophy (45). These features are associated with lung parenchymal disease, as evidenced by a loss in lung compliance (46). Removal of infant animals from the hyperoxic environment results in sustained reduction in alveoli, but recovery of some of the arterial changes (45). The administration of the elastase inhibitor, α_1-antiproteinase, is effective in reducing the damaging effects of oxygen on lung compliance, and also in the development of right ventricular hypertrophy, and the pulmonary vascular changes of extension of muscle, medial hypertrophy, and loss of vessels (46; Fig. 9). This has prompted our initiation of a double-blind clinical trial that has yielded very promising results (47). There was a trend toward reduced O_2 dependence at 28 and 36 weeks ($p = 0.06$), and a significant reduction in secondary outcomes such as pulmonary hemorrhage ($p = 0.03$).

VI. High Flow and Pressure

Chronic lung injury may be the result of high flow and pressure, resulting from a patent ductus arteriosus or from other congenital heart defects that increase pulmonary blood flow, such as a ventricular septal defect. Increased venous pressure resulting from myocardial dysfunction or from obstructed anomalous pulmonary veins also causes abnormal pulmonary artery remodeling. The arterial features are similar to those that have been described with other sources of injury (i.e., extension of muscle into peripheral arteries, medial hypertrophy of muscular arteries, and reduced peripheral arterial number, 48–51). With long-standing left-to-right shunts, there is additional neointimal formation, which progresses to oc-

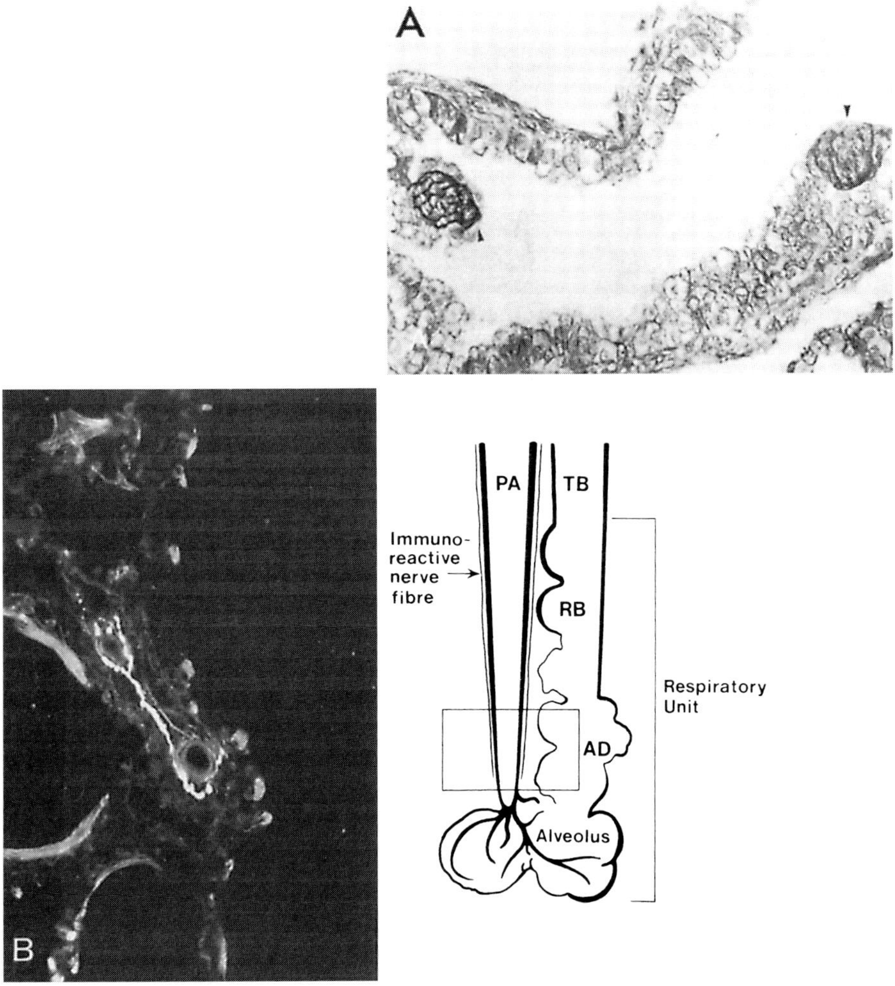

Figure 10 (A) Neuroepithelial bodies (arrowheads) are seen as dark-staining regions (immunoreactive for serotonin) in airway of a newborn infant. (Courtesy of E. Cutz.) (B) Tyrosine hydroxylase immunoreactive perivascular nerve fibers (arrow) at the adventitial–medial border of an alveolar duct artery in a child aged 2½ years; scale bar = 50 μm. Diagram on the right shows terminal bronchiolus (TB) and airways of respiratory unit accompanied by an innervated pulmonary artery (PA). RB, respiratory bronchiolus; AD, alveolar duct. Square indicates area shown in B. (From Ref. 59.)

clusion of peripheral arteries and which increases pulmonary vascular resistance to systemic or even suprasystemic levels. Although surgical correction of congenital heart defects with left-to-right shunts in early infancy is associated with regression of vascular disease (51), there is always concern that superimposition of high flow and pulmonary edema and inflammation may impair lung function, especially in the premature newborn.

Corrective cardiac surgery is also associated with heightened pulmonary vascular reactivity in the early postoperative period. The mechanism is related to endothelial injury (52), with loss of endothelial dilating capacity (53–56). In addition, an increase in von Willebrand factor activity can result in platelet aggregation (57). There is convincing data that, in addition to anesthesia, hyperventilation, nitric oxide therapy (55), and perhaps endothelin receptor blockers, will be beneficial in inhibiting this type of increased vasoreactivity. There is also considerable innervation of small peripheral arteries, and the effect of increased neuropeptide production on pulmonary vascular reactivity has been suggested (58–60; Fig. 10).

Pulmonary vein obstruction is associated with venous as well as arterial abnormalities. In the setting of obstructed anomalous veins, this is reflected in increased venous muscularity, but in the setting of isolated pulmonary venous obstruction, there is frequently severe intimal fibrosis, preventing surgical or interventional therapy (61). We carried out studies in which the pulmonary veins were banded in newborn piglets. It was interesting that the first sign of pulmonary

Figure 11 (a) Pulmonary artery pressure (P_{pa}, upper panel) and pulmonary capillary wedge pressure (P_{cw}, lower panel) in banded and sham-operated piglets at 1, 3, and 6 weeks after banding. Values are averages of mean ± SEM ($n = 6$ piglets per group at each time point). At 1 week there was no change; at 3 weeks there was a significant increase in P_{pa}, which preceded the rise in P_{cw} at 6 weeks and the further increase in P_{pa} ($^*p < 0.01$; † $p < 0.05$). (b) Transmission electron photomicrographs of representative pulmonary veins (PVs) from banded (right panel) and sham-operated (left panel) piglets at 3 weeks after banding (magnification × 14,131; inset magnification × 28,263). Both pulmonary veins show apparent injury and lifting of endothelial cells and subendothelial spaces owing to poor preservation during handling. The sham-operated PV displays an intact internal elastic lamina (IEL) and predominantly contractile-appearing smooth-muscle cells (C) in media. In contrast, PV from the banded piglet depicts complete breakdown of IEL into elastin fragments (E_{fg}), a thickened subendothelium composed of collagen, extracellular matrix (ECM), and smooth-muscle cells that appear to have migrated in from the media, many of which have a synthetic-appearing phenotype (S) exemplified by a large amount of endoplasmic reticulum and a corresponding paucity of contractile fragments. C and S smooth muscle cells are better appreciated in insets (bar = 1 μm). (From Ref. 61.)

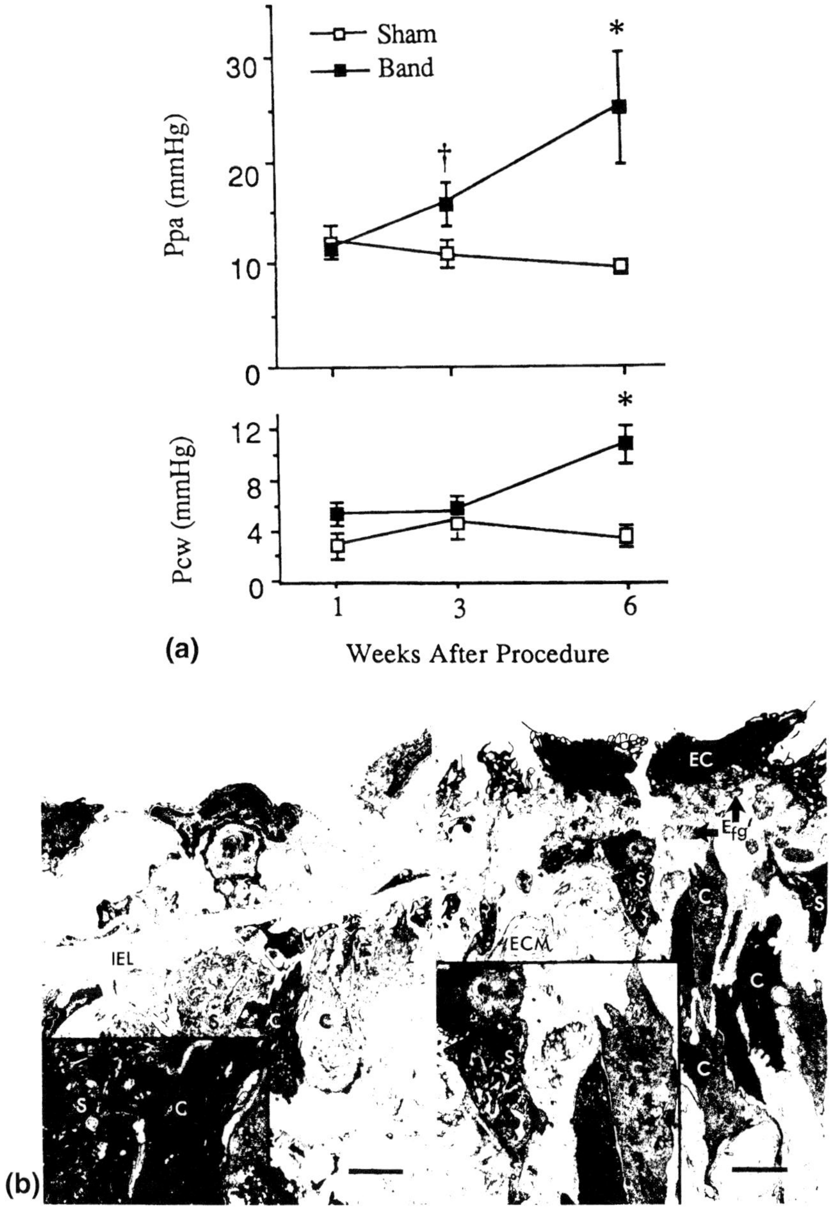
Sham
Band
Ppa (mmHg)
30
20
10
0
Pcw (mmHg)
12
8
4
0
1
3
6
(a)
Weeks After Procedure
EC
Efg
S
C
ECM
IEL
(b)

venous obstruction was an increase in pulmonary artery pressure. Later, when there was extensive intimal fibrosis of the pulmonary veins, the venous pressure began to rise (61; Fig. 11). This suggests that some of the difficulty in addressing pulmonary venous obstruction may be the lack of timely intervention.

VII. Chronic Lung Injury: Questions to Be Solved

Advances in the treatment of patients either at risk of developing chronic lung injury-related pulmonary vascular disease or with established advanced lesions will be made through a better understanding of fundamental cellular defense and remodeling mechanisms. Although we have recognized inflammatory mediators and adhesion molecules and their potential role in mediating lung vascular injury, we do not know which are the most important molecules and how they might be selectively targeted in the pulmonary vessels. Similarly, we know that controlling hemodynamic imbalance should prevent the development of pulmonary vascular abnormalities; however, we do not understand why nitric oxide may fail or whether there are even more selective pulmonary vascular mediators to target. We have described an endogenous vascular elastase in experimental models; but evidence still needs to be provided that a similar molecule plays an important clinical role, and the molecular and protein structure needs to be defined for this enzyme to be appropriately targeted. We also recognize that the pulmonary vascular changes of chronic lung injury are associated with cellular proliferation, and we need to further explore ways in which proliferating cells can be arrested and even ways in which apoptosis can be induced.

References

1. Hislop M, Reid L. Pulmonary arterial development during childhood: branching pattern and structure. Thorax 1973; 28:129–135.
2. Meyrick B, Reid L. Ultrastructural findings in lung biopsy material from children with congenital heart defects. Am J Pathol 1980; 101:527–537.
3. Jones R, Zapol WM, Reid L. Pulmonary artery remodelling and pulmonary hypertension after exposure to hyperoxia for 7 days: a morphometric and hemodynamic study. Am J Pathol 1984; 117:368–375.
4. Jones R. Ultrastructural analysis of contractile cell development in lung microvessels in hyperoxic pulmonary hypertension: fibroblasts and intermediate cells selectively reorganize nonmuscluar segments. Am J Pathol 1993; 141:1491–1505.
5. Hall SM, Haworth SG. Normal adaptation of pulmonary arterial intima to extrauterine life in the pig: ultrastructural study. J Pathol 1986; 149:55–66.
6. Merritt TA, Hallman M. Interactions in the immature lung: protease-antiprotease mechanism of lung injury. In: Merritt TA, Northway WH, Jr, eds. Bronchopulmonary Dysplasia. Palo Alto: Blackwell Scientific, 1988:117–130.

7. Li JX, Gray BM, Oliver JR, Lu CY, Philips JB III. Delayed thromboxane synthesis inhibition, but not cholinergic blockade, reverses group B streptococcus-induced pulmonary hypertension. Dev Pharmacol Ther 1992; 19:40–49.
8. Truog WE, Gibson RL, Henderson WR, Redding GJ. Tumor necrosis factor-induced neonatal pulmonary hypertension: effect of dizmagral pretreatment. Pediatr Res 1990; 27:166–171.
9. Stevens K, Janssen PL, Tucker AD. Acute and long-term TNF-alpha administration increases pulmonary vascular reactivity in isolated rat lungs. J Appl Physiol 1992; 73:708–712.
10. Meyrick B, Brigham KL. Repeated *E. coli* endotoxin induced pulmonary inflammation causes chronic pulmonary hypertension in sheep: structural and functional changes. Lab Invest 1986; 55:164–176.
11. Morelli S, Ferri C, Polettini E, et al. Plasma endothelin-1 levels, pulmonary hypertension, and lung fibrosis in patients with systemic sclerosis. Am J Med 1995; 99:255–260.
12. Voelkel NF, Tuder RM, Bridges J, Arend, WP. Interleukin-1 receptor antagonist treatment reduces pulmonary hypertension generated in rats by monocrotaline. Am J Respir Cell Mol Biol 1994; 11:664–675.
13. Clausell N, Molossi S, Rabinovitch M. Increased interleukin-1β and fibronectin expression are early features of the development of the post-cardiac transplant coronary arteriopathy in piglets. Am J Pathol 1993; 142:1772–1786.
14. Clausell N, Rabinovitch M. Upregulation of fibronectin synthesis by interleukin-1β in coronary artery smooth muscle cells is associated with the development of the post-cardiac transplant arteriopathy in piglets. J Clin Invest 1992; 92:1850–1858.
15. Clausell N, Molossi S, Sett S, Rabinovitch M. In vivo blockade of tumor necrosis factor-α in cholesterol-fed rabbits after cardiac transplant inhibits acute coronary artery neointimal formation. Circulation 1994; 89:2768–2779.
16. Molossi S, Elices M, Arrhenius T, Diaz R, Coulber C, Rabinovitch M. Blockade of very late antigen-4 integrin binding to fibronectin with connecting segment-1 peptide reduces accelerated coronary arteriopathy in rabbit cardiac allografts. J Clin Invest 1995; 95:2601–2610.
17. Molossi S, Clausell N, Sett S, Rabinovitch M. ICAM-1 and VCAM-1 expression in accelerated cardiac allograft arteriopathy and myocardial rejection are influenced differently by cyclosporine A and tumour necrosis factor-α blockade. J Pathol 1995; 176:175–182.
18. Molossi S, Elices M, Arrhenius T, Rabinovitch M. Lymphocyte transendothelial migration toward smooth muscle cells in interleukin-1β stimulated co-cultures is related to fibronectin interactions with $\alpha_4\beta_1$ and $\alpha_5\beta_1$ integrins. J Cell Physiol 1995; 164: 620–633.
19. Molossi S, Clausell N, Rabinovitch M. Reciprocal induction of tumor necrosis factor-α and interleukin-1β activity mediates fibronectin synthesis in coronary artery smooth muscle cells. J Cell Physiol 1995; 163:19–29.
20. Boudreau N, Turley E, Rabinovitch M. Fibronectin, hyaluronan and a hyaluronan binding protein contribute to increased ductus arteriosus smooth muscle cell migration. Dev Biol 1991; 143:235–247.
21. Zhu L, Wigle D, Hinek A, et al. The endogenous vascular elastase that governs

development and progression of monocrotaline-induced pulmonary hypertension in rats is a novel enzyme related to the serine proteinase adipsin. J Clin Invest 1994; 94:1163–1171.
22. Thompson K, Rabinovitch M. Exogenous leukocyte and endogenous elastases can mediate mitogenic activity in pulmonary artery smooth muscle cells by release of extracellular matrix-bound basic fibroblast growth factor. J Cell Physiol 1996; 166: 495–505.
23. Hinek A, Molossi S, Rabinovitch M. Functional interplay between interleukin-1 receptor and elastin binding protein controls fibronectin synthesis in coronary artery smooth muscle cells. Exp Cell Res 1996; 225:122–131.
24. Senior RM, Griffin G, Mecham RP, Wrenn DS, Prasad KU, Urry DW. Val-Gly-Val-Ala-Pro-Gly, a repeating peptide in elastin, is chemotactic for fibroblasts and monocytes. J Cell Biol 1984; 99:870–874.
25. Smyth MJ. Dual mechanisms of lymphocyte-mediated cytotoxicity serve to control and deliver the immune response. Bioessays 1995; 17:891–898.
26. Rosenberg HC, Rabinovitch M. Endothelial injury and vascular reactivity in monocrotaline pulmonary hypertension. Am J Physiol 1988; 255:H1484–H1491.
27. Kobayashi J, Wigle D, Childs T, Zhu L, Keeley FW, Rabinovitch M. Serum-induced vascular smooth muscle cell elastolytic activity through tyrosine kinase intracellular signalling. J Cell Physiol 1994; 160:121–131.
28. Todd L, Mullen M, Olley PM, Rabinovitch M. Pulmonary toxicity of monocrotaline differs at critical periods of lung development. Pediatr Res 1985; 19:731–737.
29. Todorovich-Hunter L, Dodo H, Ye C, McCready L, Keeley FW, Rabinovitch M. Increased pulmonary artery elastolytic activity in adult rats with monocrotaline-induced progressive hypertensive pulmonary vascular disease compared with infant rats with nonprogressive disease. Am Rev Respir Dis 1992; 146:213–223.
30. Maruyama K, Ye C, Woo M, et al. Chronic hypoxic pulmonary hypertension in rats and increased elastolytic activity. Am J Physiol 1991; 261:H1716–H1726.
31. Ye C, Rabinovitch M. Inhibition of elastolysis by SC-37698 reduces development and progression of monocrotaline pulmonary hypertension. Am J Physiol 1991; 261: H1255–H1267.
32. Sallenave J-M, Silva A. Characterization and gene sequence of the precursor of elafin, an elastase-specific inhibitor in bronchial secretions. Am J Respir Cell Mol Biol 1993; 8:439–453.
33. Jones PL, Cowan KN, Rabinovitch M. Progressive pulmonary vascular disease is characterized by a proliferative response related to deposition of tenascin-C and is preceded by subendothelial accumulation of fibronectin. Am J Pathol 1997; 150: 1349–1360.
34. Jones PL, Rabinovitch M. Tenascin-C is induced with progressive pulmonary vascular disease in rats and is functionally related to increased smooth muscle cell proliferation. Circ Res 1996; 79:1131–1142.
35. Jones PL, Crack J, Rabinovitch M. Regulation of tenascin-c, a vascular smooth muscle cell survival factor that interacts with the $\alpha v\beta 3$ integrin to promote epidermal growth factor receptor phosphorylation and growth. J Cell Biol 1997; 139:279–293.
36. Rabinovitch M, Konstam MA, Gamble WJ, et al. Changes in pulmonary blood flow affect vascular response to chronic hypoxia in rats. Circ Res 1983; 52:432–441.

37. Rabinovitch M, Mullen M, Rosenberg HC, Maruyama H, O'Brodovich H, Olley PM. Angiotensin II prevents hypoxic pulmonary hypertension and vascular changes in rats. Am J Physiol 1988; 254:H500–H508.
38. Morrell NW, Morris KG, Stenmark KR. Role of angiotensin converting enzyme and angiotensin II in the development of hypoxic pulmonary hypertension. Am J Physiol 1995; 269:H1186–H1194.
39. Prosser I, Stenmark K, Suthar M, Crouch E, Mecham R, Parks W. Regional heterogeneity of elastin and collagen gene expression in intralobar arteries in response to hypoxic pulmonary hypertension as demonstrated by in situ hybridization. Am J Pathol 1989; 135:1073–1088.
40. Durmowicz AG, Parks WC, Hyde DM, Mecham RP, Stenmark KR. Persistence, reexpression, and induction of pulmonary arterial fibronectin, tropoelastin, and type I procollagen mRNA expression in neonatal hypoxic pulmonary hypertension. Am J Pathol 1994; 145:1411–1420.
41. Frid MG, Moiseeva EP, Stenmark KR. Multiple phenotypically distinct smooth muscle cell populations exist in the adult and developing bovine pulmonary arterial media in vivo. Circ Res 1994; 75:669–681.
42. Dempsey EC, Stenmark KR, McMurtry IF, O'Brien RF, Voelkel NF, Badesch DB. Insulin-like growth factor I and protein kinase C activation stimulate pulmonary artery smooth muscle cell proliferation through separate but synergistic pathways. J Cell Physiol 1990; 144:159–165.
43. Bonvallet ST, Zamora MR, Hasunuma K, et al. BQ123, an ETA-receptor, attenuates hypoxic pulmonary hypertension in rats. Am J Physiol 1994; 266:H1327–H1331.
44. Rabinovitch M, Gamble WJ, Miettinen OS, Reid L. Age and sex influence on pulmonary hypertension of chronic hypoxia on recovery. Am J Physiol 1981; 240:H62–H72.
45. Wilson WL, Mullen M, Olley PM, Rabinovitch M. Hyperoxia-induced pulmonary vascular and lung abnormalities in young rats and potential for recovery. Pediatr Res 1985; 19:1059–1067.
46. Koppel R, Han RNN, Cox D, Tanswell AK, Rabinovitch M. α_1-Antitrypsin protects neonatal rats from pulmonary vascular and parenchymal effects of oxygen toxicity. Pediatr Res 1994; 36:763–770.
47. Stiskal J, Dunn M, Shennan AT, et al. Alpha$_1$-proteinase inhibitor therapy for the prevention of chronic lung disease of prematurity: a randomized controlled trial. Pediatrics 1998; 101:89–94.
48. Haworth SG. Pulmonary vascular disease in different types of congenital heart disease: implications for interpretation of lung biopsy findings in early childhood. Br Heart J 1984; 52:557–571.
49. Hislop A, Haworth SG, Reid L. Quantitative structural analysis of pulmonary vessels in isolated ventricular septal defects in infancy. Br Heart J 1975; 37:1014–1021.
50. Rabinovitch M, Haworth SG, Castaneda AR, et al. Lung biopsy in congenital heart disease: a morphometric approach to pulmonary vascular disease. Circulation 1978; 58:1107–1122.
51. Rabinovitch M, Keane JF, Norwood WI, Castaneda AR, Reid L. Vascular structure in lung biopsy tissue correlated with pulmonary hemodynamic findings after repair of congenital heart defects. Circulation 1984; 69:655–667.

52. Rabinovitch M, Bothwell T, Hayakawa BN, et al. Pulmonary artery endothelial abnormalities in patients with congenital heart defects and pulmonary hypertension: a correlation of light with scanning electron microscopy and transmission electron microscopy. Lab Invest 1986; 55:632–653.
53. Dinh-Xuan AT, Higgenbottam TW, Clelland C, Pepke-Zaba J, Cremona G, Wallwork J. Impairment of pulmonary endothelium-dependent relaxation in patients with Eisenmenger's syndrome. Br J Pharmacol 1990; 99:9–10.
54. Celermajer DS, Cullen S, Deanfield JE. Impairment of endothelium-dependent pulmonary artery relaxation in children with congenital heart disease and abnormal pulmonary hemodynamics. Circulation 1993; 87:440–446.
55. Wessel DL, Adatia I, Giglia TM, et al. Use of inhaled nitric oxide and acetylcholine in the evaluation of pulmonary hypertension and endothelial function after cardiopulmonary bypass. Circulation 1993; 88:2128–2138.
56. Fineman JR, Chang RS, Soifer, SJ. EDRF inhibition augments pulmonary hypertension in intact newborn lambs. Am J Physiol 1992; 262:H1365–H1371.
57. Turner-Gomes SO, Andrew M, Coles J, Trusler GA, Williams WG, Rabinovitch M. Abnormalities in von Willebrand factor and antithrombin III after cardiopulmonary bypass operations for congenital heart disease. Thorac Cardiovasc Surg 1992; 103: 87–97.
58. Heath D, Yacoub M, Gosney JR, Madden B, Caslin AW, Smith P. Pulmonary endocrine cells in hypertensive pulmonary vascular disease. Histopathology 1990; 16: 21–28.
59. Allen KM, Wharton J, Polak JM, Haworth SG. A study of nerves containing peptides in the pulmonary vasculature of healthy infants and children and of those with pulmonary hypertension. Br Heart J 1989; 62:353–360.
60. Haworth SG, Reid L. Structural study of the pulmonary circulation in total anomalous pulmonary venous return in early infancy. Br Heart J 1977; 39:80–92.
61. LaBourene JI, Coles JG, Johnson DJ, Mehra A, Keeley FW, Rabinovitch M. Alterations in elastin and collagen related to the mechanism of progressive pulmonary venous obstruction in a piglet model. A hemodynamic, ultrastructural, and biochemical study. Circ Res 1990; 66:438–456.
62. Meyrick B, Reid LM. Ultrastructural features of the distended pulmonary arteries of the normal rat. Anat Rec 1979; 193:71–97.
63. Rabinovitch M. Elastase, remodelling of the extracellular matrix, and pulmonary hypertension. Semin Respir Crit Care Med 1994; 15:119–206.

27

Pulmonary Hypertension in Chronic Lung Disease of Infancy

Pathogenesis, Pathophysiology, and Treatment

STEVEN H. ABMAN

University of Colorado School of Medicine
Denver, Colorado

I. Introduction

Nearly 30 years have passed since Northway and his colleagues provided the first clinical, radiologic, and pathological description of the chronic lung disease known as bronchopulmonary dysplasia (BPD; 228). BPD refers to the chronic lung disease of infancy that follows ventilator and oxygen therapy for neonatal respiratory distress syndrome (RDS). It was originally defined by the presence of chronic respiratory signs, abnormal chest radiographs, and persistent oxygen requirements beyond 1 month of age in newborn infants who have received intensive care. Although much has been learned about BPD since its initial description, the disease remains a "moving target," as it continues to change with time. In comparison with the original report, most infants who acquire chronic lung disease are smaller and less mature at birth, with birthweight less than 1000 g in 75% of cases (149,228,231). The "classic" clinical, radiologic, and pathological stages of BPD are often absent now because of changes in perinatal management, including the use of antenatal and postnatal steroids, surfactant therapy, improved fluid management, new ventilator strategies, and better nutritional support (9,25,40,54,70,71,149,231). As a result, the term "chronic lung disease (CLD) of infancy" has either replaced or is often used interchangeably with "BPD" as a diagnosis in many centers. Although recognizing the changing pattern of CLD from its initial descriptions, the terms BPD and CLD are used synonymously in this chapter to describe the chronic respiratory disease that often develops in neonates who are born prematurely.

Although advances in the care of premature newborns with acute RDS have improved survival, management of patients with CLD and associated cardiovascular sequelae remains an ongoing challenge. One of the most important sequelae is pulmonary hypertension. Even from the first reports of BPD, pulmonary hypertension and cor pulmonale have been recognized as contributing factors to high mortality. Early studies reported a 50% mortality rate in BPD patients with persistent echocardiographic findings of pulmonary hypertension beyond 4 months of age (110). More recent studies suggest that this association of high mortality with pulmonary hypertension still prevails in many infants with severe BPD (13,57,132). Pulmonary hypertension in BPD contributes to recurrent cyanosis and pulmonary edema, congestive heart failure, frequent respiratory exacerbations, prolonged or repeated hospitalizations, and perhaps sudden death (9,13,57,132). Infants with BPD and severe pulmonary hypertension are at greater risk for death in late infancy and severe morbidity during early childhood, especially with respiratory syncytial virus, influenza, and other lower respiratory tract infections. Unfortunately, pulmonary hypertension is often unrecognized until late in the clinical course of patients with advanced disease, and its pathogenesis, pathophysiology, and treatment are poorly understood.

The purpose of this chapter is to review the clinical problem of pulmonary hypertension in infants with CLD after premature birth. In addition to increased susceptibility to pulmonary edema, the pulmonary circulation in infants with CLD is characterized by abnormalities of lung vascular growth, structure, and tone (Fig. 1). In contrast with secondary pulmonary hypertension that occurs in association with many chronic lung diseases, such as cystic fibrosis, emphysema, interstitial lung disease, and others, the pathogenesis of pulmonary hypertension in CLD is uniquely related to how premature birth and postnatal lung injury disrupt the normal sequence of pulmonary vascular growth, development, and adaptation to postnatal life. Although often identified after the diagnosis of CLD is firmly established, pulmonary hypertension is already present earlier in the clinical course, contributing to the severity of acute RDS and progression of chronic cardiopulmonary disease. Insight into the pathophysiology and treatment of pulmonary hypertension in CLD begins with understanding normal growth and function of the pulmonary circulation, the role of pulmonary vascular disease in the pathophysiology of RDS, the adverse effects of therapeutic interventions on the lung circulation, and other issues concerning disruption of normal postnatal maturation.

Unfortunately, current knowledge about pulmonary hypertension in infants with CLD is limited to predominantly descriptive information. Little clinical data

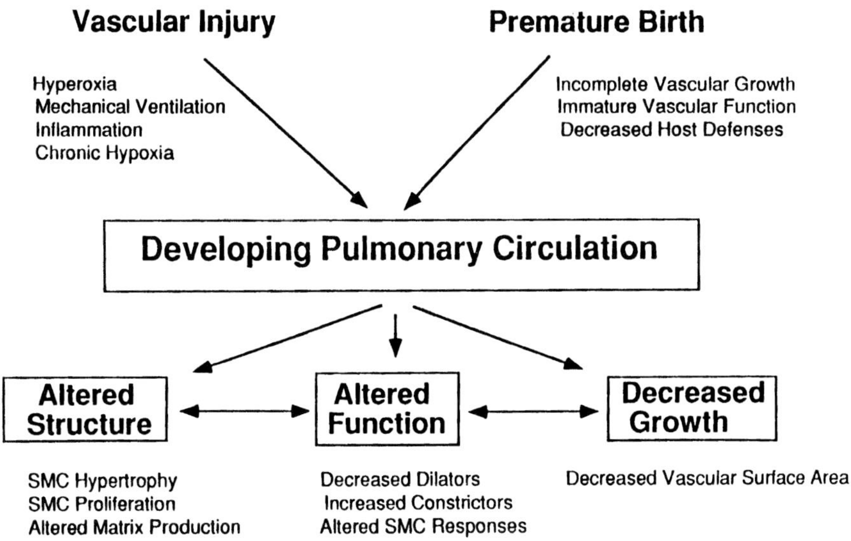

Figure 1 Potential mechanisms of injury to the pulmonary circulation in CLD.

exist on mechanisms underlying the development and resolution of pulmonary vascular disease in CLD. New laboratory studies continue to provide new insights into mechanisms that regulate pulmonary vascular growth, development, and tone; however, clinical investigations, such as studies that use human tissue, studies that prospectively assess the timing, severity, and physiological contribution of pulmonary hypertension to the clinical course and long-term outcome of CLD; and well-designed clinical interventional trials, are sorely needed. This chapter includes a brief description of normal maturation of the lung circulation and mechanisms by which lung injury may alter pulmonary vascular structure and function. Because pulmonary hypertension contributes to the severity of acute RDS early in the clinical course of premature neonates, clinical and experimental studies of pulmonary hypertension in severe RDS are briefly presented. Finally, the clinical course and diagnostic and therapeutic approaches to pulmonary hypertension in chronic lung disease of infancy and related cardiovascular sequelae are reviewed.

II. Perinatal Pulmonary Circulation: Developmental Aspects

Insight into pulmonary hypertension in premature neonates with chronic lung disease must begin with (1) an understanding of changes in vascular structure and function during normal lung growth and development; (2) mechanisms that contribute to postnatal adaptation of the premature pulmonary circulation after birth and during infancy; and (3) responses of the developing lung circulation to injury.

A. Fetal Pulmonary Circulation

Development of the pulmonary circulation in utero is characterized by early growth of large central arteries, with subsequent development of the lung microcirculation later in gestation (88,148,153,154,191). The pulmonary artery develops from the sixth branchial arch as an outgrowth of the dorsal aorta, which joins a plexus of intrapulmonary vessels that form within the lung mesenchyme by the dual processes of vasculogenesis and angiogenesis (96,147). Bronchial vessels develop from the aorta later in development (9–12 weeks; 50). By the 16th week of human gestation, all bronchial airway (or preacinar) generations have formed, along with their accompanying conducting pulmonary arteries. Intra-acinar arteries develop later in fetal life, as the pulmonary vascular surface area increases tenfold during concomitant development of alveolar ducts and alveoli in the third trimester (153). Mechanisms promoting early lung vascular differentiation and development are poorly understood, but likely include diverse paracrine and autocrine growth factors, such as transforming growth factor-β (TGF-β), insulin-like growth factor (IGF), fibroblast growth factors (FGF), vascular endothelial growth factor (VEGF), and others.

In addition to increases in pulmonary artery number, changes in pulmonary vascular structure also occur during development. In the normal late-gestation fetus, small pulmonary arteries associated with respiratory bronchioles, alveolar ducts, and saccules appear to lack muscularization, but muscularization is variable between species (88,153,154). Distal extension of smooth muscle progressively increases throughout infancy and childhood, with maximal muscularization observed in the normal adult pulmonary circulation. As the pulmonary circulation develops, pulmonary arteries acquire a muscular coat, the thickness of which is proportionate to vessel size. Thus, at birth, few intra-acinar arteries are muscularized, because vascular smooth muscle cells differentiate in distal arteries with normal postnatal growth later in infancy.

The fetal pulmonary circulation has high basal resistance and receives less than 8% of combined ventricular output, with most of the right ventricular output flowing through the ductus arteriosus to the aorta, bypassing the lungs (257,258). Although pulmonary perfusion is low during fetal life, blood flow must remain sufficient to deliver oxygen and substrates to allow lung growth in the late-gestation fetal lamb, because pulmonary artery ligation causes lung hypoplasia (299). Late in gestation, pulmonary blood flow increases in proportion to lung growth and vascular cross-sectional area, as the number of blood vessels increases more than tenfold. As blood flow increases with advancing gestation, mean pulmonary artery pressure also increases; when expressed relative to lung weight, pulmonary vascular resistance (PVR) actually increases with advancing gestation (221). Thus, despite an increase in vessel surface area, high PVR persists owing to increasing pulmonary vascular tone as the fetus nears term. Mechanisms that maintain high fetal pulmonary vascular resistance include (1) physical stimuli, such as the lack of a gas–liquid interface and rhythmic distension of the lung (61,90,91,102); (2) low oxygen tension (20–25 torr in the normal fetus); (3) decreased production of vasodilators, such as prostacyclin (PGI_2) and nitric oxide (NO; 6,52,60,80,81,210,268,270,293); (3) increased release of vasoconstrictors including endothelin-1 (ET-1; 63,64,162,165,202,307,314) and leukotrienes (LT; 62,276); or (4) altered smooth-muscle cell responsiveness (e.g., increased myogenic activity and altered calcium signaling; 33,39,83).

In addition to maturational changes in lung vascular structure, marked changes in function occur during normal development (7). For example, the acute pulmonary hemodynamic response to certain vasodilator stimuli, such as acetylcholine and oxygen, increases with advancing gestation in the ovine fetus (197,221). Maturational changes in endothelial and smooth-muscle function account for some of these changes in the regulation of pulmonary vascular tone and reactivity during fetal life. Recent observations of maturation of the NO–cGMP cascade, a potent vasodilator system in the perinatal lung, is an example of such changes. NO is produced by vascular endothelium during conversion of L-arginine to L-citrulline by the enzyme, endothelial NO synthase (eNOS; 156,219). Once produced, NO rapidly diffuses to underlying smooth-muscle cells and causes vasodilation by stimulating soluble guanylate cyclase and increasing cGMP production (24). Elevated cGMP stimulates GMP kinase, increases calcium-activated K^+-channel activity and causes membrane hyperpolarization (22,243,246). The resultant decrease of intracellular calcium content in the smooth-muscle cell leads to vasodilation. In some studies, NO directly stimulated K^+-channels independently of increased cGMP (46,290). Many investigators have demonstrated that vasodilator responses to many hemodynamic stimuli, such as increased flow or shear stress, as well as hormonal, paracrine, and pharmacological stimuli, depend on NO release (80,219,242,256). In addition, "NO activity" is dependent on multiple factors, such as eNOS content, subcellular localization (216), substrate and cofactor availability, and several smooth-muscle cell enzymes, including GMP kinase (22,199) and cGMP-specific (type V) phosphodiesterase (PDE5). PDE5 limits GMP-mediated vasodilation by hydrolysis and inactivation of cGMP, and may be especially critical for pulmonary vasoregulation in utero and in hypertensive states (34,51,75,186,199,317).

Although pulmonary vascular resistance is high in the normal fetus, basal release of NO modulates pulmonary vascular tone during fetal development (6,7). NOS activity is present in the immature lung at least as early as 75% of term, as indicated by the hypertensive response to NOS inhibition (178). NOS inhibition attenuates pulmonary vasodilation to such stimuli as acetylcholine, oxygen, and increased flow or shear stress in the normal fetal lamb (6,80,210,293). Lung NOS activity increases with postnatal maturation (7). In vitro studies suggest that pharmacological agents that cause vasodilation by stimulating NO release are less potent in fetal than in neonatal or adult pulmonary arteries. In contrast, pulmonary artery relaxation by direct stimulation of smooth muscle with sodium nitroprusside (an NO donor) is not different between fetal, newborn, or adult vessels (7). These findings suggest that maturational changes in endothelial cell function contribute to developmental changes in pulmonary vascular tone and reactivity. Parallel in vivo studies of fetal pulmonary vasoreactivity support these in vitro observations; exogenous NO or agents that directly increase smooth-muscle GMP content cause more sustained fetal pulmonary vasodilation than many endothelium-dependent agonists (2,15,178,181). Because acetylcholine and oxygen cause pulmonary vasodilation by stimulating NO release (80,210,293), maturational changes in the NO–cGMP cascade are likely to account for previous observations of progressive vasodilator responsiveness to these agents with advancing fetal age (197,221,269).

Lung eNOS mRNA and protein content progressively increase during development in fetal rat lungs, suggesting that eNOS expression is developmentally regulated (227). This may reflect the large increase in lung surface area during this time period, as intense immunostaining for eNOS appears in developing lung vessels at least as early as 30% of term in the ovine fetus (139). The significance of early expression of eNOS in the developing lung is unclear. This may include an important role of eNOS in promoting vascular growth and angiogenesis, or in limiting precocious vascular muscularization in the fetal lung (120,220,260,261,316). Alternatively, early lung eNOS expression may merely serve as a marker of growing endothelial cells (26). Given the marked pulmonary vasoconstrictor response to acute NOS inhibition in the late fetus (6), it seems likely that failure to sustain basal NO production in utero, especially in the presence of fetal hypertension, could contribute to structural vascular changes over time and resultant postnatal pulmonary hypertension (discussed later).

During late gestation, adverse intrauterine stimuli, such as decreased lung blood flow (299), chronic hypoxia (130,275), or chronic hypertension (12,196, 222), can alter lung vascular function and structure, contributing to abnormalities of postnatal adaptation (121,243,283). Mechanisms by which changes in intrauterine hemodynamic, hormonal, autocrine, and paracrine stimuli alter lung vascular growth and function are complex and remain incompletely understood. For example, pulmonary hypertension induced by early closure of the ductus arteriosus in fetal lambs alters vascular reactivity and lung structure, leading to failure of postnatal adaptation at delivery. This intervention has been used to create an experimental model of persistent pulmonary hypertension of the newborn (12, 196,222). Studies of this experimental model suggest that multiple changes in endothelial and smooth-muscle cell function and structure contribute to pulmonary vascular dysfunction, including decreased eNOS mRNA, protein, and activity (211,295), decreased sGC activity (281), high PDE cGMP hydrolytic activity (317), increased ET-1 production (163,164), and increased smooth-muscle myogenic reactivity (37). Thus, intrauterine pulmonary hypertension is characterized by changes in endothelial and smooth-muscle function, as reflected in studies of the NO–cGMP cascade, ET activity, and smooth-muscle contractility. Alterations in these mechanisms and others appear to contribute to altered structure and function of the developing lung circulation, leading to clinical disorders in postnatal cardiorespiratory adaptation (see later).

B. Transitional Pulmonary Circulation

At birth, pulmonary blood flow rapidly increases eightfold and pulmonary artery pressure decreases to roughly 50% of systemic arterial pressure in the normal-term neonate (101). Mechanisms causing the immediate fall in PVR include establishment of an air–liquid interface, rhythmic lung distension with respiration, increased oxygen tension, and altered production of vasoactive substances (90,150). Several birth-related stimuli, including increased shear stress, ventilation, and increased oxygenation, cause pulmonary vasodilation partly by stimulating the release of NO and PGI_2 (1,6,60,77,80,86,87,193,194,210,256,293). Experimental studies have demonstrated that similar mechanisms contribute to the rapid decrease in PVR at birth in premature lambs (178). As observed in near-term animals, the pulmonary vasodilator responses to ventilation with hypoxic gas mixtures (or, rhythmic distension) of the lung and increased Pao_2 are partly due to stimulation of NO release in premature lambs at least as early as 112–115 days (70% of term; 178). NO production continues to modulate pulmonary vascular tone and reactivity during the early postnatal period (87,108). In young lambs, NOS blockade increases basal PVR and augments the pulmonary vasoconstrictor response to acute hypoxia, suggesting that impaired NOS activity could potentially contribute to altered vasoreactivity in pulmonary hypertension (108). However, marked interspecies variability exists. Basal NO production modulates PVR throughout adult life in some species (sheep, pig, and dog), but not in others (rats; 85). Clinical studies suggest that basal NOS activity maintains low PVR in the human pulmonary circulation (78), and that decreased lung NOS content or activity contributes to pulmonary hypertension in children and adults with chronic lung disease (see later; 125,302,308,309).

Along with enhanced vasodilator release, decreased production of vasoconstrictors, such as LTs and ET-1, may contribute to the normal fall in PVR at birth. As infusions of LT antagonists cause pulmonary vasodilation in the ovine fetus, it has been hypothesized that high LT production in utero contributes to high PVR in the normal fetal lung (276). Although controversy exists over the physiological role of ET-1 in the perinatal lung, the preponderance of evidence supports the hypothesis that endogenous ET-1 acts primarily as a potent vasoconstrictor (63,64,162,168,298,307). ET-1 contributes to high vascular tone in the normal ovine fetal lung (165) and to the development of pulmonary hypertension in an experimental model of pulmonary hypertension after intrauterine closure of the ductus arteriosus (163,164). Thus, several endothelial-derived products, including NO, PGI_2, LTs, and ET-1, play important vasoregulatory roles in the perinatal period. Whether abnormal endothelial cell function contributes to the pathogenesis and pathophysiology of clinical pulmonary hypertension in CLD is uncertain.

In response to the marked rise in blood flow at birth, the pulmonary circulation undergoes a concomitant structural ''reorganization'' during the early postnatal period (140,146,147). Small pulmonary arteries are characterized by rapid changes in vascular dimensions immediately at birth. The external diameters of pulmonary arteries remain constant for several hours after birth, but vascular wall thickness decreases and lumen diameter increases, as endothelial cells flatten and underlying smooth muscle stretches (140,146). Progressive pulmonary vascular growth and structural adaptations cause continued decreases in PVR during late infancy, when adult values of PVR are achieved. Wall thickness in small pulmonary arteries progressively thins to adult values, as vessel diameter increases in the absence of a decrease in smooth-muscle cell number (247). During infancy, the number of arteries increases at a rate slightly greater than alveolar number, as the ratio of alveoli to arteries decreases from 20:1 at birth to 12:1 at 2 years (153,154).

Thus, successful postnatal adaptation of the pulmonary circulation is dependent on multiple and interactive changes in lung vascular tone, structure, and growth. As discussed in the following, failure of PVR to decrease after birth may contribute to the pathophysiology of severe RDS in some preterm neonates. Intrauterine or early postnatal events that disrupt normal maturation of lung vascular structure and function may set the stage for subsequent development of pulmonary hypertension during infancy and early childhood.

III. Effects of Lung Injury on the Developing Pulmonary Circulation

The pulmonary circulation is particularly susceptible to injury during the critical period of transition to postnatal life and during early infancy (204,223,289). In the immediate postnatal period, the pulmonary circulation must undergo marked vasodilation and acute structural reorganization, as described earlier. In addition, the ability to sustain low PVR is essential to allow normal lung vascular development to keep pace with lung growth during early childhood. As stated by Tomashefski and co-workers, "... there is a complex dual process of pathologic remodeling and an attempt at normal anatomic adaptation of the pulmonary vasculature to extrauterine life" (291). Pulmonary vascular disease in infants with CLD results from interactions between (1) the interruption of normal lung vascular growth and development owing to premature birth; (2) incomplete adaptation of the lung circulation at birth; (3) the effects of acute lung injury; and (4) the effects of lung repair and remodeling.

Prematurity and acute lung injury disrupts normal functional and structural adaptation of the lung circulation to postnatal life, leading to persistent elevation of pulmonary vascular resistance, altered pulmonary vasoreactivity, and structural remodeling. Lung vascular function, structure and growth are severely impaired by the mechanisms that cause injury and have been implicated in the pathogenesis of CLD: hyperoxia, barotrauma (or "volutrauma"), inflammation, and infection. Chronic hypoxia, increased blood flow owing to persistent shunt lesions, and decreased vessel number and structure can further contribute to the clinical severity of pulmonary hypertension later in the course of infants with severe CLD. Although similar stimuli alter pulmonary vascular structure and function in the adult lung, the influence of injury on the developing lung circulation has several unique features that relate directly to the timing of the injury. For example, vasodilator and vasoconstrictor mechanisms, which normally undergo prenatal and postnatal changes with maturation, are disrupted by premature birth and lung injury. In addition, fetal and neonatal smooth-muscle cells respond to injury with more marked proliferation and enhanced extracellular matrix production than adult cells, causing more striking vascular remodeling in the lung of the premature newborn (109,121). Finally, injury during this critical period inhibits subsequent alveolar and vascular development, which contributes to pulmonary hypertension in CLD.

Several animal models provide experimental support for each of these mechanisms. First, the role of pulmonary vasoconstriction has been demonstrated in studies of preterm lambs and neonates with severe RDS, including the pioneering work of Stahlman and co-workers (279,280). More recent studies of extremely premature lambs (115 days gestation) demonstrated a progressive postnatal increase of pulmonary vascular resistance during mechanical ventilation with oxygen, that was reversed with inhaled NO therapy (179). These observations suggest that preterm lambs with severe RDS do not undergo the normal postnatal decline in pulmonary vascular resistance, and that pulmonary vasoconstriction contributes to high vascular resistance, at least early in the course. Other studies have not observed high pulmonary vascular resistance in preterm animals during the early transitional period (180); this may reflect differences in species, the degree of prematurity, the severity of RDS or lung injury, experimental conditions, or other factors. As discussed later, most human neonates with mild RDS do not have high PVR, but marked pulmonary hypertension is often present in those with severe or fatal disease that has not improved with surfactant therapy (see later).

Several reports have emphasized the unique growth responses of the developing lung circulation and vascular smooth muscle cells to hypoxia and other stimuli (247–250,283,284). For example, chronic hypoxia in neonatal rats and calves causes hypertensive structural changes in the pulmonary circulation that are more striking than the adult response to hypoxia (248,250,284). Similarly, proliferative responses of cultured smooth-muscle cells from fetal and newborn calves are greater than adult bovine smooth-muscle cells (284). Thus, for each of the adverse stimuli discussed in the following sections, developmental changes in cell phenotype or behavior determine the severity of the vascular sequelae. Selected aspects of these mechanisms are now briefly described.

A. Hyperoxia

Experimental models have clearly demonstrated the adverse effects of prolonged hyperoxia on the developing lung circulation, and that these effects can occur even in the absence of mechanical ventilation (45,53,89,94,111–113,245,253,304,305). Endothelial cells are especially prone to injury, in part owing to the generation of toxic oxygen metabolites, such as superoxide anion, hydroxyl radical, and others (215). During sustained hyperoxia in adult rats, over 30% of the pulmonary vascular endothelium is destroyed, and capillary surface area is markedly decreased within 3 days (169,170). Perivascular edema, cellular debris, and thrombosis contribute to widespread, but patchy, vascular occlusion of the microcirculation. Vascular smooth-muscle cells hypertrophy and pericytes differentiate into smooth-muscle cells, thereby narrowing lumen diameter. Electron microscopy reveals generalized capillary endothelial damage, interstitial edema, proliferation of alveolar type II cells, and incorporation of hyaline membranes into septal walls. Neutrophils accumulate in the lung and augment vascular injury. As first discovered in studies of hyperoxic adult rats (111), human newborns with BPD have early and sustained increases in neutrophils in tracheal effluent samples (214,215,232). Once lung injury is established, removal from hyperoxia does not lead to rapid structural recovery (169,170). Exposure of adult rats to hyperoxia for 7 days increases medial thickness of preacinar pulmonary arteries, as vascular smooth-muscle cells hypertrophy and increase extracellular matrix production. Longer exposure to hyperoxia causes more marked structural changes with striking increases in adventitial thickness and interstitial fibrosis. The number of alveoli decreases after only 2 weeks of hyperoxia in neonatal rats, and the ratio of pulmonary arteries to alveoli decreases (253). Hyperoxia-induced inhibition of lung growth markedly decreases vascular surface area and may permanently prevent the normal postnatal decline in the ratio of alveoli to arteries.

Thus, several structural features of pulmonary vascular injury in CLD are produced in experimental models of hyperoxic lung injury.

Although few studies have examined changes in pulmonary vascular reactivity after prolonged hyperoxia, some studies suggest that sustained hyperoxia increases the pulmonary vasoconstrictor response to angiotensin II in adult rats after exposure to 87% O_2 for 7 days (133). Prolonged hyperoxia also decreases endothelium-derived relaxing factor (EDRF) activity (230), suggesting that long-term hyperoxia may impair NO production or activity, causing increased vasoconstrictor tone and pressor responses to various stimuli. Mechanisms underlying altered reactivity after long-term hyperoxia are uncertain. Oxidant stress and increased production of toxic oxygen radicals, especially superoxide anion, can alter endothelial and smooth-muscle function (74). For example, increased superoxide anion decreases NO activity (116) and impairs vasodilation in some experimental models, such as atherosclerosis. Reaction of NO and superoxide produces peroxynitrite, which may be cytotoxic and contribute to changes in vascular tone and structure during hyperoxia. Further studies are needed to define the effects of oxidant stress on vascular function in the premature lung circulation.

B. Ventilator-Induced Lung Vascular Injury

Prolonged hyperoxia alone appears sufficient to induce pulmonary vascular injury that mimics changes of CLD. Mechanical ventilation can also create significant lung vascular injury. Although much emphasis has been placed on epithelial injury during mechanical ventilation, especially with surfactant deficiency, marked injury to the pulmonary circulation has also been demonstrated (107,118,238). Ventilator-induced lung vascular injury is caused by shear stress from repetitive phasic tidal volume breaths, especially in the presence of low lung volumes (238). Mechanisms causing injury are not simply due to high peak airway pressure, but rather, to lung overdistension (58,79,95,97,98,118,301). Inappropriate ventilator strategies, especially those that promote rapid rates in the setting of inadequate alveolar recruitment, quickly promote vascular permeability and lung inflammation (225). Experimental models suggest that the use of surfactant (59) or alternative ventilator strategies, such as high-frequency oscillatory ventilation (HFOV) attenuate vascular injury, including decreased edema and inflammation, while improving gas exchange in immature animals or in models of adult RDS (ARDS) caused by surfactant washout (117,159,177,208). Recent studies suggest that ventilator-induced injury in preterm lambs can also cause persistent elevation of pulmonary artery pressure and structural lesions that mimic the pulmonary vascular changes of human CLD (18). Thus, hyperoxia and mechanical ventilation can induce acute lung vascular injury in preterm animals, and they are also likely to contribute to the development of chronic pulmonary hypertension in human neonates with CLD.

C. Inflammation

Acute lung injury caused by hyperoxia and mechanical ventilation promote lung inflammation that accelerates the development of chronic pulmonary vascular disease in premature neonates with RDS (135). Specific cellular, biochemical, and molecular mechanisms of inflammation contribute to the pathogenesis of vascular dysfunction with lung injury (17,189,240,268,292). RDS is associated with increased recruitment of neutrophils to the lung, which rapidly decrease in recovering patients, but persist in patients who acquire CLD (214,215,232). Increased inflammatory cells and their products, including eicosanoids, cytokines, elastase, and others, are recovered from tracheal effluent samples in premature infants who subsequently acquire CLD (135,214,215,285). Injury to the pulmonary vascular endothelial cell may cause changes in lung vascular function and structure in CLD. Not only are endothelial-derived products essential for regulating vascular tone during the transitional period, but lung vascular endothelium also serves other functions, such as maintenance of a nonthrombogenic, nonadhesive surface; maintenance of an intact barrier that excludes fluid, plasma proteins, and other macromolecules from the vessel wall and interstitium; metabolic activities; and others (123). Activation or injury to lung vascular endothelium profoundly affects vascular function, causing altered vasoreactivity and tone; thrombosis with platelet aggregation; neutrophil adhesion; development of edema; exposure of the vessel wall to circulating growth factors; and other effects.

Clinical studies have demonstrated elevated inflammatory products, including LTs, platelet-activating factor (PAF), ET-1, interleukin-1β (IL-1β), IL-8, and others, in tracheal effluent or serum from patients with CLD (135). In addition to chemotactic and toxic effects of inflammatory products in the premature lung, LTs, PAF, ET-1, and inflammatory cytokines also directly affect vascular tone, reactivity, and structure. Each of these agents has potent vasoactive properties that are likely to influence vascular tone and structure in CLD. For example, sulfidopeptide LTs are potent vasoconstrictor, edemogenic, and chemotaxic agents, that are elevated in tracheal effluent in patients with ARDS and BPD (284). LTs have been implicated in experimental models of pulmonary hypertension caused by chronic hypoxia (297) and monocrotaline. The source of LT production is generally from inflammatory cells, for 5-lipoxygenase (5-LO) has been localized to neutrophils and macrophages. Recently, 5-LO has also been found in lung vascular endothelium (297). Although the role of LTs in hypoxic pulmonary hypertension has been controversial, recent work suggested that inhibition of 5-lipoxygenase-activating protein (FLAP) reduced pulmonary hypertension in rats with chronic hypoxia (297). In addition, mice bred with deletion of 5-LO enzyme developed less right ventricular hypertrophy during chronic hypoxia. 5-LO is increased in lung tissue from adults with severe primary pulmonary hypertension (292a). Thus, experimental and early clinical findings suggest that inflammation, with persistent LT production, may contribute to chronic pulmonary hypertension. As with LTs, PAF is released from activated neutrophils and endothelial cells and is recovered from tracheal secretions of patients with BPD (285), perhaps contributing to pulmonary hypertension in some experimental models (235). In addition to its vasoconstrictor properties, PAF can also increase vascular permeability, stimulate smooth-muscle cell proliferation (176), and increase extracellular matrix production (292). Chronic PAF blockade attenuates the severity of pulmonary hypertension caused by chronic hypoxia in adult rats (235). Whether LT or PAF antagonists can diminish lung vascular injury and pulmonary hypertension in CLD remains unknown.

ET-1, a potent vasoconstrictor peptide with mitogenic properties, is produced from vascular endothelial cells and hypertensive smooth-muscle cells (100,314). Although several investigators have debated whether ET-1 is a marker or mediator of pulmonary hypertension (20,254,286), experimental and clinical studies have implicated ET-1 as an important contributor to the development of pulmonary hypertension. ET-1 has potent mitogenic effects on vascular smooth-muscle cells and fibroblasts (182). It contributes to pulmonary hypertension in several experimental settings, including chronic hypoxia (48,198), genetic (282), inflammatory (218), and perinatal (163,164) models. ET-1 is markedly elevated in acute lung injury in adults (99), and it may be elevated in children with CLD and pulmonary hypertension (20). Multiple mechanisms modulate ET-1 production, including cytokines (such as endotoxin, tumor necrosis factor-alpha [TNF-α], and IL-1), thrombin, hypoxia, stretch, pressure, or shear stress (131,161,173,184,206,207,311–313). NO and heparin inhibit ET production from vascular endothelium (49,158,185,195,310,315). Circulating ET-1 levels are high in adults with acute lung injury, as well as in patients with pulmonary hypertension. In patients with ARDS, plasma ET-1 levels are greater in systemic arterial blood than in pulmonary artery blood, suggesting that ET-1 may be produced within the lung in ARDS (99). The consequences of elevated lung ET-1 production may include marked pulmonary vasoconstriction, pulmonary edema, and augmented lung inflammation caused by increased neutrophil retention (201). In that extended treatment with ET-converting enzyme or receptor blockers may prevent and even reverse established pulmonary hypertension in various animal models, it is possible that ET inhibition may be useful for treating pulmonary vascular disease in infants with CLD.

Interleukins are peptide mediators that are released from inflammatory and noninflammatory cells, including epithelial and endothelial cells. They are important in signaling between cells, and they determine the type and duration of inflammatory response. IL-1β and TNF-α can induce proliferation of fibroblasts and smooth-muscle cells (66,296). Inflammatory cytokines, especially IL-1 and IL-8, appear early and persist in tracheal effluent samples from premature neonates who acquire CLD (135). These cytokines may contribute to the development of CLD primarily by increasing neutrophil recruitment to the lungs. Circulating IL-1β and IL-6 are elevated in adults with primary pulmonary hypertension (PPH; 155). Hypoxia stimulates endothelial cells to make IL-8 (172), which further amplifies lung inflammation by increasing lung neutrophil sequestration. The release of other products from activated neutrophils, including proteases and toxic oxygen radicals, can further modulate lung vascular tone and structure.

Thus, the early development of lung inflammation in RDS probably contributes to the severity of acute lung injury in premature neonates by disrupting the pulmonary vascular barrier and promoting lung edema, and by altering vasoreactivity. Persistent lung inflammation, which characterizes the transition to CLD, may lead to progressive vascular dysfunction, characterized by high pulmonary vascular tone, altered vasoreactivity, and hypertensive structural remodeling.

D. Chronic Hypoxia

Although chronic hypoxia causes pulmonary hypertension in experimental and some clinical settings, most premature neonates who acquire pulmonary hypertension with CLD are closely monitored in the neonatal intensive care unit (NICU) and infrequently are exposed to prolonged hypoxia during their early course. It appears that chronic hypoxia itself may not be a prerequisite for the development of pulmonary hypertension in BPD, but it clearly accelerates the severity of disease. Animal models suggest that sustained hypoxia for only 3 days can induce structural changes in the pulmonary circulation of adult rats (294). Even intermittent exposure to hypoxia for as little as 4 hr daily is as effective as continuous hypoxia in elevating PVR and causing right ventricular hypertrophy in rats. Exposure to intermittent hypoxia in the newborn lamb also causes sustained pulmonary hypertension (38,138,142,175). In addition, the timing of exposure to hypoxia appears to be a critical determinant of the severity of hypoxia-induced pulmonary vascular disease. Experimental studies with rats and calves suggest greater susceptibility of the neonatal pulmonary circulation in comparison with adult animals (250,284). In response to multiple growth stimuli, including hypoxia, fetal and neonatal calf pulmonary artery smooth-muscle cells undergo more striking proliferation than adult cells do (284). Hypoxia from birth slows the postnatal decline in PVR, and may increase risk for sustained pulmonary hypertension and increased vasoreactivity later in life (19,247). However, striking differences in susceptibility to hypoxia exists between species (cattle, pigs > sheep, dogs; 294). Human infants may differ from animals in their response to hypoxia; the duration and severity of hypoxia that is required for pulmonary hypertension to develop in the human neonate remains uncertain.

Chronic hypoxia can contribute to the development or persistence of pulmonary hypertension in infants with established CLD. The pulmonary vasoconstrictor response to acute hypoxia is often greater in patients with CLD than the hypoxic pressor responses in normal infants or adults (14,107). Infants with CLD may be more likely to acquire or retain pulmonary hypertension with even mild or intermittent exposure to hypoxia. Although abnormalities of the pulmonary vasculature in CLD may be caused initially by injury associated with chronic exposure to hyperoxia, "volutrauma," and inflammation, chronic hypoxia may stimulate or accelerate abnormalities of the pulmonary circulation.

IV. Pulmonary Hypertension in Premature Neonates with Severe RDS

Experimental and clinical studies of the premature newborn have demonstrated the critical role of surfactant in postnatal cardiorespiratory adaptation, and surfactant replacement therapy has dramatically altered the clinical course, management, and outcome of RDS (157,166). Historically, high PVR with low pulmonary blood flow was once considered central to the pathophysiology of severe RDS (68,69), but subsequent studies showed that the primary physiological abnormalities in RDS are related to surfactant deficiency or dysfunction (166,167). PVR drops rapidly after birth in healthy newborns or neonates with mild RDS, but sustained elevation of pulmonary artery pressure contributes to the pathophysiology of severe RDS. Echocardiographic studies of neonates with severe or fatal RDS have shown high PVR, with decreased pulmonary blood flow caused by extrapulmonary right-to-left shunting, as well as marked intrapulmonary shunting from severe parenchymal lung disease (68,69,76,144,258,279,280). Measurement of the aortopulmonary pressure gradient (APPG) across the ductus arteriosus by Doppler echocardiography has been used to assess differences in pressure between the pulmonary and systemic arterial circulations (104,105,128,266,272). The APPG normally widens during the normal transition, as pulmonary artery pressure falls and aortic pressure rises. Severe and fatal cases of RDS are associated with high pulmonary artery pressure (300). Walther and co-workers studied 79 preterm neonates with RDS, who were divided into three groups based on disease severity: absent or mild (not ventilated, $Fio_2 < 40\%$); severe (required mechanical ventilation and $Fio_2 > 60\%$); and fatal disease. Echocardiographic measurements of APPG and left pulmonary artery (LPA) velocity time integrals were serially recorded over the first few days. Changes in APPG were strikingly different between study groups. Although the APPG increased rapidly after birth in healthy term newborns and preterm neonates with mild RDS, it remained low in neonates with severe RDS, especially in fatal cases (300). Fatal RDS was characterized by low gradients that did not increase with time. Low LPA velocity further suggested that high pulmonary artery pressure was related to increased PVR and was likely associated with right-to-left extrapulmonary shunting. Thus, although left-to-right shunting is a frequent clinical problem in many premature infants with RDS, right-to-left or bidirectional shunting is characteristic of severe disease, at least over the first 3 days after birth.

In another prospective echocardiographic study of premature neonates with RDS, 50% of these patients had low APPG (266). Overall, patients with low APPG had more frequent medical complications, including pulmonary hemorrhage (19%) and a greater frequency of late detectable right-to-left shunting (bidirectional) across the ductus (81 vs. 4% in the high APPG group, at 24 hr). Although these findings suggest delayed hemodynamic adaptation with persistent elevation of pulmonary artery pressure (PAP), the neonates with low APPG also tended to have lower mean systemic arterial pressure, but there was no difference in the arterial to alveolar oxygen ratio (a/A)O_2. High PAP may occasionally be related to marked left-to-right shunting, with high pressure associated with high flow without high PVR. These physiological factors also can contribute to low APPG, complicating interpretation of echocardiographic data. Indeed, some echocardiographic studies have suggested that significant right-to-left shunting is rarely found in RDS (104). Although many preterm infants with RDS may have high PAP, it often remains subsystemic, and may not be associated with a large right-to-left shunt. Furthermore, low systemic arterial pressure can contribute to the gradient, and the presence of decreased LPA flow velocity may reflect poor myocardial function and low cardiac output. Thus, improving myocardial function and systemic hemodynamics may be more critical in this setting than is achieving pulmonary vasodilation in hypoxemic patients with severe RDS.

High pulmonary artery pressure in many neonates with severe RDS may be directly related to low lung volumes and regional hypoxia, which generally improve after surfactant therapy (171). Although surfactant therapy improves oxygenation in many premature neonates with RDS, between 6 and 24% of neonates respond poorly to surfactant replacement and have persistent hypoxemia despite treatment (65,76,129,262). Although these patients represent a smaller subgroup of neonates with RDS, those who do not respond to surfactant therapy have a disproportionately high mortality (e.g., mortality exceeds 50% in patients with a/AO_2 less than 0.12; (267). These patients often have elevated PVR, with right-to-left shunting from pulmonary vasoconstriction, as illustrated by reversal of right-to-left shunting and improved oxygenation after inhaled NO or other vasodilator therapies (10,68,69,130,209,239). Therapeutic strategies directed at lowering PVR in neonates with persistent hypoxemia, even after surfactant therapy, may improve their clinical course. Although poor outcome is often associated with high PVR in RDS, it remains uncertain whether pulmonary hypertension is a marker of disease severity or if pulmonary vasodilator therapy will improve outcome without adverse effects. Because mechanisms other than vasoconstriction can contribute to high PVR, initial therapy should be directed toward optimizing alveolar recruitment while avoiding lung overdistension, in addition to assessing myocardial function and systemic hemodynamics.

Given animal studies in experimental RDS (179) and pulmonary hypertension (114,181,252) and clinical observations (10,239), the acute hemodynamic response to inhaled NO in preterm neonates with severe RDS who failed surfactant therapy is under study. Acute and sustained clinical improvement in oxygenation with low-dose inhaled NO therapy has been reported in this subgroup of RDS patients (10,239). Clinical experience suggests that low doses (5 ppm) of inhaled NO can improve oxygenation in premature neonates by immediately lowering PVR and improving pulmonary blood flow, or by reducing intrapulmonary shunt, as demonstrated by multiple inert gas techniques in older patients with severe ARDS (253). Concern exists over potential adverse effects of inhaled NO in preterm newborns, such as oxidant lung injury, lung inflammation, surfactant inactivation, methemoglobinemia, and intracranial hemorrhage. In addition, marked increases in pulmonary blood flow owing to rapid reversal of PVR may increase left-to-right shunting across the ductus arteriosus, which could potentially increase pulmonary edema and decrease systemic perfusion. When inhaled NO is administered to neonates with severe left ventricular dysfunction owing to asphyxia, infection, or prematurity, increased pulmonary blood flow may elevate left atrial and pulmonary microvascular pressures (264). This also may decrease cardiac output and worsen systemic hypotension, further compromising the clinical course and outcome of sick premature neonates with RDS.

The potential use of inhaled NO in RDS may have important implications for the development of CLD and pulmonary hypertension. Diminished antioxidant defenses in the premature lung may make the pulmonary circulation more susceptible to oxidant injury from interactions of NO with superoxide, forming the reactive oxygen species, peroxynitrite (36,116,137), and further increase the risk for CLD. Recent observations, however, support the speculation that NO may inactivate superoxide and protect against lung vascular damage from reactive oxygen species (92,174,136,306). Experimentally, NO decreases pulmonary vascular permeability, attenuates lung inflammation by blocking neutrophil adherence to endothelium and decreasing cytokine activation of endothelium, and may stimulate epithelial clearance of alveolar edema (42,92,187,188,190). Whether NO mitigates or potentiates injury in the preterm lung with severe RDS is unknown. Low-dose (5 ppm) inhaled NO decreased lung neutrophil recruitment and myeloperoxidase activity in extremely preterm lambs with experimental RDS (177). Although data are lacking in human neonates with RDS, recent studies suggest that low-dose inhaled NO therapy reduces markers of lung inflammation (PMN activation and IL-8 content) in lavage fluid from adults with ARDS (66). Inhaled NO therapy also decreases lung leak index while lowering pulmonary capillary wedge pressure in adults with ARDS (42). Thus, inhaled NO might reduce PVR and improve ventilation–perfusion mismatch and lower intrapulmonary shunt in selected premature neonates with severe RDS. Whether inhaled NO will prove to be useful or harmful in the immediate management of severe

RDS and its influence on the incidence or severity of CLD is unknown and merits careful clinical investigation.

V. Pulmonary Hypertension in CLD of Infancy

The pulmonary circulation in CLD is characterized by abnormalites in vascular structure and function. Clinical studies have demonstrated elevated baseline pulmonary artery pressure and altered pulmonary vasoreactivity, and autopsy studies have shown hypertensive structural remodeling and decreased number of arteries associated with decreased alveolarization (''alveolar simplification''; 21,28,73,134,152,203,244,287,288,291). These features have been recognized from the earliest reports describing the course of infants with severe CLD, but the etiology, pathophysiology, and therapy of pulmonary vascular disease remains incompletely understood. Although the relative contributions of tone versus structural vascular disease to the severity of pulmonary hypertension may vary among patients, altered function and structure are both present in most infants with CLD and associated pulmonary hypertension. Functional changes in pulmonary vascular tone and vasoreactivity are closely linked with structural remodeling. For example, increased smooth-muscle growth in muscular arteries and muscularization of vessels that are normally nonmuscular, probably contribute to the high basal tone and augmented pulmonary vasoreactivity responses to constrictor stimuli, such as acute hypoxia, in patients with CLD (14). Similarly, changes in pulmonary vascular tone and vasoreactivity caused by altered endothelial or smooth-muscle function lead to sustained elevations of pulmonary artery pressure which, in turn, accelerates structural hypertensive vascular changes. Finally, abnormalities in lung growth and decreased alveolarization suggest that a restricted vascular bed will be exposed to relatively higher pulmonary blood flow, which may further accelerate abnormalities of both vessel structure and function (see Fig. 1). This also may account for the observation of more advanced pulmonary vascular disease in infants with CLD and associated patent foramen ovale or atrial septal defect. Thus, alterations of vascular tone, structure, and growth are closely linked in the pathophysiology of pulmonary hypertension in CLD.

A. Pathology

Histological abnormalities of the pulmonary circulation have been recognized in even the earliest reports describing the pathology of BPD (47,228). These findings are strikingly similar to animal models of hyperoxic or ventilator-induced lung injury in premature baboons and lambs (18,72,93). Central features include medial thickening, peripheral extension of smooth muscle to vessels that are normally only partially muscular or nonmuscular, adventitial fibrosis, occasional thromboembolic occlusion and vascular obliteration, and intimal proliferation (rarely). Although the most advanced lesions are generally found in older infants who die with BPD and cor pulmonale, infants dying at less than 1 month after birth already manifests striking histological lesions (291). Most of the early studies were descriptive, but recent studies have assessed and quantified morphological changes. Morphometric studies of eight infants with BPD who died within 2 months of birth revealed increased peripheral extension of smooth muscle to small pulmonary arteries that are usually only partially muscular or nonmuscular (291). Medial hypertrophy of muscular arteries was not striking. Occasional thromboemboli were noted, but arterial density appeared normal. The bronchial circulation was described as ''dilated and tortuous,'' readily filling with a barium–gelatin suspension after injection into the pulmonary circulation. The authors noted that their findings illustrated the interplay between the ''complex dual process of adaptation [to extrauterine life] and response to injury. . . .'' Overall, owing to the early age at death in this group, milder pulmonary vascular changes were present than reported in subsequent studies. In a description of autopsy findings in three patients with BPD and severe pulmonary hypertension who died at an older age (6 months to 3.5 years), markedly increased wall thickness of muscular pulmonary arteries, peripheral extension of muscularity, increased wall thickness of small veins, and fibrotic obliteration of some small arteries (in one patient) were present (57). Similar findings of medial hypertrophy and adventitial thickening were present at autopsy in nearly 80% of a nonselected group of older infants with BPD (age range: 3–40 months; 287).

Gorenflo and colleagues (134) compared pulmonary vascular disease in infants with BPD who died early (< 1 month) versus those who died later (1–7 months). They confirmed previous reports of abnormal distal muscularization of peripheral vessels and increased wall thickness of muscular arteries, which were more striking in patients with cor pulmonale (this correlation between cor pulmonale and severity of medial thickening was not found in another report; 152). Interestingly, the older group also had decreased arterial density by histology and postmortem angiography in comparison with younger BPD infants and normal-term infants. Alveolar number, but not arterial density, was reduced (152). Arterial number may be normal for age in infants who die with BPD at less than 1–2 months; however, marked reduction in alveolarization is found in older patients dying of BPD (203,274,287). Thus, lung injury disrupts normal postnatal alveolar and vascular growth during this critical period of rapid growth, causing decreased septation and alveolar simplification. As capillary growth parallels changes in alveolar number, these findings suggest a markedly reduced pulmonary vascular surface area. This anatomical reduction in the lung vasculature may explain persistence or late clinical problems associated with pulmonary hypertension and may limit or prevent reversal of structural vascular disease.

In conclusion, the pathology of the pulmonary circulation in many infants who die with BPD demonstrates striking vascular lesions that are predominantly characterized by marked muscularization of small pulmonary arteries and increased adventitial matrix. Signs of intimal thickening or vascular obliteration are less common. Although changes are present early, late deaths were associated with more severe changes, including decreased arterial number, partly to related abnormal lung alveolarization (103,152,203,274,287). The severity of pulmonary vascular disease may (134) or may not (152) correlate with the presence of right ventricular hypertrophy at autopsy.

B. Mechanisms Regulating Pulmonary Vascular Tone

Mechanisms contributing to the abnormal regulation of lung vascular tone and reactivity in CLD are poorly understood, but are likely to include chronic alterations in endothelial–smooth-muscle cell interactions (16,30,226,236). Experimental studies in vascular biology have demonstrated that the endothelial cell produces diverse vasoactive compounds, including dilators such as PGI_2, NO, and ''endothelium-derived hyperpolarizing factor'' (EDHF; 219,226,237). In addition, vascular endothelium is also capable of producing potent vasoconstrictors, including ET-1, LTs, and perhaps other ''endothelium-derived contracting factors.'' Persistent hemodynamic stresses (high flow, high pressure, shear stress, or stretch), hyperoxia, hypoxia, or inflammation, may alter endothelial production of these products, creating an imbalance between vasodilators and vasoconstrictors, which favors increased basal tone or heightened vasoreactivity. Altered smooth-muscle responsiveness, owing to changes in phenotype, receptor, or enzyme profiles, and myofilaments, also contribute to heightened tone. The effects of chronic vascular injury on the production of, or response to, vasoactive agents are currently under active investigation in many laboratories. Pulmonary vascular production of and responsiveness to many vasoactive substances may change with normal maturation and may vary, depending on species, postnatal age, and related factors. In addition, experimental models of chronic pulmonary hypertension caused by different mechanisms can have different effects on dilator and constrictor systems. For example, in adult rat lungs, chronic hypoxia upregulates lung eNOS mRNA, protein, and activity (160,192), whereas inflammatory (monocrotaline) and genetic (fawn hooded rat) models of pulmonary hypertension are associated with decreased eNOS protein and NO production (292b). Endothelial NOS protein and activity are decreased in developmental models of perinatal pulmonary hypertension in sheep (295) and decreased PGI_2 in hypoxic calves (27). Besides changes in eNOS expression, most studies of chronic animal models have consistently reported that elevations of ET-1, a potent vasoconstrictor, contribute to chronic pulmonary hypertension (163,164,198,218,233,282). Thus, decreased eNOS (in some models) or impaired responsiveness to NO (84) and increased ET-1 may contribute to altered vascular growth and function in various experimental models of pulmonary hypertension.

Clinical studies also suggest decreased eNOS and increased ET-1 in patients with pulmonary hypertension. In vitro studies of isolated human pulmonary arteries showed impaired endogenous NOS activity in patients with pulmonary hypertension and congenital heart disease or chronic lung disease in adults (308,309). Endothelial NOS expression in lung tissue from adults with pulmonary hypertension may be decreased in comparison with controls (125). Studies of pulmonary vasoreactivity clearly demonstrate that endogenous NOS activity contributes to basal pulmonary vascular tone in normal children and adults (78) and is impaired in pulmonary hypertension (302). In addition, increased immunoreactivity and gene expression of ET-1 is present in lung tissue from adults with severe pulmonary hypertension, suggesting that enhanced ET-1 production also may contribute to heightened vasoreactivity and hypertensive vascular remodeling in chronic pulmonary hypertension (126). Children with pulmonary hypertension, including patients with CLD, had elevated plasma concentrations of immunoreactive ET-1, which correlated with the degree of acute hypoxic pulmonary vasoconstriction (20). Thus, clinical data support the concept that an imbalance between dilator and constrictor systems, such as NO and ET-1, or thromboxane and prostacyclin (as in primary pulmonary hypertension; 67), may modulate pulmonary vascular tone and reactivity in pulmonary hypertension, but such studies are lacking in patients with CLD.

C. Physiology

Cor pulmonale, or ''pulmonary heart disease,'' represents the adaptive response of the right ventricle to increased afterload caused by pulmonary hypertension associated with lung disease. Clinical signs of overt right ventricular failure can be obscured by signs of severe CLD, leading to delays in the recognition of pulmonary hypertension. In some cases, the failing right ventricle may not be able to generate sufficient cardiac output to sustain elevated pulmonary artery pressure in the presence of high pulmonary vascular resistance. This may cause overt clinical signs of right-sided failure in some patients with only mild or moderate elevations of pulmonary artery pressure. With the gradual development of pulmonary hypertension, the right ventricle is able to adapt to increased afterload by muscle hypertrophy. Hypertrophy represents an adaptive response, which reduces ventricular compliance and increases right ventricular end-diastolic pressure and right atrial pressure. Left ventricular function is generally maintained in older patients with CLD despite pulmonary hypertension and suboptimal right ventricular function. High pulmonary vascular resistance can impair cardiac output, but normal left ventricular function is sustained until late in the clinical course. High pulmonary vascular resistance causes left ventricular dysfunction by decreasing preload and causing paradoxical interventricular septal motion (''ventricular interdependence''). Increased right ventricular dilation mechanically distorts the left ventricle, impedes left ventricular filling, and decreases cardiac output in proportion to the severity of right ventricular failure. Left ventricular hypertrophy may represent an adaptive response to increased septal wall tension, and is sometimes observed in infants with CLD and pulmonary hypertension (see later discussion). Low cardiac output can accompany severe pulmonary hypertension and is associated with poor long-term outcome.

In addition to its roles in the regulation of gas exchange, vascular tone, growth, and barrier functions, the normal pulmonary vascular endothelium serves various metabolic functions. These include activation of angiotensin, production of vasoactive substances (PGI_2, NO, LTs, endothelin, and others), and clearance or inactivation of circulating substances, including bradykinin, serotonin, and norepinephrine (NE). For example, the normal pulmonary circulation clears up to 40% of circulating NE in a single passage across the lung (277). Changes in vascular endothelial function may serve as an early and sensitive marker for pulmonary vascular injury, as in ARDS. Clinical studies show that adults with chronic obstructive pulmonary disease (COPD) and children with pulmonary hypertension owing to congenital heart disease have decreased clearance of norepinephrine (124). Similar findings have been reported in children with BPD (11). Unlike the 25% transpulmonary reduction of norepinephrine in control patients without pulmonary hypertension, infants with CLD had either no extraction or net production of norepinephrine. Possible mechanisms underlying this observation include reduced lung vascular surface area, endothelial dysfunction, or enhanced intrapulmonary production of NE. It is uncertain if the lack of NE extraction is merely a sign of pulmonary vascular abnormalities or if it contributes to physiological problems in CLD (such as systemic hypertension, LVH, high metabolic rates and poor growth, and pulmonary vasoconstriction).

D. Evaluation and Treatment

Although past studies demonstrated high mortality in prematurely born neonates with BPD and pulmonary hypertension beyond 4 months old (110), there is little information on the changes in pulmonary artery pressure that occur during the early postnatal weeks in patients who acquire CLD. Increased awareness of the high risk for pulmonary hypertension in NICU graduates with even mild lung disease may permit earlier diagnosis and a greater likelihood for successful management of pulmonary hypertension and related problems. Three recent studies have examined serial changes in echocardiographic signs of pulmonary hypertension in premature neonates with and without CLD (41,128,266). Gill and Weindling (128) studied 54 premature neonates with HMD, from birth to 1 month of age, to examine changes in pulmonary artery pressure. Echocardiographic assessment of the ratio of the time to peak velocity to the right ventricular ejection time (corrected for heart rate) was determined from the pulmonary artery Doppler waveform. CLD developed in 63% of these infants. Although estimated pulmonary artery pressure (PAP) fell over the first 14 days in both groups, the decline was less in infants with CLD, and PAP progressively increased in the CLD group during days 14–28. Infants with CLD were less mature (27 vs. 30 weeks), had lower birth weights (850 vs. 1214 g), and had worse acute lung disease (a/AO_2 0.16 vs. 0.29, on day 1) than were infants without CLD. A cross-sectional study to evaluate the prevalence and degree of pulmonary hypertension in a cohort of NICU survivors with CLD further suggested that pulmonary hypertension can be identified early by echocardiography, and that this approach may help identify those infants who are at risk for pulmonary hypertension. It is unknown if early identification and intervention alters the outcome or shortens the duration of ventilation or hospitalization in CLD.

Right ventricular dysfunction may occur at lower pulmonary artery pressures in CLD than in primary pulmonary hypertension, making problematic the diagnosis and assessment of the contribution of high pulmonary artery pressure to the clinical picture in those with CLD. Signs and symptoms of pulmonary hypertension can be nonspecific and difficult to distinguish from progression of underlying CLD. Such signs as tachypnea, fatigue, recurrent cyanotic spells, poor growth, and irritability are common in severe CLD. Pulmonary hypertension in infants is often associated with poor feeding and choking, sweating, and cyanosis. As pulmonary hypertension worsens and contributes to the underlying lung disease, progressive respiratory distress, fatigue, and other signs are often attributed to exacerbations of the primary lung disease. Physical findings of pulmonary hypertension are often subtle, especially in young infants. Neck vein distension, peripheral edema, hepatomegaly, syncope, and other signs of right ventricular failure often become apparent only late in the course. Common findings on physical examination in patients with moderate pulmonary hypertension include tachypnea, tachycardia, an accentuated second heart sound with narrow or fixed splitting, and a systolic ejection murmur at the left upper sternal border. Signs of advanced right ventricular failure include right ventricular heave, increased jugular venous distension, hepatomegaly, and peripheral edema. Although differentiating signs and symptoms from CLD versus pulmonary hypertension is difficult, awareness of the risk for pulmonary hypertension and early evaluation may lead to the diagnosis. Infants with CLD and unexplained poor growth, persistent or increased oxygen requirements, recurrent cyanotic episodes, or the lack of resolution of right ventricular hypertrophy by electrocardiogram (ECG) should undergo more thorough investigation (3,4,13).

Detection of pulmonary hypertension and assessment of its severity requires serial ECG and echocardiogram studies (41). Although ECG findings of RVH are diagnostically useful for screening most patients for pulmonary hypertension, signs of RVH are usually less pronounced in infants with CLD. The sensitivity of ECG findings of RVH in CLD is uncertain. Doppler and two-dimensional echocardiography have markedly improved noninvasive assessments of pulmonary hypertension. A major problem, however, is the technical difficulty of obtaining interpretable information in severe obstructive lung disease, for hyperinflation and large fluctuations in intrathoracic pressures with respiratory efforts may make imaging difficult. Echocardiographic signs of pulmonary hypertension include increased thickness of the right ventricular wall or increased chamber size, flattening or paradoxic motion of the interventricular septum, early closure of the pulmonic valve, and incomplete tricuspid valve closure. Increased right ventricular anterior wall thickness and interventricular septal wall thickness reflect RVH. Quantitative assessments of pulmonary hypertension include measurements of right ventricular systolic time interval (RVSTI) and tricuspid regurgitation. Although past studies used measurements of RVSTI to reflect acute changes in pulmonary artery pressure during exposure to oxygen or vasodilators (141), variability and lack of sensitivity makes this measurement inconsistent or unreliable for routine assessments of pulmonary vasoreactivity. Perhaps a more sensitive assessment of pulmonary hypertension is the measurement of peak pulmonary artery systolic pressure obtained from continuous wave Doppler measurements of the tricuspid jet, with application of the Bernouilli principle.

Although serial studies with ECG or echocardiogram are useful during long-term follow-up, early cardiac catheterization may be necessary to define more clearly the role of pulmonary vascular disease in the clinical course (14,43,44,145). Cardiac catheterization serves to quantitate the severity of pulmonary hypertension; to rule out anatomical cardiac lesions, structural pulmonary vascular lesions, thromboemboli, or significant hypertrophy of bronchial collaterals; to define optimal treatment levels for supplemental oxygen; to assess pulmonary vasoreactivity; and to test pharmacological agents for potential long-term therapy. Delays in performing cardiac catheterization in patients with CLD are common, however, potentially contributing to delays in therapy and worse outcome. Probe-patent foramen ovale may be present in many young children, suggesting that intracardiac shunt may contribute to the severity of hypoxemia in patients with CLD and pulmonary hypertension. Cardiac catheterization should include angiography to avoid missing structural lesions, such as pulmonary arterial stenosis, pulmonary venoocclusive disease, enlarged bronchial collateral vessels, and other diagnoses. Although concerns persist over the potential risks of angiography in precipitating pulmonary hypertensive crises or dysrhythmias in severe pulmonary hypertension, the use of newer contrast material (e.g., Optiray; Malinckrodt, St. Louis, MO) seems to have decreased these risks.

Assessment of pulmonary vasoreactivity, including hemodynamic measurements, is an essential part of the evaluation but is often omitted. For example, exaggerated vasoconstrictor responses to acute hypoxia in patients with only mild baseline pulmonary hypertension may help explain episodic cyanosis or progressive pulmonary hypertension in children with recurrent cyanosis, and pulmonary edema in patients with CLD. The use of anesthesia and inadvertent oversedation, hypo- or hyperventilation, and acute hypoxia can alter basal pulmonary artery pressure and reactivity during cardiac catheterization, potentially limiting the usefulness of clinical information. On the other hand, controlled hypoxic and hypercarbic challenges during catheterization may provide insight into pulmonary vascular hyperreactivity. For example, some patients require higher oxygen saturations to maintain maximal decreases in pulmonary vascular resistance and to lower the risk of intermittent increases in pulmonary artery pressure.

Whereas the vasodilator response while breathing 100% oxygen is commonly used to assess potential reversibility of pulmonary hypertension, correlation between the dilator response to oxygen and outcome is unclear. Hyperoxia is not a very potent vasodilator beyond its ability to reverse hypoxic vasoconstriction, but this assessment allows adjustment of O_2 therapy. The response to high oxygen concentration may not be sufficient to determine the relative contributions of vasoconstriction and structural remodeling to existing pulmonary hypertension. For example, it is not uncommon that pharmacological vasodilators (such as prostacyclin, sodium nitroprusside, hydralazine, and calcium channel blockers) or inhaled NO can cause greater vasodilation than can high concentrations of inspired oxygen alone. Although it remains unclear which vasodilator should be used to initially assess pulmonary vascular tone, inhaled NO may be a good choice because of its short half-life, selectivity for the pulmonary circulation (less risk for systemic hypotension, fatal dysrhythmia), and its ability to improve gas exchange, rather than worsen oxygenation, in patients with lung disease.

E. Treatment

The primary goal in the treatment of pulmonary hypertension in CLD is to optimize lung function and gas exchange. In addition to managing right heart failure, the long-term goal is to avoid the adverse effects of sustained pulmonary hypertension on progressive vascular remodeling. Mechanisms leading to reversibility of pulmonary hypertension and vascular remodeling are poorly understood, but are partly dependent on the severity of vascular remodeling at the time of diagnosis and the recognition of complicating factors that contribute to its progression. Thus, early anticipation and recognition of pulmonary hypertension in at-risk patients may improve outcome. Therapy generally targets three areas: (1) optimal management of underlying lung disease (e.g., lung inflammation and infection, and mechanical ventilation for chronic hypoventilation); (2) diagnosis and treatment of complicating or ''unsuspected'' cardiopulmonary abnormalities (such as aspiration, upper airway obstruction, or anatomical cardiac defects); and (3) treatment of the pulmonary hypertension with oxygen and pharmacological agents.

Clinical management of pulmonary hypertension in BPD entails vigilant monitoring and aggressive use of supplemental O_2 therapy (224,241). Chronic intermittent or persistent hypoxia inhibits recovery and accelerates progression of pulmonary vascular disease. At some centers, infants with CLD and pulmonary hypertension are undertreated owing to concerns of oxygen toxicity. Once persistent signs of pulmonary hypertension have been identified in older infants with CLD, even mild levels of hypoxia should not be tolerated. Reversal of hypoxia with supplemental O_2 in patients with CLD will quickly lower PVR in many patients. Although oxygen saturations below 90–92% may be well tolerated in normal children recovering from viral respiratory infections, infants with CLD require better oxygenation to minimize the adverse effects of chronic hypoxic pulmonary vasoconstriction. This recommendation is based on studies of the acute hypoxic pulmonary vasoconstrictor response in infants with CLD (14). To study pulmonary vasoreactivity and the role of O_2 therapy in the short- and long-term management of BPD, infants with BPD were studied with various levels of supplemental O_2 during cardiac catheterization. Each infant had pulmonary hypertension, despite breathing high concentrations of O_2. In contrast with the small rise in PAP during acute hypoxia in normal infants (107) or adults, infants with CLD had an exaggerated pressor response to acute hypoxia (14). This pattern is similar to infants recovering from high-altitude pulmonary edema or with symptomatic high-altitude pulmonary hypertension (107). Although the degree of rise in PAP was variable, some infants had marked elevations of PAP even with small decreases in oxygenation (14). To examine the response to low levels of supplemental O_2 therapy relevant to prolonged management, we measured the acute hemodynamic effects of supplemental O_2 delivered by nasal cannula (14). Most of the reduction in PAP achieved while breathing mixtures with high oxygen concentrations was readily achieved with low-flow O_2 at levels that corrected hypoxemia (maintained O_2 saturation >92–94%). Although occasional infants responded to higher concentrations of O_2 with a further drop in PAP, most of the response was achieved with an O_2 saturation above 94%.

Continuous long-term supplemental O_2 therapy may hasten the reduction of pulmonary hypertension in CLD by attenuating the adverse effects of intermittent or sustained hypoxia. Given these clinical studies, consistently maintaining O_2 saturations above 94% while awake, asleep, and during feeding are recommended for infants with BPD and pulmonary hypertension (4,183). Cessation of long-term O_2 therapy requires a normal ECG and prolonged monitoring with pulse oximetery, including extensive measurements with sleep and activity, for the adverse effects of O_2 withdrawal may be delayed (265). Thus, management of pulmonary hypertension in BPD remains largely supportive, with careful attention to the avoidance of the adverse effects of episodic hypoxia and hypercarbia on lung vascular remodeling and reactivity.

Resolution of pulmonary hypertension, as assessed by ECG or echocardiographic criteria, often occurs with appropriate therapy over time (4). Children with persistent RVH require more thorough and frequent evaluations of possible conditions that may be complicating their recovery. These include reassessment of oxygenation levels during prolonged pulse oximetery studies; formal sleep studies; assessment for unsuspected cardiac or lung problems contributing to the severity of the clinical course (such as aspiration, upper airway obstruction, anatomical heart disease, and large bronchial collaterals causing pulmonary edema; 3,13,263,271). Poor growth is often an indication of undertreatment with oxygen therapy, perhaps reflecting noncompliance, premature discontinuation of oxygen therapy, or unrecognized intermittent hypoxia (9). Evaluations should include sleep studies, imaging of the upper airway by flexible laryngoscopy and bronchoscopy, radiologic studies (such as barium swallow and isovue bronchograms), pulmonary function testing, and cardiac catheterization. Early identification and treatment of left-to-right shunt cardiovascular lesions may enhance long-term outcome in some patients by decreasing progressive vascular injury in a lung circulation that is already limited by decreased surface area, vascular remodeling, and vasconstriction. We speculate that even small increases in pulmonary blood flow owing to shunt lesions in the setting of a restricted pulmonary vascular bed may further accelerate structural remodeling.

The temporary response to several pharmacological agents has been examined, but there are no studies suggesting long-term benefit. Immediate hemodynamic improvement in infants with BPD and pulmonary hypertension during cardiac catheterization has been reported after brief vasodilator therapy with prostacyclin (57) and nifedipine (55). In eight patients with BPD, rapid infusion of PGI_2 did not change mean pulmonary artery pressure, but lowered pulmonary vascular resistance by 23% owing to an increase in cardiac output (64). PGI_2 did not have a selective effect on the pulmonary circulation, as systemic vascular resistance fell by 39%. Despite this apparent responsiveness to PGI_2, six patients (75%) subsequently died. Based on early studies of long-term PGI_2 therapy in primary pulmonary hypertension (PPH; 151), Barst et al. recently demonstrated improved survival and sustained clinical benefit in PPH treated with extended intravenous PGI_2 by continuous infusion pump (31,32). Long-term PGI_2 therapy has been approved for use in PPH and as a "bridge to lung transplantation." Whether long-term treatment with PGI_2 infusions could improve outcome in BPD with severe pulmonary hypertension is uncertain. In the setting of significant parenchymal lung disease, intravenous vasodilators, such as PGI_2, may worsen gas exchange by adverse effects on ventilation–perfusion matching. For example, vasodilators can effectively lower PAP in ARDS or COPD, but at a cost of decreased oxygenation (see later; 212).

Benefits from pharmacological vasodilator therapy in the long-term management of pulmonary hypertension secondary to CLD remain unproved. Long-term therapy of severe pulmonary-hypertension includes calcium channel blockers (diltiazem and nifedipine) and antiplatelet agents or anticoagulants (coumadin, heparin, or dipyridamole). Clinical studies of calcium-channel blockade in some adults with PPH have been successful, especially in combination with coumadin (251). In studies of nifedipine in infants with CLD, the fall in mean pulmonary artery pressure achieved after nifedipine treatment was similar to the response to supplemental oxygen alone (106). Because nifedipine increased cardiac output, pulmonary vascular resistance was lower after nifedipine administration than after oxygen therapy alone. Whether the combination of supplemental oxygen with long-term calcium channel blockers will enhance a sustained outcome in BPD patients with severe pulmonary hypertension has not been studied.

Assessment of the immediate response to pulmonary vasodilator therapy during cardiac catheterization is necessary to optimize treatment dose and to avoid potential adverse effects, as observed with hydralazine in patients with severe BPD and pulmonary hypertension (132). Patients with CLD and severe pulmonary hypertension acquired marked hypercarbia, with acute pulmonary edema after hydralazine infusion, perhaps owing to increased left-to-right shunting across enlarged bronchial collateral vessels (132). These observations support the need for careful assessment of the effects of vasodilator therapy on gas exchange and hemodynamic measurements before initiating long-term therapy.

Whereas various agents may be effective in briefly lowering pulmonary artery pressure, pulmonary vasodilation in the setting of parenchymal lung disease can cause severe hypoxemia by worsening ventilation–perfusion mismatch, limiting their usefulness in the presence of lung disease (212). In contrast to the potential adverse effects of most vasodilators, inhaled NO at low doses lowers PAP without worsening gas exchange, and may improve Pao_2. When administered as a gas, inhaled NO is delivered to better-aerated lung regions, causing local vasodilation, improving regional blood flow, and increasing Pao_2. This has been observed in patients with CLD treated during acute respiratory exacerbations from viral pneumonitis (8), and more recently, in other infants with CLD (200). As demonstrated in ARDS (122) and adults with COPD (29), however, high doses of inhaled NO may impair gas exchange. In these cases, the small decrements in Pao_2 with high-dose NO were likely related to worsened ventilation–perfusion matching from increased blood flow being directed toward partially aerated lung units.

The achievement of selective pulmonary vasodilation is not necessarily limited to inhaled NO. When administered by aerosolization, PGI_2 also can briefly lower PAP without causing deterioration of oxygenation in adults with ARDS. The potential for prolonged therapy with aerosolized PGI_2 or iloprost (a stable PGI_2 analogue) was recently reported in six adults with severe pulmonary hypertension (234). Aerosolized delivery of PGI_2 and iloprost allowed preferential distribution of the drug to well-ventilatred lung areas, thereby achieving selective improvement in pulmonary vasodilation and concomitant improvement of ventilation–perfusion mismatch. These agents effectively lowered PAP and had minimal systemic effects. The major problem was the transient nature of the vasodilation after PGI_2 treatment, which lasted only 10–30 min after treatment, whereas the response to iloprost persisted for up to 2 hr. Although aerosolized PGI_2 treatment may be effective in lowering PAP, long-term therapy would require frequent treatments to sustain the hemodynamic response, and such an approach may be impractical. Recent experimental studies have suggested that nebulization of an NO donor, diethylenetriamine/NO (DETA/NO), releases NO in aqueous solutions and has a long half-life. Local delivery by nebulization may provide selective pulmonary vasodilation similar to that seen with inhaled NO. In an animal model of chronic pulmonary hypertension, brief DETA/NO nebulization treatments effectively lowered PVR (143). The possibility of a selective pulmonary vasodilator therapy using intermittent nebulizer treatments is exciting. Future therapies currently under investigation are likely to provide novel approaches distinct from conventional vasodilator therapy. Such strategies may include prolonged blockade of cGMP-specific phosphodiesterases, prolonged blockade of vasoconstrictors (such as ET-1 or LTs); antiproliferative agents (such as heparin, antielastases, or ET blockade; 318); and perhaps agents that promote alveolar and capillary growth in early infancy [e.g., retinoic acid (205)].

F. Late Morbidity and Mortality

Past studies have reported mortality rates as high as 30–40% in infants with severe CLD. Most deaths (about 80%) occur during the initial hospitalization as a result of progressive respiratory failure, sepsis or pneumonia, pulmonary hypertension, and congestive heart failure. Causes of late deaths after discharge from the hospital are similar, but include severe acute respiratory failure owing to viral lower respiratory tract infections or sudden unexpected deaths (5,35,127,213,303). Many patients die with histological signs of pulmonary hypertension, but the exact role of pulmonary hypertension is often uncertain. Although pulmonary hypertension may simply be a marker of disease severity in some patients, it may contribute directly to late deaths (57,110,132). Pulmonary hypertension is often associated with other clinical features linked with high mortality, including the need for prolonged mechanical ventilation (more than 6 months), severe respiratory failure with viral infections, and frequent cyanotic episodes (5,127). Because of limited lung reserve and pulmonary vascular disease (56), infants with CLD are at high risk for profound hypoxemia and respiratory failure with viral respiratory exacerbations. Pulmonary hypertension, increased vasoreactivity, and a limited vascular bed contribute to the severity of hypoxemia owing to severe ventilation–perfusion mismatch with marked intrapulmonary shunting. Even normal infants with acute RSV infections can have transient elevation of pulmonary artery pressure. As observed in children with congenital heart disease, infants with CLD and pulmonary hypertension are likely to have a more marked rise in pulmonary artery pressure than in normal infants, which worsens pulmonary edema and contributes to high morbidity. Low-dose inhaled NO therapy can lower pulmonary artery pressure and improve intrapulmonary shunt in this setting, which may stabilize oxygenation and provide an adjuvant therapy during mechanical ventilation (8). Whether inhaled NO can shorten ventilator or PICU days, decrease ECMO use or improve survival with acute hypoxemic respiratory failure is currently under study.

Recurrent cyanotic episodes in severe BPD have been associated with late deaths (5,127). Although some episodes appear related to tracheomalacia or severe gastroesophageal reflux, mechanisms are often not identified. In severe cases, cyanosis with bradycardia persist after brief hypoxia, despite vigorous mask or endotracheal ventilation with high inspired oxygen concentrations, suggesting that the frequency of these ''spells'' or the severity of cyanosis are not simply due to persistent airways obstruction (5,119). In addition, sudden unexpected deaths can occur even in patients with tracheostomies and receiving mechanical ventilator support. Sudden deaths have been described in hospitalized infants with CLD. These deaths occurred despite continuous monitoring and aggressive cardiopulmonary resuscitation by experienced in-hospital staff. A retrospective study noted that recurrent cyanotic episodes, left and right ventricular hypertrophy, and greater use of ''polypharmacy'' (diuretics, theophylline, and β-agonists) occurred in the sudden death group (5). Whether recurrent cyanotic episodes are directly related to the high rate of so-called SIDS deaths in the outpatient setting is speculative. Abnormalities in control of breathing, cardiac dysrhythmias, and pulmonary hypertensive crises, may contribute to sudden death in infants with BPD. Southall and colleagues (278) have proposed a potential role for increased vasoreactivity and severe intrapulmonary shunting in the genesis of cyanotic spells in some children without underlying heart or lung disease. In some patients, increased pulmonary artery pressure preceded cyanosis and apnea in some infants with apparent life-threatening episodes. The exact mechanism by which abnormal control of pulmonary vascular tone can cause profound hypoxemia in these patients is unknown.

Pulmonary vascular abnormalities beyond late childhood are only beginning to be studied. Although some follow-up studies suggest that RVH is absent in older patients (229), physiological studies of late morbidity related to abnormalities of the pulmonary circulation are warranted. For example, problems may become apparent during exercise, even in the presence of minimally elevated baseline pulmonary artery pressure. The normal physiological response to exercise includes a marked increase in cardiac output associated with small increases in pulmonary artery and capillary wedge pressures, and a net fall in PVR by 60–70%. The dramatic increase in pulmonary blood flow with exercise is normally well-tolerated owing to pulmonary vascular distension, recruitment, and perhaps vasodilation. With pulmonary vascular disease, increased cardiac output can markedly elevate pulmonary artery pressure by high flow through a restricted vascular bed and an inability to distend or dilate owing to abnormal structure and reactivity. In some older children with CLD, oxygen saturation decreases during exercise, despite apparently normal oxygenation at rest, especially at altitude or with severe exercise. Studies of lung function have revealed exercise-induced bronchospasm in older patients with CLD (26,273). However, there is little information available on exercise-related cardiovascular problems. Exercise capacity in CLD patients may be limited by a restricted pulmonary vascular bed, resulting in an inability to fully accommodate increased pulmonary blood flow (217). Whether abnormalities of the pulmonary circulation will become more clinically apparent during young adulthood in some patients requires further investigation.

VI. Conclusions and Future Directions

Pulmonary hypertension contributes significantly to the morbidity and mortality of premature neonates with severe lung disease. The exact mechanisms that cause pulmonary vascular disease are incompletely understood, but as emphasized in this chapter, are related to interactions between the disruption of lung vascular growth and development by premature birth, acute lung injury, and an inability to achieve normal postnatal adaptation of the lung circulation after birth. The incidence and severity of pulmonary hypertension in established CLD is partly dependent on cardiopulmonary management in the early postnatal period. Our current therapeutic options for the management of pulmonary hypertension in CLD remain extremely limited. Recent experimental studies suggest several potential approaches that may enhance outcome in the future. In addition to vasodilator therapy, new strategies aimed at minimizing acute lung injury, directly modifying vascular structure (such as smooth-muscle hyperplasia or extracellular matrix production), or perhaps even stimulating vascular and alveolar growth, may expand our ability to more fully treat pulmonary vascular disease. Such approaches may potentially include gene transfer of NO synthase, blockade of potent vasoconstrictors and mitogens (such as ET or LTs), the use of elastase inhibitors (318), antisense oligonucleotides directed at specific growth factors, and stimulation of new alveolar and blood vessel growth (205). These experimental developments and others are likely to improve and potentially reverse structural and functional abnormalities of the pulmonary circulation in CLD.

However, our current knowledge of clinical aspects of pulmonary hypertension in infants with CLD is poor and is based primarily on anecdotal reports. Little clinical data are available to provide vital information on specific mechanisms that are associated with progressive pulmonary vascular disease in CLD or that hasten its resolution. Our current clinical approach includes close diagnostic monitoring for pulmonary hypertension; aggressive management of the underlying lung disease; careful diagnostic evaluations for ''unsuspected'' cardiac or pulmonary abnormalities that contribute to disease severity; and, maintaining high oxygen saturations using long-term supplemental oxygen therapy. Although vasodilator therapies, including hydralazine, calcium-channel blockers, prostacyclin, and inhaled NO, briefly lower pulmonary artery pressure, data that demonstrate continued efficacy with long-term therapy are lacking. The goals of vasodilator therapy are not only to improve pulmonary hemodynamics, but also to decrease the progression and to enhance recovery of hypertensive structural vascular changes by removing the adverse effects of high pressure or shear stress. Whether prolonged vasodilator therapy can achieve these goals without adverse effects, and definition of patient subgroups that may benefit from vasodilator therapy, requires further study.

More clinical investigations are needed that specifically examine early clinical events and factors that lead to the development of pulmonary hypertension in CLD. Diverse approaches are needed, including epidemiological and physiological studies that prospectively assess the contributions of timing, severity, and role of pulmonary hypertension to the clinical course and long-term outcome of CLD. Studies that apply molecular, biochemical, and histopathological techniques to human tissue may help better define the role of various vasoactive products, growth factors, and other changes in the lung circulation of patients with CLD. Finally, well-designed clinical interventional trials are needed early in the clinical course, as well as in infants with pulmonary hypertension in established CLD.

References

1. Abman SH, Accurso FJ. Acute effects of partial compression of the ductus arteriosus on the fetal pulmonary circulation. Am J Physiol 1989; 257:H626–634.
2. Abman SH, Accurso FJ. Sustained fetal pulmonary vasodilation during prolonged infusion of atrial natriuretic factor and 8-bromo-guanosine monophosphate. Am J Physiol 1991; 260:H183–192.
3. Abman SH, Accurso FJ, Bowman CM. Unsuspected cardiopulmonary abnormalities in infants with BPD. Arch Dis Child 1984; 59:966–970.
4. Abman SH, Accurso FJ, Koops BL. Experience with home oxygen in the management of infants with BPD. Clin Pediatr 1984; 23:471–476.
5. Abman SH, Burchell MF, Schaffer MS, Rosenberg AA. Late sudden unexpected deaths in hospitalized infants with BPD. Am J Dis Child 1989; 143:815–819.
6. Abman SH, Chatfield BA, Hall SL, McMurtry IF. Role of endothelium-derived relaxing factor during transition of pulmonary circulation at birth. Am J Physiol 1990; 259:H1921–1927.

7. Abman SH, Chatfield BA, Rodman DM, Hall SL, McMurtry IF. Maturation-related changes in endothelium-dependent relaxation of ovine pulmonary arteries. Am J Physiol 1991; 260:L280–285.
8. Abman SH, Griebel JL, Parker DK, Schmidt JM, Swanton D, Kinsella JP. Acute effects of inhaled NO in children with severe hypoxemic respiratory failure. J Pediatr 1994; 124:881–888.
9. Abman SH, Groothius JR. Pathophysiology and treatment of BPD. Current issues. Pediatr Clin North Am 1994; 41:277–315.
10. Abman SH, Kinsella JP, Schaffer MS, Wilkening RB. Inhaled nitric oxide therapy in a premature newborn with severe respiratory distress and pulmonary hypertension. Pediatrics 1993; 92:606–609.
11. Abman SH, Schaffer MS, Wiggins JW, Washington RL, Manco-Johnson M, Wolfe RR. Pulmonary vascular extraction of circulating norepinephrine in infants with BPD. Pediatr Pulmonol 1987; 3:386–391.
12. Abman SH, Shanley PF, Accurso FJ. Failure of postnatal adaptation of the pulmonary circulation after chronic intrauterine pulmonary hypertension in fetal lambs. J Clin Invest 1989; 83:1849–1858.
13. Abman SH, Sondheimer HM. Pulmonary circulation and cardiovascular sequelae of BPD. In: Weir. EK, Archer SL, Reeves JT, eds. Diagnosis and Treatment of Pulmonary Hypertension. Mount Kisco, NY: Futura Publishing, 1992:155–180.
14. Abman SH, Wolfe RR, Accurso FJ, Koops BL, Bowman CM, Wiggins JW. Pulmonary vascular response to oxygen in infants with severe BPD. Pediatrics 1985; 75: 80–84.
15. Accurso FJ, Alpert B, Wilkening RB, Petersen RG, Meschia G. Time-dependent response of fetal pulmonary blood flow to an increase in fetal oxygen tension. Respir Physiol 1986; 63:43–52.
16. Adnot S, Raffestin B, Eddahibi S, Braquet P, Chabrier PE. Loss of endothelium-dependent relaxant activity in the pulmonary circulation of rats exposed to chronic hypoxia. J Clin Invest 1991; 87:155–162.
17. Albelda SM, Smith CW, Ward PA. Adhesion molecules and inflammatory injury. FASEB J 1994; 8:504–512.
18. Albertine KH, Kim BI, Kullama LK, Carlton DP, Bland RD. Prolonged mechanical ventilation of preterm lambs leads to smooth muscle extension and elastin accumulation along pulmonary blood vessels. Pediatr Res 1996; 39:323A.
19. Allen K, Haworth SG. Impaired adaptation of intrapulmonary arteries to extrauterine life in newborn pigs exposed to hypoxia. an ultrastructural study. Fed Proc 1986; 45:879.
20. Allen SW, Chatfield BA, Koppenhafer SL, Schaffer MS, Wolfe RR, Abman SH. Circulating immunoreactive ET-1 in children with pulmonary hypertension: association with acute hypoxic pulmonary vasoreactivity. Am Rev Respir Dis 1993; 148: 519–522.
21. Anderson WR, Engel RR. Cardiopulmonary sequelae of reparative stages of BPD. Arch Pathol Lab Med 1983; 107:603–608.
22. Archer SL, Huang JMC, Hampl V, Nelson DP, Shultz PJ, Weir EK. NO and cGMP cause vasorelaxation by activation of a charybdotoxin-sensitive K channel by cGMP-dependent protein kinase. Proc Natl Acad Sci USA 1994; 91:7583–7587.

23. Arnal J-F, Yamin J, Dockery S, Harrison DG. Regulation of endothelial NO synthase mRNA, protein, and activity during cell growth. Am J Physiol 1994; 267: C1381–1388.
24. Arnold WP, Mittal CK, Katsuki S, Murad F. NO activates guanylate cyclase and increases guanosine 3′-5′-cyclic monophosphate levels in various tissue preparations. Proc Natl Acad Sci USA 1977; 74:3203–3207.
25. Avery GB, Fletcher AB, Kaplan M, Brudno DS. Controlled trial of dexamethasone in respirator-dependent infants with BPD. Pediatrics 1985; 75:106–111.
26. Bader D, Ramos AD, Lew CD, et al. Childhood sequelae of infant lung disease: exercise and pulmonary function abnormalities after BPD. J Pediatr 1987; 110: 693–699.
27. Badesch D, Orton E, Zapp L, Westcott J, Hester J, Voelkel N, Stenmark K. Decreased arterial wall prostaglandin production in neonatal calves with severe chronic pulmonary hypertension. Am J Respir Cell Mol Biol 1989; 1:489–498.
28. Banarjee CK, Girling WJ, Wigglesworth JS. Pulmonary fibroplasia in newborn babies treated with oxygen and artificial ventilation. Arch Dis Child 1972; 47:509–518.
29. Barbera JA, Roger N, Roca J, et al. Worsening of pulmonary gas exchange with NO inhalation in COPD. Lancet 1996; 347:436–440.
30. Barer GR, Cai Y, Russell PC, Emery CJ. Reactivity and sites of vasomotion in pulmonary vessels of chronically hypoxic rats: relation to structural changes. Am Rev Respir Dis 1989; 140:1483–1485.
31. Barst RJ, Rubin LJ, McGoon MD, Caldwell EJ, Long WA, Levy PS. Survival in primary pulmonary hypertension with long-term continuous intravenous prostacyclin. Ann Int Med 1994; 121:409–415.
32. Barst RJ, Rubin LJ, Long WA, et al. A comparison of continuous intravenous epoprostenol (prostacyclin) with conventional therapy for primary pulmonary hypertension. N Engl J Med 334:296–301, 1996.
33. Baylen BG, Emmanouillides GC, Juratsch CE, Yoshida Y, French WJ, Criley JM. Main pulmonary artery distension: a potential mechanism for acute pulmonary hypertension in the human newborn infant. J Pediatr 1980; 96:540–544.
34. Beavo JA, Reifsnyder DH. Primary sequence of cyclic nucleotide phosphodiesterase isozymes and the design of selective inhibitors. Trends Pharmacol Sci 1990; 11:150–155.
35. Beckerman RC. Unexpected deaths in infants monitored at home. Am J Dis Child 1988; 142:1033–1034.
36. Beckman JS, Beckman TW, Chen J, Marshall PA, Freeman BA. Apparent hydroxyl radical production by peroxynitrite: implications for endothelial injury from NO and superoxide. Proc Natl Acad Sci USA 1990; 87:1620–1624.
37. Belik J, Halayko AJ, Rao K, Stephens NL. Fetal ductus arteriosus ligation: pulmonary vascular smooth muscle biochemical and mechanical changes. Circ Res 1993; 72:588–596.
38. Belik J, Sienko A, Light RB. The effect of repeated intermittent hypoxia on pulmonary vasoconstriction in the newborn. Can J Physiol Pharmacol 1990; 68:355–362.
39. Belik J, Stephens NL. Developmental differences in vascular smooth muscle mechanics in pulmonary and systemic circulations. J Appl Physiol 1993; 74:682–687.

40. Bell EF, Warburton D, Stonestreet BS, Oh W. Effect of fluid administration on the development of symptomatic patent ductus arteriosus and congestive heart failure in premature infants. N Engl J Med 1980; 302:598–604.
41. Benatar A, Clarke J, Silverman M. Pulmonary hypertension in infants with chronic lung disease: noninvasive evaluation and short term effect of oxygen treatment. Arch Dis Child 1995; 72:F14–19.
42. Benzing A, Brautigan P, Geiger K, et al. Inhaled NO reduces pulmonary transvascular albumin flux in patients with acute lung injury. Anesthesiology 1995; 83:1153–1161.
43. Berman W, Yabek SM, Dillon T, Burstein R, Corlew S. Evaluation of infants with BPD using cardiac catheterization. Pediatrics 1982; 70:708–712.
44. Berman W, Katz R, Yabek SM, Dillon T, Fripp RR, Papile LA. Long term follow-up of BPD. J Pediatr 1986; 109:45–50.
45. Boat TF, Kleinerman JI, Fanaroff AA, Matthews LW. Toxic effects of oxygen on cultured human neonatal respiratory epithelium. Pediatr Res 1973; 7:607–615.
46. Bolotina VM, Najibi S, Palacino JJ, Pagano PH, Cohen RA. NO directly activates calcium-dependent potassium channels in vascular smooth muscle. Nature 1994; 368:850–853.
47. Bonikos DS, Bensch KG, Northway WH, Edwards DK. BPD: the pulmonary pathologic sequel of necrotizing bronchiolitis and pulmonary fibrosis. Hum Pathol 1976; 7:623–650.
48. Bonvallet ST, Zamoral MA, Hasunuma K, Sato K, Hanasato N, Anderson D, Sato K, Stelzner TJ. BQ123, an ET A-receptor antagonist, attenuates hypoxic pulmonary hypertension in rats. Am J Physiol 1994; 266:H1327–1331.
49. Boulanger C, Luscher TF. Release of endothelin from the porcine aorta. Inhibition by endothelium-derived nitric oxide. J Clin Invest 1990; 85:587–590.
50. Boyden EA. The time lag in the development of bronchial arteries. Anat Rec 1970; 166:611–614.
51. Braner DA, Fineman JR, Chang R, et al. M and B 22948, a cGMP phosphodiesterase inhibitor, is a pulmonary vasodilator in lambs. Am J Physiol 1993; 264:H252–258.
52. Brannon TS, North AJ, Wells LB, Shaul PW. Prostacyclin synthesis in ovine pulmonary artery is developmentally regulated by changes in cyclooxygenase-1 gene expression. J Clin Invest 1994; 93:2230–2235.
53. Bressack MA, McMillan DD, Bland RD. Pulmonary oxygen toxicity: increased microvascular permeability to protein in unanesthetized lambs. Lymphology 1979; 12:133–139.
54. Brown ER, Stark A, Sosenko I, Lawson EE, Avery ME. BPD: possible relationship to pulmonary edema. J Pediatr 1978; 92:982–984.
55. Brownlee JR, Beekman RH, Rosenthal A. Acute hemodynamic effects of nifedipine in infants with BPD and pulmonary hypertension. Pediatr Res 1988; 24:186–190.
56. Bryan MH, Hardie MJ, Reilly BJ, Swyer PR. Pulmonary function studies during the first year of life in infants recovering from respiratory distress syndrome. Pediatrics 1973; 52:169–178.
57. Bush A, Busst CM, Knight WB, Hislop AA, Haworth SG, Shinebourne EA.

Changes in pulmonary circulation in severe BPD. Arch Dis Child 1990; 65:739–745.

58. Carlton DP, Cummings JJ, Sheerer RS, et al. Lung overexpansion increases pulmonary microvascular protein permeability in young lambs. J Appl Physiol 1990; 69: 577–583.
59. Carlton DP, Cho SC, Davis P, Lont M, Bland RD. Surfactant treatment at birth reduces lung vascular injury and edema in preterm lambs. Pediatr Res 1995; 37: 265–270.
60. Cassin S. Role of prostaglandins, thromboxanes and leukotrienes in the control of the pulmonary circulation in the fetus and newborn. Semin Perinatol 1987; 11:53–63.
61. Cassin S, Dawes GS, Mott JC, Ross BB, Strang LB. Vascular resistance of the foetal and newly ventilated lung of the lamb. J Physiol 1964; 171:61–79.
62. Cassin S, Gause G, Davis T, ter Riet M, Baker R. Do inhibitors of lipoxygenase and cyclooxygenase block neonatal hypoxic pulmonary vasoconstriction? J Appl Physiol 1988; 66:1779–1784.
63. Cassin S, Kristova T, Davis T, Kadowitz P, Gause G. Tone-dependent responses to endothelin in the isolated perfused fetal sheep pulmonary circulation in situ. J Appl Physiol 1991; 70:1228–1234.
64. Chatfield BA, McMurtry IF, Hall SL, Abman SH. Hemodynamic effects of endothelin-1 on the ovine fetal pulmonary circulation. Am J Physiol 1991; 261:R182–187.
65. Charon A, Taeusch HW, Fitzgibbon C, Smith GB, Treves ST, Phelps DS. Factors associated with surfactant response in infants with severe RDS. Pediatrics 1989; 83:348–354.
66. Chollet-Martin S, Gatecel C, Kermarrec N, et al. Alveolar neutrophil functions and cytokine levels in patients with the ARDS during NO inhalation. Am J Respir Crit Care Med 1996; 153:985–990.
67. Christman BW, McPherson CD, Newman JH, King GA, Bernard GR, Groves BM, Lloyd JE. An imbalance between the excretion of thromboxane and prostacyclin metabolites in pulmonary hypertension. N Engl J Med 1992; 327:1732–1739.
68. Chu J, Clements JA, Cotton EK, Klaus MH, Sweet AY, Tooley WH. Neonatal pulmonary ischemia. Part 1. Clinical and physiologic studies. Pediatrics 1967; 40: 709–782.
69. Chu J, Clements JA, Cotton EK, Klaus MH, Sweet AY, Thomas MA, Tooley WH. The pulmonary hypoperfusion syndrome. Pediatrics 1965; 35:733–742.
70. Gerstmann DR, Minton SD, Stoddard RA, et al. The Provo Multicenter Early High Frequency Oscillatory Ventilation Trial: improved pulmonary and clinical outcome in RDS. Pediatrics 1996; 98:1044–1057.
71. Clark RH, Gerstmann DR, Null DM, deLemos RA. Prospective randomized comparison of high frequency oscillatory and conventional ventilation in respiratory distress syndrome. Pediatrics 1992; 89:5–12.
72. Coalson JJ, Kuehl TJ, Escobeda MB, et al. Baboon model of BPD. II: Pathologic features. Exp Mol Pathol 1982; 37:335–350.
73. Coalson JJ, Winter VT, deLemos RA. Decreased alveolarization in baboon survivors with BPD. Am J Respir Crit Care Med 1995; 152:640–646.

74. Coflesky JT, Jones R, Reid L, Evans JN. Mechanical properties and structure of isolated pulmonary arteries remodeled by chronic hyperoxia. Am Rev Resir Dis 1987; 136:388–394.
75. Cohen AH, Hanson K, Morris K, Fouty B, McMurtry IF, Clarke W, Rodman DM. Inhibition of cGMP-specific phosphodiesterase selectively vasodilates the pulmonary circulation in chronically hypoxic rats. J Clin Invest 1996; 97:172–179.
76. Collaborative European Multicenter Study Group. Factors influencing the clinical response to surfactant replacement therapy in babies with severe RDS. Eur J Pediatr 1991; 150:433–439.
77. Cooke JP, Rossitch E, Andon NA, Loscalzo J, Dzau VJ. Flow activates an endothelial potassium channel to release an endogenous nitrosovasodilator. J Clin Invest 1991; 88:1663–1671.
78. Cooper CJ, Landzberg MJ, Anderson TJ, et al. Role of NO in the local regulation of pulmonary vascular resistance in humans. Circulation 1996; 93:266–271.
79. Corbridge TC, Wood LDH, Crawford GP, et al. Adverse effects of large tidal volume and low PEEP in canine acid aspiration. Am Rev Respir Dis 1990; 142:311–315.
80. Cornfield DN, Chatfield BA, McQueston JA, McMurtry IF, Abman SH. Effects of birth-related stimuli on L-arginine-dependent pulmonary vasodilation in the ovine fetus. Am J Physiol 1992; 262:H1474–1481.
81. Cornfield DN, McQueston JA, McMurtry IF, Rodman DM, Abman SH. Role of ATP-sensitive K^+-channels in ovine fetal pulmonary vascular tone. Am J Physiol 1992; 263:H1363–1368.
82. Cornfield DN, Reeve HL, Tolarova S, Weir EK, Archer S. Oxygen causes fetal pulmonary vasodilation through activation of a calcium-dependent potassium channel. Proc Natl Acad Sci USA 1996; 93:8089–8094.
83. Cornfield D, Stevens T, McMurtry I, Abman S, Rodman D. Acute hypoxia causes membrane depolarization and influx in fetal pulmonary artery smooth muscle cells. Am J Physiol 1994; 266:L469–L475.
84. Crawley DE, Zhao L, Giemycz MA, Liu S, Barnes PJ, Winter RJD, Evans TW. Chronic hypoxia impairs soluble guanylate cyclase-mediated pulmonary arterial relaxation in the rat. Am J Physiol 1992; 263:L325–332.
85. Cremona G, Wood AM, Hall LW, Bower EA, Higenbottam T. Effect of inhibitors of NO release and action on vascular tone in isolated lungs of pig, sheep, dog and man. J Physiol 1994; 481.1:185–195.
86. Davidson D. Pulmonary hemodynamics at birth: effect of acute cyclooxygenase inhibition in lambs. J Appl Physiol 1988; 64:1676–1682.
87. Davidson D, Eldemerdash A. Endothelium-derived relaxing factor: evidence that it regulates pulmonary vascular resistance in the isolated newborn guinea pig lung. Pediatr Res 1991; 29:538–542.
88. Davies G, Reid LM. Growth of the alveoli and pulmonary arteries in childhood. Thorax 1970; 25:669–681.
89. Davis WB, Rennard SI, Bitterman PB, Crystal RG. Pulmonary oxygen toxicity. N Engl J Med 1983; 309:878–883.
90. Dawes GS. Foetal and Neonatal Physiology. Chicago: Year Book, 1968.

91. Dawes GS, Mott JC. The vascular tone of the foetal lung. J Physiol 1962; 164: 465–477.
92. De Caterina R, Libby P, Peng H-B, Thannickal VJ, Rajavashisth TB, Gimbrone MA, Shin WS, Liao JK. NO decreases cytokine-induced endothelial activation. NO selectively reduces endothelial expression of adhesion molecules and proinflammatory cytokines. J Clin Invest 1995; 96:60–68.
93. deLemos RA, Coalson JJ. The contribution of experimental models to our understanding of the pathogenesis and treatment of BPD. Clin Perinatol 1992; 19:521–539.
94. deLemos RA, Coalson JJ, Gerstmann DR, Keuhl TJ, Null DM. Oxygen toxicity in the premature baboon with hyaline membrane disease. Am Rev Respir Dis 1988; 136:677–682.
95. deLemos R, Wolsdorf J, Nachman R, Block AJ, Leiby G, Wolkinson HA, Allen T, Haller A, Avery ME. Lung injury from oxygen in lambs. The role of artificial ventilation. Anesthesiology 1969; 30:609–618.
96. DeRuiter MC, Grittenberger-DeGroot AC, Rammos S, Poelmann RE. The special status of the pulmonary artery in the branchial arch system of the rat. Anat Embryol 1990; 181:341–349.
97. Dreyfuss D, Basset G, Soler P, et al. Intermittent positive pressure hyperventilation with high inflation pressure produces microvascular injury in rats. Am Rev Respir Dis 1985; 132:880–884.
98. Dreyfuss D, Soler P, Basset G, et al. High inflation pressure pulmonary edema: respective effects of high airway pressure, high tidal volume and positive end-expiratory pressure. Am Rev Respir Dis 1988; 137:1159–1164.
99. Druml W, Steltzer H, Waldhausl W, Lenz K, Hammerle A, Vierhapper H, Gasic S, Wagner OF. Endothelin-1 in ARDS. Am Rev Respir Dis 1993; 148:1169–1173.
100. Dubin D, Pratt RE, Cooke JP, Dzau VJ. Endothelin, a potent vasoconstrictor, is a vascular smooth muscle mitogen. J Vasc Med Biol 1989; 1:150–154.
101. Emmanouilides GC, Moss AJ, Duffie ER, Adams FH. Pulmonary artery pressure changes in human newborn infants from birth to 3 days of age. J Pediatr 1964; 65: 327–333.
102. Enhorning G, Adams FH, Norman A. Effect of lung expansion on the fetal lamb circulation. Acta Paediatr Scand 1966; 55:441–451.
103. Erickson AM, de la Monte SM, Moore GW, Hutchins GM. Progression of morphologic changes in BPD. Am J Pathol 1987; 127:474–484.
104. Evans NJ, Archer LNJ. Doppler assessment of pulmonary artery pressure and extrapulmonary shunting in the acute phase of HMD. Arch Dis Child 1991; 66: 24–26.
105. Evans NJ, Archer LN. Postnatal circulatory adaptation in healthy term and preterm infants. Arch Dis Child 1990; 65:24–26.
106. Fanburg B, Massaro D, Cerutti P, Gail D, Beberich M. Regulation of gene expression by O_2 tension. Am J Physiol 1991; 264:L235–L241.
107. Fasules JW, Wiggins JW, Wolfe RR. Increased lung vasoreactivity in children from Leadville, Colorado, after recovery from high altitude pulmonary edema. Circulation 1985; 72:957–962.

108. Fineman JR, Heymann MA, Soifer SJ. Nitro-L-arginine attenuates endothelium-dependent pulmonary vasodilation in lambs. Am J Physiol 1991; 260:1299–1306.
109. Finkelstein JN, Horowitz S, RA Sinkin, RM Ryan. Cellular and molecular responses to lung injury in relation to induction of tissue repair and fibrosis. Clin Perinatol 1992; 19:603–620.
110. Fouron JC, LeGuennec JC, Villemont D, Bard H, Pareult G, Davignon A. Value of echocardiography in assessing the outcome of BPD. Pediatrics 1980; 65:529–535.
111. Fox RB, Hoidal JR, Brown DM, Repine JE. Pulmonary inflammation due to O_2 toxicity: involvement of chemotactic factors and PMNs. Am Rev Respir Dis 1982; 123:521–523.
112. Frank L. Oxidant injury to pulmonary endothelium. In: Said SI, ed. Pulmonary Circulation and Acute Lung Injury. New York: Futura, 1985:249–281.
113. Frank L, Bucher JR, Roberts RJ. O_2 toxicity in neonatal and adult animals of various species. J Appl Physiol 1979; 45:699–704.
114. Fratacci M-D, Frostell CG, Chen TY, Zapol WM. Inhaled NO: a selective pulmonary vasodilator of heparin–protamine vasoconstriction in sheep. Anesthesiology 1991; 75:990–999.
115. Freeman BA, Crapo JD. Biology of disease. Free radicals and tissue injury. Lab Invest 1982; 47:412–426.
116. Freeman BA, Gutierrez H, Rubbo H. NO: a central regulatory species in pulmonary oxidant reactions. Am J Physiol 1995; 268:L697–698.
117. Froese AB, McCulloch PR, Sugiura M, et al. Optimizing alveolar expansion prolongs the effectiveness of exogenous surfactant therapy in the adult rabbit. Am Rev Respir Dis 1993; 148:569–577.
118. Fu Z, Costello ML, Tsukimoto K, et al. High lung volume increases stress failure in pulmonary capillaries. Appl Physiol 1992; 73:123–133.
119. Garg M, Kurzner SI, Batista D, et al. Hypoxic arousal responses in infants with BPD. Pediatrics 1988; 82:59–63.
120. Garg UC, Hassid A. NO-generating vasodilators and 8-bromo-cGMP inhibit mitogenesis and proliferation of cultured rat vascular smooth muscle cells. J Clin Invest 1989; 83:17744–17747.
121. Geggel RL, Reid LM. The structural basis of persistent pulmonary hypertension of the newborn. Clin Perinatol, 1984; 3:525–549.
122. Gerlach H, Rossaint R, Pappert T, Falke KJ. Time course and dose-response of NO inhalation for systemic oxygenation and pulmonary hypertension in patients with ARDS. Eur J Clin Invest 1993; 23:499–502.
123. Gerritsen ME, Bloor CM. Endothelial gene expression in response to injury. FASEB J 1993; 7:523–532.
124. Gewitz MH, Pitt BR, Laks H, et al. Reversible changes in norepinephrine extraction by the lungs in children with pulmonary hypertension. Pediatr Pharmacol 1982; 2: 57–63.
125. Giaid A, Saleh D. Reduced expression of endothelial NO synthase in the lungs of patients with pulmonary hypertension. N Engl J Med 1995; 333:214–221.
126. Giaid A, Yanagasawa M, Langleben D, Michel RP, Levy R, Shennib H, Kimura

S, Masaki T, Duguid WP, Stewart DJ. Expression of endothelin-1 in the lungs of patients with pulmonary hypertension. N Engl J Med 1993; 328:1732–1739.

127. Gibson RL, Jackson JC, Twiggs GA, et al. BPD: survival after prolonged mechanical ventilation. Am J Dis Child 1988; 142:721–725.

128. Gil AB, Weindling AM. Pulmonary artery pressure changes in the very-low birthweight infant developing chronic lung disease. Arch Dis Child 1993; 68:303–307.

129. Golan E, Zalzstein E, Zmora E, Shinwell ES. Pulmonary hypertension in RDS. Pediatr Pulmonol 1995; 19:221–225.

130. Goldberg SJ, Levy RA, Siassi B. Effects of maternal hypoxia and hyperoxia upon the neonatal pulmonary vasculature. Pediatrics 1971; 48:528–533.

131. Golden CL, Kohler JP, Nick HS, Visner GA. Effects of vasoactive and inflammatory mediators on ET-1 expression in pulmonary endothelial cells. Am J Respir Cell Mol Biol 1995; 12:503–512.

132. Goodman G, Perkin RM, Anas NG, Sperling DR, Hicks DA, Rowen M. Pulmonary hypertension in infants with BPD. J Pediatr 1988; 112:67–72.

133. Gore RG, Jones R. Pulmonary vascular reactivity in hyperoxic pulmonary hypertension in the rat. J Appl Physiol 1988; 65:2617–2623.

134. Gorenflo M, Voge M, Obladen M. Pulmonary vascular changes in BPD: a clinicopathologic correlation in short- and long-term survivors. Pediatr Pathol 1991; 11: 851–866.

135. Groneck P, Speer C. Inflammatory mediators and BPD. Arch Dis Child 1995; 73: F1–3.

136. Gutierrez HH, Nieves B, Chumley P, Rivera A, Freeman BA. NO regulation of superoxide-dependent lung injury: oxidant-protective actions of endogenously produced and exogenously administered NO. Free Radic Biol Med 1996; 21:43–52.

137. Haddad IY, Ischiropoulos H, Holm BA, Beckman JS, Baker JR, Matalon S. Mechanisms of peroxynitrite-induced injury to pulmonary surfactant. Am J Physiol 1993; 265:L555–564.

138. Hakim TS, Mortola JP. Pulmonary vascular resistance in adult rats exposed to hypoxia in the neonatal period. Can J Physiol Pharmacol 1989; 68:419–424.

139. Halbower AC, Tuder RM, Franklin WA, Pollock JS, Forstermann U, Abman SH. Maturation-related changes in endothelial NO synthase immunolocalization in the developing ovine lung. Am J Physiol 1994; 267:L585–591.

140. Hall SM, Haworth SG. Normal adaptation of pulmonary arterial intima to extrauterine life in the pig. Ultrastructural studies. J Pathol 1986; 149:55–66.

141. Halliday HL, Dumpit FM, Brady JP. Effects of inspired oxygen on echocardiographic assessment of pulmonary vascular resistance and myocardial contractility in BPD. Pediatrics 1980; 65:536–540.

142. Hampl V, Herget J. Perinatal hypoxia increases hypoxic pulmonary vasoconstriction in adult rats recovering from chronic exposure to hypoxia. Am Rev Respir Dis 1990; 142:619–624.

143. Hampl V, Tristani-Firouzi M, Hutsell TC, Archer SL. Nebulized NO nucleophile adduct reduces chronic pulmonary hypertension. Cardiovasc Res 1996; 31:55–62.

144. Hansen TN, Corbet AJS, Kenny JD, Courtney JD, Rudolph AN. Effects of oxygen

and constant positive pressure breathing on AD_{CO_2} in HMD. Pediatr Res 1979; 13: 1167–1171.

145. Harrod JR, L'Heureux P, Wangensteen OD, CE Hunt. Long-term follow-up of severe respiratory distress syndrome treated with IPPB. J Pediatr 1974; 84:277–286.
146. Haworth SG. Pulmonary vascular remodeling in neonatal pulmonary hypertension: state of the art. Chest 1988; 93:133S–138S.
147. Haworth SG. Pulmonary hypertension in childhood. Perspect Pediatr Pathol 1995; 18:71–110.
148. Haworth SG, Hislop AA. Pulmonary vascular development: normal values of peripheral vascular structure. Am J Cardiol 1983; 52:578–583.
149. Hazinski TA. BPD. In: Chernick V, ed. Kendig's Disorders of the Respiratory Tract in Children, 5th ed. Philadelphia: WB Saunders, 1990:300–320.
150. Heymann MA, Soifer SJ. Control of fetal and neonatal pulmonary circulation. In: Weir EK, Reeves JT eds. Pulmonary Vascular Physiology and Pathophysiology. New York: Marcel Dekker, 1989: 33–50.
151. Higenbottam T, Wheeldon D, Wells F, Wallwork J. Longterm treatment of primary pulmonary hypertension with continuous intravenous epoprostenol (prostacyclin). Lancet 1984; 1:1046–1047.
152. Hislop AA, Haworth SG. Pulmonary vascular damage and the development of cor pulmonale following HMD. Pediatr Pulmonol 1990; 9:152–161.
153. Hislop AA, Reid L. Intrapulmonary arterial development during fetal life—branching pattern and structure. J Anat 1972; 113:35–48.
154. Hislop AA, Reid LM. Pulmonary arterial development during childhood: branching pattern and structure. Thorax 1973; 28:129–135.
155. Humbert M, Monti G, Brenot F, Sitbon O, Portier A, Graneot-Keros L, Duroux P, Galanaud P, Simmoneau G, Emllie D. Increased interleukin-1 and interleukin-6 serum concentrations in severe primary pulmonary hypertension. Am J Respir Crit Care Med 1995; 151:1628–1631.
156. Ignarro LJ, Buga GM Buga, Wood KS, Byrns RE, Chaudhuri G. Endothelium-derived relaxing factor produced and released from artery and vein is nitric oxide. Proc Natl Acad Sci USA 1987; 84:9265–9269.
157. Ikegami M, Jacobs H, Jobe A. Surfactant function in respiratory distress syndrome. J Pediatr 1983; 102:443–447.
158. Imai T, Hirata Y, Emori T, Marumo F. Heparin has an inhibitory effect on endothelin-1 synthesis and release by endothelial cells. Hypertension 1993; 21:353–358.
159. Imai Y, Kawano T, Miyasaka K, Takata M, Imai T, Okuyama R. Inflammatory chemical mediators during conventional ventilation and during high frequency oscillatory ventilation. Am J Respir Crit Care Med 1994; 150:1550–1554.
160. Isaacson T, Hampl V, Weir E, Nelson D, Archer S. Increased endothelium-derived NO in hypertensive pulmonary circulation of chronically hypoxic rats. J Appl Physiol 1994; 76:933–940.
161. Isozaki-Fukuda Y, Kojima T, Hirata Y, Ono A, Sawaragi S, Sawaragi T, Kobayashi Y. Plasma immunoreactive ET-1 concentration in human fetal blood: its relation to asphyxia. Pediatr Res 1991; 30:244–247.
162. Ivy DD, Kinsella JP, Abman SH. Physiologic characterization of endothelin A and

B receptor activity in the ovine fetal pulmonary circulation. J Clin Invest 1994; 93: 2141–2148.
163. Ivy DD, Ziegler JW, Dubus MF, Fox JJ, Kinsella JP, Abman SH. Chronic intrauterine pulmonary hypertension alters endothelin receptor activity in the ovine fetus. Pediatr Res 1995; 39:335–342.
164. Ivy DD, Parker TA, Ziegler JW, Galan HL, Kinsella JP, Abman SH. Prolonged endothelin A receptor blockade attenuates chronic intrauterine pulmonary hypertension. J Clin Invest 1997; 99:1179–1186.
165. Ivy DD, Ziegler JW, Kinsella JP, Abman SH. Endothelin blockade augments fetal pulmonary vasodilation. J Appl Physiol 1996; 81:2481–2487.
166. Jobe A. Pulmonary surfactant therapy. N Engl J Med 1993; 328:861–868.
167. Jobe A, Ikegami M, Jacobs H, Jones S, Conaway D. Permeability of premature lamb lungs to protein and the effect of surfactant on that permeability. J Appl Physiol 1983; 48:169–176.
168. Jones OW, Abman SH. Systemic and pulmonary hemodynamic effects of big endothelin-1 and phosphoramidon in the ovine fetus. Am J Physiol 1994; 266:R929–935.
169. Jones R, Zapol WM, Reid LM. Pulmonary artery remodeling and pulmonary hypertension after exposure to hyperoxia for 7 days. Am J Pathol 1984; 117:273–285.
170. Jones R, Zapol WM, Reid LM. Oxygen toxicity and restructuring of pulmonary arteries. A morphometric study. Am J Pathol 1985; 121:212–223.
171. Kaapa P, Seppanen M, Kero P, Saraste M. Pulmonary hemodynamics after synthetic surfactant replacement in neonatal RDS. J Pediatr 1993; 123:115–119.
172. Karakurum M, Shreeniwas R, Chen J, Pinsky D, Yan S-D, Anderson M, Sunouchi K, Major J, Kuwabara K, Rot A, Nowygrod R, Stern D. Hypoxic induction of interleukin-8 gene expression in human endothelial cells. J Clin Invest 1994; 93: 1564–1570.
173. Katambi T, Shimizu M, Okan K, Yano Y, Nemotol K, Ogura M, Tsukamoto T, Suzuki S, Ohira K, Yamada Y, Sekita N, Yoshida A, Someya K. Intracelluar signal transduction for interleukin-1β induced endothelin production in human umbilical vein endothelial cells. Biochem Biophys Res Commun 1992; 188:565–570.
174. Kavanaugh BP, Mouchawar A, Goldsmith J, Pearl RG. Effects of inhaled NO and inhibition of endogenous NO synthesis in oxidant-induced lung injury. J Appl Physiol 1994; 76:1324–1329.
175. Kay JM. Effect of intermittent normoxia on chronic hypoxic pulmonary hypertension, right ventricular hypertrophy, and polycythemia in rats. Am Rev Respir Dis 1980; 121:993–1001.
176. Khoury J, Langleben D. PAF stimulates lung pericyte growth in vitro. Am J Physiol 1996; 270:L298–304.
177. Kinsella JP, Halbower AC, Ziegler JW, Fox JF, Ivy DD, Abman SH. Low dose inhaled NO improves gas exchange without increasing vascular permeability in experimental HMD. Pediatr Res 1995; 37:337A.
178. Kinsella JP, Ivy DD, Abman SH. Ontogeny of NO activity and response to inhaled NO in the developing ovine pulmonary circulation. Am J Physiol 1994; 267: H1955–1961.

179. Kinsella JP, Ivy DD, Abman SH. Inhaled nitric oxide improves gas exchange and lowers pulmonary vascular resistance in severe experimental hyaline membrane disease. Pediatr Res 1994; 36:402–408.
180. Kinsella JP, Gerstmann DR, deLemos RA. Circulatory changes following premature delivery in a baboon model of HMD. Am J Physiol 1991; H1148–1154.
181. Kinsella JP, McQueston JA, Rosenberg AA, Abman SH. Hemodynamic effects of exogenous nitric oxide in ovine transitional pulmonary circulation. Am J Physiol 1992; 263:H875–880.
182. Komuro I, Kurihara H, Sugiyama T, Takaku F, Yazaki Y. ET stimulates c-*fos* and c-*myc* expression and proliferation of vascular smooth muscle cells. FEBS Lett 1988; 238:249–252.
183. Koops BL, Abman SH, Accurso FJ. Outpatient management and follow-up of BPD. Clin Perinatol 1984; 11:101–122.
184. Kourembanas S, Marsden PA, McQuillan LP, Faller DV. Hypoxia induces endothelin gene expression and secretion in cultured human endothelium. J Clin Invest 1991; 88:1054–1057.
185. Kourembanas D, McQuillan L, Leung G, Faller D. NO regulates the expression of vasoconstrictors and growth factors by vascular endothelium under normoxia and hypoxia. J Clin Invest 1993; 92:99–104.
186. Kramer GL, Wells JN. Effects of phosphodiesterase inhibitors on cyclic nucleotide levels and relaxation of pig coronary arteries. Mol Pharmacol 1979; 16:813–822.
187. Kubes P, Granger DN. NO modulates microvascular permeability. Am J Physiol 1992; 262:H611–615.
188. Kubes P, Suzuki M, Granger DN. NO: an endogenous modulator of leukocyte adhesion. Proc Natl Acad Sci USA 1991; 88:4651–4655.
189. Kunkel SL, Standiford T, Metinko AP, Streiter RM. Endothelial cell-derived novel chemotactic cytokines. In: Johnson A, Ferro TJ, eds. Lung Vascular Injury. Marcel Dekker 1992: 213–226.
190. Kurose I, Kubes P, Wolf R, Anderson DC, Paulson J, Miyasaka M, Granger DN. Inhibition of NO production: mechanisms of vascular albumin leakage. Circ Res 1993; 73:164–171.
191. Langston C, Kida K, Reed M, et al. Human lung growth in late gestation and in the neonate. Am Rev Respir Dis 1984; 129:607–613.
192. LeCras TD, Xue C, Rengesamy A, Johns RA. Chronic hypoxia upregulates endothelial and inducible NO synthase gene and protein expression in rat lung. Am J Physiol 1996; 270:L164–170.
193. Leffler CW, Hessler JR, Green RS. Mechanism of stimulation of pulmonary prostacyclin synthesis at birth. Prostaglandins 1984; 28:877–887.
194. Leffler CW, Tyler TL, Cassin S. Effect of indomethacin on pulmonary vascular response to ventilation of fetal goats. Am J Physiol 1978; 234:H346–351.
195. Lerman A, Sandok EK, Hildebrand FL, Burnett JC. Inhibition of EDRF enhances endothelin-mediated vasoconstriction. Circulation 1992; 85:1894–1898.
196. Levin DL, Hyman AI, Heymann MA, Rudolph AM. Fetal hypertension and the development of increased pulmonary vascular smooth muscle: a possible mechanism for persistent pulmonary hypertension of the newborn infant. J Pediatr 1978; 92:265–269.

197. Lewis AB, Heymann MA, Rudolph AM. Gestational changes in pulmonary vascular responses in fetal lambs in utero. Circ Res 1976; 39:536–541.
198. Li H, Chen S, Chen Y, Meng Q, Durand J, Oparil S, Elton T. Enhanced endothelin-1 and endothelin receptor gene expression in chronic hypoxia. J Appl Physiol 1994; 77:1451–1459.
199. Lincoln TM, Cornwell TL. Towards an understanding of the mechanism of action of cAMP and cGMP in smooth muscle relaxation. Blood Vessels 1991; 28:129–137.
200. Lonnquist PA, Jonsson B, Winberg P, Frostell CG. Inhaled NO in infants with developing or established chronic lung disease. Acta Paediatr 1995; 84:1188–1192.
201. Lopez-Farre A, Riesco A, Alvarez V, Egido J, Echefarreta G, Gallego MJ, Mouton M, Blum G, Gomez-Garre D, Iternando L, Sanchez-Madrid F, Casado S, Caramelo C. Endothelin stimulates human PMN adhesion to endothelial cells. Regulation by cGMP. Nephrol Dial Transplant 1992; 7:674–675A.
202. MacCumber MW, Ross CA, Glaser BM, Snyder SH. Endothelin: visualization of mRNAs by in situ hybridization provides evidence for local action. Proc Natl Acad Sci USA 1989; 86:7285.
203. Margraf LR, Tomashefski JF, Bruce MC, Dahms BB. Morphometric analysis of the lung in BPD. Am Rev Respir Dis 1991; 143:391–400.
204. Massaro D, Teich N, Maxwell S, Massaro GD, Whitney P. Postnatal development of alveoli: regulation and evidence for a critical period in rats. J Clin Invest 1985; 76:1297–1305.
205. Massaro GD, Massaro D. Postnatal treatment with retinoic acid increases the number of pulmonary alveoli in rats. Am J Physiol, 1996; 270:L305–310.
206. Malek AM, Greene AL, Izumo S. Regulation of endothelin-1 gene by fluid shear stress is transcriptionally mediated and independent of protein kinase C and cAMP. Proc Natl Acad Sci USA 1993; 90:5999–6003.
207. Marsden PA, Brenner BM. Transcriptional regulation of the endothelin-1 gene by TNFa. Am J Physiol 1992; 262:C854–861.
208. McCullough PR, Forket PG, Froese AB. Lung volume maintenance prevents lung injury during HFOV in surfactant-deficient rabbits. Am Rev Respir Dis 1988; 137: 1185–1192.
209. McIntosh N, Walters RO. Effect of tolazoline in severe HMD. Arch Dis Child 1979; 54:105–110.
210. McQueston JA, Cornfield DN, McMurtry IF, Abman SH. Effects of oxygen and exogenous L-arginine on endothelium-derived relaxing factor activity in the fetal pulmonary circulation. Am J Physiol 1993; 264:H865–871.
211. McQueston JA, Kinsella JP, Ivy DD, McMurtry IF, Abman SH. Chronic pulmonary hypertension *in utero* impairs endothelium-dependent vasodilation. Am J Physiol 1995; 268:H288–294.
212. Melot C, Hallemans R, Naije R, et al. Deleterious effects of nifedipine on pulmonary gas exchange in COPD. Am Rev Respir Dis 1984; 130:612–616.
213. Meny RG, Blackmon L, Fleischmann D, Gutberlet R, Naumberg E. Sudden infant death and home monitors. Am J Dis Child 1988; 142:1037–1040.
214. Merrit TA, Stuard ID, Puccia J, Wood B, Edwards DK, Finkelstein J, Shapiro DL. Newborn tracheal aspirate cytology: classification during respiratory distress syndrome and BPD. J Pediatr 1981; 98:949–956.

215. Merrit TA, Cochrane CG, Holcomb K, et al. Elastase and alpha-1-antiproteinase inhibitor activity in tracheal aspirates during respiratory distress syndrome. J Clin Invest 1983; 72:656–662.
216. Michel T, Li GK, Busconi L. Phosphorylation and subcellular translocation of endothelial NO synthase. Proc Natl Acad Sci USA 1993; 90:6252–6256.
217. Mitchell SH, Teague G. Reduced gas transfer at rest and during exercise in school age survivors of BPD. Am J Respir Crit Care Med 1998; 157:1406–1412.
218. Miyauchi T, Yorikane R, Sakail S, Sakurai T, Okada M, Nishikibe M, Yand M, Yamaguchi I, Sugishita Y, Goto K. Contribution of endogenous ET-1 to the progression of cardiopulmonary alterations in rats with monocrotaline-induced pulmonary hypertension. Circ Res 1993; 73:887–897.
219. Moncada S, Palmer RMJ, Higgs EA. Nitric oxide: physiology, pathophysiology, and pharmacology. Pharmacol Rev 1991; 43:109–142.
220. Morbidelli L, Chang C-H, Douglas JG, Granger HJ, Maggi CA, Geppetti P, Leddal F. NO mediates mitogenic effect of VEGF on coronary venular endothelium. Am J Physiol 1996; 270:H411–415.
221. Morin FC, Egan EA, Ferguson W, Lundgren CEG. Development of pulmonary vascular response to oxygen. Am J Physiol 1988; 254:H542–546.
222. Morin FC. Ligating the ductus arteriosus before birth causes persistent pulmonary hypertension in the newborn lamb. Pediatr Res 1989; 25:245–250.
223. Moss AJ, Emmanouilides GC, Rettori O, Higashino SM, Adams FH. Postnatal circulatory and metabolic adjustments in normal and distressed premature infants. Biol Neonate 1965; 8:177–197.
224. Moyer-Mileur LJ, Nielson DW, Pfeffer KD, Witte MK, Chapman DL. Eliminating sleep-associated hypoxemia improves growth in infants with BPD. Pediatrics 1996; 98:779–783.
225. Muscedere JG, Mullen JBM, Gaw K, Slutsky AS. Tidal ventilation at low airway pressures can augment lung injury. Am J Respir Crit Care Med 1994; 149:1327–1334.
226. Nagao T, Vanhoutte PM. Endothelium-derived hyperpolarizing factor and endothelium-dependent relaxations. Am J Respir Cell Mol Biol 1993; 8:1–6.
227. North AJ, Star RA, Brannon TS, Ujiie K, Wells LB, Lowenstein CJ, Snyder SH, Shaul PW. NO synthase type I and type III gene expression are developmentally regulated in rat lung. Am J Physiol 1994; 266:L635–641.
228. Northway WH, Rosan RC, Porter DY. Pulmonary disease following respirator therapy of HMD. N Engl J Med 1967; 276:357–368.
229. Northway WH, Moss RB, Carlisle KB, Parker BR, Popp RL, Pitlick PT, Eichler I, Lamm RL, Brown BW. Late pulmonary sequelae of BPD. N Engl J Med. 1990; 323:1793–1799.
230. Obara H, Hoshino Y, Mori M, Mikawa K, Iwai S. Endothelium-dependent relaxation in isolated pulmonary arteries from rabbits exposed to hyperoxia. Crit Care Med 1989; 17:780–785.
231. O'Brodovich HM, Mellins RB BPD. Am Rev Respir Dis 1985; 132:694–709.
232. Ogden BE, Murphy SA, Saunders GC, Pathak D, Johnson JD. Neonatal lung neutrophils and elastase/proteinase inhibitor imbalance. Am Rev Respir Dis 1984; 130: 817–821.

233. Ohlstein EH, Douglas SA. Endothelin-1 modulates vascular smooth muscle structure and vasomotion: implications in cardiovascular pathology. Drug Dev Res 1993; 29:108–128.
234. Olschewski H, Walmarth D, Schermuly R, Ghofrani A, Grimminger F, Seeger W. Aerosolized prostacyclin and iloprost in severe pulmonary hypertension. Ann Intern Med 1996; 124:820–824.
235. Ono S, Westcott JY, Voelkel NF. PAF antagonists inhibit pulmonary vascular remodeling induced by hypobaric hypoxia in rats. J Appl Physiol 1992; 73:1084–1092.
236. Packer CS, Rhoades RA. Impaired pulmonary vascular smooth muscle function in lung injury. In: Johnson A, Ferro TJ, eds. Lung Vascular Injury. New York: Marcel Dekker, 1992:227–262.
237. Palmer RMJ, Ashton DS, Moncada S. Vascular endothelial cells synthesize nitric oxide from L-arginine. Nature 1988; 333:646–666.
238. Parker JC, Hernandez LA, Longnecker GL, et al. Lung edema caused by high peak inspiratory pressures in dogs: role of increased microvascular filtration pressure and permeability. Am Rev Respir Dis 1990; 142:321–328.
239. Peliowski A, Finer NN, Etche PC, Tierney AJ, Ryan CA. Inhaled NO for premature neonates after prolonged rupture of the membranes. J Pediatr 1995; 126:450–453.
240. Phillips PG, Tsan M-F. Cytoarchitectural aspects of endothelial barrier function in reponse to oxidants and inflammatory mediators. In: Johnson A, Ferro TJ, eds. Lung Vascular Injury. New York: Marcel Dekker, 1992:113–135.
241. Pinney MA, Cotton EK Home management of BPD. Pediatrics 1978; 61:856–859.
242. Pohl U, Herlan K, Huang A, Bassenge E. EDRF-mediated shear-induced dilation opposes myogenic vasoconstriction in small rabbit arteries. Am J Physiol 1991; 261:H2016–H2023.
243. Post J, Hume J, Archer S, Weir EK. Direct role for potassium channel inhibition in hypoxic pulmonary vasoconstriction. Am J Physiol 1992; 262:C882–C890.
244. Pusey VA, MacPherson RI, Chernick V. Pulmonary fibroplasia following prolonged artificial ventilation of newborn infants. Can Med Assoc J 1969; 100:451–457.
245. Puy RJM, Hyde RW, Fisher AB, Clark JM, Dickson J, Lambertsan CJ. Alterations in the pulmonary capillary bed during early O_2 toxicity in man. J Appl Physiol 1968; 24:537–543.
246. Quast U, Guillon J-M, Cavero I. Cellular pharmacology of potassium channel openers in vascular smooth muscle. Cardiovasc Res 1994; 28:805–810.
247. Rabinovitch M. Hypoxia and pulmonary vascular development. In: Haddad GG, Lister G, eds. Tissue Oxygen Deprivation. New York: Marcel Dekker, 1996:307–333.
248. Rabinovitch M, Gamble WJ, Miettinen OS, et al. Age and sex influence on pulmonary hypertension and on recovery. Am J Physiol 1981; 240:H1462–H1472.
249. Rabinovitch M, Gamble WJ, Nadas AS, et al. Rat pulmonary circulation after chronic hypoxia: hemodynamic and structural features. Am J Physiol 1979; 236: H818–827.
250. Rabinovitch M, Konstam MA, Gamble WJ, Papanicolaou N, Aronovitz MJ, Treves

S, Reid L. Changes in pulmonary blood flow affect vascular response to chronic hypoxia in rats. Circ Res 1983; 52:432–441.

251. Rich S, Kaufmann E, Levy PS. The effect of high doses of calcium-channel blockers on survival in primary pulmonary hypertension. N Engl J Med 1992; 327:76–81.
252. Roberts JD, Chen T, Kawai N, Wain J, Dupuy P, Shimouchi A, Bloch K, Polaner D, Zapol WM. Inhaled NO reverses pulmonary vasoconstriction in the hypoxic and acidotic newborn lamb. Circ Res 1993; 72:246–254.
253. Roberts RJ, Weesner KM, Bucher JR. O_2 induced alterations in lung vascular development in the newborn rat. Pediatr Res 1983; 17:368–375.
254. Rosenberg AA, Kennaugh J, Koppenhafer SL, Loomis M, Abman SH. Increased immunoreactive endothelin-1 levels in persistent pulmonary hypertension of the newborn. J Pediatr 1993; 123:109–114.
255. Rossaint R, Falke KJ, Lopez F, Slama K, Pisonand U, Zapol WM. Inhaled NO in ARDS. N Engl J Med 1993; 328:399–405.
256. Rubanyi GM, Romero JC, Vanhoutte PM. Flow-induced release of endothelium-derived relaxing factor. Am J Physiol 1986; 250:H822–827.
257. Rudolph AM. Fetal and neonatal pulmonary circulation. Annu Rev Physiol 1979; 41:383–395.
258. Rudolph AM, Drorbaugh JE, Auld PAM, et al. Studies on the circulation in the neonatal period. The circulation in the RDS. Pediatrics 1961; 27:551–556.
259. Rudolph AM, Heymann MA, Lewis AB. Physiology and pharmacology of the pulmonary circulation in the fetus and newborn. In: Hodson W, ed. Development of the Lung. New York: Marcel Dekker, 1977:497–523.
260. Sarker R, Webb C, Stanley JC. NO inhibition of endothelial cell mitogenesis and proliferation. Surgery 1995; 118:274–279.
261. Schwartz SM, Liaw L. Growth control and morphogenesis in the development and pathology of arteries. J Cardiovasc Pharmacol 1993; 2:S31–49.
262. Segerer H, Stevens P, Schadow B, Meir R, Kattner E, Schwartx H, Curstedt T, Robertson B, Obladen M. Surfactant substitution in ventilated very low birth weight infants: factors related to response type. Pediatr Res 1991; 30:591–596.
263. Sekar KD, Duke JC. Sleep apnea and hypoxemia in recently weaned premature neonates with and without BPD. Pediatr Pulmonol 1991; 10:112–116.
264. Semigran MJ, Cockrill BA, Kacmarek R, et al. Hemodynamic effects of inhaled NO in heart failure. J Am Coll Cardiol 1994; 24:982–988.
265. Seldinger SR, Kennedy TP, Buescher P, et al. Effects of removing oxygen from patients with COPD. Am Rev Respir Dis 1987; 136:85–91.
266. Seppanen MP, Kaapa PO, Kero PO. Hemodynamic prediction of complications in neonatal respiratory distress syndrome. J Pediatr 1995; 127:780–785.
267. Shankaran S, Fanaroff AA, Wright LL, et al. Characteristics of early (< 12 hour) death among VLBW neonates. Pediatr Res 1995; 37:236A.
268. Shasby DM, Fox RB, Harada RN, Repine JE. Reduction of the edema of acute hyperoxic lung injury by granulocyte depletion. J Appl Physiol 1982; 52:1237–1244.
269. Shaul PW, Farrer MA, Zellers TM. Oxygen modulates endothelium-derived relaxing factor production in fetal pulmonary arteries. Am J Physiol 1992; 262:H355–364.

270. Shaul PW, Campbell WB, Farrer MA, Magness RR. Oxygen modulates prostacyclin synthesis in ovine fetal pulmonary arteries by an effect on cyclooxygenase. J Clin Invest 1992; 90:2147–2155.
271. Singer L, Martin RJ, Hawkins SW, Benson-Szekely LJ, Yamashita T, Carlo WA. Oxygen desaturation complicates feeding in infants with BPD after discharge. Pediatrics 1992; 90:380–384.
272. Skinner JR, Boys JR, Hunter S, Hey EN. Pulmonary and systemic arterial pressure in HMD. Arch Dis Child 1992; 67:366–373.
273. Smyth JA, Tabachnik E, Duncan WJ, Reilly RJ, Levison H. Pulmonary function and bronchial hyperactivity in long-term survivors of BPD. Pediatrics 1981; 68: 336–340.
274. Sobonya RE, Logvinoff MM, Taussig LM, Theriault A. Morphometric analysis of the lung in prolonged BPD. Pediatr Res 1982; 16:969–972.
275. Soifer SJ, Kaslow D, Roman C, Heymann MA. Umbilical cord compression produces pulmonary hypertension in newborn lambs. J Dev Physiol 1987; 9:239–252.
276. Soifer SJ, Loitz RD, Roman C, Heymann MA. Leukotriene end organ antagonists increase pulmonary blood flow in fetal lambs. Am J Physiol 1985; 249:H570–576.
277. Sole MJ, Drobac M, Schwartz L, et al. Extraction of circulating catecholamines by the lungs in normal man and in patients with pulmonary hypertension. Circulation 1979; 60:160–163.
278. Southall DP, Samuels MP, Talbert DG. Recurrent cyanotic episodes with severe arterial hypoxaemia and intrapulmonary shunting: a mechanism for sudden death. Arch Dis Child 1990; 65:953–961.
279. Stahlman M. Treatment of cardiovascular disorders of the newborn. Pediatr Clin N Am 1964; 11:363–400.
280. Stahlman M, Blankenship WJ, Shepard FM, Gray J, Young WC, Malan AF. Circulatory studies in clincal HMD. Biol Neonate 1972; 20:300–320.
281. Steinhorn RH, Russell JA, Morin FC. Disruption of cGMP production in pulmonary arteries isolated from fetal lambs with pulmonary hypertension. Am J Physiol 1995; 268:H1483–1489.
282. Stelzner T, O'Brien R, Yanagasawa M, Sakurai T, Sato K, Webb S, Zamora M, McMurtry I, Fisher J. Increased lung endothelin-1 production in rats with idiopathic pulmonary hypertension. Am J Physiol 1992; 262:L614–620.
283. Stenmark KR, Abman SH, Accurso FJ. Etiologic mechanisms of persistent pulmonary hypertension of the newborn. In: Weir EK, Reeves JT, eds. Pulmonary Vascular Physiology and Pathophysiology. New York: Marcel-Dekker, 1989:335.
284. Stenmark KR, Dempsey EC, Badesch DB, Frid M, Mecham RP, Parks WC. Regulation of pulmonary vascular wall cell growth developmental and site specific heterogeneity. Eur Respir Rev 1993; 3:629–637.
285. Stenmark KR, Eyzaguirre M, Westcott JY, et al. Potential role of eicosanoids and platelet activating factor in the pathophysiology of BPD. Am Rev Respir Dis 1987; 136:770–772.
286. Stewart DJ, Levy RD, Cernacek P, Langleben D. Increased plasma endothelin-1 in pulmonary hypertension: marker or mediator of disease. Ann Intern Med 1991; 114:464–469.
287. Stocker JT. Pathology of long-standing "healed" BPD. Hum Pathol 1986; 17:943–961.

288. Taghizadeh A, Reynolds EOR. Pathogenesis of BPD following HMD. Am J Pathol 1976; 82:241–258.
289. Tanswell AK, Freeman BA. Pulmonary antioxidant enzyme maturation in the fetal and neonatal rat. 1: developmental profile. Pediatr Res 1984; 18:584–587.
290. Tare M, Parkington HC, Coleman HA, Neild TO, Dusting GJ. Hyperpolarization and relaxation of arterial smooth muscle caused by nitric oxide derived from the endothelium. Nature 1990; 346:69–71.
291. Tomashefski JF, Opperman HC, Vawter GF. BPD: a morphometric study with emphasis on the pulmonary vasculature. Pediatr Pathol 1984; 2:469–487.
292. Tuder RM, Groves B, Badesch DB, Voelkel NF. Exuberant endothelial cell growth and elements of inflammation are present in plexiform lesions of pulmonary hypertension. Am J Pathol 1994; 144:275–285.
292a. Voelkel NF, Tuder RM, Wade K, Hoeper M, Lepley RA, Goulet JL, Koller BH, Fitzpatrick F. Inhibition of 5-lipoxygenase-activating protein reduces pulmonary vascular reactivity and pulmonary hypertension. J Clin Invest 1996; 97:2491–2498.
292b. Tyler RC, Muramatsu M, Abman SH, Stelzner TJ, Rodman DM, Bloch KD, McMurtry IF. Variable expression of endothelial NO synthase in three forms of rat pulmonary hypertension. Am J Physiol 1999; 276:in press.
293. Velvis H, Moore P, Heymann MA. Prostaglandin inhibition prevents the fall in pulmonary vascular resistance as the result of rhythmic distension of the lungs in fetal lambs. Pediatr Res 1991; 30:62–67.
294. Vender RL. Chronic hypoxic pulmonary hypertension. Chest 1994; 106:236–243.
295. Villamor E, Le Cras TD, MB Horan, AC Halbower, RM Tuder, Abman SH. Chronic intrauterine pulmonary hypertension impairs eNOS in the ovine fetus. Am J Physiol 1997; 272:L1013–1020.
296. Voelkel NF, Tuder RM. Interleukin-1 receptor antagonist inhibits pulmonary hypertension induced by inflammation. Ann NY Acad Sci 1994; 725:104–109.
297. Voelkel NF, Tuder RM, Wade K, Hoper M, Goulet J, Koller B, Fitzpatrick F. Inhibition of 5-lipoxygenase protein reduces pulmonary vascular reactivity and pulmonary hypertension in hypoxic rats. J Clin Invest 1996; 97:2491–2498.
298. Wang Y, Coceani F. Isolated pulmonary resistance vessels from fetal lambs: contractile behavior and responses to indomethacin and endothelin-1. Circ Res 1992; 71:320–330.
299. Wallen LD, Perry SF, Alston JT, Maloney JE. Morphometric study of the role of pulmonary arterial flow in fetal lung growth in sheep. Pediatr Res 1990; 27:122–127.
300. Walther FJ, Bender FJ, Leighton JO. Persistent pulmonary hypertension in premature neonates with severe RDS. Pediatrics 1992; 90:899–904.
301. Webb HH, Tierney DF. Experimental pulmonary edema due to intermittent positive pressure ventilation with high inflation pressure. Protection by PEEP. Am Rev Respir Dis 1974; 110:556–565.
302. Wessel DL, Adatia I, Giglia TM, Thompson JE, Kulik TJ. Use of inhaled NO and acetylcholine in the evaluation of pulmonary hypertension and endothelial function after cardiopulmonary bypass. Circulation 1993; 88:2128–2138.
303. Westhammer J, Brown ER, Neff RK, Taeusch HW. Sudden infant death syndrome in infants with BPD. Pediatrics 1982; 69:301–304.

304. White CW, Repine JE. Pulmonary antioxidant defense mechanisms. Exp Lung Res 1985; 8:81–96.
305. Wilson WL, Mullen M, Olley PM, Rabinovitch M. Hyperoxia-induced pulmonary vascular and lung abnormalities in young rats and potential for recovery. Pediatr Res 1985; 19:1059–1067.
306. Wink DA, Hanbauer I, Krishna MC, DeGraff W, Gamson J, Mitchell JB. NO protects against cellular damage and cytotoxicity from reactive oxygen species. Proc Natl Acad Sci USA 1993; 90:9813–9817.
307. Wong J, Fineman JR, Heymann MA. The role of endothelin and endothelin receptor subtypes in regulation of fetal pulmonary vascular tone. Pediatr Res 1994; 35:664–670.
308. Xuan ATD, Higgenbottom TW, Pepke-Zaba J, Clelland C, Wallwork J. Reduced endothelium-dependent relaxation of cystic fibrosis pulmonary arteries. Eur J Pharmacol 1989; 163:401–403.
309. Xuan ATD, Higgenbottom TW, Clelland C, Pepke-Zaba J, Cremona G, Wallwork J. Impairment of pulmonary endothelium-dependent relaxation in patients with Eisenmenger's syndrome. Br J Pharmacol 1989; 99:9–10.
310. Yokokawa K, Tahara H, Kohno M, Mandal AK, Yanagaswa M, Takeda T. Heparin regulates endothelin production through endothelium-derived NO in human endothelial cells. J Clin Invest 1993; 92:2080–2085.
311. Yoshimoto S, Ishizaki Y, Sasaki T, Murota S-I. Effect of carbon dioxide and oxygen on endothelin production by cultured porcine cerebral endothelial cells. Stroke 1991; 22:378–383.
312. Yoshizumi M, Kurihara H, Morita T, Yamashita T, Oh-hashi Y, Sugiyama T, Takaku F, Yanagisawa M, Masaki T, Yazaki Y. Interleukin-1 increases the production of ET-1 by cultured endothelial cells. Biochem Biophys Res Commun 1990; 181: 529–536.
313. Yoshizumi M, Kurihara H, Sugiyama T, Yamaoki K, Takaku F, Satoh H, Inu J, Yanagisawa M, Masakik T, Yazaki Y. Hemodynamic shear stress simulates endothelin production by cultured endothelial cells. Biochem Biophys Res Commun 1989; 161:859–864.
314. Yanagisawa M, Kurihara H, Kimura S, Tomobe Y, Kobayashi M, Mitsui Y, Yazaki Y, Goto K, Masaki T. A novel potent vasoconstrictor peptide produced by vascular endothelial cells. Nature 1988; 332:411–415.
315. Yokokawa K, Tahara H, Kohno M, Mandal AK, Yanagisawa M, Takeda T. Heparin regulates endothelin production through endothelium-derived NO in human endothelial cells. J Clin Invest 1993; 92:2080–2085.
316. Ziche M, Morbidelli L, Masini E, Amerini S, Granger HJ, Maggi CA, Geppetti P, Ledda F. NO mediates angiogenesis in vivo and endothelial cell growth and migration in vitro promoted by substance P. J Clin Invest 1994; 94:2036–2044.
317. Ziegler JW, Ivy OD, Fox J, Kinsella JP, Clarke WR, Abman SH. Dipyridamole, a cGMP phosphodiesterase inhibitor augments inhaled NO-induced pulmonary vasodilation in the ovine transitional circulation. Am J Respir Crit Care Med 1998; 157:1104–1110.
318. Zhu L, Wigle D, Hinek A, Koboyashi J, Ye C, Zuker M, Dodo H, Keeley F, Rabinovitch M. The endogenous vascular elastase that governs development and progression of monocrotaline-induced pulmonary hypertension in rats is a novel enzyme related to the serine proteinase adipsin. J Clin Invest 1994; 94:1163–1171.

28

Connective Tissues in Lung Development and Diseases in Early Infancy

DAVID J. RILEY

University of Medicine and Dentistry of New Jersey—Robert Wood Johnson Medical School
Piscataway, New Jersey

I. Introduction

Chronic lung diseases (CLD) of infants are diseases of the airways and parenchyma that progress from a phase of tissue injury and inflammation to scarring and distortion of the lung architecture. The most important disease in infants resulting in lung fibrosis is bronchopulmonary dysplasia (BPD). There is considerable circumstantial evidence that immaturity, barotrauma from mechanical ventilation, and exposure to high levels of O_2 contribute to lung fibrosis. The processes that lead to fibrous tissue formation in BPD are analogous to wound healing, and involve formation of a provisional matrix at the site of injury, followed by reconstitution of normal tissue or scar formation if the injury is severe or smoldering. If severe, scar formation leads to distortion of lung parenchyma, impaired lung function, and clinical disease.

The purpose of this chapter is to review the processes leading to fibrogenesis in chronic lung diseases of infants. It is necessary to first present an overview of the extracellular matrix (ECM) of the lung. The reader must recognize that fibrous tissue formation involves not only the ECM, but also cell proliferation, mediators, and inflammation, topics that are discussed elsewhere in this monograph. Lung injury in the neonate impairs lung development, which is possibly more important to lifetime health in survivors of BPD than the fibrosis. Therefore, ECM regulation of lung development will be reviewed. In fibrosis, diverse cells secrete a myriad of ECM proteins. The proteins orchestrate diverse biological functions, including cell migration, cell–matrix binding, expression of genes, and effects on cellular metabolism. This chapter will provide an overview of these developments in connective tissue, and describe their application to understanding lung development and the pathogenesis of interstitial lung diseases of infants.

II. Extracellular Matrix: General

The ECM is an intricate network of structurally stable macromolecules composed of a variety of polysaccharides and proteins that are secreted locally and assemble into an organized matrix. This network determines the physical characteristics of tissues: tensile strength is provided by the fiber-forming collagen, resilient properties by elastin and proteoglycans, and cell–matrix adhesion by glycoproteins. The molecular components of the ECM are a continuum, connecting the cell interior, basal lamina, and surrounding ECM. The extracellular matrix is not simply an inert supporting material; it affects cell movement, shape, metabolism, and other cellular processes. The ECM plays a role in development by controlling differentiation of cells and organization of tissues. An extensive recent literature is available on the biology and chemistry of ECM (for reviews, see 1–10).

In the lung, the organization of the matrix is highly adapted to facilitate gas exchange. Interstitial collagen enables the alveolar membrane to withstand the many deformations that occur during breathing. The meshwork of elastin fibers gives the lung its elasticity, and acts as a tether for airways and blood vessels. Type IV collagen, proteoglycans, and laminin compose basement membranes, which limit movement of macromolecules across the tissue–air interface. Proteoglycans and fibronectin mediate lung embryogenesis and development, acting as chemical signals that control proliferation, migration, and organization of cells. The extremely thin alveolar interface is elegantly designed to facilitate diffusion of gases. Alveolar diseases caused by disruption of elastin or excessive accumulation of collagen impair exchange of gases. The ECM of the lung has been reviewed in numerous publications (11–19).

A. Collagen

Molecular Collagen

Collagen is the major structural protein in the lung, composing about 10–15% of the lung's dry weight (20,21). Collagens are a family of proteins that contain repeating -Gly-X-Y- sequences, in which the X position is frequently proline and the Y position is frequently 4-hydroxyproline, that have the three chains that can

Table 1 Types of Collagen Grouped by Structure and Function

Types of collagen	Characteristics	Distribution
Fibril-forming I, II, III, V, XI	Large triple-helical domains; synthesized as precursors and secreted; assemble into fibers	Most tissues, including lung; types II and XI in cartilage
Network-forming IV, VII, X	Self-assemble to form network-like structures	Basement membranes (IV, VII); cartilage (X)
Fibril-associated with interrupted triple helices IX, XII, XIV, XVI, XIX	Short helical domains interrupted by noncollagenous sequences; attached to other fibrils	Tissues containing types I or II collagens
Beaded filament VI	Short helical domains and longer NH_2- and COOH-terminal globular domains; chain varients result from alternative splicing	Most connective tissues
Anchoring fibrils VII	Links basement membranes to type IV collagen and laminin	Many tissues
Collagens with transmembrane domains XIII, XVII	Contain a cytoplasmic transmembrane domain; type XIII undergoes alternative splicing	XIII in many tissues; XVII in skin
Family of types XV and XVIII	Large NH_2- and COOH-terminal domains; extensively glycosylated	Many tissues; XVIII expressed as high levels in liver
''Noncollagen'' collagens: Clq, acetylcholine-esterase, surfactants SP-A and SP-D, mannan-binding protein, macrophage scavenger receptors	Contain triple-helical domains, but not defined as collagens	Selective tissue distribution

potentially fold into triple-helical structures (2). At least 19 collagen types have been described and are grouped by structural and functional similarities (Table 1). Some of the more recently discovered collagen types have a variety of globular proteins with short -Gly-X-Y- repeat sequences, some of which have transmembrane domains (for reviews, see 2, 22–26). The *fiber-forming* collagens are synthesized as procollagen precursors that are secreted and exhibit large collagenous domains. Types I–III, V, and XI are included in this group. The tensile strength of type I collagen implies its importance in mechanical properties of tissue. Type III collagen is abundant in pliable tissues, such as lung. The relative amount of type III collagen is increased in early wound healing, suggesting it may be important in maintaining tissue integrity within developing or remodeling tissues. Type II collagen is found in cartilage and vitreous, in which it is a highly hydrated gel, enveloping proteoglycan molecules. Type XI collagen is thought to regulate the diameter of type II collagen. Type V collagen is widely distributed, and a variety of observations suggest it may be involved in fibrillogenesis.

The *network forming* collagens contain sequences that are frequently interrupted by noncollagenous domains. These molecules self-assemble by end-to-end interactions and intertwine to form a network. Type IV collagen is the major component of basement membranes. Type VIII and X collagen differ structurally from type IV collagen; the former form hexagonal lattices in specialized structures, and the latter is synthesized by hypertrophic chondrocytes. *Fibril-associated collagens with interrupted triple-helices* (FACIT collagen; 27) have repeat helical domains separated by non–triple-helical segments, and do not form polymers alone, but are associated with other collagen fibers. The FACIT collagens appear to serve as bridges between collagen fibers and other matrix components and cells. The *beaded filament* collagen appears as dumbbell-shaped when visualized by rotary shadowing under electron microscopy, an appearance created by short triple-helical domains separated by large globular domains. In tissues, type VI collagen forms a network, and is believed to be important in spatial separation of tissue components and in promotion of fibroblast attachment, spreading, and migration. *Anchoring fibrils* connect basement membranes to the underlying extracellular matrix. Type VII fibers are the largest collagen fibers thus far described and contain a variety of domains that are homologous with fibronectin. Recently discovered collagens with *transmembrane domains* contain both cytoplasmic and extracellular domains. Type XIII collagen undergoes extensive alternative splicing, producing numerous forms of the protein. Type XVII collagen is found predominantly in skin, and an autoimmune response to an antigenic site on this collagen is responsible for bullous pemphigoid. The *family of types XV and XVIII* collagen contain large, COOH-terminal globular domains and other domains, which suggest extensive glycosylation. These collagens are found in many tissues, and their function is not yet known. Finally, there are various *''noncollagen'' collagens* that contain collagenous sequences, but do not have a role in extracellular organization. Examples of these are the C1q component of complement, surfactant proteins SP-A and SP-D, the enzyme acetylcholinesterase, and macrophage scavenger receptors.

Collagen of the Normal Lung

The normal human lung contains at least nine types of collagen that have been identified biochemically, immunohistochemically, or by molecular techniques

Table 2 Types of Collagen Present in Normal Human Lung

Type	Comment	Ref.
I	65% of collagen in lung	28–30
II	Cartilage of trachea and larger bronchi	31
III	30% of collagen in lung	28
IV	Major component of basement membrane; NC1 domain binds to Goodpasture's antigen	33,35
V	7% of solubilized collagen	29
VI	Localized in interstitium	36
VII	Localized in bronchi, not alveolar walls	37
XIII	Alternatively spliced forms present in lung	38
XV	Present in fetal, but not adult lung; involved in embryogenesis	39,40

(Table 2). Type I collagen, which provides tensile strength, is associated with bronchi and blood vessels, and a small amount is present in interstitium (28–30). Only bronchial cartilage contains type II collagen (31). Type III collagen, localized mainly in interstitium, imparts flexibility to tissues and is more prominent in fetal tissue than in those of the adult (28–32). Type IV and V collagen are found in basement membranes, providing structural integrity to the alveolar–capillary membrane and attachment sites for alveolar epithelial cells (33). The collagens associated with basement membranes are secreted by alveolar type II cells (34). The COOH-terminal globular noncollagenous-1 (NC1) domain of type IV collagen carries an epitope that is recognized by antiglomerular basement membrane antibody in Goodpasture's syndrome (35). Type VI collagen, which serves as an anchoring element between collagen types I/III fibers and basement membrane, as well as in cell binding, is detected by immunohistochemistry at low levels in normal alveolar walls. Its turnover is too low to generate mRNA or in situ hybridization signals (36). Type VII collagen is restricted to combined stratified epithelia, as in bronchi, but is not identified in alveolar walls (37). The recently characterized type XIII collagen is expressed as varying transcripts in different tissues because of mRNA splicing of six exons (38). Another newly described collagen, type XV, is expressed in basement membranes of human fetal and adult lung (39,40).

Biosynthesis

There are type-specific differences in collagen biosynthesis. Fibril-forming collagens are secreted as precursor molecules, are not highly glycosylated, and are cross-linked extracellularly. Non–fibril-forming collagen are not secreted, so that cleavage of signal peptides does not occur; they are extensively glycosylated.

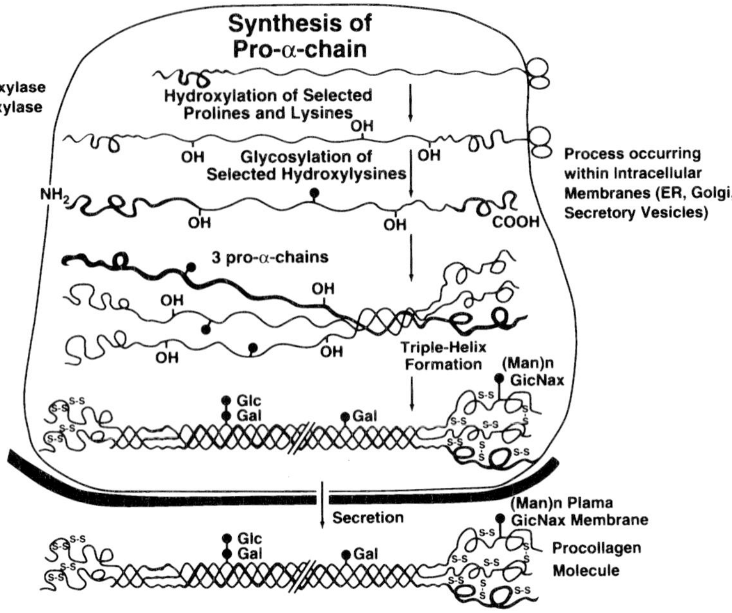

Figure 1 Sequence of steps in biosynthesis of fibril-forming collagen: After secretion of the procollagen molecule, COOH- and NH_2-terminal extensions are removed by specific peptidases to form a collagen molecule. (From Ref. 11.)

The discussion that follows pertains to biosynthesis of fiber-forming collagen, which has been well characterized (41). The fibrillar collagen genes are large (15–50 kb) and have over 50 exons, 44 of which code for the triple-helical domains (42–44). About half the triple-helical exons are 54-bp long, each of which corresponds to sequences of 18 amino acids, and the other half are a multiple of 54 bp. Following transcription, the mRNA is spliced, translocated to the cytoplasm, and translated in the rough endoplasmic reticulum (Fig. 1). A key cotranslational event is hydroxylation of prolyl and hydroxylysyl groups, which requires two enzymes, prolyl and lysyl hydroxylases, as well as cofactors, including ferrous iron, ascorbate, and α-ketoglutarate. Other posttranslational events are addition of carbohydrate residues, disulfide bond formation to join three pro-α-chains, triple-helix formation, and cleavage of signal peptides. After secretion from the cell, an enzyme cleaves the NH_2- and COOH-terminal propeptide extensions, and immunological detection of these cleaved peptides in body fluids is used as an assay for in vivo analysis of collagen synthesis (45). The soluble collagen precursors self-assemble into fibrils in which each neighboring molecule

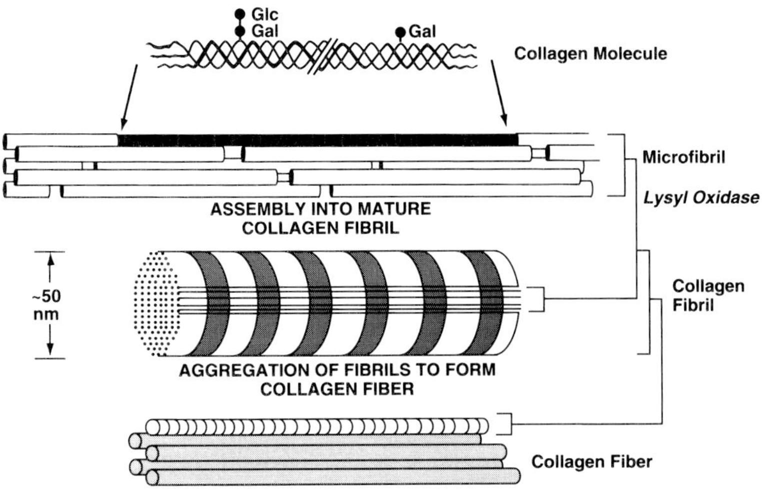

Figure 2 Formation of collagen fiber: Microfibrils each composed of five collagen molecules in lateral and end-to-end aggregation are cross-linked by lysyl oxidase to form a collagen fiber. The bands on cross-sectional view indicate the one-quarter staggered array of collagen molecules within the fibril. (From Ref. 11.)

is displaced one-quarter length, aligning in a regular array (Fig. 2). The fibrils are linked by covalent bonds at lysine and hydroxylysine residues by the enzyme lysyl oxidase.

Regulation of Collagen Synthesis and Deposition

Regulation of collagen production is of obvious relevance when considering lung development and pathological accumulation of collagen in fibrosis. At least 34 collagen genes have been described (for reviews, see 2,42–44). This subject will not be reviewed here because the regulation of the fibril-forming collagen genes is very complex and diverse, and it is likely that the other types of collagen genes have complex regulatory programs. For fibrillar collagen genes, the preponderance of studies suggest that regulation is controlled primarily at the level of mRNA, rather than by control of mRNA translation. Alternative splicing of pre-mRNAs accounts for variant forms of some types of collagen, and translational regulation of these collagens permits modulation by cytokines, growth factors, and hormones. The general mechanisms involve *cis*-acting sequences to which regulatory protein, such as *trans*-acting factors, bind. Regulation is controlled by the number and types of *trans*-acting factors. There is also evidence to suggest that there is cell-specific regulation of collagen genes during development and remodeling. The posttranslational modifications of fibril-forming collagen are regulated by cofactors and eight posttranslational enzymes that are unique to collagen biosynthesis (for review, see 41). Recently, these enzymes have been cloned and characterized, and results indicate that they have diverse functions (2).

Regulation of collagen production is modified by numerous growth factors, cytokines, hormones, and matrix peptides. The regulation by these factors is complex because they affect not only the collagen synthetic machinery, but also the proliferative capacity of collagen-producing cells and degradation of collagen (46,47). A comprehensive review of growth factors is found elsewhere in this volume (see Chap. 27). This section will highlight selected growth factors that regulate collagen synthesis. Several growth factors, some of which increase and some of which decrease collagen production, have been studied in detail.

The most potent stimulator of collagen is *transforming growth factor*-β (TGF-β), which also stimulates other ECM components (48–50). This cytokine increases collagen formation by increasing both the rate of transcription and the stability of the resulting transcripts (51,52). TGF-β simultaneously blocks matrix degradation by decreasing the synthesis of proteases and increasing the level of protease inhibitors (53). Insulin and insulin-like growth factor-1 (IGF-1) specifically stimulate collagen synthesis by a mechanism involving receptor binding and signaling through G proteins and phospholipid metabolism (54).

Several growth factors are capable of inhibiting collagen production. *Glucocorticoids* inhibit collagen synthesis in vitro, but the mechanism of this inhibition has been a matter of debate. Some studies suggest that transcriptional regulation by glucocorticoids causes decreased mRNA (55), whereas others propose a change in mRNA half-life (56). These two views were resolved by the finding that dexamethasone both decreases transcription of the collagen gene and leads to a posttranslational effect on procollagen mRNA content (57). Interferon gamma (IFN-γ) affects collagen metabolism by several mechanisms, including decreasing collagen production at the level of transcription (58) and increasing the cell surface receptors for collagen which, in turn, affects collagen deposition (59). *Prostaglandin* E_2 (PGE_2) decreases procollagen mRNA by inhibiting gene transcription in vitro (60), an effect that may be mediated through PGE_2-induced increases in cAMP levels (61). *Tumor necrosis factor*-α (TNF-α) decreases collagen formation by decreasing transcription and steady-state mRNA levels (62,63), and *interleukin-1* (IL-1) suppresses collagen expression (64). As both TNF-α and IL-1 stimulate cAMP levels (65), it is likely that they act by a mechanism similar to that of PGE_2. There are other mediators not involving growth factors that can act to modulate collagen synthesis. A pentapeptide that is cleaved from type I procollagen can induce mesenchymal cells to produce collagen through a mechanism independent of TGF-β (66). This pentapeptide might act to stimulate collagen synthesis by positive-feedback regulation. Other procollagen peptides that act to downregulate collagen synthesis have also been characterized (67,68). The true biological significance of these in vitro observations to the development of fibrosis is unclear.

Collagen Degradation

Fibrillar collagen formation is limited by intracellular and extracellular degradation of collagen. The intracellular pathway functions independently of alterations in collagen synthesis, and it involves degradation of procollagen molecules not destined for deposition in mature collagen. Approximately 15% of total collagen that is synthesized in cultured fibroblasts is degraded intracellularly (69), and labeling studies show substantial rates of collagen degradation in adult tissues (70). The major extracellular pathway of collagen resorption is through the metalloproteases (MMPs), a family of Zn^{2+}- and Ca^{2+}-dependent enzymes (71–73). Thirteen MMPs have been identified and classified into three broad groups. *Collagenases* degrade fibril-forming collagen. *Gelatinases* act on basement membrane components. *Stromelysins* have broad substrate specificity and degrade proteoglycans, laminin, fibronectin, gelatin, and basement membrane collagen. Acting together, the MMPs can completely degrade matrix components. Three levels control the activity of these enzymes: transcription, activation of latent proenzymes, and inhibition of proteolytic activity (Fig. 3). At the level of *transcription*, several cytokines and growth factors stimulate (IL-1, PDGF, TNF-α) or inhibit (glucocorticoids, TGF-β, heparin) MMPs. The second level of control is *activation of latent MMPs* by cleavage of proenzymes to the active molecule. There appears to be a cascade of events in which activated enzymes activate other proenzymes, thereby forming a positive-feedback loop. There is interaction with the plasminogen–plasmin-clotting cascade, in that plasmin cleaves and activates prostromelysin. The third level of control is *tissue inhibitors of MMPs* (TIMPs), and less specifically by α_2-macroglobulin. (α_2M) TIMPs are secreted proteins, and three TIMPs have been identified (TIMP-1, -2, and -3). TIMP-1 and -3 are inducible by cytokines and hormones, whereas TIMP-2 is constitutively expressed. There appears to be coregulation of MMPs and their inhibitors at the molecular level, forming a tightly regulated system that controls the overall composition of the ECM.

B. Elastin

Elastic fibers of the ECM give compliant tissues, such as lung, the ability to recoil after transient stretch. The main component is elastin, a highly hydrophobic molecule that is secreted into the extracellular space as the precursor tropoelastin, which subsequently forms a highly cross-linked network of elastin fibers (13,14,74,75). Elastin molecules, as are those of collagen, are rich in proline and glycine, but contain little hydroxyproline and are nonglycosylated. Because tropoelastin is hydrophobic and nonglycosylated, it requires a specific protective

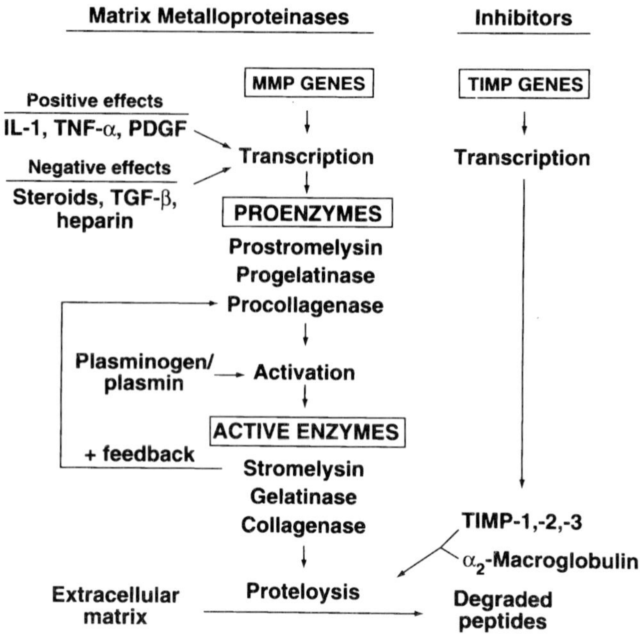

Figure 3 Regulation of extracellular matrix protein degradation: Proteolysis of extracellular matrix is regulated at the levels of gene transcription, activation of latent proenzymes, and inhibition by TIMPs and α_2-macroglobulin. (From Ref. 73.)

companion molecule (molecular chaperon) to escort it through the secretory pathways (76). Cross-links are formed extracellularly by covalent bonds between lysyl residues on adjacent molecules, a reaction catalyzed by lysyl oxidase. The cross-linked lysyl residues form desmosine, which is used as a marker for elastin in tissues and body fluids. Unlike most proteins, elastin remains unfolded as ''random coils,'' allowing the network to stretch and recoil. Elastic fibers also contain microfibrils, the exact composition of which remains to be defined. The microfibrils contain several glycoproteins (77), including fibrillin (78), a structural macromolecule that has been identified in patients with Marfan's syndrome (79). The microfibrils are secreted from cells before the elastin molecules are and are localized around immature fibers, suggesting that they may help organize the deposition of elastin fibers.

The elastin gene exists as a single copy in the human, and the structure consists of 34 small exons that code for hydrophobic and cross-link domains, interspersed between large exons (80). Unlike the fibril-forming collagen genes, the exons of elastin do not exhibit any regularity in size, and the structure permits extensive alternative splicing of the primary transcript. It is unclear, however, whether the variations produced by alternative splicing have any effect on fiber organization or biomechanical properties of elastin. Induction of elastin gene expression during development is controlled by a transcriptional mechanism, whereas cessation of expression is controlled by a posttranslational mechanism (81). Recent experiments with transgenic mice suggest that large deletions of exons coding for hydrophobic sequences can affect elastin-rich organs, producing aortic aneurysms or lesions resembling mild pulmonary emphysema (82). Although these experiments demonstrate the potential effect of mutations of the elastin gene on tissue structures, no mutations of elastin have yet been identified.

The elastin promoter contains many potential binding sites for transcriptional regulatory factors, including those for glucocorticoids, cAMP, IGF-1, and TNF-α. In upregulation by IGF-1 (83) and downregulation by TNF-α (84), evidence is compelling for transcriptional control of elastin. Reported evidence on the effects of IL-1 has been conflicting: one study found that IL-1 decreased elastin synthesis and mRNA (85), whereas another study found increased elastin gene expression (86). The effects of IL-1 may be mediated by cAMP, which regulates elastin production (87). TGF-β mainly increases elastin production by stabilization of mRNA transcripts (88). Basic fibroblast growth factor (bFGF) and TGF-α can exert negative effects on elastin production (89). Maternal administration of glucocorticoids increases lung elastin mRNA during a critical developmental period (90), suggesting that glucocorticoids regulate production of lung elastin during development. The effect could be modulated through a putative glucocorticoid response element in the promoter region of the elastin gene (80). Thus, it appears that elements in both the elastin promoter region and the posttranscriptional control region of the elastin gene regulate elastin production.

Elastin is degraded by elastases, which are proteolytic enzymes capable of solubilizing mature cross-linked elastin (91). Elastases do not form a homogeneous class of enzymes, but rather, have wide substrate specificities and are secreted from a variety of cells (91). Several elastases are pertinent to elastin degradation in the lung and are discussed in more detail in Chapter 24. Human leukocyte elastase (HLE) is a serine neutral protease found in cytoplasmic granules of polymorphonuclear neutrophils (PMNs) (92), monocytes (93), and alveolar macrophages (94). Both neutrophils and monocytes release HLE in response to a variety of stimuli (92–94). HLE binds with high affinity to sites on elastin, and the enzyme has been observed to be bound to elastin fibers in the lungs of patients with emphysema (95). Because HLE–elastin complexes retain catalytic activity for prolonged periods (96), HLE has the capacity to perpetuate elastolytic injury in vivo. More recently, cysteine proteases (97) and metalloproteases with elastolytic activity (98), derived from human alveolar macrophages, have been recognized for the potential to degrade lung elastin. The major inhibitors of elastases are members of the serpin superfamily proteins, including α_1-antitrypsin

(α_1-AT), human monocyte–neutrophil elastase inhibitor (HEI), plasminogen activator inhibitor-1 and -2, and antithrombin III (99,100). The major inhibitor of HLE in airway epithelium is secretory leukoprotease inhibitor (SLPI), also called mucous protease inhibitor (MPI), a low molecular weight protein (101). SLPI is expressed in epithelial cells (102), specifically in Clara cells and type II lung epithelial cells (103), and is thought to protect airways against neutrophil-mediated tissue destruction. The major HLE inhibitors in the lung, α_1-AT and SLPI, are slowly reversible inhibitors. α_2-Macroglobulin, which is a glycoprotein found in low concentrations in the lung, forms tight complexes with HLE and inhibits a broad spectrum of proteases (104).

C. Fibronectin

Fibronectin is an extracellular glycoprotein that exists as a soluble form in body fluids at high concentrations, and as an insoluble form in the extracellular matrix (for reviews, see 9,105–109). Extracellular fibronectin consists of highly insoluble fibronectin fibers that are organized in the fibrillar component of the ECM. Fibronectin is secreted as a dimer joined by two disulfide bonds. The molecule is composed of three regions of repeating sequences, termed I, II, and III, that are organized into distinct domains for binding to various macromolecules, such as collagen, heparin, fibrin, and cell surface receptors. The molecule is formed from a single gene product, and regions I, II, and III correspond to the exon structure of the gene (108). Alternative splicing of the gene transcript produces multiple protein isoforms, generating functional diversity that is cell-specific. Fibronectin expression is controlled principally at the level of transcription, but alternative splicing and protein secretion also regulate fibronectin production (110). Transcription is stimulated by TFG-β, cAMP, EGF, PDGF, IFN-γ, and vitamin D_3. There are cell-specific differences in fibronectin expression, which result from differential stimulation of the promoter in these cell lines (110). Fibronectin contains at least two distinct cell adhesive regions. The central, 11.5-kDa domain contains the tripeptide Arg-Gly-Asp (RGD) adhesive sequence, which binds to the classic fibronectin receptor of mesenchymal cells (111). Small peptides containing this sequence can block fibronectin-mediated cell adhesive activity in vitro and in vivo (111). The RGD sequence is not confined to fibronectin, but is a common motif in a variety of ECM proteins with cell surface receptors. Fibronectin binds to integrin receptors and modifies cell phenotype. It may play a role here by inducing MMPs, which break down ECM (112), a mechanism that plays a role in wound remodeling.

Fibronectin is primarily an adhesive glycoprotein and modulates matrix assembly. On cell surfaces, fibronectin molecules associate with each other, promoting cell–cell and cell–substratum linkages (113). Fibronectin has other diverse effects on cell function, such as promoting proliferation, differentiation, and migration of cells. For example, fibronectin can stimulate proliferation of human lung fibroblasts (114), and it can serve as a competence growth factor secreted by alveolar macrophages (115). In embryogenesis, increased amounts of fibronectin are found along pathways of migrating cells; cell migration can be inhibited by injection of RGD peptides (116). Finally, plasma fibronectin acts as a nonimmune opsonin to facilitate clearance of bacteria and cellular and extracellular matrix debris by macrophages and the reticuloendothelial system (117,118). Thus, the soluble form of fibronectin plays a role in infection, wound healing, and phagocytosis of foreign material.

D. Multifunctional Extracellular Glycoproteins: Vitronectin, SPARC, Tenascin-C, and Thrombospondin-1

In early tissue injury, cellular and plasma fibronectins and several minor components form a provisional matrix for cell migration involved in early granulation formation (for review, see 119). Among the minor components are several glycoproteins that are localized in the extracellular space and modulate cell function in early wound repair. Vitronectin, a glycoprotein found in serum and extracellular spaces, interacts with cell surfaces and ECM (120). It resembles fibronectin functionally, including the ability to mediate cell-spreading and adhesion. Vitronectin is a normal component of lung epithelial lining fluid, and increased concentrations occur in lavage fluid in idiopathic pulmonary fibrosis (IPF), in which vitronectin may have a role in fibroblast proliferation and ECM protein accumulation (121). Three glycoproteins, SPARC (secreted protein, acidic and rich in cysteine), tenascin-C, and thrombospondin-1, are chemically distinct, but function as antiadhesive proteins. During morphogenesis, all three proteins are expressed in the extracellular space, where they inhibit cell spreading, but they have no structural role in the adult (122,123). SPARC induces collagenase production when fibroblasts are in contact with collagen types I or III, but not type IV (124), suggesting an additional role in regulating remodeling the ECM. Normally, expression of these glycoproteins is limited to embryonic development. In IPF, SPARC, tenascin-C, and thrombospondin-1 are immunolocalized to the inflammatory exudates of alveoli, where they are thought to break adhesive interactions of cells allowing fibroblasts to migrate from interstitium to alveoli (125).

E. Proteoglycans

Proteoglycans are macromolecules that are composed of a core protein and glycosaminoglycans (GAGs), which are long, unbranched polysaccharide chains composed of repeating disaccharide units (10,126–129). Proteoglycans form a highly hydrated, porous ‘‘ground substance’’ in which fibrous proteins are embedded

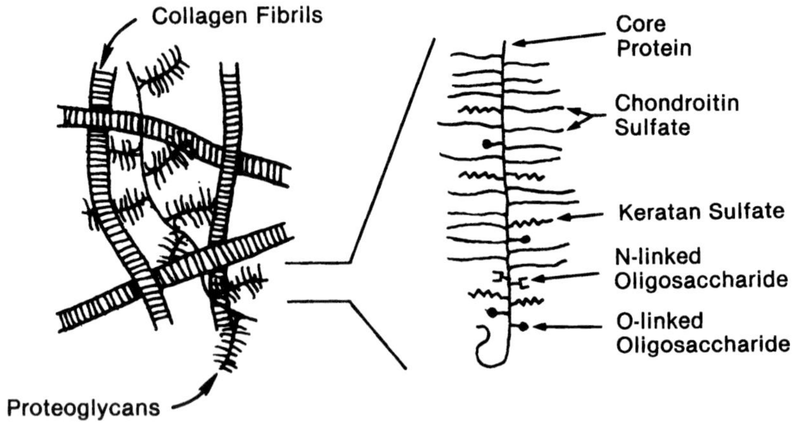

Figure 4 Scheme depicting collagen fibrils interwoven with proteoglycans in the ground substance: Proteoglycans consist of a core protein from which negatively charged glycosaminoglycans chains of chrondroitin sulfate and kertin sulfate radiate.

and through which nutrients and metabolites diffuse and cells migrate (Fig. 4). Because of their high sugar content, proteoglycans have a highly negative charge and attract cations, such as Na^+, which promotes retention of water. This hydration creates tissue turgor that enables tissues to withstand compressive forces. Proteoglycans constitute less than 10% of the weight of fibrous connective tissues.

Previously, proteoglycans were classified based on the GAG composition: hyaluronic acid (HA), chondroitin sulfate (CS), dermatin sulfate (DS), heparan sulfate (HS), heparin, and keratan sulfate (KS). They are now classified by the molecular structure of the protein core, and by functional characteristics into five large families (Table 3). *Family a* is characterized by large, aggregated proteoglycans that associate with multiple copies of different GAGs, and it is these proteoglycans that impart tissue turgor. *Family b* has smaller core proteins and many fewer GAGs. *Families c and d* play a role in the structure and composition of the ECM by modulating cell adhesion and growth factor binding. Cell–matrix adhesion by these proteoglycans supplements the more specific cell–matrix binding that occurs through integrin receptors. Among the most well studied is syndecan, a cell surface proteoglycan that binds to collagen, fibronectin, thrombospondin, and growth factors (130).

Proteoglycans in basement membranes bind and release growth factors, thereby regulating proliferation of cells involved in synthesis of ECM proteins (131). Basic and acidic FGF bind to heparan sulfate in basement membranes,

Table 3 Classification of Proteoglycans

Name	Source	Core protein size (kDa)	GAG chains	Possible functions
Family a: large extracellular proteoglycans				
Aggrecan	Cartilage	220	CS, KS	Provide support; fixed negative charge; regulate cell migration
Versican	Fibroblasts	265	CS	
Family b: small connective tissue proteoglycans				
Decorin	Many cells	36	DS	Modulates collagen fibrilogenesis
Biglycan		38	DS	
Fibromodulin		41	KS	
Family c: basement membrane heparan sulfates				
	EHS tumor	400	HS	Modulates assembly of basement membranes; provides filtration barrier
	Glomerular basement membrane	30–400	HS	
Family d: cell surface proteoglycans				
Syndecan	Mammary epithelium	31	CS, HS	Links cytoskeleton to ECM
Betaglycan	Fibroblasts	110		Receptor protein
Thrombomodulin	Endothelial cells	58–60	CS	Regulates blood coagulation
Family e: Intracellular proteoglycans				
Serglycin	Many cells	17–19	CS, DS, HS	Modulate storage and activity of granular proteases

Selected proteoglycans, grouped according to Kjellén and Lindahl (128): Abbreviation of GAG: CS, chondroitin sulfate; KS, keratin sulfate; DS, dermatin sulfate; HS, heparan sulfate.

and the heparan–FGF complex protects the FGF from degradation, thus enhancing FGF activity. Basement membrane proteoglycans concentrate TGF-β, and this interaction is complex because TGF-β regulates decorin expression, and decorin may regulate some of the growth-promoting activity of TGF-β (127). Heparan sulfate, which is released from cell surface proteoglycans, has long been known to inhibit cell proliferation, but it is also stimulates growth of certain cell types (132). *Family e* is composed of intracellular proteoglycans that govern electrostatic, osmotic, and hydration properties of cells. Thus, proteoglycans have varied functions, ranging from maintenance of mechanical properties and barrier functions, to more dynamic properties, such as cell adhesion, growth, and differentiation.

E. Basement Membrane Components

Basement membranes function in the lung to help provide structural integrity of the tissues and to regulate passage of macromolecules across the alveolar barrier. The major components of basement membranes are type IV collagen, laminin, entactin, and heparan sulfate proteoglycans (17,133,134). Laminin is a large trimeric glycoprotein that contains several functional domains that bind to other components of the basement membrane and collagen (135). Entactin is a glycoprotein that has the presumed function of facilitating basement membrane assembly by binding to collagen type IV, laminin, proteoglycans, and fibronectin (136). Basement membranes contain several forms of type IV collagen and laminin. Each component of basement membranes is biologically active, and specific cellular receptors for each component have been described (137). Among the multiple functions of basement membranes are cell proliferation, differentiation, and polarity.

F. Integrins

Integrins are a large family of heterodimeric α/β cell-surface glycoproteins (7,138,139). The family has been classified on the basis that different α-subunits, in combination with the same β-subunit, form receptors of different specificities. Multiple integrins recognize each of the ECM glycoproteins and convey information to the cell. Regulatory function through signaling by integrin–ligand interaction is extensive, and influences the expression of several genes, metabolic enzymes, and cytokines (140). This section will focus on salient points of integrin signaling and remodeling of the ECM (141). Cellular gene expression for ECM proteins is controlled, in part, by the composition of the ECM surrounding the cell. This mutual pattern of recognition between nucleus and matrix proteins produces a reciprocal interaction between cells and the surrounding ECM. The importance of this interaction is that when tissue is perturbed by injury, the altered environment produces a phenotypic change in cells that leads to processes that repair or replace injured cells, thereby healing the injury. Considerable experimental evidence supports this vital role of the ECM (141). The interaction between cells and ECM is transduced by integrins. Integrins signal the secretion of matrix metalloproteases and protease inhibitors (112). In this manner, integrin signaling mediates the synthesis, degradation, and organization of the ECM.

III. ECM Proteins in Lung Development

Extracellular matrix proteins regulate differentiated phenotypes of cells during lung development by two broad mechanisms: storage and release of growth factors that bind to ECM (reviewed in 131,142), and signaling of ECM receptors on cells by individual ECM molecules (143). Both processes contribute to the orderly anatomical changes during development. In the lung, evidence of developmental regulation by ECM proteins is derived from perturbation of cultures of embryonic lung and whole animal experiments (144–154; Table 4). New techniques have facilitated research aimed at determining control of lung development by ECM components. Immunohistological and in situ hybridization studies have shown the spatial and temporal expression of ECM proteins, and molecular probes have identified expression of several components that are normally in low

Table 4 Experimental Perturbation of Extracellular Matrix Affecting Lung Branching Morphogenesis

Component/perturbation	Ref.
Collagen	
Collagenase	144
Proline analogue	145
Fibronectin	
RGD-peptides	146
Laminin	
Antilaminin antibody	147
Cadherins	
Anticadherin antibody	148
Chondroitin sulfate proteoglycans	
β-D-Xyloside	149,150
Multiple ECM components	
TGF-β	151
Transgenic mice bearing TGF-β1 chimeric gene	152
SPARC	
Anti-SPARC antibodies	153
Tenasin-C	
Antitenascin-C antibodies	154

Abbreviations: RGD, -Arg-Gly-Asp- tripeptide; ECM, extracellular matrix; TGF-β, transforming growth factor-β; SPARC, secreted protein, acidic and rich in cysteine.

abundance. Gene knockout experiments, through homologous recombination, have shown the effects of developmental deletion of ECM proteins, ranging from lethality for type I α_1-procollagen (155) to no effect for tenascin (156). Transgenic mice overexpressing human collagenase have airspace enlargement at birth (157), and expression of a chimeric gene for TGF-β1 affects lung morphogenesis (152). The use of molecular tools, such as these, illustrate their great potential for future discovery of regulation of lung development by removing a specific ECM component.

The general features of lung growth and development (158,159), biochemistry of connective tissue development (160–163), and regulation of lung development by ECM proteins (164) have been extensively reviewed. This section will discuss a few salient points of the influence of ECM on lung development.

Expression of ECM components during lung development has been extensively characterized (32,147,153,154,165–190), and Table 5 summarizes changes in selected ECM components. *Collagen* synthesis rate is highest during fetal life and decreases shortly after birth; the total amount of collagen in lung does not change once maturity is reached (191; Fig. 5). The sites of type I collagen deposition in human fetal lung are large blood vessels, peribronchial connective tissue, and interstitium (166). Control of type I collagen expression in the developing human lung is complex, as shown by considerable heterogeneity of collagen gene expression within each of the anatomical subcompartments (166). *Elastin* production occurs during late fetal and early neonatal life; elastin production ceases when the lungs are fully mature (13,192; Fig. 6). The location of elastin expression in neonatal lungs is in vascular smooth-muscle cells and interstitial fibroblasts (170). *Proteoglycans* concentration in the lung is highest before birth and abruptly decreases to adult levels shortly after birth (175). The high levels before term may reflect a role of proteoglycans in facilitating morphogenesis. The rapid contraction of proteoglycan content after birth is consistent with a role in regulating lung fluid removal from the interstitium postnatally (175). Cellular *fibronectin* expression is ubiquitous in the developing lung, decreases in the fetus, and is at low levels in the neonate and adult (174). *Collagenase and TIMP* expression in early fetal lung is identified by reverse transcriptase–polymerase chain reaction (RT-PCR), but expression levels are too low to be localized by in situ hybridization (186). *Gelatinase* mRNA levels and activity increase in fetal lung cells before birth and then decrease at term (188,193).

Alveolar formation occurs during late fetal life by the formation of secondary septae and marked thinning of interstitial tissue. The secondary septae are composed of a central core containing fibroblasts surrounded on each side by a capillary (194; Fig. 7). The fibroblasts at the tip of the septae are rapidly dividing, causing the septum to lengthen. Elastin is deposited in the core adjacent to both lipid-laden and nonlipid-laden interstitial fibroblasts (195). The critical role of ECM in septal formation is shown by experiments using agents to block formation of collagen and elastin, which impairs alveolar development (196–198).

Table 5 Selected Examples of Expression of ECM Proteins and Enzymes by Various Methods During Lung Development

Component	Biochemistry	Immunohistology	mRNA levels	In situ hybridization	Human studies	Ref.
Collagen	X	X	X	X	X	32,165,166
Elastin	X		X	X		167–170
Fibronectin	X	X	X	X		171–174
Proteoglycans	X	X				175–177
Basement membrane components	X	X	X			178–181
Biglycan		X	X			182
Tenascin		X	X			154,183
Syndecan	X	X				184
Entactin		X	X	X		185
Laminin		X	X	X		147
Metalloproteases	X		X			186–189
TIMP			X			186
Lysyl oxidase	X					190
SPARC		X		X		153

Abbreviations: mRNA, messenger RNA; TIMP, tissue inhibitors of metalloproteases; SPARC, secreted protein, acidic and rich in cysteine. X, indicates method used to measure component in lung.

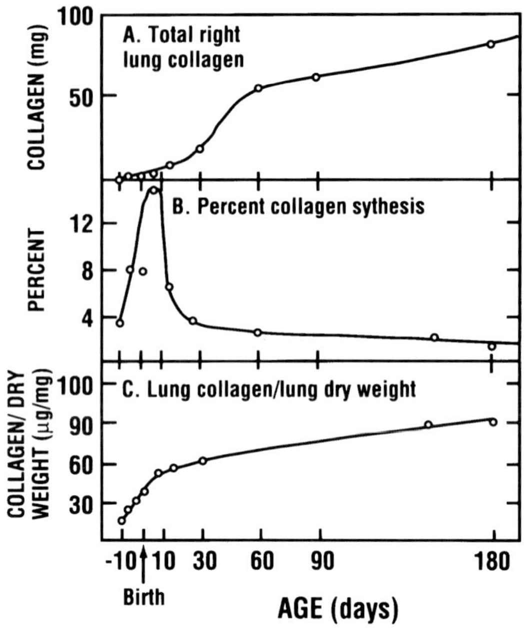

Figure 5 Changes in rabbit lung collagen with age. (From Ref. 153.)

Airway branching is dependent on the influence of mesenchyme and its associated ECM on epithelial cell differentiation. Mechanisms that modulate mesenchyme–epithelial interactions are uncertain, but involve normal synthesis of collagen, laminin, fibronectin, and syndecan. Support for this concept is derived from experiments in which branching morphogenesis in organ cultures has been perturbed using the various approaches outlined in Table 4. Taken together, these studies lend strong support to the concept that branching morphogenesis is dependent on the composition and adhesive properties of ECM molecules and their interaction with epithelial cells during development.

IV. Connective Tissue Changes in Lung Diseases of Early Infancy

A. Lung Injury and Repair as a Function of Maturation

The response of the lung to injury is complex because of the myriad cellular and molecular processes controlling tissue repair. A key event in repair of lung injury is deposition of connective tissue, a process that can lead to either reconstitution

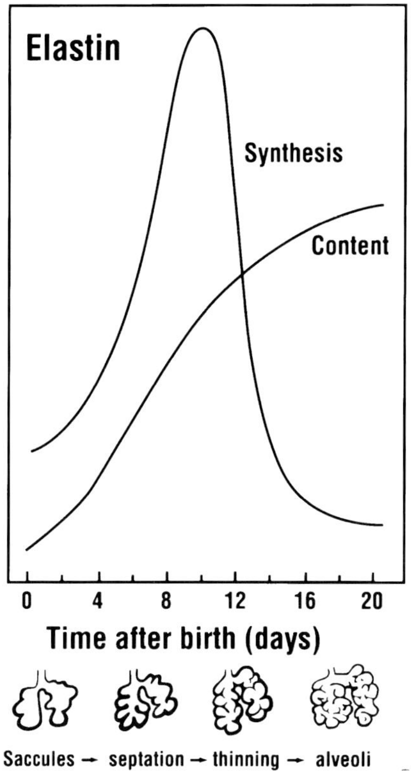

Figure 6 Profile of changing content and synthesis of elastin in the developing rat lung: No units for elastin are given, and changes represent relative changes. (From Refs. 165 and 192.)

of normal structures or replacement with scar tissue. There have been remarkable advances in unraveling the pathogenetic mechanisms of fibrotic lung diseases in adult lung tissues and animal models (199–204). Limited biochemical and immunohistochemical data are available from lungs of infants with BPD. It must be kept in mind that the generalities about lung fibrosis in adults and animal models may not apply to infants. Conditions such as hyperoxia, lung immaturity, and barotrauma may stimulate a different repair process in the infant than in the adult. A major unresolved issue in the etiology of BPD is whether hyperoxia, and various host factors in infants at risk for BPD produce a unique pattern of response to injury. There appear to be notable differences in the pathology of BPD in infants compared with pulmonary fibrosis in adults, suggesting that differ-

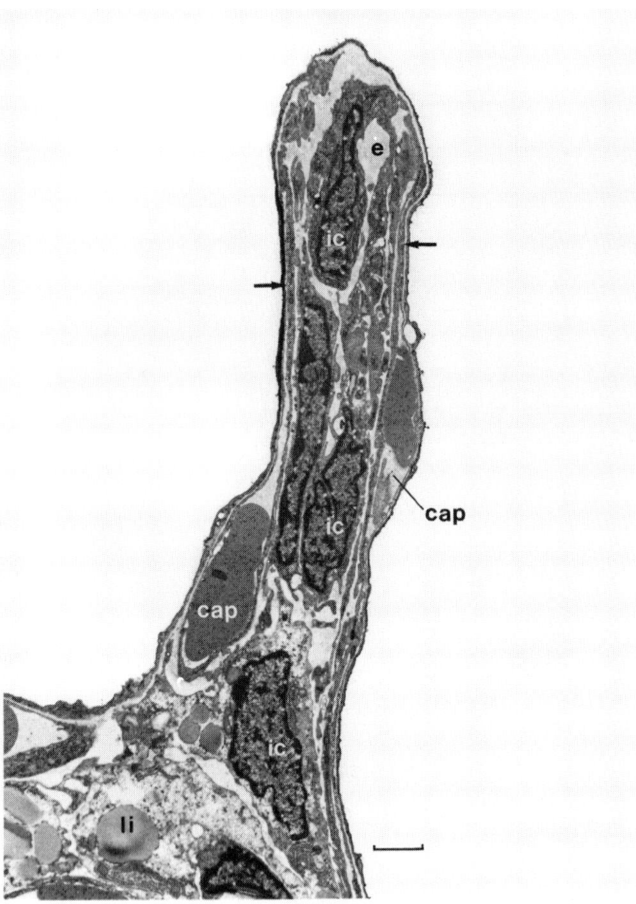

Figure 7 Electron micrograph of secondary crest of rat lung 7-days old: Capillaries (cap) on both sides of crest. Interstitial cells of two types are shown in interstitium: at base, interstitial cell containing lipid (li); toward the top, interstitial cell (ic) enfolding elastin (e). Capillary walls form extensions toward end of crest (arrows). Scale, 2 μm; × 5200. (From Ref. 194.)

ent pathogenetic processes may be involved. This section will highlight what is known of the connective tissue changes in lungs of human infants with BPD. It will also contrast the changes in BPD with those that are seen in adults with pulmonary fibrosis and animal models of this condition. As oxygen toxicity may be central to the pathogenesis of BPD, special emphasis will be given to altered connective tissue that occurs with exposure to toxic concentrations of oxygen.

B. Connective Tissue Pathology of BPD

The initial reports of the pathology of BPD reflected the most severe cases of infants who did not survive (205–210). These cases were reported in the era before antenatal glucocorticoids and exogenous surfactant and were managed without positive end-expiratory pressure and oxygen monitoring. The main features of severe BPD were extensive hyperplasia or metaplasia of the airways, interstitial fibrosis, areas of atelectasis, and airspace enlargement. The lesions evolve from an early exudative reaction (1–2 weeks), which is progressively organized by a subacute, proliferative reparative process (2–4 weeks), often leading to severe interstitial fibrosis (after 4 weeks; 210). Microscopically, alveolar walls are thickened by proliferating fibroblasts and smooth-muscle cells and scattered lymphocytes and mononuclear cells (209,210), and in advanced cases by acellular connective tissue (205). Strands of scar tissue may surround hyperexpanded areas of lung. Although most prominent in alveolar walls, fibrosis occurs around bronchi as the result of airway injury (209), and small (100-μm–diameter) pulmonary arteries have intimal hyperplasia, medial hypertrophy, and adventitial fibrosis (207). Sometimes, marked pleural fibrosis is found near large bullae (205). At the ultrastructural level, increased amounts of collagen and elastin fibers surround fibroblast-like cells (205), and the elastic fibers are thickened, tortuous, and irregularly distributed (211,212). The extent of fibrosis can vary considerably. In one study, the airspaces were replaced with fibrosis in almost one-half of the cases; fibrosis was less conspicuous in one-fifth of the cases (207). Others have reported less or no fibrosis in distal airspaces (206). Hyperoxia for longer than 50 hr (213) and mechanical ventilation using peak airway pressures greater than 35 cmH_2O (208) result in greater lung fibrosis. A feature of BPD that differs from IPF or the adult respiratory distress syndrome (ARDS) is that enlargement of airspaces predominates at an early stage of fibrosis. Morphometric analyses show airspace enlargement and fewer alveoli per lung in BPD (209,211,214), and small-airway diameters are slightly decreased or unchanged (209,211). A strikingly similar pathological picture of fibrosis and cystic spaces has been reported in a few adults with diffuse lung injury (215), raising the possibility that immaturity is not a prerequisite for the development of BPD.

Alveolar collapse as a component of lung fibrosis in BPD has been described by Reid (216). The exudative phase of BPD may affect alveoli in various ways, including absorption of the exudate, with nonresidual damage; absorption of the intra-alveolar exudate into the alveolar wall, leaving a fibrosed alveolar wall; or organization in situ such that the alveolus is obliterated. Alveolar obliteration with myofibroblasts and connective tissue is noted in IPF (217,218), and is believed to account for the ensuing restrictive lung disease (219). The ability to remove connective tissue from airspaces during the exudative phase may contribute to the lung's ability to recover from acute injury.

There is little known of the changes in basement membrane components in BPD. However, lung permeability to solutes increases in the respiratory distress syndrome (220–222), allowing an influx of plasma proteins that contain profibrotic growth factors. Fibronectin has been presumed to mediate lung injury in neonates with BPD by a variety of mechanisms (223). High levels of fibronectin in lung lavage fluid may stimulate fibrogenesis (223). Changes in lung permeability and increased lung fibronectin levels in BPD may initiate alveolar organization and lead to obliteration of alveoli.

The pathological features of BPD of infants studied in the present era, since institution of antenatal glucocorticoids and exogenous surfactant, differ somewhat from the earlier descriptions (224,225). In the cases described in the modern era, the major feature is a pattern of enlarged, simplified terminal respiratory spaces and the presence of focal fibroplasia in alveoli, without a conspicuous bronchial or bronchiolar component. Markedly abnormal arrangement of elastic fibers in alveolar walls has been noted (225). The simplified airspaces are thought to result from arrested development of the alveoli, reflecting that the human lung is normally only partially alveolarized at birth. Lung morphometric studies in these infants have shown reduced numbers of alveoli (209,211,214), and there is no compensatory growth of alveoli after this stage. Thus, there appears to be a subset of infants who have arrested alveolarization without airways disease. Although the pathogenesis of this subset is not determined, it presumably is caused by interruption of developmentally regulated genes that determine alveolar formation and growth.

C. Biochemistry of Lungs in Infants with CLD

The biochemical hallmark of pulmonary fibrosis is increased amounts of ECM proteins in lung. Analysis of ECM proteins in lungs of infants dying of BPD has been hampered by a paucity of lung specimens from patients with BPD and relevant age-matched control infants, and problems with normalizing protein concentrations in diseased tissues. Several studies have examined changes in collagen in the lungs of infants dying of BPD. Hislop and associates (214) observed increased hydroxyproline/DNA ratios in lung tissue of neonates with hyaline membrane disease compared with age-matched controls. An increased type III/I collagen ratio was observed in the lungs of neonates with BPD (226,227), a finding in accord with increased immunofluorescent type III collagen in early active fibrosis of the lung (32), and with biochemical studies of fibrotic adult human lung (28). Increased urinary excretion of hydroxyproline, a marker of increased collagen turnover, was observed in infants with BPD (228). The NH_2-terminal propeptide of type III collagen was increased in tracheal fluid and serum of infants at risk for BPD (229). This propeptide, a byproduct of type III collagen synthesis, is indicative of the active fibrosis in adult tissues (45,230). However, the interpretation of these findings is not straightforward, for the serum concentration of the NH_2-terminal propeptide of type III collagen in healthy children is normally high at birth, and declines during childhood before increasing again at puberty (231). The findings of increased type III/I collagen, elevated hydroxyproline excretion, and NH_2-terminal propeptides of type III collagen indicate increased turnover of collagen in lungs of infants who die with BPD. These biochemical markers reflect a large amount of newly synthesized collagen in the lungs of these infants.

Several studies have examined the changes in elastin turnover in BPD. Lung desmosine levels, which normally increase with age (160), tended to be higher in infants who died early of BPD (< 60 hr), but were normal in late deaths (214). The increased desmosine was restricted to a few infants with severe lung disease, and occurred during the early proliferative phase of lung injury (214). In neonates with BPD, evidence suggests increased turnover of elastin; greater urinary excretion of desmosine (232); increased elastolytic activity and desmosine in lung secretions, as well as decreased levels of antiproteases (233,234); and the appearance of degraded elastin fibers in lung tissue (235). It is not clear from these studies, however, if the increased products represent increased synthesis or degradation of elastin.

D. Pathogenesis of Airspace Enlargement in BPD

This section will discuss several observations pertinent to the genesis of airspace enlargement in BPD. At least five theories have been proposed to explain such enlargement: inhibition of formation of alveoli, barotrauma, mechanical obstruction, protease–antiprotease imbalance, and oxygen toxicity.

Inhibition of alveolarization and delay in septal formation has been observed in neonatal rats exposed to hyperoxia (233,236,237). This early period of exposure to excessive oxygen concentrations corresponds to the rapid postnatal period when alveoli form in human lungs. The lack of septal formation and loss of surface area found in humans with BPD may be due to inhibition of septation. *Barotrauma* was proposed to cause septal fibrosis by abnormal stretching of the alveolar walls by high airway pressures (207), and retraction of the septal scars was believed to produce permanent emphysema-like changes (205). The greater severity of disease in patients ventilated with higher peak airway pressures indirectly supports this theory (208). *Mechanical obstruction* as a result of obliteration of airways was proposed to lead to emphysema, air trapping, and alveolar distension, with disruption of the airspaces (205). Similarly, airway injury was thought to reduce airway growth during the rapid postnatal phase of lung development, contributing to disproportionate undergrowth of airway diameter and persistent increases in airway resistance (238). The theory of an *imbalance of proteases–antiproteases* proposes that neutrophil influx associated with lung injury leads to release of elastolytic enzymes, producing breakdown of alveolar walls (239). In addition to neutrophil influx as a source of proteolytic activity, collagenase levels may increase in the lower respiratory tract. Hyperoxia is associated with increased activities and mRNA levels for collagenase and gelatinase in lungs of newborn rats (187) and rabbits (240), but not in lungs of premature baboons (241). Increased secretion of gelatinase by lung cells has been observed in late fetal development or immediately after birth (188,193). Increased gelatinolytic activity is normally found in lungs in the perinatal period; it may reflect the remodeling of basement membranes at this time (177) and may contribute to the increased susceptibility of newborns to ECM degradation. It is unclear, however, whether the increased proteolytic activity in these studies represents simply increased turnover of ECM proteins in an injured lung, or is pathologically linked to cyst formation in BPD.

In the original description of BPD, Northway and associates proposed that *oxygen toxicity* was an important etiologic factor in modifying the acute respiratory distress syndrome, resulting in BPD (242). Hyperoxia causes lung injury by highly reactive oxyradicals, accompanied by inactivation of antioxidant enzymes. Considerable evidence indicates that an excess inflammatory response contributes to the pathogenesis of pulmonary fibrosis in O_2 toxicity (242). Histological studies demonstrate infiltration of inflammatory cells and a fibroproliferative response. Analysis of bronchoalveolar lavage fluid in oxygen toxicity shows increased concentrations of several inflammatory mediators, including proinflammatory cytokines, TNF-α, and products of inflammatory cell activation, including neutrophil elastase and collagenase, and hydrogen peroxide (243). It is recognized that certain cytokines and other agents that characterize the inflammatory response have predominately profibrotic effects. These cytokines are presumed to drive the fibroproliferative response that characterizes oxygen toxicity. Additionally, hyperoxia activates phagocytes to produce chemotactic factors that attract neutrophils into lungs (244–246). Alveolar macrophages that are exposed to high levels of O_2 release a neutrophil chemotactic substance, indicating that the alveolar macrophage might be a major source of mitogenic activity (247). Oxidants inactivate protease inhibitors (248).

It is clear that exposure of neonatal animals to hyperoxia is associated with lung fibrosis. The extent of injury, however, appears to be less in neonates than in adult animals (249,250). Premature baboons ventilated with 100% O_2 showed a reduced exudative response, with fewer hyaline membranes than adults (249), and similar differences were described in neonatal and adult rats (250). These findings are in accord with greater antioxidant protection of immature lungs. Nevertheless, high, sustained levels of hyperoxia presumably overwhelm the host defenses, and lead to oxidant-induced injury and interstitial fibrosis. Dexamethasone treatment in neonatal rats exposed to hyperoxia increased collagen deposition, suggesting that key collagen-related genes may be stimulated by dexamethasone during early hypoxic challenge (251).

Destruction of alveolar walls in hyperoxia could also be produced by direct degradation of ECM by oxyradicals. There is considerable evidence that oxidants directly degrade soluble connective tissue components and increase their susceptibility to cleavage by proteolytic enzymes (for review, see 252). Experimental observations indicate that sufficiently high concentrations of oxyradicals can directly contribute to an emphysema-like process through degradation of ECM. Two lines of evidence suggest that oxidant exposure in animals leads to airspace enlargement. First, morphometric studies have shown mild, diffuse airspace enlargement and diffuse interstitial fibrosis after recovery from exposure to 98–100% O_2. Administration of an agent that interferes with collagen deposition causes further enlargement of airspaces, suggesting that resynthesis of connective tissue is involved in the morphological changes (253). Second, acute exposure of animals to the putative oxidant cadmium chloride ($CdCl_2$) produced an intense fibrotic lesion, but if animals were treated with an agent that blocks collagen and elastin cross-linking, the lesion was converted to emphysema (254). These observations demonstrate that emphysema and fibrosis may be divergent responses to a common injury, the critical difference being the nature of the repair process (254). Fibrosis resulted if the damaged matrix components were replaced; emphysema occurred if repair or replacement was incomplete, predisposing to breakdown of alveoli and formation of enlarged airspaces. These observations in animals may explain the airspace enlargement in BPD.

V. Future Directions

It has been known for many years that the ECM regulates development and differentiation by several mechanisms. These include the composition of the ECM, binding to growth factors that affect their local concentration and biological activity, binding of individual ECM components to specific cell receptors, and signaling through cell–ECM interactions (143). These interactions affect cell differentiation, cell movement, and gene expression, processes that are essential to organ development. As impaired alveolarization is a central defect in BPD, one of the key questions is to discover how the ECM orchestrates alveolar development in the normal fetal lung. Future directions to study this question include:

1. Perturbation of lung development by exposing lung tissue in culture to specific antibodies or peptides that interfere with ECM functions.
2. Prevention of expression of specific ECM genes during late fetal devel-

opment to allow analysis of ECM proteins and receptors in lung morphological differentiation.
3. Overexpress specific ECM genes that control adhesion at critical phases of lung morphogenesis to determine whether increasing the local concentration of cell-binding sites alters structural development.
4. Downregulate genes that degrade matrix components or upregulate growth factor genes that stimulate ECM production at key times of lung morphogenesis to determine their effects on alveolar formation.

A second potentially useful future direction to pursue is the spatial and temporal changes in ECM associated with formation of alveolar capillaries during lung development. Angiogenesis that occurs in secondary crests of nascent alveoli may be key to alveolar formation. The ECM signals in mesenchyme direct angiogenesis, and these signals may be deranged in injured tissue. It is possible that inability to develop an adequate vascular supply may critically impair formation of alveoli and account for the disorganized vascular pattern found in BPD. An analysis of ECM components involved in vascularization of alveoli and experimental perturbation of the ECM components may shed light on the potential role of these components in alveolar formation.

A third direction is to use molecular approaches to study whether key ECM genes that are normally expressed in the lung during development are downregulated or upregulated following premature delivery. This approach may provide clues to developmentally regulated ECM genes that are altered by prematurity. Further study of the pattern of these genes may provide insight into their aberrant regulation during early adaptation to extrauterine life.

Finally, it is essential to explore, at a basic level, the molecular processes that control regulation of cell growth and death mediated by ECM proteins. Cell proliferation, in addition to overexpression of ECM genes, contributes to excess deposition of connective tissues in advanced BPD. The composition of ECM in contact with cells is an important determinant of their proliferative rate, and detachment of ECM triggers death of some types of mesenchymal cells. The molecular signals in ECM that are mitogenic or trigger apoptosis, and their interaction with soluble mediators, need further exploration. Lack of differentiation and proliferation of mesenchymal cells may explain failure of alveolarization in premature lungs. In addition, altered sensitivity of fibroblasts to ECM growth signals may contribute to the fibroproliferation in advanced BPD.

Acknowledgments

This work was supported in part by PHS grant HL24264 and the Barbara Wallace Cornwall Respiratory Research Laboratory. Mrs. Selena Boykin and Marcella Spioch provided expert secretarial assistance.

References

1. Hay ED. Cell Biology of Extracellular Matrix, 2nd ed. New York: Plenum Press, 1991.
2. Prockop DJ, Kivirikko KI. Collagens: molecular biology, diseases, and potentials for therapy. Annu Rev Biochem 1995; 64:403–434.
3. Mayne R, Burgeson RE. Structure and Functions of Collagen Types. Orlando, FL: Academic Press, 1987.
4. Nimni ME. Collagens: Biochemistry, Biomechanics, and Biotechnology. Vols I–III. Boca Raton, FL: CRC Press, 1988.
5. Chadwick DJ, Goode JA. The Molecular Biology and Pathology of Elastic Tissues. (Ciba Foundation Symposium 192). Chichester: John Wiley & Sons, 1995.
6. Mecham RP. Regulation of Matrix Accumulation. Orlando, FL: Academic Press, 1986.
7. Cheresh DA, Mecham RP. Integrins. Molecular and Biological Responses to the Extracellular Matrix. San Diego: Academic Press, 1994.
8. Yurchenco PD, Birk DE, Mecham RP. Extracellular Matrix Assembly and Structure. San Diego: Academic Press, 1994.
9. Hynes RO. Fibronectins. New York: Springer-Verlag, 1989.
10. Jollès P. Proteoglycans. Boston: Birkhaüser-Verlag, 1994.
11. Kelley J. Collagen. In: Massaro D, ed. Lung Cell Biology. New York: Marcel Dekker, 1989:821–866.
12. Hance A, Crystal RG. The connective tissue of the lung. Am Rev Respir Dis 1975; 112:657–709.
13. Parks WC, Pierce RA, Lee KA, Mecham RP. Elastin. In: Kleinman HK, ed. Advances in Molecular and Cell Biology. Greenwich, CT: JAI Press, 1993:133–182.
14. Mecham RP. Elastic fibers. In: Crystal RG, West JB, Weibel ER, Barnes PG, eds. The Lung: Scientific Foundations. 2nd ed. Philadelphia: Lippincott–Raven, 1997: 729–736.
15. Clark JG, Kuhn C III, McDonald JA, Mecham RP. Lung connective tissue. Int Rev Connect Tissue Res 1983; 10:249–331.
16. Goldstein RH. Control of type I collagen formation in the lung. Am J Physiol 1991; 261:L29–L40.
17. Chambers RC, Laurent GJ. Collagens. In: Crystal RG, West JB, Weibel ER, Barnes PG, eds. The Lung: Scientific Foundations. 2nd ed. Philadelphia: Lippincott–Raven, 1997:709–727.
18. Roberts CR, Wight TN, Hascall VC. Proteoglycans. In: Crystal RG, West JB, Weibel ER, Barnes PG, eds. The Lung: Scientific Foundations. 2nd ed. Philadelphia: Lippincott–Raven, 1997:757–768.
19. Crouch EC, Martin GR, Brody JS, Laurie GW. Basement membranes. In: Crystal RG, West JB, Weibel ER, Barnes PG, eds. The Lung: Scientific Foundations. 2nd ed. Philadelphia: Lippincott–Raven, 1997:769–791.
20. Bradley KH, McConnell SD, Crystal RG. Lung collagen composition and synthesis. Characterization and changes with age. J Biol Chem 1974; 249:2674–2683.
21. Pierce JA, Hocott JB. Studies on the collagen and elastin content of the human lung. J Clin Invest 1960; 39:8–14.

22. Hulmes DJS. The collagen superfamily—diverse structures and assemblies. Essays Biochem 1992; 27:49–67.
23. Mayne R, Brewton RG. New members of the collagen superfamily. Curr Opin Cell Biol 1993; 5:883–890.
24. Fleischmajer R, Olsen BR, Kühn K. Structure, molecular biology, and pathology of collagen. Ann NY Acad Sci 1990; 580:1–586.
25. Van der Rest M, Garrone R. Collagen family of proteins. FASEB J 1991; 5:2814–2823.
26. Burgeson RE, Nimni ME. Collagen types. Molecular structure and tissue distribution. Clin Orthop 1992; 282:250–272.
27. Shaw LM, Olsen BR. FACIT collagens: diverse molecular bridges in extracellular matrices. Trends Biochem Sci 1991; 16:191–194.
28. Seyer JM, Hutcheson ET, Kang AH. Collagen polymorphismn in idiopathic pulmonary fibrosis. J Clin Invest 1976; 57:1498–1507.
29. Madri JA, Furthmayr H. Collagen polymorphism in the lung. An immunohistochemical study of pulmonary fibrosis. Hum Pathol 1980; 11:353–366.
30. McLees BD, Schleiter G, Pinnell SR. Isolation of type III collagen from human adult parenchymal lung tissue. Biochemistry 1977; 16:185–190.
31. Bradley KH, McConnell-Breul SD, Crystal RG. Lung collagen heterogeneity. Proc Natl Acad Sci USA 1974; 71:2828–2832.
32. Bateman E, Turner-Warwick M, Adelmann-Grill BC. Immunohistochemical study of collagen types in human foetal and fibrotic lung. Thorax 1981; 36:645–653.
33. Kefalides NA, Denduchis B. Structural components of epithelial and endothelial basement membranes. Biochemistry 1969; 8:4613–4621.
34. Sage H, Farin FM, Striker GE, Fisher AB. Granular pneumocytes in primary culture secrete several major components of the extracellular matrix. Biochemistry 1983; 22:2148–2155.
35. Weber M, Pullig O. Different immunologic properties of globular NCl domain of collagen type IV isolated from various human basement membranes. Eur J Clin Invest 1992; 22:138–146.
36. von der Mark H, Aumailley M, Wick G, Fleischmajer R, Timpl R. Immunochemistry, genuine size and tissue localization of collagen VI. Eur J Biochem 1984; 142: 493–502.
37. Wetzels RHW, Robben HCM, Leigh IM, Schaafsma HE, Vooijs GP, Ramaekers FCS. Distribution patterns of type VIII collagen in normal and malignant human tissues. Am J Pathol 1991; 139:451–459.
38. Juvonen M, Sandberg M, Pihlajaniemi T. Patterns of expression of the six alternatively spliced exons affecting the structures of the COL1 and NC2 domains of the α1 (XIII) collagen chain in human tissues and cell lines. J Biol Chem 1992; 267: 24700–24707.
39. Kivirikko S, Saarela J, Meyers JC, Autio-Harmainen H, Pihlajaniemi T. Distribution of type XV collagen transcripts in human tissues and their production by muscle cells and fibroblasts. Am J Pathol 1995; 147:1500–1509.
40. Myers JC, Aion AS, Abraham V, Amenta PS. Type XV collagen exhibits a widespread distribution in tissues but a distinct localization in basement membrane zones. Cell Tissue Res 1996; 286:493–503.

41. Prockop DJ, Kivirikko KI, Tuderman L, Guzman NA. The biosynthesis of collagen and its disorders. N Engl J Med 1979; 301:13–23, 77–85.
42. Sandell LJ, Boyd CD. Extracellular Matrix Genes. San Diego: Academic Press, 1990.
43. Vuorio E, de Crombrugghe B. The family of collagen genes. Annu Rev Biochem 1990; 59:837–872.
44. Ramirez F, Di Liberto M. Complex and diversified regulatory programs control the expression of vertebrate collagen genes. FASEB J 1990; 4:1616–1623.
45. Rohde H, Vargas L, Hahn E, Kalbfleisch H, Bruguera M, Timpl R. Radiommunoassay for type III procollagen peptide and its application to human liver disease. Eur J Clin Invest 1979; 9:451–459.
46. Agelli M, Wahl S. Cytokines and fibrosis. Clin Exp Rheumatol 1986; 4:379–388.
47. Kovacs EJ, DiPietro LA. Fibrogenic cytokines and connective tissue production. FASEB J 1994; 8:854–861.
48. Roberts AB, Sporn MB, Assoian RK, et al. Transforming growth factor type β: rapid induction of fibrosis and angiogenesis in vivo and stimulation of collagen formation in vitro. Proc Natl Acad Sci USA 1986; 83:4167–4171.
49. Massagué J. The TGF-β family of growth and differentiation factors. Cell 1987; 49:437–438.
50. Border WA, Noble NA. Transforming growth factor-β in tissue fibrosis. N Engl J Med 1994; 332:1286–1292.
51. Ignotz RA, Massagué J. Transforming growth factor-β stimulates the expression of fibronectin and collagen and their incorporation into the extracellular matrix. J Biol Chem 1986; 261:4337–4345.
52. Penttinen RP, Kobayashi S, Bornstein P. Transforming growth factor β increases mRNA for matrix proteins both in the presence and absence of changes in mRNA stability. Proc Natl Acad Sci USA 1988; 85:1105–1108.
53. Edwards DR, Murphy G, Reynolds JJ, Whitman SE, Docherty AJ, Angel P, Heath JK. Transforming growth factor-β modulates the expression of collagenase and metalloproteinase inhibitor. EMBO J 1987; 6:1899–1904.
54. Goldstein RH, Poliks CF, Pilch PF, Smith BD, Fine A. Stimulation of collagen formation by insulin and insulin-like growth factor I in cultures of human lung fibroblasts. Endocrinology 1989; 124:964–970.
55. Cockayne D, Sterling KM Jr, Shull S, Mintz KP, Illeyne S, Cutroneo KR. Glucocorticoids decrease the synthesis of type I procollagen mRNAs. Biochemistry 1986; 25:3202–3209.
56. Hämäläinen L, Oikarinen J, Kivirikko KI. Synthesis and degradation of type I procollagen mRNAs in cultured skin fibroblasts and the effect of cortisol. J Biol Chem 1985; 260:270–275.
57. Weiner FR, Czaja MJ, Jefferson DM, Giambrone M-A, Tur-Kaspa R, Reid LM, Zern MA. The effect of dexamethasone on in vitro collagen gene expression. J Biol Chem 1987; 262:6955–6958.
58. Rosenbloom J, Feldman G, Freundlich B, Jimenez SA. Transcriptional control of human diploid fibroblast collagen synthesis by gamma-interferon. Biochem Biophys Res Commun 1984; 123:365–372.
59. Clark JG, Dedon TF, Wayner EA, Carter WG. Effects of interferon-gamma on

expression of cell surface receptors for collagen and deposition of newly synthesized collagen by cultured human lung fibroblasts. J Clin Invest 1989; 83:1505–1511.

60. Fine A, Poliks CF, Donahue LP, Smith BD, Goldstein RH. The differential effect of postaglandin E_2 on transforming growth factor-β and insulin-induced collagen formation in lung fibroblasts. J Biol Chem 1989; 264:16988–16991.
61. Baum BJ, Moss J, Breul SD, Crystal RG. Association in normal human fibroblasts of elevated levels of adenosine 3′:5′-monophosphate with a selective decrease in collagen production. J Biol Chem 1978; 253:3391–3394.
62. Kähäri V-M, Chen YQ, Su MW, Ramirez F, Uitto J. Tumor necrosis factor-α and interferon-gamma suppress the activation of human type I collagen gene expression by transforming growth factor-β_1. Evidence for two distinct mechanisms of inhibition at the transcriptional and posttranslational levels. J Clin Invest 1990; 86:1489–1495.
63. Solis-Herruzo JA, Brenner DA, Chojkier M. Tumor necrosis factor α inhibits collagen gene transcription and collagen synthesis in cultured human fibroblasts. J Biol Chem 1988; 263:5841–5845.
64. Bhatnagar R, Penfornis H, Mauviel A, Loyau G, Saklatvala J, Pujol J-P. Interleukin-1 inhibits the synthesis of collagen by fibroblasts. Biochem Int 1986; 13:709–720.
65. Zhang Y, Lin J-X, Yip YK, Vilcek J. Enhancement of cAMP levels and of protein kinase activity by tumor necrosis factor and interleukin 1 in human fibroblasts: role in the induction of interleukin 6. Proc Natl Acad Sci USA 1988; 85:6802–6805.
66. Katayama K, Armendariz-Borunda J, Raghow R, Kang AH, Seyer JM. A pentapeptide from type I procollagen promotes extracellular matrix production. J Biol Chem 1993; 268:9941–9944.
67. Aycock RS, Raghow R, Stricklin GP, Seyer JM, Kang AH. Post-transcriptional inhibition of collagen and fibronectin synthesis by a synthetic homolog of a portion of the carboxyl-terminal propeptide of human type I collagen. J Biol Chem 1986; 261:14355–14360.
68. Wu CH, Walton CM, Wu GY. Propeptide-mediated regulation of procollagen synthesis in IMR-90 human lung fibroblast cell cultures. Evidence for transcriptional control. J Biol Chem 1991; 266:2983–2987.
69. Bienkowski RS. Intracellular degradation of newly synthesized collagen. Coll Relat Res 1984; 4:399–411.
70. Laurent GJ. Dynamic state of collagen: pathways of collagen degradation in vivo and the possible role in regulation of tissue mass. Am J Physiol 1987; 252:C1–C9.
71. Birkedal-Hansen H, Moore WG, Bodden MK, Windsor LJ, Birkedal-Hansen B, DeCarlo A, Engler JA. Matrix metalloproteinases: a review. Crit Rev Oral Biol Med 1993; 4:197–250.
72. Matrisian LM. Metalloproteinases and their inhibitors in matrix remodeling. Trends Genet 1990; 6:121–125.
73. Dollery CM, McEwan JR, Henney AM. Matrix metalloproteinases and cardiovascular disease. Circ Res 1995; 77:863–868.
74. Rosenbloom J, Abrams WR, Mecham RP. Extracellular matrix 4: the elastin fiber. FASEB J 1993; 7:1208–1218.

75. Foster JA, Curtiss S. The regulation of elastin synthesis. Am J Physiol 1990; 259: L13–L23.
76. Hinek A, Rabinovich M. 67-kD elastin-binding protein is a protective "companion" of extracellular insoluble elastin and intracellular tropoelastin. J Cell Biol 1994; 126:563–574.
77. Cleary EG. The microfibillar component of elastin fibers. Morphology and biochemistry. In: Uitto J, Perejda AJ, eds. Connective Tissue Disease. Molecular Pathology of the Extracellular Matrix. New York: Marcel Dekker, 1987:55–81.
78. Sakai LY, Keene DR, Engvall EJ. Fibrillin, a new 350-kD glycoprotein, is a component of the extracellular microfibrils. J Cell Biol 1986; 103:2499–2509.
79. Dietz HC, Ramirez F, Sakai LY. Marfan's syndrome and other microfibrillar diseases. Adv Hum Genet 1994; 22:153–186.
80. Rosenbloom J, Abrams WR, Indik A, Yeh H, Ornstein-Goldstein N, Bashir MM. Structure of the elastin gene. In: Chadwick DJ, Goode JA, eds. The Molecular Biology and Pathology of Elastic Tissues (Ciba Foundation Symposium 192). Chichester: John Wiley & Sons, 1995:59–74.
81. Swee MH, Parks WC, Pierce RA. Developmental regulation of elastin production. Expression of tropoelastin pre-mRNA persists after down-regulation of steady-state mRNA levels. J Biol Chem 1995; 270:14899–14906.
82. Sechler JL, Sandberg LB, Roos PJ, Snyder I, Amenta PS, Riley DJ, Boyd CD. Elastin gene mutations in transgenic mice. In: Chadwick DJ, Goode JA, eds. The Molecular Biology and Pathology of Elastic Tissues (Ciba Foundation Symposium 192). Chichester: John Wiley & Sons, 1995:148–165.
83. Wolf BL, Rich CB, Goud HD, et al. Insulin-like growth factor-1 regulates transcription of the elastin gene. J Biol Chem 1993; 268:12418–12426.
84. Kähäri V-M, Chen YQ, Bashir M, Rosenbloom J, Uitto J. Tumor necrosis factor-α down-regulates human elastin gene expression. Evidence for the role of AP-1 in the suppression of promotor activity. J Biol Chem 1992; 267:26134–26141.
85. Berk JL, Franzblau C, Goldstein RH. Recombinant interleukin-1β inhibits elastin formation by a neonatal rat lung fibroblast subtype. J Biol Chem 1991; 266:3192–3197.
86. Mauviel A, Chen YQ, Kähäri V-M, Ledo I, Wu M, Rudnicka L, Uitto J. Human recombinate interleukin-1β up-regulates elastin gene expression in dermal fibroblasts. Evidence for transcriptional regulation in vitro and in vivo. J Biol Chem 1993; 268:6520–6524.
87. Mecham RP, Levy BD, Morris SL, Madaras JG, Wrenn DS. Increased cyclic GMP levels lead to a stimulation of elastin production in ligament fibroblasts that is reversed by cyclic AMP. J Biol Chem 1985; 260:3255–3258.
88. Kähäri V-M, Olsen DR, Rhudy RW, Carrillo P, Chen YQ, Uitto J. Transforming growth factor-β up-regulates elastin gene expression in human skin fibroblasts. Evidence for post-transcriptional modulation. Lab Invest 1992; 66:580–588.
89. Davidson JM, Zoia O, Liu JM. Modulation of transforming growth factor β-1 stimulated elastin and collagen production and proliferation in porcine vascular smooth muscle cells and skin fibroblasts by basic fibroblast growth factor, transforming growth factor-α, and insulin-like growth factor-1. J Cell Physiol 1993; 155:149–156.

90. Pierce RA, Mariencheck WI, Sandefur S, Crouch EC, Parks WC. Glucocorticoids upregulate tropoelastin expression during late stages of fetal lung development. Am J Physiol 1995; 268:L491–L500.
91. Bieth JG. Elastases: catalytic and biological properties. In: Mecham RP, ed. Regulation of Matrix Accumulation. Orlando, FL: Academic Press, 1986:217–320.
92. Havemann K, Janoff A. Neutral Proteases of Human Polymorphonuclear Leukocytes. Biochemistry, Physiology, and Clinical Significance. Baltimore: Urban & Schwarzenberg, 1978.
93. Campbell EJ, White RR, Senior RM, Rodriguez RJ, Kuhn C. Receptor-mediated binding and internalization of leukocyte elastase by alveolar macrophages in vitro. J Clin Invest 1979; 64:824–833.
94. Campbell EJ. Human leukocyte elastase, cathepsin G, and lactoferrin: family of neutrophil granule glycoproteins that bind to an alveolar macrophage receptor. Proc Natl Acad Sci USA 1982; 79:6941–6945.
95. Damiano VV, Tsang A, Kucich U, et al. Immunolocalization of elastase in human emphysematous lungs. J Clin Invest 1986; 78:482–493.
96. Morrison HM, Welgus HG, Stockley RA, Burnett D, Campbell EJ. Inhibition of human leukocyte elastase bound to elastin: relative ineffectiveness and two mechanisms of inhibitory activity. Am J Respir Cell Mol Biol 1990; 2:263–269.
97. Shi GP, Munger JS, Meara JP, Rich DH, Chapman HA. Molecular cloning and expression of human alveolar macrophage cathepsin S, an elastolytic cysteine proteinase. J Biol Chem 1992; 267:7258–7262.
98. Senior RM, Griffin GL, Fliszar CJ, Shapiro SD, Goldberg GI, Welgus HG. Human 92- and 72-kilodalton type IV collagenases are elastases. J Biol Chem 1991; 266: 7870–7875.
99. Carrell RW, Whisstock J, Lomas DA. Conformational changes in serpins and the mechanism of α_1-antitrypsin deficiency. Am J Respir Crit Care Med 1994; 150: S171–S175.
100. Potempa J, Korzus E, Travis J. The serpin superfamily of proteinase inhibitors: structure, function and regulation. J Biol Chem 1994; 269:15957–15960.
101. Thompson RC, Ohlsson K. Isolation, properties, and complete amino acid sequence of human secretory leukocyte protease inhibitor, a potent inhibitor of leukocyte elastase. Proc Natl Acad Sci USA 1986; 83:6692–6696.
102. Abe T, Kobayashi N, Yoshimura K, et al. Expression of the secretory leukoproteinase inhibitor gene in epithelial cells. J Clin Invest 1991; 87:2207–2215.
103. Sallenave J-M, Silva A, Marsden ME, Ryle AP. Secretion of mucous proteinase inhibitor and elafin by Clara cells and type II pneumocyte cell lines. Am J Respir Cell Mol Biol 1993; 8:126–133.
104. Sottrup-Jensen L. α-Macroglobulins: structure, shape, and mechanism of proteinase complex formation. J Biol Chem 1989; 264:11539–11542.
105. Hynes RO. Fibronectins. Sci Am 1986; 254:42–51.
106. Yamada KM, Aota S, Akiyama SK, LaFlamme SE. Mechanisms of fibronectin and integrin function during cell adhesion and migration. Cold Spring Harbor Symp Quant Biol 1992; 57:203–212.
107. Mosher DF, Fogerty FJ, Chernousov MA, Barry ELR. Assembly of fibronectin into extracellular matrix. Ann NY Acad Sci 1991; 614:167–180.

108. Schwarzbauer JE. Fibronectin: from gene to protein. Curr Opin Cell Biol 1991; 3: 786–791.
109. Potts JR, Campbell ID. Fibronectin structure and assembly. Curr Opin Cell Biol 1994; 6:648–655.
110. Dean DC. Expression of the fibronectin gene. Am J Respir Cell Mol Biol 1989; 1:5–10.
111. Ruoslahti E, Pierschbacher MD. New perspectives in cell adhesion: RGD and integrins. Science 1987; 238:491–497.
112. Werb Z, Tremble PM, Behrendtsen O, Crowley E, Damsky CH. Signal transduction through the fibronectin receptor induces collagenase and stromelysin gene expression. J Cell Biol 1989; 109:877–889.
113. McDonald JA. Extracellular matrix assembly. Annu Rev Cell Biol 1988; 4:183–207.
114. Bitterman PB, Rennard SI, Adelberg S, Crystal RG. Role of fibronectin as a growth factor for fibroblasts. J Cell Biol 1983; 97:1925–1932.
115. Rennard SI, Hunninghake GW, Bitterman PB, Crystal RG. Production of fibronectin by the human alveolar macrophage: mechanism for the recruitment of fibroblasts to sites of tissue injury in interstitial lung diseases. Proc Natl Acad Sci USA 1981; 78:7147–7151.
116. Duband J-L, Dufour S, Thiéry JP. The instructive role of fibronectins in cell migrations during embryonic development. Ann NY Acad Sci 1990; 588:273–280.
117. Engvall E, Rouslahti E, Miller EJ. Affinity of fibronectin to collagen of different genetic types and to fibrinogen. J Exp Med 1978; 147:1584–1595.
118. Niehaus GD, Schumacker PT, Saba TM. Influence of opsonic fibronectin deficiency on lung fluid balance during bacterial sepsis. J Appl Physiol 1980; 49:693–699.
119. Clark RAF. The Molecular and Cellular Biology of Wound Repair. 2nd ed. New York: Plenum Press, 1995.
120. Yamada KM, Akiyama SK, Hasegawa T. Recent advances in research on fibronectin and other cell attachment proteins. J Cell Biochem 1985; 28:79–82.
121. Pohl WR, Conlan MG, Thompson AB, Earl RF, Romberger DJ, Mosher DF, Rennard SI. Vitronectin in bronchoalveolar lavage fluid is increased in patients with interstitial lung disease. Am Rev Respir Dis 1991; 143:1369–1375.
122. Chiquet-Ehrismann R. Antiadhesive molecules of the extracellular matrix. Curr Opin Cell Biol 1991; 3:800–804.
123. Sage EH, Bornstein P. Extracellular proteins that modulate cell–matrix interactions: SPARC, tenascin and thrombospondin. J Biol Chem 1991; 266:14831–14834.
124. Tremble PM, Lane TF, Sage EH, Werb Z. SPARC, a secreted protein associated with morphogenesis and tissue remodeling, induces expression of metalloproteinases in fibroblasts through a novel extracellular matrix-dependent pathway. J Cell Biol 1993; 121:1433–1444.
125. Kuhn C, Mason RJ. Immunolocalization of SPARC, tenascin, and thrombospondin in pulmonary fibrosis. Am J Pathol 1995; 147:1759–1769.
126. Templeton DM. Proteoglycans in cell regulation. Crit Rev Clin Lab Sci 1992; 29: 141–184.
127. Ruoslahti E. Proteoglycans in cell regulation. J Biol Chem 1989; 264:13369–13372.

128. Kjellén L, Lindahl U. Proteoglycans: structures and interactions. Annu Rev Biochem 1991; 60:443–475.
129. Roman J, McDonald JA. Fibronectins and fibronectin receptors in lung development, injury, and repair. In: Crystal RG, West JB, Weibel ER, Barnes PG, eds. The Lung: Scientific Foundations. 2nd ed. Philadelphia: Lippincott–Raven, 1997: 737–755.
130. Bernfield M, Sanderson RD. Syndecan, a developmentally regulated cell surface proteoglycan that binds extracellular matrix and growth factors. Phil Trans R Soc Lond B Biol Sci 1990; 327:171–186.
131. Massagué J, Pandiella A. Membrane-anchored growth factors. Annu Rev Biochem 1993; 62:515–541.
132. Castellot JJ Jr, Wright TC, Karnovsky MJ. Regulation of vascular smooth muscle cell growth by heparin and heparan sulfates. Semin Thromb Haemostat 1987; 13: 489–503.
133. Timpl R. Structure and biological activity of basement membrane proteins. Eur J Biochem 1989; 180:487–502.
134. Martin GR, Timpl R, Kühn K. Basement membrane proteins: molecular structure and function. Adv Protein Chem 1988; 39:1–50.
135. Yurchenko PD, Schittny JC. Molecular architecture of basement membranes. FASEB J 1990; 4:1577–1590.
136. Chung AE, Durkin ME. Entactin: structure and function. Am J Respir Cell Mol Biol 1990; 3:275–282.
137. Kleinman HK, Schnaper HW. Basement membrane matrices in tissue development. Am J Respir Cell Mol Biol 1993; 8:238–239.
138. Pilewski JM, Albelda SM. Adhesive molecules in the lung. An overview. Am Rev Respir Dis 1993; 148:S31–S37.
139. Sheppard D. Identification and characterization of novel airway epithelial integrins. Am Rev Respir Dis 1993; 148:S38–S42.
140. Schwartz MA. Integrins as signal transducing receptors. In: Cheresh DA, Mecham RP, eds. Integrins. Molecular Biology Responses to the Extracellular Matrix. San Diego: Academic Press, 1994:33–48.
141. Ashkenas J, Damsky CH, Bissell MJ, Werb Z. Integrins, signalling, and the remodeling of the extracellular matrix. In: Cheresh DA, Mecham RP, eds. Integrins. Molecular Biology Responses to the Extracellular Matrix. San Diego: Academic Press, 1994:79–100.
142. Nathan C, Sporn M. Cytokines in context. J Cell Biol 1991; 113:981–986.
143. Adams JC, Watt FM. Regulation of development and differentiation by the extracellular matrix. Development 1993; 117:1183–1198.
144. Wessells NK, Cohen JM. Effects of collagenase on developing epithelia in vitro: lung, ureteric bud, and pancreas. Dev Biol 1968; 18:294–309.
145. Alescio T. Effect of proline analogue, azetidine-2-carboxylic acid, on the morphogenesis in vitro of mouse embryonic lung. J Embryol Exp Morphol 1973; 29:439–451.
146. Roman J, Little CW, McDonald JA. Potential role of RGD-binding integrins in mammalian lung branching morphogenesis. Development 1991; 112:551–558.
147. Schuger L, O'Shea S, Rheinheimer J, Varani J. Laminin in lung development: effects of anti-laminin antibody in murine lung morphogenesis. Dev Biol 1990; 137: 26–32.

148. Hirai Y, Nose A, Kobayashi S, Takeichi M. Expression and role of E- and P-cadherin adhesion molecules in embryonic histogenesis. I. Lung epithelial morphogenesis. Development 1989; 105:263–270.
149. Smith CI, Hilfer SR, Searls RL, Nathanson MA, Allodoli MI. Effects of β-D-xyloside on differentiation of the respiratory epithelium of the fetal mouse lung. Dev Biol 1990; 138:42–52.
150. Smith CI, Webster EH, Nathanson MA, Searls RL, Hilfer SR. Altered patterns of proteoglycan deposition during maturation of the fetal mouse lung. Cell Differ Dev 1990; 32:83–96.
151. Serra R, Pelton RW, Moses HL. TGF-β1 inhibits branching morphogenesis and N-*myc* expression in lung bud organ cultures. Development 1994; 120:2158–2161.
152. Zhou L, Dey CR, Wert SE, Whitsett JA. Arrested lung morphogenesis in transgenic mice bearing an PS-C–TGF-β1 chimeric gene. Dev Biol 1996; 175:227–238.
153. Strandjord TP, Sage EH, Clark JG. SPARC participates in the branching morphogenesis of developing fetal rat lung. Am J Respir Cell Mol Biol 1995; 13:279–287.
154. Young SL, Chang L-Y, Erickson HP. Ontogeny of tenascin in rat lung and evidence for its function in branching morphogenesis. Dev Biol 1994; 161:615–625.
155. Schnieke A, Harbers K, Jaenisch R. Embryonic lethal mutation in mice induced by retrovirus insertion into the α1(I) collagen gene. Nature 1983; 304:315–320.
156. Saga Y, Yagi T, Ikawa Y, Sakakura T, Aizawa S. Mice develop normally without tenascin. Genes Dev 1992; 6:1821–1831.
157. D'Armiento J, Dalal SS, Okada Y, Berg RA, Chada K. Collagenase expression in lungs of transgenic mice causes pulmonary emphysema. Cell 1992; 71:955–961.
158. Langston C, Thurlbeck WM. Lung growth and development in late gestation and early postnatal life. Perspect Pediatr Pathol 1982; 7:203–235.
159. Burri PH. Postnatal development and growth. In: Crystal RG, West JB, Weibel ER, Barnes PG, eds. The Lung: Scientific Foundations. 2nd ed. Philadelphia: Lippincott–Raven, 1997:1013–1026.
160. Franzblau C, Hayes JA, Snider GL. Biochemical insights into the development of connective tissue. In: Hodson WA, ed. Development of the Lung. New York: Marcel Dekker, 1977; 367–397.
161. Crouch EC, Parks WC. Comparative biochemistry and molecular biology of pulmonary connective tissues. In: Parent RA, ed. Comparative Biology of the Normal Lung. Boca Raton, FL: CRC Press, 1992; 451–483.
162. Guzowski DE, Blau H, Bienkowski RS. Extracellular matrix in developing lung. In: Scarpelli EM, ed. Pulmonary Physiology: Fetus, Newborn, Child, and Adolescent. Philadelphia: Lea & Febiger, 1990:83–105.
163. Bienkowski RS, Gotkin MG. Control of collagen deposition in mammalian lung. Proc Soc Exp Biol Med 1995; 209:118–140.
164. McGowan SE. Extracellular matrix and the regulation of lung development and repair. FASEB J 1992; 6:2895–2904.
165. Cowan MJ, Crystal RG. Lung growth after unilateral pneumonectomy: quantitation of collagen synthesis and content. Am Rev Respir Dis 1975; 111:267–277.
166. Davila RM, de Mello D, Crouch EC. Ontogeny of type I procollagen expression during human fetal lung development. Am J Physiol 1995; 286:L309–L320.
167. Dubick MA, Rucker RB, Cross CE, Last J. Elastin metabolism in rodent lung. Biochim Biophys Acta 1981; 672:303–306.

168. Meyers B, Dubick M, Last JA, Rucker RB. Elastin synthesis during perinatal lung development in the rat. Biochim Biophys Acta 1983; 761:17–22.
169. Shabahara S, Davidson JM, Smith K, Crystal RG. Modulation of tropoelastin production and elastin messenger ribonucleic acid activity in developing sheep lung. Biochemistry 1981; 20:6577–6584.
170. Bruce MC. Developmental changes in tropoelastin mRNA levels in rat lung: evaluation by in situ hybridization. Am J Respir Cell Mol Biol 1991; 5:344–350.
171. Chen WT, Chen JM, Mueller SC. Coupled expression and colocalization of 140K cell adhesion molecules, fibronectin, and laminin during morphogenesis and cytodifferentiation in chick lung. J Cell Biol 1986; 103:1073–1090.
172. Plumb DJ, Dubaybo BA, Thet LA. Changes in lung tissue fibronectin content and synthesis during postnatal lung growth. Pediatr Pulmonol 1987; 3:413–419.
173. Roman J, McDonald JA. Expression of fibronectin, the integrin α-5, and smooth muscle actin in heart and lung development. Am J Respir Cell Mol Biol 1992; 6:472–480.
174. Sinkin RA, Sanders RS, Horowitz S, Finkelstein JN, Lomonaco MB. Cell-specific expression of fibronectin in adult and developing rabbit lung. Pediatr Res 1995; 37:189–195.
175. Allen SJ, Sedin GE, Jonzon A, Wells AF, Laurent TC. Lung hyaluronan during development: a quantitative and morphological study. Am J Physiol 1991; 260:H1449–H1454.
176. Sannes PL, Burch KK, Khosla J, McCarthy KJ, Couchman JR. Immunohistochemical localization of chondroitin sulfate, chondroitin sulfate proteoglycan, heparan sulfate proteoglycan, entactin, and laminin in basement membranes of postnatal developing and adult rat lungs. Am J Respir Cell Mol Biol 1993; 8:245–251.
177. Ferrara TB, Fox RB. Effects of oxygen toxicity on cuprolinic blue-stained proteoglycans in alveolar basement membrane. Am J Respir Cell Mol Biol 1992; 6:219–224.
178. Horowitz AL, Crystal RG. Content and synthesis of glycosaminoglycans in the developing lung. J Clin Invest 1975; 56:1312–1318.
179. Radhakrishnamurthy B, Williams J, Berenson GS. The composition of glycosaminoglycans in developing rabbit lungs. Proc Soc Exp Biol Med 1980; 164:287–291.
180. Brody JS, Vaccaro CA, Gill PJ, Silbert JE. Alterations in alveolar basement membrane during postnatal lung growth. J Cell Biol 1982; 95:394–402.
181. Boot-Handford RO, Kurkinen M, Prockop DJ. Steady-state levels of mRNAs coding for the type IV collagen and laminin polypeptide chains of basement membranes exhibit marked tissue-specific stoichiometric variations in the rat. J Biol Chem 1987; 262:12475–12478.
182. Veness-Meechan KA, Rhodes DN, Stiles AD. Temporal and spatial expression of biglycan in chronic oxygen-induced lung injury. Am J Respir Cell Mol Biol 1994; 11:509–516.
183. Zhao Y, Young SL. Tenascin in rat lung development: in situ localization and cellular sources. Am J Physiol 1995; 269:L481–L491.
184. Brauker JH, Trautman MS, Bernfield M. Syndecan, a cell surface proteoglycan, exhibits a molecular polymorphism during lung development. Dev Biol 1991; 147:285–292.

185. Senior RM, Griffin GL, Mudd MS, Moxley MA, Longmore WJ, Pierce RA. Entactin expression by rat lung and rat alveolar epithelial cells. Am J Respir Cell Mol Biol 1996; 14:239–247.
186. Brenner CA, Adler RR, Rappolee DA, Pederson RA, Werb Z. Genes for extracellular matrix degrading metalloproteinases and their inhibitor, TIMP-1, are expressed during early mammalian development. Genes Dev 1989; 3:848–859.
187. Devaskar UP, Taylor W, Govindrajan R, Malicdem M, Heyman S, de Mello DE. Hyperoxia induces interstitial (type I) and increases type IV collagenase mRNA expression and increases type I and IV collagenolytic activity in newborn rat lung. Biol Neonate 1994; 66:76–85.
188. Delacourt C, D'Ortho M-P, Macquin-Mavier I, Pezet S, Harf A, Lafuma C. Increased 92 kD gelatinase activity from alveolar macrophages in newborn rats. Am J Respir Crit Care Med 1995; 151:1939–1945.
189. Malicdem M, Taylor W, Goerke M, Devaskar U. Ontogeny of rat lung type IV collagenase mRNA expression and collagenolytic activity during the perinatal period. Biol Neonate 1993; 64:376–381.
190. Brody JJ, Kagen H, Manalo A. Lung lysyl oxidase activity: relation to lung growth. Am Rev Respir Dis 1979; 120:1289–1295.
191. Hance AJ, Crystal RG. Collagen. In: Crystal RG, ed. The Biochemical Basis of Pulmonary Function. New York: Marcel Dekker, 1976:215–271.
192. Powell JT, Whitney PL. Postnatal development of the rat lung. Changes in lung lectin, elastin, acetylcholinesterase, and other enzymes. Biochem J 1980; 188:1–8.
193. Arden MG, Spearman MA, Adamson IY. Degradation of type IV collagen during the development of fetal rat lung. Am J Respir Cell Mol Biol 1993; 9:99–105.
194. Burri PM. Development and growth of the human lung. In: Fishman AP, Fisher AB, eds. Handbook of Physiology. The Respiratory System. Vol. 1. Bethesda, MD: American Physiological Society, 1985:1–46.
195. Brody JS, Kaplan NB. Proliferation of alveolar interstitial cells during postnatal lung growth. Evidence for two distinct populations of pulmonary fibroblasts. Am Rev Respir Dis 1983; 127:763–770.
196. Fisk DE, Kuhn C III. Emphysema-like changes in the lung of the blotchy mouse. Am Rev Respir Dis 1976; 113:787–797.
197. O'Dell BL, Kilburn KH, McKenzie WN. The lung of the copper deficient rat. A model for developmental pulmonary emphysema. Am J Pathol 1978; 91:431–442.
198. Kida K, Thurlbeck WM. The effects of β-aminopropionitrile on the growing rat lung. Am J Pathol 1980; 101:693–710.
199. Phan SH, Thrall RS. Pulmonary Fibrosis. New York: Marcel Dekker, 1995.
200. Crouch E. Pathobiology of pulmonary fibrosis. Am J Physiol 1990; 259:L159–L184.
201. Wolff G, Crystal RG. Biology of pulmonary fibrosis. In: Crystal RG, West JB, Weibel ER, Barnes PG, eds. The Lung: Scientific Foundations. 2nd ed. Philadelphia: Lippincott–Raven, 1997:2509–2524.
202. Fine A, Goldstein, RH. Animal models of pulmonary fibrosis. In: Crystal RG, West JB, Weibel ER, Barnes PG, eds. The Lung: Scientific Foundations. 2nd ed. Philadelphia: Lippincott–Raven, 1997:2525–2536.

203. Raghu G, Striker LJ, Hudson LD, Striker GE. Extracellular matrix in normal and fibrotic human lungs. Am Rev Respir Dis 1985; 131:281–289.
204. Clark JG. The molecular pathology of pulmonary fibrosis. In: Uitto J, Perejda AJ, eds. Connective Tissue Disease. Molecular Pathology of the Extracellar Matrix. New York: Marcel Dekker, 1987:321–343.
205. Bonikos DS, Bensch KG, Northway WH Jr, Edwards DK. Bronchopulmonary dysplasia: the pulmonary pathologic sequel of necrotizing bronchiolitis and pulmonary fibrosis. Hum Pathol 1976; 7:643–666.
206. Erickson AM, de la Monte SM, Moore GW, Hutchins GM. The progression of morphologic changes in bronchopulmonary dysplasia. Am J Pathol 1987; 127:474–484.
207. Stocker JT. Pathologic features of long-standing ‘‘healed’’ bronchopulmonary dysplasia: a study of 28 3- to 40-month-old infants. Hum Pathol 1986; 17:943–961.
208. Taghizadeh A, Reynolds EO. Pathogenesis of bronchopulmonary dysplasia following hyaline membrane disease. Am J Pathol 1976; 82:241–264.
209. Sobonya RE, Logvinoff MM, Taussig LM, Theirault A. Morphometric analysis of the lung in prolonged bronchopulmonary dysplasia. Pediatr Res 1982; 16:969–972.
210. Anderson WR, Engel RR. Cardiopulmonary sequelae of reparative stages of bronchopulmonary dysplasia. Arch Pathol Lab Med 1983; 107:603–608.
211. Margraf LR, Tomashefski JF Jr, Bruce MC, Dahms BB. Morphometric analysis of the lung in bronchopulmonary dysplasia. Am Rev Respir Dis 1991; 143:391–400.
212. Nakamura Y, Fukuda S, Hashimoto T. Pulmonary elastic fibers in normal human development and in pathological conditions. Pediatr Pathol 1990; 10:689–706.
213. Anderson WR, Strickland MB. Pulmonary complications of oxygen therapy in the neonate. Arch Pathol 1971; 91:506–514.
214. Hislop AA, Wigglesworth JS, Desai R, Aber V. The effects of preterm delivery and mechanical ventilation on human lung growth. Early Hum Dev 1987; 15:147–164.
215. Churg A, Golden J, Fligiel S, Hogg JC. Bronchopulmonary dysplasia in the adult. Am Rev Respir Dis 1983; 127:117–120.
216. Reid LM. Bronchopulmonary dysplasia: pathology. J Pediatr 1979; 95:836–841.
217. Basset F, Ferrans VJ, Soler R, Takemura T, Fukuda Y, Crystal RG. Intraluminal fibrosis in interstitial lung disorders. Am J Pathol 1986; 122:443–461.
218. Kuhn C III, Boldt, J, King TE, Crouch E, Vartio T, McDonald JA. An immunohistochemical study of architectural remodeling and connective tissue synthesis in pulmonary fibrosis. Am Rev Respir Dis 1989; 140:1693–1703.
219. Crystal RG, Bitterman PB, Rennard SI, Hance AJ, Keogh BA. Interstitial lung diseases of unknown cause. Disorders characterized by chronic inflammation of the lower respiratory tract. N Engl J Med 1984; 310:154–166, 235–244.
220. Brown ER, Stark A, Sosenko I, Lawson EE, Avery ME. Bronchopulmonary dysplasia: possible relationship to pulmonary edema. J Pediatr 1978; 92:982–984.
221. Jefferies AL, Coates G, O’Brodovich H. Pulmonary epithelial permeability in hyaline-membrane disease. N Engl J Med 1984; 311:1075–1080.
222. Bressack MA, McMillen DD, Bland RP. Pulmonary oxygen toxicity: increased microvascular permeability to protein in unanesthetized lambs. Lymphology 1979; 12:133–139.

223. Watts CL, Fanaroff AA. Fibronectin: role in respiratory distress syndrome and bronchopulmonary dysplasia. Semin Perinatol 1992; 16:162–169.
224. Chambers HM, Van Velzen D. Ventilator-related pathology in the extremely immature lung. Pathology 1989; 21:79–83.
225. Van Lierde S, Cornelis A, Devlieger H, Moerman P, Lauweryns J, Eggermont E. Different patterns of pulmonary sequelae after hyaline membrane disease: heterogeneity of bronchopulmonary dysplasia? Biol Neonate 1991; 60:152–162.
226. Shoemaker CT, Reiser KM, Goetzman BW, Last JA. Elevated ratios of type I/III collagen in lungs of chemically ventilated neonates with respiratory distress. Pediatr Res 1984; 18:1176–1180.
227. Togari H, Hashimoto Y, Wada Y, Hayakawa T. Increased type III/I collagen and alpha 1(I)/alpha 2(I) chain in a bronchopulmonary dysplastic lung. Acta Paediatr Jpn 1993; 35:101–107.
228. Co E, Chari G, McCulloch K, Vidyasagar D. Dexamethasone treatment suppresses collagen synthesis in infants with bronchopulmonary dysplasia. Pediatr Pulmonol 1993; 16:36–40.
229. Heikinheimo M, Halila R, Marttinen E, Raivo K. N-terminal propeptide of type III collagen in tracheal fluid and serum in preterm infants at risk for bronchopulmonary dysplasia. Pediatr Res 1992; 31:340–343.
230. Cantin AM, Boileau R, Bégin R. Increased procollagen III aminoterminal peptide-related antigens and fibroblast growth signals in lungs of patients with idiopathic pulmonary fibrosis. Am Rev Respir Dis 1988; 137:572–578.
231. Danne I, Grüters A, Schuppan D, Quantas N, Enders I, Weber B. Relationship of procollagen type III propeptide-related antigens in serum to somatic growth in healthy children and patients with growth disorders. J Pediatr 1989; 114:257–260.
232. Bruce MC, Wedig K, Jentoft N, Martin RJ, Cheng P-W, Boat TF, Fanaroff A. Altered urinary excretion of elastin crosslinks in premature infants who developed bronchopulmonary dysplasia. Am Rev Respir Dis 1985; 131:568–572.
233. Bruce MC, Schuyler M, Martin RJ, Starcher BC, Tomashefski JF Jr, Wedig KE. Risk factors for the degradation of lung elastic fibers in the ventilated neonate. Implications for impaired lung development in bronchopulmonary dysplasia. Am Rev Respir Dis 1992; 146:204–212.
234. Bruce MC, Martin RJ, Boat TF. Concentrations of α_1-proteinase inhibitor and α_2-macroglobulin in serum and lung secretions of intubated infants. Pediatr Res 1984; 18:35–40.
235. Bruce MC, Pawlowski R, Tomashefski JF Jr. Changes in lung elastic fiber structure and concentration associated with hyperoxic exposure in the developing rat lung. Am Rev Respir Dis 1989; 140:1067–1074.
236. Randell SH, Mercer RR, Young SL. Postnatal growth of pulmonary acini and alveoli in normal and oxygen exposed rats studied by serial section reconstruction. Am J Anat 1989; 186:55–68.
237. Bucher JR, Roberts RJ. The development of the newborn rat lung in hyperoxia: a dose response study of lung growth, maturation, and changes in antioxidant enzyme activities. Pediatr Res 1981; 15:999–1008.
238. Northway WH Jr, Moss RB, Carlisle KB, et al. Late pulmonary sequelae of bronchopulmonary dysplasia. N Engl J Med 1990; 323:1793–1799.

239. Merritt TA, Cochrane CG, Holcomb K, et al. Elastase and α_1-proteinase inhibitor activity in tracheal aspirates during respiratory distress syndrome. Role of inflammation in the pathogenesis of bronchopulmonary dysplasia. J Clin Invest 1983; 72: 656–666.
240. Horowitz S, Shaprio DL, Finklestein JN, Notter RH, Johnston CJ, Quible DJ. Changes in gene expression in hyperoxia-induced neonatal lung injury. Am J Physiol 1990; 258:L107–L111.
241. Minoo P, Penn R, deLemos DM, Coalson JJ, deLemos RA. Tissue inhibitor of metalloproteinase-1 in mRNA is specifically induced in lung tissue after birth. Pediatr Res 1993; 34:729–734.
242. Northway WH Jr, Rosan RC, Porter DY. Pulmonary disease following respiratory therapy of hyaline-membrane disease. N Engl J Med 1967; 276:357–368.
243. Deneke SM, Fanburg BL. Normobaric oxygen toxicity to the lung. N Engl J Med 1980; 303:76–86.
244. Fox RB, Hoidal JR, Brown DM, Repine JE. Pulmonary inflammation due to oxygen toxicity: involvement of chemotactic factors and polymorphonuclear leukocytes. Am Rev Respir Dis 1981; 123:521–523.
245. Merritt TA. Oxygen exposure in the newborn guinea pig lung lavage cell populations, chemotactic and elastase response: a possible relationship to neonatal bronchopulmonary dysplasia. Pediatr Res 1982; 16:798–805.
246. Newman JH, Loyd JE, English OK, Ogletree ML, Fulkerson WJ, Brigham KL. Effects of 100% oxygen on lung vascular function in awake sheep. J Appl Physiol 1983; 54:1379–1386.
247. Harada RM, Vatter AE, Repine JE. Macrophage effect or function in pulmonary oxygen toxicity: hyperoxia damages and stimulates alveolar macrophages to make and release chemotaxins for polymorphonuclear leukocytes. J Leuckoc Biol 1984; 35:373–383.
248. Johnson D, Travis J. The oxidative inactivation of human α_1-proteinase inhibitor. Further evidence for methionine at the reactive site. J Biol Chem 1979; 254:4022–4026.
249. Coalson JJ, Kuehl TJ, Prihoda TJ, DeLemos RA. Diffuse alveolar damage in the evolution of bronchopulmonary dysplasia in the baboon. Pediatr Res 1988; 24:357–366.
250. Hellström B, Nergårdh A. The effect of high oxygen concentration and hypothermia on the lung of the newborn mouse. Acta Paediatr Scand 1965; 54:457–466.
251. Chen YW, Martinez MA, Frank L. Prenatal dexamethasone administration to premature rats exposed to prolonged hyperoxia: a new rat model of pulmonary fibrosis (bronchopulmonary dysplasia). J Pediatr 1997; 130:409–416.
252. Riley DJ, Poiani GJ. Hyperoxia and oxidants in pulmonary fibrosis. In: Phan SH, Thrall RS, eds. Pulmonary Fibrosis. New York: Marcel Dekker, 1995:293–317.
253. Riley DJ, Berg RA, Edelman NH, Prockop DJ. Prevention of collagen deposition following pulmonary oxygen toxicity in the rat by *cis*-4-hydroxy-L-proline. J Clin Invest 1980; 65:643–651.
254. Niewoehner DE, Hoidal JR. Lung fibrosis and emphysema: divergent responses to a common injury? Science 1982; 217:359–360.

29

Pulmonary Edema After Premature Birth

Progression from Acute to Chronic Lung Disease

RICHARD D. BLAND

University of Utah School of Medicine
Salt Lake City, Utah

DAVID P. CARLTON

University of Utah Health Sciences Center
Salt Lake City, Utah

I. Introduction

Pulmonary edema is a consistent pathological feature of both the acute and chronic respiratory distress syndromes that occur after premature birth. In acute respiratory distress syndrome, or hyaline membrane disease (HMD), the lungs typically are heavy and have a widened interstitium between airspaces and blood vessels; accumulation of fluid within dilated lymphatic channels and the connective tissue space surrounding large pulmonary blood vessels and airways; and abundant deposits of plasma proteins within the terminal respiratory units (1). These signs of abnormal vascular and epithelial permeability usually disappear as the respiratory distress resolves, either spontaneously or after treatment with surfactant and assisted ventilation. Sometimes, however, the need for prolonged mechanical ventilation persists because of continuing respiratory failure, either from residual lung diseasc, chest wall instability, apnea, or infection. Long-term exposure to repetitive lung inflation with positive pressure and supplemental oxygen often leads to chronic lung disease (CLD). This condition was described by Northway et al. (2) as bronchopulmonary dysplasia (BPD), the pathology of which includes edema, prominent lymphatics, inflammation, and subsequent fibrosis (Fig. 1) (3).

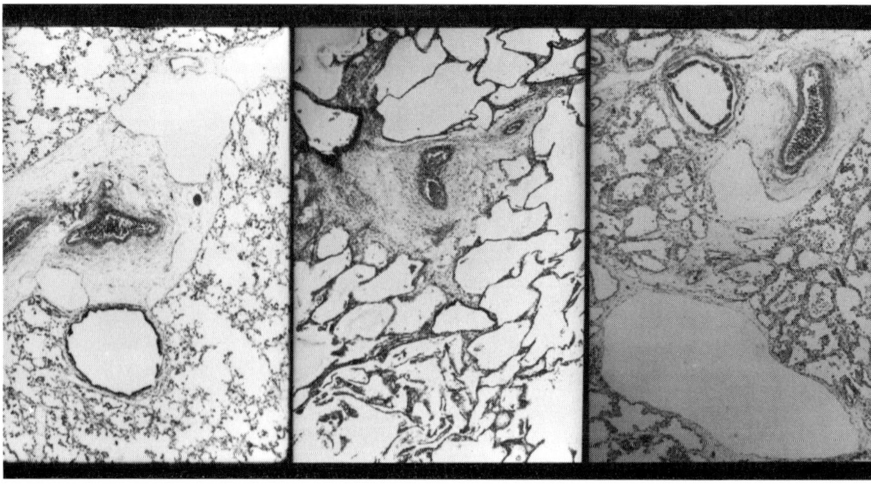

Figure 1 Histological sections of lung obtained from infants who were mechanically ventilated after premature birth until death at 1 month (left), 2 months (center), or 6 months (right): Perivascular cuffs of fluid and dilated lung lymphatics are indicative of interstitial pulmonary edema, progressing to perivascular fibrosis, and distorted lung architecture with cyst formation.

The relation between excess fluid intake soon after birth and the development of this persistent form of respiratory distress was reported two decades ago (4). Subsequent studies have provided evidence that early postnatal restriction of fluid and salt intake might lessen the incidence or severity of CLD (5–7). Although the clinical course and lung pathology of this condition have changed in recent years as a consequence of prenatal glucocorticoid administration, surfactant replacement therapy, better nutrition, and progress in respiratory care practices that have reduced the need for supplemental oxygen and high inflation pressures, pulmonary edema remains an important component of the current version of CLD after premature birth (8).

Before presenting what is known about pulmonary edema in CLD after premature birth, we will briefly review normal fluid balance in the developing lung and discuss some of the characteristics of the immature lung that make it especially vulnerable to excess fluid accumulation and resultant respiratory failure. Several conditions that often prevail after premature birth probably contribute to the frequency with which pulmonary edema occurs in infants who are born too soon (Table 1). Some of these conditions are specifically related to the long-term ventilatory support that such infants often require. One purpose of this chapter is to present experimental evidence documenting the presence of these condi-

Table 1 Features of the Immature Lung, Compared with the Mature Lung, That Make It Vulnerable to Postnatal Edema

Excess fetal lung liquid per unit lung mass
Fewer sodium channels and less Na,K-ATPase activity in lung epithelium
Greater lung vascular filtration pressure
Increased lung epithelial protein leak, associated with postnatal ventilation
Increased lung vascular protein permeability, associated with postnatal ventilation

tions and their role in edema formation after premature birth and prolonged mechanical ventilation. Much of our knowledge about the pathogenesis of neonatal lung edema derives from experiments performed with fetal and newborn animals, to which we will refer often. Because respiratory distress in newborn infants frequently has a prenatal origin, and because preterm lungs contain more water at birth than term lungs do, this chapter includes a brief discussion of fetal lung liquid and its removal near the time of birth.

II. Lung Fluid Balance During Fetal Development

Before birth the lungs are filled with liquid that flows from the pulmonary circulation into potential airspaces as a result of chloride secretion across the respiratory tract epithelium (9). This liquid drains through the conductive airways into the oropharynx, from which it is either swallowed or expelled into the amniotic sac. Normal intrauterine lung growth depends largely on the balance between adequate production and controlled drainage of luminal liquid (10). Thus, conditions that inhibit production of fetal lung liquid, such as pulmonary artery occlusion (11,12), diaphragmatic hernia (13,14), and uterine compression of the fetal chest from chronic leakage of amniotic liquid (15,16), also inhibit lung growth. These observations emphasize the importance of liquid expansion of potential airspaces in the development of normal lung structure before birth which, in turn, may affect lung function after birth.

Both the rate of liquid formation and the liquid volume within the lumen of the fetal lung normally decrease before birth (17–21). Thus, lung water content is approximately 25% greater after preterm delivery than it is at term (22), and newborn animals that are delivered by cesarean section without prior labor have significantly more liquid in their lungs than do animals that are delivered vaginally or by cesarean section after the onset of labor (17,23). In studies done with fetal sheep, extravascular lung water was about 45% less in mature fetuses that were killed during labor than it was in fetuses that had no labor, and there was a further 38% reduction in extravascular lung water measured in lambs that were studied 6 hr after birth (17). Morphometric analysis of sections of frozen lung obtained from fetal lambs with and without prior labor showed that the reduction in lung water content that occurs before birth is the result of a decrease in the volume of liquid in potential airspaces relative to the volume in the interstitium. Diminished secretion, and perhaps absorption, of luminal liquid before birth decreases lung water by about 15 mL/kg body weight, leaving a residual volume of approximately 6 mL/kg (17), which must be removed from potential airspaces soon after birth to permit effective pulmonary gas exchange.

A. Hormonal Influences on Lung Liquid Absorption Near Birth

What causes the reduction in fetal lung liquid secretion before birth? Various studies have shown that hormonal changes that occur in the fetus just before and during labor may have an important role in triggering this adaptive process. Several studies have examined the influence of catecholamines on the formation of fetal lung liquid. Studies done with fetal lambs late in gestation showed that intravenous infusion of epinephrine or isoproterenol, but not norepinephrine, caused reabsorption of liquid from potential airspaces, an effect that β-adrenergic blockade with propranolol prevented (24,25). A subsequent report showed that intraluminal administration of amiloride, a sodium transport inhibitor, blocked the effect of epinephrine on fetal lung liquid absorption (26). This finding indicates that β-adrenergic agonists stimulate sodium uptake by the lung epithelium which, in turn, drives liquid from the lung lumen into the interstitium, where it can be absorbed into the bloodstream.

Tracheal instillation of a cyclic adenosine monophosphate analogue (db-cAMP) also caused absorption of lung liquid in fetal lambs late in gestation (27). The inhibitory effects of both intrapulmonary db-cAMP and intravenous epinephrine on net production of lung luminal liquid in fetal sheep increase with advancing gestational age, and both responses are attenuated by prior removal of the thyroid gland (28). Replacement therapy with triiodothyronine (T_3) after thyroidectomy restored the inhibitory effect of epinephrine on lung liquid formation in fetal sheep (29). Moreover, treatment of preterm fetal sheep with triiodothyronine and hydrocortisone, when given together, may stimulate early maturation of epinephrine-induced absorption of lung liquid (30). There is a synergistic effect of terbutaline, a β-adrenergic agonist, and aminophylline, a phosphodiesterase inhibitor, in switching lung liquid secretion to absorption in fetal lambs (31). Addition of the sodium transport inhibitor amiloride to the lung liquid prevented liquid absorption. These findings support the notion that as birth approaches, conditions that stimulate production of cAMP in the lung may trigger absorption of luminal liquid through a sodium-dependent epithelial transport process.

The decrease in fetal lung liquid production that occurs before birth may be related to a rise in plasma epinephrine concentration late in labor (18). In fetal sheep, however, lung water content often decreases before there is any detectable release of catecholamines (17,19). The concentration of β-adrenergic receptors in lung tissue increases late in gestation (32–34), which may make the lungs more responsive to the effects of epinephrine during labor (18). Other reports have suggested that lung liquid absorption near birth may not depend on epinephrine. In fetal rabbits, irreversible blockade of β-adrenergic receptors did not prevent the normal decrease in lung water that occurs during parturition (35), and with fetal lambs that were experiencing labor, inhibition of β-adrenergic activity with propranolol did not prevent absorption of lung liquid (19). Other hormones, including vasopressin (36–41), inhibit production of liquid in the fetal lung, and at least one study provided evidence that release of both epinephrine and vasopressin at birth may be additive in stimulating lung liquid absorption (38).

Recent observations indicate that nitric oxide and surfactant, which are important modulators of lung function during and soon after birth, may inhibit lung liquid production by apparently different mechanisms that are yet to be defined (42–44). Whereas, the sodium-transport inhibitor amiloride partially blocks the decrease in lung liquid production that occurs with bovine surfactant administration in immature fetal sheep (44), amiloride had no such effect on the decrease in lung liquid production associated with nitric oxide administration (42). It is possible that these and other biologically active substances that are released in the lungs close to the time of birth may have important effects in shifting liquid from the lung lumen into the interstitium during and after birth.

B. Birth-Related Changes in Lung Epithelial Ion Transport

Active sodium transport across the mature pulmonary epithelium drives liquid from the lung lumen into the interstitium, with subsequent absorption into the vasculature (19,26,45–47). Thus, the lung epithelium switches from a predominantly chloride-secreting membrane before birth to a predominantly sodium-absorbing membrane after birth. In vitro studies of ion transport and the bioelectric properties of cultured alveolar epithelial cells harvested from fetal and adult rats have shown that the same cells which secrete surfactant into the airspaces also may pump sodium in the opposite direction, thereby generating the driving force for absorption of liquid from the lung lumen (48–53). In these studies, monolayers of cultured distal lung epithelial cells (type II cells), when mounted in an Ussing-type chamber, maintained a transepithelial electrical potential difference (luminal side negative) that increased in response to β-adrenergic stimulation with terbutaline and decreased in response to luminal amiloride or albuminal ouabain. Although type II cells occupy only a small portion of the surface area of terminal airspaces, numerous microvilli on the luminal aspect of these cells greatly increase their absorptive surface area (54). In addition, morphometric

Table 2 Lung Epithelial Cell Na,K-ATPase Activity and Extravascular Lung Water in Preterm and Term Newborn Rabbits

Gestational age	Ouabain-sensitive $^{86}Rb^+$ (K^+) uptake[a,b] (nmol/10^6 cells)/hr	Extravascular lung water[b] (g/g dry lung)
Preterm (28 days)	5 ± 1	10.5 ± 0.5
Term (31 days)	15 ± 2*	8.0 ± 0.4*
Numbers are mean ± SE		

[a]Index of Na,K-ATPase activity.
[b]Lung epithelial cell Na,K-ATPase activity is less and extravascular lung water is greater after premature birth than at term.
*Significant difference, term versus preterm, $p < 0.05$.
Source: Refs. 56 and 61.

studies indicate that there are almost three times as many type II cells per unit tissue mass lining the interior of the newborn lung as there are lining the interior of the adult lung (55). Thus, it is reasonable to postulate that sodium-transport by type II cells probably is important in liquid clearance during and after birth.

Several studies have shown that Na,K-ATPase of distal lung epithelial cells increases close to the time of birth (56–60). Studies using freshly isolated distal lung epithelial cells from fetal, newborn, and adult rabbits showed that sodium-pump turnover number increased fourfold during labor, followed by a threefold increase in sodium pump number between the newborn and adult stages of lung development (56,58). Turnover number, an index of Na,K-ATPase activity, was not significantly different in newborn and adult cells. Thus, sodium pump activity in distal lung epithelium of rabbits increases at birth, and the number of sodium pumps increases after birth. In related studies, sodium pump activity was similar in cells harvested from fetal rabbits and from newborn pups that had respiratory distress after premature birth (56). These findings indicate that the stress of premature birth and subsequent respiratory failure does not increase lung epithelial cell cation flux, an observation that may help explain the lung liquid retention that often occurs with premature birth (Table 2; 22,61).

At least two studies have shown that mRNA abundance for the α_1- and β_1-isoforms of Na,K-ATPase in fetal rat lungs increases just before birth (57,59). These changes are associated with parallel increases in the expression of epithelial sodium and water channels in perinatal rat lung (62–65). Other studies suggest that glucocorticoids may increase mRNA abundance for the α_1- and β_1-isoforms of Na,K-ATPase in rat lungs during early development (66), and glucocorticoids also may help regulate the expression of sodium channels and of aquaporins in the developing rat lung (67,68). Thus, hormones that are released into the circulation near the time of birth may have important effects on lung epithelial ion transport and related removal of liquid from the lungs during and immediately after birth. Recent reports also indicate that the increase in pulmonary oxygen tension that occurs near the time of birth may play an important role in signaling the switch from chloride secretion to sodium absorption in the respiratory epithelium near birth (69,70). The observation that mice rendered deficient in epithelial sodium channels die soon after birth from inability to remove fetal lung liquid underscores the importance of lung epithelial sodium transport in successful adaptation at birth (71).

C. Routes of Lung Liquid Removal at Birth

When liquid is displaced from the lung lumen into the interstitium by the aforementioned epithelial sodium-transport mechanism, potential routes for removal of this liquid at birth include lung lymphatics, the circulation, the pleural space, the mediastinum, and the upper airway. Studies done with catheterized fetal and newborn lambs showed that the postnatal increase in lung lymph flow is transient and small, accounting for no more than about 15% of the amount of excess liquid that drains from the lungs postnatally (17,72,73). These studies showed that lymph protein concentration decreases with the start of ventilation, as protein-poor luminal liquid enters the interstitium and decreases the protein concentration of lung lymph. With subsequent uptake of this liquid into the bloodstream, the concentration of protein in lymph returns to its baseline level. These studies showed that at term gestation lung lymphatics normally drain only a small fraction of liquid in potential airspaces. Other studies conducted in the same laboratory showed that either elevated left atrial pressure or reduction of plasma protein concentration slows the rate at which liquid from potential airspaces leaves the lungs of healthy, mature lambs (72,73). These findings support the view that the pulmonary circulation absorbs most of the residual liquid present in potential airspaces at birth. It is also possible that some liquid enters the bloodstream through the mediastinum and pleural cavity, although other studies indicate that in normal lambs very little luminal liquid drains by way of the pleural space.

How important is the upper airway as a pathway for liquid drainage from the lung lumen at birth? Karlberg et al. (74) measured changes in thoracic pressure and volume in human infants during birth and concluded that chest compression associated with vaginal delivery drives liquid from the lungs into the oropharynx. Other studies, however, indicate that thoracic squeeze during spontaneous birth may have little effect on clearance of fetal lung liquid. Animals that are delivered by cesarean section during labor have no more water in their lungs than do animals that are born vaginally (17,23). Studies of lung liquid dynamics in near term fetal lambs have shown that late in labor, as luminal liquid is absorbed across the epithelium, the upper airway functions as a one way valve, inhibiting entry of amniotic liquid into the lung lumen, but allowing outward flow of pulmonary liquid into the oropharynx (18). Thus, although the conducting airways may serve as an escape route for lung liquid during delivery without prior labor, they probably play a minor role in liquid clearance during the normal birth process.

In fetal sheep, less than 10% of the combined ventricular output of blood from the heart flows through the lungs (75). At the time of birth, when respiratory gas exchange switches from the placenta to the lungs, pulmonary blood flow increases between five- and tenfold (75–77). Hydraulic pressure in the pulmonary artery is greater before birth than it is after birth, and protein osmotic pressure in plasma is less before birth than it is after birth, so that net filtration pressure in the pulmonary microcirculation is greater during fetal life than it is postnatally (78). Lung lymph flow, expressed per gram of dry lung tissue, is not significantly different before birth than it is after birth (17), and there is no apparent difference in lung vascular protein permeability in the preterm fetal lung compared with the mature postnatal lung of sheep (78). In preterm lambs with respiratory distress, the postnatal increase in lung lymph flow lasts for several hours and is accompanied by a substantial increase in protein clearance, indicative of abnormal lung vascular protein permeability (79).

III. Postnatal Lung Fluid Balance

Figure 2 depicts the fluid compartments of the normal newborn lung and the principal forces that regulate fluid filtration in the pulmonary microcirculation. The epithelium, consisting of surfactant-producing, columnar-shaped type II cells and expansive type I cells connected by tight junctions, separates airspaces from the interstitium and it is virtually impermeable to protein (80,81). Protein leaks may occur across the epithelium when the transpulmonary pressure exceeds 35–40 cmH_2O (82), as it often does after premature birth, when surface tension at the air–liquid interface makes the lungs stiff and vulnerable to injury. The vascular endothelium, which separates the microcirculation from the interstitium, allows macromolecules to pass through it, but restricts passage of large molecules more than it restricts small ones (83). Thus, the concentration of albumin within the interstitium of the newborn lung averages about 75–80% of the concentration of albumin in plasma, whereas the concentration of globulins in interstitial fluid averages about 50–55% of the concentration of globulins in plasma (84). These tissue proteins yield an osmotic pressure of more than 10 cmH_2O (85), which inhibits the flow of fluid into the airspaces. In addition, active sodium transport by lung epithelial cells helps prevent accumulation of excess fluid within the airspaces (19,45,46,56,58,59,62).

Liquid flow across the microvascular membrane largely depends on the

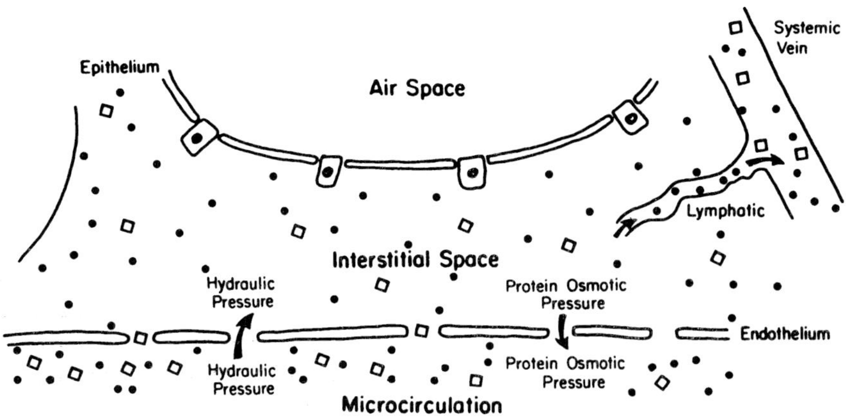

Figure 2 Cartoon showing the fluid compartments in the newborn lung and variables that affect filtration in the pulmonary microcirculation; namely, the transvascular differences in hydraulic and protein osmotic pressures. Solid circles represent albumin molecules, open squares indicate globulin molecules. (From Ref. 212.)

balance between differences in (1) intravascular and extravascular hydraulic pressures and (2) intravascular and extravascular protein osmotic pressures (see Fig. 2). Conditions that either increase the transmural hydraulic pressure difference or decrease the transmural difference in protein osmotic pressure hasten liquid flow from the circulation into the interstitium, whereas conditions that reduce the sum of these filtration forces decrease fluid movement, thereby inhibiting edema formation. Other variables that influence lung water balance are microvascular surface area, endothelial and epithelial protein permeability, and the capacity of pulmonary lymphatics to drain liquid from the lungs into the bloodstream.

A. Hemodynamic Forces and Fluid Balance in the Newborn Lung

Fluid filtration pressure in the pulmonary circulation and microvascular surface area per unit lung mass are greater in the newborn lung than in the adult lung (84,86,87). These developmental differences in the pulmonary circulation may reflect the fact that blood flow per unit lung mass is considerably greater in newborn lungs than it is in adult lungs (88). Moreover, because the newborn lung is about one-quarter the size of the mature lung (84), it is likely that left atrial pressure exceeds alveolar pressure (West zone III; 89) throughout a greater fraction of the pulmonary circulation in the newborn lung, when compared with the adult lung. Measurements of alveolar liquid pressure in excised lungs of newborn and adult animals have provided evidence that hydraulic pressure in the pulmonary interstitium may be less soon after birth than it is later in life (90,91). In addition, plasma protein concentration of newborn animals is significantly less than it is in adult animals, so that the difference in protein osmotic pressure between plasma and lung interstitial fluid is less soon after birth than it is later in life (92). Thus, net lung fluid filtration is greater per unit lung mass in newborns than it is in adults (84,86).

Studies performed with newborn and adult sheep have yielded strong evidence that permeability to plasma proteins in the pulmonary microcirculation is not appreciably different as a function of postnatal age (86,92). Two groups of investigators have shown that, in newborn lambs, increased pulmonary blood flow through a vascular shunt also increases lung fluid filtration, probably by expanding the perfused surface area of the pulmonary microcirculation (93,94). In studies designed to examine the effect of a patent ductus arteriosus on pulmonary hemodynamics and lung fluid balance in preterm lambs that were mechanically ventilated for several hours after birth, ductal patency doubled pulmonary blood flow and increased lung vascular pressures, with a resultant 70% increase in lung lymph flow and a significant reduction in the lymph/plasma protein concentration ratio (95). These findings may help explain why some infants who are born prematurely experience respiratory failure in the presence of a large left-to-right shunt through a patent ductus arteriosus.

Other conditions that increase filtration pressure in the pulmonary circulation may contribute to edema formation in the newborn lung. When the lung vascular bed fails to develop normally before birth, as in pulmonary hypoplasia, or when the lung's circulation is reduced in size because of fibrosis or partial lung resection, an increase in pulmonary perfusion is likely to elevate microvascular pressure and cause edema. Excessive intravascular infusions of fluid may also overload the pulmonary circulation and cause fluid to accumulate in the lungs (85). Intravenous infusion of lipid emulsion increases pulmonary microvascular pressure and transvascular filtration of fluid in the lungs of newborn lambs (96), an effect that presumably results from lipid-induced release of arachidonic acid metabolites, as inhibitors of thromboxane synthesis prevented the pulmonary vasoconstrictor response to lipid infusion in these studies.

When pulmonary microvascular pressure increases, net filtration of fluid into the lungs increases, and the concentration of protein in interstitial fluid decreases. Associated increases in lymph flow and in the protein osmotic pressure difference between plasma and tissue fluid protect the lungs from edema until the drainage capacity of lymphatics is overwhelmed by the increased rate of fluid filtration.

B. Effect of Hypoproteinemia on Fluid Balance in the Newborn Lung

A decrease in plasma protein osmotic pressure may substantially increase fluid filtration in the pulmonary circulation of adult animals of various species (97–

100). Newborn animals have lower concentrations of protein in their plasma than do mature animals. Studies of plasma protein reduction in catheterized, awake lambs showed that a 50% reduction in intravascular protein osmotic pressure led to an increase in lung lymph flow that averaged close to 50% (92). With development of hypoproteinemia, the average difference in plasma protein osmotic pressure between plasma and lymph decreased by approximately 2 mmHg at normal left atrial pressure and by about 5 mmHg in the presence of induced left atrial hypertension. When applied to the Starling equation governing microvascular fluid filtration, these changes in liquid-driving pressure were sufficient to account for the observed increases in lung fluid filtration. Thus, small changes in transvascular protein osmotic pressure have a substantial effect on the flow of fluid from the microcirculation into the interstitium of the lungs. This shift in fluid from the vasculature into the lung tissue might be attributable to the presence of specific water channels, or aquaporins, which have been localized to the pulmonary endothelium during early lung development (63). Reduction of plasma protein concentration in newborn lambs did not affect net protein clearance from the lungs, nor did it accentuate the increase in lymph flow that was associated with left atrial pressure elevation. Tracer studies done with radiolabeled albumin injected intravenously before and after protein drainage showed that there was no change in lung vascular protein permeability. Moreover, pulmonary edema did not develop in these hypoproteinemic lambs, even when their left atrial pressure was increased to nearly 16 mmHg for 4 hr, demonstrating the capacity of lung lymphatics to keep pace with transvascular fluid filtration and thereby inhibit edema formation.

In another series of experiments, however, pulmonary edema did develop in newborn lambs that received rapid intravenous infusion of isotonic saline (85). In addition to increasing lung microvascular pressure and decreasing plasma protein osmotic pressure, acute fluid overload also enhances pulmonary blood flow and elevates systemic venous pressure, which may impair lymphatic drainage from the lungs (101,102). This may help explain why pulmonary edema occurred in newborn lambs that received excessive intravascular fluid, whereas it did not occur in hypoproteinemic lambs with mechanically induced left atrial hypertension. Impaired lymphatic drainage may contribute to lung edema in some cases of right-sided heart failure, or when there is blockage of the superior vena cava, such that lung lymphatics must pump against a very high central venous pressure. Following lymphatic obstruction, edema persists until new channels form, or until the damaged lymphatics heal (103).

C. Effect of Hypoxia on Fluid Balance in the Newborn Lung

In studies performed with adult sheep, hypoxia causes pulmonary hypertension without affecting lung lymph flow or lymph protein concentration, indicating that hypoxia has no significant effect on net fluid filtration in the adult lung (104). In newborn lambs, however, pulmonary vasoconstriction from hypoxia increased lung lymph flow, with an associated reduction in lymph protein concentration (86,88,105). These changes in lymph flow and lymph protein concentration are similar to those that occur when a balloon catheter in the left atrium is filled with saline to raise lung microvascular pressure in lambs (86,92). Thus, hypoxia in newborn sheep appears to constrict lung vessels distal to sites of fluid exchange. An alternative explanation is that neonatal hypoxia may cause intense pulmonary vasoconstriction, redirecting the increased blood flow that occurs during hypoxia to fewer lung vessels, thereby, transmitting to fluid-exchange sites a greater fraction of the pressure in the pulmonary artery.

Previously published studies have provided evidence supporting both of these explanations. Direct micropuncture measurement of microvascular pressures in isolated, perfused lungs of newborn lambs showed an increase in pulmonary venular as well as arterial pressure during hypoxia (106). Other studies done with newborn lambs before and during hypoxia showed that hypoxia shifts blood flow from the lower to the upper portions of the newborn lung (107). This finding supports the hypothesis that redistribution of perfusion in young animals with high pulmonary blood flow may account for the increase in lung fluid filtration that occurs in hypoxic lambs. Other investigators found a significant increase in lung lymph flow and a decrease in lymph protein concentration in adult sheep after extensive lung resection, also suggesting a threshold of pulmonary blood flow per unit lung mass above which lung fluid filtration increases even in the mature lung (108). Hypoxia does not alter lung microvascular protein permeability in either newborn or adult sheep (86,104,105,109–111).

D. Effect of Hyperoxia on Fluid Balance in the Newborn Lung

Pulmonary edema sometimes occurs as a result of lung microvascular injury, in which damage to the pulmonary endothelium allows protein-rich liquid to leak at an increased rate from the microcirculation into the lung interstitium. If there is coexisting epithelial injury, proteinaceous liquid enters airspaces and interferes with respiratory gas exchange. One source of neonatal lung microvascular injury is prolonged hyperoxia. Studies of lung fluid balance in awake, newborn lambs showed increased pulmonary microvascular protein permeability within 3–4 days of sustained hyperoxia (112). Lung lymph flow began to increase on the third day of oxygen breathing, and the concentration of protein in lymph increased progressively from the third to the fifth day of hyperoxia, with no appreciable change in lung vascular pressures. These changes in lung lymph flow and lymph protein concentration are indicative of abnormal vascular permeability to protein. Radioactive protein tracer studies in these animals also demonstrated an increase in permeability within 5 days, when all of the lambs were suffering respiratory failure from oxygen toxicity. Extravascular lung water content and histology confirmed the presence of severe pulmonary edema. In a subsequent study, lambs pretreated with large doses of vitamin E, an antioxidant, acquired the same degree of oxygen-induced lung vascular injury as did lambs that did not receive vitamin E (113).

Granulocytes may contribute to the development of various types of lung microvascular injury (114–117), including endothelial damage and edema from prolonged hyperoxia (118,119). In studies designed to assess the importance of neutrophils as possible mediators of pulmonary oxygen toxicity, rabbits and lambs were rendered neutropenic by treatment with either nitrogen mustard (rabbits) or hydroxyurea (lambs) before they were placed in 100% oxygen for several days (120). Neutrophil depletion had no effect on survival time nor on lung water content of either adult rabbits or newborn lambs that continuously breathed pure oxygen at 1-atm pressure. Neutropenia also had no influence on lung lymph protein clearance in lambs with sustained hyperoxia. Thus, granulocytes are not essential for the development of oxygen-induced lung microvascular injury. Other cells within the lung, including alveolar macrophages (121,122) and other pulmonary parenchymal cells (123), are capable of generating toxic oxygen metabolites that may contribute to the development of lung injury, particularly if endogenous antioxidant enzymes are deficient, as they may be following premature birth (124).

Several experimental approaches have been used to try to prevent or lessen the severity of oxygen-induced lung vascular injury in newborn animals. One study showed that intraperitoneal injection of liposomes, containing superoxide dismutase and catalase, decreased mortality among newborn rats that were placed in 100% oxygen (125). Although the rate of survival was greater among rats that received antioxidant enzymes, it was unclear whether this treatment reduced the severity of lung injury. A single dose of bacterial endotoxin prolonged survival and reduced lung injury in hyperoxic adult rats, a response that seemed to be related to increased pulmonary antioxidant enzyme activity following injection of endotoxin (126). Low doses of endotoxin afforded partial protection to newborn sheep when they were exposed to prolonged hyperoxia (127). Lambs that received endotoxin before oxygen exposure had delayed onset of lung vascular protein leak and pulmonary edema, and these lambs survived longer in oxygen than did lambs that received no endotoxin. Unlike the studies with adult rats, however, treatment of lambs with endotoxin did not increase lung antioxidant enzyme activity. These findings, coupled with a higher ratio of reduced to oxidized glutathione in the lungs of endotoxin-treated lambs, led the authors to speculate that endotoxin pretreatment may have reduced the oxidant stress of prolonged hyperoxia by inhibiting production of toxic oxygen metabolites within the lung, possibly by blocking the activity of cytochrome P-450 (127). In a subsequent report, the same group of investigators (128) showed that treatment of newborn lambs with cimetidine, a noncompetitive inhibitor of cytochrome P-450 activity, slowed the progression of oxygen-induced lung microvascular injury and increased the ratio of reduced to oxidized glutathione in the lungs. Cimetidine also inhibited the increase in pulmonary microsomal P-450 activity that was associated with prolonged oxygen breathing. These observations indicate that improved understanding of the mechanisms responsible for oxygen-induced lung injury may provide the basis for effective treatment, or possibly prevention, of this and other conditions that cause neonatal respiratory failure.

At least two groups of investigators have examined the influence of dietary fat on oxygen-induced lung injury in newborn animals. In one study, there was less lung vascular protein leak and longer survival of hyperoxic lambs for which milk feedings were supplemented with sunflower oil (rich in polyunsaturated fatty acids) compared with lambs that received milk alone (129). Other investigators reported a protective effect of unsaturated fatty acids in the diet of newborn rats exposed continuously to pure oxygen (130). The specific mechanism by which these dietary modifications may alter susceptibility to pulmonary oxygen toxicity remains to be determined. A clinical trial of early treatment of preterm infants with intravenous lipids had no significant effect on the incidence or the severity of subsequent CLD (131). These observations demonstrate the importance of carefully designed clinical trials to test the potential benefits or harmful effects of therapeutic interventions that are supported by data from animal experiments.

E. Effect of Group B Streptococcal Sepsis on Fluid Balance in the Newborn Lung

In adult animals bacterial sepsis and endotoxemia may induce increased lung vascular protein permeability (116,132). Neonatal infection with group B, β-hemolytic *Streptococcus* species often leads to respiratory failure from pulmonary edema associated with lung microvascular injury. An elegant series of studies conducted with newborn sheep showed the pathophysiology of this condition (133–136). Intravenous infusion of live bacteria (group B, β-hemolytic streptococci, type III) or their polysaccharide toxin caused a biphasic reaction, with an initial period of fever, shaking, and tachypnea, accompanied by pulmonary hypertension, granulocytopenia, and increased flow of protein-poor lymph, followed by a period of increased lymph protein clearance, indicative of lung endothelial injury (133). Pretreatment with indomethacin prevented the initial phase of pulmonary hypertension and fever, but did not modify the granulocytopenia or the apparent increase in lung vascular protein permeability that occurred between 2 and 6 hr after the infusion of bacteria or toxin (134). Lung morphology showed dilated capillaries with disrupted and fragmented basement membranes, numerous granulocytes both within and around the pulmonary microcirculation, and extensive interstitial edema (135). Treatment with large doses of methylprednisolone before and after injection of the bacterial toxin did not prevent the early febrile response or pulmonary hypertension, but such treatment completely blocked the granulocytopenia and the increase in lung vascular permeability to protein. A subsequent study by the same group showed that the pulmonary vascular response to group B *streptococcal* toxin was virtually the same in young lambs as it was in older sheep (137). Increased total lung resistance and decreased lung compliance during the early phase of the response coincided with increased concentrations of thromboxane B_2 measured in lung lymph. These observations support the notion that both lipid mediators and granulocyte products probably contribute to the lung vascular response and injury that often develop in infants with systemic bacterial infection.

F. Effect of Pulmonary Microembolism on Fluid Balance in the Newborn Lung

Pulmonary microembolism, a well-recognized cause of respiratory failure and lung edema in adults, is considered a rare event in infants and children. In the presence of deep vein thrombosis, notably after trauma or major surgery, embolization may lead to acute pulmonary hypertension and rapid accumulation of protein-rich fluid in the lungs. These life-threatening complications also can occur as a result of air microembolism associated with open-heart surgery or with inadvertent delivery of air through intravenous infusion of fluid. The frequency with which these mishaps occur is unknown, but they may be more common than appreciated in infants and children who are managed in intensive care units.

Continuous intravenous infusion of air in adult sheep causes reproducible and reversible injury of the pulmonary microcirculation, leading to increased flow of protein-rich lung lymph, sometimes progressing to interstitial pulmonary edema (138,139). Air microemboli lodge in small pulmonary arteries, with accumulation of neutrophils at the air–liquid interface. When neutrophils are activated, as they may be in the presence of circulating complement or when exposed to platelet-activating factor, they may produce acute endothelial injury, either by secretion of proteolytic enzymes or by production of toxic oxygen metabolites, or both (114,140). Electron microscopy shows gaps between endothelial cells through which neutrophils migrate into the interstitium, with disruption of the basal lamina (139). Granulocyte depletion attenuates this injury (115), implying that inflammatory cells have an important role in the development of the increased lung vascular protein permeability that occurs during air microembolism.

In mature newborn lambs, continuous intravenous infusion of tiny air bubbles for 8 hr led to a sustained increase in pulmonary arterial pressure, as left atrial pressure and lung blood flow did not change significantly (141). Lung lymph flow and lymph protein clearance nearly tripled, although surface area for liquid filtration probably decreased because of mechanical obstruction of the vascular bed by the air bubbles. These findings are consistent with a change in pulmonary microvascular permeability to protein, during which there was a significant reduction in arterial oxygenation that probably resulted from a mismatch of ventilation and perfusion, perhaps from bronchoconstriction and nonuniform distribution of blood flow within the lungs, which typically occur in pulmonary microembolism (142,143). Treatment of these lambs with furosemide led to a significant decrease in lung lymph flow, indicative of reduced fluid filtration in the pulmonary microcirculation (141). These experimental observations may provide an explanation for the respiratory deterioration that sometimes accompanies inadvertent injection of air in infants receiving intravenous fluids, and the apparent benefit of diuretics in reducing lung dysfunction associated with abnormal lung vascular protein leaks.

G. Effects of Furosemide on Fluid Balance in the Newborn Lung

Diuretics are the mainstay in the management of infants and children with pulmonary edema. Effective diuresis decreases pulmonary microvascular pressure and increases protein osmotic pressure in plasma. These two changes inhibit fluid filtration into the lungs and hasten the entry of water into the pulmonary microcirculation from the interstitium.

In newborn lambs, intravenous furosemide caused an increase in plasma protein concentration and a decrease in pulmonary vascular pressures, with resultant reduction in lung fluid filtration, indicated by a decrease in lung lymph flow (144). These changes occurred both in the presence and absence of lung microvascular injury (141,144). Furosemide also has an effect on lung fluid balance that is independent of the drug's diuretic action. In lambs without kidneys, intravenous infusion of furosemide consistently led to a small decrease in lung lymph flow, without any change in pulmonary vascular pressure or plasma protein concentration. This nondiuretic influence of furosemide may derive from increased capacitance of peripheral systemic veins (145), with diminished pulmonary blood flow and resultant reduction in lung microvascular surface area for fluid exchange (141). The depressant effect of furosemide on cardiac output probably limits its usefulness in the early postnatal management of respiratory distress in preterm infants (146–149). However, effective diuresis with furosemide or other diuretic agents may have a beneficial effect in infants with persistent respiratory distress from chronic lung disease after premature birth (150–154).

H. Effect of Overinflation on Fluid Balance in the Newborn Lung

The lung epithelium normally forms a tight barrier against protein movement between the interstitium and airspaces, but epithelial leaks and alveolar edema may occur when excessive transpulmonary pressure overinflates the lungs (82). In studies performed with mechanically ventilated lambs that were delivered prematurely, a direct relation was noted between the peak airway pressure used to inflate the lungs during the first 3 hr after birth and subsequent epithelial protein leak (155). These changes in epithelial protein permeability probably reflect overexpansion of at least some areas of the lung, with distortion of intercellular junctions and resultant transudation of protein from the interstitium into the airspaces (156). Lung immaturity appears to increase the vulnerability of the pulmonary epithelium to protein leaks associated with lung overinflation (157). The presence of plasma-derived fibrin in the terminal air sacs of infants with respiratory distress syndrome (158) is indicative of epithelial injury.

Lung overinflation causes vascular injury and edema in lungs of adult animals (159–162). One report showed that application of positive end-expiratory pressure decreased diffuse alveolar damage in adult rats that were mechanically ventilated with high-volume ventilation for a period of 20 min (161). Studies performed with lungs from young rabbits showed that positive-pressure ventilation for 1 hr, with peak inflation pressures of up to 45 cmH_2O, also increased lung vascular filtration coefficient (163). In these experiments, restriction of chest wall movement with a plaster cast inhibited the increase in filtration coefficient.

In vivo studies of lung overinflation in catheterized newborn lambs showed that high inflation pressure, coupled with lung overexpansion, on average caused a sevenfold increase in lung lymph flow and lymph protein flow, indicative of increased pulmonary microvascular permeability to protein (164). In a related series of experiments, high-inflation pressure without lung overexpansion did not increase either lymph flow or protein flow. These observations may have important implications for the clinical management of patients with respiratory failure. For example, in the presence of nonuniform lung inflation, which is common in many types of newborn and adult respiratory disease, overexpansion of relatively normal regions of lung might contribute to the development of endothelial injury and edema.

Mechanical stress and release of vasoactive substances and oxygen radicals within the lung probably play an important role in the pathogenesis of this type of pulmonary injury. Proteolytic enzymes released from inflammatory and lung parenchymal cells also may contribute to the development of neonatal pulmonary edema. Newborn infants with respiratory distress, especially those who are born prematurely, are deficient in protease inhibitors, both in their plasma (165–169) and in their lungs (170–174). At least three groups of investigators have demonstrated an increase in the number of neutrophils, macrophages, and neutrophil-derived elastase activity in liquid suctioned from the airways of infants with respiratory distress (170,171,173). These investigators also showed that both elastase inhibitory capacity and α_1-protease inhibitor activity were reduced in infants with

CLD following acute neonatal lung injury. Hence, these early inflammatory changes may contribute to the development of CLD of early infancy (175).

I. Vulnerability to Pulmonary Edema After Premature Birth

Several features of the immature lung make it vulnerable to postnatal edema (see Table 1). Because the volume of liquid within the lumen of the fetal lung normally decreases late in gestation (17,20,21), premature birth is often associated with an excess amount of liquid in potential airspaces (22). Reduced numbers of sodium channels, sodium pumps, and sodium pump activity on epithelial cells of the immature lung may retard normal clearance of this liquid, thereby contributing to postnatal respiratory distress (46,56,58). The burden of this excess retained fetal lung liquid, most of which must drain from the lungs through the pulmonary circulation, may be further complicated by persistent elevation of lung vascular filtration pressure that often prevails after premature birth (79).

In newborn lambs, some of which were delivered prematurely and others at term, the hydraulic pressure within the pulmonary circulation was greater after premature birth than it was at term (Table 3; 79,84,86,92). This increased intravascular pressure is at least partly the result of greater blood flow per kilogram body weight and per unit lung mass in the immature versus the mature lung (see Table 3). Greater hydraulic pressure within the pulmonary circulation, coupled with less plasma protein osmotic pressure and a lower interstitial hydraulic pressure (91), causes increased transvascular fluid filtration, detected as increased lung lymph flow, with a low lymph/plasma protein ratio and more extravascular lung water in the preterm compared with the term neonatal lung (see Table 3).

These differences in fluid filtration forces are further accentuated by the presence of severe respiratory failure (79) or by excessive pulmonary blood flow through a large patent ductus arteriosus (95). In respiratory failure from inadequate surfactant in the airspaces, assisted ventilation with high inflation pressures and high concentrations of supplemental oxygen may further contribute to lung edema by increasing both lung vascular and epithelial protein leaks (79,155, 157).

These effects on protein permeability across the pulmonary endothelial–epithelial barrier may be attenuated by immediate postnatal treatment with surfactant (155,176). Surfactant also increases lung epithelial cell Na,K-ATPase activity and inhibits lung liquid secretion in fetal sheep (44). Prenatal glucocorticoid treatment also may reduce lung vascular and epithelial protein leaks and reduce vulnerability to air leaks (177,178). Prenatal glucocorticoids also increase expression of lung epithelial cell sodium channels (67) and Na,K-ATPase in the developing lung (66), in addition to increasing epinephrine-induced absorption of lung liquid in fetal sheep (30). Thus, the combination of prenatal glucocorticoid treatment and surfactant replacement at birth may have important beneficial effects

Table 3 Variables Related to Fluid Balance in the Immature and Mature Newborn Lung

Gestation	Vascular pressure (mmHg) Pulmonary artery	Left atrium	Lung interstitial pressure[a] (mmHg)	Protein concentrations (g/dL) Lymph	Plasma	L/P	Pulmonary blood flow (mL/min)/kg	Lung lymph flow (mL/h)/kg	Extravascular lung water (g/g dry lung)
Preterm	36	4	2	1.54	3.22	0.48	381	0.79	4.8
	±5	±2	±1	±0.24	±0.45	±0.02	±153	±0.29	±0.5
Term	20*	4*	6*	3.59*	5.80*	0.62*	314*	0.34*	4.3*
	±3	±1	±1	±0.40	±0.30	±0.05	±40	±0.10	±0.2

Numbers are mean ± SD.

[a]Relative to pleural pressure at inflation pressure of 25 cmH_2O.

*Significant difference, term versus preterm, $p < 0.05$.

Source: Refs. 17, 79, 84, 91, 92, 95.

in hastening postnatal clearance of lung liquid and preventing postnatal protein leaks and fluid accumulation in the lungs after premature birth.

J. Effects of Mechanical Ventilation on Lung Fluid Balance After Premature Birth

Lambs that are delivered prematurely often die of respiratory failure from a condition that mimics the clinical, physiological and histological features observed in human infants with HMD (79,179–181). Studies done with catheterized lambs that were delivered prematurely by cesarean section at 130 days gestation (term = 147 days) showed that severe respiratory failure developed in six of ten lambs that were mechanically ventilated with 100% O_2 for 8 hr after birth (79). These six lambs required peak inflation pressures that averaged greater than 50 cmH_2O between 4 and 8 hr after birth. They had severe hypoxemia and pulmonary hypertension, with a progressive increase in hematocrit and a reduction in plasma protein concentration secondary to generalized protein loss from the circulation. In contrast with previous studies performed with more mature lambs (17), lymph flow and lymph protein flow remained high for the entire study. The postnatal tripling of lymph flow and lymph protein flow clearly showed that lung vascular permeability to protein increased in these preterm lambs with severe respiratory distress (Fig. 3). Lung histological studies and postmortem measurement of extravascular lung water confirmed the presence of severe pulmonary edema (Fig. 4). In the four lambs that did not have respiratory distress, lung lymph flow and protein clearance decreased to values that were no greater than prenatal measurements, and their postmortem lung water measurements were significantly less than they were in lambs that had respiratory distress. Thus, abnormal leakage of protein-rich liquid from the lung microcirculation into the interstitium constitutes a major component in the pathogenesis of neonatal respiratory distress in preterm lambs (79). This lung vascular injury can be inhibited by surfactant administration at birth (176), probably by reducing the need for high-inflation pressures to achieve adequate ventilation and oxygenation and by yielding uniform inflation of distal respiratory units in the immature lung (182).

Mechanically ventilated preterm lambs with severe respiratory failure had a significant reduction in circulating neutrophils within 30 min of birth, and this was associated with neutrophil accumulation within the lungs. The magnitude of the early postnatal decrease in circulating neutrophils correlated with the degree of lung vascular protein leak and pulmonary edema (183). When lambs were made neutropenic from prenatal treatment with nitrogen mustard, lung vascular injury and edema did not occur postnatally. These and earlier observations of neutrophil abundance in airway secretions of infants with severe respiratory distress indicate that circulating neutrophils and their secretory products, specifically proteolytic enzymes and toxic oxygen metabolites, may play an important role

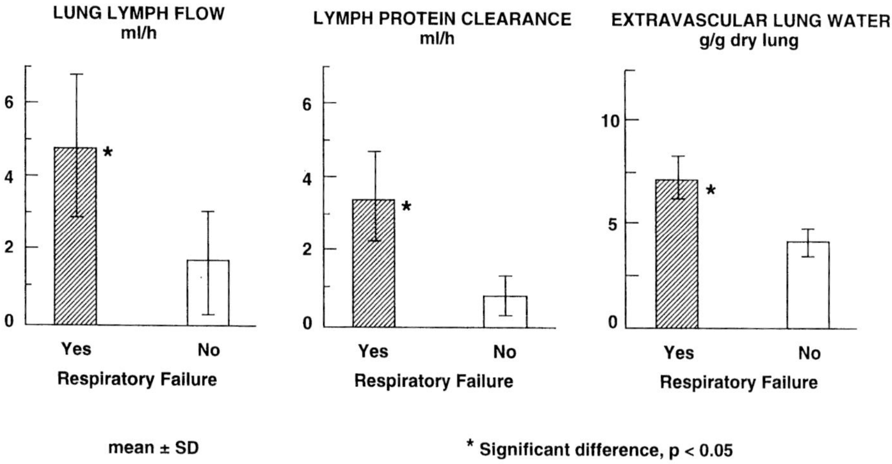

Figure 3 Studies of lung vascular protein permeability done with ten lambs (birth weight 3.6 ± 0.7 kg) that were delivered prematurely by cesarean section at 133 ± 1 days gestation (term = 147 days) and mechanically ventilated for 6 hr after birth. Six lambs (hatched bars) had respiratory failure, as judged by severe hypoxemia in 100% oxygen and need for peak inflation pressures > 50 cmH_2O. Four lambs (open bars) had no respiratory failure. Lung lymph flow and lymph protein flow during the last 2 hr of study and postmortem extravascular lung water were significantly greater ($p < .05$) in the lambs that had respiratory failure versus those that did not.

in the pathogenesis of acute lung vascular protein leak and edema in HMD (170,173,183,184). The mechanisms by which neutrophils are recruited into the lungs after premature birth and mechanical ventilation are unclear, but it is likely that a variety of chemoattractants, including interleukin-8 (IL-8; 185), are released in response to the pulmonary stresses associated with increased blood flow and pressures within the lung circulation, and increased gas flow and pressures within the airways and distal airspaces.

The early postnatal inflammatory changes that accompany acute respiratory failure after premature birth and positive-pressure ventilation may be associated with increased accumulation of hyaluronan in the lungs (186). The hydrophilic nature of this large extracellular matrix proteoglycan may contribute to water retention in the lungs of infants with HMD (187).

K. Lung Fluid Balance in Chronically Ventilated Preterm Lambs

Sustained mechanical ventilation of lambs for 3–4 weeks after premature birth leads to a chronic form of lung injury that closely mimics the pathophysiology

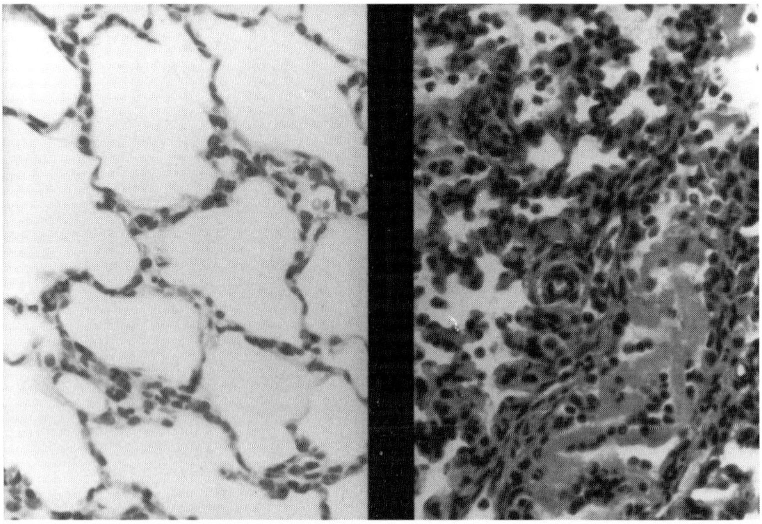

Figure 4 Histological sections of lung obtained from lambs that were delivered by cesarean section at 128 days gestation (term = 147 days) and mechanically ventilated for 8 hr after birth: The lungs were cross-clamped at the hilum and fixed in formalin at the prevailing peak inflation pressure. (Left panel) lung from a lamb that did not have respiratory failure, showing well-inflated airspaces and thin interstitium. (Right panel) lung from a lamb that had respiratory failure, showing atelectasis, proteinaceous fluid within open airspaces, and abundant neutrophils, indicative of inflammation and edema from abnormal lung vascular and epithelial protein permeability.

and histopathology of BPD, including pulmonary vascular dysfunction and edema (188,189). To test the importance of different ventilation strategies in causing such chronic lung injury, we compared the effects of two patterns of assisted breathing, slow and deep versus rapid and shallow lung inflation, on respiratory and pulmonary vascular variables in 16 lambs that were delivered operatively at 125 ± 3 days gestation (term = 147 days) and mechanically ventilated for 3–4 weeks postnatally (190). Ten lambs were ventilated at a rate of 20 breaths per minute with a tidal volume that averaged approximately 15 ± 5 mL/kg with an inspiratory time of 0.75 sec; and 6 lambs were ventilated at a rate of 60 breaths per minute, with a tidal volume of 6 ± 2 mL/kg and an inspiratory time of 0.25 sec. Peak inflation pressure was adjusted to keep the $Paco_2$ between 35 and 45 mmHg, with sufficient supplemental oxygen to keep the Pao_2 between 60 and 90 mmHg. Each lamb had vascular catheters placed before delivery for subsequent monitoring of arterial blood pressure, pH, and blood gas tensions, and for delivery of intravenous nutrition. They received calf lung surfactant (Infasurf, 350 mg) at birth and, in the first few days after birth, they had surgery for ligation of their ductus arteriosus and placement of catheters to allow serial measurements of pulmonary vascular resistance and lung lymph flow. Vascular pressures, cardiac output, lung lymph flow, and protein concentrations in lymph and plasma were measured for 4–8 hr at weekly intervals. After 3 weeks of study, peak (30 ± 8 vs. 17 ± 1 cmH_2O) and mean (10 ± 1 vs. 7 ± 1 cmH_2O) airway pressures were greater in lambs that were ventilated at 20 breaths per minute than in those that were ventilated at 60 breaths per minute. From the first to the last week of study, pulmonary vascular resistance did not change significantly with either ventilation pattern. In contrast, pulmonary vascular resistance decreased by 43 ± 14% between weeks 1 and 3 in control lambs that were born at term gestation.

Lung lymph flow, an index of net transvascular fluid filtration, increased over time in lambs that were ventilated at 20 breaths per minute, but not in lambs that were ventilated at 60 breaths per minute. Lymph protein concentration decreased relative to plasma protein concentration in all lambs, consistent with increased filtration pressure in the pulmonary microcirculation, rather than abnormal protein permeability. Postmortem extravascular lung water showed pulmonary edema (6.4 ± 1.9 g/g dry lung; normal 4.6 ± 0.2), with no significant difference related to ventilation pattern. Postmortem histopathology of lung tissue that was fixed at the prevailing peak inflation pressure showed nonuniform inflation, abundant macrophages, and edema (Fig. 5), as well as increased elastin deposition in distal lung of both groups compared with control term lambs that were killed at the same postconception age (<1-day-old) or the same postnatal age (3-week-old) as chronically ventilated preterm lambs (191,192). These observations provide physiological, histological, and biochemical evidence that prolonged mechanical ventilation of preterm lambs leads to chronic lung injury that closely resembles BPD in human infants (193–195).

Some of these chronically ventilated preterm lambs had episodes of generalized bacterial infection, during which their lung lymph flow and lymph protein concentration increased, indicative of increased pulmonary vascular protein permeability. When their infection resolved in response to appropriate antibiotic therapy, however, lung lymph flow returned to baseline values, and lymph protein concentration invariably decreased to low levels, consistent with increased lung vascular filtration pressure. Thus, the pulmonary edema that typically occurs in chronic lung injury after premature birth and prolonged mechanical ventilation appears to be the result of increased lung vascular filtration pressure rather than increased vascular permeability to protein.

Increased smooth-muscle mass around small pulmonary arteries and diminished numbers of vessels within the lung are characteristic findings in both preterm animals (188,196–198) and human infants with CLD (3,194,199). These vascular abnormalities increase fluid filtration pressure in the pulmonary micro-

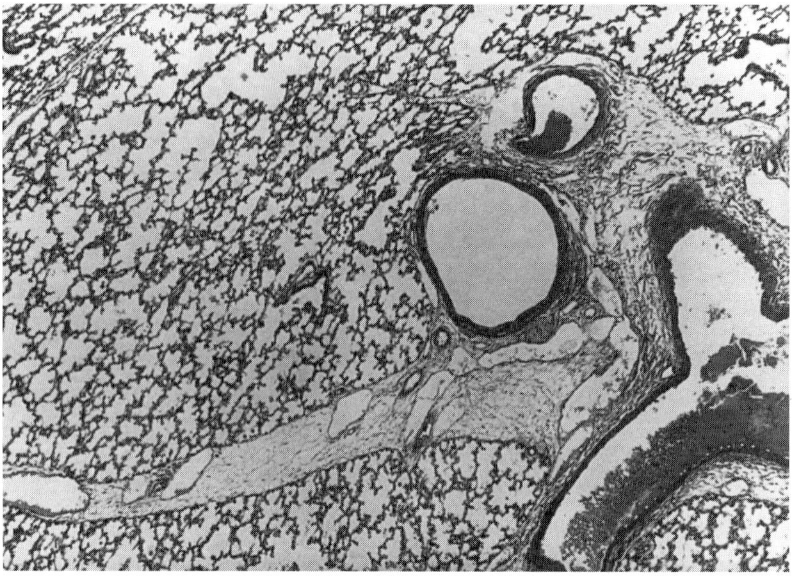

Figure 5 Histological section of lung obtained from a lamb that was delivered prematurely at 125 days gestation (term = 147 days) and mechanically ventilated at a rate of 20 breaths per minute for 3 weeks after birth. Note the perivascular cuffs of fluid, dilated lymphatics and thickened interlobar fissure, indicative of interstitial edema.

circulation and thereby contribute to edema formation. Besides the pulmonary hypertension that often accompanies CLD after premature birth and long-term mechanical ventilation, increased lung microvascular pressure may result from left ventricular dysfunction associated with intermittent episodes of hypoxia, nutritional deficiencies, or the systemic hypertension that sometimes occurs in infants with CLD (200). Intravenous lipid administration and injection of drugs, such as sodium pentobarbital, can also increase lung vascular pressure and, thereby, hasten fluid entry into the lungs. Other conditions that may contribute to pulmonary edema in CLD include recurrent infection, as well as impaired lymphatic drainage associated with interstitial fibrosis or central venous hypertension from long-standing parenteral nutrition through a catheter in the subclavian vein or superior vena cava.

L. Summary

There is abundant experimental work to help explain why infants who are born prematurely have a high incidence of respiratory distress associated with pulmonary edema (1–3,201). Animal studies have shown that the lungs contain more fluid per unit tissue mass after premature birth than after birth at term (17,22). In addition, the lung epithelium has fewer sodium channels, fewer sodium pumps, and less Na,K-ATPase activity after preterm than after term birth (56–59,62), such that postnatal absorption of fetal lung liquid may be slower after premature birth than it is after birth at term (22,61). Compared with infants who are born at term, those who are delivered prematurely have greater filtration pressure in their pulmonary circulation (200,202–205), particularly if they experience hypoxia or if they have increased pulmonary blood flow from persistent patency of the ductus arteriosus. Protein osmotic pressure in their plasma is low (206,207), especially if they receive too much fluid and salt postnatally. Because the airspaces of their lungs are often unstable from insufficient surfactant, a large transpulmonary pressure often develops, with considerable heterogeneity of lung expansion. Chemoattractants in the lung draw neutrophils from the pulmonary circulation into the airspaces, with subsequent release of inflammatory mediators (170,171,173,183–185). These developments may cause leaks in the epithelium (158,208) and endothelium (79), and reduce interstitial pressure around extra-alveolar vessels (91), which may contribute to edema formation (209,210).

Infants with respiratory distress often require mechanical ventilation with high concentrations of inspired oxygen, which may injure the lungs, cause release of toxic oxygen metabolites, and proteolytic enzymes, and possibly interfere with lymphatic drainage, particularly in the presence of interstitial emphysema or fibrosis. These events may cause fluid accumulation and an abnormal distribution of protein in the lungs, with impaired respiratory gas exchange.

Subsequent prolonged mechanical ventilation, often with recurrent episodic hypoxemia and intermittent infections, yields persistent elevation of pulmonary vascular resistance (200,204), with resultant increase in lung fluid filtration and subsequent pulmonary edema. Use of milk formulas with high caloric density (up to 30 cal/oz) to feed such infants, coupled with cautious administration of diuretics and avoidance of hypoxia and other noxious stimuli that increase vascular pressures and blood flow, may be useful in reducing lung fluid filtration and lessening the severity of pulmonary edema in these infants.

IV. Lingering Questions

Despite recent progress in our understanding of normal fluid balance in the developing lung, especially of respiratory epithelial ion transport and related fluid movement before and after birth, information is lacking on what initiates acute lung injury and associated changes in lung vascular and epithelial protein permeability after premature birth and mechanical ventilation. It is also unclear how and where large molecular weight proteins enter the airspaces from the vasculature and interstitium of the lungs to produce hyaline membranes, and it is unknown how these proteinaceous deposits are removed from the lungs during the healing phase of acute respiratory distress syndrome. Clarification of how inflammatory cells, including neutrophils and macrophages, gain access to the lung parenchyma and affect membrane permeability, perhaps by release of secretory products, could pave the way for effective therapeutic interventions or even preventive measures. The mechanisms by which endothelial and epithelial cells become disengaged to allow fluid and protein leaks after premature birth remain unknown, and there is virtually no information on how barrier function of the respiratory epithelium and vascular endothelium is restored during repair from acute lung injury after premature birth. The importance of aquaporins and endocytotic vesicles in transporting water and solutes between the pulmonary microcirculation and terminal air sacs during edema formation and its resolution is yet to be defined. The role of extracellular matrix proteins in storing and removing excessive lung fluid needs further study. The possible roles of surfactant, nitric oxide, and various hormones, including glucocorticoids, in regulating lung fluid balance after birth warrant further inquiry. We need to learn more about how various growth factors influence alveolar and capillary proliferation during early lung development and during recovery from lung injury. The pathogenesis of pulmonary fibrosis and excessive elastin deposition in the lungs of persistently ventilated preterm animals and humans needs to be clarified. Because pulmonary edema associated with chronic lung disease after premature birth and prolonged mechanical ventilation appears to be related to abnormal lung vascular resistance, better understanding of what controls angiogenesis and vascular smooth-muscle growth should provide valuable insight into the mechanisms by which lung edema occurs during long-term repetitive inflation and stretching of an incompletely developed lung.

Answers to these and many other important questions on fluid balance in the developing lung and during injury and repair will require a wide array of experimental approaches. An enormous amount of information can be derived from basic studies at the cellular and molecular level, including the use of gene modification techniques coupled with relevant physiological, histological, and biochemical assessment of transgenic animals. There is still much to be learned from in vitro studies of lung cell structure and function, including the influence of various growth factors and proinflammatory mediators. In vivo studies using relevant animal models of acute and chronic lung injury after premature birth and mechanical ventilation can be extremely useful in defining the time course of lung pathology and in probing possible mechanisms of injury and repair, including assessment of therapeutic interventions. And finally, there is a crucial need for carefully designed clinical studies of human infants with evolving and established CLD to help validate basic laboratory findings and to test the efficacy of promising therapeutic or preventive measures.

To maximize chances for success in transferring important laboratory discoveries to effective bedside applications, basic scientists and clinicians need to share ideas and collaborate on research related to early lung growth and development and mechanisms of injury and repair. Successful development and application of prenatal glucocorticoid and postnatal surfactant therapies in preventing or reducing the severity of acute respiratory distress after premature birth (211) clearly illustrates the enormous benefits that can derive from such a broad, integrated approach to investigating a challenging and long-standing clinical problem.

References

1. Lauweryns JM. Hyaline membrane disease: a pathological study of 55 infants. Arch Dis Child 1965; 40:618–625.
2. Northway WH Jr, Rosan RC, Porter DY. Pulmonary disease following respiratory therapy of hyaline membrane disease: bronchopulmonary dysplasia. N Engl J Med 1967; 276:357–368.
3. Bonikos DS, Bensch KG, Northway WH Jr, et al. Bronchopulmonary dysplasia: the pulmonary pathologic sequel of necrotizing bronchiolitis and pulmonary fibrosis. Hum Pathol 1976; 7:643–666.
4. Brown ER, Stark A, Sosenko I, et al. Bronchopulmonary dysplasia: possible relationship to pulmonary edema. J Pediatr 1978; 92:980–984.
5. Accurso F. Relation of fluid intake to BPD. J Pediatr 1979; 94:681–682.
6. Costarino AT, Baumgart S. Controversies in fluid and electrolyte therapy for the premature infant. Clin Perinatol 1988; 15:863–878.
7. Costarino AT, Gruskay JA, Corcoran L, et al. Sodium restriction versus daily maintenance replacement in very low birth weight premature neonates: a randomized, blind therapeutic trial. J Pediatr 1992; 120:99–106.
8. Bland RD. Persistent respiratory distress syndromes. In: Rudolph AM, ed. Pediatrics. Norwalk CT: Appleton & Lange, 1996:1619–1625.
9. Olver RE, Strang LB. Ion fluxes across the pulmonary epithelium and the secretion of lung liquid in the foetal lamb. J Physiol 1974; 241:327–357.
10. Harding R, Hooper SB. Regulation of lung expansion and lung growth before birth. J Appl Physiol 1996; 81:209–224.
11. Wallen LD, Perry SF, Alston JT, et al. Morphometric study of the role of pulmonary arterial flow in fetal lung growth in sheep. Pediatr Res 1990; 27:122–127.
12. Wallen LD, Kulisz E, Maloney JE. Main pulmonary artery ligation reduces lung fluid production in fetal sheep. J Dev Physiol 1991; 16:173–179.
13. Harrison MR, Bressack MA, Churg AM, et al. Correction of congenital diaphragmatic hernia in utero. II. Simulated correction permits fetal lung growth survival at birth. Surgery 1980; 88:260–268.
14. Pringle KC, Turner JW, Schofield JC, et al. Creation and repair of diaphragmatic hernia in fetal lamb: lung development and morphology. J Pediatr Surg 1984; 19: 131–140.

15. Adzick NS, Glick PL, Villa RL, et al. Experimental pulmonary hypoplasia and oligohydramnios: relative contributions of lung fluid and fetal breathing movements. J Pediatr Res 1984; 19:658–665.
16. Dickson KA, Harding R. Decline in lung liquid volume and secretion rate during oligohydramnios in fetal sheep. J Appl Physiol 1989; 67:2401–2407.
17. Bland RD, Hansen TN, Haberkern CM, et al. Lung fluid balance in lambs before and after birth. J Appl Physiol 1982; 53:992–1004.
18. Brown MJ, Olver RE, Ramsden CA, et al. Effects of adrenaline and of spontaneous labour on the secretion and absorption of lung liquid in the fetal lamb. J Physiol 1983; 344:137–152.
19. Chapman DL, Carlton DP, Nielson DW, et al. Changes in lung liquid during spontaneous labor in fetal sheep. J Appl Physiol 1994; 76:523–530.
20. Dickson KA, Maloney JE, Berger PJ. Decline in lung liquid volume before labor in fetal lambs. J Appl Physiol 1986; 61:2266–2272.
21. Kitterman JA, Ballard PL, Clements JA, et al. Tracheal fluid in fetal lambs: spontaneous decrease prior to birth. J Appl Physiol 1979; 47:985–989.
22. Bland RD. Dynamics of pulmonary water before and after birth. Acta Paediatr Scand Suppl 1983; 305:12–20.
23. Bland RD, Bressack MA, McMillan DD. Labor decreases the lung water content of newborn rabbits. Am J Obstet Gynecol 1979; 135:364–367.
24. Walters DV, Olver RE. The role of catecholamines in lung liquid absorption at birth. Pediatr Res 1978; 12:239–242.
25. Lawson EE, Brown ER, Torday JS, et al. The effect of epinephrine on tracheal fluid flow and surfactant efflux in fetal sheep. Am Rev Respir Dis 1978; 118:1023–1026.
26. Olver RE, Ramsden CA, Strang LB, et al. The role of amiloride-blockable sodium transport in adrenaline-induced lung liquid reabsorption in the fetal lamb. J Physiol 1986; 376:321–340.
27. Walters DV, Ramsden CA, Olver RE. Dibutyryl cyclic AMP induces a gestation-dependent absorption of fetal lung liquid. J Appl Physiol 1990; 68:2054–2059.
28. Barker PM, Brown MJ, Ramsden CA, et al. The effect of thyroidectomy in the fetal sheep on lung liquid reabsorption induced by adrenaline or cyclic AMP. J Physiol 1988; 407:373–383.
29. Barker PM, Walters DV, Strang LB. The role of thyroid hormones in maturation of the adrenaline-sensitive lung-liquid reabsorption mechanism in the fetal sheep. J Physiol 1990; 424:473–485.
30. Barker PM, Walters DV, Markiewicz M, et al. Development of the lung liquid reabsorptive mechanism in fetal sheep; synergism of triiodothyronine and hydrocortisone. J Physiol 1991; 433:435–449.
31. Chapman DL, Carlton DP, Cummings JJ, et al. Intrapulmonary terbutaline and aminophylline decrease lung liquid in fetal lambs. Pediatr Res 1991; 29:357–361.
32. Cheng JB, Goldfein A, Ballard PL, et al. Glucocorticoids increase pulmonary β-adrenergic receptors in fetal rabbit. Endocrinology 1980; 107:1646–1648.
33. Warburton DL, Parton L, Buckley S, et al. β-Receptors and surface active material flux in fetal lamb lung: female advantage. J Appl Physiol 1987; 63:828–833.
34. Whitsett JA, Manton MA, Carovec-Beckerman C, et al. β-Adrenergic receptors in the developing rabbit lung. Am J Physiol 1981; 240:E351–E357.

35. McDonald JV, Gonzales LW, Ballard PL, et al. Lung β-adrenergic blockade affects perinatal surfactant release but not lung water. J Appl Physiol 1986; 60:1727–1733.
36. Perks AM, Cassin S. The effects of arginine vasopressin and other factors on the production of lung liquid in fetal goats. Chest 1982; 81:63S–65S.
37. Perks AM, Cassin S. The rate of production of lung liquid in fetal goats, and the effect of expansion of the lungs. J Dev Physiol 1985; 7:149–160.
38. Perks AM, Cassin S. The effects of arginine vasopressin and epinephrine on lung liquid production in fetal goats. Can J Physiol Pharmacol 1989; 67:491–498.
39. Wallace MJ, Hooper SB, Harding R. Regulation of lung liquid secretion by arginine vasopressin in fetal sheep. Am J Physiol 1990; 258:R104–R111.
40. Cassin S, Perks AM. Amiloride inhibits arginine vasopressin-induced decrease in fetal lung liquid secretion. J Appl Physiol 1993; 75:1925–1929.
41. Cummings JJ, Carlton DP, Poulain FR, et al. Vasopressin effects on lung liquid volume in fetal sheep. Pediatr Res 1995; 38:30–35.
42. Cummings JJ. Nitric oxide decreases lung liquid production in fetal lambs. J Appl Physiol 1997; 83:1538–1544.
43. Carlton DP, Bolshoun PA. Nitric oxide reduces Na-K-2Cl cotransport in distal lung epithelial cells from fetal sheep. Pediatr Res 1998; 42:277A.
44. Carlton DP, Davis PL, Gismondi PA, et al. Surfactant alters lung liquid production and epithelial ion transport in fetal sheep. Pediatr Res 1996; 39:327A.
45. O'Brodovich H, Hannam V, Rafii B. Sodium channel but neither Na^+-H^+ nor Na-glucose symport inhibitors slow neonatal lung water clearance. Am J Respir Cell Mol Biol 1991; 5:377–384.
46. O'Brodovich H, Hannam V, Spear M, et al. Amiloride impairs lung liquid clearance in newborn guinea pigs. J Appl Physiol 1990; 68:1758–1762.
47. Cotton CU, Boucher RC, Gatzy JT. Paths of ion transport across canine fetal tracheal epithelium. J Appl Physiol 1988; 65:2376–2382.
48. Mason RJ, Williams MC, Widdicombe JH, et al. Transepithelial transport by pulmonary alveolar type II cells in primary culture. Proc Natl Acad Sci USA 1982; 79:6033–6037.
49. Cheek JM, Kim KJ, Crandall ED. Tight monolayers of rat alveolar epithelial cells: bioelectric properties and active sodium transport. Am J Physiol 1989; 256:C688–C693.
50. O'Brodovich H, Rafii B, Post M. Bioelectric properties of fetal alveolar epithelial monolayers. Am J Physiol 1990; 258:L201–L206.
51. Rao AK, Cott GR. Ontogeny of ion transport across fetal pulmonary epithelial cells in monolayer culture. Am J Physiol 1991; 261:L178–L187.
52. Barker PM, Stiles AD, Boucher RC, et al. Bioelectric properties of cultured epithelial monolayers from distal lung of 18-day fetal rat. Am J Physiol 1992; 262:L628–L636.
53. Pitkänen OM, Tanswell AK, O'Brodovich HM. Fetal lung cell-derived matrix alters distal lung epithelial ion transport. Am J Physiol 1995; 268:L762–L771.
54. Weibel ER, Gehr P, Haies D, et al. The cell population of the normal lung. In: Bouhuys A, ed. Lung Cells in Disease. Amsterdam: Elsevier/North-Holland, 1976: 3–16.
55. Randell SH, Silbajoris R, Young SL. Ontogeny of rat lung type II cells correlated

with surfactant lipid and surfactant apoprotein expression. Am J Physiol 1991; 266: L562–L570.
56. Bland RD, Boyd CAR. Cation transport in lung epithelial cells derived from fetal, newborn and adult rabbits. Influence of birth, labor and postnatal development. J Appl Physiol 1986; 62:507–515.
57. O'Brodovich H, Staub O, Rossier BC, et al. Ontogeny of α_1- and β-isoforms of Na^+-K^+-ATPase in fetal distal rat lung epithelium. Am J Physiol 1993; 264:C1137–C1143.
58. Chapman DL, Widdicombe JH, Bland RD. Developmental differences in rabbit lung epithelial cell Na-K-ATPase. Am J Physiol 1990; 259:L481–L487.
59. Ingbar DH, Weeks CB, Gilmore-Hebert M, et al. Developmental regulation of Na,K-ATPase in rat lung. Am J Physiol 1996; 270:L619–L629.
60. Crump RG, Askew GR, Wert SE, et al. In situ localization of sodium–potassium ATPase mRNA in developing mouse lung epithelium. Am J Physiol 1995; 269: L299–L308.
61. Bland RD. Pathogenesis of pulmonary edema after premature birth. Adv Pediatr 1987; 34:175–222.
62. O'Brodovich H, Cannessa C, Ueda J, et al. Expression of the epithelial Na^+ channel in the developing rat lung. Am J Physiol 1993; 265:C491–C496.
63. Umenishi F, Carter EP, Yang B, et al. Sharp increase in rat lung water channel expression in the perinatal period. Am J Respir Cell Mol Biol 1996; 15:673–679.
64. Ruddy MK, Drazen JM, Pitkänen OM, et al. Modulation of aquaporin 4 and the amiloride-inhibitable sodium channel in perinatal rat lung epithelial cells. Am J Physiol 1998; 274:L1066–L1072.
65. Lee MD, King LS, Nielsen S, et al. Genomic organization and developmental expression of aquaporin-5 in lung. Chest 1997; 111(suppl 6): 111S–113S.
66. Celsi G, Wang ZM, Akusjarvi G, et al. Sensitive periods for glucocorticoids' regulation of Na,K-ATPase mRNA in the developing lung and kidney. Pediatr Res 1993; 33:5–9.
67. Tchepichev S, Ueda J, Canessa C, et al. Lung epithelial Na channel subunits are differentially regulated during development and by steroids. Am J Physiol 1995; 269:C805–C812.
68. King LS, Nielsen S, Agre P. Aquaporin-1 water channel protein in lung. J Clin Invest 1996; 97:2183–2191.
69. Barker PM, Gatzy JT. Effect of gas composition on liquid secretion by explants of distal lung of fetal rat in submersion culture. Am J Physiol 1993; 265:L512–L517.
70. Pitkänen O, Tanswell AK, Downey G, et al. Increased Po_2 alters the bioelectric properties of fetal distal lung epithelium. Am J Physiol 1996; 270:L1060–L1066.
71. Hummler E, Barker P, Gatzy J, et al. Early death due to defective neonatal lung liquid clearance in αENaC-deficient mice. Nature Genet 1996; 12:325–328.
72. Cummings JJ, Carlton DP, Poulain FR, et al. Hypoproteinemia slows lung liquid clearance in young lambs. J Appl Physiol 1993; 74:153–160.
73. Raj JU, Bland RD. Lung luminal liquid clearance in newborn lambs. Am Rev Respir Dis 1986; 134:305–310.
74. Karlberg P, Adams FH, Beubelle F, et al. Alteration of the infant's thorax during vaginal delivery. Acta Obstet Gynecol Scand 1962; 41:223–229.

75. Rudolph AM, Heymann MA. Circulatory changes during growth in the fetal lamb. Circ Res 1970; 26:289–299.
76. Iwamoto HS, Teitel D, Rudolph AM. Effects of birth-related events on blood flow distribution. Pediatr Res 1987; 22:634–640.
77. Teitel DF, Iwamoto HS, Rudolph AM. Effects of birth-related events on central blood flow patterns. Pediatr Res 1987; 22:557–566.
78. Carlton DP, Cummings DP, Scheerer R, et al. Lung vascular protein permeability in preterm fetal and mature newborn sheep. J Appl Physiol 1994; 77:782–788.
79. Bland RD, Carlton DP, Scheerer RG, et al. Lung fluid balance in lambs before and after premature birth. J Clin Invest 1989; 84:568–576.
80. Normand ICS, Reynolds EOR, Strang LB. Passage of macromolecules between alveolar and interstitial spaces in foetal and newly ventilated lungs of the lamb. J Physiol 1970; 210:151–164.
81. Normand ICS, Olver RE, Reynolds EOR, et al. Permeability of lung capillaries and alveoli to non-electrolytes in the foetal lamb. J Physiol 1971; 219:303–330.
82. Egan EA, Olver RE, Strang LB. Changes in non-electrolyte permeability of alveoli and the absorption of lung liquid at the start of breathing in the lamb. J Physiol 1975; 244:161–179.
83. Boyd RDH, Hill JR, Humphreys PW, et al. Permeability of lung capillaries to macromolecules in fetal and newborn lambs and sheep. J Physiol 1969; 201:567–588.
84. Bland RD, McMillan DD. Lung fluid dynamics in awake newborn lambs. J Clin Invest 1977; 60:1107–1115.
85. Bland RD, Bressack MA. Lung fluid balance in awake newborn lambs with pulmonary edema from rapid intravenous infusion of isotonic saline. Pediatr Res 1979; 13:1037–1042.
86. Bland RD, Hansen TN, Hazinski TA, et al. Studies of lung fluid balance in newborn lambs. Ann NY Acad Sci 1982; 384:126–145.
87. Sundell HW, Brigham KL, Harris TR, et al. Lung water and vascular permeability surface area in newborn lambs delivered by cesarean section compared with the 3–5-day-old lamb and adult sheep. J Dev Physiol 1980; 2:191–204.
88. Bland RD, Bressack MA, Haberkern CM, et al. Lung fluid balance in hypoxic, awake newborn lambs and mature sheep. Biol Neonate 1980; 38:221–228.
89. West JB, Dollery CT, Naimark A. Distribution of blood flow in isolated lung: relation to vascular and alveolar pressures. J Appl Physiol 1964; 19:713–724.
90. Fike CD, Lai-Fook SJ, Bland RD. Alveolar liquid pressures in newborn and adult rabbit lungs. J Appl Physiol 1988; 64:1629–1635.
91. Raj JU. Alveolar liquid pressure measured by micropuncture in isolated lungs of mature and immature fetal rabbits. J Clin Invest 1987; 79:1579–1588.
92. Hazinski TA, Bland RD, Hansen TN, et al. Effect of hypoproteinemia on lung fluid balance in awake newborn lambs. J Appl Physiol 1986; 61:1139–1148.
93. Teague WG, Berner ME, Bland RD. Effect of pulmonary perfusion on lung fluid filtration in young lambs. Am J Physiol 1988; 255:H1336–H1341.
94. Feltes TF, Hansen TH. Effects of an aorticopulmonary shunt on lung fluid balance in the young lamb. Pediatr Res 1989; 26:94–97.
95. Alpan G, Scheerer R, Bland R, et al. Patent ductus arteriosus increases lung fluid filtration in preterm lambs. Pediatr Res 1991; 30:616–621.

96. Teague WG, Raj JU, Braun D, et al. Lung vascular effects of lipid infusion in awake lambs. Pediatr Res 1987; 22:714–719.
97. Guyton AC, Lindsey AW. Effect of elevated left atrial pressure and decreased plasma protein concentration on the development of pulmonary edema. Circ Res 1959; 7:649–657.
98. Kramer G, Harms B, Gunther R, et al. The effects of hypoproteinemia on blood-to-lymph fluid transport in sheep lung. Circ Res 1981; 49:1173–1180.
99. Kramer GC, Harms BA, Bodai BI, et al. Effects of hypoproteinemia and increased vascular pressure on lung fluid balance in sheep. J Appl Physiol 1983; 55:1514–1522.
100. Zarins CK, Rice CL, Peters RM, et al. Lymph and pulmonary response to isobaric reduction in plasma oncotic pressure in baboons. Circ Res 1978; 43:925–930.
101. Drake R, Giesler M, Laine G, et al. Effect of outflow pressure on lung lymph flow in unanesthetized sheep. J Appl Physiol 1985; 58:70–76.
102. Laine GA, Allen SJ, Katz J, et al. Effect of systemic venous pressure elevation on lymph flow and lung edema formation. J Appl Physiol 1986; 61:1634–1638.
103. Cowan GSM Jr, Staub NC, Edmunds LG Jr. Changes in the fluid compartments and dry weights of reimplanted dog lungs. J Appl Physiol 1976; 40:962–970.
104. Bland RD, Demling RH, Selinger SL, et al. Effects of alveolar hypoxia on lung fluid and protein transport in unanesthetized sheep. Circ Res 1977; 40:269–274.
105. Bressack MA, Bland RD. Alveolar hypoxia increases lung fluid filtration in unanesthetized newborn lambs. Circ Res 1980; 46:111–116.
106. Raj JU, Chen P. Micropuncture measurements of microvascular pressures in isolated lamb lungs during hypoxia. Circ Res 1986; 59:398–404.
107. Hansen TN, LeBlanc AL, Gest AL. Hypoxia and angiotensin II infusion redistribute lung blood flow in lambs. J Appl Physiol 1985; 58:812–818.
108. Landolt CC, Matthay MA, Albertine KH, et al. Overperfusion, hypoxia and increased pressure cause only hydrostatic pulmonary edema in anesthetized sheep. Circ Res 1986; 52:335–341.
109. Hansen TN, Hazinski TA, Bland RD. Effects of asphyxia on lung fluid balance in baby lambs. J Clin Invest 1984; 74:370–376.
110. Hansen TN, Hazinski TA, Bland RD. Effects of hypoxia on transvascular fluid filtration in newborn lambs. Pediatr Res 1984; 18:434–440.
111. Raj JU, Hazinski TA, Bland RD. Effect of hypoxia on lung lymph flow in newborn lambs with left atrial hypertension. Am J Physiol 1988; 254:H487–H493.
112. Bressack MA, McMillan DD, Bland RD. Pulmonary oxygen toxicity; increased microvascular permeability to protein in unanesthetized lambs. Lymphology 1979; 12:133–139.
113. Hansen TN, Hazinski TA, Bland RD. Vitamin E does not prevent oxygen-induced lung injury in newborn lambs. Pediatr Res 1982; 16:583–587.
114. Craddock PR, Fehr J, Brigham KL, et al. Complement and leukocyte-mediated pulmonary dysfunction in hemodialysis. N Engl J Med 1977; 296:769–774.
115. Flick M, Perel A, Staub N. Leucocytes are required for increased lung microvascular permeability after microembolization in sheep. Circ Res 1981; 48:344–351.
116. Heflin AC, Brigham KL. Prevention by granulocyte depletion of increased vascular

permeability of sheep lung following endotoxemia. J Clin Invest 1981; 68:1253–1260.
117. Johnson A, Malik AB. Pulmonary edema after glass bead microembolization: protective effect of granulocytopenia. J Appl Physiol 1982;52:155–161.
118. Fox RB, Hoidal JR, Brown DM, et al. Pulmonary inflammation due to oxygen toxicity: involvement of chemotactic factors and polymorphonuclear leukocytes. Am Rev Respir Dis 1981; 123:521–523.
119. Shasby DM, Fox RB, Harada RN, et al. Reduction of the edema of acute hyperoxic lung injury by granulocyte depletion. J Appl Physiol 1982; 52:1237–1244.
120. Raj JU, Hazinski TA, Bland RD. Oxygen-induced lung microvascular injury in neutropenic rabbits and lambs. J Appl Physiol 1985; 58:921–927.
121. Hoidal JR, Beall GD, Repine JE. Production of hydroxyl radical by human alveolar macrophages. Infect Immunol 1979; 26:1088–1092.
122. Clement A, Chadelat K, Sardet A, et al. Alveolar macrophage status in bronchopulmonary dysplasia. Pediatr Res 1988; 23:470–473.
123. Freeman BA, Crapo JD. Hyperoxia increases oxygen radical production in rat lungs and lung mitochondria. J Biol Chem 1981; 256:10986–10992.
124. Frank L, Sosenko IRS. Prenatal development of lung antioxidant enzymes in four species. J Pediatr 1987; 110:106–110.
125. Tanswell AK, Freeman BA. Liposome-entrapped antioxidant enzymes prevent lethal O_2 toxicity in the newborn rat. J Appl Physiol 1987; 63:347–352.
126. Frank L, Summerville J, Massaro D. Protection from oxygen toxicity with endotoxin. J Clin Invest 1980; 65:1104–1110.
127. Hazinski TA, Kennedy KA, France ML, et al. Pulmonary O_2 toxicity in lambs: physiological and biochemical effects of endotoxin infusion. J Appl Physiol 1988; 65:1579–1585.
128. Hazinski TA, France ML, Kennedy KA. Cimetidine reduces hyperoxic lung injury in lambs. J Appl Physiol 1989; 67:1586–1592.
129. McMillan DD, Boyd GN. The role of antioxidants and diet in the prevention or treatment of oxygen-induced lung microvascular injury. Ann NY Acad Sci 1982; 384:535–543.
130. Sosenko IRS, Innis SM, Frank L. Polyunsaturated fatty acids and protection of newborn rats from oxygen toxicity. J Pediatr 1988; 112:630–637.
131. Sosenko IRS, Rodriguez-Pierce K, Bancalari E. Effect of early initiation of intravenous lipid administration on the incidence and severity of chronic lung disease in premature infants. J Pediatr 1983; 123:975–982.
132. Brigham KL, Woolverton WC, Blake LH, et al. Increased sheep lung vascular permeability caused by pseudomonas bacteremia. J Clin Invest 1974; 54:792–804.
133. Rojas J, Green RS, Hellerqvist CG, et al. Studies on group B β-hemolytic *Streptococcus*. II. Effects on pulmonary hemodynamics and vascular permeability in unanesthetized sheep. Pediatr Res 1981; 15:899–904.
134. Rojas J, Larsson LE, Ogletree ML, et al. Effects of cyclooxygenase inhibition on the response to group B streptococcal toxin in sheep. Pediatr Res 1983; 17:107–110.
135. Rojas J, Larsson LE, Hellerqvist CG, et al. Pulmonary hemodynamic and ultrastructural changes associated with group B streptococcal toxemia in adult sheep and newborn lambs. Pediatr Res 1983; 17:1002–1008.

136. Rojas J, Palme C, Ogletree ML, et al. Effects of methylprednisolone on the response to group B streptococcal toxin in sheep. Pediatr Res 1984; 18:1141–1144.
137. Sandberg K, Engelhardt B, Hellerqvist C, et al. Pulmonary response to group β streptococcal toxin in young lambs. J Appl Physiol 1987; 63:2024–2030.
138. Ohkuda K, Nakahara K, Binder A, et al. Venous air emboli in sheep: reversible increase in lung microvascular permeability. J Appl Physiol 1981; 51:887–894.
139. Albertine KH, Wiener-Kronish JP, Koike K, et al. Quantification of damage by air emboli to lung microvessels in anesthetized sheep. J Appl Physiol 1984; 57:1360–1368.
140. Henson PM, McArthy K, Larsen GL, et al. Complement fragments, alveolar macrophages and alveolitis. Am J Pathol 1979; 97:93–110.
141. Berner ME, Teague WG Jr, Scheerer RG, et al. Furosemide reduces lung fluid filtration in lambs with lung microvascular injury from air emboli. J Appl Physiol 1989; 67:1990–1996.
142. Malik AB. Pulmonary microembolism. Physiol Rev 1983; 63:1114–1207.
143. Nadel JA, Colebatch HJH, Olsen CR. Location and mechanism of airway constriction after barium sulfate microembolism. J Appl Physiol 1964; 19:387–394.
144. Bland RD, McMillan DD, Bressack MA. Decreased pulmonary transvascular fluid filtration in awake newborn lambs after intravenous furosemide. J Clin Invest 1978; 62:601–609.
145. Dikshit K, Vyden JK, Forrester JS. Renal and extrarenal hemodynamic effects of furosemide in congestive heart failure after acute myocardial infarction. N Engl J Med 1978; 288:1087–1090.
146. Green TP, Thompson TR, Johnson DE, et al. Diuresis and pulmonary function in premature infants with respiratory distress syndrome. J Pediatr 1983; 103:618–623.
147. Green TP, Johnson DE, Bass JL, et al. Prophylactic furosemide in severe respiratory distress syndrome: blinded prospective study. J Pediatr 1988; 112:605–612.
148. Marks KH, Berman W, Friedman Z, et al. Furosemide in hyaline membrane disease. Pediatrics 1978; 62:785–788.
149. Savage MO, Wilkinson AR, Baum JD, et al. Furosemide in respiratory distress syndrome. Arch Dis Child 1975; 50:709–713.
150. Kao LC, Warburton D, Cheng MH, et al. Effect of oral diuretics on pulmonary mechanics in infants with chronic bronchopulmonary dysplasia: results of a double-blind crossover sequential trial. Pediatrics 1984; 74:37–44.
151. Albersheim SG, Solimano AG, Sharma AK, et al. Randomized, double-blind, controlled trial of long-term diuretic therapy for bronchopulmonary dysplasia. J Pediatr 1989; 115:615–620.
152. Rush MG, Engelhardt B, Parker RA, et al. Double-blind, placebo-controlled trial of alternate-day furosemide therapy in infants with chronic bronchopulmonary dysplasia. J Pediatr 1990; 117:112–188.
153. McCann EM, Lewis K, Deming DD, et al. Controlled trial of furosemide therapy in infants with chronic lung disease. J Pediatr 1985; 106:957–962.
154. Engelhardt B, Elliott S, Hazinski TA. Short- and long-term effects of furosemide on lung function in infants with bronchopulmonary dysplasia. J Pediatr 1986; 109: 1034–1039.
155. Jobe A, Ikegami M, Jacobs H, et al. Permeability of premature lamb lungs to protein

and the effect of surfactant on that permeability. J Appl Physiol 1983; 55:169–176.
156. Nilsson R, Grossman G, Robertson B. Lung surfactant and the pathogenesis of neonatal bronchiolar lesions induced by artificial ventilation. Pediatr Res 1978; 12:249–255.
157. Jobe A, Jacobs H, Ikegami M, et al. Lung protein leaks in ventilated lambs: effect of gestational age. J Appl Physiol 1985; 58:1246–1251.
158. Gitlin D, Craig JM. The nature of the hyaline membrane in asphyxia of the newborn. Pediatrics 1956; 17:64–71.
159. Parker JC, Townsley MI, Rippe B, et al. Increased microvascular permeability in dog lungs due to high peak airway pressures. J Appl Physiol 1984; 57:1809–1816.
160. Dreyfuss D, Basset G, Soler P, et al. Intermittent positive-pressure hyperventilation with high inflation pressures produces pulmonary microvascular injury in rats. Am Rev Respir Dis 1985; 132:880–884.
161. Dreyfuss D, Soler P, Basset G, et al. High inflation pressure pulmonary edema. Respective effects of high airway pressure, high tidal volume, and positive end-expiratory pressure. Am Rev Respir Dis 1988; 137:1159–1164.
162. Dreyfuss D, Saumon G. Ventilator-induced lung injury. Lessons from experimental studies. Am J Respir Crit Care Med 1998; 157:294–323.
163. Hernandez LA, Peevy KJ, Moise AA, et al. Chest wall restriction limits high airway pressure-induced lung injury in young rabbits. J Appl Physiol 1989; 66:2364–2368.
164. Carlton DP, Cummings JJ, Scheerer RG, et al. Lung overexpansion increases pulmonary microvascular protein permeability in young lambs. J Appl Physiol 1990; 69:577–583.
165. Evans HE, Levi M, Mandl I. Serum enzyme inhibitor concentrations in the respiratory distress syndrome. Am Rev Respir Dis 1970; 101:359–363.
166. Evans HE, Keller S, Mandl I. Serum trypsin inhibitory capacity and the idiopathic respiratory distress syndrome. J Pediatr 1982; 81:588–592.
167. Kotas RV, Fazen LE, Moore TE. Umbilical cord serum trypsin inhibitor capacity and the idiopathic respiratory distress syndrome. J Pediatr 1982; 81:593–599.
168. Makram WE, Johnson AM. Serum proteinase inhibitors in infants with hyaline membrane disease. J Pediatr 1972; 81:579–587.
169. Mathis RK, Freier EF, Hunt CE, et al. alpha$_1$-Antitrypsin in the respiratory distress syndrome. N Engl J Med 1973; 288:59–64.
170. Merritt TA, Cochrane CG, Holcomb K, et al. Elastase and α-proteinase inhibitor activity in tracheal aspirates during respiratory distress syndrome. J Clin Invest 1983; 72:656–666.
171. Speer CP, Ruess D, Harms K, et al. Neutrophil elastase and acute pulmonary damage in neonates with severe respiratory distress syndrome. Pediatrics 1993; 91:794–799.
172. Watterberg KL, Carmichael DF, Gerdes JS, et al. Secretory leukocyte protease inhibitor and lung inflammation in developing bronchopulmonary dysplasia. J Pediatr 1994; 125:264–269.
173. Ogden BE, Murphy SA, Saunders GC, et al. Neonatal lung neutrophils and elastase/proteinase inhibitor imbalance. Am Rev Respir Dis 1984; 130:817–821.
174. Groneck P, Speer CP. Inflammatory mediators and bronchopulmonary dysplasia. Arch Dis Child 1995; 73:F1–F3.

175. Groneck P, Gotze-Speer B, Oppermann M, et al. Association of pulmonary inflammation and increased microvascular permeability during the development of bronchopulmonary dysplasia: a sequential analysis of inflammatory mediators in respiratory fluid of high-risk preterm neonates. Pediatrics 1994; 93:712–718.
176. Carlton DP, Cho SC, Davis P, et al. Surfactant treatment at birth reduces lung vascular injury and edema in preterm lambs. Pediatr Res 1995; 37:265–270.
177. Ikegami M, Berry D, Elkady T, et al. Corticosteroids and surfactant change lung function and protein leaks in the lungs of ventilated premature rabbits. J Clin Invest 1987; 79:1371–1378.
178. Elkady T, Jobe A. Corticosteroids and surfactant increase lung volumes and decrease rupture pressures of preterm rabbit lungs. J Appl Physiol 1987; 63:1616–1621.
179. Normand ICS, Reynolds EOR, Strang LB, et al. Flow and protein concentration of lymph from lungs of lambs developing hyaline membrane disease. Arch Dis Child 1968; 43:334–339.
180. Reynolds EOR, Jacobson HN, Motoyama EK, et al. The effect of immaturity and prenatal asphyxia on the lungs and pulmonary function of newborn lambs: the experimental production of respiratory distress. Pediatrics 1965; 35:382–392.
181. Stahlman M, LeQuire VS, Young WC, et al. Pathophysiology of respiratory distress in newborn lambs. Am J Dis Child 1964; 108:375–393.
182. Carlton DP, Cho S-C, Davis P, et al. Inflation pressure and lung vascular injury in preterm lambs. Chest 1994; 105:115S–116S.
183. Carlton DP, Albertine KH, Cho SC, et al. Role of neutrophils in lung vascular injury and edema after premature birth in lambs. J Appl Physiol 1997; 83:1307–1317.
184. Jackson JC, Chi EY, Wilson CB, et al. Sequence of inflammatory cell migration into lung during recovery from hyaline membrane disease in premature newborn monkeys. Am Rev Respir Dis 1987; 135:937–940.
185. Jones CA, Cayabyab RG, Kwong KY, et al. Undetectable interleukin (IL)-10 and persistent IL-8 expression early in hyaline membrane disease: a possible developmental basis for the predisposition to chronic lung inflammation in preterm newborns. Pediatr Res 1996; 39:966–975.
186. Juul SE, Kinsella MG, Jackson JC, et al. Changes in hyaluronan deposition during early respiratory distress syndrome in premature monkeys. Pediatr Res 1994; 35: 238–243.
187. Allen SJ, Sedin EG, Jonzon A, et al. Lung hyaluronan during development: a quantitative and morphological study. Am J Physiol 1991; 260:H1449–H1454.
188. Albertine KH, Carlton DP, Cho S, et al. Histopathology of chronic lung injury in preterm lambs. FASEB J 1995; 9:A275.
189. Bland RD, Cho SC, Carlton D, et al. Chronic lung injury in mechanically ventilated preterm lambs. FASEB J 1995; 9:A275.
190. Bland R, Kullama L, Carlton D, et al. Chronic lung injury in preterm lambs: effect of ventilation rate and tidal volume. Pediatr Res 1996; 39:327A.
191. Pierce RA, Albertine KH, Starcher BC, et al. Chronic lung injury in preterm lambs: disordered pulmonary elastin deposition. Am J Physiol 1997; 272:L452–L460.
192. Albertine KH, Kim BI, Kullama LK, et al. Chronic lung injury in preterm lambs. Disordered respiratory tract development. Am J Respir Crit Care Med 1998; March.
193. Bonikos DS, Bensch KG, Northway WH Jr. Oxygen toxicity in the newborn: the

effect of chronic continuous 100% oxygen on the lungs of newborn mice. Am J Pathol 1976; 85:623–635.

194. Margraf LR, Tomashefski JF, Bruce MC, et al. Morphometric analysis of the lung in bronchopulmonary dysplasia. Am Rev Respir Dis 1991; 143:391–400.
195. Van Lierde S, Cornelis A, Devlieger H, et al. Different patterns of pulmonary sequelae after hyaline membrane disease: heterogeneity of bronchopulmonary dysplasia? Biol Neonate 1991; 60:152–162.
196. Coalson JJ, Winter V, deLemos RA. Decreased alveolarization in baboon survivors with bronchopulmonary dysplasia. Am J Respir Crit Care Med 1995; 152:640–646.
197. Coalson JJ, Winter VT, Gerstmann DR, et al. Pathophysiologic, morphometric, and biochemical studies of the preterm baboon with bronchopulmonary dysplasia. Am Rev Respir Dis. 1992; 145:872–881.
198. Bland R, Carlton D, Albertine K, et al. Pulmonary vascular effects of nitric oxide and cGMP in preterm lambs with chronic lung injury. FASEB J 1998; 12:A645.
199. Hislop A, Haworth S. Pulmonary vascular damage in the development of cor pulmonale following hyaline membrane disease. Pediatr Pulmonol 1990; 9:152–161.
200. Abman SA, Warady BA, Lum G, et al. Systemic hypertension in infants with BPD. J Pediatr 1984; 104:929–931.
201. DeSa DJ. Pulmonary fluid content in infants with respiratory distress. J Pathol 1969; 97:469–479.
202. Rudolph AM, Drorbaugh JE, Auld PAM, et al. Studies on the circulation in the neonatal period. The circulation in the respiratory distress syndrome. Pediatrics 1961; 27:551–566.
203. Abman SH, Wolfe RR, Accurso FJ, et al. Pulmonary vascular response to oxygen in infants with severe BPD. Pediatrics 1985; 75:80–84.
204. Berman W, Yabek SM, Dillon T, et al. Evaluation of infants with BPD using cardiac catheterization. Pediatrics 1982; 70:708–712.
205. Albertine KH, Kim BI, Kullama LK, et al. Prolonged mechanical ventilation of preterm lambs leads to smooth muscle extension and elastin accumulation along pulmonary blood vessels. Pediatr Res 1996; 39:323A.
206. Bland RD. Cord-blood total protein level as a screening aid for the idiopathic respiratory distress syndrome. N Engl J Med 1972; 287:9–13.
207. Wu PYK. Colloid oncotic pressure: current status and clinical applications in neonatal medicine. Clin Perinatol 1982; 9:645–657.
208. Jefferies AL, Coates G, O'Brodovich H. Pulmonary epithelial permeability in hyaline membrane disease. N Engl J Med 1984; 311:1075–80.
209. Albert RK, Lakshminarayan S, Hildebrandt J, et al. Increased surface tension favors pulmonary edema formation in anesthetized dogs' lungs. J Clin Invest 1979; 63: 1015–1018.
210. Clements JA. Pulmonary edema and permeability of alveolar membranes. Arch Environ Health 1961; 2:280–283.
211. Jobe AH, Mitchell Br, Gunket JH. Beneficial effects of the combined use of prenatal corticosteroids and postnatal surfactant. Am J Obstet Gynecol 1993; 168:508–513.
212. Bland RD. Edema formation in the newborn lung. Clin Perinatol 1982; 9:593–611.

30

Molecular Mechanisms of Oxygen-Induced Lung Injury

CHARLES VINCENT SMITH and STEPHEN E. WELTY

Baylor College of Medicine
Houston, Texas

I. Introduction

Although there appears to be a general consensus that developmental immaturity, mechanical ventilation, and often, infection are major contributors to the development of bronchopulmonary dysplasia (BPD), or chronic lung disease of early infancy (CLD), available evidence indicates that effects arising from exposure to elevated oxygen tensions are also important in the etiology of the disease (1–4). Although the hypothesis that hyperoxia contributes significantly to the development of CLD has not been proved with certainty, the support for a causal relation is sufficient to warrant the use of this working hypothesis.

A critical aspect of the importance of immaturity in the development of CLD is the immaturity of the premature infant's antioxidant defense mechanisms (see Chap. 12; 5–7). Oxidant mechanisms can participate in the initiation of the inflammatory response that is the hallmark of CLD (1,8–14). Recent studies (15–17) have shown that oxidative mechanisms contribute to the lung injury that results from acute blast overpressure, as occurs during detonation of explosives. The mechanical ventilation component of risk for development of CLD may represent a chronic expression of similar mechanisms that differ in magnitude and

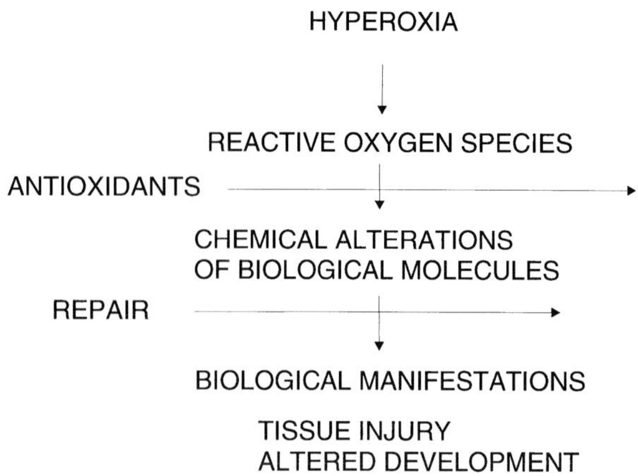

Figure 1 Overview of working hypothesis for the role of oxidative processes in hyperoxic lung injury.

chronicity of the insult, the developmental immaturity of the subject, and the developmental expression of the injury.

The established or likely contributions of reactive oxygen species to the conditions related to the individual risk factors for the development of CLD, including lung immaturity, tissue trauma associated with mechanical ventilation, and infection, underscore the importance of research designed to improve understanding of the mechanisms by which reactive oxygen species cause injury to lung tissue and contribute to the development of CLD. That the effects of hyperoxia are mediated by increased generation of reactive oxygen species and resultant oxidative modification of critical biological molecules by these chemically reactive intermediates is a central working hypothesis in ongoing efforts to unravel the complex molecular mechanisms that produce CLD (Fig. 1). In this chapter we will focus on some of the important studies that have examined the chemical transformations involved in the pathogenesis of hyperoxic lung injury and other models of cell damage.

II. Possible Roles of Hyperoxic Lung Injury in CLD

The effects of exposure of experimental animals to concentrations of O_2 higher than 95% have been studied extensively for several decades in an effort to delineate the mechanisms of tissue injury. The mechanisms by which hyperoxia causes acute lung injury may not be completely identical with the mechanisms by which hyperoxia and the other relevant insults contribute to CLD's development, but the mechanisms involved in both acute and chronic injury need to be defined before meaningful comparisons can be made. Many aspects in the progression of the effects of hyperoxia in different species of experimental animals have been described (5,6,18–22), but the molecular events responsible for the mechanisms of injury are still poorly understood. Careful morphometric studies of various species, including humans, demonstrate similar alterations of lung cells, resulting from exposure to hyperoxia (23,24). The earliest evidence of toxicity includes subtle changes in endothelial cells that subsequently lead to increased protein permeability and pulmonary edema (23–27). Shortly after changes are noted in endothelial cells, inflammatory cells accumulate in the pulmonary capillaries and interstitium, after which there is accelerated destruction of endothelial cells and increased edema. Studies by Crapo and colleagues showed that the first blood cells to accumulate in lungs with hyperoxia are platelets (24), although the potential significance of this finding has not been explored adequately. Alveolar epithelial cells are damaged at about the same time, with type I cell destruction and type II cell hyperplasia. Hence, the destructive phase of pulmonary oxygen toxicity is characterized by a combination of endothelial cell injury and interstitial and alveolar edema through a damaged alveolar epithelial cell layer.

The physiological consequences of these morphological findings have been well characterized in the ovine model of pulmonary oxygen toxicity, in which there is an abrupt increase in lung lymph flow, indicative of increased fluid filtration across the pulmonary circulation (25). The particularly striking feature of the effects of hyperoxic exposure is the time-dependent decay of pulmonary function, as a consequence of florid pulmonary edema (26–29) and death of the animal (23,30–32). This course of events matches the progression that sometimes occurs clinically, in which the patient dies of systemic hypoxia caused by pulmonary edema and resultant respiratory failure while being ventilated with 100% O_2.

The relatively sudden onset of endothelial and epithelial cell injury, followed quickly by lung edema, occurs after several days of exposure to hyperoxia. This delayed, abrupt response suggests the continuous production of potentially damaging intermediates that are detoxified efficiently until the animal is depleted of a critical substrate, whereupon the reactive oxygen species begin to initiate tissue damage. Superoxide ($O_2^{\bullet -}$), hydrogen peroxide (H_2O_2), and hydroxyl radical ($HO^{\bullet}$) are the reactive metabolites of oxygen that are usually considered, and increased production of hydrogen peroxide in response to elevated oxygen tensions has been reported (33). Cellular glutathione (γ-glutamylcysteinylglycine; GSH) represents a logical candidate for the protective substrate, the depletion of which determines the onset of irreversible tissue damage (Fig. 2). In concordance with this hypothesis, manipulation of experimental animals' ability to maintain their GSH concentrations, as by feeding animals diets deficient in sulfur-containing amino acids, potentiates hyperoxic lung injury (34–36). In apparent conflict with this hypothesis, however, are data showing that lung GSH concentra-

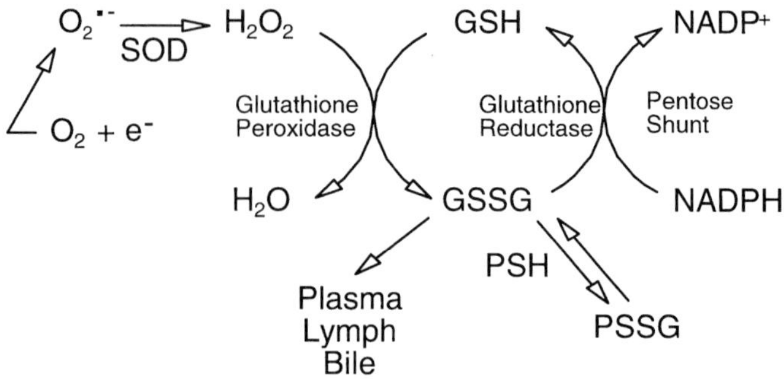

Figure 2 Glutathione cycle: Increased generation of superoxide and hydrogen peroxide resulting from hyperoxia or other oxidant exposure increases utilization of GSH for reduction of hydroperoxides. Most of the GSSG produced in this process is reduced back to GSH by glutathione reductase, at the expense of oxidation of NADPH. Some cells actively export GSSG, but GSSG can also undergo thiol–disulfide exchange reactions to *S*-thiolate proteins. The formation of disulfides in critical proteins may account for some of the physiological consequences of exposure to hyperoxia.

tions are not depleted significantly before the onset of respiratory failure in animals that are subjected to prolonged hyperoxia (34).

The effects of oxidation of GSH would be expected to be mediated through generation of increased steady-state concentrations of glutathione disulfide (GSSG), resulting in *S*-thiolation reactions with critical thiol groups on proteins, and changes in the functions of these proteins (see Fig. 2). It is possible, however, that depletion of GSH or accumulation of GSSG and *S*-thiolation reactions are critical events in the initiation of pulmonary failure, but the absence of marked changes in these parameters in experimental animals exposed to hyperoxia (37,38) indicate that any biologically critical depletion and oxidation would be limited to a particular cell type or subcellular organelle; if so, the compartmentalized depletion or oxidation of GSH would not necessarily be detected by measurements made with whole tissue (39).

The oxidation of proteins is not limited to shifts in thiol–disulfide status, and the formation of ''protein carbonyls,'' so termed because they have been studied primarily through derivatization with 2,4-dinitrophenylhydrazine (DNPH), has attracted increasing attention in several studies (40–43). Studies with living animals and airway secretions obtained from premature infants indicate that these protein modifications occur and may provide useful biomarkers of molecular damage from hyperoxia (44–47). Unlike the oxidation of thiols to disulfides, the oxidation of proteins to form the DNPH-reactive species does not require increased production of H_2O_2 (48,49).

Cells exposed to high concentrations of oxygen may increase production and leakage of superoxide and hydrogen peroxide in mitochondria and endoplasmic reticulum (50,51). Superoxide can be dismutated to hydrogen peroxide in a reaction that is catalyzed by superoxide dismutase, and superoxide may reduce ferric iron (Fe^{3+}) to ferrous iron (Fe^{2+}). Hydrogen peroxide can be reduced to water by the GSH system or converted to water and molecular oxygen by the peroxisomal enzyme catalase. Conversely, hydrogen peroxide can react with Fe^{2+} to produce the highly reactive hydroxyl radical ($HO^{\bullet}$), or ferryl or perferryl intermediates that exhibit reactivities that are comparable with $HO^{\bullet}$ (52). Physiological steady states are defined by a balance between the rate of production of cellular reactive oxygen species and the orderly reduction of these species to nonreactive molecules. Most efforts to ameliorate the effects of hyperoxia exposure in animals have been directed at augmenting the GSH-dependent defense mechanisms and enhancing the activities of superoxide dismutase (53–56). Less effort has been directed at decreasing the rates of production of reactive oxygen species (57,58).

An alternative hypothesis on the origin of the time-dependent onset of hyperoxia-induced pulmonary failure is that this phase of the injury is mediated by neutrophils, which are recruited to the lungs and activated, consequently injuring adjacent tissue by releasing intracellular proteases and reactive oxygen species (59–69). Careful histological analyses of neutrophil accumulation in hyperoxic lungs and the temporal relation of neutrophil accumulation to the acceleration of lung injury support the neutrophil recruitment hypothesis. Some investigators have used pharmacological methods to deplete circulating neutrophils in vivo in animals exposed to hyperoxia (70,71). The results of these studies are variable and, occasionally, directly contradict one another. More recent investigations with monoclonal antibodies to key elements of the cellular machinery involved in inflammatory responses support the hypothesis that neutrophil accumulation in the lung contributes to the pathophysiology of hyperoxic lung injury (72). However, the molecular mechanisms leading to the neutrophil recruitment and the facets of hyperoxic, lung injury that are caused by neutrophil activities remain poorly understood.

III. Reactive Oxygen Species in Hyperoxic Lung Injury

It is reasonable to assume that the initial steps in hyperoxic lung injury are mediated by chemically reactive oxygen metabolites. Despite much research, however, the mechanisms by which these initial alterations are expressed remains unclear. Efforts to ameliorate hyperoxic lung injury by administration of vitamin E, GSH, or other antioxidants, with the intent of shifting a balance between prooxidants and antioxidants, have been used and occasionally show modest improvements.

Table 1 Reactive Oxygen Species in Biological Systems

Species	Name	Reactant	Product
O_2	Oxygen	$R^\bullet$	$ROO^\bullet$
$^1O_2$	Singlet oxygen		
$O_2^{\bullet-}$	Superoxide	$O_2^{\bullet-}$	$H_2O_2 + O_2$
		Fe^{3+}	$Fe^{2+} + O_2$
		$NO^\bullet$	$OONO^-$
H_2O_2	Hydrogen peroxide	GSH	GSSG
		Fe^{2+}	$Fe^{3+} + HO^\bullet$ or $Fe\text{-}O^\bullet$
$HO^\bullet$	Hydroxyl radical	Many compounds	Oxidation, HOH
H_2O	Water	Epoxides	Diols
HOCl	Hypochlorous acid	RNH_2; RSH	RNHCl; RSCl
$NO^\bullet$	Nitric oxide	$O_2^{\bullet-}$	$OONO^\bullet$
HOONO	Peroxynitrous acid		
NO_2	Nitrogen dioxide		
α-toco-OH	α-Tocopherol	$ROO^\bullet$	ROOH + α-toco-$O^\bullet$
$ROO^\bullet$	Alkylperoxyl radical	RH	R + ROOH
$RO^\bullet$	Alkoxyl radical	RH	$R^\bullet$ + ROH
		(β-scission)	RCHO
RCHO	Aldehydes	RNH_2	RN=CHR
RCH=CHCHO	α,β-Unsaturated aldehydes	RSH	RS-adduct
O_3	Ozone	RCH=CHR	RCHO + others

The frequent failure of therapeutic approaches based on relatively simple hypotheses to provide satisfactory protection, however, indicates that the critical mechanisms are more complex (26,73–75). A greater appreciation of the differences in reactivities of specific reactive oxygen species and radicals (Table 1) may help resolve apparent inconsistencies in the results of studies examining hyperoxic lung injury.

IV. Biomarkers of Reactive Oxygen Species in Biological Systems

A. Thiol–Disulfide Alterations

Glutathione is found in relatively high concentrations (1–10 mM) in virtually all mammalian cells and is found in lower concentrations in extracellular fluids, including plasma and lymph (1–10 μM), alveolar lining fluid (200–800 μM), and bile (2 mM and greater in the rat; 76–83). GSH serves various functions, including transfer of reducing equivalents, providing a storage and transport form of cysteine, and conjugation with electrophilic intermediates, usually leading to excretion of the corresponding mercapturic acids. The transfer of reducing equivalents is a critical aspect of the interaction of GSH with hydrogen peroxide and other oxidants and products of peroxidation, and of the management of protein thiol–disulfide transformations and steady states. The diverse biological uses of GSH are essential to normal physiological functions, and sustaining these capabilities is equally essential to optimal health and development. In addition, study of the specific alterations of GSH following toxicant exposure or imposition of a physiological stress offers a useful approach to characterization of the chemically reactive intermediates that are often proposed as contributors to observed tissue injury or disease processes (84).

Low concentrations of GSH have been observed in the plasma of premature infants, suggesting that many premature infants are inadequately prepared developmentally to cope with the oxidant stresses imposed by the extrauterine environment and the consequent increased exposures to hydrogen peroxide or other peroxides (85). In addition, premature infants show relatively high plasma concentrations of GSSG, suggesting increased rates of oxidation of GSH or decreased effectiveness of reduction of GSSG by cellular glutathione reductase in these individuals. That the highest plasma concentrations of GSSG were observed in the most premature infants, many of whom were being ventilated with room air, suggests that even air may constitute an oxidant stress for very premature infants. In addition, hepatic cystathionase activities are low in premature infants, indicating that cysteine may be a conditionally essential amino acid in these individuals (86–88).

Synthesis and utilization of GSH generate a dynamic steady state that can be perturbed in many ways. The most frequently encountered alterations of normal steady state are caused by increased consumption of GSH secondary to exposure to or generation of one or more electrophilic species, including oxidants and some alkylating intermediates. Increased basal concentrations of GSH probably are not as important as is sustaining GSH synthesis in the presence of oxidant stresses (89,90). Decreased availability of amino acid precursors, usually cysteine, can exacerbate the effects of a metabolic stress. Limitations of substrate for GSH synthesis, and perhaps for GSSG reduction, may account for a significant portion of the effects of dietary deprivations on hyperoxic lung injury (30,53,91). Under normal situations, GSH synthesis is probably regulated intracellularly by the feedback inhibition of γ-glutamylcysteine synthase (γ-GCS) by GSH itself (92). Diminished activities of γ-GCS appear to bc responsible for the low plasma concentrations of GSH observed in adults and children infected with the human immunodeficiency virus (HIV; 39,93). Despite frequent claims that oxidative stresses have an important mechanistic role in the pathology of HIV, increases in GSSG concentrations in plasma and bronchoalveolar lavage (BAL) fluids have not been observed in infected individuals (39,94,95). Inhibition of γ-GCS can be accomplished in experimental models by administration of L-buthionine-S-sulfoximine (BSO; 78). Decreased cellular ATP availability is a potential mechanism for limitation of GSH synthesis. Although γ-GCS and glutathione synthetase are ATP-dependent, as are other transformations in GSH homeostasis, the effect of ATP limitations on GSH metabolism has received little attention.

Extracellular concentrations of GSH are determined by the competitive processes of cellular synthesis, export, and clearance, for which γ-glutamyl transpeptidase (γ-GT) is a major factor (78). The basic determinants of input, disposition, and turnover of GSH and related thiols and disulfides in the plasma are not yet adequately understood. Synthesis and export of GSH by the liver, with extrahepatic uptake and utilization, primarily through hydrolysis by γ-GT, acquisition of the precursor amino acids, and intracellular utilization for resynthesis of GSH or synthesis of proteins is probably the dominant process in most circumstances (78,96). Evidence supporting direct cellular uptake of GSH has been reported, however, in some circumstances (97,98).

Increased GSSG contents or GSSG/GSH ratios can arise from changes in any of the many factors that are involved in generation, distribution, and reduction of GSSG, and clearance of either form (see Fig. 2). Reduction of H_2O_2 by GSH does not alter the quantitative capacity for protein thiol *S*-thiolation. Reduction back to GSH by glutathione reductase (GR) is required, and reducing equivalents, supplied through NADPH, are required for this process. Many cell types export GSSG by active transport. As a result, oxidant stress responses by the glutathione system are often most marked in the extracellular fluids (99). Few examples of intracellular accumulation of high concentrations of GSSG have been reported, particularly from studies in vivo. In the absence of evidence for GSSG receptors, the simplest hypotheses for effects of shifts in thiol–disulfide status are increased *S*-thiolation of critical proteins (100–102) or limitation of other GSH-dependent functions. This latter mechanism should be accompanied by marked depletion of GSH and the expression of other changes, such as oxidations that are not mediated by thiol–disulfide exchange reactions.

Thiol–disulfide exchange reactions are implicit in the notion that increased

Figure 3 Thiol–disulfide exchange reactions: At equilibrium, the fraction of a protein thiol (PSH) that is *S*-thiolated in exchange reactions with GSSG would be determined by the ratios of the concentrations of GSH and GSSG, and the equilibrium constant K_1. The graph shows a plot for this relation for $K_1 = 1$, as a function of the GSH/GSSG ratio. In most tissues in vivo, the GSH/GSSG ratio is greater than 100, and as can be seen, very large changes in the GSH/GSSG ratio are needed to alter the percentage of the PSH/PSSG couple that is in the reduced state. Also note that PSH/PSSG is not a function of the absolute concentration of GSH. For proteins that form intramolecular disulfide bonds, the fraction of protein in the fully reduced state is dependent on the absolute concentrations of GSH.

A. Simple protein thiol S-thiolation by GSSG

$$PSH + GSSG \rightleftharpoons PSSG + GSH \qquad (1)$$

$$K_1 = \frac{[PSSG]\ [GSH]}{[PSH]\ [GSSG]}$$

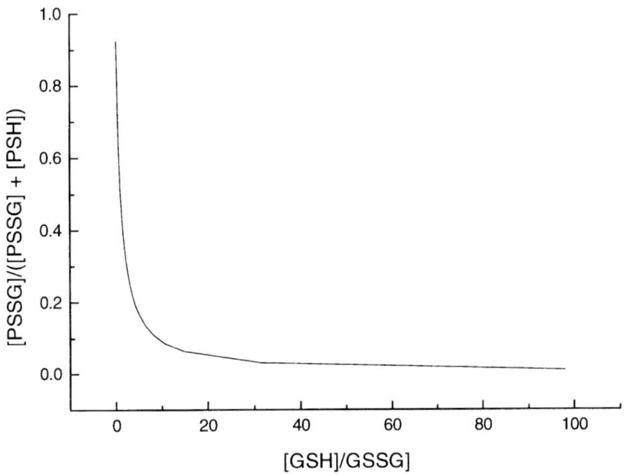

B. GSSG-driven formation of intramolecular disulfides

$$P(SH)_2 + GSSG \rightleftharpoons P(SS) + 2\ GSH$$

$$K_2 = \frac{[P(SS)]\ [GSH]^2}{[P(SH)_2]\ [GSSG]} \qquad (2)$$

Note that equation 1 is not a function of absolute [GSH], whereas equation 2 is.

levels of GSSG or decreased GSH/GSSG ratios mediate oxidant injury. The chemistry of exchange reactions with protein thiols has been reviewed (103,104). Physiologically, such reactions are important in protein folding in the endoplasmic reticulum (105), but strong evidence for the contributions of protein thiol *S*-thiolation reactions in examples of oxidant-mediated pathology has not been presented. Although biological systems, for the most part, strive to avoid chemical equilibria, studies of chemical equilibria offer useful insights into these proposals. First, *S*-thiolation of an isolated protein thiol (PSH) to form the corresponding mixed disulfide with GSH (PSSG) would be a function of the GSH/GSSG ratio, and would be independent of the absolute concentrations (Fig. 3). In most tissues, the GSH/GSSG ratio exceeds 100:1, so that protein thiols with a K_{eq} of 1 would require massive changes in GSH/GSSG ratios and equilibration with the new steady state to manifest significant alteration in PSH/PSSG status. The formation of protein–protein disulfides would be expected to be influenced by absolute GSH concentrations, but direct experimental tests of this proposal are needed.

We have studied the effects of hyperoxia and other examples of oxidant stresses in vivo on protein thiol status of experimental animals. In these studies, we have employed the reagent monobromobimane (mBBr), which forms highly fluorescent thioether derivatives with free thiols, but is unreactive with disulfides and most other functional groups (Fig. 4). Tissue protein thiol status of experimental animals in vivo is resistant to oxidation from hyperoxia or other oxidant stresses (38,102,106,107). We have observed a marked loss of thiol-dependent fluorescence in a single mitochondrial protein in the livers of mice treated with hepatotoxic doses of acetaminophen, and have characterized this protein as carbamyl phosphate synthetase-I (101). This effect is paralleled by loss of enzyme activity, as measured in tissue homogenates and by hyperammonemia, but the absence of recovery of thiol status or of enzyme activity with treatment of homogenates with the disulfide-reducing agent dithiothreitol (DTT) suggests that there is alkylation, rather than *S*-thiolation, of the thiol(s).

The use of mBBr has significant limitations, some of which are minimized by the use of the method developed by Thomas and his colleagues (Fig. 5; 108–111). This method, which involves the use of cycloheximide to inhibit protein synthesis and [^{35}S]cysteine to label the cellular GSH pool, is not readily adaptable for use in vivo and in human studies. In addition to problems associated with interpretation of experimental models in vitro, the method of Thomas is limited by artifacts that are associated with cycloheximide and by inhibition of protein synthesis and the inability to detect protein–protein disulfides.

An additional limitation of the method described by Thomas is that it assesses changes only in cellular compartments in which the GSH pool is labeled adequately, whereas there is strong evidence that mitochondrial GSH is substantively compartmentalized from the cytosolic pool (Fig. 6). Olafsdottir and Reed

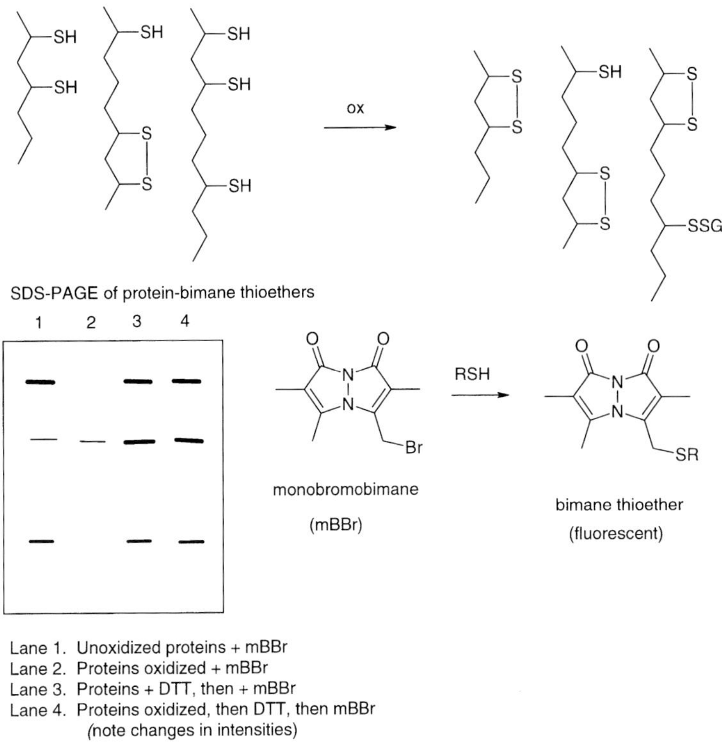

Figure 4 Determination of protein thiol status using monobromobimane (mBBr): The approach is illustrated in schematic fashion. The chain-like structures are not intended to depict carbon–carbon bonds, but to represent unspecified peptide segments of undetermined length and composition. Free thiols are alkylated by mBBr, yielding highly fluorescent thioethers, which are separated by electrophoresis and detected by fluorescence. *S*-Thiolation diminishes the fluorescence, but this effect can be reversed with dithiothreitol (DTT) or other disulfide-reducing agents. Irreversible oxidation, such as to the sulfonic acid, or alkylation to form a thioether, would cause loss of fluorescence that would not be reversed by DTT.

(112) observed no increase in GSSG in the media from isolated mitochondria exposed to *tert*-butylhydroperoxide (t-BuOOH), indicating that mitochondria may not have an effective GSSG efflux system. Their data are consistent with the finding that the human protein associated with multidrug resistance, or ATP-dependent glutathione *S*-conjugate pump, which also can export GSSG as a substrate, is located at the plasma membrane, but is not found associated with mitochondrial membranes (113,114). Accumulation of GSSG within mitochondria,

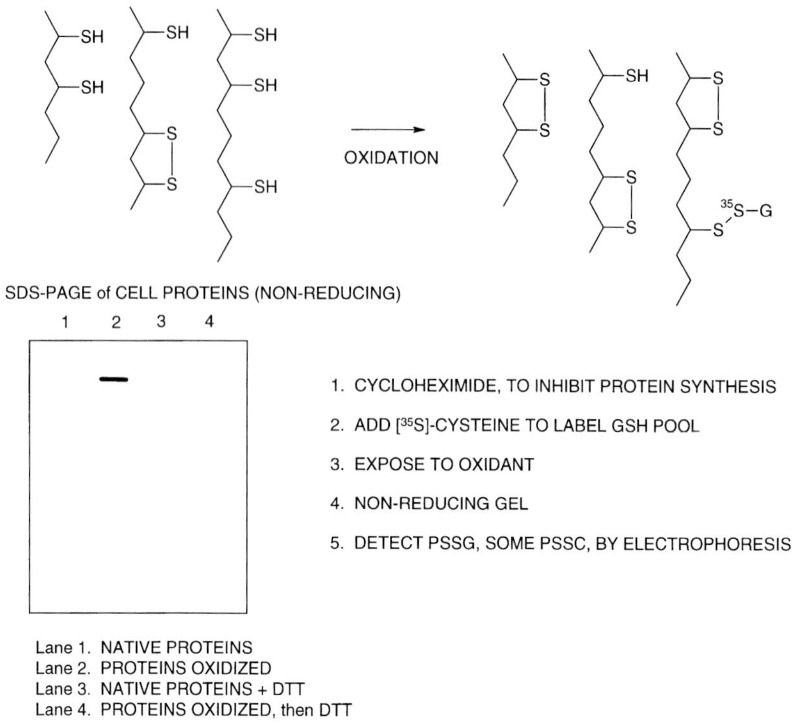

Figure 5 Determination of protein *S*-glutathiolation: In this approach to the study of protein oxidation, cells are treated with cycloheximide to inhibit protein synthesis, [^{35}S] Cysteine is added to label the cellular GSH pool, and cells exposed to the oxidant to be studied. Proteins are separated by electrophoresis and *S*-glutathiolation detected by autoradiography. As can be seen, this method gives lower background, but does not detect the formation of protein–protein disulfides and would be difficult to use in vivo.

therefore, may be more likely than are increases in whole-cell or tissue GSSG concentrations during oxidant stresses. The lack of an effective GSSG efflux system in mitochondria would place additional emphasis on glutathione reductase activities in mitochondria relative to cellular resistance to oxidant stress, for the absence of an effective GSSG efflux system would mean that only the reduction of GSSG by glutathione reductase would be active in maintaining appropriate GSH/GSSG ratios.

Mitochondrial GSH/GSSG ratios may function in regulating the thiol–disulfide status of mitochondrial protein thiol groups, such as the mitochondrial permeability transition (MPT) pore. The MPT pore is a voltage-dependent,

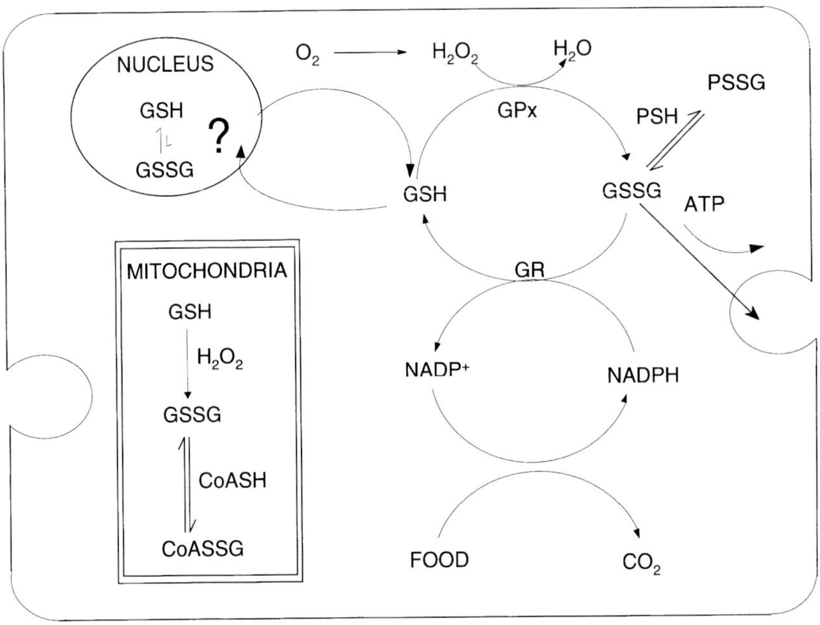

Figure 6 Compartmentation of GSH: Cellular GSH is not distributed homogeneously, and significant compartmentation of mitochondrial GSH has been observed. Mitochondrial thiol–disulfide status appears to be particularly important for cell survival, but mitochondria represent 10% or less of the total cellular mass and GSH, which makes assessment of the thiol–disulfide redox status of mitochondria in live animal models difficult. We have employed measurements of CoASH/CoASSG ratios as markers of intramitochondrial redox status.

cyclosporine-inhibitable channel that allows solutes of less than 1500 molecular weight to equilibrate across the mitochondrial inner membrane, and is responsible for the rapid efflux of solutes such as GSH and Ca^{2+}. Blockage of the opening of the MPT pore by cyclosporine protects cells from oxidant-mediated lethal injury, and the redox status of vicinal thiol groups in a mitochondrial protein appears to play a crucial role in determining the gating potential of the transition (115–117).

Mitochondria constitute about 10% of a cell's mass, and a comparable fraction of cellular GSH. Changes in mitochondrial GSH and GSSG status are difficult to determine, particularly in vivo, partly because of the difficulty in isolating mitochondria under conditions that do not permit significant changes in thiols and disulfides (118). Mitochondrial GSH exchanges with cytosolic GSH, but is regulated separately (78). Mitochondria do not appear to export GSSG (112).

Coenzyme A (CoASH), which is located principally in the mitochondria, and CoASSG (the mixed disulfide of CoASH with GSH) exchange with GSH and GSSG (103,104). Thus, levels of CoASH and CoASSG, which can be measured by high-performance liquid chromatography (HPLC) in acid supernatants of rapidly frozen tissues, can provide an estimate of intramitochondrial thiol–disulfide redox status (119).

In addition to redox modulation of pore function and enzyme activity, oxidation–reduction effects of gene expression have been reported (120). Redox control of gene transcription has been suggested to be expressed through formation and disassembly of iron–sulfur clusters (121). According to this hypothesis, the formation of [2Fe-2S] and [4Fe-4S] clusters and assembly into protein-bound configurations with the appropriate apoproteins, such as the iron-regulatory protein, offers a means for control of gene expression by what amounts to a redox-sensing mechanism. A similar interaction of the [2Fe-2S] cluster in ferrochelatase with nitric oxide has been proposed (122) along with the hypothesis that the anemia frequently observed in individuals with chronic infections may be partly due to inactivation of ferrochelatase, upregulation of heme oxygenase, and increased translation of mRNA for transferrin receptor protein, all in response to actions on [Fe-S] clusters by nitric oxide produced by inducible nitric oxide synthetase in activated macrophages.

B. Protein Carbonyls

In recent years, proteins have received increasing attention as targets for free radical and oxidant damage (123). Protein oxidation can lead to a loss of critical sulfhydryl groups, in addition to modifications of amino acids, leading to the formation of carbonyls and other oxidized moieties (Fig. 7). One important point illustrated in Figure 7 is that, in the absence of redox-active iron chelates or direct sources of other reactive oxygen species, increased generation of H_2O_2 will result almost exclusively in formation of GSSG, and perhaps of PSSG. The oxidations of proteins and other biomolecules to different types of products, illustrated here as the oxidation of proteins to aldehydes, depends on active catalysts. The protein carbonyls are frequently investigated through derivatization with DNPH, presumably through formation of the corresponding hydrazones. Oxidized proteins are much more susceptible to proteolysis (124), but at the same time, oxidatively modified proteins or oxidized regions of these proteins are degraded less effectively by proteolysis (123,125). The accumulation of protein carbonyl groups appears to increase with age (41). Increases in oxidized proteins may be involved with age-related losses of selected biochemical and physiological functions, and may reflect unrepaired damage to other cellular macromolecules, such as DNA. As with lipids, the removal of oxidized proteins is an ongoing process, and it is only when the rate at which they are produced exceeds their rates of removal or

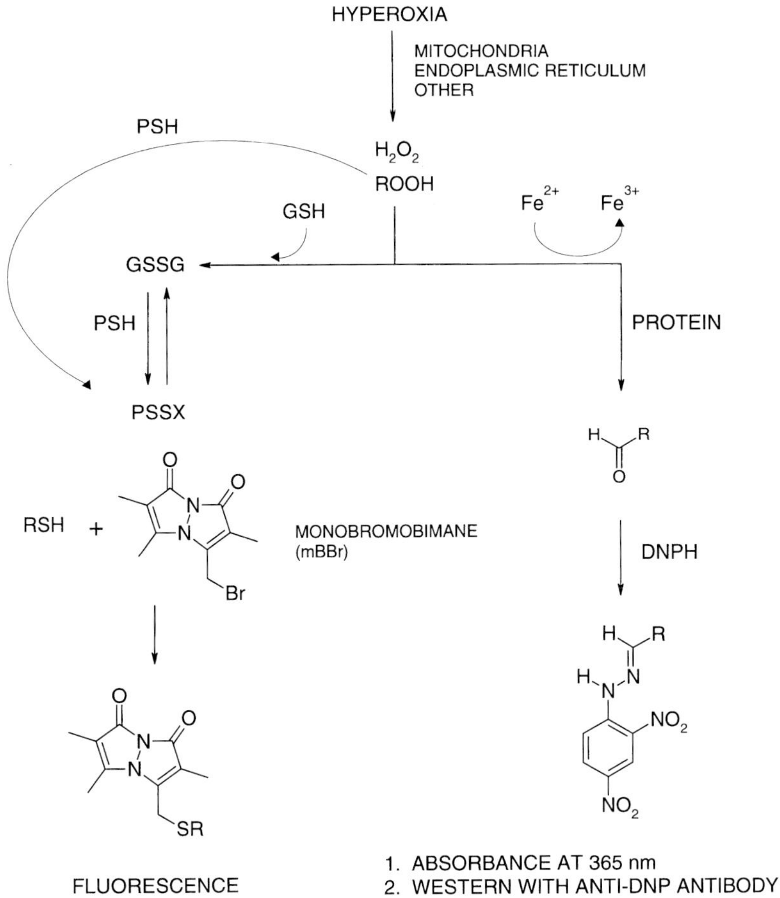

Figure 7 Biomarker competition in assessing the effects of oxidant stress: Although in some cases multiple biomarkers of oxidant exposure change in unison, there are examples in which one parameter changes in discordance with another. Illustrated here is the disposition of hydroperoxides that, in the absence of redox-active iron chelates, drive formation of GSSG, and perhaps of PSSG. In the presence of redox-active transition metal chelates—in this example iron—direct oxidations of proteins to different types of products, illustrated here as the oxidation of proteins to aldehydes (protein carbonyls). These "protein carbonyls" frequently are investigated through derivatization with DNPH.

replacement with fresh, fully functional molecules that cell injury becomes evident (126).

A recent study in prematurely delivered infants correlated the need for more than 40% oxygen in the first few days of life, and the need for ventilation after 3 days, with increased protein oxidation in BAL samples (44). This study documents that although there is some relation between the oxygen concentration administered and protein oxidation, there is also an association between oxidative events and duration of ventilation, independent of the concentration of supplemental inspired oxygen. Studies in experimental animals have shown increases in DNPH reactivities of proteins in BAL fluids (45). In this study, β-casein was identified as having been oxidized to a DNPH-reactive form. This observation not only implicates this irreversible oxidation in the effects of hyperoxia, but also indicates that the participation of cytotoxic T lymphocytes, the most likely source of the β-casein, needs to be investigated in hyperoxic lung injury.

C. Lipid Peroxidation Products

The peroxidation of lipids (Fig. 8) has been studied extensively, partly because of the structural and functional importance of lipids in cell membranes, partly because many of the products and intermediates formed as a result of the oxidation of lipids exhibit potent biological activities, and partly because of the ease with which some products of lipid peroxidation can be measured. Unfortunately, the simplicity of some lipid peroxidation assays (particularly the measurement of thiobarbituric acid-reactive species, frequently called TBARS, and many times inappropriately equated with malondialdehyde) has yielded many published reports that do not take into consideration the numerous limitations of the individual assays (127–131). Furthermore, the issue of cause and effect is often ignored, as are distinctions between mechanisms of initiation of injury versus those responsible for propagation of the lesion. Cellular lipids are likely to become much more susceptible to peroxidation after cell death, which is an important consideration when assessing peroxidation as a cause, rather than a marker, of cell death. The peroxidation of lipids as a consequence of cell death may also lead to additional cell killing or organ dysfunction.

Analytical methods have been developed that assess the concentrations of specific products of lipid peroxidation (9,132–135). Application of these methods to studies of relevant biological models has frequently led to observations that may seem surprising, if the effects of competitive pathways for peroxidation and secondary reactions are not given appropriate consideration (127). These chemically specific methods of analysis, when applied to studies of hyperoxic lung injury, can provide critical information on the nature of the oxidative processes that are operative in hyperoxia. In addition, many of the individual products of

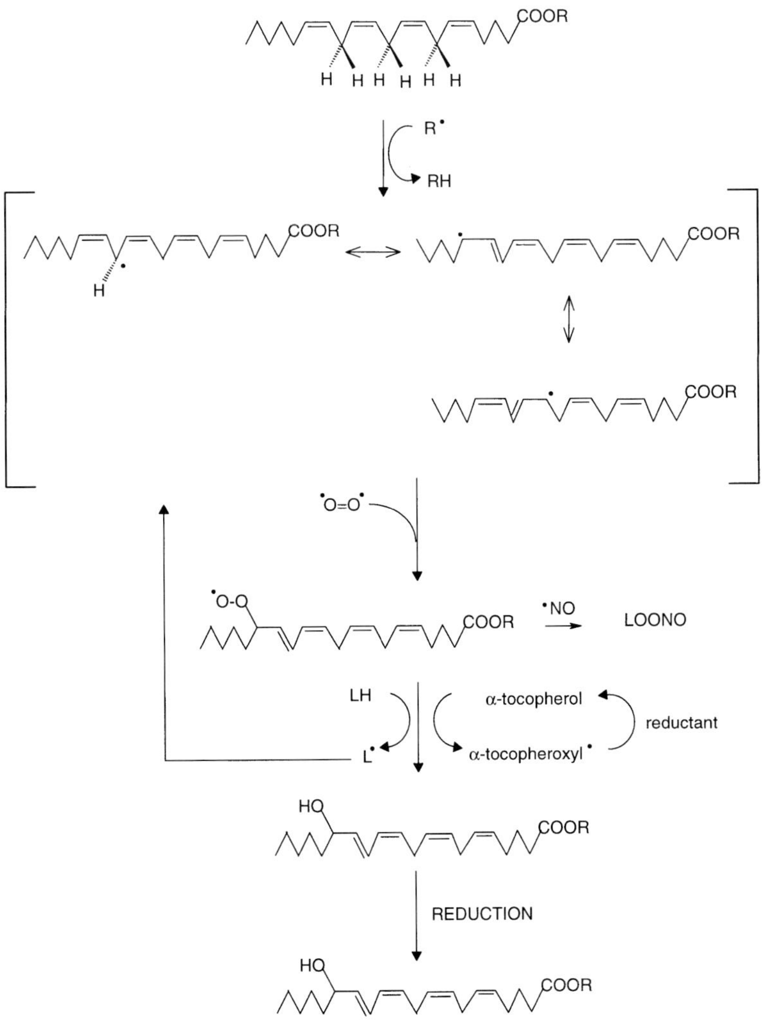

Figure 8 Lipid peroxidation: Radicals react with arachidonic acid primarily by abstraction of one of the six bis-allylic H atoms. The resulting pentadienyl radicals, one of which is shown in its three principal resonance forms, reacts rapidly with dioxygen at either terminus of the conjugated system to form the corresponding peroxyl radicals. The peroxyl radicals can propagate the overall reaction by abstraction of a bis-allylic H atom from another lipid molecule, unless reduced by α-tocopherol or other antioxidant. The product hydroperoxide can be reduced to the hydroxy acid, or can mediate oxidation of other biomolecules. This scheme is highly simplified.

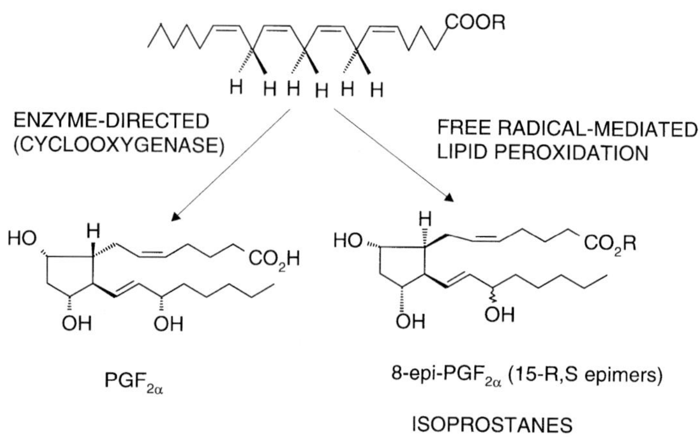

Figure 9 Comparison of structures of prostaglandins produced enzymatically through cyclooxygenase and of isoprostanes produced by chemical oxidation: The 8-epi-$PGF_{2\alpha}$, produced by chemical oxidation of arachidonic acid, differs only in the stereochemistry at the 8-position and possesses potent physiological properties. Although the enzymatic oxidation is specific, the analogous chemical process can produce numerous isomeric products.

lipid oxidation exhibit potent biological activities that are likely to contribute to the overall pathology of oxidant exposure, despite that some products of lipid peroxidation are formed in rather low efficiencies. For example, 8-epi prostaglandin-$F_{2\alpha}$ ($PGF_{2\alpha}$), which is formed by the chemical oxidation of arachidonic acid in phospholipids (Fig. 9), is an exceedingly potent vasoconstrictor (135). Quantitative assessments of the efficiency with which this product is formed during lipid peroxidation have estimated that more than 100,000 molecules of arachidonate are oxidized for every molecule of 8-epi-$PGF_{2\alpha}$ produced (136). The low yield of formation does not necessarily mean that the processes leading to the formation of 8-epi-$PGF_{2\alpha}$ and related products are not relevant physiologically or pathologically, because of the potent physiological activities. The data indicate, however, that other specific products of lipid peroxidation that are formed in much larger quantities also need to be considered (127). For example, certain peroxidized phospholipids form, through β-scission reactions (9), highly active platelet-activating factor (PAF)-like lipids. Not all radical species stimulate lipid peroxidation. Rubbo et al. (137) have reported that nitric oxide forms derivatives of lipid oxidation products, apparently through radical–radical-coupling reactions, the net effects of which would be termination of the radical chain propagation (see Fig. 8) and formation of LONO and LOONO species. The significance of these reactions and the biological activities of these products, if any, are still poorly understood.

D. Oxidation of Nucleic Acids

One possible mechanism that has been proposed to explain cell death after exposure to reactive oxygen species (ROS) involves the enzyme poly(ADP-ribose) polymerase, which is activated following peroxide-mediated DNA damage (138). Once activated, poly(ADP-ribose) polymerase uses large amounts of NAD to repair DNA damaged by ROS. Depletion of NAD has been proposed as a possible mechanism by which a cell's ability to produce ATP is impaired, thereby leading to energy deficiency, changes in calcium homeostasis, and ultimately, in cell death. Although this mechanism may not be sufficient to explain the effects of oxidant injury (139), oxidant processes can disrupt pathways that are critical for the maintenance of normal adenine and pyridine nucleotide status. Because these nucleotides are necessary for viability, affected cells, if not overtly damaged, are at least likely to be more susceptible to other stresses.

With ^{32}P-postlabeling analyses of DNA that was exposed to H_2O_2 and Fe(II) or Ni(II) in vitro, we recently detected a series of DNA alterations that we called type II I-compounds (140). Studies using synthetic oligomers of known structure indicated the formation of intrastrand cross-links, such that one major product formed only if dAdA were present, whereas other products were found only following oxidation of oligodeoxyribonucleotides containing AC or CA sequences, respectively. Other adducts were observed that appeared to be independent of the identity of the 3′-base, suggesting the formation of $5' \rightarrow 3'$ purine–sugar cross-links. Some of the modified products characterized by these studies of oxidation of synthetic DNA comigrate with products isolated from renal DNA of rats treated with ferric nitrilotriacetate in vivo, supporting the potential relevance of related transformations in disease processes. These observations imply considerable potential significance of these processes in human health and disease, but elucidation is needed of the structures of these products of DNA oxidation, their metabolic dispositions, and the biological consequences of their formation.

E. Oxidation of Carbohydrates

Very little is known about the oxidation of carbohydrate moieties, hyperoxia, lung injury, and chronic lung disease (CLD) of early infancy. Carbohydrates can be oxidized nonenzymatically, and the primary expectation for biological manifestations of such oxidations would be altered function of adhesion molecules. These transformations are likely to be complex and difficult to study, and commercially available kits for their analysis are not expected in the near future.

V. Roles of Iron Metabolism in Reactive Oxygen-Mediated Tissue Injury

A substantial body of experimental evidence indicates that the availability of chemically redox-active iron chelates can be a major determinant of cellular responses to reactive oxygen species (45,141–144). The scheme presented in Figure 10 suggests a framework within which the mechanisms responsible for these observations can be considered. Intracellular iron is normally sequestered in redox-inactive forms, such as in ferritin, so that very little chemically "free" iron is available. Reduction of ferritin-bound ferric iron (Fe^{3+}) to ferrous iron, which is bound less avidly to ferritin, can result in release of the iron. This iron, released from ferritin or other physiological pools, will bind to available ligands and, in the presence of reactive peroxides, can catalyze oxidation at or near the site of binding, depicted in the present example as formation of a protein carbonyl.

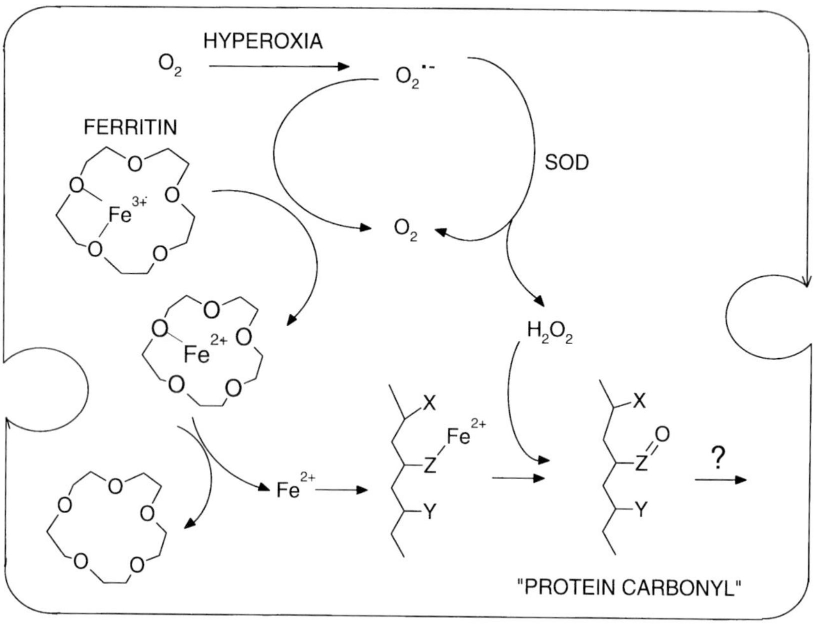

Figure 10 Possible source of redox-active iron chelates in hyperoxia: Intracellular iron normally is sequestered carefully in redox-inactive forms, such as in ferritin. Reduction of ferritin-bound ferric iron (Fe^{3+}) to ferrous iron, which is bound less avidly, can result in release of the iron. This iron will bind to available ligands and, in the presence of reactive peroxides, can catalyze oxidation at or near the site of binding, depicted in the present example as formation a protein carbonyl.

Some prematurely born infants are not as efficient in sequestration of iron (145), which may present problems. In studies reported by Revenis and Kaliner (146), prematurely born infants with hyaline membrane disease who recovered without subsequent CLD had higher concentrations of lactoferrin in their tracheal aspirates than did a comparable group of infants with subsequent CLD. This finding suggests that lactoferrin might have an important role related to inflammatory lung disease of early infancy. Another study, however, showed marked toxic effects of the iron chelator desferrioxamine in premature baboons that were exposed to hyperoxia (147). This latter report indicates that pharmacological interventions designed to modulate iron homeostasis in prematurely born infants or experimental animals must be based on a more complete understanding of the complex mechanisms of oxidation and lung injury than is now available.

VI. Summary and Conclusions

It is our interpretation of the evidence now available that the oxidative injury component of CLD is not the result of a relatively simple alteration in a balance between oxidants and antioxidants. Understanding the complex mechanisms by which reactive oxygen species induce biochemical alterations, thereby leading to cellular dysfunction, and integrating these insights with whole animal and human physiological responses, are essential for the rational design of approaches to prevent and treat the adverse effects of hyperoxia which, in turn, should reduce the incidence and severity of CLD.

References

1. Zimmerman JJ. Bronchoalveolar inflammatory pathophysiology of bronchopulmonary dysplasia. Clin Perinatol 1995; 22:429–456.
2. Abman SH, Groothius JR. Pathophysiology and treatment of bronchopulmonary dysplasia. Pediatr Clin North Am 1994; 41:277–315.
3. Northway WH Jr. An introduction to bronchopulmonary dysplasia. Clin Perinatol 1992; 19:489–495.
4. Northway WH Jr. Bronchopulmonary dysplasia: twenty-five years later. Pediatrics 1992; 89:969–973.
5. Frank L, Sosenko IRS. Development of lung antioxidant enzyme system in late gestation: possible implications for the prematurely born infant. J Pediatr 1987; 110:9–14.
6. Frank L, Sosenko IRS. Prenatal development of lung antioxidant enzymes in four species. J Pediatr 1987; 110:106–110.
7. Loeb GA, Skelton DC, Forman HJ. Dependence of mixed disulfide formation in alveolar macrophages upon production of oxidized glutathione: effect of selenium depletion. Biochem Pharmacol 1989; 38:3119–3121.

8. Cantin AM, Begin R. Glutathione and inflammatory disorders of the lung. Lung 1991; 169:123–138.
9. Zimmerman GA, Prescott SM, McIntyre TM. Oxidatively fragmented phospholipids as inflammatory mediators: the dark side of polyunsaturated lipids. J Nutr 1995; 125:1661S–1665S.
10. Contreras M, Hariharan N, Lewandoski JR, Ciesielski W, Kosick R, Zimmerman JJ. Bronchoalveolar oxyradical inflammatory elements herald bronchopulmonary dysplasia. Crit Care Med 1996; 24:29–37.
11. Groneck P, Gotze-Speer B, Oppermann M, Eiffert H, Speer CP. Association of pulmonary inflammation and increased microvascular permeability during the development of bronchopulmonary dysplasia: a sequential analysis of inflammatory mediators in respiratory fluids of high-risk preterm neonates. Pediatrics 1994; 93: 712–718.
12. Pierce MR, Bancalari E. The role of inflammation in the pathogenesis of bronchopulmonary dysplasia. Pediatr Pulmonol 1995; 19:371–378.
13. Shi MM, Godleski JJ, Paulauskis JD. Regulation of macrophage inflammatory protein-1a mRNA by oxidative stress. J Biol Chem 1996; 271:5878–5883.
14. Watterberg KL, Demers LM, Scott SM, Murphy S. Chorioamnionitis and early lung inflammation in infants in whom bronchopulmonary dysplasia develops. Pediatrics 1996; 97:210–215.
15. Elsayed NM. Toxicology of blast overpressure. Toxicology 1997; 121:1–15.
16. Elsayed NM, Gorbunov NV, Kagen VE. A proposed biochemical mechanism involving hemoglobin for blast overpressure-induced injury. Toxicology 1997; 121: 81–90.
17. Pittet JF, Mackersie RC, Martin TR, Matthay MA. Biological markers of acute lung injury: prognostic and pathogenetic significance. Am Rev Respir Dis 1997; 155:1187–1205.
18. Frank L, Bucher JR, Roberts RJ. Oxygen toxicity in neonatal and adult animal of various species. J Appl Physiol 1978; 45:699–704.
19. Yam J, Frank L, Roberts RJ. Oxygen toxicity: comparison of lung biochemical responses in neonatal and adult rats. Pediatr Res 1978; 12:115–119.
20. Frank L, Sosenko IS. Failure of premature rabbits to increase antioxidant enzymes during hyperoxic exposure: increased susceptibility to pulmonary oxygen toxicity compared with term rabbits. Pediatr Res 1991; 29:292–296.
21. Sosenko IR, Frank L. Guinea pig lung development: antioxidant enzymes and premature survival in high O_2. Am J Physiol 1987; 252:R693–R698.
22. Sosenko IR, Frank L. Lung development in the fetal guinea pig: surfactant, morphology, and premature viability. Pediatr Res 1987; 21:427–431.
23. de Lemos R, Wolfsdorf J, Nachman R, et al. Lung injury from oxygen in lambs. Anesthesiology 1969; 30:609–618.
24. Crapo JD, Barry BE, Foscue HA, Shelburne J. Structural and biochemical changes in rat lungs occurring during exposures to lethal and adaptive doses of oxygen. Am Rev Respir Dis 1980; 122:123–143.
25. Bressack MA, McMillan DD, Bland RD. Pulmonary oxygen toxicity: increased microvascular permeability to protein in unanesthetised lambs. Lymphology 1979; 12:133–139.

26. Hansen TN, Hazinski TA, Bland RD. Vitamin E does not prevent oxygen-induced lung injury in newborn lambs. Pediatr Res 1982; 16:583–587.
27. Newman JH, Loyd JE, English DK, Ogletree ML, Fulderson WJ, Brigham KL. Effects of 100% oxygen on lung vascular function in awake sheep. J Appl Physiol 1983; 54:1379–1386.
28. Fukushima M, King LS, Kang K, Banerjee M, Newmann JH. Lung mechanics and airway reactivity in sheep during development of oxygen toxicity. J Appl Physiol 1990; 69:1779–1785.
29. Hazinski TA, Kennedy KA, France ML, Hansen TN. Pulmonary O_2 toxicity in lambs: physiological and biochemical effects of endotoxin infusion. J Appl Physiol 1988; 65:1579–1585.
30. Smith LJ, Friedman H, Anderson J. Hyperoxic lung injury in mice: effect of neutrophil depletion and food deprivation. J Lab Clin Med 1988; 111:449–458.
31. Smith LJ. Hyperoxic lung injury: biochemical, cellular, and morphologic characterization in the mouse. J Lab Clin Med 1985; 106:269–278.
32. Berg JT, Allison RC, Taylor AT. Endotoxin extends survival of adult mice in hyperoxia. Proc Soc Exp Biol Med 1990; 90:167–170.
33. Turrens JF, Freeman BA, Crapo JD. Hyperoxia increases H_2O_2 release by lung mitochondria and microsomes. Arch Biochem Biophys 1982; 217:411–421.
34. Deneke SM, Gershoff SN, Fanburg BL. Potentiation of oxygen toxicity in rats by dietary protein or amino acid deficiency. J Appl Physiol 1983; 54:147–151.
35. Deneke SM, Lynch BA, Fanburg BL. Effects of low protein diets or feed restriction on rat lung glutathione and oxygen toxicity. J Nutr 1985; 115:726–732.
36. Fanburg BL, Deneke SM. Protein deficiency potentiates oxygen toxicity. Exp Lung Res 1988; 14:911–919.
37. Stenzel JD, Welty SE, Benzick AE, Smith EO, Smith CV, Hansen TN. Hyperoxic lung injury in Fischer-344 and Sprague-Dawley rats in vivo. Free Radic Biol Med 1993; 14:531–539.
38. Awasthi S, Gyurasics A, Knight SA, Welty SE, Smith CV. Protein oxidation biomarkers in hyperoxic lung injury in rats: effects of U-74389. Toxicol Lett 1998; 95:47–61.
39. Smith CV, Jones DP, Guenthner TM, Lash LH, Lauterburg BH. Compartmentation of glutathione. Implications for the study of toxicity and disease. Toxicol Appl Pharmacol 1996; 140:1–12.
40. Levine RL. Oxidative modification of glutamine synthetase. I. Inactivation is due to loss of one histidine residue. J Biol Chem 1983; 258:11823–11827.
41. Stadtman ER. Protein oxidation and aging. Science 1992; 257:1220–1224.
42. Levine RL, Williams JA, Stadtman ER, Shacter E. Carbonyl assays for determination of oxidatively modified proteins. Methods Enzymol 1994; 233:346–357.
43. Shacter E, Williams JA, Lim M, Levine RL. Differential susceptibility of plasma proteins to oxidative modification: examination by Western blot immunoassay. Free Radic Biol Med 1994; 17:429–437.
44. Gladstone IM, Levine RL. Oxidation of proteins in neonatal lungs. Pediatrics 1994; 93:764–768.
45. Knight SA, Smith CV, Welty SE. Iron and oxidized β-casein in the lavages of hyperoxic Fischer-344 rats. Life Sci 1997; 62:165–176.

46. Wearden ME, Dzdic N, Rogers LK, Smith CV. Oxidation of lung proteins in rats exposed to inhaled nitric oxide and hyperoxia [abstr]. Pediatr Res 1998; 43:202A.
47. Wearden ME, Hegemier SE, Dzdic N, et al. Protein oxidation and nitrotyrosine formation in tracheal aspirate fluids of mechanically ventilated neonates exposed to hyperoxia and/or inhaled nitric oxide [abstr]. Pediatr Res 1998; 43:203A.
48. Yang C-Y, Gu Z-W, Yang H-X, Gotto AM Jr, Smith CV. Oxidative modifications of apoB-100 by exposure of low density lipoproteins to HOCl in vitro. Free Radic Biol Med 1997; 23:82–89.
49. Smith CV, Rogers LK, Garcia-Prats AJ, Gu ZW, Yang C-Y. Oxidation of cysteine residues in proteins by myeloperoxidase (MPO) or HOCl in vitro produces sulfenyl or sulfonyl chloride intermediates [abstr]. Pediatr Res 1998; 43:196A.
50. Freeman BA, Topolosky MK, Crapo JD. Hyperoxia increases oxygen radical production in rat lung homogenates. Arch Biochem Biophys 1982; 216:477–484.
51. Kiezka H, Kappus H. Oxygen dependence of CCl_4-induced lipid peroxidation in vitro and in vivo. Toxicol Lett 1980; 5:191–196.
52. Ortiz de Montellano PR. Catalytic sites of hemoprotein peroxidases. Annu Rev Pharmacol Toxicol 1992; 32:89–107.
53. Frank L. Developmental aspects of experimental pulmonary oxygen toxicity. Free Radic Biol Med 1991; 11:463–494.
54. Frank L. Antioxidants, nutrition, and bronchopulmonary dysplasia. Clin Perinatol 1992; 19:541–562.
55. Freeman BA, Young SL, Crapo JD. Liposome-mediated augmentation of superoxide dismutase in endothelial cells prevents oxygen injury. J Biol Chem 1983; 258: 12534–12542.
56. Oury TD, Chang L-Y, Marklund SL, Day BJ, Crapo JD. Immunocytochemical localization of extracellular superoxide dismutase in human lung. Lab Invest 1994; 70:889–898.
57. Hazinski TA, France M, Kennedy KA, Hansen TN. Cimetidine reduces hyperoxic lung injury in lambs. J Appl Physiol 1989; 67:2586–2592.
58. Gonder JC, Proctor RA, Will JA. Genetic differences in oxygen toxicity are correlated with cytochrome P-450 inducibility. Proc Natl Acad Sci USA 1985; 82:6315–6319.
59. Ogden BE, Murphy SA, Saunders GC, Pathak D, Johnson JD. Neonatal lung neutrophils and elastase/proteinase inhibitor imbalance. Am Rev Respir Dis 1984; 130: 817–821.
60. Harlan JM, Schwartz BR, Reidy MA, Schwartz SM, Ochs HD, Harker LA. Activated neutrophils disrupt endothelial monolayer integrity by an oxygen radical-independent mechanism. Lab Invest 1985; 52:141–150.
61. Pontremoli S, Melloni E, Michetti M, et al. Cytolytic effects of neutrophils: role for a membrane-bound neutral proteinase. Proc Natl Acad Sci USA 1986; 83:1685–1689.
62. Tsaka T, Herkner KR. Polymorphonuclear elastase in neonatal sepsis. Clin Chim Acta 1990; 193:103–112.
63. Simchowitz L, Spilberg I. Chemotactic factor-induced generation of superoxide radicals by human neutrophils: evidence for the role of sodium. J Immunol 1979; 123:2428–2435.

64. Thomas EL, Learn DB, Jefferson MM, Weatherred W. Superoxide-dependent oxidation of extracellular reducing agents by isolated neutrophils. J Biol Chem 1988; 263:2178–2186.
65. Carden DL, Smith JK, Korthius RJ. Oxidant-mediated, CD 18-dependent microvascular dysfunction induced by complement-activated granulocytes. Am J Physiol 1991; 260:H1144–H1152.
66. Nathan CF. Neutrophil activation on biological surfaces. J Clin Invest 1987; 80: 1550–1560.
67. Nathan CF. Respiratory burst in adherent human neutrophils: triggering by colony-stimulating factors CSF-GM and CSF-G. Blood 1989; 73:301–306.
68. Nathan C, Srimal S, Farber C, et al. Cytokine-induced respiratory burst of human neutrophils: dependence on extracellular matrix proteins and CD11/CD18 integrins. J Cell Biol 1989; 109:1341–1349.
69. Shappell SB, Toman C, Anderson DC, Taylor AA, Entman ML, Smith CW. Mac-1 (CD11b/CD18) mediates adherence-dependent hydrogen peroxide production by human and canine neutrophils. J Immunol 1990; 144:2702–2711.
70. Shasby DM, Fox RB, Harada RN, Repine JE. Reduction of the edema of acute hyperoxic lung injury by granulocyte depletion. J Appl Physiol 1982; 52:1237
71. Raj U, Hazinski TA, Bland RD. Oxygen-induced lung microvascular injury in neutropenic rabbits and lambs. J Appl Physiol 1985; 58:921–927.
72. Wegner CD, Wolyniec WW, LaPlante AM, et al. Intracellular adhesion molecule-1 contributes to pulmonary oxygen toxicity in mice: role of leukocytes revisited. Lung 1992; 170:267–279.
73. Walther FJ, Kuipers IM, Pavlova Z, Willebrand D, Abuchowski A, Viau AT. Mitigation of pulmonary oxygen toxicity in premature lambs with intravenous antioxidants. Exp Lung Res 1990; 16:177–189.
74. Patterson CE, Butler JA, Byrne FD, Rhodes ML. Oxidant lung injury: intervention with sulfhydryl reagents. Lung 1985; 1985; 163:23–32.
75. Richards IM, Griffin RL, Fidler SF, Jacobsen EJ. Effect of the 21-aminosteroid, U-74389F, on hyperoxic lung injury in rats. Agents Actions 1993; 39:C136–C138.
76. Larsson A, Orrenius S, Holmgren A, Mannervik B, eds. Functions of Glutathione: Biochemical, Physiological, Toxicological, and Clinical Aspects. New York: Raven Press, 1983.
77. Dolphin D, Avramovic O, Poulson R, eds. Glutathione: Chemical, Biochemical, and Medical Aspects. III. New York: John Wiley & Sons, 1989.
78. Meister A. Glutathione deficiency produced by inhibition of its synthesis, and its reversal; applications in research and therapy. Pharm Ther 1991; 51:155–194.
79. Reed DJ. Glutathione: toxicological implications. Annu Rev Pharmacol Toxicol 1990; 30:603–631.
80. Jenkinson SG, Black RD, Lawrence RA. Glutathione concentrations in rat lung bronchoalveolar lavage fluid: effects of hyperoxia. J Lab Clin Med 1988; 112:345–351.
81. Kennedy KA, Lane NL. Effect of in vivo hyperoxia on the glutathione system in neonatal rat lung. Exp Lung Res 1994; 20:73–83.
82. Pacht ER, Timerman AP, Lykens MG, Merola AJ. Deficiency of alveolar fluid

glutathione in patients with sepsis and the adult respiratory distress syndrome. Chest 1991; 100:1397–1403.

83. Smith CV, Mitchell JR. Pharmacological aspects of glutathione in drug metabolism. In: Dolphin D, Poulson R, Avramovic O, eds. Coenzymes and Cofactors. New York: John Wiley & Sons, 1989:1–44.
84. Smith CV, Hughes H, Lauterburg BH, Mitchell JR. Chemical nature of reactive metabolites determines their biological interactions with glutathione. In: Larsson A, Orrenius S, Holmgren A, Mannervik B, eds. Functions of Glutathione: Biochemical, Physiological, Toxicological, and Clinical Aspects. New York: Raven Press, 1983:125–138.
85. Smith CV, Hansen TN, Martin NE, McMicken HW, Elliott SJ. Oxidant stress responses in premature infants during exposure to hyperoxia. Pediatr Res 1993; 34: 360–365.
86. Rollins D, Larsson A, Steen B, et al. Glutathione and gamma-glutamyl cycle enzymes in human fetal liver. J Pharmacol Exp Ther 1981; 217:697–700.
87. Zlotkin SH, Anderson GH. Sulfur balances in intravenously fed infants: effects of cysteine supplementation. Am J Clin Nutr 1982; 36:862–867.
88. Zlotkin SH, Anderson GH. The development of cystathionase activity during the first year of life. Pediatr Res 1982; 16:65–68.
89. Corcoran GB, Racz WJ, Smith CV, Mitchell JR. Effects of *N*-acetylcysteine on acetaminophen covalent binding and hepatic necrosis in mice. J Pharmacol Exp Ther 1985; 232:864–872.
90. Corcoran GB, Todd EL, Racz WJ, Hughes H, Smith CV, Mitchell JR. Effects of *N*-acetylcysteine on the disposition and metabolism of acetaminophen in mice. J Pharmacol Exp Ther 1985; 232:857–863.
91. Smith LJ, Horcher P, Anderson J, Shamsuddin M. Effect of fasting on the lung glutathione redox cycle in air- and oxygen-exposed mice: beneficial effects of sugar. J Lab Clin Med 1990; 116:717–723.
92. Huang C-S, Chang L-S, Anderson ME, Meister A. Catalytic and regulatory properties of the heavy subunit of rat kidney γ-glutamylcysteine synthetase. J Biol Chem 1993; 268:19675–19680.
93. Helbling G, Von Overbeck J, Lauterburg BH. Decreased release of glutathione into the systemic circulation of patients with HIV infection. Eur J Clin Invest 1996; 26: 38–44.
94. Buhl R, Holroyd KJ, Mastrangeli A, et al. Systemic glutathione deficiency in symptom-free HIV-seropositive individuals. Lancet 1989; 2:1294–1298.
95. Smith CV, Rogers LK, Rabin RL, Maldonado YA, Herzenberg LA, Petru A. Effects of human immunodeficiency virus (HIV) infection on plasma glutathione status in children [abstr]. Pediatr Res 1994; 35:392A.
96. Lauterburg BH, Adams JD, Mitchell JR. Hepatic glutathione homeostasis in the rat: efflux accounts for glutathione turnover. Hepatology 1984; 4:586–590.
97. Ookhtens M, Mittur AV. Developmental changes in plasma thiol–disulfide turnover in rats: a multicompartmental approach. Am J Physiol 1994; 36:R415–R425.
98. Bai C, Brown LAS, Jones DP. Glutathione transport by type II cells in perfused rat lung. Am J Physiol 1994; 267:L447–L455.
99. Lauterburg BH, Smith CV, Hughes H, Mitchell JR. Biliary excretion of glutathione

and glutathione disulfide in the rat: regulation and response to oxidative stress. J Clin Invest 1984; 73:124–133.
100. Weis M, Cotgreave IC, Moore GA, Norbeck K, Moldeus P. Accessibility of hepatocyte protein thiols to monobromobimane. Biochim Biophys Acta 1993; 1176:13–19.
101. Gupta S, Rogers LK, Taylor SK, Smith CV. Inhibition of carbamyl phosphate synthetase-I and glutamine synthetase by hepatotoxic doses of acetaminophen in mice. Toxicol Appl Pharmacol 1997; 146:317–327.
102. Gupta S, Kleiner HE, Rogers LK, Lau SS, Smith CV. Redox stress and hepatic DNA fragmentation induced by diquat in vivo are not accompanied by increased 8-hydroxydeoxyguanosine contents. Redox Rep 1997; 3:31–39.
103. Gilbert HF. Molecular and cellular aspects of thiol–disulfide exchange. Adv Enzymol 1990; 63:69–172.
104. Gilbert HF. Thiol/disulfide exchange equilibria and disulfide bond stability. Methods Enzymol 1995; 251:8–28.
105. Walker KW, Gilbert HF. Scanning and escape during protein–disulfide isomerase-assisted protein folding. J Biol Chem 1997; 272:8845–8848.
106. Moorthy B, Nguyen UT-L, Stewart KD, Welty SE, Smith CV. Induction and decline of hepatic cytochromes P4501A1 and 1A2 in rats exposed to hyperoxia are not paralleled by changes in glutathione *S*-transferase-α. Toxicol Lett 1997; 90: 67–75.
107. Adcock LM, Yamashita Y, Goddard-Finegold J, Smith CV. Cerebral hypoxia–ischemia increases microsomal iron in newborn piglets. Metab Brain Dis 1996; 11: 359–367.
108. Rokutan K, Thomas JA, Sies H. Specific *S*-thiolation of a 30-kDa cytosolic protein from rat liver under oxidative stress. Eur J Biochem 1989; 179:233–239.
109. Seres T, Ravichandran V, Moriguchi T, Rokutan K, Thomas JA, Johnston RB Jr. Protein *S*-thiolation and dethiolation during the respiratory burst in human monocytes. J Immunol 1996; 156:1973–1980.
110. Ravichandran V, Seres T, Moriguchi T, Thomas JA, Johnston RB Jr. *S*-Thiolation of glyceraldehyde-3-phosphate dehydrogenase by the phagocytosis-associated respiratory burst in blood monocytes. J Biol Chem 1994; 269:25010–25015.
111. Lii C-K, Chai Y-C, Zhao W, Thomas JA, Hendrich S. *S*-Thiolation and irreversible oxidation of sulfhydryls on carbonic anhydrase III during oxidative stress: a method for studying protein modification in intact cells and tissues. Arch Biochem Biophys 1994; 308:231–239.
112. Olafsdottir K, Reed DJ. Retention of oxidized glutathione by isolated rat liver mitochondria during hydroperoxide treatment. Biochim Biophys Acta 1988; 964:377–382.
113. Evers R, Zaman GJR, van Deemeter L, et al. Basolateral localization and export activity of the human multidrug resistance-associated protein in polarized pig kidney cells. J Clin Invest 1996; 97:1211–1218.
114. Almquist KC, Loe DW, Hipfner DR, Mackie JE, Cole SPC, Deeley RG. Characterization of the M_r 190,000 multidrug resistance protein (MRP) in drug-selected and transfected human tumor cells. Cancer Res 1995; 55:102–110.
115. Petronilli V, Costantini P, Scorrano L, Colonna R, Passamonti S, Bernardi P. The

voltage sensor of the mitochondrial permeability transition pore is tuned by the oxidation–reduction state of vicinal thiols. J Biol Chem 1994; 269:16638–16642.
116. Constantini P, Chernyak BV, Petronilli V, Bernardi P. Selective inhibition of the mitochondrial permeability transition pore at the oxidation–reduction sensitive dithiol by monobromobimane. FEBS Lett 1995; 362:239–242.
117. Constantini P, Chernyak BV, Petronilli V, Bernardi P. Modulation of the mitochondrial permeability transition pore by pyridine nucleotides and dithiol oxiation at two separate sites. J Biol Chem 1996; 271:6746–6751.
118. Smith LJ, Anderson J. Oxygen-induced lung damage. Relationship to lung mitochondrial glutathione levels. Am Rev Respir Dis 1992; 146:1452–1457.
119. Gyurasics A, Kelley DK, Rogers LK, Welty SE, Hansen TN, Smith CV. Mitochondrial compartmentalization of hyperoxic stresses investigated by measurement of coenzyme A (CoASH) and CoASSG in rat lungs [abstr]. Pediatr Res 1994; 35: 392A.
120. Guyton KZ, Xu Q, Holbrook NJ. Induction of the mammalian stress response gene *GADD153* by oxidative stress: role of AP-1 element. Biochem J 1996; 314:547–554.
121. Beinert H, Kiley P. Redox control of gene expression involving iron–sulfur proteins. Change of oxidation-state or assembly/disassembly of Fe–S clusters? FEBS Lett 1996; 382:218–219.
122. Sellers VM, Johnson MK, Dailey HA. Function of the [2Fe–2S] cluster in mammalian ferrochelatase: a possible role as a nitric oxide sensor. Biochemistry 1996; 35: 2699–2704.
123. Dean RT, Fu S, Stocker R, Davies MJ. Biochemistry and pathology of radical-mediated protein oxidation. Biochem J 1997; 324:1–18.
124. Pacifici RE, Davies KJA. Protein, lipid and DNA repair systems in oxidative stress: the free-radical theory of aging revisited. Gerontology 1991; 37:166–180.
125. Grant AJ, Jessup W, Dean RT. Inefficient degradation of oxidized regions of protein molecules. Free Radic Res Commun 1993; 18:259–267.
126. De Duve C, Wattiaux R. Functions of lysosomes. Annu Rev Physiol 1966; 28: 435–492.
127. Smith CV. Correlations and apparent contradictions in assessment of oxidant stress status in vivo. Free Radic Biol Med 1991; 10:217–224.
128. Janero DR. Malondialdehyde and thiobarbituric acid-reactivity as diagnostic indices of lipid peroxidation and peroxidative tissue injury. Free Radic Biol Med 1990; 9:515–540.
129. Kosugi H, Kikugawa K. Potential thiobarbituric acid-reactive substances in peroxidized lipids. Free Radic Biol Med 1989; 7:205–207.
130. Kojima T, Kikugawa K, Kosugi H. Is the thiobarbituric acid-reactivity of blood plasma specific to lipid peroxidation? Chem Pharm Bull 1990; 38:3414–3418.
131. Kikugawa K, Kojima T, Yamaki S, Kosugi H. Interpretation of the thiobarbituric acid reactivity of rat liver and brain homogenates in the presence of ferric ion and ethylenediaminetetraacetic acid. Anal Biochem 1992; 202:249–255.
132. Hughes H, Smith CV, Mitchell JR. Quantitation of lipid peroxidation products by gas chromatography–mass spectrometry. Anal Biochem 1986; 152:107–112.
133. Hughes H, Smith CV, Horning EC, Mitchell JR. HPLC and GC–MS determina-

tion of specific lipid peroxidation products in vivo. Anal Biochem 1983; 130:431–436.

134. Smith CV, Reilly MH. Formation of pentane versus 1-pentanol in the ferrous sulfate initiated decomposition of 15-hydroperoxyeicosatetraenoic acid in hypoxic and hyperoxic conditions. Biochem Pharmacol 1989; 38:1362–1364.
135. Morrow JD, Roberts LJI. The isoprostanes. Current knowledge and directions for future research. Biochem Pharmacol 1996; 51:1–9.
136. Longmire AW, Swift LL, Roberts LJI, Awad JA, Burk RF, Morrow JD. Effect of oxygen tension on the generation of F_2-isoprostanes and malondialdehyde in peroxidizing rat liver microsomes. Biochem Pharmacol 1994; 47:1173–1177.
137. Rubbo H, Parthasarathy S, Barnes S, Kirk M, Kalyanaraman B, Freeman BA. Nitric oxide inhibition of lipoxygenase-dependent liposome and low-density lipoprotein oxidation: termination of radical chain propagation reactions and formation of nitrogen-containing oxidized lipid derivatives. Arch Biochem Biophys 1995; 324:15–25.
138. Schraufstatter IU, Hyslop PA, Hinshaw DB, Spragg RG, Sklar LA, Cochrane CG. Hydrogen peroxide-induced injury of cells and its prevention by inhibitors of poly(ADP-ribose) polymerase. Proc Natl Acad Sci USA 1986; 83:4908–4912.
139. Andreoli SP. Mechanisms of endothelial cell ATP depletion after oxidant injury. Pediatr Res 1989; 25:97–101.
140. Randerath K, Randerath E, Smith CV, Chang J. Structural origins of bulky oxidative DNA adducts (type II I-compounds) as deduced by oxidation of oligonucleotides of known sequence. Chem Res Toxicol 1996; 9:247–254.
141. Ryan TP, Aust SD. The role of iron in oxygen-mediated toxicities. Crit Rev Toxicol 1992; 22:119–141.
142. Balla G, Vercellotti GM, Eaton JW, Jacob HS. Iron loading of endothelial cells augments oxidant damage. J Lab Clin Med 1990; 116:546–554.
143. Smith CV. Evidence for the participation of lipid peroxidation and iron in diquat-induced hepatic necrosis in vivo. Mol Pharmacol 1987; 32:417–422.
144. Gupta S, Rogers LK, Smith CV. Biliary excretion of lysosomal enzymes, iron, and oxidized protein in Fischer-344 and Sprague-Dawley rats and the effects of diquat and acetaminophen. Toxicol Appl Pharmacol 1994; 125:42–50.
145. Lentjes EGWM, Lindeman JHN, van de Bent W, Berger HM. Measured versus calculated latent iron binding capacity in plasma of newborns. Ann Clin Biochem 1995; 32:478–481.
146. Revenis ME, Kaliner MA. Lactoferrin and lysozyme deficiency in airway secretions: association with the development of bronchopulmonary dysplasia. J Pediatr 1992; 121:262–270.
147. deLemos RA, Roberts RJ, Coalson JJ, deLemos JA, Null DM, Gerstmann DR. Toxic effects associated with the administration of deferoxamine in the premature baboon with hyaline membrane disease. Am J Dis Child 1990; 144:915–919.

31

Assessment of Tissue Injury from Reactive Oxygen Metabolites

MICHAEL J. THOMAS

Bowman Gray School of Medicine
Wake Forest University
Winston-Salem, North Carolina

HENRY JAY FORMAN

University of Southern California
Los Angeles, California

TIMOTHY W. ROBISON

Food and Drug Administration
Bethesda, Maryland

I. Introduction

Chronic lung diseases of the newborn may result from inflammation or oxygen therapy, a procedure aimed at maintaining adequate oxygen delivery to the brain and other organs. Both of these causes of chronic lung disease would be expected to involve injury from reactive oxygen metabolites. The literature abounds with reviews on the production of reactive oxygen species by inflammatory cells and pulmonary oxygen toxicity as a consequence of oxygen therapy. Inflammatory cells produce reactive oxygen species as part of their microbicidal action. This can unfortunately injure normal tissue as collateral damage in the war against bacteria. Oxygen toxicity likely originates from increased generation of hydrogen peroxide by the mitochondria and perhaps other organelles at high oxygen concentrations. In this chapter, we have described methods for evaluating the involvement of reactive oxygen species. As the reader will find inherent difficulties in measurement of reactive oxygen species makes assessment of the contribution of these species to diseases, such as bronchopulmonary dysplasia, a monumental task. Fortunately, some of the newer methods described below may lead the way toward a more rigorous evaluation of cause and effect between chronic diseases of early infancy and production of reactive oxygen species.

The participation of free radical reactions is usually inferred from the isolation of trace amounts of characteristic products left behind by a free radical process. In this chapter we will first describe the chemistry of free radical oxidation and then describe methods for detecting products that are characteristic of radical oxidation. Several recent articles review techniques that are used to detect oxidation products from lipids, proteins, and nucleic acids (1–4). Only a few of the newer, more specific methods for measuring aldehydes, hydroperoxides, isoprostanes, oxidatively modified DNA bases, and oxidized protein will be covered in this chapter.

In the presence of sufficient concentrations of oxygen, reactive oxygen species, ultraviolet light, or high-energy radiation can initiate free radical chain reactions. The chain-carrying radical under these conditions is usually the hydroperoxyl radical, $ROO^{\bullet}$. A variety of cellular components can be oxidized during free radical autoxidation. However, the free radical oxidations of lipids and DNA are the best understood (5–9) and will be the focus of this chapter. The primary products from free radical autoxidation of polyunsaturated fatty acids (PUFA; fatty acid constituents of lipids), are hydroperoxides. Their decomposition gives secondary products that can diffuse from the site of formation and react with proteins, DNA, and such, causing loss of essential biochemical functions. Radical reactions involving DNA give rise to structurally modified DNA bases, cause the formation of stable cross-links between DNA bases and between DNA and protein, or cause DNA strand breaks (10). These modifications to DNA may cause incorrect base substitution or completely block replication (11,12).

Lipid peroxidation is probably the best understood of all of the free radical chain reactions that can take place in vivo. Figure 1 depicts a free radical chain autoxidation of PUFA, one of the most easily oxidized constituents of the cell membrane. The radical that starts the first step, called initiation, is often difficult to define because it is usually present at virtually undetectable concentrations. Some typical initiators include nitrogen dioxide (NO_2), a stable free radical; hydroxyl radical, generated by the reaction of a reduced transition metal with H_2O_2, and the conjugate acid of superoxide (O_2^-), $HO_2^{\bullet}$. The second step, called the propagation step, amplifies the first step and may yield 1000 hydroperoxide molecules for each initiating event. Because radical species react rapidly with one another, the process is self-limiting through a step called termination.

The small amounts of hydroperoxides detected in the tissues and body fluids of healthy organisms suggest that these products are formed in low yield, or that they are rapidly converted into other products, or both. Tissues of aerobic organisms contain enzymes that destroy oxidants, small molecules that inhibit autoxidation, and enzymes that repair damage to complex molecules such as DNA. Antioxidant enzymes include the superoxide dismutases, catalases, and glutathione peroxidases, that decompose O_2^-, H_2O_2, and peroxides, respectively. In addition, tissues and body fluids contain proteins that sequester transition metal ions, making them unavailable for reaction with O_2^-, H_2O_2, and lipid hydroperoxides. It has been suggested that peroxidized PUFA are selectively removed from

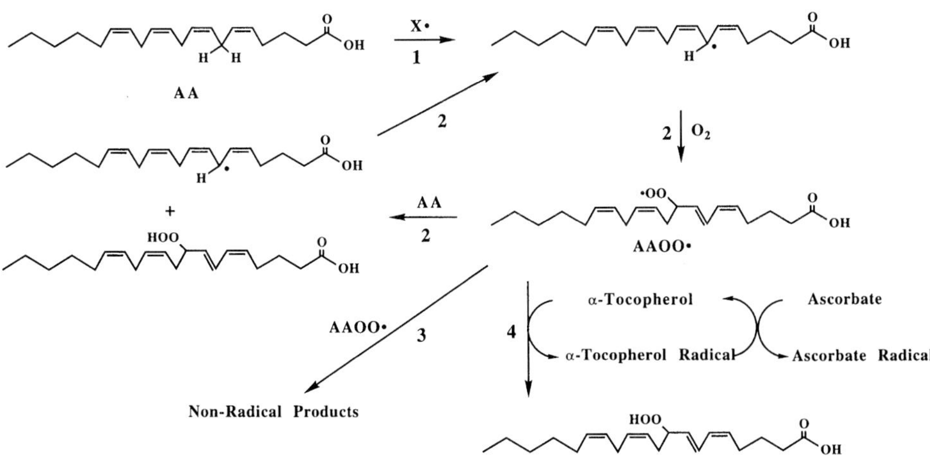

Figure 1 Scheme showing the steps in free radical autoxidation of the polyunsaturated fatty acids arachidonic acid: X$^•$ is the usually unknown initiating radical and step 1 is called initiation. Step 2 is the step that generates large amounts of hydroperoxide, called propagation. Step 3 shows the reaction of two radicals to yield nonradical products. Step 4 shows how α-tocopherol functions as an antioxidant and how ascorbate may regenerate α-tocopherol from the radical. Only 1 of the 12 possible hydroperoxide isomers is shown.

membranes by phospholipases to facilitate catabolism (13). Cells contain several small molecules called antioxidants (e.g., α-tocopherol and ascorbate) that inhibit free radical chain autoxidation by intercepting hydroperoxyl radicals. It has been suggested that α-tocopherol and ascorbate act in concert to protect lipid membranes from autoxidation: α-tocopherol intercepts the lipid hydroperoxyl radical, giving α-tocopheroxyl radical and one molecule of hydroperoxide, and then ascorbate reduced α-tocopheroxyl radical back to α-tocopherol (14).

The small amounts of hydroperoxide (e.g., those formed when α-tocopherol breaks a free radical chain) that escape reduction by glutathione peroxidase can break down to form toxic products. Figure 2 shows a typical autoxidation and several pathways for hydroperoxide decomposition. The formation of ethane and pentane is characteristic of *n*-3 and *n*-6 PUFA autoxidation (15), respectively. The mechanism, called β-scission, that gives these hydrocarbon gases also gives aldehydes (16). Although aldehydes are readily metabolized (17–20), in many instances, they are saved from catabolism by dilution into the surrounding medium. The toxic aldehydes, such as 4-hydroxynonenal (21,22), are more likely to be deactivated by several different enzymes (18,23).

For many years malondialdehyde (MDA), measured as a thiobarbituric acid-reactive substance (TBARS), has been used to quantify in vivo lipid autoxidation. Malondialdehyde is formed in low yield from PUFA hydroperoxides con-

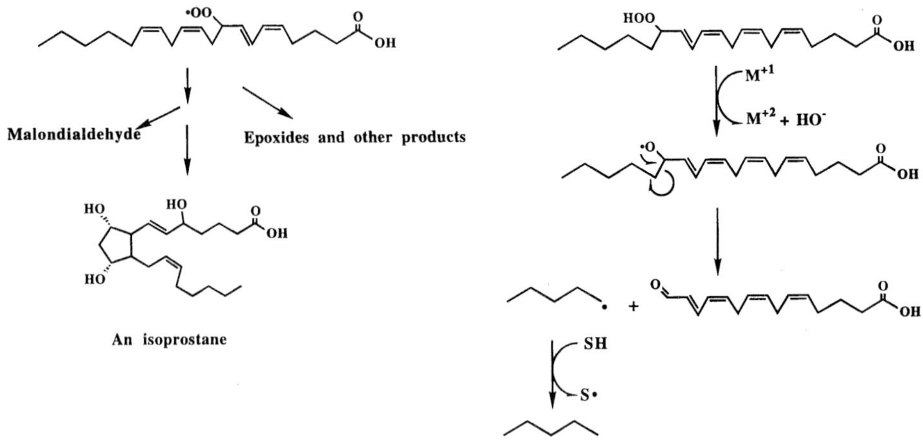

Figure 2 Other products formed by free radical autoxidation: The first panel shows the generation of an isoprostane and malondialdehyde from the hydroperoxyl radical. The second panel shows how a hydroperoxide should break down to form an aldehyde and pentane.

taining three or more double bonds (24), but it is formed by a pathway that branches from the path that gives the monohydroperoxides (16). Accurate measurement of TBARS requires precise protocols, such as that reported by Esterbauer and Cheeseman (25). Because MDA may be generated by the analysis procedure, gentle analysis methods, such as the technique that employs gas chromatography–mass spectrometry (GC–MS) of the pentafluorohydrazine derivative (26), should be contemplated. Recently, Morrow and Robert (27) demonstrated that a proposed MDA precursor (28) was converted into a diasterimeric mixture of prostaglandin-F_2 (PGF_2) isomers, called isoprostanes. Quantitation of isoprostanes may be one of the most precise measures of in vivo free radical autoxidation (29).

Glutathione (GSH), present in cells at a concentration of 1–10 mM, is a substrate for a group of peroxide-reducing enzymes, the glutathione peroxidases. The oxidized form of glutathione, the disulfide (GSSG), increases when glutathione peroxidase is actively reducing peroxides. Glutathione disulfide is rapidly reduced by glutathione reductase and normally represents less than 1% of total glutathione. However, when GSSG is formed, it can exchange with protein sulfhydryls to produce protein–glutathione mixed disulfides (30): GSSG + protein–SH $\rightleftarrows$ GSH + protein-S–S-G. The mixed disulfides have a longer half-life than GSSG and may be a sensitive indicator of basal oxidative stress (30,31). It has been suggested that the concentration of GSH in plasma and lung lavage can be used as a measure of oxidative stress. Problems in measurement are the result of a low (<10-μM) plasma concentration and small volume (despite high GSH concentration) of the lung lining fluid. In pulmonary oxidative stress, alveolar edema can significantly lower GSH concentration without consuming GSH. In contrast, the small amount of cell breakage that inevitably occurs during phlebotomy or bronchoalveolar lavage (BAL) will make GSH measurement artificially high owing to contamination from the large intracellular pool.

Protein oxidation is a normal physiological process that marks proteins for degradation by proteolytic systems. Oxidative damage to proteins, however, can increase turnover and decrease enzymatic function, and is associated with several pathological processes (32). Protein modification may occur by metal-catalyzed oxidation, oxidations mediated by ozone, or from attack of oxides of nitrogen on susceptible amino acids, such as tyrosine (33,34). Direct oxidation may introduce carbonyl groups into proteins. The increase in carbonyl groups, or the concomitant decrease in primary amines, can be taken as evidence of oxidative modification (32). Oxidation or radical attack on a protein may generate tyrosine radicals. These radicals readily dimerize to form the stable, easily detected dityrosines (34). In addition to the direct oxidation, aldehydes produced by the oxidation of PUFA may react with certain function groups on proteins (e.g., the reaction of 4-hydroxynonenal with thiols and unique lysyl residues).

II. Methods

A. Aldehydes

Detection sensitivity is increased if the aldehydes are converted into stable derivatives. 2,4-Dinitrophenylhydrazones have been the derivatives of choice because reliable methods for separating the various aldehyde classes and individual aldehyde derivatives are available (36,37). Because the dinitrophenylhydrazone (DNP) derivatives are colored, it is easy to monitor the development of thin-layer chromatography (TLC) and high performance liquid chromatography (HPLC) separations. However, to detect the small amounts of aldehydes released in vivo, other derivatives have been used with more sensitive detection methods [e.g., fluorescence spectroscopy (38–40) and mass spectrometry (MS; 41–46)]. Recently, Thomas et al. (47) demonstrated that DNP derivatives can be quantified at a concentration of 10 pg per injection, using gas chromatography (GC) coupled to negative-ion MS. This GC–MS method has been used to identify the aldehydes released into the medium by alveolar macrophages exposed to nitrogen dioxide (NO_2; (17), to determine the aldehyde distribution in the brain tissue of rats maintained on an ethanol diet (48), and to identify the aldehydes formed from ozonolysis of arachidonic acid (49).

B. Isoprostanes

Isoprostane is the name given to a class of compounds that are formed by the free radical cyclization of arachidonic acid. In 1990, Morrow et al. (50,51) reported the detection of isoprostanes in plasma. These compounds were detected in plasma as free acids and also esterified in complex lipids. In vitro studies of low-density lipoprotein (LDP) oxidation have demonstrated that isoprostanes are formed during free radical chain autoxidation induced by copper ions (52–54), azo initiators (54,55), and cultured cells (56,57). Isoprostanes have been detected in plasma and urine (58) and in lipid extracts of atherosclerotic lesions from nonhuman primates (55). In humans, plasma isoprostanes were higher in patients who smoked (e.g., 448 pmol/L in nonsmokers and 816 pmol/L in smokers; 59). In rats, iron overload (60), diquat administration (61,62), vitamin E deficiency (63), carbon tetrachloride administration (64,65), and ischemia–reperfusion (66) were associated with increased isoprostane levels. 8-Epi-PGF$_{2\alpha}$, a powerful vasoconstrictor in rats (67,68), is one of the isoprostanes that is formed by autoxidation (51–53,57,65), and it has been detected in vivo (69). Isoprostanes are measured using GC–MS negative-ion detection techniques after conversion to pentafluorobenzyl ester trimethylsilyl ethers (70).

C. Lipid Hydroperoxides

Two new methods have recently been applied to rapidly quantify hydroperoxides. The first employs the oxidation of ferrous ion to ferric ion, followed by chelation to xylenol orange (71–74). Results obtained using this method compare favorably with other measures of oxidation, including TBARS, iodometric methods, and the formation of conjugated dienes (72). The level of sensitivity is approximately 1 μM. When used to measure lipid hydroperoxides in human plasma, this method gives a mean value of 3.02 ± 1.85 μM (71), in reasonable agreement with iodometric methods (75,76).

The second method employs the oxidation by hydroperoxides of the nonfluorescent diphenyl-1-pyrenylphosphine to the fluorescent diphenyl-1-pyrenylphosphine oxide (77–80). The method has been used for direct measurement of extracted peroxides, with a detection limit of 200 pmol, and for postcolumn detection of HPLC effluent, with a sensitivity of approximately 1–3 pmol (77). When the HPLC method was used to measure of hydroperoxides in plasma, cholesteryl ester hydroperoxides were detected at 24.5 ± 9.6 nM and phosphatidylcholine hydroperoxides from 20 to 55 nM (77,80). Plasma triacylglycerols contributed negligible amounts of hydroperoxide. This method is as sensitive as methods that measure chemiluminescence from microperoxidase-catalyzed oxidation of isoluminol (81). The levels of plasma hydroperoxides reported using these methods were significantly lower than those from iodometry or xylenol orange.

D. DNA Base Damage Products

The most common techniques for measuring DNA base damage are GC–MS and HPLC analysis after the bases have been released by digestion. Products commonly measured by GC–MS techniques include thymine glycol, 8-hydroxyguanine, and 8-hydroxy-2-deoxyguanosine. Typical GC–MS methods for quantifying base damage have employed acid hydrolysis and derivatization to give *t*-butyldimethylsilyl derivatives (82). The GC–MS technique is more informative than other techniques, because it gives both characteristic ion(s) and a characteristic retention time for each product. Oxidative damage by radicals has been detected at levels that are biologically relevant (83,84). Conventional HPLC techniques approach the sensitivity of GC–MS methods when the more sensitive detection techniques, such as on-line electrochemical detection, are employed (85). HPLC and GC–MS techniques do not always give the same results, an issue that was addressed in a review article (86). Both the HPLC and GC–MS methods can detect 1 damaged base per 10^5 or 10^6 undamaged bases. The use of ^{32}P-postlabeling techniques has increased the sensitivity of the HPLC method to a level that equals or slightly exceeds that of MS methods (87). Two new methods may provide increased sensitivity and selectivity for quantifying damaged bases. These techniques are called immuno polymerase chain reaction (PCR; 88) and sequencing by hybridization (89,90). Both techniques use PCR to amplify low levels of products. The specificity of the first method comes from antigen binding to monoclonal antibodies, whereas the specificity of the second method comes from enhanced stringency during DNA hybridization.

E. Protein Modification

Generation of nitrotyrosine and dityrosine in protein may be measured using HPLC methods (33–35,91). Two methods that show approximately equal sensitivity for measuring protein carbonyls employ either the reduction of carbonyls to alcohols with [^{3}H]$NaBH_4$ or the formation of dinitrophenylhydrazones followed by HPLC separation with optical detection (32,92). Protein carbonyls can be measured in mixtures by preparing DNP-derivatives (32,93) and then performing Western blot analysis with antidinitrophenyl antisera.

Protein thiols react with glutathione disulfide or with other compounds (e.g., α,β-unsaturated aldehydes) by Michael addition (94), to form stable adducts. The most common methods for quantifying mixed disulfides employ reagents, such as *N*-iodoacetyl-3-[^{125}I]iodotyrosine or fluorodinitrobenzene (95,96), that react rapidly with "free" protein thiols. The measurements are usually reported relative to an "unoxidized" control sample. A more direct measure of glutathione mixed disulfides is obtained by performic acid oxidation and cleavage of the mixed disulfide to sulfonic acids, followed by HPLC quantitation of the phenylisothiocyanate derivative (97).

F. Summary

This chapter describes the chemistry of free radical oxidation. Free radical oxidation does not leave a well-marked trial for the investigator to follow. Therefore, the participation of radical processes must be inferred from the small amounts of characteristic oxidation products left behind in tissues. Because radical oxidation may be a "natural" process, the small changes in the levels of oxidation products during oxidative stress are measured against a background of these same products (98–100). Several of the newer methods for detecting the participation of radical oxidation are based on well-established chemical or chromatographic principles. They all gave good results when applied to in vitro samples. However, some of the methods gave conflicting results when used with in vivo samples that contain trace amounts of the compound(s) under investigation. These conflicts suggest that a better understanding of the chemistry behind the methods or of the biological process is required to validate the methods.

III. Future Directions

So what are the future directions for the assessment of tissue injury by reactive oxygen metabolites? The most obvious question is can one determine whether oxidation of tissue components is a primary event in the development of diseases, such as bronchopulmonary dysplasia? This requires the ability to match early diagnosis of the disease with methods that are sensitive enough to determine low levels of oxidized products. Results of such investigation could provide correlative evidence for the involvement of oxidation. If such a correlation can be established, one possible strategy for determining a cause-and-effect relation would be intervention with antioxidants. If an antioxidant simultaneously decreases production of oxidized tissue components, while further development of the disease is slowed, then there is reasonable evidence supporting the hypothesis of an underlying oxidative mechanism in the disease. Although such an approach may seem to be straightforward, delivery of antioxidants to the required site of action is not always possible. In such cases, a false-negative result can occur. It is also possible that oxidants may be involved in a more subtle matter than can be determined by measuring oxidized products. For example, low concentrations of hydrogen peroxide can stimulate the production of cytokines, while not producing any measurable oxidized tissue products. Here, an antioxidant may be effective, although the rationale for its use may not be as obvious. As we learn more about the role oxidants play in normal physiology and pathology, new approaches for assessing their role in disease will certainly develop.

Acknowledgments

The authors wish to thank Dr. Qirui Chen for technical assistance in preparing this manuscript. HJF and TWR were supported by Grants HL37556 and HL46493 from the National Institutes of Health.

References

1. Packer L. Oxygen radicals in biological systems, part D. Methods Enzymol 1994; 234.

2. Packer L. Oxygen radicals in biological systems, part C. Methods Enzymol 1994; 233.
3. Packer L, Glazer AN. Oxygen radicals in biological systems, part B. Methods Enzymol 1990; 186.
4. Cadet J, Weinfeid M. Detecting DNA damage. Anal Chem 1993; 65:675A–682A.
5. Bateman L. Olefin oxidation. Q Rev 1954; 8:147–167.
6. Bolland JL. Kinetic studies in the chemistry of rubber and related materials. I. The thermal oxidation of ethyl linoleate. Proc R Soc Lond A 1946; 186:218–236.
7. Porter NA, Weber BA, Weenen H, Khan JA. Autoxidation of polyunsaturated lipids. Factors controlling the stereochemistry of product hydroperoxides. J Am Chem Soc 1980; 102:5597–5601.
8. Steenken S. Purine bases, nucleosides, and nucleotides: aqueous solution redox chemistry and transformation reactions of their radical cations and e^- and OH adducts. Chem Rev 1989; 89:503–520.
9. Loidl-Stahlhofen A, Hannemann K, Spiteller G. Generation of α-hydroxyaldehydic compounds in the course of lipid peroxidation. Biochim Biophys Acta 1994; 1213: 140–148.
10. Saul RL, Ames BN. Background levels of DNA damage in the population. Basic Life Sci 1986; 38:529–535.
11. Ide H, Kow YW, Wallace SS. Thymine glycol and urea residues in M13 DNA constitute replicative blocks in vitro. Nucleic Acids Res 1985; 13:8035–8052.
12. Cheng KC, Cahill DS, Dasai H, Nishimura S, Loeb LA. 8-Hydroxyguanine, an abundant form of oxidative DNA damage, causes GT and AC substitutions. J Biol Chem 1992; 267:166–172.
13. van Kuijk FJGM, Sevanian A, Handelman GJ, Dratz EA. Trends Biochem Sci 1987; 12:31–34.
14. Packer LE, Slater TF, Willson RL. Direct observation of a free radical interaction between vitamin E and vitamin C. Nature 1979; 278:737–738.
15. Dumelin EE, Tappel AL. Hydrocarbon gases produced during in vitro peroxidation of polyunsaturated fatty acids and decomposition of preformed hydroperoxides. Lipids 1977; 12:894–900.
16. Gardner HW. Oxygen radical chemistry of polyunsaturated fatty acids. Free Radic Biol Med 1989; 7:65–86.
17. Robison TW, Forman HJ, Thomas MJ. Release of aldehydes from rat alveolar macrophages exposed in vitro to low concentrations of nitrogen dioxide. Biochim Biophys Acta 1995; 1256:334–340.
18. Danielson UH, Esterbauer H, Mannervik B. Structure–activity relationships of 4-hydroxyalkenals in the conjugation catalyzed by mammalian glutathione transferases. Biochem J 1987; 247:707–713.
19. Spitz DR, Sullivan SJ, Malcom RR, Roberts RJ. Glutathione dependent metabolism and detoxification of 4-hydroxy-2-nonenal. Free Radic Biol Med 1991; 11:415–423.
20. Poli G, Dianzani MU, Cheeseman KH, Slater TF, Lang J, Esterbauer H. Separation and characterization of the aldehydic products of lipid peroxidation stimulated by carbon tetrachloride or ADP–iron in isolated rat hepatocytes and rat liver microsomal suspensions. Biochem J 1985; 227:629–638.
21. Comporti M. Lipid peroxidation and cellular damage in toxic liver injury. Lab Invest 1985; 53:599–623.

22. Esterbauer H, Weger W. Action of aldehydes on normal and malignant cells. III. Synthesis of homologous 4-hydroxy-2-alkenals. 2. Monatshr Chem 1967; 98:1994–2000.
23. Sellin S, Holmquist B, Mannervik B, Vallee BL. Oxidation and reduction of 4-hydroxyalkenals catalyzed by isozymes of human alcohol dehydrogenase. Biochemistry 1991; 30:2514–2518.
24. Dahle LK, Hill EG, Holman RT. The thiobarbituric acid reaction and the autoxidations of polyunsaturated fatty acid methyl esters. Arch Biochem Biophys 1962; 8:253–261.
25. Esterbauer H, Cheeseman KH. Determination of aldehydic lipid peroxidation products: malonaldehyde and 4-hydroxynonenal. Methods Enzymol 1990; 186:407–421.
26. Yeo HC, Helbock HJ, Chyu DW, Ames BN. Assay of malondialdehyde in biological fluids by gas chromatography–mass spectrometry. Anal Biochem 1994; 220: 391–396.
27. Morrow JD, Roberts LJ. Quantification of noncyclooxygenase derived prostanoids as a marker of oxidative stress. Free Radic Biol Med 1991; 10:195–200.
28. Pryor WA, Stanley JP, Blair E. Autoxidation of polyunsaturated fatty acids: II. A suggested mechanism for the formation of TBA-reactive material from prostaglandin-like endoperoxides. Lipids 1976; 11:370–379.
29. Roberts JL, Morrow JD. Isoprostanes, novel markers of endogenous lipid peroxidation and potential mediators of oxidant injury. Ann NY Acad Sci 1994; 744:237–242.
30. Brigelius R, Muckel C, Akerboom TPM, Sies H. Identification and quantitation of glutathione and its relationship to glutathione disulfide. Biochem Pharmacol 1983; 32:2529–2534.
31. Loeb GA, Skelton DC, Forman HJ. Dependence of mixed disulfide formation in alveolar macrophages upon production of oxidized glutathione: effect of selenium depletion. Biochem Pharmacol 1989; 38:3119–3121.
32. Levine RL, Williams JA, Stadtman ER, Shacter E. Carbonyl assays for determination of oxidatively modified proteins. Methods Enzymol 1994; 233:346–357.
33. Kikugawa K, Kato T, Okamoto Y. Damage of amino acids and proteins induced by nitrogen dioxide, a free radical toxin in air. Free Radic Biol Med 1994; 16:373–382.
34. Haddad IY, Crow JP, Hu P, Ye Y, Beckman J, Matalon S. Concurrent generation of nitric oxide and superoxide damages surfactant protein A. Am J Physiol 1994; 267:L242–L249.
35. Giulivi C, Davies KJA. Dityrosine: a marker for oxidatively modified proteins and selective proteolysis. Methods Enzymol 1994; 233:363–371.
36. Esterbauer H, Zollner H. Methods for determination of aldehydic lipid peroxidation products. Free Radic Biol Med 1989; 7:197–203.
37. Esterbauer H, Cheeseman KH, Dianzani MU, Poli G, Slater TF. Separation and characterization of the aldehydic products of lipid peroxidation stimulated by ADP–Fe^{+2} in rat liver microsomes. Biochem J 1982; 208:129–140.
38. Holley AE, Walker MK, Cheeseman KH, Slater TF. Measurement of *n*-alkanals and hydroxyalkenals in biological samples. Free Radic Biol Med 1993; 15:281–289.

39. Yoshino K, Matsuura T, Sano M, Saito S, Tomita I. Fluorimetric liquid chromatographic determination of aliphatic aldehydes arising from lipid peroxides. Chem Pharm Bull (Tokyo) 1986; 34:1694–1700.
40. Beckman JK, Morley SA, Greene HL. Analysis of aldehydic lipid peroxidation products by TLC/densitometry. Lipids 1991; 26:155–161.
41. van Kuijk FJGM, Thomas DW, Stevens RJ, Dratz EA. Occurrence of 4-hydroxyalkenals in rat tissues determined as pentafluorobenzyl oxime derivative by gas chromatography–mass spectrometry. Biochem Biophys Res Commun 1986; 139:144–149.
42. Kinter M, Sullivan S, Roberts J, Spitz D. Trace quantitation of 4-hydroxy-2-nonenal in biological samples as its oxime-bis-*tert*-butyldimethylsilyl derivative using 3-hydroxynonenal as an internal standard. J Chromatogr 1992; 578:9–16.
43. van Kuijk FJGM, Siakotos AN, Fong LG, Stephens RJ, Thomas DW. Quantitative measurement of 4-hydroxyalkenals in oxidized low-density lipoprotein by gas chromatography–mass spectrometry. Anal Biochem 1995; 224:420–424.
44. Selley ML, Bartlett MR, McGuiness JA, Hapel AJ, Ardlie NG. Determination of the lipid peroxidation product *trans*-4-hydroxy-2-nonenal in biological samples by high-performance liquid chromatography and combined capillary column gas chromatography–negative-ion chemical ionisation mass spectrometry. J Chromatogr 1989; 488:329–340.
45. Bringmann G, Gassen M, Schneider S. Toxic aldehydes formed by lipid peroxidation I. Sensitive, gas chromatography-based stereoanalysis of 4-hydroxyalkenals, toxic products of lipid peroxidation. J Chromatogr 1994; A670:153–160.
46. Luo XP, Yazdanpanah M, Bhooi N, Lehotay DC. Determination of aldehydes and other lipid peroxidation products in biological samples by gas chromatography–mass spectrometry. Anal Biochem 1995; 228:294–298.
47. Thomas MJ, Robison TW, Samuel M, Forman HJ. Detecting and identifying volatile aldehydes as dinitrophenylhydrazones using gas chromatography mass spectrometry. Free Radic Biol Med 1995; 18:553–557.
48. Thomas MJ, Robison TW, Forman HJ, Cunningham CC. Detecting aldehydes as dinitrophenylhydrazones using GC/MS [abstr]. J Free Radic Biol Med 1994; 2:M/O13.
49. Kzumbo WJ, Hanley NM, Agarwal S, Thomas MJ, Madden MC. Products of ozonized arachidonic acid potentiate the formation of DNA single strand breaks in cultured human lung cells. Environ Mol Mutagen 1996; 27:185–195.
50. Morrow JD, Harris TM, Roberts LJ. Noncyclooxygenase oxidative formation of a series of novel prostaglandins: analytical ramifications for measurement of eicosanoids. Anal Biochem 1990; 184:1–10.
51. Morrow JD, Hill KE, Burk RF, Nammour TM, Badr KF, Roberts LJ. A series of prostaglandin F_2-like compounds are produced in vivo in humans by a noncyclooxygenase, free radical-catalyzed mechanism. Proc Natl Acad Sci USA 1990; 87:9383–9387.
52. Gopaul NK, Nourosz-Zadeh J, Mallet AI, Ånggärd EE. Formation of PGF_2-isoprostanes during the oxidative modification of low density lipoprotein. Biochem Biophys Res Commun 1994; 200:338–343.
53. Proudfoot JM, Beilin LJ, Croft KD. PGF_2-isoprostanes formed during copper-

induced oxidation of low-density lipoproteins are the prostaglandins that cross-react with PGE_2 antibodies. Biochem Biophys Res Commun 1995; 206:455–461.
54. Lynch SM, Morrow JD, Roberts LJ, Frei B. Formation of non-cyclooxygenase-derived prostanoids (F_2-isoprostanes) in plasma and low density lipoprotein exposed to oxidative stress in vitro. J Clin Invest 1994; 93:998–1004.
55. Thomas MJ, Chen Q, Rudel LL. The correlation between isoprosane levels and the extent of atherosclerosis. Fourth Annual Meeting of the Oxygen Society, San Francisco, CA, 1997, Abstr. 3-32.
56. Marchant CE, Bottoms MA, Law N, Mitchinson MJ, Hunt JV. Lipid peroxidation, lipoprotein cell-associated and ceroid accumulation in P388D1 macrophage-like cells. Biochim Biophys Acta 1994; 1215:267–274.
57. Gopaul NK, Nourooz-Zadeh J, Mallet AI, Ånggärd EE. Formation of F_2-isoprostanes during aortic endothelial cell-mediated oxidation of low density lipoprotein. FEBS Lett 1994; 348:297–300.
58. Awad JA, Morrow JD, Takahashi K, Roberts LJ. Identification of non–cyclooxygenase-derived prostanoid (F_2-isoprostane) metabolites in human urine and plasma. J Biol Chem 1993; 268:4161–4169.
59. Morrow JD, Frei B, Longmire AW, Gaziano JM, Lynch SM, Shyr Y, Strauss WE, Oates JA, Roberts LJ. Increase in circulating products of lipid peroxidation (F_2-isoprostanes) in smokers. N Engl J Med 1995; 332:1198–1203.
60. Dabbagh HJ, Mannion T, Lynch SM, Frei B. The effect of iron overload on rat plasma and liver oxidant status in vivo. Biochem J 1994; 300:799–803.
61. Burk RF, Hill KE, Award JA, Morrow JD, Kato T, Cockell KA, Lyons PR. Pathogenesis of diquat-induced liver necrosis in selenium-deficient rats: assessment of the roles of lipid peroxidation and selenoprotein P. Hepatology 1995; 21:561–569.
62. Awad JA, Burk RF, Roberts LJ. Effect of selenium deficiency and glutathione-modulating agents on diquat toxicity and lipid peroxidation in rats. J Pharmacol Exp Ther 1994; 270:858–864.
63. Awad JA, Morrow JD, Hill KE, Roberts LJ, Burk RF. Detection and localization of lipid peroxidation in selenium- and vitamin E-deficient rats using F_2-isoprostanes. J Nutr 1994; 124:810–816.
64. Morrow JD, Awad JA, Kato T, Takahashi K, Badr KF, Roberts LJ, Burk RF. Formation of novel non–cyclooxygenase-derived prostanoids (F_2-isoprostanes) in carbon tetrachloride hepatotoxicity. J Clin Invest 1992; 90:2502–2507.
65. Morrow JD, Minton TA, Mukundan CR, Campbell MD, Zackert WE, Daniel VC, Badr, KF, Blair IA, Roberts LJ. Free radical-induced generation of isoprostanes in vivo. J Biol Chem 1994; 269:4317–4326.
66. Mathews WR, Guido DM, Fisher MA, Jaeschke H. Lipid peroxidation as molecular mechanism of liver cell injury during reperfusion after ischemia. Free Radic Biol Med 1994; 16:763–770.
67. Morrow JD, Minton TA, Roberts LJ. The F_2-isoprostane, 8-epi-prostaglandin $F_{2\alpha}$, a potent agonist of the vascular thromboxane/endoperoxide receptor, is a platelet thromboxane/endoperoxide receptor antagonist. Prostaglandins 1992; 44:155–163.
68. Fukunaga M, Makita N, Roberts LJ, Morrow JD, Takahashi K, Badr KF. Evidence for the existence of F_2-isoprostane receptors on rat vascular smooth muscle cells. Am J Physiol 1993; 264:C1619–C1624.

69. Morrow JD, Minton TA, Badr KF, Roberts LJ. Evidence that the F_2-isoprostane, 8-epi-prostaglandin $F_{2\alpha}$, is formed in vivo. Biochim Biophys Acta 1994; 1210:244–248.
70. Morrow JD, Roberts LJ. Mass spectrometry of prostanoids: F_2-isoprostanes produced by non-cyclooxygenase free radical-catalyzed mechanism. Methods Enzymol 1994; 233:163–174.
71. Nourooz-Azdeh J, Tajaddini-Sarmadi J, Wolff SP. Measurement of plasma hydroperoxide concentrations by the ferrous oxidation–xylenol orange assay in conjunction with triphenylphosphine. Anal Biochem 1994; 220:403–409.
72. Jiang Z-Y, Hunt JV, Wolff SP. Ferrous ion oxidation in the presence of xylenol orange for detection of lipid hydroperoxide in low density lipoprotein. Anal Biochem 1992; 202:384–389.
73. Jiang A-Y, Woollard ACS, Wolff SP. Lipid hydroperoxide measurement by oxidation of Fe^{2+} in the presence of xylenol orange. Comparison with the TBA assay and an iodometric method. Lipids 1991; 26:853–856.
74. Jaeger J, Sorensen K, Wolff, SP. Peroxide accumulation in detergents. J Biochem Biophys Methods 1994; 29:77–81.
75. Thomas SM, Jessup W, Gebicki JM, Dean RT. A continuous-flow automated assay for iodometric estimation of hydroperoxides. Anal Biochem 1989; 176:353–359.
76. Cramer GL, Miller JF, Pendleton RB, Lands WEM. Iodometric measurement of lipid hydroperoxides in human plasma. Anal Biochem 1991; 193:204–211.
77. Meguro H, Akasaka K, Ohrui H. Determination of hydroperoxides with fluorometric reagent diphenyl-1-pyrenylphosphine. Methods Enzymol 1990; 186:157–161.
78. Akasaka K, Ijichi S, Watanabe K, Ohrui W, Meguro H. High-performance liquid chromatography and postcolumn derivatization with diphenyl-1-pyrenylphosphine for fluorimetric determination of triacylglycerol hydroperoxides. J Chromatogr 1992; 596:197–202.
79. Akasaka K, Ohrui H, Meguro H. Simultaneous determination of hydroperoxides of phosphatidylcholine, cholesterol esters and triacylglycerols by column-switching high-performance liquid chromatography with a post-column detection system. J Chromatogr 1993; 622:153–159.
80. Akasaka K, Ohrui H, Meguro H. Determination of triacylglycerol and cholesterol ester hydroperoxides in human plasma by high-performance liquid chromatography with fluorometric postcolumn detection. J Chromatogr 1993; 617:205–211.
81. Frei B, Yamamoto Y, Niclas D, Ames B. Evaluation of an isoluminol chemiluminescence assay for the detection of hydroperoxides in human blood plasma. Anal Biochem 1988; 175:120–130.
82. Dizdaroglu M. The use of capillary gas chromatography mass spectrometry for identification of radiation-induced DNA base damage and DNA base–amino acid cross-links. J Chromatogr 1984; 295:103–121.
83. Dizdaroglu M, Bergtold DS. Characterization of free radical-induced base damage in DNA at biologically relevant levels. Anal Biochem 1990; 156:182–188.
84. Dizdaroglu M, Olinski R, Doroshow JH, Akman SA. Modification of DNA bases in chromatin of intact target human cells by activated human polymorphonuclear leukocytes. Cancer Res 1993; 53:1269–1272.
85. Wagner JR, Hu C-C, Ames B. Endogenous oxidative damage of deoxycytidine in DNA. Proc Natl Acad Sci USA 1992; 89:3380–3384.

86. Halliwell B, Dizdaroglu M. The measurement of oxidative damage to DNA by HPLC and GC/MS techniques. Free Radic Res Commun 1992; 16:75–87.
87. Weinfeld M, Soderlind K-JM. ^{32}P-postlabeling detection of radiation-induced DNA damage: identification and estimation of thymine glycols and phosphoglycolate termini. Biochemistry 1991; 30:1091–1097.
88. Sano T, Smith CL, Cantor CR. Immuno-PCR: very sensitive antigen detection by means of specific antibody–DNA conjugates. Science 1992; 258:120–122.
89. Broude NE, Sano T, Smith CL, Cantor CR. Enhanced DNA sequencing by hybridization. Proc Natl Acad Sci USA 1994; 91:3072–3076.
90. Gao S, Drouin R, Holmquist GP. DNA repair rates mapped along the human PGK1 gene at nucleotide resolution. Science 1994; 263:1438–1440.
91. Malencik DA, Zao Z, Anderson SR. Determination of dityrosine, phosphotyrosine, phosphothreonine, and phosphoserine by high-performance liquid chromatography. Anal Biochem 1990; 184:353–359.
92. Levine RL, Garland D, Oliver CN, Amici A, Climent I, Lenz A-G, Ahn B-W, Shaltiel S, Stadtman ER. Determination of carbonyl content in oxidatively modified proteins. Methods Enyzmol 1990; 186:464–478.
93. Keller RJ, Halmes NC, Hinson JA, Pumford NR. Immunochemical detection of oxidized proteins. Chem Res Toxicol 1993; 6:430–433.
94. Uchida K, Stadtman ER. Quantitation of 4-hydroxynonenal protein adducts. Methods Enzymol 1994; 233:371–381.
95. Gitler C, Mogyoros M, Kalef E. Labeling of protein vicinal dithiols: role of protein–S_2 to protein–$(SH)_2$ conversion in metabolic regulation and oxidative stress. Methods Enzymol 1994; 233:403–415.
96. Reed DJ, Babson JR, Beatty PW, Brodie AE, Ellis WW, Potter DW. High-performance liquid chromatography analysis of nanomole levels of glutathione, glutathione disulfide, and related thiols and disulfides. Anal Biochem 1980; 106:55–62.
97. Kumari K, Khanna P, Ansari NH, Srivastava SK. High performance liquid chromatography method for the determination of protein–glutathione mixed disulfides. Anal Biochem 1994; 220:374–376.
98. Ames BN, Shigenaga MK, Park E-M. DNA damage by endogenous oxidants as a cause of aging and cancer. In: Davies KJA, ed. Oxidative Damage and Repair. New York: Pergamon Press, 1991:181–185.
99. Kosugi H, Kojima T, Kikugawa K. Characteristics of the thiobarbituric acid reactivity of human urine as a possible consequence of lipid peroxidation. Lipids 1993; 28:337–343.
100. Agarwal S, Wee JJ, Hadley M, Draper HH. Identification of a deoxyguanosine–malondialdehyde adduct in rat and human urine. Lipids 1994; 29:429–432.

32

Chronic Lung Disease of Early Infancy
Role of Neutrophils

DIANE E. LORANT, KURT ALBERTINE, and JOHN F. BOHNSACK

University of Utah Health Sciences Center
Salt Lake City, Utah

I. Introduction

Despite the introduction of surfactant therapy and improved methods of ventilation, bronchopulmonary dysplasia (BPD), or chronic lung disease (CLD) of prematurity, continues to be a significant problem for preterm infants recovering from hyaline membrane disease (HMD), or acute lung injury of prematurity. In this chapter, we review the mechanisms by which neutrophils are recruited to the lung and mediate tissue injury, and the clinical and experimental evidence that neutrophils contribute to the progression of HMD to chronic lung disease. Several lines of evidence support a role for neutrophil-mediated injury early in the development of BPD. Determining the mechanism(s) by which neutrophils are recruited to the lung and exacerbate acute lung injury in the ventilated newborn could lead to the development of therapeutic interventions that attenuate the neutrophil-mediated damage that contributes to BPD.

II. Mechanisms of Neutrophil-Mediated Injury and Recruitment to the Lung

Neutrophils have the potential to mediate lung injury through several mechanisms that usually contribute to the neutrophil's role in host defense, particularly the release of proteolytic enzymes and toxic oxygen radicals (1,2). Human neutrophils store at least six proteases in their granules, including neutrophil elastase, cathepsin G, collagenase, gelatinase, proteinase-3, and plasminogen activator. These enzymes are released into the extracellular space following neutrophil activation and may contribute to acute and chronic lung injury by their ability to injure endothelial or epithelial cells and to degrade extracellular matrix. Neutrophils may also mediate lung injury through their ability to produce toxic oxygen metabolites. Following activation, neutrophils markedly increase their oxygen consumption and produce superoxide anions. When two superoxide molecules interact, one is oxidized and the other is reduced in a dismutation reaction, with the formation of oxygen and hydrogen peroxide (H_2O_2). Both superoxide and H_2O_2 mediate oxidative damage to biological targets, and intrapulmonary instillation of enzymes that produce superoxide and H_2O_2 produce lung injury independent of neutrophil proteases (3). In fact, immune complex injury in the lung is inhibited by the H_2O_2 scavenger catalase, but not by known potent inhibitors of neutrophil neutral proteases (4). In addition, the action of neutrophil-derived myeloperoxidase and halides on H_2O_2 increases the toxicity of H_2O_2 by forming toxic products that include hypohalous acids, halogens, long-lived oxidants such as chloramines or aldehydes, and possibly hydroxyl radicals and singlet oxygen (5). These products are powerful toxins, primarily because of their ability to oxidize essential cell constituents, and experimental data indicate that the presence of myeloperoxidase intensifies the lung injury caused by superoxide and H_2O_2 (3). The oxidants generated by the myeloperoxidase system can also functionally inactivate antiproteases in the lung. Intratracheal instillation of myeloperoxidase and H_2O_2 in guinea pigs results in a loss of half the α_1-antiprotease inhibitor in bronchoalveolar lavage liquid compared with control animals (6). Destruction of antiprotease by oxidants may produce elastase–antielastase imbalance in vivo and contribute to the development of acute and chronic lung injury.

Neutrophil recruitment and activation in the lung are essential for neutrophils to mediate lung damage. Until recently, neutrophil recruitment to inflammatory sites was largely believed to result from directed migration of the neutrophil out of the bloodstream toward chemoattractants generated at the site of inflammation. Neutrophil recruitment is now better understood to result from the sequential interaction between several classes of adhesion molecules expressed on both the endothelium and the neutrophil (Fig. 1; 7,8). The first step in adhesion involves the arrest of the neutrophil through a "tethering" mechanism that causes the freely circulating neutrophil to roll along the vessel wall. This rolling phenomenon slows the velocity of the circulating neutrophil and is mediated by a class of three adhesion molecules, termed the selectins (7–16; L-selectin, E-selectin, and P-selectin). L-selectin is constitutively expressed on the neutrophil surface and is briefly upregulated and then rapidly shed following neutrophil activation (17,18). P-selectin and E-selectin are expressed on the surface of activated endo-

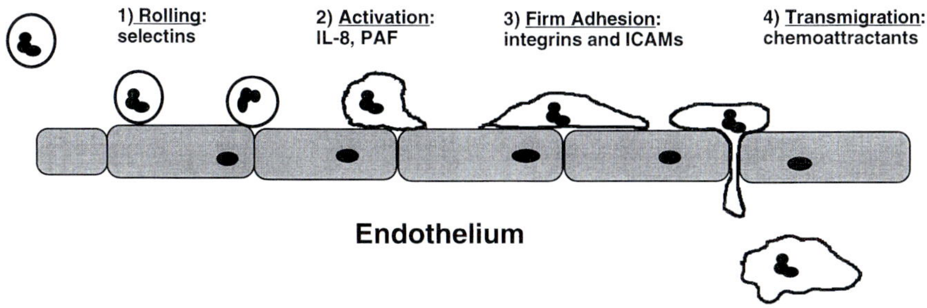

Figure 1 Steps in neutrophil extravasation: (1) The circulating neutrophil is slowed by a tethering through selectin-mediated interactions with the endothelium, a process that leads to rolling of the neutrophil along the vessel wall and juxtaposition of the neutrophil to the endothelium. (2) Neutrophils are then activated by endothelial cell-derived agonists, such as PAF and IL-8. (3) Activation of the neutrophil causes the neutrophil to spread and adhere firmly to the endothelium, leading to arrest of the neutrophil. (4) Neutrophils migrate across the endothelium and into the extravascular compartment in response to chemoattractants produced by endothelium and parenchymal cells.

thelial cells. P-selectin is stored in Weibel-Palade bodies in endothelial cells and is rapidly expressed on the endothelial cell surface when these cells are stimulated with certain agonists (histamine, thrombin, C5a) or oxidants (19–22). E-selectin is expressed on the surface of endothelial cells after stimulation with certain cytokines, such as tumor necrosis factor (TNF) and interleukin-1 (IL-1). The expression of E-selectin requires protein synthesis; therefore, its expression is delayed until 2–4 hr after stimulation (23).

As neutrophils roll along the endothelial cell surface, they are activated by endothelial cell-derived agonists, such as IL-8 or platelet activating factor (PAF; 24–28: see Fig. 1). Activation of neutrophils causes upregulation of their surface integrins CD11b/CD18 ($\alpha M\beta 2$) and CD11a/CD18 ($\alpha L\beta 2$; 29). Activation of the CD11/CD18 integrins results in firm adhesion of neutrophils to the endothelial cell surface through the binding of the neutrophil integrins to their counterreceptors on endothelial cells, intercellular adhesion molecule-1 (ICAM-1) and intercellular adhesion molecule-2 (ICAM-2; 29). Neutrophil sequestration in the pulmonary circulation may also result from physical trapping of the activated neutrophil within the lumen of the pulmonary capillaries. Because the diameter of pulmonary capillaries (8–10 μm) is similar to that of a circulating neutrophil (7 μm), neutrophils must have the ability to deform to pass through capillaries (30,31). Chemoattractants cause rapid polymerization of the neutrophil actin cytoskeleton, causing the neutrophil to become less deformable. In some situations, chemoattractant-induced decreases in deformability cause neutrophil sequestration in the pulmonary vasculature without any apparent contribution from specific adhesion receptors (32).

Arrest of activated neutrophils at the endothelial cell interface may cause injury to the pulmonary vasculature, leading to increased permeability of the blood vessels to water and proteins. Neutrophil adhesion to the blood vessel wall may also be followed by extravasation of the neutrophil into the lung parenchyma and airspaces, presumably under the influence of chemoattractants produced by the endothelium and cells such as alveolar macrophages. Activation of neutrophils outside the vasculature can cause further tissue injury.

The molecular mechanisms that mediate neutrophil recruitment to lung appears to depend on the nature of the inciting injury. Mulligan et al. reported (33) that anti-P-selectin antibody reduces lung vascular endothelial injury caused by intravenous infusion of cobra venom factor, an agent that causes systemic activation of complement. Also, anti-E-selectin monoclonal antibodies block immune–complex-mediated pulmonary vascular injury (34). Monoclonal antibody directed against CD18 integrins blocks neutrophil migration into rabbit lungs in vivo in response to experimental *Streptococcus pneumoniae* infection, but does not block neutrophil migration in response to infection with *Escherichia coli* or intratracheal instillation of lipopolysaccharide (35,36). In some experimental models, neutrophil extravasation in the lung in response to an inciting agent is mediated by adhesion molecules different from those that mediate neutrophil extravasation in the systemic circulation in response to the same inciting agent. For example, neutrophil migration into the peritoneum in response to experimental infection with *S. pneumoniae* is completely absent in mice they are doubly deficient in P-selectin and ICAM-1, whereas neutrophil migration into the alveoli in response experimental *S. pneumoniae* pneumonia is not affected. The results of these experiments imply novel P-selectin, ICAM-1, and CD18-independent mechanisms for neutrophil extravasation within the lung (37). Some of the differences between mechanisms that mediate neutrophil recruitment in the systemic and pulmonary circulation may be related to the different sites at which neutrophil extravasation occurs in the systemic and pulmonary circulation. Emigration of neutrophils in the systemic circulation takes place through postcapillary venules, whereas emigration in the lung occurs through the capillary bed (38).

III. Pathological and Clinical Studies of Neutrophil Involvement in BPD

Although it has been proposed that processes of inflammation contribute to the destruction of capillary beds and alveolar walls in chronic lung injury of prematurity (39), most histopathological studies that describe the abnormal pulmonary architecture in neonatal chronic lung disease do not comment on the presence or absence of neutrophils in the lungs (40–46). It is possible that neutrophil-mediated damage to the lungs occurred before the time of death and that neutrophils are no longer conspicuous at the time of most postmortem examinations of infants with BPD. Bonikos et al., however, described neutrophils in the lungs in a detailed histopathological study of 21 infants who died with BPD (47). These authors described damage to the bronchial and bronchiolar ciliary apparatus and mucous membranes, severe necrotizing bronchiolitis, and marked bronchiolar and alveolar fibrosis. The necrosis was associated with a severe acute and chronic inflammatory reaction. Neutrophils were identified among the mucosal cells, particularly in the deep layer of the altered epithelium of segmental and subsegmental bronchi. There was a qualitative increase in the number of septal neutrophils in infants in whom the overall pulmonary damage was most severe, and especially in those with the longest survival in high oxygen concentrations. This study did not identify the infants who had pneumonia.

Several clinical studies have reported a correlation between the presence of neutrophils in the airways of infants with hyaline membrane disease and subsequent development of chronic lung disease. D'Ablang et al. (48) noted the presence of neutrophils in tracheal aspirates of patients with stage II–IV bronchopulmonary dysplasia (Northway classification; 46), but did not quantify neutrophil number nor correlate the presence of neutrophils with the severity of the BPD. Subsequently, Merritt et al. (49) characterized the cell population in the tracheobronchial washings of newborns undergoing artificial ventilation for HMD. These investigators noted a temporal progression in the appearance of inflammatory cells in the tracheal aspirates, with neutrophils first appearing at a mean postnatal age of 3 days, followed by the appearance of macrophages at a mean postnatal age of 11 days. Four of seven infants with HMD who did not subsequently acquire BPD did not have neutrophils (or macrophages) in their tracheal aspirates, whereas all patients with subsequent BPD had both neutrophils and macrophages present (49). This same group of investigators later reported that the number of neutrophils in tracheobronchial washings on postnatal day 3 was tenfold higher in infants who subsequently had BPD than it was in infants who did not have BPD (50). The difference in total number of inflammatory cells persisted at postnatal day 7, but the relative proportion of neutrophils in tracheal aspirates at this time was not given. Moreover, the infants who did not acquire BPD were no longer receiving assisted ventilation by postnatal day 7. Therefore, correlative analyses could not be made between the presence of inflammatory cells and the development of chronic lung disease at or after postnatal day 7. Ogden et al. (51) performed a prospective study in 41 intubated infants to determine whether the inflammatory cell content of bronchoalveolar lavage fluid (BAL) was predictive of the development of BPD. Thirty-one infants were initially intubated for hyaline membrane disease, while the remaining ten infants with normal lungs were intubated for other reasons. In infants with hyaline membrane disease, inflammatory cells at younger than 24 hr of life were similar to inflammatory cells of infants who were intubated but had normal lungs. By 48 and 96 hr, however, bronchoalveolar lavage fluid retrieved from infants with hyaline membrane disease showed a marked increase in neutrophils. By 1 week after birth, infants who did not go on to acquire BPD had normal numbers of neutrophils in bronchoalveolar lavage fluid, whereas in infants who subsequently had BPD, bronchoalveolar lavage neutrophil counts remained significantly elevated throughout the 5-week study period. Several more recent studies confirmed that neutrophil number is increased in tracheobronchial washings obtained from infants during the first week who subsequently have BPD, compared with infants who do not (52–54). None of these studies, however, compared the number of neutrophils in the tracheobronchial washings of the BPD group beyond the first week of life with an age-matched control group because infants without subsequent BPD generally have their endotracheal tubes removed within a week. Thus, it is impossible to conclude definitively that neutrophil numbers remained elevated after the first week in infants with BPD compared with intubated controls. In one study, the number of neutrophils in the BPD group was no different from the control group in the second week after birth, suggesting that prolonged intubation alone may cause neutrophils to appear in tracheal aspirates; however, the control group during this time period was small (54).

A problem with the interpretation of data from studies performed on tracheobronchial washings is that the samples are more likely to reflect the contents of the proximal, rather than the distal airways, where much of the characteristic histopathology of BPD is found (45). Furthermore, only 1–2% of cells in the airspace are actually recovered by bronchoalveolar lavage, even under ideal experimental conditions (38). In a more recent study, Ferriera et al. (55) hypothesized that neutrophil localization in the lung during lung injury in preterm infants should be reflected in lower circulating neutrophil counts. In a retrospective review of 332 preterm infants less than 34 weeks gestation, this group found that patients with significant neutropenia (neutrophil concentration < 25th percentile within 2 hr after birth) required significantly more ventilatory support at 12 hr than did patients without neutropenia. Additionally, patients with early neutropenia were significantly less likely to be extubated and on room air at 1 week and at 1 month after birth (55). It is uncertain, however, that the neutropenia noted in these patients was the result of recruitment of neutrophils to the lungs.

Taken together, the clinical studies cited here suggest that neutrophils contribute to the acute lung injury in hyaline membrane disease, and that the greater the neutrophil-mediated damage that occurs early in the process (in the first week), the greater the risk of subsequent BPD. An alternative hypothesis that must be considered is that neutrophils are not the cause of the acute injury, but rather, a response to the pathophysiological process that actually causes BPD.

Neutrophil elastase has been proposed to contribute to several forms of lung injury, including adult respiratory distress syndrome, cystic fibrosis, and emphysema, either through excessive elastase secretion in the lung, or from an imbalance between the amount of elastase and naturally occurring elastase inhibitors (56). Orderly synthesis of elastin appears to be necessary for normal alveolar development during late fetal and postnatal life because elastin is synthesized at the tip of the secondary crest, the structure from which newly formed anatomical alveoli evolve (57). Postmortem examination of lungs from patients with BPD characteristically reveals decreased lung alveolarization and disordered elastin fibers in the alveolar walls (58). These findings, along with increased levels of the elastin-specific product desmosine, in the urine of infants who acquire BPD (59), supports the hypothesis that elastinolysis is an important pathophysiological mechanism underlying the disordered lung architecture found in BPD.

Various investigators have attempted to correlate neutrophil elastase activity in the tracheobronchial lavage fluid of infants with HMD with progression to BPD. In the study by Merritt et al. (50), infants who later acquired BPD had significantly elevated tracheobronchial elastase activity on days 3–8, compared with infants with HMD or control infants without HMD. The elastase activity remained elevated in the patients with BPD through postnatal day 14, but age-matched controls were not available after 8 days. The elastase was felt to be of neutrophil origin because most of the elastase activity was inhibited by a serine esterase inhibitor. In this study, the percentage of tracheal α_1-antiprotease that was inactive (due to oxidation, proteolytic cleavage, or being complexed with protease) increased between day 1 and day 4 both in infants with HMD alone and in infants who later had BPD, but the infants with subsequent BPD had greater α_1-antiproteinase inactivation than did infants with HMD alone. These data suggest that an imbalance between elastase and its major pulmonary inhibitor, α_1-antiprotease, may contribute to the injury that occurs in BPD. Other investigators reported similar results. Ogden et al. (51) found that elastase activity in tracheobronchial lavage samples increased during the first week in babies with HMD alone and in babies who later had BPD, but elastase activity in babies that acquired BPD did not return to normal, whereas elastase activity in babies with HMD alone returned to normal at 1 week. Infants with subsequent BPD also had higher ratios of tracheal elastase to α_1-antiprotease at days 2, 4, and 7 than did infants with respiratory distress syndrome (RDS) alone. Watterberg et al. (54) also found that infants who acquired BPD had greater elastase activity in tracheobronchial lavage specimens recovered during the first week of life compared with infants who did not acquire BPD. The sensitivity of the elastase activity to serine esterase inhibitors was not determined in the latter two studies, thus, making it more difficult to infer that neutrophils were the source of the elastase activity. Another study compared elastase activity in tracheobronchial washings from patients with BPD with that of infants without BPD who required mechanical ventilation in postnatal weeks 4 through 9 (60). Although there was no significant difference in elastase activity between the two groups, a significant increase was found in the ratio of elastase activity to α_1-antiprotease in BPD patients compared with control infants without BPD, suggesting that a protease–antiprotease imbalance persisted in the patients who acquired BPD. In contrast with these studies, Bruce et al. (61) did not detect any elastase activity in 26 of 65 tracheobronchial washings of ventilated premature infants. Correlation between the presence of elastase activity and the development of BPD was not specifically examined in the latter study. Taken together, the finding of increased tracheobronchial elastase activity and elastase–antielastase imbalance in these studies supports the notion that ongoing elastinolysis contributes to the disordered architecture and decreased alveolarization that are characteristic of BPD.

Although it is clear that neutrophils are found in the tracheobronchial aspirates of infants who acquire BPD, nothing is known about the molecular mechanisms, particularly the specific adhesion receptors that are involved in recruitment of the neutrophils to the airspaces of these infants. There is an increase in chemotactic activity that accompanies the elevated number of neutrophils in tracheobronchial fluid specimens of neonates with signs of early chronic lung disease (52). Specifically, the levels of C5a, leukotriene-B_4 (LTB_4), and IL-8 are elevated and associated with greater numbers of neutrophils (52). It is unclear whether these chemotactic agents stimulate the initial migration of neutrophils, or if they are present as a result of transmigration of activated neutrophils. LTB_4 and IL-8 are synthesized by activated neutrophils, and C5a may be generated by proteases that are secreted by activated neutrophils (62–64). Production of these chemotactic agents by neutrophils may serve to amplify neutrophil recruitment and activation. Alveolar macrophages that synthesize LTB_4, Il-8, and a variety of functionally active complement components may also be a source of chemoattractant activity (65). Macrophages exposed to hyperoxia release substances that activate neutrophils (66), and activated pulmonary macrophages have been described in infants with BPD (67).

If neutrophils and their products contribute to chronic lung injury in neonates, then reducing neutrophil influx into the lungs should reduce the injury. Several studies have demonstrated an improvement in BPD following administration of dexamethasone (68). In one study, treatment of infants with BPD (mean age 39 days) with dexamethasone significantly reduced the number of neutrophils and amount of elastase in tracheobronchial lavage fluid; a control group of infants treated with placebo did not have a reduction in either neutrophils or elastase in the tracheobronchial lavage fluid (69). Another study (70) reported that treatment with dexamethasone caused a reduction in tracheobronchial aspirate elastase in infants with BPD (mean age 25 days), whereas administration of placebo did not cause a reduction in tracheobronchial elastase. Thus, the improvement in pulmonary status seen in BPD patients after treatment with dexamethasone appears to correspond to a reduction in tracheobronchial neutrophil number and levels of elastase. Although these data indirectly support a role for neutrophils in the pathogenesis of BPD, it is clear that corticosteroids are not selective inhibitors of neutrophil recruitment. Dexamethasone treatment reduces a variety of other potentially injurious mediators in the lung that might contribute to the pathophysiology of BPD (68).

IV. The Role of Neutrophils in Animal Models of BPD

Several animal models of neonatal lung injury provide insight into the contribution that neutrophils may make to the pathophysiology of BPD. Prolonged exposure of neonatal rats to hyperoxic conditions results in decreased alveolarization and disordered elastin in the alveolar walls, histopathological changes that resemble those observed in human BPD (68). In vitro and in vivo experimental observations suggest a role for neutrophils in the lung injury caused by hyperoxia. Hyperoxic damage to lung cells (lung epithelial cells, lung fibroblasts, and pulmonary artery endothelial cells) in vitro is exacerbated by the coincubation of these cells with activated neutrophils (71), demonstrating that release of inflammatory mediators by activated neutrophils could contribute to pulmonary oxygen toxicity in animals exposed to hyperoxia. Bowman et al. (72) showed that neutrophil adhesion to pulmonary artery endothelial cells exposed to hyperoxia in vitro is increased compared with endothelial cells exposed to normoxia. The adhesion molecules and agonists involved in this neutrophil adhesion, however, were not identified.

One possible mechanism for hyperoxia-induced neutrophil adhesion is expression of P-selectin on the plasma membrane of endothelium, and endothelial cell production of the neutrophil agonist PAF. Exposure of human umbilical vein endothelial cells to oxidants in vitro induces prolonged (several hours) expression of P-selectin on the surface, and synthesis of PAF by the endothelial cells (22,73). The PAF produced by endothelial cells remains associated with the cell membrane (74,75), but oxidant treatment of endothelial cells also induces the shedding of membrane vesicles containing oxidized phospholipids that activate neutrophils by binding to the PAF receptor (76). Studies carried out in vivo also suggest the importance of cell adhesion molecules in the pathogenesis of hyperoxic lung injury. Rinaldo et al. (77) induced pulmonary endothelial injury in vivo by exposing rats to 100% oxygen for 36 hr. Although there was no histological evidence of lung injury or inflammation in exposed rats, a significantly greater number of systemically injected radiolabeled neutrophils accumulated in the lungs of rats that were exposed to hyperoxia compared with control rats (77). The molecular mechanisms of the pulmonary sequestration of neutrophils were not identified. In another study, inhalation of an oxygen concentration higher than 95% for up to 72 hr in adult rats caused marked upregulation of mRNA for both P-selectin and E-selectin (78). There was also a marked increase of lung weight of accumulation of fluid in the thorax and of neutrophils in the bronchial lumen.

The role of neutrophils in hyperoxic lung injury has been examined more directly in vivo in several different animal species. An increased number of neutrophils was found in the lung interstitium of adult rats after exposure to 100% oxygen for 60 hr, or 85% oxygen for 7 days compared with control animals maintained in normoxic conditions (79). In another study, Fox et al. (80) described increased numbers of neutrophils and neutrophil chemotactic factors in the alveolar lavage fluid of adult rats exposed to oxygen concentrations higher than 95% for 66 hr, when compared with rats kept in 21% oxygen. Merritt et al. (81) found increased numbers of neutrophils in lung lavage of neonatal guinea pigs exposed to 100% oxygen for 72 hr compared with control animals that were exposed to room air. Lung injury, as assessed by protein concentration in the lung lavage fluid, was also evident by 48 hr, but continued to increase between 72 and 144 hr, after the largest neutrophil influx (81).

To further determine the role of neutrophils in lung injury, investigators have induced neutropenia or attempted to prevent neutrophil recruitment in animals before exposure to hyperoxia. Shasby et al. (82) made rabbits neutropenic by administering nitrogen mustard, and reported that neutropenic rabbits had less lung edema after exposure to hyperoxia for 72 hr than did control (normoxic) animals or hyperoxic animals that were treated with nitrogen mustard but that did not become neutropenic. They also found that the number of neutrophils in lung lavages correlated with the degree of edematous lung injury, as assessed by albumin concentration in lung lavage and the ratio of lung weight to body weight. In another study, a monoclonal antibody to ICAM-1 inhibited the acute lung dysfunction induced in mice by inhalation of pure oxygen, and the attenuated lung damage was accompanied by decreased neutrophil infiltration in the lungs (83). In contrast, Raj et al. (84) induced neutropenia in rabbits with nitrogen mustard and found that decreasing the number of neutrophils in the lungs by more than 90% did not influence survival time or extravascular lung water content. In the same study, newborn lambs were rendered neutropenic with hydroxyurea, after which they breathed 100% oxygen for up to 5 days. Lung injury, as assessed by measurement of lung lymph flow and protein flow, was the same in control lambs as it was in lambs that were made neutropenic before exposure to hyperoxia. The reason for the discrepancy between results of the neutrophil depletion studies is unclear. Conflicting results may be secondary to the means by which lung injury is induced, how lung injury is measured, and the time course over which the study is performed.

Although these studies suggest that neutrophils might play a role in the development of hyperoxic lung injury, their relevance to lung injury in preterm infants is unclear, as these experiments addressed the role of neutrophils in lung injury in adult or mature newborn animals. Thus, surfactant deficiency, the major factor predisposing the preterm human infant to acute lung injury, does not contribute to the lung injury in these models, nor were the animals subjected to the barotrauma caused by mechanical ventilation. In a study that somewhat more closely models preterm lung injury, adult rabbits were lavaged to deplete the lung of surfactant, after which they were mechanically ventilated with 100% oxygen for 4 hr to induce lung injury (85). Rabbits made neutropenic by treatment with nitrogen mustard had decreased lung injury as assessed by respiratory gas exchange, protein leak, and the presence or absence of hyaline membranes. Repletion of neutrophils into neutropenic rabbits resulted in impaired respiratory gas exchange and hyaline membranes, similar to those that were observed in rabbits with normal neutrophil counts (85). In another study, guinea pigs that were delivered 3 days prematurely were exposed for 96 hr to either 95% oxygen or air. The hyperoxic animals acquired acute lung injury with pulmonary edema and intra-alveolar fibrin deposition. Histological postmortem examination showed larger numbers of neutrophils in the lung parenchyma of the hyperoxic animals compared with air-breathing controls (86). In a model of acute preterm lung injury, Tabor et al. (87) administered a PAF receptor antagonist intravenously to preterm rabbits and ventilated the animals for 30 min with 100% oxygen. They found that protein leak into the airspace was significantly reduced in rabbits that were treated with the PAF-receptor antagonist compared with control animals. The mechanism by which PAF contributed to protein leak in this model was not explored and could have been independent of PAF effects on neutrophil activation.

The aforementioned studies of hyperoxic lung injury were mostly studies of acute lung injury. Experimental investigation of the contribution of neutrophils to chronic lung injury requires better animal models of chronic lung disease of newborns. Such animal models should fulfill several criteria, including preterm delivery, surfactant deficiency, a requirement for mechanical ventilation, and exposure to hyperoxia commensurate with that used in the care of premature human infants. In one such model, premature baboons (delivered on day 140 of a 180 day gestation) are exposed to prolonged hyperoxia and mechanical ventilation. The preterm baboons acquire chronic lung disease that resembles mild to moderate human BPD after 7–14 days of mechanical ventilation with high concentrations of inspired oxygen (88). An increased number of neutrophils are found in the bronchoalveolar lavage fluid obtained on day 6 from the group of baboons that acquired BPD, although the predominant cell type found at that time is the macrophage (89). The authors also described an increased number of neutrophils in the alveolar septa of the animals that have BPD (89). These data are consistent with the results of the clinical studies in infants, described earlier in this chapter, in which increased numbers of neutrophils are found in tracheobronchial lavage specimens obtained postnatally from infants who subsequently have BPD. However, no significant difference was found after 14 days between the number of neutrophils found in lung lavage or in tissue sections of airspaces of baboons with BPD compared with a control group that did not have BPD (88).

Lambs have acute and chronic lung injury following preterm delivery and prolonged mechanical ventilation (90,91). With this model of hyaline membrane disease, Carlton et al. (92) reported that circulating neutrophil numbers fall during the first 30–90 min following preterm delivery of lambs, and that the amount of reduction in circulating neutrophil number correlates with the degree of neutrophil accumulation in the lung at postmortem examination performed 8 hr after birth (Fig. 2). Lung vascular injury in the preterm lambs, as assessed by postmortem extravascular water content and by lung lymph liquid volume and protein concentration 6–8 hr after delivery, was also directly proportional to the fall in circulating neutrophils and accumulation of neutrophils in the airspaces (92). The finding of early neutrophil accumulation in the lung is consistent with the results of studies by Jackson et al. (93), who observed increased numbers of neutrophils in the lung vasculature, interstitiums and alveoli early in the course of acute lung injury in premature *Macaca nemestrina* monkeys that, similar to the preterm lambs, also underwent artificial ventilation. These data also lend credence to the hypothesis that the neutropenia observed within 2 hr after birth in human preterm neonates with acute lung injury (55; described earlier) results from neutrophil localization in the lung. To further test the hypothesis that neutrophils contribute to the acute lung injury of prematurity, Carlton et al. (92) induced neutropenia prenatally in fetal lambs with nitrogen mustard and found significantly less lung vascular damage following preterm delivery. The decreased vascular injury was accompanied by a marked decrease in neutrophil accumulation in the airspaces (see Fig. 2). These data support a role for neutrophils in acute lung injury of prematurity, but do not address whether the neutrophil-mediated damage contributes to chronic lung injury that develops in these preterm animals following prolonged mechanical ventilation.

V. Conclusions

Given the results of clinical and experimental studies, we speculate that a contribution of neutrophils to chronic lung injury in human neonates occurs early, during the process of acute lung injury that accompanies mechanical ventilation and exposure to the elevated concentrations of oxygen required for treatment of lung disease that is associated with surfactant deficiency. Although the recent studies in preterm lambs suggest a rapid, and perhaps transient, neutrophil sequestration in the lungs shortly after birth, it is likely that continued trauma induced by mechanical ventilation and tissue injury that is associated with hyperoxia results in neutrophil recruitment into the lung. Despite certain shortcomings, the

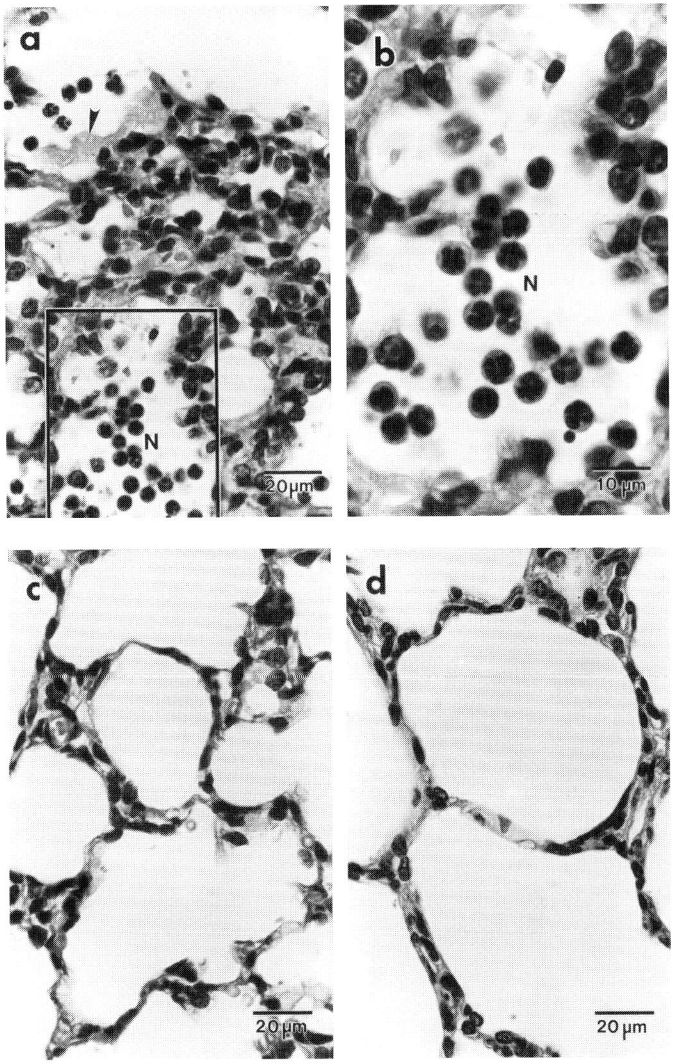

Figure 2 Histopathology of acute lung injury of premature lambs at 126 days approximate gestation (term is 148 days) that were mechanically ventilated for 8 hr with 100% oxygen: None of the lambs received surfactant replacement. (a, b) Neutrophil accumulation and hyaline membrane formation (arrowhead) in the distal airspaces of the lung. The blocked area in a is shown at higher magnification in b to demonstrate that the leukocytes in the airspaces are predominantly neutrophils. (c) Preterm lambs that did not develop acute lung injury had inflated distal airspaces that lacked neutrophils and hyaline membranes. (d) In utero treatment of preterm lambs with nitrogen mustard to eliminate neutrophils before operative delivery also resulted in uninjured lungs, suggesting a role for neutrophils in the pathogenesis of acute lung injury of prematurity.

results of the clinical studies suggest that a larger number of neutrophils accumulate in the first week in the proximal airways of infants who later acquire BPD, a finding corroborated by evidence derived from the premature baboon model of BPD. Neutrophils that migrate into lung parenchyma are likely to be activated and thereby mediate lung damage by the release of proteases and oxidants. A cause-and-effect relation between neutrophil influx during the first week of life and acute and subsequent chronic lung injury in preterm infants, however, remains to be established. The contribution made to chronic lung disease by neutrophils that are present in the lung after the first week of life is far less clear. Further analyses of neutrophil localization, activation, and degranulation, and the molecular mechanisms governing neutrophil sequestration and extravasation in the pulmonary circulation of preterm animals with evolving chronic lung injury will be necessary to delineate the role of the neutrophil in chronic lung disease of prematurity.

References

1. Weissmann G, Smolen JE, Korchak HM. Release of inflammatory mediators from stimulated neutrophils. N Engl J Med 1980; 303:27.
2. Fantone JC, Ward PA. Polymorphonuclear leukocyte-mediated cell and tissue injury: oxygen metabolites and their relations to human disease. Hum Pathol 1985; 16:973.
3. Johnson KJ, Fantone JC III, Kaplan J, Ward PA. In vivo damage of rat lungs by oxygen metabolites. J Clin Invest 1981; 67:983.
4. Johnson KJ, Ward PA. Role of oxygen-metabolites in immune complex injury of lung. J Immunol 1981; 126:2365.
5. Rosen GM, Pou S, Ramos CL, Cohen MS, Britigan BE. Free radicals and phagocytic cells. FASEB J 1995; 9:200.
6. Zaslow MC, Clark RA, Stone PJ, Calore J, Snider GL, Franzblau C. Myeloperoxidase-induced inactivation of α_1-antiprotease in hamsters. J Lab Clin Med 1985; 105: 178.
7. Springer TA. Traffic signals for lymphocyte recirculation and leukocyte emigration: the multistep paradigm. Cell 1994; 76:301.
8. Hynes RO, Lander AD. Contact and adhesive specificities in the associations, migrations, and targeting of cells and axons. Cell 1992; 68:303.
9. Ley K, Tedder TF, Kansas GS. L-selectin can mediate leukocyte rolling in untreated mesenteric venules in vivo independent of E- or P-selectin. Blood 1993; 82:1632.
10. Ley K, Bullard DC, Arbones ML, Bosse R, Vestweber D, Tedder TF, Beaudet AL. Sequential contribution of L- and P-selectin to leukocyte rolling in vivo. J Exp Med 1995; 181:669.
11. Kansas GS, Ley K, Munro M, Tedder TF. Regulation of leukocyte rolling and adhesion to high endothelial venules through the cytoplasmic domain of L-selectin. J Exp Med 1993; 177:833.
12. Mayadas TN, Johnson RC, Rayburn H, Hynes RO, Wagner DD. Leukocyte rolling

and extravasation are severely compromised in P-selectin-deficient mice. Cell 1993; 74:541.

13. Dore M, Korthuis RJ, Granger DN, Entman ML, Smith CW. P-selectin mediates spontaneous leukocyte rolling in vivo. Blood 1993; 82:1308.
14. Asako H, Kurose I, Wolf R, DeFrees S, Zheng Z-L, Phillips ML, Paulson JC, Granger N. Role of H_1 receptors and P-selectin in histamine-induced leukocyte rolling and adhesion in postcapillary venules. J Clin Invest 1994; 93:1508.
15. Lawrence M, Springer T. Leukocytes roll on a selectin at physiologic flow rates: distinction from and prerequisite for adhesion through integrins. Cell 1991; 65:859.
16. Abbassi O, Kishimoto TK, McIntire LV, Anderson DC, Smith CW. E-selectin supports neutrophil rolling in vitro under conditions of flow. J Clin Invest 1993; 92: 2719.
17. Kishimoto TK, Jutila MA, Berg EL, Butcher EC. Neutrophil Mac-1 and MEL-14 adhesion proteins are inversely regulated by chemotactic factors. Science 1989; 245:1238.
18. Spertini O, Kansas GS, Munro JM, Griffin JD, Tedder TF. Regulation of leukocyte migration by activation of the leukocyte adhesion molecule-1 (LAM-1) selectin. Nature 1991; 349:691.
19. McEver R, Beckstead J, Moore K, Marshall-Carlson L, Bainton D. GMP-140, a platelet α-granule membrane protein, is also synthesized by vascular endothelial cells and is localized in Weibel-Palade bodies. J Clin Invest 1989; 84:92.
20. Geng J-G, Bevilacqua MP, Moore KL, McIntyre TM, Prescott SM, Kim JM, Bliss GA, Zimmerman GA, McEver RP. Rapid neutrophil adhesion to activated endothelium mediated by GMP-140. Nature 1990; 343:757.
21. Foreman KE, Vaporciyan AA, Bonish BK, Jones ML, Johnson KJ, Glovsky MM, Eddy SM, Ward PA. C5a-induced expression of P-selectin in endothelial cells. J Clin Invest 1994; 94:1147.
22. Patel KD, Zimmerman GA, Prescott SM, McEver RP, McIntyre TM. Oxygen radicals induce human endothelial cells to express GMP-140 and bind neutrophils. J Cell Biol 1991; 112:749.
23. Bevilacqua MP, Pober JS, Mendrick DL, Cotran RS, Gimbrone MA. Identification of an inducible endothelial–leukocyte adhesion molecule. Proc Nat Acad Sci USA 1987; 84:9238.
24. Zimmerman GA, McIntyre TM, Mehra M, Prescott SM. Endothelial cell-associated platelet-activating factor: a novel mechanism for signaling intercellular adhesion. J Cell Biol 1990; 110:529.
25. Lorant DE, Patel KD, McIntyre TM, McEver RP, Prescott SM, Zimmerman GA. Coexpression of GMP-140 and PAF by endothelium stimulated by histamine or thrombin: a juxtacrine system for adhesion and activation of neutrophils. J Cell Biol 1991; 115:223.
26. Detmers PA, Lo SK, Olsen-Egbert E, Walz A, Baggiolini M, Cohn ZA. Neutrophil-activating protein 1/interleukin 8 stimulates the binding activity of the leukocyte adhesion receptor CD11b/CD18 on human neutrophils. J Exp Med 1990; 171:1155.
27. Huber AR, Kunkel SL, Todd RF, Weiss SJ. Regulation of transendothelial neutrophil migration by endogenous interleukin-8. Science 1991; 254:99.
28. Carveth HJ, Bohnsack JF, McIntyre TM, Baggiolini M, Prescott SM, Zimmerman GA. Neutrophil activating factor (NAF) induces polymorphonuclear leukocyte ad-

herence to endothelial cells and to subendothelial matrix proteins. Biochem Biophys Res Commun 1989; 162:387.
29. Hynes RO. Integrins: versatility, modulation, and signaling in cell adhesion. Cell 1992; 69:11.
30. Albertine K, Rosolia D, Peters S, Gee M. Physical and cytochemical properties of neutrophils activated in situ in the lung during ZAP infusion in sheep. J Appl Physiol 1993; 74:1361.
31. Staub N, Schultz E, Albertine K. Leukocytes and pulmonary microvascular injury. Ann NY Acad Sci 1982; 384:332.
32. Worthen GS, Schwab B III, Elson EL, Downey GP. Mechanics of stimulated neutrophils: cell stiffening induces retention in capillaries. Science 1989; 245:183.
33. Mulligan MS, Polley MJ, Bayer RJ, Nunn MF, Paulson JC, Ward PA. Neutrophil-dependent acute lung injury. Requirement for P-selectin (GMP-140). J Clin Invest 1992; 90:1600.
34. Mulligan MS, Varani J, Dame MK, Lane CL, Smith CW, Anderson DC, Ward PA. Role of endothelial-leukocyte adhesion molecule 1 (ELAM-1) in neutrophil-mediated lung injury in rats. J Clin Invest 1991; 88:1396.
35. Doerschuk CM, Winn RK, Coxson HO, Harlan JM. CD-18-dependent and -independent mechanisms of neutrophil emigration in the pulmonary and systemic microcirculation of rabbits. J Immunol 1990; 144:2327.
36. Winn RK, Mileski WJ, Kovach NL, Doerschuk CM, Rice CL, Harlan JM. Role of protein synthesis and CD11/CD18 adhesion complex in neutrophil emigration into the lung. Exp Lung Res 1993; 19:221.
37. Bullard DC, Qin L, Lorenzo I, Quinlin WM, Doyle NA, Bosse R, Vestweber D, Doerschuk CM, Beaudet AL. P-selectin/ICAM-1 double mutant mice: acute emigration of neutrophils into the peritoneum is completely absent but is normal into pulmonary alveoli. J Clin Invest 1995; 95:1782.
38. Downey GP, Worthen GS, Henson PM, Hyde DM. Neutrophil sequestration and migration in localized pulmonary inflammation. Am Rev Respir Dis 1993; 147: 168.
39. Reid L. Bronchopulmonary dysplasia—pathology. J Pediatr 1979; 95:836.
40. Wigglesworth JS. Pathology of the lung in the fetus and neonate, with particular reference to problems of growth and maturation. Histopathology 1987; 11:671–689.
41. Oppermann HC, Wille L, Bleyl U, Obladen M. Bronchopulmonary dysplasia in premature infants. A radiological and pathological correlation. Pediatr Radiol 1977; 5: 137.
42. Taghizadeh A, Reynolds EOR. Pathogenesis of bronchopulmonary dysplasia following hyaline membrane disease. Am J Pathol 1976; 82:241.
43. Boss JH, Craig JM. Reparative phenomena in lungs of neonates with hyaline membranes. Pediatrics 1962; 29:890.
44. Banerjee CK, Girling DJ, Wigglesworth JS. Pulmonary fibroplasia in newborn babies treated with oxygen and artificial ventilation. Arch Dis Child 1972; 47:509.
45. Chambers HM, van Velzen D. Ventilator-related pathology in the extremely immature lung. Pathology 1989; 21:79.
46. Northway WH Jr, Rosan RC, Porter DY. Pulmonary disease following respirator therapy of hyaline-membrane disease. N Engl J Med 1967; 276:357.

47. Bonikos DS, Bensch KG, Northway WH, Edwards DK. Bronchopulmonary dysplasia: the pulmonary pathologic sequel of necrotizing bronchiolitis and pulmonary fibrosis. Hum Pathol 1976; 7:643.
48. D'Ablang GB, Bernard B, Saharov I, Barton L, Kaplan B, Schwinn C. Neonatal pulmonary cytology and bronchopulmonary dysplasia. Acta Cytol 1975; 19:21.
49. Merritt TA, Stuard ID, Puccia J, Wood B, Edwards DK, Finkelstein J, Shapiro DL. Newborn tracheal aspirate cytology: classification during respiratory distress syndrome and bronchopulmonary dysplasia. J Pediatr 1981; 98:949.
50. Merritt TA, Cochrane CG, Holcomb K, Bohl B, Hallman M, Strayer D, Edwards DK III, Gluck L. Elastase and α_1-proteinase inhibitor activity in tracheal aspirates during respiratory distress syndrome. Role of inflammation in the pathogenesis of bronchopulmonary dysplasia. J Clin Invest 1983; 72:656.
51. Ogden BE, Murphy SA, Saunders GC, Pathak D, Johnson JD. Neonatal lung neutrophils and elastase/proteinase inhibitor imbalance. Am Rev Respir Dis 1984; 130: 817.
52. Groneck P, Gotze-Speer B, Oppermann M, Eiffert H, Speer CP. Association of pulmonary inflammation and increased microvascular permeability during the development of bronchopulmonary dysplasia: a sequential analysis of inflammatory mediators in respiratory fluids of high-risk preterm neonates. Pediatrics 1994; 93: 712.
53. Arnon S, Grigg J, Silverman M. Pulmonary inflammatory cells in ventilated preterm infants: effect of surfactant treatment. Arch Dis Child 1993; 69:44.
54. Watterberg KL, Carmichael DF, Gerdes JS, Werner S, Backstrom C, Murphy S. Secretory leukocyte protease inhibitor and lung inflammation in developing bronchopulmonary dysplasia. J Pediatr 1994; 125:264.
55. Ferreira PJ, Albertine KH, Carlton DP. Early postnatal neutropenia and respiratory distress in preterm infants. J Invest Med 1996; 44:133A.
56. Janoff A. Proteases and lung injury. State of the art minireview. Chest 1984; 545:54S.
57. Burri PH. Postnatal development and growth. In: Crystal RG, West JB, eds. The Lung. Scientific Foundations. New York: Raven Press, 1991:677.
58. Hislop AA, Wigglesworth JS, Desai R, Aber V. The effects of preterm delivery and mechanical ventilation on human lung growth. Early Hum Dev 1987; 15:147.
59. Bruce MC, Wedig KE, Jentoft N, Martin RJ, Cheng PW, Boat TF, Fanaroff AA. Altered urinary excretion of elastin cross-links in premature infants who develop bronchopulmonary dysplasia. Am Rev Respir Dis 1985; 131:568.
60. Walti H, Tordet C, Gerbaut L, Saugier P, Moriette G, Reliet JP. Persistent elastase/proteinase inhibitor imbalance during prolonged ventilation of infants with bronchopulmonary dysplasia: evidence for the role of nosocomial infections. Pediatr Res 1989; 26:351.
61. Bruce MC, Schuyler M, Martine RJ, Starcher BC, Tomashefski JF Jr, Wedig KE. Risk factors for the degradation of lung elastic fibers in the ventilated neonate. Implications for impaired lung development in bronchopulmonary dysplasia. Am Rev Respir Dis 1992; 146:204.
62. Samuelsson B. Leukotrienes: mediators of immediate hypersensitivity reactions and inflammation. Science 1983; 220:568.
63. Wright DG, Gallin JL. Modulation of the inflammatory response by products re-

leased from human polymorphonuclear leukocytes during phagocytosis. Generation and inactivation of chemotactic factor C5a. Inflammation 1975; 1:23.
64. Cassatella MA, Bazzoni F, Ceska M, Ferro I, Baggiolini M, Berton G. IL-8 production by human polymorphonuclear leukocytes. J Immunol 1992; 148:3216–3220.
65. Reynolds HY. Lung inflammation: role of endogenous chemotactic factors in attracting polymorphonuclear granulocytes. Am Rev Respir Dis 1983; 127:S16.
66. Harda RN, Vatter AE, Repine JE. Macrophage effector function in pulmonary oxygen toxicity: hyperoxia damages and stimulates alveolar macrophages to make and release chemotaxins for polymorphonuclear leukocytes. J Leukoc Biol 1984; 35:373.
67. Irving LB, Jordana M, O'Brodovich H, Gauldie J. Alveolar macrophage activation in bronchopulmonary dysplasia. Am Rev Respir Dis 1986; 133:A207.
68. Silverman M. Chronic lung disease of prematurity: are we too cautious with steroids? Eur J Pediatr 1994; 153(suppl 2):S30.
69. Yoder MC, Chua R, Tepper R. Effect of dexamethasone on pulmonary inflammation and pulmonary function of ventilator-dependent infants with bronchopulmonary dysplasia. Am Rev Respir Dis 1991; 143:1044.
70. Gerdes JS, Harris MC, Polin RA. Effects of dexamethasone and indomethacin on elastase, alpha$_1$-proteinase inhibitor, and fibronectin in bronchoalveolar lavage fluid from neonates. J Pediatr 1988; 113:727.
71. Suttorp N, Simon LM. Lung cell oxidant injury. Enhancement of polymorphonuclear leukocyte-mediated cytotoxicity in lung cells exposed to sustained in vitro hyperoxia. J Clin Invest 1982; 70:342.
72. Bowman CM, Butler EN, Vatter AE, Repine JE. Hyperoxia injures endothelial cells in culture and causes increased neutrophil adherence. Chest 1983; 83:33S.
73. Lewis MS, Whatley RE, Cain P, McIntyre TM, Prescott SM, Zimmerman GA. Hydrogen peroxide stimulates the synthesis of platelet-activating factor by endothelium and induces endothelial cell-dependent neutrophil adhesion. J Clin Invest 1988; 82: 2045.
74. Prescott SM, Zimmerman GA, McIntyre TM. Human endothelial cells in culture produce platelet-activating factor (1-alkyl-2-acetyl-*sn*-glycero-3-phosphocholine) when stimulated with thrombin. Proc Natl Acad Sci USA 1984; 81:3534.
75. McIntyre TM, Zimmerman GA, Satoh K, Prescott SM. Cultured endothelial cells synthesize both platelet-activating factor and prostacyclin in response to histamine, bradykinin, and adenosine triphosphate. J Clin Invest 1985; 76:271.
76. Patel KD, Zimmerman GA, Prescott SM, McIntyre TM. Novel leukocyte agonists are released by endothelial cells exposed to peroxide. J Biol Chem 1992; 267:15168.
77. Rinaldo JE, English D, Levine J, Stiller R, Henson J. Increased intrapulmonary retention of radiolabeled neutrophils in early oxygen toxicity. Am Rev Respir Dis 1988; 137:345.
78. Griffin RL, Krzesicki RF, Fidler SF, Rosenbloom CL, Auchampach JA, Manning AM, Haas JV, Cammarata SK, Chim JE, Richards IM. Attenuation of oxidant-induced lung injury by 21-aminosteroids (lazaroids): correlation with the mRNA expression for E-selectin, P-selectin, ICAM-1, and VCAM-1. Environ Health Perspect 1994; 102(suppl 10):193.
79. Crapo JD, Barry BE, Foscue HA, Shelburne J. Structural and biochemical changes

in rat lungs occurring during exposures to lethal and adaptive doses of oxygen. Am Rev Respir Dis 1980; 122:123.
80. Fox RB, Hoidal JR, Brown DM, Repine JE. Pulmonary inflammation due to oxygen toxicity: involvement of chemotactic factors and polymorphonuclear leukocytes. Am Rev Respir Dis 1981; 123:521.
81. Merritt TA. Oxygen exposure in the newborn guinea pig lung lavage cell populations, chemotactic and elastase response: a possible relationship to neonatal bronchopulmonary dysplasia. Pediatr Res 1982; 16:798.
82. Shasby DM, Fox RB, Harada RN, Repine JE. Reduction of the edema of acute hyperoxic lung injury by granulocyte depletion. J Appl Physiol 1982; 52:11237.
83. Wegner CD, Wolyniec WW, LaPlante AM, Marschman K, Lubber K, Haynes N, Rothlein R, Letts LG. Intercellular adhesion molecule-1 contributes to pulmonary oxygen toxicity in mice: role of leukocytes revised. Lung 1992; 170:267.
84. Raj JU, Hazinski TA, Bland RD. Oxygen-induced lung microvascular injury in neutropenic rabbits and lambs. J Appl Physiol 1985; 53:921.
85. Kawano T, Mori S, Cybulsky M, Burger R, Ballin A, Cutz E, Bryan AC. Effect of granulocyte depletion in a ventilated surfactant-depleted lung. J Appl Physiol 1987; 62:27.
86. Kelly FJ, Town GI, Phillips GJ, Holgate ST, Roche WR, Postle AD. The pre-term guinea-pig: a model for the study of neonatal lung disease. Clin Sci 1991; 81:439.
87. Tabor BL, Lewis JF, Ikegami M, Jobe AH. Platelet-activating factor antagonists decrease lung protein leak in preterm ventilated rabbits. Am J Obstet Gynecol 1992; 167:810.
88. Coalson JJ, Winter VT, Gerstmann DR, Idell S, King RJ, Delemos RA. Pathophysiologic, morphometric, and biochemical studies of the premature baboon with bronchopulmonary dysplasia. Am Rev Respir Dis 1992; 145:872.
89. Jenkinson SG, Roberts RJ, DeLemos RA, Lawrence RA, Coalson JJ, King RJ, Null DM, Gerstmann DR. Allopurinol-induced effects in premature baboons with respiratory distress syndrome. J Appl Physiol 1991; 70:1160.
90. Bland RD, Chos S, Carlton DP, Albertine K, Davis P. Chronic lung injury in mechanically ventilated preterm lambs. FASEB J 1995; 9:A275.
91. Albertine KH, Carlton DP, Cho S, Davis PL, Bland RD. Histopathology of chronic lung injury in preterm lambs. FASEB J 1995; 9:A275.
92. Carlton DP, Cho SC, Albertine KH, Davis P, Bland RD. Role of neutrophils in lung vascular injury edema after premature birth in lambs. J Appl Physiol 1997; 83:1307–1317.
93. Jackson JC, Chi EY, Wilson CB, Truog WE, Teh EC, Hodson WA. Sequence of inflammatory cell migration into lung during recovery from hyaline membrane disease in premature newborn monkeys. Am Rev Respir Dis 1987; 135:937.

33

The Role of Pulmonary Macrophages in Chronic Lung Disease of Early Infancy

MICHAEL P. SHERMAN

University of California
Davis, California

WILLIAM E. TRUOG

University of Missouri
Kansas City, Missouri

I. Introduction

Chronic lung disease (CLD) of early infancy is a multifaceted disease that is caused by prolonged oxygen therapy or the barotrauma of assisted ventilation (1–4). Although endothelium, type II pneumonocytes, fibroblasts, and neutrophils have major roles in the pathophysiology of CLD, pulmonary macrophages are arguably the major cell type responsible for the initiation, regulation, and resolution of inflammation in this disease. The role of pulmonary macrophages is one that reaches far beyond the inflammatory responses of the immature lung to hyperoxia or physical injury. This chapter will address the pathophysiology of CLD as it relates to pulmonary macrophages. Recently reviewed subject areas include (1) the emergence of the pulmonary macrophage populations during fetal and neonatal life, (2) the role that macrophages and pulmonary infections play in the pathogenesis of chronic lung disease of early infancy, (3) the interactions of lung macrophages have with other pulmonary cells by cell-to-cell communication or mediator release, (4) the importance that macrophages have in clearing inflammatory neutrophils from the alveoli, (5) the limitations of studying lung macrophages in human neonates, and (6) future recommendations for understanding macrophages as important participants in the causation and resolution of acute lung injury during the neonatal period. Each topic will summarize our current knowledge related to clinical and basic research on lung macrophages of newborns, and indicate additional investigations needed to facilitate new therapeutic and preventive strategies for CLD.

II. Emergence of Pulmonary Macrophage Populations and the Pathophysiology of CLD of Early Infancy

This section reviews the presence of macrophages in different lung compartments and their roles in the lung. The emergence of these different macrophage subpopulations in the lung before and after birth is described. Finally, the importance of a nascent lung macrophage population as a component in the pathophysiology of chronic lung disease of early infancy is discussed.

A. Compartmental Characteristics of Pulmonary Macrophages

Over 100 years ago, Metchnikoff described ameba-like phagocytes that were easily identified in mammals, the lineage of which extended throughout phylogeny to invertebrates (5). The presence of these phagocytes in almost all tissues and organs has resulted in extensive investigations of the mononuclear phagocytic system. Compared with studies of adult animals and humans, however, knowledge of the mononuclear phagocytic system of newborns is limited. The first in vitro and in vivo reports investigating macrophages of newborns appeared 20 years ago and used pulmonary alveolar macrophages (6–9). The ease of obtaining alveolar macrophages by lung lavage has resulted in a greater understanding of these mononuclear phagocytes compared with their counterparts in other lung locations. Pulmonary macrophages, by their specialized functions in different locations, have been divided into bronchial, alveolar, interstitial, intravascular, and pleural types (10,11). The alveolar macrophage is the resident phagocyte of the alveolar space in newborns and adults (reviewed in Ref. 12). Subpopulations of alveolar macrophages express different receptors, have varying cytological and phagocytic characteristics, and manifest distinct mediator release, depending on the disease state (13–15). The properties of alveolar macrophage subpopulations have not been studied during the course of CLD using either a premature animal model or human subjects. Although bronchial macrophages partially represent macrophages leaving the more distal pulmonary airspaces through the mucociliary escalator, there are identifiable bronchial macrophages that are tightly adherent to tracheobronchial epithelium. These phagocytes remove foreign material from the large airways (16). The relative contributions made by tracheobronchial versus alveolar macrophages in clearing damaged and shed epithelia and apoptotic neutrophils has not been examined. Interstitial macrophages are located in the lung's connective tissue and are recovered by digesting minced pulmonary tissue (17). The numbers of interstitial macrophages can change during the course of different lung diseases (18). These phagocytes share some characteristics with alveolar macrophages, such as particulate ingestion, release of oxygen intermediates, and receptors for the Fc fragment of immunoglobulins (19,20).

The ability of interstitial macrophages to synthesize DNA and replicate has suggested that they function to renew the alveolar macrophage population (21). Interstitial macrophages of newborn lungs have not been investigated. In addition to alveolar and interstitial macrophages, newborns in the order Artiodactyla (hoofed animals) have pulmonary intravascular macrophages (22). The presence of pulmonary intravascular macrophages has also been demonstrated in adult humans (23). These macrophages appear to function as an accessory reticuloendothelial clearance system separate from that of liver and spleen (24,25). Neither the numbers, the function, nor the propensity of pulmonary intravascular macrophages to injure pulmonary endothelium have been studied in newborn infants. Nevertheless, it is interesting to speculate that these macrophages may damage endothelium and amplify pulmonary inflammation when newborns require intensive care caused by bacteremia or infections related to indwelling vascular catheters. The final macrophage compartment in the lung is that of the pleural macrophage. These macrophages have similarities to peritoneal macrophages (26). Their presence and role in initiating pleural fibrosis during the course of neonatal lung diseases has not been reported in thc literature.

B. The Origins of Pulmonary Macrophages in Newborns and the Association Between Population Kinetics and CLD of Early Infancy

The origins of macrophage precursors begin in the lung of fetal rats during the bronchial bud stage (27–30). As lung development progresses, the pulmonary interstitium, and to a lesser extent the free airspaces, have replicating cells with surface markers and intracellular histochemical characteristics of macrophages. In neonatal rabbits, these cells are not blood monocytes, but immature macrophages. These cells can be distinguished from a second source of monocytic phagocytes that originate in the bone marrow and enter the alveoli from blood just before, and following parturition (6). All mammalian species studied (6,31–33), including man (34,35), appear to have this intra-alveolar influx of monocytic-appearing phagocytes at close to the time of birth. Near the time of birth, monocytic-appearing cells entering the alveoli from blood are capable of at least one more cell division (36), a phenomenon similar to macrophage renewal described in adults (37). Cellular replication is largely responsible for the increasing alveolar macrophage numbers between postnatal days 1 and 5 (33,36). In postnatal pigs, pulmonary intravascular macrophages also proliferate within the lung's capillaries (38). The expansion of interstitial, bronchial, and pleural macrophage subpopulations has not been studied in the newborn.

The influx and replication of alveolar macrophages following birth appears to be mediated by negatively charged phospholipids. Phosphatidylglycerol (PG) strongly stimulates migration and replication of macrophages (39,40). In premature monkeys, increased alveolar macrophage numbers were related to the quantity of phospholipid present and the absence of hyaline membrane disease (32). Human premature infants who received surfactant replacement also have higher macrophage numbers between 3 and 7 days of age compared with untreated newborns (41). Increased polymorphonuclear (PMN) leukocytes and diminished macrophages are an early and consistent finding in the bronchial aspirates of premature infants who acquire CLD (39,41). Taken together, these findings suggest that surfactant has a major role in the emergence of the alveolar macrophage population. As the acute lung injury phase of CLD resolves, macrophages become more prominent in tracheal aspirates of human premature newborns (42). Jackson and colleagues, using a premature monkey model of hyaline membrane disease, concluded that the influx of macrophages during recovery would modulate neutrophil activity for "better or worse" (43). One can speculate that the premature human lung withstands prolonged hyperoxia and ventilator barotrauma to a greater extent than the adult lung because it is macrophage-deficient. For example, reduced numbers of macrophages in the lungs of extremely premature infants might mean there are lower concentrations of macrophage-derived proinflammatory and fibrosis-initiating cytokines and growth factors. This assumption is supported by a study using rats that were depleted of macrophages and then exposed to hyperoxia (44). Rats with alveolar macrophages were very susceptible to O_2 toxicity, with a 100% mortality after 74 hr, whereas 20% of macrophage-depleted rats survived beyond that point. Thus, it might be anticipated that an excess of macrophages in neonatal lungs might enhance death from hyperoxia or increase pulmonary fibrosis during the recovery phase of acute lung injury. The interrelations between macrophages and hyperoxic lung injury might be tested by comparing the outcome of normal neonatal mice versus a recently described transgenic mouse bearing a tissue-specific surfactant protein C–granulocyte–macrophage colony-stimulating factor (GM–CST) chimeric gene which causes marked increases in pulmonary macrophages (45). It might be expected that the increased alveolar macrophage population in this transgenic strain of mice would hasten neonatal death during hyperoxia. Certainly, the relation between the population kinetics of macrophages in the lungs of prematurely born infants and the pathogenesis of CLD deserves further study.

III. The Role of Pulmonary Macrophages and Lung Infection in the Pathophysiology of CLD of Early Infancy

This section briefly outlines neonatal susceptibility to pneumonia based on maturational deficiencies in alveolar macrophage microbicidal activity. The potential contribution of pulmonary infections to the pathogenesis of CLD of early infancy is also reviewed. Lastly, neonatal treatments are discussed that may alter the antimicrobial functions of macrophages, thereby rendering the neonate at risk for pulmonary infection and the amplification of lung inflammation.

A. Maturation of Microbicidal Mechanisms in Newborn Alveolar Macrophages

Congenital and hospital-acquired lung infections are common in intensive care nurseries (46–48). Despite a high incidence, little information exists to help clarify if congenital pneumonia increases the risk of CLD. Regardless of the role that congenital pneumonia has in the pathophysiology of CLD, it is well established that nosocomial pneumonia heightens morbidity and mortality in infants with this disease (48). Several physiological events explain the increased susceptibility of newborns to pulmonary infection. As cited previously (6,32,35), pulmonary alveolar macrophages are markedly reduced in the lungs of preterm animals and humans. The absence of these phagocytes can result in severe neonatal pneumonia if amniotic fluid infection results in bacterial colonization of the fetal lung (49). With term parturition, the intra-alveolar macrophage population increases expeditiously unless clinical conditions, such as hyperoxia exist (50). A second explanation for neonatal susceptibility to pneumonia is that newborn macrophages have immature antibacterial mechanisms, including decreased complement receptors (51), impaired respiratory burst activity (52), and diminished lysosomal microbicides (7,53). Conversely, it is reported that macrophages recovered from the lungs of infants with established CLD have increased production of H_2O_2 compared with macrophages lavaged from ventilator-dependent infants without CLD (54). Because infants who acquire CLD are more susceptible to nosocomial pneumonia than their nonafflicted counterparts in the intensive care nursery, the increased production of H_2O_2 by macrophages may be a marker of their activation and associated with lung injury, rather than a heightened host defense. Thus, maturational events in alveolar macrophages, the lung's innate phagocytic system, increase the risk for pulmonary infections and, in turn, add to the occurrence or severity of CLD.

B. Pulmonary Infection and Its Role in the Pathogenesis of CLD in Early Infancy

The importance of pulmonary infections in the pathogenesis of CLD is illustrated by the exclusion of infants with congenital pneumonia from surfactant replacement studies when the outcome variables included the incidence of CLD (55–57). This approach may be based on the observation that infants with pneumonia have higher concentrations of elastase and leukocyte protease inhibitor in bronchoalveolar lavage fluid than do those with respiratory distress syndrome (RDS;

58). Increased elastase content and reduced protease inhibitor levels in bronchoalveolar lavage fluid during the first week of life predict the development of bronchopulmonary dysplasia (59,60). Furthermore, pulmonary infections should amplify the concentration of mediators that enhance lung inflammation. Despite the assumption that congenital pneumonia might increase a premature infant's susceptibility to CLD, only *Ureaplasma urealyticum* infections have been implicated in the pathogenesis of CLD (61,62). Experimental studies have shown mechanisms wherein pulmonary *U. urealyticum* infections would cause CLD (63,64). Pulmonary infections with *U. urealyticum* as an initiator of CLD is controversial, however, as logistic regression analyses have identified the degree of immaturity as being the more important inciting factor, compared with infection (65,66). Excluding studies of *U. urealyticum*, chorioamnionitis, and the presence of interleukin-1β(IL-1β) in pulmonary secretions of preterm infants, is strongly associated with the development of bronchopulmonary dysplasia (67). The role of intrauterine infection or congenital pneumonia as cofactors that enhance the lung's inflammatory response in CLD certainly deserves attention in future studies.

C. Clinical Conditions Affecting Macrophage Function and Their Relation to the Pathogenesis of CLD of Early Infancy

Added to the maturational abnormalities of macrophages that augment the newborn's risk for congenital pneumonia are various postnatal therapies that also may affect macrophage competence. Commonly used treatments that are applied to the care of preterm infants include oxygen, surfactant replacement, and dexamethasone. These treatments might be expected to increase the infant's susceptibility to nosocomial lung infection and to amplify inflammation. First among these interventions is prolonged hyperoxia, which not only suppresses macrophage replication in the pulmonary alveoli after birth (50), but also impairs the macrophage's bactericidal activity (68). A diminished macrophage population and damaged antimicrobial mechanisms of macrophages would certainly contribute to the development of nosocomial pneumonia, a disease seen frequently in newborns who acquire CLD. Prolonged exposure to hyperoxia also causes an excessive release of phospholipids into the alveoli. Alveolar macrophages then engulf the phospholipid (lamellar bodies) and can develop a defect in their ability to kill inhaled *Escherichia coli* (69). This abnormality is akin to a bactericidal defect of macrophages recovered from humans with alveolar proteinosis and can be simulated by instilling phospholipid vesicles down the trachea of term newborn rabbits (70). Nevertheless, premature rabbits infected with group B streptococcal aerosols do not have excessive intrapulmonary bacterial proliferation after commercially available surfactant preparations are instilled into their macrophage-deficient lungs (71). Thus, surfactant preparations do not act as a growth medium in vivo and, in fact, some of the surfactant preparations used in the clinical setting may actually restrict bacterial growth.

Inhaled nitric oxide (iNO) has been used successfully in treating pulmonary hypertension in term neonates (72). Clinical trials are now being formulated to treat premature infants with respiratory distress syndrome (Wearden ME, personal communication). Issues remain, however, concerning the safety of iNO, for breathing NO along with hyperoxia has the potential to generate highly oxidative, nitrogen-centered species such as NO_2 and N_2O_3 (73). In adult studies, these nitrogen-centered species were potent oxidants that readily damaged alveolar macrophages and other airway cells. To study this potential, we exposed 2-week-old piglets to either 5 or 50 parts per million (ppm) of iNO and 94+% oxygen for 24 hr and then ascertained the toxic effects in lavaged alveolar macrophages (74,75). After 24 hr, 50 ppm of NO and hyperoxia caused significant neutrophil influx when the NO_2 formed in the chamber was maintained at 2 ppm or higher (Table 1). When procedures were used to diminish the formation of or eliminate NO_2, so that concentrations of NO_2 were less than 1 ppm in the exposure chamber, neutrophil influx was significantly reduced. Furthermore, inhaling 94+% O_2 and 50 ppm NO for 24 hr resulted in a significantly enhanced ability of lavaged macrophages to kill nonopsonized group B streptococci (GBS) when compared with room air-exposed macrophages (Fig. 1A). The same exposure had no detrimental effect on the antibacterial activity of macrophages toward GBS opsonized with piglet serum (see Fig. 1B). Because 24 hr of exposure to 50 ppm of iNO and hyperoxia was associated with some augmentation of GBS ingestion, enhanced

Table 1 Leukocyte Composition of Bronchoalveolar Lavage Fluid Following Exposure to Hyperoxia and Inhaled Nitric Oxide

	Leukocyte composition[a]		
Type of exposure	Macrophages ($\times 10^6$)	Neutrophils ($\times 10^6$)	Lymphocytes ($\times 10^6$)
$FIO_2 = 0.21$	44.9 ± 2.5 [95.3]	0.9 ± 0.5 [1.8]	0.7 ± 0.2 [1.5]
$FIO_2 \geq 0.94$	58.9 ± 2.9 [97.1]	0.2 ± 0.2 [0.3]	1.1 ± 0.5 [1.8]
$FIO_2 \geq 0.94$ + 5 ppm NO	50.0 ± 8.2 [95.0]	0.5 ± 0.2 [1.8]	1.8 ± 1.3 [2.8]
$FIO_2 \geq 0.94$ + 50 ppm NO (charcoal present)	68.3 ± 11.5 [87.5]	10.7 ± 9.9 [9.3]	1.9 ± 0.8 [2.3]
$FIO_2 \geq 0.94$ + 50 ppm NO (no charcoal)	66.6 ± 13.4 [48.8]	69.0 ± 21.6* [46.3]	3.8 ± 2.1 [2.8]

[a]Results are expressed as cells per kilogram body weight ($\times 10^6$) and presented as mean ± SEM ($n = 6$ animals per group). The numbers in brackets show the mean percentage of that cell type based on all cells identified. The $FIO_2 = 0.21$, $FIO_2 \geq 0.94$, and $FIO_2 \geq 0.94$ + 5 ppm NO groups were also exposed in the presence of activated charcoal.

*$p < 0.05$ vs. the $FIO_2 = 0.21$, $FIO_2 \geq 0.94$, and $FIO_2 \geq 0.94$ + 5 ppm NO groups using repeated-measures analysis of variance.

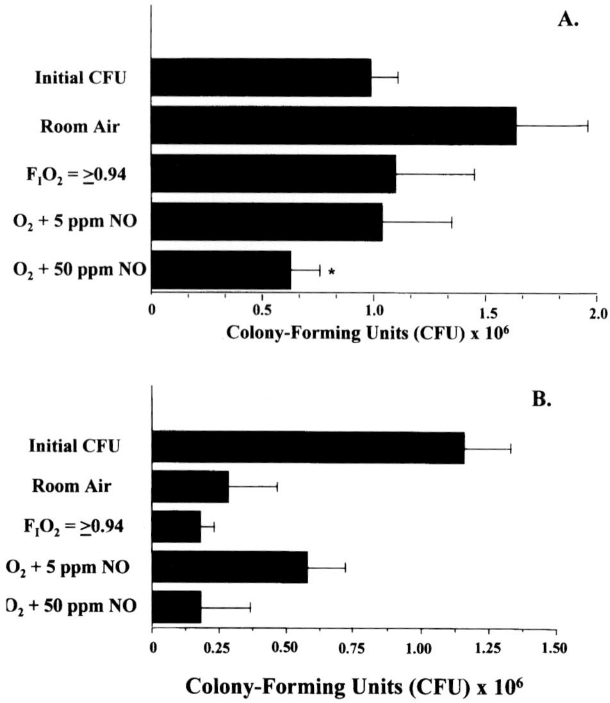

Figure 1 The effect of inhaled nitric oxide and hyperoxia on the killing of nonopsonized and opsonized group B streptococci (GBS) by lavaged bronchoalveolar macrophages: (A) The results of incubating lavaged bronchoalveolar macrophages with nonopsonized GBS; (B) the findings when GBS were preopsonized with piglet serum. The columns represent the mean, and the error bars are the SEM (no. of animals = 6 per treatment group). Differences among the groups were ascertained by the Kruskal-Wallis test. The asterisk signifies a $p < 0.05$ vs. the room air group.

respiratory burst activity, and increased killing of nonopsonized GBS by alveolar macrophages (75), we suspected that the macrophages were ''activated.'' Therefore, we examined macrophages lavaged from exposed piglets for markers of macrophage activation. Early growth response-1 (*Egr-1*) gene is an immediate early gene that encodes a zinc-finger transcription factor and is essential for macrophage differentiation and activation (76). Northern analysis of macrophages lavaged from piglets exposed to 50 ppm of iNO and hyperoxia shows *Egr-1* induction as compared with macrophages recovered from normal piglets, piglets exposed to hyperoxia alone, or piglets treated with 5 ppm of iNO and hyperoxia (74; Fig. 2). Thus, iNO may have beneficial or detrimental effects on the functions

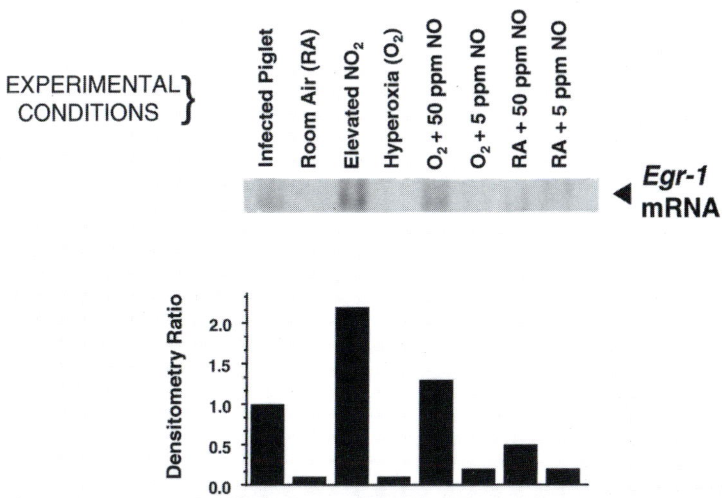

Figure 2 The effect of inhaled nitric oxide or hyperoxia on the expression of early growth response-1 (*Egr-1*) mRNA in bronchoalveolar macrophages of piglets. The type of inhaled gas exposure is shown above the Northern analyses. As a positive control, mRNA was isolated from bronchoalveolar macrophages of a nonexposed piglet with known pulmonary infection. Because no porcine cDNA probes exist, Northern blot analyses used a human probe (77) to demonstrate the induction of *Egr-1* mRNA.

of pulmonary alveolar macrophages. Because iNO is being used with increasing frequency in premature infants, the alterations in macrophages engendered by iNO or hyperoxia deserve further study relative to the pathogenesis of CLD.

Lastly, for more than a decade, dexamethasone has been a frequently used agent that decreases pulmonary inflammation and promotes ventilator weaning in infants with CLD (78). In newborn rats, however, dexamethasone reduces the number and phagocytic activity of macrophages in the lung (79). Thus, the effects of dexamethasone may be complex and difficult to predict. Dexamethasone reduces leukotriene secretion in premature infants with CLD, and this presumably reduces neutrophil recruitment to the lung and diminishes lung injury (80). Conversely, macrophage-related killing of microorganisms is impaired by hyperoxia; therefore, macrophages would need to release leukotrienes and other chemoattractants to recruit neutrophils as a second line of phagocytic defense. Besides potentially impairing the recruitment of neutrophils, therapy with dexamethasone may hinder the clearance of bacteria by macrophages (69). As we move from microbicidal characteristics of macrophages to describing the other functions of macrophages associated with the pathophysiology of CLD, it is noteworthy that macrophages secrete mediators that promote lung healing by fibrosis. Dexamethasone suppresses collagen synthesis in infants with CLD (81).

IV. Interactions of Lung Macrophages with Other Pulmonary Cells by Direct Cell-to-Cell Communication and Secretory Activity

Macrophages play an important role in the initiation of inflammation after a pulmonary insult, and also in the resolution and repair of the lung after injury. This section discusses the role of macrophages in (1) cell signaling through adhesion molecules, (2) their release of proinflammatory cytokines and chemoattractants, (3) the remodeling of extracellular matrix and secretion of growth factors by macrophages, and (4) the role of macrophages in the clearance of apoptotic neutrophils from the alveoli. These actions are the most compelling relative to the role of macrophages in the initiation and the resolution of CLD during early infancy. Most of this information is extrapolated, however, from reports associated with adult respiratory distress syndrome or other pulmonary inflammatory diseases, rather than studies performed in neonatal animals or humans who have disorders consistent with CLD.

A. Expression of Adhesion Molecules by Alveolar Macrophages: Their Role in CLD

The expression, regulation, and interactions of cell surface proteins that mediate adherence between cells, and between cells and the extracellular matrix, is a rapidly expanding area of investigation and new information. Current understanding of this complex system proposes the presence of three classes of proteins: integrins, selectins, and immunoglobulin-related molecules. Perhaps best studied of these are the integrins, which are large glycoproteins that influence both cell–cell and cell–matrix interactions. They are classified into subfamilies, based on a common β-subunit. Various subunit β-integrins function preferentially as receptors for collagen, laminin, fibronectin, and vitronectin. β_2-Integrins serve primarily in cell–cell interactions. By contrast, the selectin family comprises groups of proteins that participate in leukocyte–endothelial interactions. Selectins help regulate the first stage of granulocyte and macrophage attachment to the underlying endothelium. The integrins then help produce tighter adherence between cell types. There is evidence that monocytic cells, including macrophages, require adhesion to become activated. It is only during the activated state that phagocytosis, tissue recruitment and, perhaps most important for CLD, the production of inflammatory mediators occurs.

In 1992, Albert and associates (82) evaluated β_2-integrins on alveolar macrophages obtained from healthy adult human and nonhuman primates. They studied both expression of the CD11/CD18 integrin subunits on alveolar macrophages and their role in chemotaxis and adherence to alveolar epithelial cell monolayers in culture. They concluded (1) that alveolar macrophages constitutively express CD11a/CD18 surface antigen and its mRNA, (2) that chemotaxis of alveolar macrophages is CD18-dependent, and (3) that adhesion of alveolar macrophages to an epithelial cell monolayer is partly, but not completely, dependent on the β_2-integrins. More recently, Prieto et al. (83) evaluated multiple adhesion molecules by comparing results using peripheral blood monocytes and alveolar macrophages. They discovered that the β_1-integrin subunit was expressed on more than one-half of alveolar macrophages, and that α_3- and α_5-subunits were also present. Constitutive expression of CD11b, L-selectins, and other substances in the alveolar macrophage was significantly lower when compared with peripheral blood monocytes. This would be consistent with the fact that these cells are resident phagocytes, which need to exist in a nonactivated state. Because they were obtained by alveolar lavage, these macrophages would not have been tightly bound to underlying epithelial cells. It is difficult to draw inferences about the activated state of macrophages obtained by lung lavage because activated cells may be tightly bound to the epithelium. Both Albert et al. (82) and Prieto et al. (83) specifically studied nonstimulated cells from healthy nonsmoking adults. The surface to which the alveolar macrophage is attached may influence what factors are produced by the alveolar macrophage. Collagen peptides stimulate alveolar macrophages to release chemotaxis factors for neutrophils (84). In a separate report, Kang and colleagues (85) used in vitro studies to show that endotoxin stimulation of bronchoalveolar macrophages produce time-dependent regulation of the expression, first up and then down, of the very late-activating (VLA) class of adhesive substances and of fibronectin. Very late-activating (VLA) integrins are thought to be particularly important in macrophage adherence to the extracellular matrix (85). Prolonged exposure to endotoxin may impede VLA integrin-mediated migration and result in altered accumulation of macrophages in the lung. These findings are compatible with a prolonged inflammatory state in the lung and with increased expression and production of fibronectin, a glycoprotein that is associated with inflammation and fibrosis. Surprisingly, there are no reports showing the presence of endotoxin in airway secretions of patients either with evolving or established CLD. Endotoxin could be both a marker for and a participant in the processes leading to the activation of inflammatory cells in the lung.

Kojima and associates (86) measured soluble intracellular adhesion molecule (sICAM-1) in preterm infants who did and who did not acquire CLD. This substance serves as a ligand for antigens that are expressed on many inflammatory cells. Serial measurements were made at postnatal days 2–4, 6–7, and 12–14.

In those infants who later had CLD, concentrations of sICAM-1 in tracheal aspirates were increased by postnatal days 6–7 and 12–14. Low levels of sICAM-1 were found consistently, however, in tracheal aspirates of infants who did not acquire CLD. The authors suggested that increased numbers of pulmonary macrophages and neutrophils might lead to augmented production and release of sICAM-1. Alveolar macrophages also secrete the proinflammatory cytokine, interleukin-1 (IL-1). This cytokine can induce and increase production of sICAM-1 in several cell types. This, in turn, would increase the adhesion of neutrophils within the lung, and promotes their release of toxic substances that attracts other inflammatory cells to the pulmonary alveoli and causes additional lung injury. This assumption is supported by the increased tissue expression of ICAM-1 in mice that have hyperoxic lung injury and associated inflammation (87,88). The increasing availability of specific monoclonal antibodies against cell adhesion proteins will help improve our understanding of the pathophysiology of CLD of early infancy. The use of anti-CD18 antibodies suppresses alveolar macrophage production of $O_2^{\bullet-}$ and tumor necrosis factor in a rat model of lung injury that is induced by cobra venom factor or hyperoxia (89). It remains unknown whether specific monoclonal antibodies against specific cell adhesion antigens, if given during the first week after birth, will ameliorate the pulmonary injury seen during CLD. The field of adhesive protein biology and protective immunotherapy against these cell determinants merits future attention either as investigative or therapeutic agents.

B. The Secretion of Proinflammatory Cytokines by Lung Macrophages: Their Role in CLD

Macrophages secrete a plethora of mediators that enhance pulmonary inflammation (reviewed in 90,91). During a study of hyperoxic injury to alveolar macrophages using newborn rabbits, we noted that animals became ill only when neutrophils migrated across the endothelial–epithelial barrier (68). Neutrophil influx was concurrent with the appearance of a defect in antibacterial activity of alveolar macrophages. Alveolar macrophages release chemoattractants following hyperoxic damage and recruit neutrophils so that a second line of phagocytic defense is available in the pulmonary alveoli (68,92,93). Studies exposing lungs or macrophages to hyperoxia (64,94) have shown the following chemoattractants for neutrophils: (1) C-C and C-X-C chemokines (especially interleukin-8; IL-8), (2) complement components (especially C5a), (3) interleukin-1β (IL-1β), (4) interleukin-6 (IL-6), (5) tumor necrosis factor-α (TNF-α), and (6) leukotrienes (especially LTB_4). It is known, however, that IL-6 activity remains elevated in infants with CLD (95). Unfortunately, there is no consensus about the predominant chemoattractant in the lungs of premature infants who acquire CLD. Such knowledge might result in a therapeutic agent to prevent its secretion or action. Interestingly, alveolar macrophages from newborn rabbits secrete more IL-1 when they are exposed to lipopolysaccharide (96). Nevertheless, our knowledge concerning the secretion of proinflammatory mediators by macrophages and other pulmonary cells is nearly nonexistent in newborn infants. The most notable recent finding is that dexamethasone attenuates IL-8 release by human alveolar macrophages, a finding that is relevant to treating oxygen- and ventilator-dependent infants with CLD (97).

C. Lung Repair After Injury: Tissue Remodeling and Growth Factor Secretion by Pulmonary Macrophages

Normal development of the lung must include development of the extracellular matrix (ECM). In the lung, the structural demands of the ECM are unique because of the need for both elastic and contractile elements, as well as constituents that provide stiffness. In addition, lung growth during the late second and third trimesters involves rapid proliferation of acinar spaces and small vessels. This normal process requires expression of both adhesive and antiadhesive elements (98). Proteins with antiadhesive properties that have been recognized recently include secreted protein, acidic and rich in cystine (SPARC) and tenascin. Disruption of the metabolism that is responsible for producing extracellular matrix further impairs alveolar maturation in infants with CLD. The result may be permanent impairment of septation and alveolarization and a secondary disruption of pulmonary vascular development.

At some point in the evolution of CLD, the bronchiolitis, alveolitis, interstitial and alveolar edema, and the other signs of acute inflammatory reaction resolve. There is indirect evidence that alveolar and interstitial macrophages induce the fibrosis seen in CLD. This evidence is inferred from studies of alveolar macrophages in adult animal and human models of fibrosing conditions. Macrophages participate in this process by their synthesis and secretion of growth factors (99). These growth factors, in turn, initiate the chemotaxis and activation of fibroblasts, which secrete collagens and other substances to form the fibrotic regions. Macrophages also appear to be involved in the metabolism of hyaluronan and other large complex molecules that form the structure on which fibrotic tissue is deposited. Current reports do not provide information on the time course over which the alveolar macrophage initiates fibrosis, nor do we understand the degree of alveolar macrophage upregulation necessary to initiate the process.

Macrophages are assumed to participate in pulmonary fibrosis, in part because they synthesize and secrete basic fibroblast growth factor (bFGF). This potent stimulator of fibroblast growth has been linked with fibroproliferative processes in adults (100). Immunohistochemical studies of lung tissue from patients who died following acute lung injury showed numerous alveolar macrophages that were immunoreactive for bFGF. In addition, the alveolar macrophage appears to be a source of bFGF in the fibroproliferative disorder of intra-alveolar fibrosis following acute lung injury. Macrophages obtained by bronchoalveolar lavage (BAL) reveal the presence of mRNA for two forms of bFGF (100). These findings have not been extended to neonates. Other growth factors that are associated with fibroblast proliferation—namely, platelet-derived growth factor (PDGF) and transforming growth factor-beta (TGF-β)—also are released by pulmonary macrophages (90). Both PDGF and TGF-β have a major role in initiating pulmonary fibrosis. Given the excess of activated alveolar macrophages that are found in lungs of infants with established CLD (101), it seems likely that macrophages participate in the fibroproliferative process. To our knowledge, no study has examined neonatal macrophages for the presence of immunoreactive bFGF, PDGF, or TGF-β, particularly when there is a risk of developing CLD.

There is evidence that alveolar macrophages also release a family of large extracellular matrix antiadhesive molecules, collectively called the tenascins. These glycoproteins are expressed abundantly in fetal tissues and in more restricted fashion in adult tissues (102). One member of this glycoprotein family, tenascin-C, is found in large concentrations in the rat lung in the early postnatal period, with reduced expression in the adult. With immunohistochemical techniques, Young and associates (103) demonstrated by electron microscopy that neonatal lungs of rats express tenascin-C during branching morphogenesis. Tenascin also plays a role in the developing lung by epithelial cell–matrix interactions. How the disruption of normal lung morphogenesis contributes to the final appearance of bronchopulmonary dysplasia, and the role of alveolar macrophages in this process, remains to be established.

Alveolar macrophages also may participate in the more chronic pattern of lung fibrotic injury through their interaction with the large molecular weight substance hyaluronan. This complex glycoprotein is found in lung interstitial areas. Underhill et al. (104) demonstrated that the amount of hyaluronan in relation to lung protein content decreased as lung development progressed in the mouse. During development, much of the relatively large amount of interstitial hyaluronan diminished, and in the adult, hyaluronan was restricted to the regions surrounding major blood vessels, bronchi, and bronchioles. Hyaluronan acts as a ligand for the CD44 receptor, and its interaction with this receptor mediates both normal development and repair. Underhill and associates (104) found that the expression and distribution of the cell surface receptor CD44 was associated with macrophages. As development progresses, macrophages in the lungs of mice express more CD44 receptors, and this increase is temporally correlated with the decrease in hyaluronan content. There is immunohistochemical evidence that hyaluronan has been internalized into alveolar macrophages. In summary, there is evidence to support the theory that macrophages in the lung during normal development regulate both the total amount of hyaluronan present in the lung and its intrapulmonary distribution during development.

Extracellular matrix components, including hyaluronan, which are present at different stages during lung development and which are generated at inflammatory sites, may influence tissue remodeling by their effects on leukocyte adherence and local cytokine production. Noble et al. (105) showed that macrophages derived from murine bone marrow when stimulated with soluble hyaluronic acid produced a variety of cytokines, including IL-1β, TNF-α, and IGF-1. There is evidence that hyaluronan activates the CD44 surface receptor on macrophages to induce the expression and production of these cytokines. These studies are relevant because of the previous finding that hyaluronan production by macrophages precedes the tissue fibrotic response (106).

Juul and associates (107) showed, in a premature primate model of RDS, that hyaluronan concentrations increased with the length of mechanical ventilation and with the severity of illness in preterm primates. Hyaluronan was identified using a biotinylated probe in freeze-dried lung sections. The authors concluded that hayluronan in lungs of prematurely delivered primates with RDS is increased, relative to normal lungs, within 6 hr after birth and that these increased quantities of hyaluronan were decreased by surfactant treatment. More prolonged evaluation was not performed, and it is not possible to infer from the published studies what the content or the metabolism of hyaluronan is in chronic lung injury. Excess hyaluronan could increase the stiffness of the lung, lowering compliance and increasing the work of breathing. An adequate macrophage population would act to engulf excess hyaluronan and diminish abnormalities of pulmonary mechanics. Thus, emergence of the lung's interstitial macrophage subpopulation may be critical to resolving this aspect of pulmonary damage in neonates.

Fibronectin is an additional component of the extracellular matrix that is distributed throughout pulmonary connective tissue and the basement membrane. It is associated with native procollagen molecules and other matrix components throughout the alveolar interstitium. Because there is increased fibronectin deposition in the lungs of patients with idiopathic pulmonary fibrosis, its relation to the development of chronic pulmonary injury in neonates needs to be explored further. The potentially important role of fibronectin in the pathogenesis and pathophysiology of CLD has been reviewed by Watts and Fanaroff (108). These investigators found that the airway aspirate samples from babies with CLD showed increased quantities of fibronectin when compared with age-matched control infants without CLD (109). Importantly, the fibronectin concentrations in tracheal aspirates were standardized using the free secretory component of IgA, a peptide for which the concentration in airways is independent of capillary leakage. Studies on the response of macrophages to hyperoxic pulmonary injury have included demonstration of the acquisition and enhanced expression of the surface fibronectin receptor on alveolar macrophages recovered from guinea pigs exposed to hyperoxia (110). In addition, Sinkin et al. (111) demonstrated increased mRNA for fibronectin in alveolar macrophages recovered from adult rabbits that were exposed to 100% oxygen for up to 64 hr. These findings suggest that one of the ways oxygen may disrupt pulmonary function and architecture is by altering macrophage-mediated fibronectin metabolism, as hyperoxia would reduce the number of macrophages at a time when they are needed for fibronectin recycling.

One of the major products of activated macrophages, the proinflammatory cytokine TNF-α, is involved in both pulmonary inflammation and fibrosis. The mechanisms by which TNF-α promotes fibrosis are unclear, and it is unknown whether these mechanisms apply to the 25- to 30-week–postconceptual aged infant. One possibility, which has been suggested in adults (105), is that TNF-α promotes the generation of growth factors that stimulate fibroblast proliferation and collagen deposition. The interaction between the production and release of inflammatory cytokines by macrophages and the secretion of proteases from neutrophils are potentially important pathways in the pathogenesis of macrophage-associated pulmonary injury.

Several enzymes that degrade extracellular matrix are produced by macrophages and neutrophils (90). Under normal conditions (normoxia), alveolar macrophages of newborn rats have increased secretion of the 92-kDa type IV gelatinase (collagenase; 112). Exposure of neonatal alveolar macrophages of rats to phorbol myristate acetate (PMA), stimulates release of reactive oxygen intermediates, and produces a four- to fivefold rise in gelatinase activity. No secretion of the tissue inhibitor of metalloproteases (TIMP) by neonatal alveolar macrophages of rats was observed in the first 24 hr of life. Other investigators have found a marked increase in TIMP-1 expression in the lungs of baboons following birth (113). The disparity between these two reports emphasizes the importance of species differences when conducting research on neonatal lung injury and repair. Furthermore, Devaskar and associates (114) found increased activity of type I and type IV collagenase in the lungs of newborn rats that were exposed to hyperoxia. Reports indicate that zinc metalloproteases that are produced by alveolar macrophages degrade several biologically active substrates, including bradykinin, neurotensin, and substance P (115). The activity of zinc metalloproteases has not been studied in newborns. Given the importance of different digestive enzymes that are secreted by pulmonary macrophages during lung injury and repair, this should be a fruitful area of investigation as it relates to CLD.

Lastly, pulmonary macrophages may release growth factors, namely, hepatocyte growth factor (HGF) and keratinocyte growth factor (KGF), that are important not only for fibroblast growth, but for the proliferation of type II pneumocytes (116–118). Again, important species differences may exist, as the production of HGF mRNA was detected in rat alveolar macrophages, but not in human alveolar macrophages (116). Hepatocyte growth factor production as it relates to macrophages also may be difficult to interpret because the secretory products of macrophages—namely, bFGF, PDGF, and TGF-β—upregulate expression of HGF in fibroblasts (119). Secretion by lung parenchymal macrophages of an epidermal growth-like molecular species has also been reported and appears to be under the control of interferon-gamma (IFN-γ; 120). This factor could be blocked partially by incubation with heparin, and the investigators speculate that this factor represents a substance by which macrophages activate T lymphocytes, resulting in pulmonary fibrosis. The panoply of growth factors produced and released by pulmonary macrophages, and their complex interactions with different lung cells, has not been studied during the progression of CLD. This would be extremely useful information as it relates to repair of the lung in neonates.

In summary, macrophages throughout the lung are in an ideal position to modify and perhaps exacerbate pulmonary fibrosis in response to any toxic stimulus, particularly persistent or prolonged hyperoxia. The end result of fibrosis that occurs in severe chronic lung injury of neonates may represent a persistent overstimulation of macrophages by toxic stimuli. If this is true, it will be a challenge to discover ways to modulate the responses of macrophages and to calm their synthesis and secretion of substances that, if produced in excess, lead to inflammation and subsequent fibrosis within the lung. Understanding the activity of the activated macrophage during the early prefibrosis stages of CLD remains an extremely ripe area for investigations, in both human infants with CLD and appropriate animal models of CLD.

D. Removal of Apoptotic Neutrophils by Alveolar Macrophages: A Critical Event in Preventing Lung Injury

Damaged alveolar macrophages secrete mediators that recruit neutrophils to the alveoli. The recruitment and death of neutrophils in the pulmonary alveoli is thought to be a major factor associated with acute lung injury in newborns, children and adults (121). Because neutrophils generally have a short life span (perhaps only 12–24 hr), they undergo either necrosis and lysis or apoptosis and clearance in the pulmonary alveoli (122,123). During neutrophil necrosis, many cytotoxic contents (proteases, cationic proteins, myeloperoxidase, hydrolases, and DNA) are released. During neutrophil apoptosis, these ''toxins'' may be contained. Containing the toxins of neutrophils in the alveoli requires the participation of alveolar macrophages. During morphogenesis, macrophages are ''croquemorts'' or the catchers of death, and they are essential to organ development and tissue remodeling (124). After birth, this function of macrophages extends to alveolar inflammation where human monocytes–macrophages employ specific receptor mechanisms (CD44) to ingest apoptotic neutrophils (125). A major function of tissue macrophages is engulfing and safely degrading apoptotic cells during tissue repair (126). Ingestion of apoptotic, alveolar neutrophils by alveolar macrophages is known to occur in human newborns (127), a process essential to resolving inflammation (122,123,126). Novel treatments must be discovered that diminish macrophage injury, increase macrophage population expansion, and enhance macrophage functions during the clinical setting of hyperoxia and assisted ventilation. Cytoprotective therapies that would attain the three aforementioned goals are necessary if alveolar macrophages are to accomplish their task of clearing apoptotic neutrophils from pulmonary alveoli during acute lung injury.

V. Limitations to the Study of Alveolar Macrophages in CLD of Early Infancy and Future Research Directions

There are substantial limitations to the study of the alveolar or interstitial macrophage in the development, progression, exacerbation, and healing of chronic pulmonary injury in prematurely born infants. The most important limitation is the difficulty in extrapolating data from in vitro or in vivo studies that cannot control for all the underlying factors that may contribute to the development of lung injury in humans. Among these factors are species differences; variations in activation and function of macrophages obtained from newborns versus adults; and distinctions between bronchoalveolar macrophages obtained from preterm compared with term newborns.

An appropriate model for assessing the role of macrophages in contributing to or defending against the development of chronic inflammatory injury requires very specific characteristics. Such a model would need to be controlled for the degree of prematurity and for the development of an RDS-like illness that would require exposure to supplemental oxygen and positive-pressure ventilation in varying degrees and doses. The model would need sufficient vigor to survive long enough to develop chronic pulmonary changes. The animal model would need to demonstrate ontogeny of the pulmonary macrophage system similar to, if not identical with, that of the preterm, human newborn. It is hazardous to equate macrophage function in adult humans or animals with respiratory distress syndrome (ARDS), asthma, or inhalation injury (e.g., silicosis or asbestosis) to a meaningful understanding of lung macrophage physiology in preterm infants. Nevertheless, that is where our knowledge about lung injury has for the most part been derived. Few studies in appropriate animal models, or in human neonates with CLD, have addressed the specifics of macrophage number, macrophage function, or macrophage interactions with other lung cells.

It is also important to recognize that the disorder labeled ''chronic lung disease of early infancy'' has changed since its initial characterization in 1967

(1). Chronic lung injury no longer commonly arises as a continuum of severe respiratory distress syndrome in infants of 30–36 weeks gestation, or in term infants who have suffered severe meconium aspiration or other forms of pneumonia. Chronic lung injury is almost exclusively limited to babies less than 30 weeks gestation and less than 1250 g birthweight (128). Thus, the injury develops in profoundly immature lungs, ones that have been infrequently exposed to the potential beneficial, but also confounding, effects of antenatal treatments, including corticosteroid therapy either alone or in combination with other modulators of lung maturation. The macrophage population in these extremely premature infants has not been investigated to any extent.

Even as the 21st century approaches, there is still only fragmentary evidence for the role of lung macrophages in neonates with evolving CLD. Relevant data obtained either from preterm human newborns at risk for or with established CLD (34,35,41,42,59,60), or from appropriate animal models (e.g., prematurely delivered primates and other newborn animals, such as rabbit pups; 43,71), are available. Even in the animal models that can be controlled for prematurity, interpretation is obscured because prematurity was associated with cesarean-section delivery, rather than with vaginal delivery, with or without labor. This fact is relevant because of the possible contribution of vaginal colonization with organisms of low pathogenicity that some authors (61,62,67) have identified as contributing to the severity, if not the initiation, of chronic pulmonary injury in very low birthweight infants.

There are many questions relevant to the relation between newborn pulmonary macrophages and the pathogenesis of neonatal lung injury that must be addressed in the future. Among those questions are, what is the effect of administering supplemental oxygen on (1) the numbers of lung macrophages in premature neonates and on (2) their state of activation, including up- or downregulation of key enzyme systems? What cytokine products or proinflammatory lipid substances are produced by lung macrophages of preterm infants as a result of exposure to hyperoxia? Given this scenario, what is the degree and duration of hyperoxia necessary to induce changes in macrophage function? In premature infants, what are the combined effects of oxygen and different periods and modes of positive-pressure ventilation on macrophage function? In the prematurely born infant, what are the consequences of other therapies on macrophage function, most importantly, the effects of surfactant replacement at birth or the administration of corticosteriods on postnatal days 1, 7, or 28, and their abilities to mitigate lung inflammation? What is the importance for each of the aforementioned conditions, either alone or in combination, on the secretory components of macrophages or their contact interactions with other pulmonary cells? Each effector and its effect must be assessed using better biochemical and molecular markers of injury and repair in the immature lung. At present, we have only touched the surface of the role of pulmonary macrophages in the pathophysiology of CLD. Future investigations will have formidable challenges if the pathophysiology of CLD is to be defined correctly and appropriate new therapies are to be instituted.

Acknowledgment

This work was supported in part by HL 52079 (MPS) from the National Heart, Lung, and Blood Institute.

References

1. Northway WH Jr, Rosan RC, Porter DY. Pulmonary disease following respirator therapy of hyaline membrane disease. N Engl J Med 1967; 276:357–668.
2. Philip AGS. Oxygen plus pressure plus time: the etiology of bronchopulmonary dysplasia. Pediatrics 1975; 55:44–50.
3. DeLemos RA, Coalson JJ, Gerstmann DR, Kuehl TJ, Null DM Jr. Oxygen toxicity in the premature baboon with hyaline membrane disease. Am Rev Respir Dis 1987; 136:677–682.
4. Lee RMKW, O'Brodovich H. Airway epithelial damage in premature infants with respiratory failure. Am Rev Respir Dis 1988; 137:450–457.
5. Metchnikoff II. Lecons sur la pathologie comparée de l'inflammation. Paris, 1892. (English translation reprinted by Dover, New York, 1968).
6. Zeligs BJ, Nerurkar LS, Bellanti JA, Zeligs JD. Maturation of the rabbit alveolar macrophage during animal development. I. Perinatal influx into alveoli and ultrastructural differentiation. Pediatr Res 1977; 11:197–208.
7. Nerurkar LS, Zeligs BJ, Bellanti JA. Maturation of the rabbit alveolar macrophage during animal development. II. Biochemical and enzymatic studies. Pediatr Res 1977; 11:1202–1207.
8. Zeligs BJ, Nerurkar LS, Bellanti JA. Maturation of the rabbit alveolar macrophage during animal development. III. Phagocytic and bactericidal functions. Pediatr Res 1977; 11:1208–1211.
9. Sherman M, Goldstein E, Lippert W, Wennberg R. Neonatal lung defense mechanisms: a study of the alveolar macrophage system in neonatal rabbits. Am Rev Respir Dis 1977; 116:433–440.
10. Reasor MJ, Ogle CL, Walker ER, Kacew S. Amiodarone-induced phospholipidosis in rat alveolar macrophages. Am Rev Respir Dis 1988; 137:510–518.
11. Brain JD. Lung macrophages: how many kinds are there? What do they do? Am Rev Respir Dis 1988; 137:507–509.
12. Sherman MP, Ganz T. Host defense in pulmonary alveoli. Annu Rev Physiol 1992; 54:331–350.
13. Shellito J, Kalreider HB. Heterogeneity of immunological function among subfractions of normal rat alveolar macrophages. Am Rev Respir Dis 1984; 129:747–753.
14. Hance AJ, Douches S, Winchester RJ, Ferrans VJ, Crystal RG. Characterization

of mononuclear phagocyte subpopulations in the human lung by using monoclonal antibodies: changes in alveolar macrophage phenotype associated with pulmonary sarcoidosis. J Immunol 1985; 134:284–292.

15. Brannen AL, Chandler DB. Alveolar macrophage subpopulations responsiveness to chemotactic stimuli. Am J Pathol 1988; 132:161–166.
16. Brain JD, Gehr P, Kavet RI. Airway macrophages. The importance of the fixation method. Am Rev Respir Dis 1984; 129:823–826.
17. Holt PG, Degebrodt A, Venaille T, et al. Preparation of interstitial lung cells by enzymatic digestion of tissue slices: preliminary characterization by morphology and performance in functional assays. Immunology 1985; 54:139–147.
18. Thet LA, Wrobel DJ, Crapo JD, Shelburne JD. Morphologic aspects of the protection by endotoxin against acute and chronic oxygen-induced lung injury in adult rats. Lab Invest 1983; 48:448–457.
19. Lehnert BE, Valdez YE, Holland LM. Pulmonary macrophages: alveolar and interstitial populations. Exp Lung Res 1985; 9:177–190.
20. Warren JS, Kunkel RG, Johnson KJ, Ward PA. Comparative O_2^- responses of lung macrophages and blood phagocytic cells in the rat. Possible relevance to IgA immune complex induced lung injury. Lab Invest 1987; 57:311–320.
21. Bowden DH, Adamson IYR. The pulmonary interstitial cell as immediate precursor of the alveolar macrophage. Am J Pathol 1972; 68:521–528.
22. Longworth KE, Westgate AM, Grady MK, Westcott JY, Staub NC. Development of pulmonary intravascular macrophage function in newborn lambs. J Appl Physiol 1992; 73:2608–2615.
23. Dehring DJ, Wismar BL. Intravascular macrophages in pulmonary capillaries of humans. Am Rev Respir Dis 1989; 139:1027–1029.
24. Warner AE, Molina RM, Brain JD. Uptake of bloodborne bacteria by pulmonary intravascular macrophages and consequent inflammatory responses in sheep. Am Rev Respir Dis 1987; 136:683–690.
25. Warner AE, Brain JD. The cell biology and pathogenic role of pulmonary intravascular macrophages. Am J Physiol 1990; 258:L1–L12.
26. Zlotnik A, Vatter A, Hayes RL, Blumenthal E, Crowle AJ. Mouse pleural macrophages: characterization and comparison with mouse alveolar and peritoneal macrophages. J Reticulendothel Soc 1982; 31:207–220.
27. Sorokin SP, McNelly NA, Hoyt RF Jr, Svoboda KK. Precursors of macrophages in embryonic rat lungs fail to exhibit granulocyte-forming potential. Anat Rec 1994; 240:387–397.
28. Sorokin SP, Hoyt RF Jr, McNelly NA. Factors influencing fetal macrophage development: I. Reactions of the tumor necrosis factor-alpha cascade and their inhibitors. Anat Rec 1996; 246:481–497.
29. Sorokin SP, McNelly NA, Hoyt RF Jr. Factors influencing fetal macrophage development: II. Effects of the PDGF subfamily of protein–tyrosine kinase receptor ligands as studied in organ-cultured rat lungs. Anat Rec 1996; 246:498–506.
30. Sorokin SP, Hoyt RF Jr, Reenstra WR, McNelly NA. Factors influencing fetal macrophage development: III. Immunocytochemical localization of cytokines and time-resolved expression of differentiation markers in organ-cultured rat lungs. Anat Rec 1997; 248:93–103.

31. Rothlein R, Gallily R, Kim YB. Development of alveolar macrophages in specific pathogen-free and germ-free Minnesota miniature swine. J Reticuloendothel Soc 1981; 30:483–495.
32. Jacobs RF, Wilson CB, Palmer S, et al. Factors related to the appearance of alveolar macrophages in the developing lung. Am Rev Respir Dis 1985; 131:548–553.
33. Weiss RA, Chanana AD, Joel DD. Postnatal maturation of pulmonary antimicrobial defense mechanisms in conventional and germ-free lambs. Pediatr Res 1986; 20: 496–504.
34. Ogden BE, Murphy S, Saunders GC, Johnson JD. Lung lavage of newborns with respiratory distress syndrome. Prolonged neutrophil influx is associated with bronchopulmonary dysplasia. Chest 1983; 83:31S–33S.
35. Alenghat E, Esterly JR. Alveolar macrophages in perinatal infants. Pediatrics 1984; 74:221–223.
36. Evans MJ, Sherman MP, Campbell LA, Shami SG. Proliferation of pulmonary alveolar macrophages during postnatal development of rabbit lung. Am Rev Respir Dis 1987; 136:384–387.
37. Van Furth R. Cellular biology of pulmonary macrophages. Int Arch Allergy Appl Immunol 1985; 76(suppl 1):21–27.
38. Winkler GC, Cheville NF. Monocytic origin and postnatal mitosis of intravascular macrophages in porcine lung. J Leukoc Biol 1985; 38:471–480.
39. Lynn WS, Mukherjee C. Motility of rabbit alveolar cells. Role of unsaturated fatty acids. Am J Pathol 1979; 96:663–671.
40. Yui S, Yamazaki M. Relationship of ability of phospholipids to stimulate growth and bind to macrophages. J Leukoc Biol 1987; 41: 392–399.
41. Arnon S, Grigg J, Silverman M. Pulmonary inflammatory cells in ventilated preterm infants: effects of surfactant treatment. Arch Dis Child 1993; 69:44–48.
42. Merritt TA, Stuard ID, Puccia JM, et al. Newborn tracheal aspirate cytology: classification during respiratory distress syndrome and bronchopulmonary dysplasia. J Pediatr 1981; 98:949–956.
43. Jackson JC, Chi EY, Wilson CB, Truog WE, Teh EC, Hodson WA. Sequence of inflammatory cell migration into lung during recovery from hyaline membrane disease in premature newborn monkeys. Am Rev Respir Dis 1987; 135:937–940.
44. Berg JT, White JE, Tsan MF. Response of alveolar macrophage-depleted rats to hyperoxia. Exp Lung Res 1995; 21:175–185.
45. Huffman JA, Wert SE, Dranoff G, Mulligan RC, Whitsett JA. Macrophages accumulate in lungs of transgenic mice bearing a tissue-specific SP-C–GM-CSF chimeric gene. Pediatr Res 1995; 37:392A.
46. Hemming VG, Overall JC Jr, Britt MR. Nosocomial infections in a newborn intensive-care unit. Results of forty-one months of surveillance. N Engl J Med 1976; 294:1310–1316.
47. Sherman MP, Chance KH, Goetzman BW. Gram's stains of tracheal secretions predict neonatal bacteremia. Am J Dis Child 1984; 138:848–850.
48. Stoll BJ, Gordon T, Korones SB, Shankaran S, Tyson JE, Bauer CR, Fanaroff AA, Lemons JA, Donovan EF, Oh W, Stevenson DK, Ehrenkranz RA, Papille L-A, Verter J, Wright LL. Late-onset sepsis in very low birth weight neonates: a report

from the National Institute of Child Health and Human Development Neonatal Research Network. J Pediatr 1996; 129:63–71.
49. Sherman MP, Johnson JT, Rothlein R, Hughes BJ, Smith CW, Anderson DC. Role of phagocytes in host defense against group B streptococci in preterm versus term rabbit lung. J Infect Dis 1992; 166:818–826.
50. Sherman MP, Evans MJ, Campbell LA. Prevention of pulmonary alveolar macrophage proliferation in newborn rabbits by hyperoxia. J Pediatr 1988; 112:782–786.
51. Hall SL, Sherman MP. Intrapulmonary bacterial clearance of type III group B *Streptococcus* is reduced in preterm compared with term rabbits and occurs independent of antibody. Am Rev Respir Dis 1992; 145:1172–1177.
52. Sherman MP, Lehrer RI. Oxidative metabolism of neonatal and adult rabbit lung macrophages stimulated with opsonized group B streptococci. Infect Immun 1985; 47:26–30.
53. Kradin RL, McCarthy KM, Preffer FI, Schneeberger EE. Flow-cytometric and ultrastructural analysis of alveolar macrophage maturation. J Leukoc Biol 1986; 40: 407–417.
54. Clement A, Chadelat K, Sardet A, Grimfeld A, Tourier G. Alveolar macrophage status in bronchopulmonary dysplasia. Pediatr Res 1988; 23:470–473.
55. Ten Centre Study Group. Ten centre trial of artificial surfactant (artificial lung expanding compound) in very premature babies. Br Med J 1987; 294:991–996.
56. Kendig JW, Notter RH, Cox C, et al. Surfactant replacement therapy at birth: final analysis of a clinical trial and comparisons with similar trials. Pediatrics 1988; 82: 756–762.
57. Bose C, Corbet A, Bose G, et al. Improved outcome at 28 days of age for very low birth weight infants treated with a single dose of a synthetic surfactant. J Pediatr 1990; 117:947–953.
58. Ohlsson K, Sveger T, Svenningsen N. Protease inhibitors in bronchoalveolar lavage fluid from neonates with special reference to secretory leukocyte protease inhibitor. Acta Paediatr 1992; 81:757–759.
59. Merritt TA, Cochrane CG, Holcomb K, et al. Elastase and alpha$_1$-proteinase inhibitor activity in tracheal aspirates during respiratory distress syndrome. Role of inflammation in the pathogenesis of bronchopulmonary dysplasia. J Clin Invest 1983; 72:656–666.
60. Ogden BE, Murphy SA, Saunders GC, Pathak D, Johnson JD. Neonatal lung neutrophils and elastase/proteinase inhibitor imbalance. Am Rev Respir Dis 1984; 130: 817–821.
61. Ollikainen J, Heikkaniemi H, Korppi M, Sarkkinen H, Heinonen K. *Ureaplasma urealyticum* infection associated with acute respiratory insufficiency and death in premature infants. J Pediatr 1993; 122:756–760.
62. Wang EE, Cassell GH, Sanchez PJ, Regan JA, Payne NR, Liu PP. *Ureaplasma urealyticum* and chronic lung disease of prematurity: critical appraisal of the literature on causation. Clin Infect Dis 1993; 17(suppl 1):S112–S116.
63. Crouse DT, Cassell GH, Waites KB, Foster JM, Cassady G. Hyperoxia potentiates *Ureaplasma urealyticum* pneumonia in newborn mice. Infect Immun 1990; 58: 3487–3493.

64. Walsh WF, Butler J, Coalson J, Hensley D, Cassell GH, deLemos RA. A primate model of *Ureaplasma urealyticum* infection in the premature infant with hyaline membrane disease. Clin Infect Dis 1993; 17(suppl 1):S158–S162.
65. Smyth AR, Shaw NJ, Pratt BC, Weindling AM. *Ureaplasma urealyticum* and chronic lung disease. Eur J Pediatr 1993; 152:931–932.
66. Jonsson B, Karell AC, Ringertz S, Rylander M, Faxelius G. Neonatal *Ureaplasma urealyticum* colonization and chronic lung disease. Acta Paediatr 1994; 83:927–930.
67. Watterberg K, Demers LM, Scott SM, Murphy S. Chorioamnionitis and early lung inflammation in infants in whom bronchopulmonary dysplasia develops. Pediatrics 1996; 97:210–215.
68. Sherman MP, Condiotti R. Hyperoxia damages phagocytic defenses of neonatal rabbit lung. J Appl Physiol 1987; 62:684–690.
69. Sherman MP, Campbell LA, Aeberhard EE, Barrett CT. Hyperoxia (H), dexamethasone (D) and newborn alveolar macrophage (AM) function. Pediatr Res 1987; 21: 376A.
70. Sherman MP, D'Ambola JB, Aeberhard EE, Barrett CT. Surfactant therapy of newborn rabbits impairs lung macrophage bactericidal activity. J Appl Physiol 1988; 65:137–145.
71. Sherman MP, Campbell LA, Merritt TA, et al. Effect of different surfactants on pulmonary group B streptococcal infection in premature rabbits. J Pediatr 1994; 125:939–947.
72. Abman SH, Kinsella JP, Schaffer MS, Wilkenking RB. Inhaled nitric oxide in the management of a premature newborn with severe respiratory distress and pulmonary hypertension. Pediatrics 1993; 92:606–609.
73. Gaston B, Drazen JM, Loscalzo J, Stamler JS. The biology of nitrogen oxides in the airways. Am J Respir Crit Care Med 1994; 149:538–551.
74. Sherman MP, Moise SL, Norberg M, Weatherstone KB, Truog WE. Pulmonary phagocyte responses to inhaled nitric oxide and hyperoxia. Pediatr Res 1995; 37: 349A.
75. Sherman MP, Truog WE. Inhaled nitric oxide and hyperoxia activate bronchoalveolar macrophages for group B streptococcal killing. Pediatr Res 1997; 41:178A.
76. Liebermann DA, Hoffman B. Differentiation primary response genes and proto-oncogenes as positive and negative regulators of terminal hematopoietic cell differentiation. Stem Cells (Dayt) 1994; 12:352–369.
77. Weatherstone KB, Moise S, Fu K, Andrews G, Sherman MP. Early gene expression and regulation of monocyte maturation in the cord blood. J Invest Med 1996; 44: 368A.
78. Avery GB, Fletcher AB, Kaplan M, Brundo DS. Controlled trial of dexamethasone in respirator-dependent infants with bronchopulmonary dysplasia. Pediatrics 1985; 75:106–111.
79. Lortie C, King GM, Adamson IYR. Effects of dexamethasone on macrophages in fetal and neonatal rat lung. Pediatr Pulmonol 1990; 8:138–144.
80. Davidson D, Drafta D, Wilkens BA. Elevated urinary leukotriene E_4 in chronic lung disease of extreme prematurity. Am J Respir Crit Care Med 1995; 151:841–850.

81. Co E, Chari G, McCulloch K, Vidyasagar D. Dexamethasone treatment suppresses collagen synthesis in infants with bronchopulmonary dysplasia. Pediatr Pulmonol 1993; 16:36–40.
82. Albert RK, Embree LJ, McFeely JE, Hickstein DD. Expression and function of β_2 integrins on alveolar macrophages from human and non-human primates. Am J Respir Cell Mol Biol 1992; 7:182–189.
83. Prieto J, Eklund A, Patarroyo M. Regulated expression of integrins and other adhesion molecules during differentiation of monocytes into macrophages. Cell Immunol 1994; 156:191–211.
84. Laskin DL, Soltys RA, Berg RA, Riley DJ. Activation of neutrophils by factors released from alveolar macrophages stimulated with collagen-like polypeptides. Am J Respir Cell Mol Biol 1990; 2:463–470.
85. Kang Y-H, Lee C-H, Brummel SE, Newball HH, Forrester J. Effects of endotoxin on expression of VLA integrins by human bronchoalveolar lavage macrophages. J Leukoc Biol 1995; 57:624–634.
86. Kojima T, Sasai M, Kobayashi Y. Increased soluble ICAM-1 in tracheal aspirates of infants with bronchopulmonary dysplasia. Lancet 1993; 342:1023–1024.
87. Wegner CD, Wolyneic WW, LaPlante AM, et al. Intercellular adhesion molecule-1 contributes to pulmonary oxygen toxicity in mice: role of leukocytes revisited. Lung 1992; 170:267–279.
88. Welty SE, Rivera JL, Elliston JF, et al. Increases in lung tissue expression of intercellular adhesion molecule-1 are associated with hyperoxic lung injury and inflammation in mice. Am J Respir Cell Mol Biol 1993; 9:393–400.
89. Mulligan MS, Varani J, Warren JS, et al. Roles of beta 2 integrins of rat neutrophils in complement- and oxygen radical-mediated acute lung injury. J Immunol 1992; 148:1847–1857.
90. Sibille Y, Reynolds HY. Macrophages and polymorphonuclear neutrophils in lung defense and injury. Am Rev Respir Dis 1990; 141:471–501.
91. Kelley J. Cytokines of the lung. Am Rev Respir Dis 1990; 141:765–788.
92. Bowman CM, Harada RN, Repine JE. Hyperoxia stimulates alveolar macrophages to produce and release a factor which increases neutrophil adherence. Inflammation 1983; 7:331–338.
93. Harada RN, Vatter AE, Repine JE. Macrophage effector function in pulmonary oxygen toxicity: hyperoxia damages and stimulates alveolar macrophages to make and release chemotaxins for polymorphonuclear leukocytes. J Leukoc Biol 1984; 35:373–383.
94. Mikawa K, Nishina K, Maekawa N, Obara H. Attentuation of hyperoxic lung injury in rabbits with superoxide dismutase: effects on inflammatory mediators. Acta Anaethesiol Scand 1995; 39:317–322.
95. Bagchi A, Viscardi RM, Taciak V, Ensor JE, McCrea KA, Hasday JD. Increased activity of interleukin-6 but not tumor necrosis factor-alpha in lung lavage of premature infants associate with the development of bronchopulmonary dysplasia. Pediatr Res 1994; 36:244–252.
96. Rozycki HJ. Elevated production of interleukin-1-beta from alveolar macrophages isolated from newborn rabbits. Biol Neonate 1994; 66:93–99.
97. Deaton PR, McKellar CT, Culbreth R, Veal CF, Cooper JA Jr. Hyperoxia stimulates

interleukin-8 release from alveolar macrophages and U937 cells: attenuation by dexamethasone. Am J Physiol 1994; 267:L187–L192.

98. Strandjord TP, Sage EH, Clark JG. SPARC participates in the branching morphogenesis of developing fetal rat lung. Am J Respir Cell Mol Biol 1995; 13:279–287.
99. Brandes ME, Finkelstein JN. The production of alveolar macrophage-derived growth regulating proteins in response to lung injury. Toxicol Lett 1990; 54:3–22.
100. Henke C, Marineli W, Jessurun J, et al. Macrophage production of the basic fibroblast growth factor in fibroproliferative disorder of alveolar fibrosis after lung injury. Am J Pathol 1993; 143:1189–1199.
101. Jacobson JD, Truog WE, Benjamin DR. Increased expression of human leukocyte antigen-DR on pulmonary macrophages in bronchopulmonary dysplasia. Pediatr Res 1993; 34:341–344.
102. Erickson HP, Bourdon MA. Tenascin: an extracellular matrix protein prominent in specialized embryonic tissues and tumors. Annu Rev Cell Biol 1989; 5:71–92.
103. Young SL, Chang LY, Erickson HP. Tenascin-C in rat lung: distribution, ontogeny and role in branching morphogenesis. Dev Biol 1994; 161:615–625.
104. Underhill CB, Nguyen HA, Shizari M, Culty M. CD44 positive macrophages take up hyaluronan during lung development. Dev Biol 1993; 155:324–336.
105. Noble PW, Lake FR, Henson PM, Riches DW. Hyaluronate activation of CD44 induces insulin-like growth factor-1 expression by a tumor necrosis factor-α-dependent mechanism in murine macrophages. J Clin Invest 1993; 91:2368–2377.
106. Teder P, Nettelbladt O, Heldin P. Characterization of the mechanism involved in bleomycin-induced increased hyaluronan production in rat lung. Am J Respir Cell Mol Biol 1995; 12:181–189.
107. Juul SE, Kinsella MG, Jackson JC, et al. Changes in hyaluronan deposition during early respiratory distress syndrome in premature monkeys. Pediatr Res 1994; 35: 238–243.
108. Watts CL, Fanaroff AA. Fibronectin: role in respiratory distress syndrome and bronchopulmonary dysplasia. Semin Perinatol 1992; 16:162–169.
109. Watts CL, Fanaroff AA, Bruce MC. Elevation of fibronectin levels in lung secretions of infants with respiratory distress syndrome who develop bronchopulmonary dysplasia. J Pediatr 1992; 120:614–620.
110. Kradin RL, Zhu Y, Hales CA, et al. Response of pulmonary macrophages to hyperoxic pulmonary injury: acquisition of surface fibronectin and fibrinogen and enhanced expression of a fibronection receptor. Am J Pathol 1986; 125:349–357.
111. Sinkin RA, LoMonaco MB, Finkelstein JN, et al. Increased fibronection mRNA in alveolar macrophages following in vivo hyperoxia. Am J Respir Cell Mol Biol 1992; 7:548–555.
112. Delacourt C, D'Ortho MP, Macquin-Mavier I, Pezet S, Harf A, Lafuma C. Increased 92 kD gelatinase activity from alveolar macrophages in newborn rats. Am J Respir Crit Care Med 1995; 151:1939–1945.
113. Minoo P, Penn R, deLemos DM, Coalson JJ, deLemos RA. Tissue inhibitor of metalloproteinase-1 mRNA is specifically induced in lung tissue after birth. Pediatr Res 1993; 34:729–734.
114. Devaskar UP, Taylor W, Govindrajan R, et al. Hyperoxia induces interstitial (type

I) and increased type IV collagenase mRNA expression and increases type I and II collagenolytic activity in newborn rat lung. Biol Neonate 1994; 66:76–85.

115. Lesser M, Fung K, Choi HS, Yoo OH, Cardozo C. Identification of two zinc metalloproteinases in alveolar macrophages of rats, guinea pigs, and human beings. J Lab Clin Med 1992; 120:597–603.
116. Mason RJ, Leslie CC, McCormick-Shannon K, et al. Hepatocyte growth factor is a growth factor for rat alveolar type II cells. Am J Respir Cell Mol Biol 1994; 11: 561–567.
117. Panos RJ, Rubin JS, Aaronson SA, Mason RJ. Keratinocyte growth factor and hepatocyte growth factor/scatter factor are heparin-binding growth factors for alveolar type II cells in fibroblast-conditioned medium. J Clin Invest 1993; 92:969–977.
118. Shimamoto A, Kimura T, Matsumoto K, Nakamura T. Hepatocyte growth-like protein is identical to macrophage stimulating protein. FEBS Lett 1993; 333:61–66.
119. Gohda E, Matsunaga T, Kataoka H, Takebe T, Yamamoto I. Induction of hepatocyte growth factor in human skin fibroblasts by epidermal growth factor, platelet-derived growth factor, and fibroblast growth factor. Cytokine 1994; 6:633–640.
120. Kumar RK, O'Grady R, Li W, Rajkovic I. Secretion of epidermal growth factor-like molecular species by lung parenchymal macrophages: induction by interferon-gamma. Growth Factors 1993; 9:223–230.
121. Weiss SJ. Tissue destruction by neutrophils. N Engl J Med 1989; 320:365–376.
122. Savil JS, Wyllie AH, Henson JE, Walport MJ, Henson PM, Haslett C. Macrophage phagocytosis of aging neutrophils in inflammation. Programmed cell death in the neutrophil leads to its recognition by macrophages. J Clin Invest 1989; 83:865–875.
123. Cox G, Crossley J, Xing Z. Macrophage engulfment of apoptotic neutrophils contributes to the resolution of acute pulmonary inflammation in vivo. Am J Respir Cell Mol Biol 1995; 12:232–237.
124. Franc NC, Dimarcq J-L, Lagueux M, Hoffmann, Ezekowitz RAB. Croquemort, a novel *Drosophila* hemocyte/macrophage receptor that recognizes apoptotic cells. Immunity 1996; 4:431–443.
125. Hart SP, Dougherty GJ, Haslett C, Dransfield I. CD44 regulates phagocytosis of apoptotic neutrophil granulocytes, but not apoptotic lymphocytes, by human macrophages. J Immunol 1997; 159:919–925.
126. Bellingan GJ, Caldwell H, Howie SEM, Dransfield I, Haslett C. In vivo fate of the inflammatory macrophage during resolution of inflammation. Inflammatory macrophages do not die locally, but emigrate to the draining lymph nodes. J Immunol 1996; 157:2577–2585.
127. Grigg JM, Savill JS, Sarraf C, Haslett C, Silverman M. Neutrophil apoptosis and clearance from neonatal lungs. Lancet 1991; 338:720–722.
128. Truog WE, Jackson JC. Alternative modes of ventilation in the prevention and treatment of bronchopulmonary dysplasia. Clin Perinatol 1992; 19:621–647.

34

Oxidants and Antioxidants

What Role Do They Play in Chronic Lung Disease?

H. LEE FRANK and ILENE R.S. SOSENKO

University of Miami School of Medicine
Miami, Florida

I. Introduction

The infant who is born prematurely must face multiple hardships, including those associated with shortened gestation, interrupted development, and dramatic environmental transition. Could Shakespeare have been aware of these adverse circumstances facing the premature infant when he described the prematurely born Richard II as ''rudely stamped . . . deformed, unfinished, sent before my time into this breathing world 'scarce' made up''? With incompletely developed antioxidant defenses and having been denied the final trimester's acquisition of a number of crucial nutrients, the premature infant leaves behind the relatively hypoxic intrauterine environment and is forced to adapt to the relatively hyperoxic extrauterine environment. The immature antioxidant defenses coupled with an oxidant environment and nutritional inadequacies may play a crucial role in the development of chronic lung disease (CLD) in the preterm neonate.

This chapter will summarize several topics, including general principles of oxidants and antioxidants, the association of oxidant processes and CLD in the premature infant, the role of protective antioxidant mechanisms in the lung, the gestational development of antioxidant protection, and the vulnerability of the prematurely born in terms of antioxidant defenses. Finally, the chapter will conclude by presenting potential therapeutic interventions, as well as controversies, unanswered questions, and possibilities for future research using antioxidant augmentation to protect the vulnerable premature infant from the development of CLD.

II. General Principles of Oxidants and Antioxidants

Oxygen itself is essentially nonreactive. During normal metabolism, however, aerobic cells produce a variety of highly reactive metabolic oxygen by-products, especially by the mitochondrial respiratory chain of enzymes and the microsomal cytochrome P-450 system. These reactive oxygen species have the potential for significant cytotoxicity because they have the ability to react with and ultimately alter all of the principal cellular components. Specifically, interaction of toxic oxygen metabolites with cell proteins results in oxidation and inactivation of enzymes; interaction with lipids produces lipid peroxidation of unsaturated bonds, especially of cellular and organelle membranes, leading to disruption of cellular function and integrity; interaction with carbohydrates can cause depolymerization; and finally, interaction with the genetic material can result in DNA cross-linkage and scission of DNA strands (1–4).

The major reactive species that produce these cytotoxic effects include the superoxide anion ($O_2^{\cdot-}$), hydrogen peroxide (H_2O_2), the extremely reactive hydroxyl free radical (OH^-), singlet oxygen ($^1O_2$), and various lipid-based free radicals that are formed when oxygen free radicals attack polyunsaturated fatty acid bonds in lipid components of the cell. Under conditions of hyperoxia, the rate of free radical production increases progressively with increasing oxygen tensions (5–9). For example, in conditions of 95% O_2, mitochondrial and microsomal free radical generation may increase tenfold or more compared to 21% O_2 conditions (8). Furthermore, the availability of transition metal ions increases the production of free radicals and toxic oxygen metabolites, such as the generation of highly reactive hydroxyl radicals from superoxide anion by the iron-catalyzed Haber–Weiss reaction (10). In addition, free radicals are formed from enzymatic reactions involving the xanthine dehydrogenase–xanthine oxidase enzyme system. When xanthine oxidase is converted from xanthine dehydrogenase by such conditions as endotoxin exposure or activated neutrophils, this enzyme catalyzes the breakdown of adenosine monophosphate (AMP) to uric acid, with the generation of superoxide anion and hydrogen peroxide (11).

To handle the normal flux of potentially cytotoxic O_2 species, aerobic cells have evolved a formidable system of antioxidant defenses to effectively scavenge and detoxify most of the reactive O_2 free radicals before damaging interactions with vital cell components can take place. Table 1 lists the major enzymatic catalytic defenses, the antioxidant enzymes (AOE)s; Table 2 lists the secondary

Table 1 Antioxidant Defense Systems and Their Role in Prevention of Cell Damage by Cytotoxic O_2 Species: The Chemical or Stoichiometric Antioxidant Defense System

Reactive O_2 species	Antioxidant enzymes	Cell components attacked by reactive O_2 species
O_2^- Superoxide radical	$O_2^- + O_2^- + 2\ H \xrightarrow{(SOD)} O_2 + H_2O_2$	Lipids: peroxidation of unsaturated fatty acids in cell membranes.
H_2O_2 Hydrogen peroxide	$2\ H_2O_2 \xrightarrow[(GP)]{(CAT)} O_2 + 2\ H_2O$	Proteins: oxidation of sulfhydryl-containing enzymes (enzyme inactivation)
$ROO^{\cdot}$ Peroxyl radical	$2\ ROO^{\cdot} + 2\ H^+ \xrightarrow{(GP)} O_2 + 2\ ROH$	Carbohydrates: depolymerization of polysaccharides
$^1O_2$ Singlet oxygen	$^1O_2$ (scavenged by β-carotene)	Nucleic Acids: base hydroxylation, cross-linkage, DNA strand scission
$OH^{\cdot}$ Hydroxyl radical	$OH^{\cdot}$ [scavenged by vitamin E(?), GSH(?), Ascorbate(?)]	(Also, inhibition of protein, nucleotide, fatty acid biosynthesis).

Table 2 Antioxidant Defense Systems and Their Role in Prevention of Cell Damage by Cytotoxic O_2 Species: The Chemical or Stoichiometric Defense System

Principal Components:	
Lipid Soluble	
Vitamin E (tocopherol)	Reduces chain-reaction lipid peroxidation in cell membranes, may directly convert O_2^- and $OH^\bullet$ radicals to less reactive forms.
β-carotene (precursor to Vitamin A)	Scavenges O_2^- and $^1O_2$; may also react directly with peroxyl radicals.
Water Soluble	
Vitamin C (Ascorbate)	Directly scavenges O_2^- and $OH^\bullet$ radicals; contributes to regeneration (reduction) of oxidized Vitamin E.
Glutathione (GSH)	Substrate for glutathione peroxidase; may react directly with O_2^-, $OH^\bullet$ radicals and may also regenerate oxidized vitamin E.

Abbreviations: SOD = superoxide dismutase; CAT = catalase; GP = glutathione peroxidase; GSH = glutathione; R = lipid; ROH = nontoxic lipid alcohol.
From Ref. 27 with permission.

chemical antioxidants, such as tocopherol, ascorbate, glutathione, and others. Although this secondary antioxidant defense system is believed to play an important role in the overall antioxidant armamentarium of aerobic cells, the primary cellular defense system against oxidant stress involves the AOEs, specifically superoxide dismutase (SOD), catalase, and the glutathione peroxidase (GP) redox enzyme complex.

According to the ''oxygen free radical theory of oxygen toxicity,'' basal levels of the cellular antioxidant defense system are adequate to maintain oxidant–antioxidant equilibrium in aerobic cells under normoxic conditions. However, under hyperoxic conditions, the marked increase in cellular O_2 free radical generation may overwhelm the basal antioxidant detoxifying capacity, leading to a state of oxidant–antioxidant disequilibrium and of O_2 free radical-mediated cell toxicity. When cells have the capacity to respond to increased oxidant stress with augmented levels of the primary antioxidant protective system—the AOEs—the state of oxidant–antioxidant equilibrium may be reestablished, with subsequent ''tolerance'' to the lethal effects of hyperoxic exposure. Evidence supporting the crucial protective role of the pulmonary AOEs includes a multitude of experiments in which relative resistance to pulmonary oxygen toxicity is associated with elevated levels of pulmonary AOE activity in response to hyperoxic exposure; conversely, vulnerability of the lung to the damaging effects of hyperoxia has been associated with deficient AOE activity or chemical inhibition of the AOEs (12–21).

III. Evidence Linking Oxygen Radicals and CLD

Epidemiological studies have demonstrated an increased incidence of CLD in preterm versus term neonates (22). Furthermore, the incidence of CLD increases with decreasing gestational age. Several recent studies have linked free radical formation or antioxidant indices with prematurity and CLD. When the rate of lipid peroxidation associated with free radicals was studied in premature infants by measuring expired ethane and pentane, these measurements suggested that lipid peroxidation correlated with gestational age and birthweight. Furthermore, infants with the highest amounts of expired ethane and pentane had an increased risk of dying or acquiring CLD (23). A second study, using a different marker of free radical generation—namely, plasma allantoin concentration—demonstrated an increase in this measurement within the first 1–2 days after birth in premature infants who required significant exposure to supplemental oxygen and subsequently had CLD, compared with infants who had less oxygen exposure and who did not acquire CLD (24). Similarly, when plasma allantoin and allantoin/uric acid ratios were used as markers of oxidative stress and examined in tracheal aspirates on the first day after birth, these measurements were elevated in those infants who acquired CLD and correlated with oxygen therapy (25). Finally, *plasma antioxidant ability*, defined as the quantity of plasma required to inhibit lipid peroxidation in vitro, predicts mortality in the premature infant (26). These findings suggest that toxic oxygen metabolites may contribute to the development of poor neonatal outcome, including death or CLD.

IV. Development of the AOE System in the Fetal Lung

At birth the newborn faces a host of new challenges. At the time of birth, the newborn will encounter a much more O_2-enriched world than the one encountered as a fetus, with changes from the in utero oxygen milieu (producing arterial oxygen tensions of 20–30 mmHg) to the extrauterine milieu (with arterial oxygen tensions of >80 mmHg), representing a severalfold increase in ambient O_2 tension (27,28). Studies examining "preparation for birth" phenomena—namely, fetal development of the pulmonary AOE system and the surfactant system late in gestation—have demonstrated a developmental pattern of pulmonary basal AOE activities in the lungs of several species, including rat, rabbit, guinea pig, hamster, and sheep, with a maturational pattern similar to that for surfactant DSPC (29–34; Fig. 1). Furthermore, Figure 2 depicts the overall magnitude of the prenatal changes in pulmonary AOE activities.

In addition to these parallel developmental patterns of the pulmonary AOE and surfactant systems, these two lung systems demonstrate certain similarities in hormonal regulation. For example, glucocorticoids appear to accelerate the

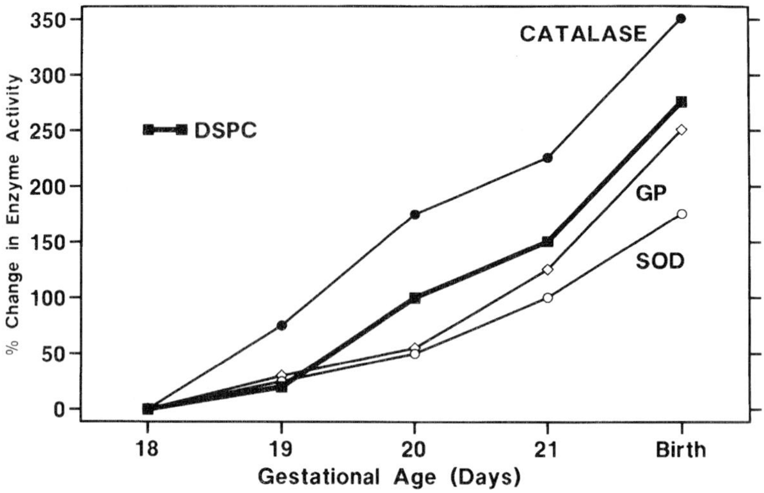

Figure 1 Changes in pulmonary antioxidant enzyme (AOE) activities in late gestation in the fetal rat (day 18 to term): superoxide dismutase (SOD), glutathione peroxidase (GP), and catalase (CAT). Note parallel time course of late gestational elevation in AOEs and lung surfactant disaturated phosphatidylcholine (DSPC). (From Ref. 99.)

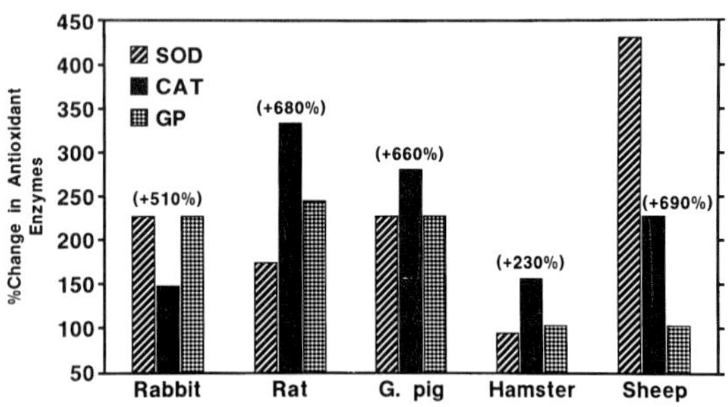

Figure 2 Total pulmonary AOE activity increases in the last 15–20% of gestation in five different species: SOD, superoxide dismutase; CAT, catalase; GP, glutathione peroxidase. Note average magnitude of maturational increases of AOEs before birth of 500–600%. (From Ref. 12.)

late gestational development of both the AOEs and surfactant. When pregnant rats were treated with dexamethasone in late gestation, the offspring demonstrated advancement in both surfactant and AOE development (35); conversely, maternal rats that were treated with metyrapone, which blocked endogenous glucocorticoid production, had offspring that manifested delays in both surfactant and AOE development (36). However, a second hormonal regulatory system—namely, the thyroid—appears to have different effects on the surfactant and AOE systems, with acceleration of surfactant phospholipid development and delay of AOE development (37). The inhibition of AOE development by thyroid hormone occurred with either triiodothyronine (T_3) or thyrotropin-releasing hormone (TRH) administration to pregnant rats, and was confirmed by studies of pharmacological thyroid blockade (38,39).

Data pertaining to AOE development in the human fetal lung are relatively sparse, but generally consistent with the animal studies. Three studies that measured activities or mRNA expression in lung tissue obtained from autopsies of human fetuses that ranged in gestation from 18–20 weeks to term have reported progressive increases in catalase, CuZn SOD (predominantly cytosolic), and Mn SOD (predominantly mitochondrial) during fetal development (40–42). The time course of AOE system maturation appears more protracted in the human fetus, occurring during the last 40% of gestation and coinciding with the longer period of surfactant development in the human fetal lung, compared with the shorter time course (during the final 10–15% of gestation) found for the animal species that have been studied (43,44).

V. Vulnerability of the Premature Infant Relative to Antioxidant Defenses

Because oxygen toxicity and premature birth are both important factors in the pathogenesis of CLD (22,45,46), it is logical to consider the relation between premature birth and the development of antioxidant defenses. Premature birth is associated with interruption of transplacental delivery of the secondary or chemical system of antioxidants (see Table 2), including vitamins A and C, glutathione, sulfur-containing amino acids, ceruloplasmin, transferrin, and trace metals that serve as cofactors for the AOEs, all of which are normally transferred from the maternal to the fetal circulation in the latter part of the third trimester (47–53). Paradoxically, vitamin C, although capable of serving an antioxidant function, may actually compromise antioxidant mechanisms and worsen oxidant damage in the premature infant. Plasma of premature infants has high concentrations of total vitamin C; plasma ascorbate levels are greater in premature infants compared with term infants (54). In vitro studies report that vitamin C inhibits the ferroxidase activity of ceruloplasmin, with the degree of inhibition related to the ratio of ascorbate to ceruloplasmin, suggesting that vitamin C may inhibit the antioxidant capacity of plasma in premature infants and thereby negatively influence outcome (55).

The premature infant may have increased vulnerability to chronic lung damage because of the incomplete development of the pulmonary AOE defense system. Yet, despite the likely insufficiency of basal AOE levels in premature infants, the ability to increase lung AOE activities in response to hyperoxic exposure is a more accurate predictor of vulnerability to oxidant stress. When AOE activities and lung pathology were assessed in both term and prematurely delivered rabbit pups exposed to prolonged hyperoxia, preterm rabbits had an impaired ability to mount an increased AOE response, decreased survival, and lung pathology showing intra-alveolar edema and focal hemorrhage. In contrast, term rabbit pups had significant increases in AOE activities following hyperoxic exposure (Fig. 3), greater survival in oxygen, and less lung pathology than did preterm pups (56.) AOE mRNA expression in the lungs in response to hyperoxia was also greater in term than in preterm rabbits (57). Furthermore, in the premature baboon model of BPD (58,59), no changes in the activities of any of the AOEs were found even after 6 days of breathing 95% O_2 (60). Although prematurely delivered baboons were able to increase both MnSOD mRNA and protein when challenged with oxygen and mechanical ventilation, baboons that acquired BPD had a significant decrease in MnSOD mRNA compared with oxygen-ventilated controls that did not have lung pathology consistent with BPD (61).

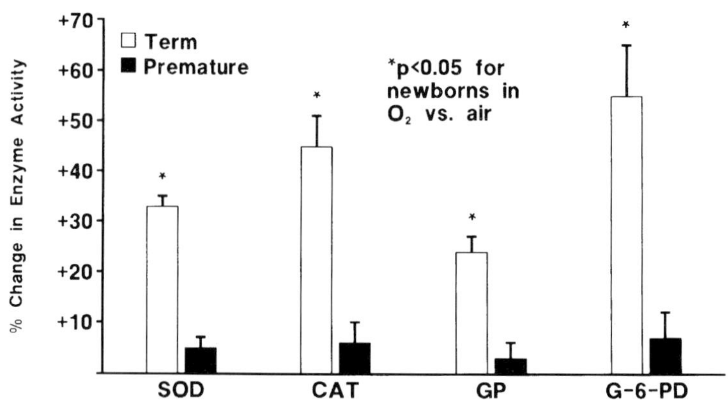

Figure 3 Comparative AOE responses to 48 hr of hyperoxia in premature versus term rabbits: Note the significant increases in pulmonary AOE activities [superoxide dismutase (SOD), catalase (CAT), glutathione peroxidase (GP), and glucose-6-phosphate dehydrogenase (G-6-PD)] in the full-term rabbit pups (*), and the lack of lung AOE increases in the premature rabbit pups (29 days of a 31.5 days of gestation). (From Ref. 56.)

Thus, the combination of immaturity of basal AOE development, the blunted ability to mount a protective AOE response to hyperoxia, and inadequacies of chemical antioxidants and trace metal cofactors may make the premature infant lung vulnerable to increased oxygen exposure after birth. It is even possible that exposure of the extremely immature lung to 21% oxygen may represent a formidable cytotoxic challenge.

VI. Experimental and Potential Therapeutic Modification of Antioxidant Defenses

Four potential experimental and therapeutic approaches might benefit the vulnerable premature infant who has inadequate antioxidant defenses and increased risk for chronic lung damage: antenatal stimulation of AOE development during late gestation; administration of missing antioxidant enzymes or chemical antioxidants; genetic manipulations to increase AOEs; and pharmacological stimulation of the capacity to mount a protective hyperoxic AOE response.

In terms of antenatal stimulation of AOE development, studies of prenatal glucocorticoid administration in experimental animals have shown acceleration of the normal maturational pattern of the pulmonary AOE system (35). Thus, the commonly used clinical practice of prenatal betamethasone treatment to increase pulmonary surfactant and thereby enhance lung development in cases of threatened premature delivery may also yield protection against oxidant stress in the prematurely delivered neonate which, in turn, might contribute to a positive respiratory outcome (62). In terms of antenatal thyroid hormone intervention, experimental animal studies would suggest a positive influence on surfactant development, but a negative influence on AOE development (37–39). Whereas early clinical trials of antenatal TRH administration reported improved respiratory outcome (63), the Australian collaborative trial data showed an increased risk of RDS and need for mechanical ventilation in the TRH-treated group (64), findings that could relate to the negative influence of thyroid hormones on AOE development (37–39).

Further studies of hormonal treatment or other measures to stimulate AOE system development in utero could have an important clinical effect. For example, various well-characterized growth factors, such as epidermal growth factor (EGF), platelet-derived growth factor (PDGF), acidic fibroblast growth factor (a-FGF), transforming growth factor-alpha (TGF-α), and keratinocyte growth factor (KGF), stimulate maturation and proliferation of pulmonary epithelial type II cells (65–68). Because the type II cell produces surfactant and is relatively resistant to oxygen toxicity (perhaps reflecting a high complement of AOEs), prenatal exposure to the aforementioned growth factors might accelerate maturation of pulmonary surfactant or AOEs and, thereby, protect the vulnerable preterm lung from chronic damage. This possibility is worthy of further investigation.

The second potential therapeutic approach to improve the antioxidant defenses in the preterm lung involves exogenous administration of antioxidants, either the AOEs themselves or chemical antioxidant substances. The first series of experimental and clinical studies examining exogenous AOE administration used bovine SOD preparations that were administered either parenterally or intratracheally (69–72). These studies failed to demonstrate a significant protective effect against pulmonary oxygen toxicity, but did reveal two major problems related to drug delivery. When SOD was delivered into the trachea and its distribution was examined using radiolabeling, the distribution of the SOD was patchy, rather than homogeneous. Second, very little of the administered SOD was actually taken up by lung cells, probably because the large AOE proteins were unable to penetrate cells. Moreover, the half-life of free SOD in plasma is short, with rapid clearance through the kidneys (73,74).

A recent report has provided more encouraging evidence that exogenous AOE treatment might be successful. When a novel approach was employed, that of premixing the free AOE preparation with a clinically available surfactant preparation, the radiolabeled and fluorescent-labeled SOD and catalase that were delivered intratracheally had a uniform distribution in the lungs, which the investigators attributed to the spreading properties of the surfactant preparation (75). Mixing the AOE with the surfactant preparation enabled better lung uptake of the SOD and catalase, such that AOE activities were increased in lung homogenates as early as 1 hr after treatment, and the observed increases in pulmonary AOE activities persisted for at least 24 hr after treatment (75).

The ability of this new method of exogenous AOE delivery to successfully achieve a meaningful degree of protection from oxygen-induced lung damage was subsequently confirmed in several in vivo studies. For example, newborn piglets that were treated with the AOE–surfactant preparation and subsequently ventilated with supplemental oxygen for several days had less hyperoxic lung damage than did control piglets (76). Treated piglets had decreased pulmonary edema and decreased protein yield in bronchoalveolar lavage fluid. In addition, lung lipid peroxidation products were significantly increased only in the untreated group of newborn piglets. The availability of human recombinant AOE preparations provides a particularly exciting prospect for future clinical testing. A recent study on the safety and pharmacokinetics of recombinant human CuZn SOD administered intratracheally to premature infants with RDS who were at risk for acquiring CLD demonstrated significantly increased SOD activity and concentration in serum, tracheal fluid, and urine. These changes in SOD lasted 2–3 days and were associated with reductions of inflammatory markers in tracheal fluid (77).

Exogenous administration of different chemical agents that serve an antioxidant function may have the potential to provide protection against oxidant lung damage. Studies in experimental animals suggest that iron-chelating agents may have a protective effect. Young rabbits that received intratracheal iron-free transferrin (with the capacity to bind free iron and, thereby reduce iron-catalyzed free radical formation) followed by hyperoxia, had decreased lipid peroxidation, as assessed by the amount of malondialdehyde in bronchoalveolar lavage (78). In a similar fashion, newborn rats that were treated with the iron chelator deferoxamine and then exposed to prolonged hyperoxia demonstrated decreased evidence of lung growth inhibition related to hyperoxia and decreased lung conjugated diene levels than untreated oxygen-exposed controls (79). Deferoxamine, currently in use therapeutically for clinical hematological disorders (80), eventually may have application for treating human infants at risk for oxidant lung injury. Another chemical agent with potential antioxidant function is allopurinol, which serves as an inhibitor of xanthine oxidase (which catalyzes reactions that generate superoxide). When allopurinol was administered to premature baboons that were exposed to prolonged hyperoxia, these treated animals demonstrated decreased lung injury and increased antioxidant defenses, including lung glutathione concentrations (60). In rats, allopurinol treatment decreased the number of neutrophils that entered the lungs with exposure to hyperoxia, but it failed to decrease lung injury, as assessed by the amount of LDH or protein within the airspaces (81). Similar results were obtained from a prospective, randomized controlled trial designed to determine whether allopurinol would have a protective effect on complications of prematurity suspected to be related to oxidant injury. Treatment of preterm infants with allopurinol failed to protect against periventricular leukomalacia, retinopathy of prematurity, or CLD (82).

For genetic manipulation of AOE in the lung, molecular biology has increased our understanding of gene expression under both normal and abnormal conditions, including hyperoxia. Molecular biologists have been able to successfully manipulate normal gene expression for a variety of important cellular proteins. In recent years the tools of molecular biology have been used to investigate the role of AOEs in protection against hyperoxic exposure. For example, in transgenic mice that express increased pulmonary activity and mRNA abundance of a single AOE (an increase of MnSOD of about 50%), a marked improvement in hyperoxic survival was found in the transgenic mice, compared with control mice (LT_{50} of 230 hr vs. 130 hr, respectively) (83). Also, in experiments involving lung epithelial cells in culture, investigators have used a replication-deficient adenovirus vector (attached to the cDNA of the specific enzyme) to achieve gene transfer of specific enzymes into the cultured cells. When cultured lung epithelial cells were transfected with genetic material encoding for catalase or SOD, these manipulations resulted in significantly elevated cellular catalase or SOD concentrations and significantly improved lung cell survival when the cells were subsequently exposed to hyperoxia (84,85). Transfection studies are presently being explored for possible in vivo application, in which adenoviral vectors attached to genetic material encoding for vital lung protein products could be delivered directly to the lungs (86,87). Preliminary work using direct lung transfection of the cDNA encoding for catalase and SOD demonstrated substantially increased activities of catalase and SOD in rat lung homogenates 3 days after transfection (88). This preliminary investigation indicated that not only did the transfected cDNA for the AOE enter the lung cells and penetrate the nuclei, but also that the inserted cDNA was effectively transcribed and translated into new catalase and SOD protein. The successful transfection was associated with improved hyperoxic survival of the transfected versus control animals (88).

A final potential therapeutic approach to protection against free radical-induced lung damage would involve a method to stimulate the induction of a protective AOE response to hyperoxic exposure. Whereas neonatal animals have the ability to respond to an increase in ambient oxygen exposure by a protective increase in AOE levels, prematurely delivered newborns and adult animals do not have this capability; therefore, they are unable to tolerate hyperoxia. When adult experimental animals, however, are treated with a low dose of bacterial lipopolysaccharide (endotoxin), they respond in a fashion that is similar to neonatal animals, wherein they are able to mount a protective hyperoxic AOE response; hence, they are effectively protected from pulmonary oxygen toxicity (89,90). The mechanism by which endotoxin treatment produces this effect is only partially understood (91,92), and it may be associated with specific cytokines, including interleukin-1 (IL-1) and TNF-α (93,94). A recent study that examined the gene expression of insulin-like growth factor (IGF-1 and -2) in lungs of newborn rats exposed to hyperoxia demonstrated a ''reemergence'' of a fetal pattern of gene expression of IGF-1 and IGF-2 during hyperoxic exposure. Whether any of the AOE activity responses to hyperoxia were associated with the increases in lung IGF was not explored in this study (95).

VII. Oxygen Toxicity, Antioxidant Enzymes, and CLD: Unanswered Questions and Future Clinical Applications

In summary, data on the late gestational time course of maturation of the protective AOE system and clinical studies linking indices of free radical formation, prematurity, and CLD, all provide evidence that CLD in premature infants is, at least partly, related to oxygen free radical damage. Therefore, one or more of the four discussed categories of intervention to augment antioxidant defenses; that is (1) antenatal stimulation of AOE development, (2) exogenous administration of AOE or chemical antioxidants, (3) genetic manipulation of AOE in the lung, and (4) stimulation of the ability to induce a protective hyperoxic increase in AOE, could potentially reduce or ameliorate the development of chronic lung damage in premature infants. The availability of such models as the premature baboon model of CLD (58,59) or the prematurely delivered rat model of lung fibrosis (96) provide a potent means of exploring not only potential mechanisms related to oxidant lung damage, but also potentially protective therapeutic interventions. In addition, results of human clinical trials involving antioxidant intervention are beginning to appear in the literature. For example, a study examining whether allopurinol could protect against oxidant-related complications of prematurity yielded results indicating a lack of protection (82). Studies are presently in progress assessing the role of intratracheally administered recombinant human SOD to prevent chronic lung damage in premature infants at risk.

Recent epidemiological data suggest that antioxidant augmentation alone may not be adequate in eradicating CLD from premature infant populations. Specifically, CLD occurs with significant frequency in very low birth weight infants without preceding RDS and with minimal early supplemental oxygen exposure (97). Similar studies have found, however, an association between persistent patency of the ductus arteriosus (PDA), nosocomial infection, and the development of CLD (98). Thus, the previously discussed therapeutic modalities to augment antioxidant defenses may provide partial, but not complete, efficacy in protecting against CLD. It may, therefore, require additional therapeutic strategies besides augmentation of antioxidant capacity, including early PDA closure, prevention of infection, or delivery of anti-inflammatory agents, to protect the premature infant from chronic lung damage and its sequelae.

References

1. Freeman BA, Crapo JD. Biology of disease. Free radicals and tissue injury. Lab Invest 1982; 47:412–426.
2. Halliwell B, Gutteridge JMC. Protection against oxidants in biological systems: the superoxide theory of oxygen toxicity. In: Halliwell B, Gutteridge JMC, eds. Free Radicals in Biology and Medicine. Oxford: Clarendon Press, 1989:86–187.
3. Jackson RM. Molecular, pharmacologic, and clinical aspects of oxygen-induced lung injury. Clin Chest Med 1990; 11:73–86.
4. Heffner JE, Repine JE. Pulmonary strategies of antioxidant defense. Am Rev Respir Dis 1989; 140:531–554.
5. Zweier JL, Duke SS, Kuppusamy P, et al. Electron paramagnetic resonance evidence that cellular oxygen toxicity is caused by generation of superoxide and hydroxy free radicals. FEBS Lett 1989; 252:12–16.
6. Freeman BA, Crapo JD. Hyperoxia increases oxygen free radical production in rat lung and lung mitochondria. J Biol Chem 1981; 256:10986–10992.
7. Freeman BA. Topolsky MK, Crapo JD. Hyperoxia increases oxygen radical production in rat lung homogenates. Arch Biochem Biophys 1982; 216:477–484.
8. Turrens JF, Freeman BA, Crapo JD. Hyperoxia increases H_2O_2 release by lung mitochondria and microsomes. Arch Biochem Biophys 1982; 217:411–421.

9. Yusa T, Crapo JD, Freeman BA. Hyperoxia enhances lung and liver nuclear superoxide generation. Biochim Biophys Acta 1984; 793:167–174.
10. Aust SD, Chignell CF, Bray TM, Kalyanaraman B, Mason RP. Free radicals in toxicology. Toxicol Appl Pharmacol 1993; 120:168–178.
11. Brigham KL, Meyrick B, Berry LC Jr, et al. Antioxidants protect cultured bovine endothelial cells from injury by endotoxin. J Appl Physiol 1987; 63:840–850.
12. Frank L. Developmental aspects of experimental pulmonary oxygen toxicity. Free Radical Biol Med 1991; 11:463–494.
13. Jamieson D. Oxygen toxicity and reactive oxygen metabolites in mammals. Free Radical Biol Med 1989; 7:87–108.
14. White CW. Pulmonary oxygen toxicity: cellular mechanisms of oxidant injury and antioxidant defenses. In: Bancalari E, Stocker JT, eds. Bronchopulmonary Dysplasia. Cambridge, MA: Hemisphere, 1988:22–41.
15. Sies H. Strategies of antioxidant defense. Eur J Biochem 1993; 215:213–219.
16. Yam J, Frank L, Roberts RJ. Oxygen toxicity: comparison of lung biochemical response in neonatal and adult rats. Pediatr Res 1978; 12:115–119.
17. Turrens JF, Crapo JD, Freeman BA. Protection against oxygen toxicity by intravenous injection of liposome entrapped catalase and superoxide dismutase. J Clin Invest 1984; 73:87–95.
18. Briscoe P, Caniggia I, Graves A, et al. Delivery of superoxide dismutase to pulmonary epithelium via pH-sensitive liposomes. Am J Physiol 1995; 268:L374–L380.
19. Frank L, Yam J, Roberts RJ. The role of endotoxin in protection of adult rats from high oxygen lung toxicity. J Clin Invest 1978; 61:269–275.
20. Frank L, Summerville J, Massaro D. Protection from oxygen toxicity with endotoxin: role of the endogenous antioxidant enzymes of the lung. J Clin Invest 1980; 65: 1104–1111.
21. Frank L, Wood DL, Roberts RJ. The effect of diethyldithiocarbamate (DDC) on oxygen toxicity and lung enzyme activity in immature and adult rats. Biochem Pharmacol 1978; 27:251–254.
22. Palta M, Gabbert D, Weinstein MR, et al. Multivariate assessment of traditional risk factors for chronic lung disease in very low birth weight infants. J Pediatr 1991; 119:285–292.
23. Varsila E, Pitkanen O, Hallman M, et al. Immaturity-dependent free radical activity in premature infants. Pediatr Res 1994; 36:55–59.
24. Ogihara T, Okamoto R, Kim HS, et al. New evidence for the involvement of oxygen radicals in triggering neonatal chronic lung disease. Pediatr Res 1996; 39:117–119.
25. Moison RM, de Beaufort AJ, Haasnoot AA, et al. Uric acid and ascorbic redox ratios in plasma and tracheal aspirate of preterm babies with acute and chronic lung disease. Free Radic Biol Med 1997; 23:226–234.
26. Silvers KM, Gibson AT, Powers HJ. High plasma vitamin C concentrations at birth associated with low antioxidant status and poor outcome in premature infants. Arch Dis Child Fetal Ed 1994; 71:40–44.
27. Dejours P. Principles in Comparative Respiratory Physiology. 2nd ed. Amsterdam: Elsevier North Holland, 1981:147–171.
28. Towell ME, Johnson J, Smedstad K, et al. Fetal blood and tissue po_2 during maternal oxygen breathing. J Dev Physiol 1984; 5:177–185.

29. Frank L, Groseclose EE. Preparation for birth into an O_2-rich environment: the antioxidant enzymes in the developing rabbit lung. Pediatr Res 1984; 18:240–244.
30. Tanswell AK, Freeman BA. Pulmonary antioxidant enzyme maturation in the fetal and neonatal rat. I. Developmental profiles. Pediatr Res 1984; 18:584–587.
31. Gerdin E, Vyden O, Eriksson UJ. The development of antioxidant enzymatic defense in the perinatal rat lung: activities of superoxide dismutase, glutathione peroxidase, and catalase. Pediatr Res 1985; 19:687–691.
32. Walther FJ, Wade AB, Warburton D, et al. Ontogeny of antioxidant enzymes in the fetal lamb lung. Exp Lung Res 1991; 17:39–45.
33. Frank L, Sosenko IRS. Prenatal development of lung antioxidant enzymes in four species. J Pediatr 1987; 110:106–110.
34. Frank L, Sosenko IRS. Development of lung antioxidant enzyme system in late gestation: possible implications for the prematurely-born infant. J Pediatr 1987; 110: 9–14.
35. Frank L, Lewis PL, Sosenko IR. Dexamethasone stimulates fetal rat lung antioxidant enzyme activity in parallel with surfactant stimulation. Pediatrics 1985; 75:569–574.
36. Sosenko IRS, Lewis PL, Frank L. Metyrapone delays surfactant and antioxidant enzyme maturation in developing rat lung. Pediatr Res 1986; 20:672–675.
37. Sosenko IRS, Frank L. Thyroid hormone depresses antioxidant enzyme maturation in fetal rat lung. Am J Physiol 1987; 253:R292–R598.
38. Rodriguez MP, Sosenko IR, Antigua MC, et al. Prenatal hormone treatment with thyrotropin releasing hormone and with thyrotropin releasing hormone plus dexamethasone delays antioxidant enzyme maturation but does not inhibit a protective antioxidant enzyme response to hyperoxia in newborn rat lung. Pediatr Res 1991; 30:522–527.
39. Sosenko IRS, Frank L. Thyroid inhibition and developmental increases in fetal rat lung antioxidant enzymes. Am J Physiol 1989; 257:L94–L99.
40. Autor AP, Frank L, Roberts RJ. Developmental characteristics of pulmonary superoxide dismutase: relationship to idiopathic respiratory distress syndrome. Pediatr Res 1976; 10:154–158.
41. Dobashi K, Asayama K, Hayashibe H, et al. Immunologic study of copper–zinc and manganese superoxide dismutases in the lungs of human fetuses and newborn infants. Developmental profile and alterations in hyaline membrane disease and bronchopulmonary dysplasia. Virchows Archiv A. Pathol Anat Histopathol 1993; 423: 177–189.
42. Asikainen TM, Saksela M, Heikinheimo M, et al. Expression of antioxidant enzymes during human lung development. Pediatr Res 1997; 41:40A.
43. Floros J. Sixty years of surfactant research. Am J Physiol 1990; 259:L238–L240.
44. Rooney SA. The surfactant system and lung phospholipid biochemistry. Am Rev Respir Dis 1985; 131:439–460.
45. Bancalari E. Pathogenesis of bronchopulmonary dysplasia: an overview. In: Bancalari E, Stocker JT, eds. Bronchopulmonary Dysplasia. Washington, DC: Hemisphere, 1988:3–15.
46. Rosenfeld W. Clinical evidence of oxidant injury in bronchopulmonary dysplasia. In: Bancalari E, Stocker JT, eds. Bronchopulmonary Dysplasia. Washington, DC: Hemisphere, 1988:42–48.

47. Hustead VA, Gutcher GR, Anderson SA, et al. Relationships of vitamin A (retinol) status to lung disease in the preterm infant. J Pediatr 1984; 105:610–615.
48. Gutcher GR, Raynor WJ, Farrell PM. An evaluation of vitamin E status in premature infants. Am J Clin Nutr 1984; 40:1078–1089.
49. Huijbers WAR, Schrijver J, Speek AJ, et al. Persistent low plasma vitamin E levels in premature infants surviving respiratory distress syndrome. Eur J Pediatr 1986; 145:170–171.
50. Omene JA, Longe AC, Ihongbe JC, et al. Decreased umbilical cord serum ceruloplasmin concentrations in infants with hyaline membrane disease. J Pediatr 1981; 99: 136–138.
51. Rosenfeld W, Concepcion L, Evans H, et al. Serial trypsin inhibitory capacity and ceruloplasmin levels in prematures at risk for bronchopulmonary dysplasia. Am Rev Respir Dis 1986; 134:1229–1232.
52. Walravens PA. Nutritional importance of copper and zinc in neonates and infants. 1980; 26:185–189.
53. Van Caille-Bertand M, Degenhart HJ, Fernandes J. Selenium status of infants on nutritional support. Acta Paediatr Scand 1984; 73:816–821.
54. Gopinathan V, Miller NJ, Milner AD, Rice-Evans CA. Bilirubin and ascorbate antioxidant activity in neonatal plasma. FEBS Lett 1994; 349:197–200.
55. Powers HJ, Loban A, Silvers K, Gibson AT. Vitamin C at concentrations observed in premature babies inhibits the ferroxidase activity of ceruloplasmin. Free Radic Res 1995; 22:57–65.
56. Frank L, Sosenko IRS. Failure of premature rabbits to increase antioxidant enzymes during hyperoxic exposure: increased susceptibility to pulmonary oxygen toxicity compared to term rabbits. Pediatr Res 1991; 29:292–296.
57. Sosenko IRS, Chen Y, Price LT, et al. Failure of premature rabbits to increase lung antioxidant enzyme activities following hyperoxic exposure: antioxidant enzyme gene regulation and pharmacologic intervention with endotoxin and dexamethasone. Pediatr Res 1995; 37:469–475.
58. Escobedo MB, Hilliard JL, Smith F, et al. A baboon model of bronchopulmonary dysplasia. I. Clinical features. Exp Mol Pathol 1982; 37:323–334.
59. Coalson JJ, Kuehl TJ, Escobedo MB, et al. A baboon model of bronchopulmonary dysplasia. II. Pathological features. Exp Mol Pathol 1982; 37:335–350.
60. Jenkinson SG, Roberts RJ, DeLemos RA, et al. Allopurinol-induced effects in premature baboons with respiratory distress syndrome. J Appl Physiol 1991; 70:1160–1167.
61. Clerch LB, Wright AE, Coalson JJ. Lung manganese superoxide dismutase protein expression increases in the baboon model of bronchopulmonary dysplasia and is regulated at a posttranscriptional level. Pediatr Res 1996; 39:253–258.
62. Crowley PA. Antenatal corticosteroid therapy: a meta-analysis of the randomized trials 1972–1994. Am J Obstet Gynecol 1995; 173:322–335.
63. Ballard RA, Ballard PL, Creasy RK, et al. The TRH Study Group: respiratory disease in very low birth weight infants after prenatal TRH and glucocorticoid. Lancet 1992; 339:510–515.
64. Crowther CA, Hiller JE, Haslam RR, et al. Australian collaborative trial of antenatal TRH: adverse effects at 12 month follow-up. Pediatrics 1997; 99:311–317.
65. Panos RJ, Rubin JS, Csaky KG, et al. Keratinocyte growth factor and hepatocyte

growth factor/scatter factor are heparin-binding growth factors for alveolar type II cells in fibroblast-conditioned medium. J Clin Invest 1993; 92:969–977.
66. Leslie CC, McCormick-Shannon K, Robinson PC, et al. Stimulation of DNA synthesis in cultured rat alveolar type II cells. Exp Lung Res 1985; 8:53–66.
67. Catterton WZ, Escobedo MB, Sexson WR, et al. Effect of epidermal growth factor on lung maturation in fetal rabbits. Pediatr Res 1979; 13:104–108.
68. King RJ, Jones MB, Minoo P. Regulation of lung cell proliferation by polypeptide growth factors. Am J Physiol 1989; 257:L23–L38.
69. Rosenfeld W, Evans H, Concepcion L, et al. Prevention of bronchopulmonary dysplasia by administration of bovine superoxide dismutase in preterm infants with respiratory distress syndrome. J Pediatr 1984; 105:781–786.
70. Rosenfeld W, Concepcion L. Pharmacologic intervention: use of the antioxidant superoxide dismutase. In: Merritt TA, Northway WH Jr, Boynton BR, eds. Bronchopulmonary Dysplasia. Boston: Blackwell, 1988:365–374.
71. Shaffer SG, O'Neill DH, Thibeault BW. Administration of bovine superoxide dismutase fails to prevent chronic pulmonary sequelae of neonatal oxygen exposure in the rat. Pediatrics 1987; 141:942–946.
72. Crapo JD, DeLong DM, Sjostrom K, et al. The failure of aerosolized superoxide dismutase to modify pulmonary oxygen toxicity. Am Rev Respir Dis 1977; 122: 1027–1033.
73. Huber W, Saifer MGP, Williams LD. Superoxide dismutase pharmacology and orgotein efficacy: new perspectives. In: Bannister WH, Bannister JV, eds. Biological and Clinical Aspects of Superoxide and Superoxide Dismutase. Amsterdam: Elsevier/North Holland, 1980:395–407.
74. Michelson AM, et al. Penetration of erythrocytes by superoxide dismutase. In: Bannister WH, Bannister JV, eds. Biological and Clinical Aspects of Superoxide and Superoxide Dismutase. Amsterdam: Elsevier/North Holland, 1980:348–366.
75. Nieves-Cruz B, Rivera A, Cifuentes J, et al. Clinical surfactant preparations mediate SOD and catalase uptake by type II cells and lung tissue. Am J Physiol 1996; 270: L659–L667.
76. Davis JM, Rosenfeld WN, Sanders RJ, et al. Prophylactic effects of recombinant human superoxide dismutase in neonatal lung injury. J Appl Physiol 1993; 74:2234–2241.
77. Rosenfeld WN, Davis JM, Parton L, et al. Safety and pharmacokinetics of recombinant human superoxide dismutase administered intratracheally to premature neonates with respiratory distress syndrome. Pediatrics 1996; 97:811–817.
78. Hallman M, Chundu V, Barsotti M, Bry K. Transferrin modifies surfactant responsiveness in acute respiratory failure: role of iron-free transferrin as an antioxidant. Pediatr Pulmonol 1996; 22:14–22.
79. Frank L. Hyperoxic inhibition of newborn rat lung development: protection by deferoxamine. Free Radic Biol Med 1991; 11:341–348.
80. Verhasselt B, Delangle J, Verstraete A, Leroux-Roels G. Colorimetric quantification of urinary iron during deferoxamine therapy. Clin Chem 1994; 40:497–498.
81. Bryan CL. Lewis RE, Owens SL, Emmanuel B, Jenkinson SG. Allopurinol inhibition of neutrophilic alveolar response during hyperoxia. J Appl Physiol 1993; 75:357–363.

82. Russell GA, Cooke RW. Randomized controlled trial of allopurinol prophylaxis in very preterm infants. Arch Dis Child 1995; 73:F27–F31.
83. Wispe JR, Warner BB, Clark JC, et al. Human Mn-superoxide dismutase in pulmonary epithelial cells of transgenic mice confers protection from oxygen injury. J Biol Chem 1992; 267:23937–23941.
84. Huang T-T, Carlson EJ, Leadon SA, et al. Relationship of resistance to oxygen free radicals to Cu, Zn superoxide dismutase activity in transgenic, transfected, and trisomic cells. FASEB J 1992; 6:903–910.
85. Erzunum SC, Lemarchand P, Rosenfeld MA, et al. Protection of human endothelial cells from oxidant injury by adenovirus-mediated transfer of the human catalase cDNA. Nucleic Acids Res 1993; 21:1607–1612.
86. Mastrangeli A, Danel C, Rosenfeld MA, et al. Diversity of airway epithelial cell targets for in vivo recombinant adenovirus-mediated gene transfer. J Clin Invest 1993; 91:225–234.
87. McCray PB Jr, Amstrong K, Zabner J, et al. Adenovirus-mediated gene transfer to the fetal pulmonary epithelium. Pediatr Res 1994; 35:72A.
88. Prayssac P, Erzurum SC, Donel C, et al. Adenovirus-mediated transfer to the lungs of catalase and superoxide dismutase cDNAs prevents hyperoxia toxicity but not ischemia–reperfusion injury in rats. Am J Respir Crit Care Med 1997; 155:265A.
89. Frank L, Yam J, Roberts RJ. The role of endotoxin in protection of adult rats from high oxygen toxicity. J Clin Invest 1978; 61:269–275.
90. Frank L, Summerville J, Massaro D. Protection from oxygen toxicity with endotoxin: role of the endogenous antioxidant enzymes of the lung. J Clin Invest 1980; 65: 1104–1111.
91. Hass MA, Massaro D. Differences in Cu/Zn superoxide dismutase induction in lungs of neonatal and adult rats. Am J Physiol 1987; 253:C66–C70.
92. Visner GA, Dougall WC, Wilson JM, et al. Regulation of manganese and copper–zinc superoxide dismutase mRNA levels in pulmonary cells by endotoxin and oxygen. Am Rev Respir Dis 1989; 139:368A.
93. White C. Molecular mechanisms of cytokine-induced tolerance to acute oxidant lung injury. In: Johnson A, Ferro TJ, eds. Lung Vascular Injury. New York: Marcel Dekker, 1992:191–211.
94. White CW, Ghezzi P, McMahon S, et al. Cytokines increase rat lung antioxidant enzymes during exposure to hyperoxia. J Appl Physiol 1989; 66:1003–1007.
95. Veness-Meehan KA, Moats-Staat BM, Price WA, et al. Re-emergence of a fetal pattern of insulin-like growth factor expression during hyperoxic rat lung injury. Am J Respir Crit Care Med 1997; 16:538–548.
96. Chen Y, Martinez MA, Frank L. Prenatal dexamethasone administration to premature rats exposed to prolonged hyperoxia: a new rat model of pulmonary fibrosis (bronchopulmonary dysplasia). J Pediatr 1997; 130:409–416.
97. Horbar JD, McAuliffe TL, Adler SM, et al. Variability in 28-day outcomes for very low birth weight infants: an analysis of 11 neonatal intensive care units. Pediatrics 1988; 82:554–559.
98. Rojas M, Gonzalez A, Bancalari E, et al. Changing trends in the epidemiology and pathogenesis of neonatal chronic lung disease. J Pediatr 1995; 126:605–610.
99. Frank L. Antioxidants, nutrition and bronchopulmonary dysplasia. In: Holtzman RB, Frank L, eds. Bronchopulmonary Dysplasia. Clin Perinatol 1992; 19:541–562.

35

Proteolytic Enzymes and Their Inhibitors in Lung Health and Disease

JOHN R. HOIDAL and MARI K. HOIDAL

University of Utah
Salt Lake City, Utah

I. Introduction

Proteases play a central role in the degradation of proteins by hydrolyzing peptide bonds. Originally thought to fulfill primarily digestive functions, it is now believed that these enzymes are the principal regulators of many crucial and diverse physiological processes, and that they have a central role in pathological tissue destruction of many organs. Their role in tissue destruction has been investigated in greatest detail in the lungs, especially in relation to the pathogenesis of emphysema. Recent investigations suggest prominent roles for proteases in growth and development and in neonatal lung injury, making a review of the actions of proteases and the factors controlling their expression important when discussing lung diseases in infants. In this chapter we will review the classification of proteases, examine the principal regulatory mechanisms whereby the actions of the enzymes are controlled, and consider their physiological and pathological roles, particularly in relation to pulmonary health and disease. We will end with a discussion of what the future holds in this rapidly advancing field.

At the outset, a review of the terminology that is commonly used to describe proteolytic enzymes is in order (reviewed in 1). The term referring to any of the enzymes that hydrolyze peptide bonds is *peptidase*. Peptidases are divided into two groups. Those that cleave polypeptide chains in their inner regions are referred to as *proteases* or *endopeptidases*. Those that act only near the amino (NH_2)- or carboxy (COOH)-terminal are referred to as *exopeptidases*. *Oligopeptidases* comprise a subgroup of proteases that act on peptides of up to 20 or 30 amino acid residues. This review focuses primarily on proteases.

II. Classification of Proteases

Proteases are usually classified based on the chemical groupings responsible for their catalytic activities. They act through four distinct catalytic mechanisms; hence, they are subdivided into four major classes according to the active groups: serine, metallo-, cysteine, or aspartic. There are multiple evolutionary origins of proteases, so that each major class is represented by several families (1). Members of an evolutionary family are recognized by similarities in their amino acid residues, especially in the vicinity of the catalytic residue. Several proteases have been identified that do not fall into the four classes. Included in this group of unclassified proteases are the membrane-bound signal peptidases (2) and the proteases present in proteasomes (3). Recently, classification of proteases based on structural and evolutionary relationships has been proposed as an extension of the classification by catalytic type (4). This approach has not yet received widespread acceptance. Thus, this review of proteases is based on their catalytic class.

A. Serine Proteases

Serine proteases make up two superfamilies of proteolytic enzymes: the chymotrypsin superfamily and the subtilisin superfamily (5). Within these two superfamilies, over 20 families have been recognized. The families are from at least four separate evolutionary origins.

In humans, serine proteases are primarily members of the chymotrypsin superfamily. They include digestive, lysosomal, coagulation, fibrinolytic, and immune cell secretory enzymes. Examples of digestive serine proteases are chymotrypsin, trypsin, and elastase that are released from the pancreas into the duodenum and cleave dietary proteins. The coagulation, fibrinolysis (tissue plasminogen activator, urokinase-type plasminogen activator, and plasmin), and complement systems also consist of serine proteases. Of particular importance to immune and inflammatory processes in the lung are the granule-associated serine proteases that are expressed in cells of bone marrow origin, including polymorphonuclear leukocytes (PMNLs), mast cells, and cytotoxic lymphocytes. The granule-associated proteases are major constituents of these cells, and not only are they a physiological necessity, but they are also a potential hazard. That is, if they are uncontrolled, they may destroy the protein components of cells and tissues. PMNLs contain three major serine proteases: elastase (HLE), proteinase

3 (PR-3), and cathepsin G (Cat G). These enzymes are involved in the movement of PMNLs through the basement membrane at sites of inflammation (6), degradation of phagocytosed materials (7), and microbial killing (8). Granules found in natural killer (NK) cells, cytotoxic T lymphocytes, and lymphokine-activated killer cells contain multiple serine proteases called granzymes that are involved in target cell destruction, including tumor cell cytotoxicity and apoptosis (9,10). Mast cell granules contain two types of serine proteases: chymase and tryptase. These proteases are released from mast cells during allergic reactions and are likely involved in neurogenic inflammation (11), submucosal gland secretion (12), and vasoactive peptide metabolism (13).

In humans, the subtilisin superfamily of serine proteases is represented by a newly discovered group of endoproteases that carry out intracellular processing of protein precursors. These enzymes differ from the chymotrypsin family, in that the His, Asp, and Ser charge-transfer triad involved in catalysis is ordered differently, suggesting that the two groups arose through convergent evolution. The subtilisin group includes the furins that are involved in processing of NH_2-terminal propeptides from numerous proteins and the recently discovered prohormone-converting enzymes, that in humans include PC-1/3 and PC-2 (14). The furins are expressed in most tissues, whereas the prohormone-converting enzymes are expressed primarily in endocrine tissues (15). The characteristics of the subtilisin superfamily, including their tissue-specific expression, subcellular localization, and cleavage site selectivity are just beginning to be determined.

The mechanism of hydrolysis of peptide bonds by serine proteases has been studied extensively (reviewed in 16). Hydrolysis depends on a uniquely reactive serine residue for catalytic activity, and a common ''catalytic triad'' of serine (Ser; nucleophile), aspartate (Asp; electrophile), and histidine (His; base). These residues are part of a hydrogen-bonding system. Peptide bond cleavage involves an initial nucleophilic attack by the serine residue on the carbonyl carbon of the susceptible peptide bond of the substrate. This is followed by formation of an ester between the serine and the substrate, resulting in release of the amino portion of the peptide bond. Finally, following the addition of a water molecule, the acyl enzyme is hydrolyzed, the acyl portion of the peptide bond is released, and the active serine protease is regenerated.

B. Matrix Metalloproteases

The metalloproteases constitute the most diverse of the catalytic classes of proteases. In humans this class is represented by matrix metalloproteases (matrixins) and the astracin-like protease, P-aminobutyric acid (PABA)-peptide hydrolase, which is found on brush border membranes of the intestine and kidney. The matrixins constitute a single evolutionary superfamily of extracellular proteases of closely related primary structure and include collagenases, gelatinases, stromelysins, and their activators. These enzymes are believed to be primary mediators of the physiological and pathological degradation of extracellular matrix that occurs during morphogenesis, involution, wound healing, and cancer (17). Matrixins share a common domain structure composed of propeptide, catalytic, hinge, and hemopexin-like domains (an exception is MMP-7 or matrilysin that lacks a hemopexin-like domain). The 12 identified human matrixins are each encoded by a different gene, and each has a different substrate specificity against extracellular matrix macromolecules. Ten of the matrixins are produced by cells as soluble zymogens and are secreted by most cells immediately after synthesis. Inflammatory cells, however, store the matrixins in their secretory granules. For example, PMNLs store collagenase (MMP-8) and gelatinase b (MMP-9) in their specific (18) or gelatinase granules (19). Three of the human matrixins (MMP-1, MMP-8, and collagenase 3) belong to the collagenase subgroup (20–22). The gelatinase subclass is composed of two members, 72-kDa (MMP-2) and 92-kDa (MMP-9) type IV collagenases (23,24). The stromelysin subclass includes stromelysins-1, -2, -3, and matrilysin (25–27). Two recently discovered matrixins have transmembrane domains at the COOH-terminus and are expressed as ectoenzyme membrane proteins (28). All matrixins contain a zinc-binding domain at the active site that is coordinated to three histidine residues (29). The zinc ion acts as an electrophile, assisting in the attack on the carbonyl carbon of the substrate peptide bond by the oxygen of a water molecule.

C. Cysteine Proteases

The cysteine proteases are a class of enzymes that depend on a catalytic dyad of cysteine and histidine (30). In humans, the two major groups of cysteine proteases are the lysomal proteases, cathepsin B, H, L, S, and dipeptidylpeptidase-I (DPP-I or cathepsin C), and the cytosolic calpains, I and II. Given the functional inhibition and evolutionary relationships, the recently described interleukin-1 β–converting enzyme (ICE) is classified as a cysteine protease. The cathepsins are found widely distributed in many tissues, but their levels vary significantly from one tissue to another, and from one cell type to another. Cathepsins B, H, L, O, S, and DPP-I are contained within lysosomes and are involved in terminal degradation of intracellular proteins. An expanded physiological role for these enzymes has been suggested recently by the demonstration that cathepsin B is a processing enzyme for prorenin and for the activation of prourokinase-type plasminogen activator (31,32). The cathepsins are also capable of directly degrading structural elements of the lung, such as collagen, elastin, fibronectin, and laminin, over a wide range of pH (33), suggesting a possible role in lung destruction.

Calpains, a special group of cytosolic cysteine proteases that are present in most cells, require calcium for activity (34). Calpains, through their ability to activate intracellular proteases and phosphatases and to induce specific cytoskeletal rearrangements, are believed to be important in signaling, vesicular trafficking, and structural stabilization within the cell. The mechanism of catalytic action of the cysteine proteases is similar to that of the serine proteases except that a nucleophilic sulfur of the active-site cysteine replaces the serine residue.

D. Aspartic Proteases

Aspartic proteases were the first known enzymes (chymosin), the first described protease type (pepsin), and the second protein crystallized (pepsin; 35). In humans, the major proteases in this class are cathepsins D and E, renin, and the digestive enzymes pepsin and gastricin. Most of the aspartic proteases are single-chain enzymes, with a molecular mass of 35,000. Cathepsin D exists in a two-chain form. The zymogens of aspartic proteases have an NH_2-terminal propeptide of up to 50 amino acids long, that is cleaved at activation. This group of proteases is directly dependent on aspartic acid residues for catalytic activity. The catalytic aspartic residues are located centrally in the substrate-binding cleft of the mature enzymes. The substrate specificity of the aspartic proteases spans from the exclusive cleavage by renin of the Leu10–Val11 bond of angiotensinogen to a broad peptide bond specificity for most other enzymes in this catalytic group.

III. Control of Proteolytic Enzymes

Proteolytic activity in tissues is controlled at multiple levels. Three principal regulatory mechanisms have been devised by nature to control protease activity: (1) regulation of their gene expression; (2) activation of their inactive precursors (zymogens) by limited proteolysis; and (3) inactivation by complexing with inhibitors. The relative importance of these various mechanisms differs for different proteases. In addition to the principal regulatory mechanisms, several factors may modify protease activity, including phosphorylation and glycosylation, storage in vesicles, localization on membranes, pH, and the concentrations of calcium ions and ATP.

The first level of protease control is through regulation of gene expression. The expression of various protease genes is regulated throughout prenatal and postnatal development, aging, and wound healing. Similar to the synthesis of most proteins, the synthesis of proteases is controlled by regulatory elements in the gene. The absence of a TATA box in some protease genes suggests that they are "housekeeping" genes. Most proteases have a variety of regulatory elements. Thus, some proteases are constitutively synthesized by cells, whereas others are synthesized only after stimulation. Certain proteases have multiple transcription initiation sites and are constitutively synthesized by one mechanism, and synthesized on stimulation by another mechanism. For example, cathepsin D, an aspartic protease, is constitutively synthesized from one mRNA transcript and induced by estrogen stimulation from a longer mRNA transcript (36). Cytokines, polypeptide hormones, steroid hormones, and other growth regulators influence the synthesis of proteases through signal transduction pathways or by direct binding to nuclear receptors. The effect of these modulatory factors is frequently cell-specific and differs between the various proteases. In addition, cytokines may act synergistically or in opposition to each other in inducing protease gene expression.

One of the most important controls of proteolytic activity is the synthesis and storage of proteases as inactive zymogens (16). Most of these enzymes are stored and transported in a zymogen form and activated when their enzymatic activity is needed, usually on secretion from a cell. Activation of zymogens involves the cleavage of one or more peptide bonds that are usually in the NH_2-terminal portion of the proenzymes. Zymogen activation is of particular interest and importance when it occurs in a series of consecutive reactions or cascades as, for example, in blood coagulation, fibrinolysis, and complement activation. The physiological importance of zymogen activation has been demonstrated in several disease states that are related to deficiencies of functional zymogens. As examples, several types of familial hemophilias are due to deficiencies of plasma proteases that normally activate zymogens in the blood coagulation cascade.

Zymogen activation is a carefully regulated process. The basic principles of the chemical changes in covalent structure that are responsible for zymogen activation have been known for decades. However, the structural changes that accompany the zymogen–enzyme conversion were delineated only recently. In general, it has become apparent that zymogens lack the structural attributes required for formation of the enzyme–substrate complexes. These attributes are acquired by removal of the activation peptide. Often, several mechanisms are used to regulate zymogen activation.

Exceptions to this general scheme of zymogen activation at secretion are the granule-associated serine proteases of immune and inflammatory cells. These enzymes, including monocyte–neutrophil elastase (HLE), Cat G, and PR-3 of PMNL, the lymphocyte granzymes, and mast cell tryptase and chymase, are of critical importance in various pulmonary disorders. These granule-associated enzymes are stored in fully active forms, rather than as zymogens. Nevertheless, based on their known cDNA sequences, they are initially translated as zymogens. The granule-associated protease zymogens are processed at unusual amino acid residues, compared with other protease zymogens. Pancreatic digestive enzymes, and members of the blood-clotting cascade and the complement pathway, all include proteases that are initially produced as zymogens and that require removal of NH_2-terminal segments to be activated. These traditional zymogens are activated by clipping the propeptide at a basic residue (typically an arginine) or, occasionally, at an aromatic residue. In the granule-associated proteases of immune and inflammatory cells, activation typically occurs by clipping the peptide at an acidic residue (37). The cysteine protease dipeptidyl peptidase-I appears to catalyze the removal of the activation dipeptide from many of the granule-associated proteases (38).

Another principal regulatory mechanism that controls proteolytic activity is inactivation of proteases by complex formation with inhibitors. Protease inhibitors are present within cells, in the extracellular matrix, and in blood and secreted fluids. These proteins prevent access of substrates to the catalytic sites of proteases by steric hindrance, either by binding directly to the catalytic site, in a substrate- or product-like manner, or by binding to surface sites adjacent to the catalytic residues of the cognate proteases. The importance of inhibitors as a regulatory mechanism to control proteolytic activity is demonstrated by familial deficiency of α_1-protease inhibitor, a genetic disorder that is associated with the development of emphysema, resulting from abnormally low plasma and tissue concentrations of the inhibitor, and by antithrombin III deficiency, an inherited cause of venous thromboembolism, of which the homozygous state is lethal to the fetus.

The action of most inhibitors is restricted to a specific catalytic class. Exceptions are α_2-macroglobulin inhibitors that can inhibit proteases of all catalytic classes, according to a ''molecular trap'' mechanism, by virtue of a promiscuous ''bait region,'' and recently described members of the ovalbumin family of serine protease inhibitors that also inhibit cysteine proteases (39).

Inhibitors of each proteolytic class will now be considered, focusing primarily on those that are present in humans.

A. Serine Protease Inhibitors

Most protease inhibitors characterized in humans are directed toward serine proteases. Serpins (the acronym denotes *ser*ine *p*rotease *in*hibitors) are the most prevalent serine protease inhibitors in humans (40). They constitute a superfamily of single-chain proteins that typically range between 40 and 60 kDa in molecular mass and include α_1-protease inhibitor, α_1-antichymotrypsin, antithrombin III, heparin cofactor II, C1-inhibitor, α_2-antiplasmin, plasminogen activator inhibitor I and II, protein C inhibitor, protease nexin-I, and human monocyte–neutrophil elastase inhibitor (HEI). Serpins contain a conserved domain of 350- to 370-amino–acid residues, usually flanked by unique NH_2- and COOH-terminal extensions for individual inhibitors, as well as variable degrees of glycosylation (41). Most inhibitory serpins are found in an active form under physiological conditions. Inhibitory serpins interact at a 1 : 1 stoichiometry with their target protease at a reactive site located within a loop structure 30- to 40-amino–acid residues from the COOH-terminus. This area is exposed on the surface of the protein. The inhibitor reacts with cognate proteases by a substrate-like mechanism, forming stable complexes. For many serpin–protease complexes, the inhibitory molecules are cleaved, resulting in a major conformational change and a more stable complex. Cleavage of the serpin occurs at the "reactive center" between two amino acids designated P_1 and $P_{1'}$. The P_1 residue largely dictates the fidelity of the interaction of the inhibitor and the protease, although amino acid residues immediately surrounding the cleavage site also contribute to the affinity and specificity of the interaction (40).

A second class of serine protease inhibitors is the low molecular weight mucous protease inhibitors. The major inhibitor of this group, secretory leukocyte protease inhibitor (SLPI), also called mucous protease inhibitor (MPI), antileukoprotease (ALP), or bronchial inhibitor (BrI) is found in a variety of mucous secretions and cartilage (42,43). It is a two-domain structure, containing 107-amino–acid residues, that is acid-stable and cysteine-rich. Its inhibitory site is in the COOH-terminal domain. SLPI inhibits HLE, Cat G, trypsin, chymotrypsin, and chymase (44), and is the main serine protease inhibitor in upper respiratory tract secretions. Recently, a second inhibitor of this group has been described, elafin or elastase-specific inhibitor (ESI; 45,46). Elafin is smaller than SLPI (6 kDa compared with 12 kDa), with homology to SLPI at the inhibitory site. Elafin inhibits pancreatic elastase, HLE, and PR-3, but not trypsin, plasmin, chymotrypsin, or Cat G. To date, it has been found in bronchial secretions and the skin of psoriasis patients.

A third class of serine protease inhibitors is the Kunitz-type inhibitors, found in tissues and body fluids (16,47). Members of this group include the basic pancreatic trypsin inhibitor bikunin, inter–α-trypsin inhibitor, pre–α-trypsin inhibitor, lipoprotein-associated coagulation inhibitor, the α_3-chain of type VI collagen, and one form of the amyloid β-precursor protein that has been observed to be increased in amyloid deposits within the brain of Alzheimer patients. All of these inhibitors contain either bikunin, the inhibitor subunit, or a homologous inhibitory subunit. The physiological target of either bikunin or inter–α-trypsin is unknown. These molecules inhibit trypsin, chymotrypsin, HLE, Cat G, and plasmin (48). Given their K_i values and the ability of the proteases to transfer from bikunin or inter–α-trypsin inhibitor to other inhibitors, such as α_1-protease inhibitor, these inhibitors may serve as "shuttle" inhibitors (49).

B. Matrix Metalloprotease Inhibitors

The tissue inhibitors of metalloproteases (TIMPs) are the major local inhibitors of the matrixins. Three forms have been identified (50). All active forms of matrixins are inhibited by TIMP-1, a 28.5-kDa glycoprotein that is synthesized by connective tissue cells and macrophages, and by TIMP-2, a 23-kDa nonglycosylated protein that is found in lower concentrations than TIMP-1 in most tissues. TIMP-3, a 21-kDa protein, is less well characterized, but is unique in its avid binding to extracellular matrix. The human mRNA for TIMP-3 is widely expressed in connective tissue. The individual TIMPs show considerable structural similarity owing to the conservation of cysteine residues that form disulfide bonds. All TIMPs form high-affinity, noncovalent, and essentially irreversible complexes with the active forms of the matrixins, with a 1:1 stoichiometry. TIMP inhibition of the matrixins largely occurs as a result of binding the catalytic (NH_2-terminal) domains of the enzymes to the NH_2-terminal domain of the two domain TIMPs. However, the mechanism of TIMP action is complex, involving numerous points of interaction with the active enzymes. For example, the TIMP COOH-terminal domain has several enzyme-binding sites that differ according to the particular matrixin, and act to increase the rate of inhibition. The mechanism of this rate enhancement is by an increase of the probability of interaction of the two NH_2-terminal domains.

C. Cysteine Protease Inhibitors

The major cysteine protease inhibitors include the cystatins that inhibit cathepsins B, H, L, O, and S, and the calpastatins that inhibit the calpains. Four types or families of cystatins have been recognized: the stefins, cystatins, kininogens, and cathelins (51). The stefins, which include human stefin A and B, are single-chain nonglycosylated molecules of about 11 kDa that are widely distributed in tissues and extracellular fluids. They are reversible competitive inhibitors of cathepsins B, H, and L. The cystatins are slightly larger, with molecular masses close to 13 kDa. Included in this family are human cystatins C, D, S, SN, and SA. The kininogens are multipurpose molecules that are precursors of the vasoactive kinins and act as high molecular cofactors for the intrinsic coagulation system and cysteine protease inhibitors. The last family, cathelins, inhibits cathepsin L, but not other cysteine proteases.

Two specific inhibitors of calpains, calpastatin I and II, are produced in many cells (16,52). Similar to the proteolytic activity of calpains, their inhibition is calcium-dependent. Calpastatins inhibit the autolytic activation of calpains as well as the proteolytic activity.

D. Aspartic Protease Inhibitors

No specific naturally occurring human aspartic inhibitors have been identified. However, the propeptide of the aspartic protease cathepsin D inhibits aspartic proteases (53). Whether this is a physiological mechanism of inhibition is unknown. The aspartic proteases also are susceptible to inhibition by pepstatins that are pentapeptides produced by various species of *Actinomyces* (35). The development of synthetic aspartic protease inhibitors is being pursued, in view of the importance of renin in the pathobiology of systemic hypertension and the demonstration that human immunodeficiency virus type 1 (HIV-1) uses an aspartic protease to cleave functional core proteins from larger proteins (54). The first drugs that were designed to treat AIDS by blocking aspartic proteases were recently marketed.

E. α_2-Macroglobulin

α_2-Macroglobulin reacts with proteases of all four catalytic classes and is the only known mammalian inhibitor of aspartic proteases (55). It is composed of four identical subunits with a total molecular mass of 718 kDa. Proteases initially cleave α_2-macroglobulin in a 25-amino–acid residue-exposed loop, called the *bait region*, that is present on each subunit. This cleavage alters the conformation of the macroglobulin subunits to trap the protease. Each trapped molecule binds through multiple cross-links to one or more of the macroglobulin subunits. Most bound proteases retain activity toward small substrates, but not toward large substrates. This provides a mechanism to convert proteases from endopeptidases to oligopeptidases. Protease-activated α_2-macroglobulin can bind other molecules in addition to proteases, including growth factors and cytokines. The physiological importance of this is largely unknown.

IV. Functions of Proteolytic Enzymes

The growing realization of the physiological importance of proteases, together with technological advances in approaches to their detection and characterization, has generated renewed intensity in the study of these enzymes. Proteases serve a variety of functions at the cellular, tissue, and systemic levels. Proteolytic processes occur in each of the functionally distinct intracellular compartments of the cell. The lysosomal system is a particularly rich source of intracellular proteases. It likely evolved from the digestive system of a unicellular organism that secreted proteolytic enzymes into its surrounding medium (56). Lysosomes have several acid peptidases that carry out the comprehensive degradation of proteins. In the endoplasmic reticulum, Golgi apparatus, and secretory vesicles, proteins are processed by proteases to remove the signal and sometimes propeptides. Mitochondrial proteases also process newly synthesized proteins that they import from the cytoplasm. The proteolytic enzymes of the soluble phase of the cytoplasm include the large multimolecular complexes of the ATP- and ubiquitin-dependent system, and the multicatalytic endopeptidase complex. Under normal conditions, specific intracellular proteases process hormones and cytokines. Substantial progress has been made recently in identifying and characterizing the proteases responsible for prohormone and cytokine processing. The proteolytic enzymes that are present in the extracellular environment on the external face of the plasma membrane, adherent to extracellular matrix, or in body fluids, vary greatly between different environments. Although generally perceived as regulators of clotting and fibrinolytic cascades, or as mediators of extracellular matrix remodeling, these extracellular proteases are emerging as important modulators of all the aspects of competent physiological responses (reviewed in 57). Through the signaling properties of highly regulated membrane receptors, proteases influence general physiological reactions, such as chemotaxis and intercellular adhesion, and specialized mechanisms, such as cytotoxicity and apoptosis. As examples, the participation of serine proteases in the mechanism of target cell lysis has been postulated for more that two decades (58–60). The earlier reports suggested that protease activity was required for cellular cytoxicity. A more direct participation of proteases in the lytic process was postulated by the identification of granzymes, a family of serine protases that are stored in secretory granules of cytolytic T lymphocytes and NK cells. Recent observations suggest that granzymes participate in cellular cytotoxicity by activating an endogenous pathway of programmed apoptosis in target cells (61–64). Surprisingly, granzymes have also been implicated in lymphocyte proliferation (65). As one example, granzyme A induces antigen-dependent B-cell proliferation (66). Potent mitogenic effects have been observed with several other serine proteases, including mast cell tryptases (66), thrombin (67), and urokinase-type plasminogen activator (68).

Morphogenesis of the lung and postnatal lung growth occur within the architectural framework of the extracellular matrix. Although lung development and postnatal lung growth involve remodeling of the extracellular matrix, little information is available about matrix turnover during this period or the role of specific proteases. In the rat, rapid collagen synthesis and degradation, particularly of type IV collagen, was observed in the earliest phases of postnatal lung growth (69). The source and type of enzymes responsible for the degradation have not been determined. Also of note, the major inhibitor of matrixins in baboons, TIMP-1, undergoes a marked increase in abundance shortly after birth (70). This response to parturition is specific to the lung. When taken collectively, these data suggest that the expression of proteases and their inhibitors is highly regulated during lung development, and that these molecules play an important role in the process.

Of particular relevance to pulmonary function in the newborn is the recently developed information that a neutral serine protease is required for extracellular metabolism of pulmonary surfactant (71). It appears that this enzyme, termed surfactant convertase, is required for the conversion of tubular myelin to the small vesicular form of surfactant. Characterization of the biochemical nature of the convertase has been explored by Gross and colleagues, who initially identified the protease (72). Studies to date suggest that the protease has a molecular mass of approximately 75 kDa, that it is inhibited by a wide range of serpins, including α_1-protease inhibitor, and that it is likely synthesized by alveolar type II cells. Experiments suggest that the physiological action of the convertase in converting tubular myelin to small vesicles is not at the level of making tubular myelin into a surface-active monomolecular film, but rather, at a stage that is distal to the formation of the monomolecular film, perhaps by facilitating the reorientation of phospholipid from the surface into small vesicles. Although the study of surfactant convertase is at a preliminary stage, the potential importance of the enzyme to neonatal lung disease is substantial.

V. Proteases and Pulmonary Diseases

Proteases have been implicated in several specific pulmonary disorders. The best-studied pulmonary pathological condition in which a relative protease excess has been assigned a central pathobiochemical role is emphysema. The protease most implicated in this disorder is HLE. Studies 30 years ago showed that an inherited deficiency of α_1-protease inhibitor predisposes individuals to early-onset emphysema (73). It was subsequently demonstrated that intratracheal insufflation of HLE caused an emphysema-like condition in experimental animals. As a result of this information, a central role for HLE was suggested for all forms of pulmonary emphysema (74,75); however, the evidence that HLE plays a pivitol role in emphysema remains circumstantial. Studies showing increased tissue levels of HLE related to tissue pathology are controversial (76), as are studies of HLE concentrations and activity in bronchoalveolar lavage (BAL) fluids from normal subjects, and in cigarette smokers with and without emphysema. Moreover, other PMNL enzymes (e.g., PR-3 and Cat G) were recently implicated, as were proteases from macrophages, including the matrixins and thiol proteases (33,77,78). From currently available information, it is likely that there are several different proteases and different pathological processes involved in the development of pulmonary emphysema.

Particularly relevant to pediatrics is the potential role of proteases in the pathobiochemistry of cystic fibrosis (CF). Proteolytic destruction of lung tissue is thought to be central to the progression of the airways disease in CF. The major focus has been on serine proteases, particularly HLE. The sputum of CF subjects have markedly elevated elastolytic activity and increased urinary excretion of desmosine, a biochemical marker of elastin destruction (79). Moreover, elastic fibers in the airways of CF subjects are irregular and abruptly terminated, as opposed to the usual delicate morphology in normal subjects. The major source of elastolytic activity in bronchial secretions of patients with CF is HLE (80,81). Proteases likely contribute to the pathogenesis of CF lung disease, not only by causing destruction of the normal lung architecture, but also in at least two other ways. First, proteases likely contribute to the mucous hypersecretion that is a prominent pathological feature of CF. HLE and Cat G are the most potent known stimuli of mucous secretion from airway submucosal glands, both from the standpoint of threshold concentration and the magnitude of response (82). Second, these same enzymes cleave immunoglobulins in vitro and in CF secretions (83).

The immune fragments resulting from proteolytic cleavage fail to support phagocytosis and may actually inhibit the process. The PMNLs present in bronchial secretions of patients with CF had decreased expression of CR1, the receptor for the complement component C3b (84). The decreased expression was attributed to the proteolytic action of HLE. Thus, both immunoglobulin- and complement-mediated phagocytosis is impaired in CF airways. This could contribute to the inability of CF subjects to eradicate chronic lung infections. Recent studies suggest that metalloproteases also may participate in the proteolytic processes in CF. High levels of active collagenase and gelatinase have been detected in the sputum from CF subjects. Most of the matrixins present were of PMNL origin (85,86). Lung damage, as assessed by increased type IV collagen degradation products in sputum, was correlated with concentrations of active gelatinase (86), supporting a significant role for this enzyme in the airway damage that occurs in CF.

A third pulmonary disease in which proteases may have important pathogenic roles is asthma. Because of the strong circumstantial evidence implicating inflammation in the pathogenesis of asthma, investigators have sought to find mediators derived from inflammatory cells that might account for the increased responsiveness of airway smooth muscle, the abnormal mucous secretion, and the increased vascular permeability that are characteristic of the disease. There is considerable evidence that the granule-associated serine proteases play a significant role in these processes. The proteases that reside in mast cells, eosinophils, PMNL, T lymphocytes, and subsets of monocytes, all have been implicated in the various phases of the inflammatory responses in asthma. As one example, chymases and tryptase, which account for up to 25% of the total protein within mast cells (87), likely play a central role in asthma. Biological effects of mast cell chymases that are relevant to asthma include (1) their marked potentiation of histamine-induced vascular permeability in ragweed-allergic dogs (88); (2) their capacity to degrade extracellular matrix molecules, including collagen and proteoglycans (89–91); (3) their potent secretagogue activity for airway submucosal gland cells (12); (4) their ability to cleave surface glycoconjugates from the glycocalyx of airway epithelial cells (92); (5) their ability to cleave vasoactive intestinal peptide (VIP) (13), a principal relaxant of human airway smooth muscle; and (6) their capacity to activate the vasodilating peptides bradykinin and kallidin (93). Tryptase, in addition to sharing many of these same actions, also potentiates airway smooth-muscle contraction in response to agonists, such as histamine (94), suggesting an important role in the hyperresponsiveness of airways in asthma. As a second example, serine proteases in PMNL granules are important constituents of the inflammatory response in asthma, particularly during acute exacerbations (95). HLE and Cat G are potent stimulants for secretion of proteoglycans from airway gland serous cells (82). In addition, HLE activates IL-8 gene transcription, synthesis, and secretion by bronchial epithelial cells (96). Because IL-8 has potent chemoattractive and activating properties for PMNL and

T lymphocytes, this provides a self-perpetuating mechanism for the inflammatory process in asthma. Finally, the chymase residing in the granules of eosinophils, in addition to sharing properties with mast cell chymases, stimulates release of histamine and peroxidase from eosinophils (97).

Proteases have also been implicated in pulmonary disorders that are characterized by parenchymal fibrosis. The most noteworthy of these disorders is the adult respiratory distress syndrome (ARDS). This syndrome is associated with a prominent influx of PMNL; also, elevated HLE in bronchoalveolar lavage fluid from patients with ARDS has been shown (98,99). PMNL-derived collagenase has also been detected in lavage aspirates from patients with ARDS (100,101). It is possible that the fibrotic process that is characteristic of the late stages of ARDS occurs in response to lung injury, mediated, in part, by inflammatory cell proteases. Bronchoalveolar lavage aspirates from individuals with pulmonary fibrosis of varying etiologies contain high concentrations of collagenase that is thought to be of PMNL origin (102,103). The biological relevance of proteases in fibrotic lung disorders remains to be determined. Because these disorders are characterized by disruption of extracellular matrix, in particular collagen and elastin, a likely scenario is an initial proteolytic attack, followed by disorderly repair, resulting in fibrosis. Tryptase is also increased in the bronchoalveolar lavage aspirates of subjects with pulmonary fibrosis (100). Tryptase is a potent stimulus for fibroblast proliferation (104) and enhances the mitogenic potential of other growth factors. Thus, proteases may be involved in both matrix destruction and the ensuing exuberant repair observed in lung fibrotic disorders.

VI. Proteases and Chronic Lung Diseases of Early Infancy

Premature infants with acute neonatal lung injury, usually RDS, may develop chronic pulmonary disease, the most common form being bronchopulmonary dysplasia (BPD). The pathogenesis of BPD is uncertain. Several reports, however, emphasize the importance of inflammatory events. Many of these studies have focused on the role of proteases, in particular HLE, in the development of BPD. Several studies have detected elevated HLE activity in tracheal aspirates from intubated neonates with BPD (105–109). In some studies, an imbalance has been reported between elastase and the elastase inhibitors, α_1-protease inhibitor and SLPI, both in patients with RDS who progressed to BPD (105,106,110) and in patients with established BPD (108). The results of these studies suggest that neither of these two antiproteases increases sufficiently to compensate for the increased inflammatory burden. However, other studies have demonstrated increased elastase concentrations in tracheal aspirates of only a few patients with BPD (111). The explanation for this disparity is unknown, but may relate to the difference in the assays used to detect HLE or elastase inhibitory activity, or to the site of origin of the secretions (tracheal secretions are from airways, not distal lung). As with all studies of this type, analysis of tracheal aspirate does not necessarily indicate localized areas of proteolytic imbalance. Therefore, increased elastase load without free elastase in the aspirate, especially in association with low SLPI levels, could represent local imbalance sufficient to cause proteolytic injury.

The protease imbalance hypothesis in BPD has recently been extended to include mast cell-derived proteases. Lyle and colleagues have demonstrated significantly increased tryptase-containing mast cells in bronchial and peribronchiolar regions of the lungs from patients with long-standing BPD, when compared with controls (112). The precise role of the mast cell and its tryptase is unclear, but tryptase is a potent mitogen for fibroblasts and enhances the mitogenic potential of other growth factors (104).

Thus, as in other fibrotic disorders, serine proteases may play a role not only in the tissue destruction associated with BPD, but also in the ensuing fibroproliferative response. This raises the possibility that therapy with exogenous protease inhibitors might prevent the development of BPD. The potential for this approach was demonstrated in rat pups subjected to hyperoxia (113). Administration of α_1-protease inhibitor prevented the right ventricular hypertrophy, increased pulmonary arterial muscularity, and decreased lung compliance that developed in control animals exposed to hyperoxia. Recently, a randomized, placebo-controlled, prospective study of treatment with α_1-protease inhibitor was conducted in 106 infants with RDS (114). The incidence of BPD was less in the treated infants, but the difference did not reach statistical significance. However, the incidence of pulmonary hemorrhage was significantly less in the treated group. Further work is needed to determine if these findings were due to the effect of the medication or chance events.

VII. What Lies Ahead?

The ultimate fate of most proteins is degradation by proteases. Although initially perceived as extracellular regulators of digestive, clotting, fibrinolytic, and complement cascades, and as mediators of matrix remodeling, it is now clear that proteases play crucial roles in the life processes of all mammalian cells. Through the signaling properties of highly regulated membrane receptors, proteases influence a wide range of activities, including cellular movement, adhesion, and programmed cell death. A challenge for future investigations will be to dissect the structure–function requirements of protease–cellular interactions. This will involve further characterization of recently described proteases, identification and characterization of new proteases and their inhibitors, delineation of the receptors used by specific proteases to activate cells, and elucidation of the intracellular-signaling pathways regulating this novel aspect of the cellular response. The result will be an improved understanding of the evolution of proteolytic enzymes and their partners. As one example of the types of advances to expect, the concept of a gene family of protease-activated receptors was recently underscored by isolation and cloning of the genes for the thrombin receptor and the highly homologous PAR-2 (115).

Evidence is rapidly accumulating that growth and differentiation involves the coordinated actions of proteolytic enzymes. The recent discovery of novel precursor-processing endoproteases has greatly accelerated progress in understanding the complex mechanisms underlying the maturation of growth factors, cytokines, prohormones, neuropeptides, and many other precursor-derived proteins. The continued elucidation of the proteolytic components required for protein processing will provide new insights into the molecular mechanisms of human development and disease.

The future will witness the continued development of novel therapeutic strategies that employ specific protease inhibitors that will be applicable to a wide variety of disciplines, extending from developmental biology, to oncology, to aging. It is highly likely that in the near future we will understand the crystal structure of many proteases of all catalytic classes and their complexes with protease inhibitors. When this occurs, it will be possible to design smaller inhibitors that are just as effective as their natural counterparts to regulate a wide variety of proteases. Knowledge about protease inhibitors has helped us understand the pathogenesis of many experimental models of lung disease and will be even more useful in the future. To date, the use of protease inhibitors in human therapy has been restricted to mainly aprotinin and angiotensin-converting enzyme (ACE) inhibitors. However, the success of ACE inhibitors as pharmacological tools in hypertension has been a strong stimulant for new approaches to therapy with protease inhibitors. The development of HIV-1 protease inhibitors presents an exceptional opportunity to pursue effective agents in the treatment of AIDS. The self-assembly of two identical monomers into a symmetrical structure in HIV-1 protease is not only an elegant way to create an active enzyme, while encoding a minimal amount of genetic information, but is also in concordance with the bilobular active-site found in mammalian aspartic proteases.

New technologies will greatly facilitate elucidation of the biological and pathobiological roles of proteases and their inhibitors. Two more recently developed technologies, gene targeting and gene transfer, will allow more definitive characterization of the in vivo role of gene products. The consequences of gain or loss of function of proteolytic systems on reproduction, development, health, survival, and on hemostasis, thrombosis, neointima formation, tissue remodeling, brain function, malignancy, and neovascularization can be determined by these technologies. In addition, the possible use of transgenic mice to study gene regulation or to generate monoclonal antibodies against conserved epitopes in the targeted proteins is now possible.

In conclusion, it is not possible to determine the limits of the biological systems in which proteases may be involved, but it is clear that a multitude of additional roles will be identified. The challenge will be to control the pathological effects of proteolytic enzymes without disrupting their vital physiological functions.

References

1. Barrett AJ. Classification of peptidases. In: Barrett AJ, ed. Methods in Enzymology, Proteolytic Enzymes: Serine and Cysteine Peptides. San Diego: Academic Press, 1994.
2. Dalbey RE, von Heinje G. Signal peptidases in prokaryotes and eukaryotes—a new protease family? Trends Biol Sci 1992; 17:474.
3. Rechsteiner M, Hoffman L, Dubiel W. The multicatalytic and 26S proteases. J Biol Chem 1993; 268:6065.
4. Rawlings ND, Barrett AJ. Evolutionary families of peptides. Biochem J 1993; 290: 205.
5. Rawlings ND, Barrett AJ. Families of serine peptidases. In: Barrett AJ, ed. Methods in Enzymology, Proteolytic Enzymes: Serine and Cystein Peptidases. San Diego: Academic Press, 1994.
6. Henson PM, Johnston JRB. Tissue injury in inflammation: oxidants, proteinases and cationic proteins. J Clin Invest 1987; 79:669–674.
7. Janoff A. Elastase in tissue injury. Annu Rev Med 1985; 36:207–216.
8. Gabay JE. Antimicrobial proteins with homology to serine proteases. Ciba Found Symp 1994; 186:237–247.
9. Masson D, Tschopp J. A family of serine esterases in lytic granules of cytolytic T lymphocytes. Cell 1987; 49:679–685.
10. Bleackley RC, Lobe CG, Duggan B, Ehrman N, Fregeau C, Mier M, Letellier M, Havele C, Shaw J, Paetkau V. The isolation and characterization of a family of serine protease genes in activated cytotoxic T lymphocytes. Immunol Rev 1988; 103:5–19.
11. Brian SD, Williams TJ. Substance P regulates the vasodilator activity of calcitonin gene-related peptide. Nature 1988; 335:73–75.
12. Sommerhoff CP, Caughey GH, Finkbeiner WE, Lazarus SC, Basbaum CB, Nadel JA. Mast cell chymase: a potent secretagogue for airway gland serous cells. J Immunol 1989; 142:2450–2456.
13. Caughey GH, Leidig F, Vino NF, Nadel JA. Substance P and vasoactive intestinal peptide degradation by mast cell tryptase and chymase. J Pharmacol Exp Ther 1988; 244:133–137.
14. Steiner DF, Smeekens SP, Ohagi S, Chan SJ. The new enzymology of precursor processing endoproteases. J Biol Chem 1992; 267:23435–23438.
15. Seidah NG, Chretien M, Day R. The family of subtilisin/kexin like pro-protein and pro-hormone convertases: divergent or shared functions. Biochimie 1994; 76:197–209.

16. Twining SS. Regulation of proteolytic activity in tissues. Crit Rev Biochem Mol Biol 1994; 29:315–383.
17. Woessner JFJ. The family of matrix metalloproteinases. Ann NY Acad Sci 1994; 732:11–21.
18. Hibbs MS, Bainton DF. Human neutrophil gelatinase is a component of specific granules. J Clin Invest 1989; 84:1395.
19. Kjeldsen L, Bainton DF, Sengelov H, Borregaard N. Structural and functional heterogeneity among peroxidase-negative granules in human neutrophils: identification of a distinct gelatinase-containing granule subset by combined immunocytochemistry and subcellular fractionation. Blood 1993; 82:3183–3191.
20. Goldberg GI, Wilhelm SM, Kronberger A, Bauer EA, Grant GA, Eisen AZ. Human fibroblast collagenase. Complete primary structure and homology to an oncogene transformation-induced rat protein. J Biol Chem 1986; 261:6600–6605.
21. Hasty KA, Pourmotabbed TF, Goldberg GI, Thompson JP, Spinella DG, Stevens RM, Mainardi CL. Human neutrophil collagenase. A distinct gene product with homology to other matrix metalloproteinases. J Biol Chem 1990; 265:11421–11424.
22. Freije JMP, Diez-Itza I, Balbin M, Sanchez LM, Blasco R, Tolivia J, Lopez-Otin C. Molecular cloning and expression of collagenase-3, a novel human matrix metalloproteinase produced by breast carcinomas. J Biol Chem 1994; 269:16766–16773.
23. Collier IE, Wilhelm SM, Eisen AZ, Marmer BL, Grant GA, Seltzer JL, Kronberger A, He CS, Bauer EA, Goldberg GI. H-*ras* oncogene-transformed human bronchial epithelial cells (TBE-1) secrete a single metalloprotease capable of degrading basement membrane collagen. J Biol Chem 1988; 267:6579–6587.
24. Wilhelm SM, Collier IE, Marmer BL, Eisen AZ, Grant GA, Goldberg GI. SV40-transformed human lung fibroblasts secrete a 92-kDa type IV collagenase which is identical to that secreted by normal human macrophages. J Biol Chem 1989; 264:17213–17221.
25. Whitham SE, Murphy G, Angel P, Rahmsdorf HJ, Smith BJ, Lyons A, Harris TJ, Reynolds JJ, Herrlich P, Docherty AJ. Comparison of human stromelysin and collagenase by cloning and sequence analysis. Biochem J 1986; 240:913–916.
26. Muller D, Quantin B, Gesnel MC, Millon-Collard R, Abecassis J, Breathnach R. The collagenase gene family in humans consists of at least four members. Biochem J 1988; 253:187–192.
27. Basset P, Bellocq JP, Wolf C, Stoll I, Hutin P, Limacher JM, Podhajcer OL, Chenard MP, Rio MC, Chambon P. A novel metalloproteinase gene specifically expressed in stromal cells of breast carcinomas. Nature 1990; 348:699–704.
28. Takino T, Sato H, Shinagawa A, Seiki M. Identification of the second membrane-type matrix metalloproteinase (MT-MMP-2) gene from a human placenta cDNA library. MT-MMPs form a unique membrane-type subclass in the MMP family. J Biol Chem 1995; 260:23103–23020.
29. Lovejoy B, Cleasby A, Hassell AM, Inogley K, Luther MA, Wigl D, McGeehan G, McElroy AB, Drewry D, Lambert MH, Jordan SR. Structure of the catalytic domain of fibroblast collagenase complexed with an inhibitor. Science 1994; 263:375.

30. Rawlings ND, Barrett AJ. Families of cysteine peptidases. In: Barrett AJ, ed. Methods in Enzymology. Proteolytic enzymes: Serine and Cysteine Peptidases. San Diego: Academic Press, 1994.
31. Shinagawa T, Do YS, Baxter JK, Carilli C, Schilling J, Hsueh WA. Identification of an enzyme in human kidney that correctly processes prorenin. Proc Natl Acad Sci USA 1990; 87:1927–1933.
32. Kobayashi H, Schmitt M, Goretzki L, Chucholowski N, Calvete J, Kramer M, Gunzaler WA, Janicke F, Graeff H. Cathepsin B efficiently activates the soluble and the tumor cell receptor-bound form of the proenzyme urokinase type plasminogen activator (pro-uPA). J Biol Chem 1991; 266:5147–5152.
33. Chapman HAJ, Munger JS, Shi G-P. The role of thiol proteases in tissue injury and remodeling. Am J Respir Crit Care Med 1994; 150:5155–5159.
34. Saido T, Sorimachi H, Suzuki K. Calpain: new perspectives in molecular diversity and physiological–pathological involvement. FASEB J 1994; 8:814.
35. Szecsi PB. The aspartic proteases. Scan J Clin Lab Invest 1992; 52:5–22.
36. Cavailles V, Augereau P, Rochefort H. Cathepsin D gene is controlled by a mixed promoter, and estrogens stimulate only TATA-dependent transcription in breast cancer cells. Proc Natl Acad Sci USA 1993; 90:203.
37. Dikov MM, Springman EB, Yeola S, Serafin WE. Processing of procarboxypeptidase A and other zymogens in murine mast cells. J Biol Chem 1994; 269:25897–25904.
38. McGuire MJ, Lipsky PE, Thiele DL. Generation of active myeloid and lymphoid granule serine proteases requires processing by the granule thiol protease dipeptidyl peptidase I. J Biol Chem 1993; 268:2458–2467.
39. Komiyama T, Ray CA, Pickup DJ, Howard AD, Thornberry NA, Peterson EP. Inhibition of interleukin-1 beta converting enzyme by the cowpox virus serpin CrmA. An example of cross-class inhibition. J Biol Chem 1994; 269:19331–19337.
40. Potempa J, Korzus E, Travis J. The serpin superfamily of proteinase inhibitors: structure, function, and regulation. J Biol Chem 1994; 269:15957–15960.
41. Huber R, Carrell RW. Implications of the three-dimensional structure of alpha 1-antitrypsin for structure and function of serpins. J Biochem 1989; 28:8951–8966.
42. Thompson RC, Ohlsson K. Isolation, properties, and complete amino acid sequences of human secretory leukocyte protease inhibitor, a potent inhibitor of leukocyte elastase. Proc Natl Acad Sci USA 1986; 83:6692–6696.
43. Fritz H. Human mucus proteinase inhibitor (human MPI). Biol Chem Hoppe Seyler 1988; 369:79–82.
44. Boudier C, Bieth JG. The proteinase: mucus proteinase inhibitor binding stoichiometery. J Biol Chem 1992; 267:4370–4375.
45. Wiedow O, Schroder JM, Gregory H, Young JA, Christophers E. Elafin, an elastase-specific inhibitor from human skin. J Biol Chem 1990; 265:14791–14795.
46. Sallenave JM, Marsden MD, Ryle AP. Isolation of elafin and elastase-specific inhibitor (ESI) from bronchial secretions: evidence of sequence homology and immunological cross-reactivity. Biol Chem Hoppe Seyler 1992; 373:27–33.
47. Salier JP. Inter-alpha-trypsin inhibitor: emergence of a family within the Kunitz-

type protease inhibitor superfamily [review]. Trends Biochem Sci 1990; 15:435–439.
48. Potempa J, Kwon K, Chawla R, Travis J. Inter-alpha-trypsin inhibitor. Inhibition spectrum of native and derived forms. J Biol Chem 1989; 264:109.
49. Pratt CW, Roche PA, Pizzo SV. The role of inter-alpha-trypsin inhibitor and other proteinase inhibitors in the plasma clearance of neutrophil elastase and plasmin. Arch Biochem Biophys 1987; 258:591.
50. Willenbrock F, Murphy G. Structure–function relationships in the tissue inhibitors of metalloproteinases. Am J Respir Crit Care Med 1994; 150:S165–S170.
51. Turk V, Bode W. The cystatins: protein inhibitors of cysteine proteinases. FEBS Lett 1991; 285:213–219.
52. Pontremoli S, Melloni E, Viotti PL, Michetti M, Salamino F, Horecker BL. Identification of two calpastatin forms in rat skeletal muscle and their susceptibility to digestion by homologous calpains. Arch Biochem Biophys 1991; 288:646–652.
53. Fusek M, Mares M, Vagner J, Voburka Z, Baudys M. Inhibition of aspartic proteinases by propart peptides of human procathepsin D and chicken pepsinogen. FEBS Lett 1991; 287:160–162.
54. Roberts NA, Martin JA, Kinchington D, Broadhurst AV, Craig JC, Duncan IB, Galpin SA, Handa BK, Kay J, Krohn A. Rational design of peptide-based HIV proteinase inhibitors. Science 1990; 248:358–361.
55. Borth W. alpha 2-Macroglobulin, a multifunctional binding protein with targeting characteristics. FASEB J 1992; 6:3345–3353.
56. Barrett AJ. Cellular proteolysis. An overview. Ann NY Acad Sci 1992; 674:1–15.
57. Altieri DC. Proteases and protease receptors in modulation of leukocyte effector functions. J Leukoc Biol 1995; 58:120–127.
58. Trinchieri G, DeMarchi M. Antibody-dependent cytotoxicity in humans. III. Effect of protease inhibitors and substrates. J Immunol 1972; 116:885–891.
59. Matter A. A study of proteolysis as a possible mechanism for T-cell mediated target cell lysis. Scand J Immunol 1975; 4:349–356.
60. Chang TW, Eisen HN. Effect of $N\alpha$-tosyl-L-lysl-chloromethylketone on the activity of cytoxic T lymphocytes. J Immunol 1980; 124:1028–1033.
61. Shi L, Kam CM, Powers JC, Aebersold R, Greenberg AH. Purification of three cytotoxic lymphocyte granule serine proteases that induce apoptosis through distinct substrate and target cell interactions. J Exp Med 1992; 176:1521–1529.
62. Shiver JW, Su L, Henkart PA. Cytotoxicity with target DNA breakdown by rat basophilic leukemia cells expressing both cytolsin and granzyme A. Cell 1992; 71: 315–322.
63. Heusel JW, Wesselschmidt RL, Shresta S, Russel JH, Ley TJ. Cytoxic lymphocytes require granzyme B for the rapid induction of DNA fragmentation and apoptosis in allogenic target cells. Cell 1994; 76:977–987.
64. Trapani JA, Smyth MJ, Apostolidis VA, Dawson M, Browne KA. Granule serine proteases are normal nuclear constituents of natural killer cells. J Biol Chem 1994; 269:18359–18365.
65. Simon MM, Hoschutzky H, Furth V, Simon HG, Kramer MD. Purification and characterization of a T-cell specific serine protease (TSP-1) from clone cytolytic T lymphocytes. EMBO J 1986; 5:3267–3274.

66. Ruoss SJ, Hartmann T, Caughey GH. Mast cell tryptase is a mitogen for cultured fibroblasts. J Clin Invest 1991; 88:493–499.
67. Chen LB, Teng NNH, Buchanan JM. Mitogenicity of thrombin and surface alterations on mouse splenocytes. Exp Cell Res 1976; 60:219–230.
68. Cohen SD, Israel E, Spiess-Meier B, Wainberg MA. Plasminogen activator is an apparent lymphocyte mitogen. J Immunol 1981; 126:1415–1420.
69. Arden MG, Adamson IY. Collagen degradation during postnatal lung growth in rats. Pediatr Pulmonol 1992; 14:95–101.
70. Minoo P, Penn R, deLemos DM, Coalson JJ, deLemos RA. Tissue inhibitor of metalloproteinase-1 mRNA is specifically induced in lung tissue after birth. Pediatr Res 1993; 34:729–734.
71. Gross NJ. Extracellular metabolism of pulmonary surfactant: the role of a new serine protease. Annu Rev Physiol 1995; 57:135–150.
72. Gross NJ, Schultz RM. Requirements for extracellular metabolism of pulmonary surfactant: tentative identification of serine protease. Am J Physiol 1992; 262: L446–L453.
73. Laurell CB, Eriksson S. The electrophoretic alpha-1-globulin pattern of serum in alpha-1-antitrypsin deficiency. Scand J Clin Lab Invest 1963; 15:132–140.
74. Janoff A, Sloan BGW, Damiano V, Sandhaus RA, Elias J, Kimbel P. Experimental emphysema induced with purified human neutrophil elastase: tissue localization of the instilled protease. Am Rev Respir Dis 1977; 115:461–478.
75. Senior RM, Tegner H, Kuhn C, Ohlsson K, Starcher BC, Pierce JA. The induction of pulmonary emphysema with human leukocyte elastase. Am Rev Respir Dis 1977; 116:469–475.
76. Damiano VV, Tsang A, Kucich U, Abrams WR, Rosenbloom J, Kimbel P, Fallahnejad M, Weinbaum G. Immunolocalization of elastase in human emphysematous lungs. J Clin Invest 1986; 78:482–493.
77. Kao RC, Wehner NG, Skubitz KM, Gray BH, Hoidal JR. Proteinase 3: a distinct human polymorphonuclear leukocyte proteinase which produces emphysema in hamsters. J Clin Invest 1988; 82:1963–1973.
78. Shaprio SD. Elastolytic metalloproteinases produced by human mononuclear phagocytes. Potential roles in destructive lung disease. Am J Respir Crit Care Med 1994; 150:S160–S164.
79. Bruce MC, Ponca L, Klinger JC, Stern RC, Tomashefski JFJ, Dearborn DG. Biochemical and pathological evidence for proteolytic destruction of lung connective tissue in cystic fibrosis. Am Rev Respir Dis 1985; 132:529–535.
80. Suter S, Schaad UB, Roux L, Nydegger UE, Waldvogel FA. Granulocyte neutral proteases and *Pseudomonas* elastase as possible causes of airway damage in patients with cystic fibrosis. J Infect Dis 1984; 149:523–531.
81. Goldstein W, Doring G. Lysosomal enzymes from polymorphonuclear leukocytes and proteinase inhibitors in patients with cystic fibrosis. Am Rev Respir Dis 1986; 134:49–56.
82. Sommerhoff CP, Nadel JA, Basbaum CB, Caughey GH. Neutrophil elastase and cathepsin G stimulate secretion from cultured bovine airway gland serous cells. J Clin Invest 1990; 85:682–689.
83. Fick RB, Naegel GP, Squier SV, Wood RE, Bernard J, Gee L, Reynolds HY. Pro-

teins of the cystic fibrosis respiratory tract. Fragmented immunoglobulin G opsonic antibody causing defective opsonophagocytosis. J Clin Invest 1984; 74:236–248.
84. Berger M, Sorensen RU, Tosi MR, Dearborn DG, Doring G. Complement receptor expression on neutrophils at an inflammatory site, the *Pseudomonas*-infected lung in cystic fibrosis. J Clin Invest 1989; 84:1302–1313.
85. Power C, O'Connor CM, MacFarlane D, O'Mahoney S, Gaffney K, Hayes J, Fitz-Gerald MX. Neutrophil collagenase in sputum from patients with cystic fibrosis. Am J Respir Crit Care Med 1994; 150:818–822.
86. Delacourt C, LeBourgeois M, D'Ortho MP, Doit C, Scheinmann P, Navarro J, Harf A, Hartmann DJ, Lafuma C. Imbalance between 95 kDa type IV collagenase and tissue inhibitor of metalloproteinases in sputum of patients with cystic fibrosis. Am J Respir Crit Care Med 1995; 152:765–774.
87. Schwartz LB, Lewis RA, Austen KF. Tryptase from human pulmonary mast cells. Purification and characterization. J Biol Chem 1981; 256:1939–1943.
88. Rubinstein I, Nadel JA, Graf PD, Caughey GH. Mast cell chymase potentiates histamine-induced wneal formation in the skin of ragweed-allergic dogs. J Clin Invest 1990; 86:555–559.
89. Sage H, Bornstein RG, Bornstein P. Structural studies of human type IV collagen. J Biol Chem 1967; 254:9893–9900.
90. Seppa H, Vaananen D, Korhonen K. Effect of mast cell chymase of rat skin on intracellular matrix: a histochemical study. Acta Histochem (Jenna) 1979; 64:64–70.
91. Briggaman RA, Schechter NM, Fraki J, Lazarus GS. Degradation of the epidermal–dermal junction by proteolytic enzymes from human skin and human polymorphonuclear leukocytes. J Exp Med 1984; 160:1027–1042.
92. Varsano S, Basbaum CB, Forsberg LS, Borson DB, Caughey GH, Nadel JA. Dog tracheal epithelial cells in culture synthesize sulfated macromolecular glycoconjugates and release them from the cell surface upon exposure to extracellular proteinases. Exp Lung Res 1987; 13:157–183.
93. Reilly DF, Schechter NB, Travis J. Inactivation of bradykinin and kallidin by cathepsin G and mast cell chymase. Biochem Biophys Res Commun 1985; 127:443–449.
94. Sekizawa K, Caughey GH, Lazarus SC, Gold WM, Nadel JA. Mast cell tryptase causes airway smooth muscle hyperresponsiveness in dogs. J Clin Invest 1989; 83: 175–179.
95. Fahy JV, Kim KW, Liu J, Boushey HA. Prominent neutrophilic inflammation in sputum from subjects with asthma exacerbation. J Allergy Clin Immunol 1995; 95: 843–852.
96. Nakamura H, Yoshimura K, McElvaney NG, Crystal RG. Neutrophil elastase in respiratory epithelial lining fluid of individuals with cystic fibrosis induces interleukin-8 gene expression in a human bronchial epithelial cell line. J Clin Invest 1992; 89:1478–1484.
97. Matsunaga Y, Kido H, Kawaji K, Kamoshita K, Katunuma N, Ogura T. Inhibitors of chymotrypsin-like proteases inhibit eosinophil peroxidase release from activated human eosinophils. Arch Biochem Biophys 1994; 312:67–74.
98. Lee CT, Fein AM, Lippmann M, Holtzman H, Kimbel P, Weinbaum G. Elastolytic

activity in pulmonary lavage fluid from patients with adult respiratory-distress syndrome. N Engl J Med 1981; 304:192–196.
99. Suter PM, Suter S, Girardin E, Roux-Lambard P, Grau GE, Dayer JM. High bronchoalveolar levels of tumor necrosis factor and its inhibitors, interleukin-1, interferon, and elastase, in patients with adult respiratory distress syndrome after trauma, shock, or sepsis. Am Rev Respir Dis 1992; 145:1016–1022.
100. Christner P, Fein A, Goldberg S, Lippmann M, Abrams W, Weinbaum G. Collagenase in the lower respiratory tract of patients with adult respiratory distress syndrome. Am Rev Respir Dis 1985; 131:690–695.
101. Weiland JE, Davis WB, Holter JF, Mohammed JR, Dorinsky PM, Gadek JE. Lung neutrophils in the adult respiratory distress syndrome. Clinical and pathophysiologic significance. Am Rev Respir Dis 1986; 133:218–225.
102. Gadek JE, Kelman JA, Fells G. Collagenase in the lower respiratory tract of patients with idiopathic pulmonary fibrosis. N Engl J Med 1979; 301:737–742.
103. Chanez P, Lacoste J, Guillot B, Giron J, Barneion G, Enhander I, Godard P, Michel FB, Bousqet J. Mast cells' contribution to the fibrosing alveolitis of the scleroderma lung. Am Rev Respir Dis 1993; 147:1497–1502.
104. Hartmann T, Ruoss SJ, Raymond WW, Seuwen K, Caughey GH. Human tryptase as a potent, cell-specific mitogen: role of signaling pathways in synergistic responses. Am J Physiol 1992; 6:L528–L534.
105. Merritt TA, Chochrane CG, Holcomb K. Elastase and α_1-proteinase inhibitor activity in tracheal aspirates during respiratory distress syndrome. J Clin Invest 1983; 72:656–666.
106. Ogden BE, Murphy SA, Saunders GC, Pathak D, Johnson JD. Neonatal lung neutrophils and elastase/proteinase inhibitor imbalance. Am Rev Respir Dis 1984; 130: 817–821.
107. Gerdes JS, Harris MC, Polin RA. Effects of dexamethasone and indomethacin on elastase, a_1-proteinase inhibitor and fibronectin in bronchoalveolar lavage fluid from neonates. J Pediatr 1988; 113:727–731.
108. Walti H, Tordet C, Gerbaut L, Saugier P, Moriette G, Relier JP. Persistent elastase/proteinase inhibitor imbalance during prolonged ventilation of infants with bronchopulmonary dysplasia: evidence for the role of nosocomial infections. Pediatr Res 1989; 26:351–355.
109. Gerdes JS, Whitsett J, Long W. Elastase activity and surfactant protein concentration in tracheal aspirates from neonates receiving synthetic surfactant. J Pediatr 1992; 120:S34–S39.
110. Watterberg KL, Carmichael DF, Gerdes JS, Werner S, Backstro C, Murphy S. Secretory leukocyte protease inhibitor and lung inflammation in developing bronchopulmonary dysplasia. J Pediatr 1994; 125:264–269.
111. Sluis KB, Darlow BA, Vissers MCM, Winterbourn CC. Proteinase–antiproteinase balance in tracheal aspirates from neonates. Eur Respir J 1994; 7:251–259.
112. Lyle RE, Tryka AF, Griffin WS, Taylor BJ. Tryptase immunoreactive mast cell hyperplasia in bronchopulmonary dysplasia. Pediatr Pulmonol 1995; 19:336–343.
113. Koppel R, Han RNH, Cox D, Tanswell AK. α_1-Antitrypsin protects neonatal rats from pulmonary vascular and parenchymal effects of oxygen toxicity. Pediatr Res 1995; 36:763–770.

114. Stiskal JA, Dunn MS, Shennan AT, O'Brien KKE, Kelly EN, Koppel RI, Cox DW, Ito S, Chappel SL, Rabinovitch M. α_1-Proteinase inhibitor therapy for the prevention of chronic lung disease of prematurity: a randomized, controlled trial. Pediatrics 1998; 101:89–94.
115. Schmidt VA, Vitale E, Bahou WF. Genomic cloning and characterization of the human thrombin receptor gene. J Biol Chem 1996; 271:9307–9312.

36

Site- and Mechanism-Targeted Interventions for Tissue Free Radical Injury

WILLIAM R. BERRINGTON, MARGARET M. TARPEY, and BRUCE A. FREEMAN

University of Alabama at Birmingham
Birmingham, Alabama

BRUCE R. PITT

University of Pittsburgh School of Medicine
Pittsburgh, Pennsylvania

I. Introduction

Since the discovery of the biological existence of reactive oxygen species (e.g., free radicals or oxidants) in 1969, there has been a proliferation of reports on the chemical nature, production, and reactions of these species, as well as the description of defense mechanisms and pharmacological approaches to preventing oxidant tissue injury. There is extensive evidence that reactive species contribute to pulmonary and vascular injury in the critical care setting, but little success has been enjoyed in the application of antioxidant interventions. We will make the point in the present chapter that only recently are key mechanisms for free radical-mediated tissue injury being described. This is mainly due to the limitations imposed by the high reactivity of free radical species in preventing their tissue measurement and the only recent establishment of incisive cause-and-effect relations between oxidant stress and tissue injury. This dilemma, in turn, has impeded the development of tissue site-directed and reaction mechanism-directed strategies for potent pharmacological interventions.

With new information in hand on the importance of free radical reactions in the interstitial matrix, the description of key intracellular sites of radical production and reaction, and the realization that the free radical signal transduction mediator nitric oxide (•NO) plays a central role in regulating tissue redox reactions, the pursuit of more efficacious antioxidant therapies for oxidant lung and vascular injury is moving forward by leaps and bounds. This is a timely advance, because it is now appreciated that redox reactions not only contribute to the regulation of intermediary metabolism, but also to gene expression of inflammatory mediators, such as chemokines and integrins. The following pages will review these recent advances, identify gaps in our present understanding of key issues, and present examples of both novel and potent site- and mechanism-directed strategies for limiting free radical injury to target molecules and tissues.

II. Oxidant-Protective Reactions of Nitric Oxide

A. The Dual Actions of Nitric Oxide in Tissue Free Radical Injury

Chemical reaction systems, cell and animal models, and clinical studies have recently revealed an ability of •NO to modulate reactions and pathological processes long associated with the excess production and biological effects of reactive oxygen species (Fig. 1). These species play an essential role in many metabolic processes that require the transfer of single electrons. Free radicals may be toxic in two ways: First, they can interact with metal or organic redox centers, promoting irreversible oxidation reactions outside normal catalytic cycles and inactivation of the target metabolic process. Second, free radicals have the capacity to initiate reactions that then become self-sustaining through the regeneration of propagating radicals. In either event, this results in deleterious effects on the cell. The most effective protection against these processes is to terminate the radicals that sustain propagation or to scavenge the initiating radical. Several such antioxidant protective systems have been identified in the cell and in this section the hypothesis that •NO also plays a key role in these processes is reviewed.

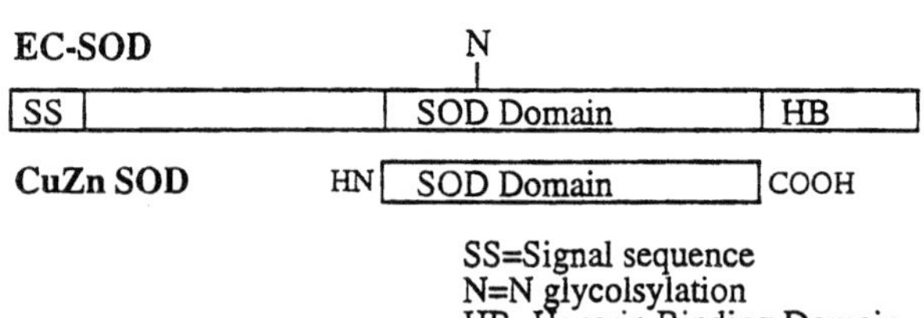

Figure 1 Key sites of nitric oxide prooxidant and antioxidant action on various pathways of reaction of partially reduced oxygen species.

Nitric oxide is an ubiquitous signal transduction molecule and mediator of tissue injury because of its chemical properties, which include (1) relatively low reactivity for a free radical species, resulting in a biological half-life in the range of seconds; (2) charge neutrality; (3) a small molecular radius; (4) hydrophobicity, allowing facile transmembrane diffusion; (5) selective reactivity with heme and iron–sulfur proteins; and (6) facile reaction with molecular oxygen and oxygen-derived free radical species (e.g., superoxide anion, $O_2^{\bullet-}$, and organic-derived free radicals). The latter reactivity of $^{\bullet}NO$ provides tissues with a nonenzymatic method for modulating the local concentration of $^{\bullet}NO$ and leads to many of the toxic and cytoprotective actions of $^{\bullet}NO$.

B. Nitric Oxide as a Prooxidant

During the initial description of endothelial-dependent relaxation, now known to be due to $^{\bullet}NO$, it was noted that strategies that enhanced tissue rates of $O_2^{\bullet-}$ production inhibited the action of endothelial-derived relaxation factor (EDRF) and, conversely, inhibition of $O_2^{\bullet-}$ production or reactions enhanced EDRF activity (1). This revealed that oxygen radicals can serve critical roles as modulators of the biological reactions of $^{\bullet}NO$. We now know that $^{\bullet}NO$ reacts with radical species including $O_2^{\bullet-}$ and lipid peroxyl radicals ($LOO^{\bullet}$) at almost diffusion-limited rate constants (1,2). A critical reaction that $^{\bullet}NO$ undergoes in oxygenated biological media is direct bimolecular reaction with $O_2^{\bullet-}$, yielding peroxynitrite ($ONOO^-$) at almost diffusion-limited rates (6.7×10^9 mol^{-1} sec^{-1}; Ref. 2). This rate constant is about 3.5 times faster than the enzymatic disproportionation of $O_2^{\bullet-}$ catalyzed by superoxide dismutases (SOD) at neutral pH ($k_{SOD} = 2 \times 10^9$ mol^{-1} sec^{-1}). Thus, $ONOO^-$ formation represents a major potential pathway of $^{\bullet}NO$ reactivity that depends on both rates of tissue $^{\bullet}NO$ and $O_2^{\bullet-}$ production and scavenging (e.g., local superoxide dismutase and oxyhemoglobin concentrations). Peroxynitrite has a half-life of less than 1 sec under physiological conditions, owing to proton-catalyzed decomposition of peroxynitrous acid (ONOOH) and competing target molecule reactions of ONOOH (3–7). The mechanisms and extents of $ONOO^-$ reaction will be strongly influenced by the presence of CO_2/H_2CO_3, which is typically 25 mM in biological tissues and can significantly exceed this concentration during pathological processes (8). Nitric oxide thus can potentiate $O_2^{\bullet-}$-mediated tissue damage, leading to $ONOO^-$ formation and represents a major potential pathway of $^{\bullet}NO$ reactivity. In many instances, it is also becoming apparent that $ONOO^-$ serves as a mediator in oxidative actions originally attributed to $^{\bullet}NO$ or other oxygen-derived species, as noted for lipoprotein oxidation and aconitase inhibition (9,10). Peroxynitrite is now being exposed as a key contributing reactive species in pathological events associated with stimulation of tissue production of $^{\bullet}NO$ (e.g., systemic hypotension, inhibition of intermediary metabolism, ischemia–reperfusion injury, immune complex-stimulated pulmonary edema, cytokine-induced oxidant lung injury, and inflammatory cell-mediated pathogen-killing/host injury; 9–19). There is growing evidence that $^{\bullet}$NO-mediated production of $ONOO^-$ readily occurs in vivo, underscoring the importance of understanding the target molecule reactions that occur during the coordinated production of oxygen and nitrogen-containing reactive species (18–20).

Nitric oxide has been recognized as a crucial macrophage-derived effector molecule, with its cytotoxic reactions defending the host against bacteria, tumor cells, and parasites (13–15). However, excess endogenous tissue $^{\bullet}$NO production may lead to pathological responses that occur during such diverse events as allograft transplant rejection, tissue ischemia–reperfusion phenomena, excitatory amino acid-induced brain injury, and immune complex-stimulated pulmonary edema (11,12). Metal- and thiol-containing proteins serve as major target sites for $^{\bullet}$NO reaction (21). The toxicity of $^{\bullet}$NO has principally been attributed to direct $^{\bullet}$NO reaction with thiol and iron–sulfur-containing mitochondrial enzymes (17,22–24) and the inhibition of DNA synthesis by inactivation of the nonheme iron-containing enzyme ribonucleotide reductase (25). Nitric oxide also mediates inhibition of mitochondrial cytochrome *c* oxidase and deenergizes mitochondria at low $^{\bullet}$NO and oxygen concentrations (26–29). Thiol-containing enzymes are also critical targets for $^{\bullet}$NO, by as yet poorly defined pathways, for $^{\bullet}$NO does not directly react with sulfhydryls to yield *S*-nitrosothiols (30). Because tissue $^{\bullet}$NO concentrations are low, reaching a maximum of about 1 μM during acute events (reperfusion of ischemic organs or inflammation; 30,31), significant reactivity with nonheme iron, iron–sulfur complex, and thiol-containing proteins often requires high concentrations of $^{\bullet}$NO, $^{\bullet}$NO-generating agents, or the reactant. This point was recently made by the observation that $^{\bullet}$NO has minimal direct inhibitory action toward aconitase isoenzymes, which are dependent on cubane iron–sulfur centers (4Fe–4S) for catalytic activity (16). Aconitase was long thought to be a key toxic target molecule reaction during monocyte $^{\bullet}$NO-mediated host defense processes. This observation is consistent with the hypothesis that $^{\bullet}$NO must first react with monocyte or target cell-derived $O_2^{\bullet -}$ to yield $ONOO^-$, which then reacts with and inhibits aconitase at a much greater rate. These pivotal reports reaffirm that when a diverse spectrum of reactive species are being produced, relative rates of production of individual reactants, the chemical nature of nearby target molecules, and local concentrations of antioxidant defenses will profoundly affect outcome.

C. Nitric Oxide as an Oxidant-Protective Species

As the reaction of $^{\bullet}$NO with $O_2^{\bullet -}$ yields the potent oxidant $ONOO^-$, from a purely chemical point of view it would follow that (1) an even broader array of target molecules would become susceptible to the toxic effects of reactive oxygen species when ·NO is present and (2) ·NO will potentiate the toxicity of reactive oxygen species. Although this is sometimes true, it is evident that ·NO also exerts direct or indirect antioxidant actions in biological systems subjected to concomitant oxidant stress from excess production of reactive oxygen species, implying antioxidant qualities for this molecule. There are various explanations for this chemical trait that are summarized in the following.

First, nitric oxide undergoes a facile reaction with lipid epoxyallylic and peroxyl radicals (3). Nitric oxide has been observed to play a critical role in regulating lipid oxidation induced by reactive oxygen and nitrogen species ($O_2^{\bullet-}$, hydrogen peroxide (H_2O_2), ·OH, and $ONOO^-$) and activated reticuloendothelial cells (7,9,32,33). Nitric oxide (in some conditions) will stimulate $O_2^{\bullet-}$-induced lipid and lipoprotein oxidation and under other conditions mediate protective reactions in membranes by inhibiting $O_2^{\bullet-}$ and $ONOO^-$-induced lipid oxidation. The latter actions require higher (but still biologically relevant) rates of ·NO production. The prooxidant versus antioxidant outcome of lipid oxidation reactions sensitive to ·NO regulation are critically dependent on relative concentrations of individual reactive species (33–34). For example, the continuous infusion of ·NO at various rates into liposome suspensions exposed to xanthine oxidase first stimulated and then inhibited formation of 2-thiobarbituric acid (TBA)-reactive products at rates of ·NO infusion greater than 1 $\mu M\ min^{-1}$ (32). Nitric oxide stimulated only $O_2^{\bullet-}$-dependent lipid peroxidation when production rates of ·NO were less than or equivalent to rates of $O_2^{\bullet-}$ production. Thus, there is a dynamic competition between $O_2^{\bullet-}$ and lipid radicals for reaction with ·NO. When available for reaction with lipid radicals, ·NO can act as an inhibitor of chain propagation reactions by radical–radical reaction with at least lipid peroxyl radicals at near diffusion-limited rates (for LOO·, $k = 1.3 \times 10^9\ M^{-1}\ sec^{-1}$; 3).

Second, nitric oxide will modulate levels of lipophilic antioxidants (such as α-tocopherol) during lipid oxidation processes. α-Tocopherol, a lipophilic chain-breaking antioxidant in biological membranes and lipoproteins, acts by donating hydrogen atoms to chain-propagating peroxyl radical species (LOO·) to form the corresponding hydroperoxide (35). As the reaction of LOO· with α-tocopherol occurs at a rate three orders of magnitude less than for the reaction of LOO· with ·NO, ·NO could act more readily than or in concert with α-tocopherol, lycopene, retinyl derivatives, and β-carotene as an antioxidant defense against oxygen radical and lipoxygenase-derived oxidized lipid species. Nitric oxide crosses cell membranes and can concentrate in lipophilic milieu by virtue of its low molecular mass, volatility, free radical nature, and high lipid partition coefficient. Based on comparison of relative rate constants, it is predicted that the termination of LOO· by ·NO will be significantly more facile than both the reaction of LOO· with α-tocopherol ($k = 2.5 \times 10^6\ M^{-1}\ sec^{-1}$) and the initiation of secondary peroxidation propagation reactions by LOO· with nearby unsaturated lipids ($k = 30 - 200\ M^{-1}\ sec^{-1}$). In support of this argument, introduction of ·NO into lipid oxidation systems containing α-tocopherol results in preferential reaction of $^{\bullet}NO$ with lipid-derived radical species and prevents oxidation of α-tocopherol (57,67). One mechanism explaining the protection of α-tocopherol from oxidation by oxidizing lipids, until $^{\bullet}NO$ falls to a limiting concentration, can be the preferential reaction of $^{\bullet}NO$ with $LO^{\bullet}$ and $LOO^{\bullet}$ at significantly greater rates than α-tocopherol to yield nitrogen-containing radical–radical termination products (36,37). The mobility of α-tocopherol in the lateral plane of the membrane and its exact positioning in the membrane may restrict its antioxidant actions. This, in part, explains why $^{\bullet}NO$ can be much more facile at terminating lipid peroxyl radical species. Thus, because of a high reactivity with other radical species, a relatively lower reactivity of lipid radical–$^{\bullet}NO$ termination products and an ability of $^{\bullet}NO$ to readily traverse membranes and lipoproteins, $^{\bullet}NO$ can effectively terminate radical species throughout all aspects of membrane and lipoprotein microenvironments. This can also help maintain other tissue antioxidant defenses during periods of oxidant stress.

Third, it is important to place the reactivity of $^{\bullet}NO$ within the context of cell biological issues, where it displays diverse mechanisms of oxidant protection. This includes modulation of cell adhesion, migration, proliferation, and gene expression, in addition to its radical termination properties. Endogenous cell $^{\bullet}NO$ production was cytoprotective toward exogenously and endogenously generated reactive oxygen species in cultures of pulmonary epithelial cells (38). If rates of $^{\bullet}NO$ production in the culture medium were less than for $O_2^{\bullet-}$, then $ONOO^-$ production was favored and caused $^{\bullet}NO$ to increase, not decrease, oxidant injury induced by xanthine oxidase-derived $O_2^{\bullet-}$ and its secondary dismutation and metal reaction products. A number of model systems for inflammation that include a pathogenic role for oxidant injury indicate that either endogenous $^{\bullet}NO$ biosynthesis or exogenous supplementation with sources of $^{\bullet}NO$ inhibit oxidant-dependent damage at both molecular and tissue functional levels. Many, if not all, of these studies have inflammatory injury as a common denominator. In the initial stages of inflammation, $O_2^{\bullet-}$ synthesis is stimulated and appears to exceed the rate of $^{\bullet}NO$ formation, which may be necessary to remove the inhibitory effects of $^{\bullet}NO$ on the recruitment of inflammatory cells (39). Later in the process, nitric oxide syntheses are induced that are capable of generating more $^{\bullet}NO$ than $O_2^{\bullet-}$ (40). Ultimately, the resolution of inflammation requires the restoration of the relative rates of $^{\bullet}NO$ and $O_2^{\bullet-}$ formation that prevailed before the process started. Failure to normalize may be an important factor predisposing to chronic inflammation, and this may occur when detoxification pathways become overwhelmed. Investigation of the effects of $^{\bullet}NO$ on neutrophil and macrophage $O_2^{\bullet-}$ production have produced some important results, as well as yielding some highly questionable data, mostly a result of artifacts in $O_2^{\bullet-}$ quantitation in the presence of $^{\bullet}NO$. The main problem with many of these studies (41–43) is that introduction of exogenous $^{\bullet}NO$ or enhancement of rates of endogenous $^{\bullet}NO$ production in test systems relying on cytochrome *c*-mediated $O_2^{\bullet -}$ detection, creates a number of analytical pitfalls.

Finally, the proof of concept regarding the oxidant-protective qualities of $^{\bullet}$NO can be found from its actions in pulmonary disease. Inhaled $^{\bullet}$NO, at concentrations similar to those produced in vivo, has been clinically administered in the gas phase for up to several weeks when treating pulmonary hypertension, providing an informative test system for the toxicological properties of $^{\bullet}$NO (44). This use of inhaled $^{\bullet}$NO as a selective pulmonary vasodilator is possible because it will react with oxyhemoglobin before reaching the systemic circulation. Inhaled $^{\bullet}$NO is frequently administered in the presence of hyperoxic gas mixtures, as many of the pulmonary pathologies indicating use of $^{\bullet}$NO as a pulmonary vasodilator involve impaired pulmonary gas exchange and hypoxemia. The lungs of those receiving inhaled $^{\bullet}$NO are also suffering from oxidative stress owing to active inflammatory processes and exposure to hyperoxia, known to stimulate lung tissue production of reactive oxygen species at rates directly proportional to oxygen concentration (45). Hyperoxia will also increase rates of gas-phase oxidation of $^{\bullet}$NO to nitrogen dioxide ($^{\bullet}NO_2$), N_2O_3, and N_2O_4. The first indication that $^{\bullet}$NO was protective in oxidant-induced lung injury came from the observation that lungs, perfused ex vivo with purine plus xanthine oxidase as a source of $O_2^{\bullet -}$, H_2O_2, and $^{\bullet}$OH, showed protection from oxidant-induced increases in vascular resistance and reduced injury to alveolar–capillary barrier function on ventilation with 90–120 ppm $^{\bullet}$NO (46). In vivo studies of rats exposed to 100% oxygen plus ~50 ppm $^{\bullet}$NO showed an $^{\bullet}$NO-dependent increase in survival time to the normally lethal hyperoxia, confirming the isolated lung observation (38). A clinical study of patients suffering from adult respiratory distress syndrome, long associated with inflammatory cell and oxidant stress-mediated lung injury, showed that inhalation of 18 ppm $^{\bullet}$NO for 4 days resulted in decreased indices of pulmonary lavage neutrophil activation (H_2O_2 production) and indices of inflammation (b_2 integrin CD11b/CD18 expression and lavage IL-6 and IL-8 content; 47).

In summarizing this section, although many observations suggest that $^{\bullet}$NO can act in an oxidant-inhibitory manner in acute lung injury, the caveat should be added that more subtle toxic reactions can occur at the same time, including inhibition of mitochondrial respiration, damage to alveolar interstitial components (48), inhibition of surfactant function (49), formation of $ONOO^-$ and nitrated aromatic acid derivatives (50), and above 40 ppm, significant formation of methemoglobin, a particular risk for methemoglobin reductase-deficient infants (51). The clinical experiences of critical care physicians studying this therapeutic modality also suggests that it is sometimes difficult to ''wean'' patients from the $^{\bullet}$NO inhaled with other ventilator air/oxygen blends, in terms of the patient being able to autoregulate pulmonary blood flow. This observation provides possible in vivo evidence for the ability of $^{\bullet}$NO to inhibit endogenous nitric oxide synthases by coordination at the catalytic heme iron of the enzyme (52). In spite of these qualifiers, however, these data indicate that ˙NO can exert oxidant-protective effects. In the next sections, we present strategies for beneficially modulating the balance of tissue ˙NO, $O_2^{\bullet -}$ H_2O_2, and ˙OH concentrations to encourage the salutary actions of these mediators of tissue metabolic homeostasis and inflammation.

III. Targeting Catalytic Radical Scavengers to the Extracellular Compartment

A. Rationale for Targeting the Extracellular Milieu with Superoxide Dismutase

Many pathological situations are initially characterized by impairment of several ˙NO-mediated physiological functions including impaired endothelial-dependent relaxation, increased smooth-muscle cell proliferation and increased transendothelial inflammatory cell migration. In the vascular wall, this can result from one of three possible scenarios: (1) lack of endothelial production of ˙NO because of biosynthetic enzyme inhibition or cell damage, (2) inability of smooth-muscle cells to respond to ˙NO signaling, or (3) a decrease in ˙NO half-life and shorter diffusion distances of ˙NO in the extracellular matrix. Although pathological conditions may act by any or all of these steps, it is becoming increasingly evident that loss of ˙NO bioactivity and inhibition of ˙NO diffusion are early features in many disease processes. For example, central to the pathogenesis of atherosclerosis is the early development of vascular unresponsiveness to ˙NO-mediated vasorelaxation, even though vascular ˙NO production may be enhanced (53,54). Likewise, ventilation/perfusion ratio (V/Q) mismatches found in respiratory distress syndromes (55) and high-altitude pulmonary edema (HAPE; 56), are partly due to either impaired production of ˙NO or impaired diffusibility of ˙NO to sites of action, thus contributing to the pathogenesis of these diseases. In vivo, ˙NO has limited reactivity and, for the most part, is ''scavenged'' by either oxyhemoglobin (oxyHb) or $O_2^{\bullet -}$. Nitric oxide reacts with oxyHb to produce nitrate and methemoglobin (metHb). This reaction prevents steady-state concentrations of ˙NO from reaching effective levels in blood and allows for ˙NO diffusion from the site of synthesis, vascular endothelium, to be directed abluminally where it can exert its effect on smooth-muscle cell guanylate cyclase activity.

It has been known for more than a decade that modulation of ˙NO activity is dependent on tissue rates of $O_2^{\bullet -}$ production (1). Nitric oxide reacts at near diffusion-limited rates (rate constant $= 6.7 \times 10^9$) with $O_2^{\bullet -}$ to produce the highly reactive peroxynitrite ($ONOO^-$) that, when protonated, forms a potent oxidizing species similar to the hydroxyl radical (2,5). Peroxynitrite is capable of oxidizing thiols, methionine, DNA, and lipids (6,57–59). Therefore, decreasing steady-state concentrations of $O_2^{\bullet -}$ in the extracellular matrix facilitates access of ${}^{\bullet}NO$ to its physiological target (soluble guanylate cyclase) without its reacting through pathways that yield potentially damaging oxidative effects. Extracellular SOD (EC-SOD) thus may serve to create protective zones or channels for the efficient diffusion of ${}^{\bullet}NO$ from one site to another. We strongly hold the view that to be effective in scavenging sometimes ubiquitous and always highly reactive free radical species, antioxidant interventions should be catalytic (e.g., enzymatic or enzyme mimetic). By virtue of their high rate constants for reacting with and detoxifying free radical species, catalytic scavengers will be much more potent in lowering steady-state concentrations of reactive species than small radical-scavenging molecules.

B. Extracellular Superoxide Dismutase

Recently, it has been appreciated that, for tissues in which ${}^{\bullet}NO$ is an important signal transduction mediator (vessel wall, lung), there is also a high specific activity of extracellular superoxide dismutase (EC-SOD; 60,61). Extracellular SOD in baboon and human aortas may approach 70% of total SOD in the tissues (62). Even though the nucleotide sequence of EC-SOD lacks homology with cytoplasmic CuZnSOD, the amino acid sequence of the active site of EC-SOD is homologous, suggesting an early gene duplication event in the evolutionary appearance of EC-SOD. Extracellular SOD, unlike dimeric CuZnSOD, is secreted by cells as a tetramer into the extracellular space. The primary amino acid sequence of both EC-SOD and CuZnSOD show a region of high homology, flanked by both a lengthy nonhomologous NH_2-terminus and a short region of nonhomology at the COOH-end (Fig. 2). Mutational studies conclude that the COOH-terminus is important by ionically anchoring the molecule to heparan sulfate proteoglycans in the extracellular matrix (ECM) owing to a region of nine positively charged amino acid residues (63). The nonhomologous NH_2-terminus is thought to be important in tetramerization based on cross species studies done in the rat, in which EC-SOD is found in the dimeric form. EC-SOD, unlike CuZnSOD, is *N*-glycosylated on asparagine 89. Although removal of this carbohydrate does not affect the ability of the enzyme to scavenge $O_2^{\bullet -}$, it may affect enzyme half-life in plasma and also alter enzyme solubility (64). This can be important when considering production of EC-SOD in recombinant systems, such as bacteria and insects, that differ from mammalian systems in protein glycosylation extents and mechanisms. EC-SOD isolated from humans is heterogeneous in its affinity for heparin. Enzyme displaying high heparin affinity has been termed EC-SOD C, whereas EC-SOD B and EC-SOD A have less affinity for heparin immobilized on Sepharose. The variability of heparin affinity in isolated EC-SOD results from posttranslational proteolytic cleavage and subsequent removal of the heparin-binding domains from the catalytic molecule (65).

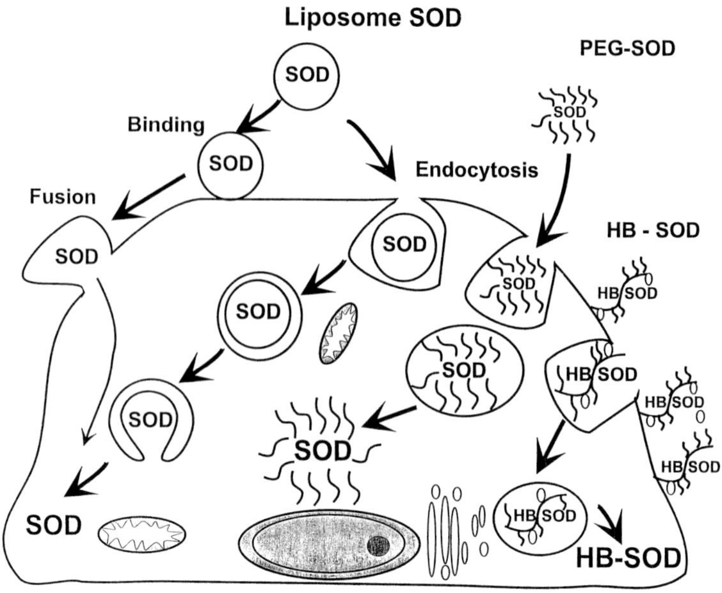

Figure 2 Comparison of the functional domains in the primary amino acid sequence of EC-SOD and CuZnSOD.

C. Regulation of EC-SOD in Inflammation and Disease

Inflammatory conditions are associated with an influx of neutrophils and macrophages that are capable of synthesizing large quantities of both $O_2^{\bullet-}$ and $^{\bullet}NO$. Neutrophils produce $O_2^{\bullet-}$ by activation of a membrane-bound NADPH oxidase and can also produce large quantities of nitric oxide by expression of an inducible nitric oxide synthase (66,67). Protection of surrounding tissues from both $O_2^{\bullet-}$ and its secondary products ($ONOO^-$) thus may be an important role for EC-SOD in inflammation. EC-SOD expression in fibroblasts is upregulated in the presence of cytokines, such as interferon-γ (IFN-γ) and markedly downregulated by transforming growth factor-β (TGF-β), suggesting that increased expression of EC-SOD is an important ingredient in the inflammatory response (68). Localization of EC-SOD also may protect key target molecules from the damaging effects of $O_2^{\bullet-}$. For example, EC-SOD coats collagen I molecules in the lung (69). Collagen is sensitive to breakdown by $O_2^{\bullet-}$ and, likewise, collagen fragments are potent chemoattractants in inflammation (70,71). In support of these concepts, mice lacking EC-SOD are more susceptible to hyperoxia and ozone-induced inflammation (135). The ability of EC-SOD to be protective in inflammatory conditions, as well as its ability to restore normal physiological functions of •NO, has made EC-SOD a conceptually interesting and, in practice, an important strategy for site-directed antioxidant therapy.

D. Recombinant EC-SOD and Chimeric EC-SOD–CuZnSOD Fusion Proteins

Large-scale production of EC-SOD and its use in tissue supplementation during pathological events may become an important therapy. Acute conditions, such as respiratory distress and organ transplantation, as well as more chronic conditions, such as atherosclerosis and rheumatoid arthritis, may benefit from EC-SOD supplementation therapy. Insolubility of the nonglycosylated enzyme, however, makes large-scale recombinant production of EC-SOD by prokaryotic and insect systems difficult to manage. Attachment of a murine whey acidic protein regulatory sequence upstream from the human EC-SOD nucleotide-coding sequence has made isolation of glycosylated protein from murine milk a possibility for isolation of large quantities of EC-SOD (72). An alternative approach to isolation of native EC-SOD, is the construction of recombinant fusion proteins that link the highly soluble CuZnSOD with the heparin-binding sequence of EC-SOD or other proteins that contain heparin-binding regions (73,74). CuZnSOD, because of its low molecular weight (32-kDa dimeric molecular weight), is rapidly cleared from the plasma on intravenous injection. Attachment of a heparin-binding sequence not only helps localize SOD activity to critical compartments, but also may significantly increase the half-life of the molecule on intravenous administration. For example, only 1% of injected chimeric heparin-binding SOD is found in the urine 20 min after injection, whereas 70% of CuZnSOD is filtered by the kidney and excreted (75). Immunohistochemistry showed that following intravenous injection of chimeric heparin-binding SOD, the enzyme concentrated on the surface and subendothelial matrix of vessels where it could readily enhance endothelial-dependent vasorelaxation. Therefore, immobilization of heparin-binding SOD activity to the ECM helps protect the enzyme from rapid clearance and targets important superoxide-scavenging potential to physiologically critical compartments.

E. Tissue Protection Induced by Administration of Heparin-Binding Forms of Superoxide Dismutase

Extracellular SOD supplementation has been beneficial in treating reperfusion injury in ischemic rat hearts, and also protects vessels from superoxide radical challenge (76,77). Localized scavenging of superoxide anion may have a profound effect on vascular function. In rats made hypertensive with angiotensin II, injection of chimeric SOD rapidly normalized blood pressure, implicating elevated superoxide production as an important determinant of angiotensin-induced hypertension (74). Treatment with heparin-binding SODs (HB-SODs) may become beneficial in improving normal physiological function of $^{\bullet}$NO in the vascular system. Studies outlining HB-SOD as treatment for other tissue insults are ongoing.

IV. Targeting Catalytic Radical Scavengers to the Intracellular Compartment

A. Rationale for Modification of Antioxidant Enzyme Delivery Systems to Mediate Intracellular Delivery

Cytosolic supplementation with antioxidant enzymes in disease processes associated with enhanced intracellular reactive oxygen species formation has been proposed as a therapeutic modality to limit tissue injury. Additionally, increased antioxidant enzyme activity can be used as a tool to probe the contributions of individual reactive oxygen species in models of disease and injury. However, implementation of such an approach has been limited by the physicochemical properties of biological macromolecules. Novel strategies have been developed to address the problem of delivery of enzymatically active protein to sites of reactive species formation (Fig. 3).

In settings where injury is known to be caused by excess formation of reactive species, addition of native oxidant-scavenging enzymes is often ineffective. For example, when SOD (CuZnSOD) is administered systemically, the circulating half-life is less than 10 min, with rapid excretion of the intact protein in the urine. Additionally, intracellular access is limited both by the size of the SOD molecule (32 kDa), and its electronegative charge, resulting in repulsion from the anionic cell membrane. Several methods have been devised to enhance delivery of antioxidant enzymes. Chemical modification of protein resulting in net positive charge, while maintaining enzymatic activity, results in enhanced cytoprotection following oxidant injury (78–80).

B. Polyethylene Glycol-Derivatized Antioxidant Enzymes

Conjugation of enzymes with polyethylene glycol or pyran increases the molecular weight of the complex three- to tenfold; renal clearance of SOD and catalase is thus reduced, resulting in enhanced circulating half-life of the enzyme (81,82). Such covalent modification also reduces antigenicity and diminishes hydrolysis by proteases (83,84). It is unlikely that polyethylene glycol-derivatized enzymes

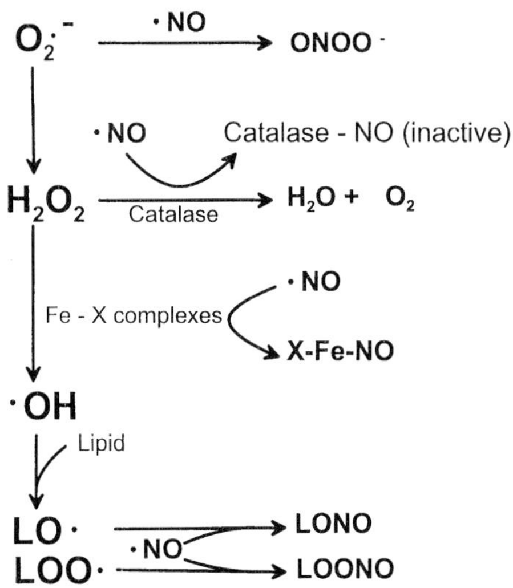

Figure 3 Potential mechanisms of cellular interactions of liposome-entrapped and heparin-binding forms of superoxide dismutase.

are soluble within aliphatic lipid bilayers, preventing direct movement across cell membranes. Rather, intracellular access is achieved by adsorption to cell surfaces and subsequent endocytosis. Polyethylene glycol associates with membrane phospholipid head groups (85), possibly allowing anchorage of polyethylene glycol-conjugated proteins to the cell surface before endocytosis. Consequently, treatment of endothelial cells in vitro with polyethylene glycol-conjugated antioxidant enzymes results in enhanced intracellular antioxidant enzyme activity. When endocytosis is augmented, as can occur with some cell injury processes, uptake of polyethylene glycol-conjugated enzymes was enhanced even further, suggesting that reversibly injured tissue may accumulate more modified antioxidant enzyme than would control tissue (86).

Numerous studies, both in vitro and in vivo, have demonstrated improved intracellular uptake and resistance to disease states following administration of polyethylene glycol-conjugated antioxidant enzymes compared with native proteins. Models have included pulmonary oxygen toxicity (85–88), ischemic brain injury (89), viral myocarditis (90), acute ischemic renal failure (91), as well as partially restoring endothelial-dependent vascular relaxation in an animal model of atherosclerosis (92). Such encouraging animal data have prompted clinical trials of polyethylene glycol–SOD in the treatment of severe closed head injury. Although overall outcome differences were not statistically significant, there were more favorable neurological outcomes in the treated groups. Interestingly, there was a decreased incidence of adult respiratory distress syndrome in the group receiving low-dose polyethylene glycol–SOD compared with the placebo group (93).

C. Liposome-Entrapped Antioxidant Enzymes

In an attempt to more precisely target delivery of antioxidant enzymes to cellular sites of oxidant generation, entrapment within unilamellar lipid vesicles or liposomes has been employed. Liposomes, composed of amphiphilic molecules, such as cholesterol and phospholipids, have been used extensively to increase the efficiency of drug delivery. A variety of macromolecules can be entrapped within the aqueous phase, and hydrophobic radical scavengers (e.g., tocopherols or carotenoids) can be intercalated into the liposomal membrane. Several factors determine site-specific delivery of liposomes and their contents. These include the physical state of the liposomes, delivery route, and interactions with nontarget tissues. Physical characteristics of liposomal preparations greatly influence subsequent behavior in biological systems. Lipid composition, surface charge, membrane fluidity, overall size, and presence of targeting molecules at the surface influence liposome stability, circulating half-life, and cell-specific as well as organ-specific recognition.

A major sink for uptake of liposomes has been the reticuloendothelial system, particularly the liver and spleen. Despite this capacity of the reticuloendothelial system to retain a large portion of the administered dose of liposomes, circulating half-times and tissue enzyme-specific activities have increased following intravenous and intraperitoneal administration of antioxidant-containing liposomes, compared with native enzymes. Lung catalase and SOD activities can be increased 3.1- and 1.7-fold, respectively, 2 hr following a single injection of enzyme–liposome mixture composed of cholesterol, dipalmitoylphosphatidylcholine, and stearylamine, prepared by reverse-phase evaporation (94). Similar preparations of SOD and catalase have resulted in diminished pulmonary oxygen toxicity when injected intravenously (95) or intratracheally (96,97). Additionally, in vitro models have demonstrated enhanced antioxidant enzyme activities in both endothelial cells and alveolar epithelium, with concomitant resistance to oxidant stress (98,99).

Although some success has been achieved with liposomes prepared by reverse-phase evaporative processes, there are limitations to the technique. Reverse-phase evaporation subjects enzymes to denaturing solvents and results in inconsistent preparations that tend to aggregate, thereby limiting therapeutic potential (100). Another approach is to utilize pH-sensitive liposomes as vectors. These liposomes are formed by extrusion under N_2 gas, resulting in small, uniform (180 ± 77 nm when using a 600-nm pore size filter) liposomes that are stable for 1 week at 4°C (100). Following endocytosis, these liposomes fuse with or destabilize the endosome on acidification, allowing liposomal contents access to the cytoplasm with limited proteolysis within the lysosome (101). This method has been used to enhance SOD delivery to alveolar epithelial cells in culture (100). pH-sensitive liposomal delivery of antioxidant enzymes has also been employed to inhibit oxygen radical attenuation of nitric oxide-dependent signal transduction and to improve vasorelaxation responses in models of atherosclerosis and hypertension. Intravenous administration of 1500 U/kg liposomal SOD daily for 5 days, resulted in a twofold increase in SOD activity of rabbit aortic homogenates (102). Electron microscopic immunocytochemistry demonstrated enzyme delivery to the cytoplasm of both vascular endothelium and underlying smooth muscle as well as in the interstitial matrix. This augmentation of enzyme activity was associated with improvement in impaired endothelial-dependent relaxation responses. Similar restoration of endothelial-dependent relaxation was observed when aortas from angiotensin II-induced hypertensive rats were incubated ex vivo with pH-sensitive liposomal SOD (103). Treatment with pH-sensitive liposomal SOD also restored vasorelaxant responses in a model of chronic nitroglycerin tolerance (104).

Further refinements in liposomal delivery technique include the addition of molecules to specifically target liposomal contents to specific organs or cell types. For example, the inclusion of surfactant protein A in antioxidant enzyme–liposome preparations enhances alveolar epithelial antioxidant enzyme activity twofold over enzyme–liposomes lacking surfactant protein A (100,105). The addition of amphiphilic polyethylene glycol lipid derivatives to liposomes results in sterically stabilized liposomes with long circulating half-lives and diminished uptake by the reticuloendothelial system (106). The combination of these methods thus may result in the delivery of antioxidant enzymes to specific sites of reactive species formation while minimizing total doses of proteins.

In addition to enhancing cell targeting and uptake of liposomal preparations, surfactant itself also can be used as a vector to enhance pulmonary delivery of antioxidant enzymes. Intratracheal instillation of surfactant that was obtained by bronchoalveolar lavage and contained 90% phospholipid and 10% protein resulted in a significant increase in alveolar type II cellular SOD activity, whereas surfactant preparations composed primarily of phospholipid with minimal protein content, demonstrated virtually no antioxidant enzyme capacity (107). Emulsions composed of the clinically available surfactant, Survanta, and SOD and catalase, increased antioxidant enzyme activity of fetal lung epithelial cells in vitro, and intratracheal administration resulted in enhanced enzyme activities in rat lung homogenates. Confocal microscopy revealed the presence of enzyme in lung epithelium cytoplasm following in vivo treatment (108).

These studies demonstrate the usefulness of liposomes as vectors for enzyme delivery to study the potential role of oxidants in pulmonary and vascular disease processes.

V. Gene Therapy Strategies for Enhancing Pulmonary Antioxidant Defenses

A. Rationale for Gene Therapy to the Developing Lung in Oxidant-Mediated Lung Injury

Extraordinary advances in molecular biology and techniques of somatic gene transfer have made gene therapy to lung an important clinical issue. Recent reviews have outlined issues surrounding somatic gene transfer to the lung, including limitations of current vectors and clinical conditions in which postnatal gene therapy may be applicable (109,110). Although the focus of such efforts has been directed toward cystic fibrosis (111), application of gene therapy for acquired pulmonary diseases, including neoplasms and ARDS, is apparent (109). In addition, several reviews have discussed issues of gene therapy to the developing lung for inherited and acquired lung disease (112,113). Several physiological and anatomical features of the fetal and neonatal lung suggest that pulmonary somatic gene transfer during development may be more effective than our current experience with mature lungs. The fluid-filled future airspaces of the fetal lung contain considerably fewer macrophages, less complex surface-lining material, and lower protein content than mature lung, thereby facilitating delivery of macromolecules, including DNA, to lung tissue targets. The significantly greater number of dividing cells during lung development (114) and the potential for an expanding stem cell population are advantageous when cell division is required for accommodation of several types of integrating viral vectors. A limited immune response at critical times in development of the fetal lung may minimize adverse host responses, while enhancing transgene expression with currently available replication-defective adenoviral vectors that still possess cytotoxic and immunostimulatory gene products. In the specific case of antioxidant gene therapy, lower expression of native antioxidant genes in the premature lung makes overexpression of these transgene products a plausible therapeutic strategy.

B. Vectors for Gene Transfer to the Developing Lung

In contrast with mature lung, only a few vectors expressing the reporter gene, β-galactosidase (LacZ), have been studied in preclinical trials of somatic gene transfer to developing lung. Although it is likely that many forms of oxidant-mediated lung injury will require only transient expression; nonetheless, it is conceivable that longer-term transgene expression may also be therapeutic. Both nonintegrating and integrating vectors have been studied. All work to date has been limited to introduction of vectors into the future airspaces. Thus, the possibility of intravascular gene delivery remains untested.

Nonintegrating vectors, including adenoviruses (AdV) and liposomes, have been reported to produce significant, but transient, gene expression in the lungs of developing mammals. When AdV–LacZ was introduced in the amniotic fluid of fetal rats at 16 days gestation, high-level expression was noted over the subsequent 2-week period (115). In contrast, intra-amniotic administration of AdV–LacZ was extremely inefficient in transducing airway cells of fetal mice or sheep (116,117). It appears that for most species, intrabronchial administration of AdV vectors into the fetus is more likely to result in significant airway transgene expression (117,118) than after intra-amniotic delivery. In both of these studies, unexpected pulmonary inflammatory responses resulted in loss of transgene expression and significant intrapulmonary pathology. The surprising cellular and humoral-mediated response to AdV suggests that fetal sheep are not immunotolerant to this form of the virus. Accordingly, other periods in development may be better suited for AdV-mediated gene transfer; alternatively, newer generations of AdV vectors, with larger portions of the viral genome deleted, will be necessary. An encouraging preliminary report suggests that AdV may be administered in the ventilatory line of premature baboons with no significant toxicity (119). Preliminary results (120) in neonatal piglets with the other major nonintegrating vector, liposome, also appear promising. Cationic liposomes have been noted by several investigators to produce remarkable, but transient, transgene expression in mature lungs of mice (121) and rat (122). It remains to be determined if efficacy is sufficient to inhibit oxidant-mediated lung injury.

Integrating vectors for somatic gene transfer to the lung are of particular interest for treating inherited disorders, such as cystic fibrosis and α_1-antitrypsin or surfactant apoprotein B deficiencies. Nonetheless, it is conceivable that long-term expression of transgenes may be required in oxidant-mediated neonatal lung injury. Pitt et al. (113) reported expression of LacZ in the lungs of developing sheep 3–4 weeks after replication-deficient Moloney murine leukemia retrovirus was injected into the trachea of permanently catheterized fetal sheep. In this study, unexpected pulmonary toxicity, along with early fetal death, suggests that alternative retroviral constructs or delivery systems may be required. Pseudotype retroviruses with the G protein of vesicular stomatitis virus produced significant and long-lasting gene expression in the liver of neonatal mice after intrahepatic injection (136). Recombinant adenoassociated virus (AAV) vectors produce long-term expression in mature rabbit lung (123). The same group of investigators recently demonstrated successful transduction of alveolar type II cells after instillation of recombinant AAV in newborn rabbit lungs (124). It appears from this latter study that AAV, unlike its wild-type counterpart that undergoes high-frequency stable integration in a site-specific fashion in quiescent cells has a propensity for dividing cells.

C. Candidate Genes for Somatic Transfer for Oxidant-Mediated Injury in the Developing Lung

In general, candidate genes for somatic transfer in oxidant-mediated injury in the developing lung should have the following characteristics: (1) they should complement a constitutive gene for which expression is low during lung development; and (2) they should be used when small-molecule or protein-based antioxidant therapy has significant pharmacokinetic limitations. Gene therapy may be considered in lieu of treatment with traditional antioxidants that are unstable in the extracellular environment of the lung and do not cross plasma membranes readily when intracellular antioxidant defense requires augmentation. Strategies have involved overexpression of traditional antioxidants, including catalase (125), superoxide dismutase (126), heat-shock protein 70 (127), and metallothionein (128) in cultured cells. Progress has been made in reducing the inflammatory response of mature intact lungs after somatic gene transfer of cyclooxygenase (129), α_1-antitrypsin (130), and TNF-R decoy (131) in vivo.

D. Potential for Gene Transfer to Developing Human Lung

Major ethical and technical issues remain before clinical trials using gene therapy to developing human lung are implemented. Nonetheless, it is encouraging that several investigators have noted efficient gene transfer to human fetal airways that are maintained in various xenograft models (132). Alternatively, successful gene transfer with adenoviruses was noted in organotypic culture of human lung (133,134).

VI. Summary

There has been a revolutionary increase in our understanding and appreciation of the multifaceted roles that reactive species play in the maintenance of tissue metabolic homeostasis and during processes of cell and organ injury. Acquisition of this knowledge has been assisted by the development and application of more incisive and quantitative means for detecting the nature and rates of biological production of inherently evanescent free radical and oxidizing species. The significance of reactive species in biological and pathological events continues to grow, as we learn more about the critical actions that reactive species play in regulation of metabolism and gene expression, as well as the interdependency between oxygen radicals and the functions and reactions of the signal transduction mediator nitric oxide. For all of these reasons, a means to effectively modulate steady-state concentrations of reactive oxygen species and nitric oxide is crucial, because it facilitates mechanistic studies of metabolism and pathological processes and provides more efficacious avenues for pharmacological intervention. The present discussion of the targeted modulation of tissue antioxidant defenses has focused on current knowledge of potentially beneficial approaches to solving these problems.

Acknowledgments

This work was supported by NIH grants R01 HL32154 (BRP), PO1 HL48676, RO1 HL40458 (BAF), and K08 HL03457 (MMT).

References

1. Gryglewski R, Palmer R, Moncada S. Superoxide anion is involved in the breakdown of endothelium-derived vascular relaxing factor. Nature 1986; 320:454–456.
2. Huie RE, Padmaja S. Reaction of NO with $O_2^{\bullet -}$. Free Radic Res Commun 1993; 18:195–199.
3. Padmaja S, Huie RE. The reaction of nitric oxide with organic peroxyl radicals. Biochem Biophys Res Commun 1993; 195:539–544.
4. Pryor WA, Squadrito GL. The chemistry of peroxynitrite: a product from the reaction of nitric oxide with superoxide. Am J Physiol 1995; 268:L699–L722.
5. Beckman JS, Beckman TW, Chen J, Marshall PA, Freeman BA. Apparent hydroxyl radical production by peroxynitrite: implications for endothelial injury from nitric oxide and superoxide. Proc Natl Acad Sci USA 1990; 87:1620–1624.
6. Radi R, Beckman JS, Bush K, Freeman BA. Peroxynitrite oxidation of sulfhydryls: the cytotoxic potential of endothelial-derived superoxide and nitric oxide. J Biol Chem 1991; 266:4244–4250.
7. Van der Vliet A, Smith D, O'Neill CA, Kaur H, Darley-Usmar VM, Cross CE, Halliwell B. Interactions of peroxynitrite with human plasma and its constituents. Oxidative damage and antioxidant depletion. Biochem J 1994; 303:295–301.
8. Radi R, Cosgrove T, Beckman JS, Freeman BA. Peroxynitrite-induced luminol chemiluminescence. Biochem J 1993; 290:51–57.
9. Hogg N, Darley-Usmar VM, Wilson MT, Moncada S. The oxidation of α-tocopherol in human low density lipoprotein by the simultaneous generation of superoxide and nitric oxide. FEBS Lett 1993; 326:199–203.
10. Castro L, Rodriguez M, Radi R. Aconitase is readily inactivated by peroxynitrite, but not by its precursor, nitric oxide. J Biol Chem 1994; 269:29409–29415.
11. Matheis G, Sherman MP, Buckberg GD, Haybron DM, Young HH, Ignarro LJ. Role of L-arginine–nitric oxide pathway in myocardial reoxygenation injury. Am J Physiol 1992; 262:H616–H620.
12. Mulligan MS, Warren JS, Smith CW, Anderson DC, Yeh CG, Rudolph AR, Ward PA. Lung injury after deposition of IgA immune complexes. Requirements for CD18 and L-arginine. J Immunol 1992; 148:3086–3092.
13. Zhu L, Gunn C, Beckman JS. Bactericidal activity of peroxynitrite. Arch Biochem Biophys 1992; 298:452–457.
14. Denicola A, Rubbo H, Rodriguez D, Radi R. Peroxynitrite-mediated cytotoxicity to *Trypanosoma cruzi*. Arch Biochem Biophys 1993; 304:279–286.
15. Carreras MC, Pargament GA, Catz SD, Poderoso JJ, Boveris A. Kinetics of nitric oxide and hydrogen peroxide production and formation of peroxynitrite during the respiratory burst of human neutrophils. FEBS Lett 1994; 341:65–68.

16. Radi R, Rodriguez M, Castro L, Telleri R. Inhibition of mitochondrial electron transport by peroxynitrite. Arch Biochem Biophys 1994; 308:89–95.
17. Haddad IY, Ischiropoulos H, Holm BA, Beckman JS, Baker JR, Matalon S. Mechanism of peroxynitrite-induced injury to pulmonary surfactants. Am J Physiol 1993; 265:L555–L564.
18. Beckman JS, Ye YZ, Anderson PG, Chen J, Accavitti MA, Tarpey MM, White CR. Extensive nitration of protein tyrosines in human atherosclerosis detected by immunohistochemistry. Biol Chem Hoppe-Seyler 1994; 375:81–88.
19. White R, Brock T, Chang L, Crapo J, Briscoe P, Ku D, Bradley W, Gianturco S, Gore J, Freeman BA, Tarpey MM. Superoxide and peroxynitrite in atherosclerosis. Proc Natl Acad Sci USA 1994; 91:1044–1048.
20. Kooy NW, Royall JA. Agonist-induced peroxynitrite production from endothelial cells. Arch Biochem Biophys 1994; 310:352–359.
21. Wink DA, Osawa Y, Darbyshire J, Jones CR, Eshenaur S, Nims RW. Inhibition of cytochromes P450 by nitric oxide and a nitric oxide-releasing agent. Arch Biochem Biophys 1993; 300:115–123.
22. Schmidt HH, Walter U. NO at work. Cell 1994; 78:919–925.
23. Snyder SH. Nitric oxide: first in a new class of neurotransmitters? Science 1993; 257:494–496.
24. Hibbs JB, Taintor RR, Vavrin Z, Rachlin EM. Nitric oxide: a cytotoxic activated macrophage effector molecule. Biochem Biophys Res Commun 1988; 157:87–94.
25. Lepoivre M, Flaman J, Bobe P, Lemaire G, Henry Y. Quenching of the tyrosyl free radical of ribonucleotide reductase by nitric oxide: relationship to cytostasis induced in tumor cells by cytotoxic macrophages. J Biol Chem 1994; 269:21891–21897.
26. Cleeter MWJ, Cooper JM, Darley-Usmar VM, Moncada S, Schapira AHV. Reversible inhibition of cytochrome *c* oxidase, the terminal enzyme of the mitochondrial respiratory chain, by nitric oxide. Implications for neurodegenerative diseases. FEBS Lett 1994; 345:50–54.
27. Schweizer M, Richter C. Nitric oxide potently and reversibly deenergizes mitochondria at low oxygen tension. Biochem Biophys Res Commun 1994; 204:169–175.
28. Takehara Y, Kanno T, Yoshioka T, Inoue M, Utsumi K. Oxygen dependent regulation of mitochondrial energy metabolism by nitric oxide. Arch Biochem Biophys 1995; 323:27–32.
29. Brown GC, Cooper CE. Nanomolar concentrations of nitric oxide reversibly inhibit synaptosomal respiration by competing with oxygen at cytochrome *c* oxidase. FEBS Lett 1994; 356:295–298.
30. Loscalzo J, Welch G. Nitric oxide and its role in the cardiovascular system. Prog Cardiov Dis 1995; 38:87–104.
31. Albina JE, Reichner JS. Nitric oxide in inflammation and immunity. N Horizons 1995; 3:46–64.
32. Rubbo H, Radi R, Trujillo M, Telleri R, Kalyanaraman B, Barnes S, Kirk M, Freeman BA. Nitric oxide regulation of superoxide and peroxynitrite-dependent lipid peroxidation: formation of novel nitrogen-containing oxidized lipid derivatives. J Biol Chem 1994; 269:26066–26075.

33. Rubbo H, Parthasarathy S, Kalyanaraman B, Barnes S, Kirk M, Freeman BA. Nitric oxide inhibition of lipoxygenase-dependent liposome and low density lipoprotein oxidation: termination of radical chain propagation reactions and formation of nitrogen-containing oxidized lipid derivatives. Arch Biochem Biophys 1995; 324:15–25.
34. Chumley P, Rubbo H, Gutierrez HH, Freeman BA. Nitric oxide regulation of superoxide, hydrogen peroxide, and peroxynitrite-dependent injury to vascular endothelium. Free Radic Biol Med 1997; (submitted).
35. Liebler DC. The role of metabolism in the antioxidant function of vitamin E. Crit Rev Toxicol 1993; 23:147–169.
36. Goss SP, Hogg N, Kalyanaraman B. The antioxidant effect of spermine NONOate in human low density lipoprotein. Chem Res Toxicol 1995; 8:800–806.
37. Rubbo H, Paler-Martinez A, Chumley P, Kirk M, Barnes B, Freeman BA. Nitric oxide and α-tocopherol react to inhibit lipid oxidation: termination of propagation reactions and recovery of reduced α-tocopherol. J Biol Chem 1996; (submitted).
38. Gutierrez H, Chumley P, Rivera A, Freeman BA. Nitric oxide regulation of superoxide-dependent lung cell injury: oxidant-protective actions of endogenously produced and exogenously administrated nitric oxide. Free Radic Biol Med 1996; 21: 43–52.
39. Miller RA, Britigan BE. The formation and biologic significance of phagocyte-derived oxidants. J Invest Med 1995; 43:39–49.
40. Albina JE, Reichner JS. Nitric oxide in inflammation and immunity. N Horizons 1995; 3:46–64.
41. Clancy RM, Leszczynska J, Abramson SB. Nitric oxide, an endothelial cell relaxation factor, inhibits neutrophil superoxide anion production via a direct action on the NADPH oxidase. J Clin Invest 1992; 90:1116–1121.
42. Wiedermann CJ, Sitte B, Zilian U, Reinisch N, Beimpold H, Finkenstedt G, Braunsteiner H. Inhibition of superoxide anion release from circulating neutrophils by L-arginine in man. Clin Invest 1993; 71:985–989.
43. Rubanyi GM, Ho E, Cantor E, Lumma W, Parker LH. Cytoprotective function of nitric oxide: inactivation of superoxide radicals produced by human leukocytes. Biochem Biophys Res Commun 1991; 181:1392–1397.
44. Rossaint R, Gerlach H, Falke KJ. Inhalation of nitric oxide—a new approach in severe ARDS. Eur J Anesthesiol 1994; 11:43–51.
45. Freeman BA, Crapo JD. Hyperoxia increases oxygen radical production in rat lungs and lung mitochondria. J Biol Chem 1981; 256:10986–10992.
46. Kavanagh BP, Mouchawar A, Goldsmith J, Pearl RG. Effects of inhaled nitric oxide and inhibition of endogenous nitric oxide synthesis in oxidant-induced acute lung injury. J Appl Physiol 1994; 76:1324–1329.
47. Chollet-Martin S, Gatecel C, Kermarrec N, Gougerot-Pocidalo MA, Payen DM. Alveolar neutrophil functions and cytokine levels in patients with the adult respiratory distress syndrome during nitric oxide inhalation. Am J Respir Crit Care Med 1996; 153:985–990.
48. Mercer RR, Costa DL, Crapo JD. Effects of prolonged exposure to low doses of nitric oxide or nitrogen dioxide on the alveolar septa of the adult rat lung. Lab Invest 1995; 73:20–28.

49. Haddad IY, Crow J, Hu P, Ye Y, Beckman JS, Matalon S. Concurrent generation of nitric oxide and superoxide damages surfactant protein A. Am J Physiol 1994; 267:L242–L249.
50. Kooy N, Royall J, Ye Y, Kelly D, Beckman JS. Evidence for in vivo peroxynitrite production in human acute lung injury. Am J Respir Crit Care Med 1995; 151: 1250–1254.
51. Ahluwalia JS, Kelsall A, Raine J, Rennie JM, Mahmoo, Oduro A, Latimer R, Pickett J, Higenbottam TW. Safety of inhaled nitric oxide in premature neonates. Acta Pediatr 1994; 83:347–348.
52. Griscavage JM, Fukuto J, Komori Y, Ignarro LJ. Nitric oxide inhibits neuronal nitric oxide synthase by interacting with the heme prosthetic group. J Biol Chem 1994; 269:21644–21649.
53. Harrison DG, Freiman PC, Armstrong ML, Marcus ML, Heistad DD. Alterations in vascular reactivity in atherosclerosis. Circ Res 1987; 61:74–80.
54. Jayakody L, Senaratne M, Thomson A, Kappagoda T. Endothelium-dependent relaxation in experimental atherosclerosis in the rabbit. Circ Res 1987; 60:251–264.
55. Rossaint R, Falke K, Lopez F, Slama K, Pison U, Zapol W. Inhaled nitric oxide for the adult respiratory distress syndrome. N Engl J Med 1993; 328:399–405.
56. Scherrer U, Vollenweider L, Delabays A, Savcic M, Eichenberger U, Kleger G, Fikrle A, Ballmer P, Nicod P, Bartsch P. Inhaled nitric oxide for high-altitude pulmonary edema. N Engl J Med 1996; 334:624–629.
57. Pryor WA, Jin X, Squadrito GL. One- and two-electron oxidations of methionine by peroxynitrite. Proc Natl Acad Sci USA 1994; 91:11173–11177.
58. Salgo MG, Stone K, Squadrito GL, Battista JR, Pryor WA. Peroxynitrite causes DNA nicks in plasmid pBR322. Biochem Biophys Res Commun 1995; 210:1025–1030.
59. Darley-Usmar VM, Hogg N, O'Leary VJ, Moncada S. The simultaneous generation of superoxide and nitric oxide can initiate lipid peroxidation in human low-density lipoproteins. Free Radic Res Commun 1993; 17:19–20.
60. Carlsson LM, Jonsson J, Edlund T, Marklund SL. Mice lacking extracellular superoxide dismutase are more sensitive to hyperoxia. Proc Natl Acad Sci USA 1995; 92:6264–6268.
61. Stralin P, Karlsson K, Johansson BO, Marklund SL. The interstitium of the human arterial wall contains very large amounts of extracellular-superoxide dismutase. Arterioscler Thromb Vasc Biol 1995; 15:2032–2036.
62. Oury TD, Day BJ, Crapo JD. Extracellular superoxide dismutase in vessels and airways of humans and baboons. Free Radic Biol Med 1996; 20:957–965.
63. Sandström J, Carlsson L, Marklund S, Edlund T. The heparin-binding domain of extracellular superoxide dismutase C and formation of variants with reduced heparin affinity. J Biol Chem 1992; 267:18205–18209.
64. Edlund A, Edlund T, Hjalmarsson K, Marklund SL, Sandström J, Strömqvist M, Tibell L. A non-glycosylated extracellular superoxide dismutase variant. Biochem J 1992; 288:451–456.
65. Karlsson K, Edlund A, Sandström J, Marklund SL. Proteolytic modification of the heparin-binding affinity of extracellular superoxide dismutase. Biochem J 1993; 290:623–626.

66. Maridonneau-Parini I, Tringale SM, Tauber AI. Identification of distinct activation pathways of the human neutrophil NADPH-oxidase. J Immunol 1986; 137:2925–2929.
67. McCall TB, Boughton-Smith NK, Palmer RMJ, Whittle BJR, Moncada S. Synthesis of nitric oxide from L-arginine by neutrophils: release and interaction with superoxide anion. Biochem J 1989; 261:293–296.
68. Marklund SL. Regulation by cytokines of extracellular superoxide dismutase and other superoxide dismutase isoenzymes in fibroblasts. J Biol Chem 1992; 267: 6696–670.
69. Oury TD, Chang L-Y, Marklund SL, Day BJ, Crapo JD. Imunohistochemical localization of extracellular superoxide dismutase in human lung. Lab Invest 1994; 889–898.
70. Monboisse J-C, Gardes-Albert M, Randoux A, Borel J-P, Ferradini C. Non-enzymatic degradation of acid-soluble calf skin collagen by superoxide ion: protective effect of flavonoids. Biochem Pharmacol 1983; 32:53–58.
71. Riley DJ, Kerr JS, Laskin DL, Guss HN, Curran SF, Berg RA. Intratracheal instillation of collagen peptides induces a neutrophil influx in rat lungs. Trans Assoc Am Physicians 1984; 97:290–295.
72. Hansson L, Edlund M, Edlund A, Johansson T, Marklund SL, Fromm S, Strömqvist M, Törnell J. Expression and characterization of biologically active human extracellular superoxide dismutase in milk of transgenic mice. J Biol Chem 1994; 269: 5358–5363.
73. Boissinot M, Kuhn LA, Lee P, Fisher CL, Wang Y, Hallewell RA, Tainer JA. Rational design and expression of a heparin-targeted human superoxide dismutase. Biochem Biophys Res Commun 1993; 190:250–256.
74. Münzel T, Kurz S, Rajagopalan S, Thoenes M, Berrington WR, Thompson JA, Freeman BA, Harrison DG. Hydralazine prevents nitroglycerin tolerance by inhibiting activation of a membrane-bound NADH oxidase: a new action for an old drug. J Clin Invest 1996; 98:1465–1470.
75. Inoue M, Watanabe N, Matsuno K, Sasaki J, Tanaka Y, Hatanaka H, Amachi T. Expression of a hybrid Cu/Zn-type superoxide dismutase which has high affinity for heparin-like proteoglycans on vascular endothelial cells. J Biol Chem 1991; 266:16409–16414.
76. Abrahamsson T, Brandt U, Marklund SL, Sjoqvist P-O. Vascular bound recombinant extracellular superoxide dismutase type C protects against the detrimental effects of superoxide radicals in endothelium-dependent arterial relaxation. Circ Res 1992; 70:264–271.
77. Sjöquist P-O, Marklund SL. Endothelium bound extracellular superoxide dismutase type C reduces damage in reperfused ischaemic rat hearts. Cardiovasc Res 1992; 26:347–350.
78. Kohen R, Kakunda A, Rubinstein A. The role of cationized catalase and cationized glucose oxidase in mucosal oxidative damage induced in the rat jejunum. J Biol Chem 1992; 267:21349–21354.
79. Salin ML, McCord JM. Free radicals and inflammation. Protection of phagocytosing leukocytes by superoxide dismutase. J Clin Invest 1975; 56:1319–1323.
80. Schalkwijk J, van den Berg WB, van de Putte LB, Joosten LA, van den Bersselaar

L. Cationization of catalase, peroxidase, and superoxide dismutase. Effect of improved intraarticular retention on experimental arthritis in mice. J Clin Invest 1985; 76:198–205.

81. White CW, Jackson JH, Abuchowski A, Kazo GM, Mimmack RF, Berger EM, Freeman BA, McCord JM, Repine JE. Polyethylene glycol-attached antioxidant enzymes decrease pulmonary oxygen toxicity in rats. J Appl Physiol 1989; 66:584–590.
82. Pyatak PS, Abuchowski A, Davis FF. Preparation of a polyethylene glycol: superoxide dismutase adduct, and an examination of its blood circulation life and anti-inflammatory activity. Res Commun Chem Pathol Pharmacol 1980; 29:113–127.
83. Abuchowski A, McCoy JR, Palczuk NC, van Es T, Davis FF. Effect of covalent attachment of polyethylene glycol on immunogenicity and circulating life of bovine liver catalase. J Biol Chem 1977; 252:3582–3586.
84. Abuchowski A, van Es T, Palczuk NC, Davis FF. Alteration of immunological properties of bovine serum albumin by covalent attachment of polyethylene glycol. J Biol Chem 1977; 252:3578–3581.
85. Boni LT, Hah JS, Hui SW, Mukherjee P, Ho JT, Jung CY. Aggregation and fusion of unilamellar vesicles by poly(ethylene glycol). Biochim Biophys Acta 1984; 775: 409–418.
86. Beckman JS, Minor RL Jr, White CW, Repine JE, Rosen GM, Freeman BA. Superoxide dismutase and catalase conjugated to polyethylene glycol increases endothelial enzyme activity and oxidant resistance. J Biol Chem 1988; 263:6884–6892.
87. Tang G, White JE, Gordon RJ, Lumb PD, Tsan MF. Polyethylene glycol-conjugated superoxide dismutase protects rats against oxygen toxicity. J Appl Physiol 1993; 74:1425–1431.
88. Walther FJ, Nunez FL, David-Cu R, Hill KE. Mitigation of pulmonary oxygen toxicity in rats by intratracheal instillation of polyethylene glycol-conjugated antioxidant enzymes. Pediatr Res 1993; 33(pt 1):332–335.
89. Liu TH, Beckman JS, Freeman BA, Hogan EL, Hsu CY. Polyethylene glycol-conjugated superoxide dismutase and catalase reduce ischemic brain injury. Am J Physiol 1989; 256(pt 1):H589–H593.
90. Hiraoka Y, Kishimoto C, Takada H, Kurokawa M, Ochiai H, Shiraki K, Sasayama S. Role of oxygen derived free radicals.
91. Mihara K, Oka Y, Sawai K, Takakura Y, Hashida M. Improvement of therapeutic effect of human recombinant superoxide dismutase on ischemic acute renal failure in the rat via cationization and conjugation with polyethylene glycol. J Drug Target 1994; 2:317–321.
92. Mugge A, Elwell JH, Peterson TE, Hofmeyer TG, Heistad DD, Harrison DG. Chronic treatment with polyethylene-glycolated superoxide dismutase partially restores endothelium-dependent vascular relaxations in cholesterol-fed rabbits. Circ Res 1991; 69:1293–1300.
93. Young B, Runge JW, Waxman KS, Harrington T, Wilberger J, Muizelaar JP, Boddy A, Kupiec JW. Effects of pegorgotein on neurologic outcome of patients with severe head injury. A multicenter, randomized controlled trial. JAMA 1996; 276: 538–543.
94. Turrens JF, Crapo JD, Freeman BA. Protection against oxygen toxicity by intrave-

nous injection of liposome-entrapped catalase and superoxide dismutase. J Clin Invest 1984; 73:87–95.

95. Freeman BA, Turrens JF, Mirza Z, Crapo JD, Young SL. Modulation of oxidant lung injury by using liposome-entrapped superoxide dismutase and catalase. Fed Proc 1985; 44:2591–2595.
96. Padmanabhan RV, Gudapaty R, Liener IE, Schwartz BA, Hoidal JR. Protection against pulmonary oxygen toxicity in rats by the intratracheal administration of liposome-encapsulated superoxide dismutase or catalase. Am Rev Respir Dis 1985; 132:164–167.
97. Walther FJ, David-Cu R, Lopez SL. Antioxidant-surfactant liposomes mitigate hyperoxic lung injury in premature rabbits. Am J Physiol 1995; 269(pt 1):L613–L617.
98. Buckley BJ, Tanswell AK, Freeman BA. Liposome-mediated augmentation of catalase in alveolar type II cells protects against H_2O_2 injury. J Appl Physiol 1987; 63: 359–367.
99. Beckman JS, Minor RL Jr, Freeman BA. Augmentation of antioxidant enzymes in vascular endothelium. J Free Radic Biol Med 1986; 2:359–365.
100. Briscoe P, Caniggia I, Graves A, Benson B, Huang L, Tanswell AK, Freeman BA. Delivery of superoxide dismutase to pulmonary epithelium via pH-sensitive liposomes. Am J Physiol 1995; 268(pt 1):L374–L380.
101. Collins D, Litzinger DC, Huang L. Structural and functional comparisons of pH-sensitive liposomes composed of phosphatidylethanolamine and three different diacylsuccinylglycerols. Biochim Biophys Acta 1990; 1025:234–242.
102. White CR, Brock TA, Chang LY, Crapo JD, Briscoe P, Ku DD, Bradley WA, Gianturco SH, Gore J, Freeman BA, Tarpey MM. Superoxide and peroxynitrite in atherosclerosis. Proc Natl Acad Sci USA 1994; 91:1044–1048.
103. Rajagopalan S, Kurz S, Munzel T, Tarpey M, Freeman BA, Griendling KK, Harrison DG. Angiotensin II-mediated hypertension in the rat increases vascular superoxide production via membrane NADH/NADPH oxidase activation. Contribution to alterations of vasomotor tone. J Clin Invest 1996; 97:1916–1923.
104. Munzel T, Sayegh H, Freeman BA, Tarpey MM, Harrison DG. Evidence for enhanced vascular superoxide anion production in nitrate tolerance: a novel mechanism underlying tolerance and cross tolerance. J Clin Invest 1995; 95:187–194.
105. Walther FJ, David-Cu R, Supnet MC, Longo ML, Fan BR, Bruni R. Uptake of antioxidants in surfactant liposomes by cultured alveolar type II cells is enhanced by SP-A. Am J Physiol 1993; 265:L330–L339.
106. Woodle MC, Lasic DD. Sterically stabilized liposomes [review]. Biochim Biophys Acta 1992; 1113:171–199.
107. Matalon S, Holm BA, Baker RR, Whitfield MK, Freeman BA. Characterization of antioxidant activities of pulmonary surfactant mixtures. Biochim Biophys Acta 1990; 1035:121–127.
108. Nieves-Cruz B, Rivera A, Cifuentes J, Pataki G, Matalon S, Carlo WA, Tanswell AK, Freeman BA. Clinical surfactant preparations mediate SOD and catalase uptake by type II cells and lung tissue. Am J Physiol 1996; 270:L659–L667.
109. Curiel DT, Pilewski JM, Albelda SM. Gene therapy approaches for inherited and acquired lung disease. Am J Respir Mol Cell Biol 1996; 14:1–18.

110. Crystal RG. Transfer of genes to humans: early lessons and obstacles to success. Science 1995; 270:404–410.
111. Alton EW, Geddes DM. Gene therapy for cystic fibrosis: a clinical perspective. Gene Ther 1995; 2:88–95.
112. Coutelle C, Douar A-M, Colledge WH, Proster U. The challenge of fetal gene therapy. Nature Med 1995; 1:864–866.
113. Pitt BR, Robbins PD. Fetal gene therapy. Retrovirus-mediated gene therapy to fetal lung. Hum Mol Reprod 1996; 2:467–469.
114. McCray PB Jr, Thomas P, Faasee T, Wang G, O'Brien L, Davidson BL. Proliferation indices of pulmonary epithelia during human lung development: targeting gene transfer with integrating vectors [abstr]. Am J Respir Crit Care Med 1996; 153: A115.
115. Sekhorn HS, Larson JE. In utero gene transfer into the pulmonary epithelium. Nature Med 1995; 1:1201–1203.
116. Holzinger A, Trapnell BC, Weaver TE, Whitsett JA, Iwamoto HS. Intra-amniotic administration of an adenoviral vector for gene transfer to fetal sheep and mouse tissues. Pediatr Res 1995; 38:844–850.
117. McCray PB Jr, Armstrong K, Zabner J, Miller DW, Koretzky GA, Couture L, Robillard JE, Smith AE, Welsh MJ. Adeno-viral mediated gene transfer to fetal pulmonary epithelial in vitro and in vivo. J Clin Invest 1995; 95:2622–2632.
118. Vincent MC, Trapnell BC, Baughman RP, Weret SE, Whitsett JA, Iwamoto HS. Adenovirus-mediated gene transfer to the respiratory tract of fetal sheep in utero. Hum Gene Ther 1995; 6:1019–1028.
119. Katkin J, Seidner S, Langston C, Welty S. Delivery of a recombinant adenovirus to the lungs of premature primates: safety and efficacy [abstr]. Am J Respir Crit Care Med 1996; 153:A113.
120. Niu J, Perry R, Siddig M, Davis J, Horowitz S, Simon S, Langenback E, Parton L. Aerosolized gene delivery to piglets with cationic liposomes [abstr]. Am J Respir Crit Care Med 1996; 153:A765.
121. Stribling R, Brunette E, Liggett D, Gaensler K, Debs R. Aerosol gene delivery in vivo. Proc Natl Acad Sci USA 1992; 89:11277–11281.
122. Logan JL, Bebok Z, Walker LC, Peng S, Felgner PL, Siegal GP, Frizzell RA, Dong J, Howard M, Matalon S, Lindsey JR, DuVall M, Sorscher EJ. Cationic lipids for reporter gene and CFTR transfer to rat pulmonary epithelium. Gene Ther 1995; 2: 38–49.
123. Flotte TR, Afione SC, Conrad C, McGrath SA, Solow R, Oka H, Zeitlin PL, Guggino WB, Carter BJ. Stable in vivo expression of the cystic fibrosis transmembrane conductance regulator with an adeno-associated virus vector. Proc Natl Acad Sci USA 1993; 90:10613–10617.
124. Zeitlin PL, Chu S, McVeigh U, Ferguson K, Flotte TR, Guggino WB. Alveolar stem cell transduction by an adenovirus-associated viral vector. Gene Ther 1995; 2:623–631.
125. Ezurum SC, Lemarchand P, Rosenfeld MA, Yoo JH, Crystal RG. Protection of human endothelial cells from oxidant injury by adenovirus-mediated transfer of the human catalase cDNA. Nucleic Acids Res 1993; 21:1607–1612.
126. Tzeng E, Kim Y-M, Pitt BR, Lizonova A, Kovesdi L, Billiar TR. Adenoviral trans-

fer of the inducible nitric oxide synthase gene blocks endothelial cell apoptosis. Surgery 1997; 122:255–263.
127. Wong HR, Mannix RJ, Rusnak JM, Boota A, Zar H, Watkins SC, Lazo JS, Pitt BR. The heat shock response attenuates lipopolysaccharide-mediated apoptosis in cultured sheep pulmonary artery endothelial cells. Am J Respir Mol Cell Biol 1996; 15:745–751.
128. Schwarz MA, Lazo JS, Yalowich JC, Allen WP, Whitmore M, Bergonia HA, Tzeng E, Billiar TR, Robbins PD, Lancaster JR Jr, Pitt BR. Metallothioncin protects against the cytotoxic and DNA damaging effects of nitric oxide. Proc Natl Acad Sci USA 1995; 92:4452–4456.
129. Conary JT, Parker RE, Christman BW, Faulks RD, King GA, Meyrick BO, Brigham KL. Protection of rabbit lungs from endotoxin injury by in vivo hyperexpression of the prostaglandin G/H synthase gene. J Clin Invest 1994; 93:1834–1840.
130. Canonico AE, Brigham KL, Carmichael LC, Plitman JD, King GA, Blackwell TR, Christman JW. Plasmid–liposome transfer of an α_1 antitrypsin gene to cystic fibrosis bronchial epithelial cells prevents elastase-induced cell detachment and cytokine release. Am J Respir Cell Mol Biol 1996; 14:348–355.
131. Kolls J, Peppel K, Silva M, Beutler B. Prolonged and effective blockade of tumor necrosis factor activity through adenovirus-mediated gene transfer. Proc Natl Acad Sci USA 1994; 91:215–219.
132. Peault B, Tirouvanziam R, Sombardier M-N, Chen S, Perricaudet M, Gaillard D. Gene transfer to human fetal pulmonary tissue developed in immunodeficient SCID mice. Hum Gene Ther 1994; 5:1131–1137.
133. Deutsch GH, Wright E, Robbins PD, DeLuca NA, Pitt BR, Pilewski JM. Gene transfer to adult and fetal human airway epithelia using replication-deficient pseudotyped retrovirus and herpes simplex virus-1 [abstr]. Am J Respir Crit Care Med 1996; 153:A115.
134. Ballard PL, Zepeda ML, Schwartz M, Lopez N, Wilson JM. Adenovirus-mediated gene transfer to human fetal lung, ex vivo. Am J Physiol 1995; 268:L839–L845.
135. Carlsson LM, Jonsson J, Edlund T, Marklund SL. Mice lacking extracellular superoxide dismutase are more sensitive to hyperoxia. Proc Natl Acad Sci USA 1995; 92:6264–6268.
136. Miyanohara A, Yee J-K, Bouic K, Laporte P, Friedmann T. Efficient in vivo transduction of the neonatal mouse liver with pseudotyped retroviral vectors. Gene Ther 1995; 2:138–142.

37

Genetic Models for the Study of Autocrine–Paracrine Signaling in Lung Development and Repair

JEFFREY A. WHITSETT and THOMAS R. KORFHAGEN

University of Cincinnati College of Medicine
and Children's Hospital Medical Center
Cincinnati, Ohio

I. Introduction

The transgenic mouse is being actively applied to the study of lung morphogenesis and repair providing the ability to assess the function of regulatory molecules, cell matrix, and cell–cell interactions in vivo (1). In the mouse lung, morphogenesis begins on day 9 postconception as evagination of the foregut endoderm into the splanchnic mesenchyme. Thereafter, epithelial cells of the lung invade the mesenchyme, undergo branching morphogenesis and form the bronchi, bronchioles, and terminal airspaces. Underlying mesenchymal cells must also proliferate and differentiate to form the underlying stromal tissues, including cartilage, pulmonary vessels and supporting smooth muscle, capillaries, and other complex structures characteristic of the mature lung. Postnatally, these structures provide stable conducting airways and gas-exchange areas, protected by complex host defenses that keep the postnatal lung free of invading organisms. Although in vitro systems have been useful in the analysis of lung cell differentiation and gene expression, the application of transgenic mice to add or mutate genes in the developing lung in vivo has become useful in defining mechanisms that determine lung morphogenesis and repair. In the present chapter, we will discuss findings from experiments with transgenic mouse models used to study lung morphogenesis and repair, focusing on fibroblast growth factor-7 (FGF-7), transforming growth factor-α (TGF-α), and their receptors.

II. Role of Fibroblast Growth Factors

As in other organs systems undergoing branching morphogenesis, a critical role of the mesenchyme in formation of the respiratory tract was inferred from organ culture experiments in which removal of the mesenchyme from the epithelium of lung buds blocked branching morphogenesis (2). Soluble factors and direct cell–cell interactions have been postulated as providing the critical information required for lung growth and differentiation. The fibroblast growth factor (FGF) family of polypeptides has been recognized as important mesenchymal factors involved in the morphogenesis of various organs, including the lung.

The acidic fibroblast growth factor system consists of more than a dozen polypeptides and associated receptors that are increasingly recognized as playing an important role in organogenesis and in tissue repair (3,4). Of these, acidic FGF-7 (also termed KGF; keratinocyte growth factor), and the KGF receptor (also termed FGF-receptor 2; FGF-R2) have been implicated in epithelial proliferation or branching morphogenesis in the lung. FGF-7 is expressed in the mesenchyme of the developing lung throughout morphogenesis in close proximity to the invading respiratory epithelial cells of the lung buds (5). It interacts preferably with the FGF-R2. The FGF-R2–IIIb splice variant is the predominant FGF-R2 expressed in adult mouse lung. The FGF-R2 is expressed at high levels in the epithelial cells at the tips of lung buds throughout branching morphogenesis of the mouse lung (6). FGF-7 and acidic FGF bind to the FGF receptors and are potent mitogens for type II cells in vitro (7). Addition of FGF-7 to fetal epithelial cell cultures supports both growth and differentiation and maintains branching of lung buds in the absence of lung mesenchyme in vitro (8,9).

A. Expression of a Dominant–Negative FGF-R2 Receptor in the Developing Lung

The FGF receptors consist of an extracelluar ligand-binding domain, a transmembrane domain, and an intracellular kinase domain (3,4). Dimerization of the FGF receptor is induced by ligand binding. Phosphorylation of the intracellular, cytoplasmic domain occurs in response to dimer formation. Because of the homodimeric structures, these tyrosine kinase-mediated receptor systems are amenable to mutations that inactivate the receptor complex by formation of heterodimers of the mutated and wild-type receptor. The mutated receptor acts in a dominant–negative fashion to inhibit signaling of the normal receptor (10). Thus, deletion or mutation of the cytoplasmic domain creates a dominant–negative FGF receptor, capable of binding ligand and dimerizing with endogenous wild-type receptors, but incapable of signal transduction because phosphorylation of the cytoplasmic domains of the wild-type receptor is blocked by the mutant receptor. Inhibition of FGF-R2 signaling can be accomplished by high-level, cell-specific expression of the FGF-R2 dominant–negative receptor. Peters et al. employed the FGF-R2–IIIb splice variant to create an FGF dominant–negative receptor (Fig. 1). The mutant receptor was expressed under control of the surfactant protein C (SP-C) promoter to inhibit FGF signaling in the developing respiratory epithelium (11).

B. SP-C–FGF-R II D/N Transgenic Mice

Because of its colocalization with the expression of the FGF-R2, the SP-C promoter element from the human gene was used to inhibit FGF receptor signaling in the developing lung of transgenic mice. The human SP-C promoter is transcriptionally active as early as day 10 postconception, being expressed in the tips of developing lung buds (12) in a pattern similar to that of the FGF-R2. The SP-C

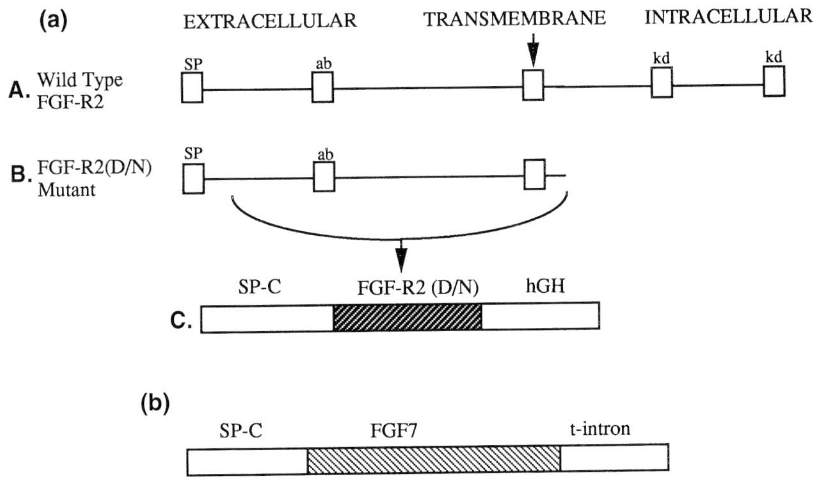

Figure 1 Transgenic constructs used to express the FGF-R2(D/N) receptor: (a) The FGF-R2 protein is represented by A. SP designates the signal peptide; ab, the acidic domain, and kd, the intracellular domains containing phosphorylation sites. The deleted receptor, consisting of the extracellular and transmembrane domains is illustrated by B. The transgene construct, illustrated in C, encodes the mutated FGF-R2. Termination signals from human growth hormone (hGH) were included to correctly terminate transcription. Vector sequences were deleted before microinjection of oocytes. (b) The SP-C–FGF-7 transgene directs the expression of the active FGF-7 (KGF) polypeptide in the developing respiratory epithelium. The plasmid was linearized to remove vector DNA and microinjected into oocytes to generate the SP-C–FGF-7 transgenic mice.

promoter is expressed throughout lung organogenesis and postnatally, when its transcriptional activity is restricted to distal bronchiolar and type II epithelial cells. The human SP-C promoter (3.7 kb) was used to generate a chimeric gene construct bearing the FGF-R D/N mutation (see Fig. 1). SP-C-FGF-R D/N plasmid DNA was injected into the male pronucleus of oocytes that were transferred to pseudopregnant foster mice.

Mice bearing the SP-C–FGF-R D/N died of respiratory failure at birth. SP-C–FGF-R (D/N)-bearing transgenic mice lacked distal pulmonary structures, the lungs consisting of a trachea and mainstem bronchi lined by columnar epithelial cells expressing CC10 (Fig. 2). Distal parenchymal tissues, including bronchioles and alveolar type II cells, were entirely lacking from these mice (Fig. 3). Likewise, the lungs of these transgenic mice lacked significant pulmonary vascular structures. In situ hybridization analysis of the transgenic mice using the CC10 as a probe demonstrated the presence of the conducting airways and lack of parenchymal compartments. Of interest, one transgenic SP-C–FGF-R2(D/N) mouse (with a partial defect in receptor signaling) produced hypoplastic lungs containing residual cells expressing SP-C mRNA. In contrast, most SP-C–FGF-R2(D/N)-bearing transgenic mice entirely lacked cells expressing endogenous SP-C mRNA. This partial defect is likely related to mosaicism, leading to partial inhibition of FGF-R2 signaling. Mosaicism occurs relatively frequently in transgenic mice and has limited expression of the transgene to only a subset of respiratory epithelial progenitor cells.

The findings of Peters et al. support the critical role of the FGF-R2 in branching morphogenesis and proliferation of the distal subsets of cells in the respiratory epithelium (11). The virtually complete loss of alveolar structures suggests a critical role of FGF receptors in proliferation of progenitor cells of the distal respiratory epithelium. The maintenance of the trachea and bronchi in the SP-C–FGF-R2(D/N) mice supports the possibility that a subset of cells of the foregut endoderm, distinct from those dependent on FGF signaling (or those expressing SP-C), is established before the activation of the SP-C promoter. Alternatively, cells of the proximal conducting airway, including the trachea and mainstem bronchi, may not require the function of the FGF receptor, or are responsive to growth factors other than FGF-7. The experiments with the FGF-D/N receptor supports the concept that FGF-7, produced by the lung mesenchyme, stimulates mitotic activity of progenitor cells in the developing respiratory epithelium. This conclusion is supported by the observation that FGF-7 activates proliferation of type II epithelial cells (7,8). Thus, the precise temporal–spatial expression of FGF-7 by mesenchymal cells near the tips of the branching lung buds is likely required for normal-branching morphogenesis of the lung. The finding that FGF-7 suffices to maintain branching and proliferation of fetal respiratory epithelial cells in the absence of mesenchyme in vitro (8,9) supports its fundamental role in lung morphogenesis.

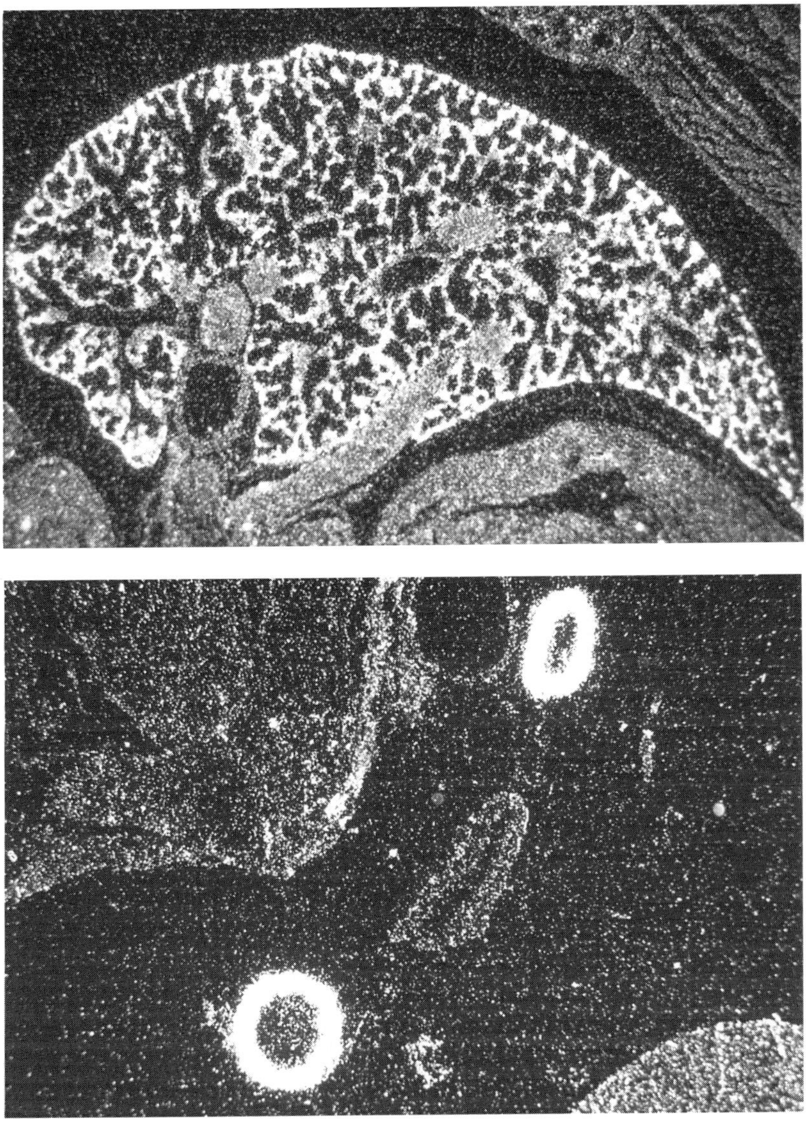

(a)

(b)

Figure 2 In situ hybridization of SP-C and CC10 mRNA in lungs from newborn SP-C–FGF-R2(D/N) transgenic mice: (a) The distribution of SP-C mRNA in lungs from a wild-type littermate. SP-C mRNA was entirely lacking in SP-C–FGF-R2(D/N) mice (not shown). (b) The distribution of CC10 mRNA (a marker of the conducting airway epithelium) in the SP-C–FGF-R2(D/N) mice, demonstrating the lack of parenchymal tissues and the simple bronchial tubules characteristic of these mice.

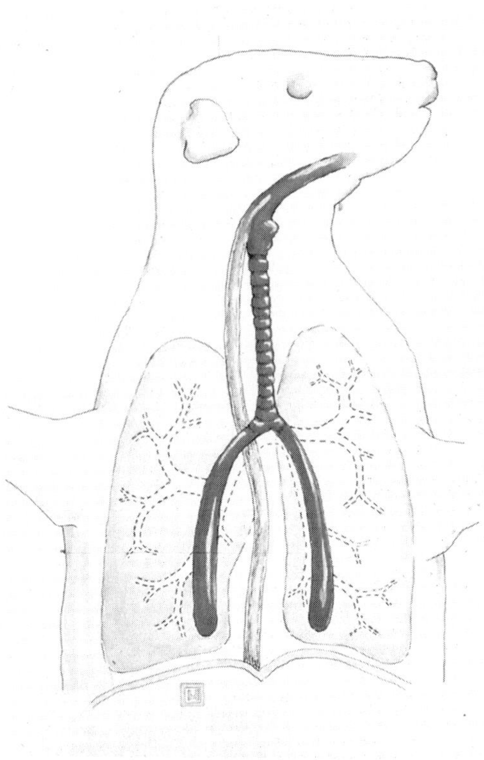

Figure 3 Reconstruction of residual lung tissue in the SP-C–FGF-R2(D/N) mice. (From Ref. 11.)

C. Expression of FGF-7 in the Lungs of Transgenic Mice

To assess the role of FGF-7 in the developing respiratory epithelium, Simonet et al. (13) produced transgenic mice in which the polypeptide was expressed under control of the SP-C promoter throughout lung development. This experiment was based on the hypothesis that precise temporal–spatial expression of FGF-7 in the lung is a critical determinate of branching morphogenesis. Human FGF-7 ligand was expressed in the respiratory epithelium under control of the SP-C promoter (see Fig. 1b). In initial experiments, transgenic mice bearing the SP-C–FGF-7 transgene were not readily identified in the offspring of the injected oocytes, suggesting the potential prenatal lethality of the construct. Transgenic mice were therefore obtained by hysterotomy on day 15–17 of gestation. Fetal mice bearing the SP-C–FGF-7 chimeric gene succumbed between days 15 and

17 of gestation; pathological findings were confined to the lung (Fig. 4). Although growth and organogenesis of the mouse pups appear to be normal, marked disruption of lung parenchyma was noted in the FGF-7 transgenic mice. SP-C–FGF-7 mice developed lung lesions histologically similar to cystadenomatoid malformations (CAM) of the lung. Marked cystic changes were observed in lung from most of the transgenic mice. The lesions were bilateral and the pathology of lung tissue varied from nearly solid lesions to fluid-filled cysts. Lung tissue lacked the normal-branching pattern of the fetal lung. Histopathological findings were confined to the lung and were consistent with the sites of expression of FGF-7 in the developing respiratory epithelium, as assessed by in situ hybridization. The level of expression of epithelial cell markers, such as SP-C, CC10, and SP-B mRNAs were not significantly altered in the transgenic mice; however, the orderly pattern of branching morphogenesis was markedly disrupted. These studies support the concept that precise temporal–spatial control of FGF-7 expression is required for the process of branching morphogenesis. The profound effects of altered FGF receptor signaling on fetal lung growth and branching morphogenesis support the important role of FGF-7 (produced by the stromal cells) and the FGF receptors present in respiratory epithelial cells (Fig. 5). The findings of Ullrich et al., demonstrating a marked proliferative effect of FGF-7 after intratracheal administration to adult rats in vivo (14), provides strong support for the importance of FGF receptor signaling in the respiratory epithelium in the postnatal lung, where it likely plays a role in regeneration of the respiratory epithelium following injury. Epithelial–mesenchymal interactions, mediated by FGF receptor activity are, therefore, likely to play an important role in the repair of lung parenchyma associated with bronchopulmonary dysplasia in infants recovering from respiratory distress syndrome.

The dilation of lung saccules in the lungs of fetal SP-C–FGF-7 mice suggests that FGF-7 activates ion transport and, in particular, Cl^-dependent fluid secretion (Zhou et al., unpublished observations). FGF-7 enhanced Cl^- transport and lung liquid production by the respiratory tract, a finding that may be relevant to the pathogenesis and therapy of cystic fibrosis.

III. TGF-α and EGF-R Signaling and Pulmonary Fibrosis and Airspace Remodeling

Transforming growth factor-alpha (TGF-α) is a member of the polypeptide growth factor family, including epidermal growth factor (EGF), heparin-binding EGF, and TGF-α. EGF family members bind to and activate EGF receptors in target tissues. Binding of EGF to its receptors activates dimerization and autophosphorylation of the cytoplasmic domain of the EGF receptors. Activation of EGF receptors induces a variety of cellular responses in target tissues, including

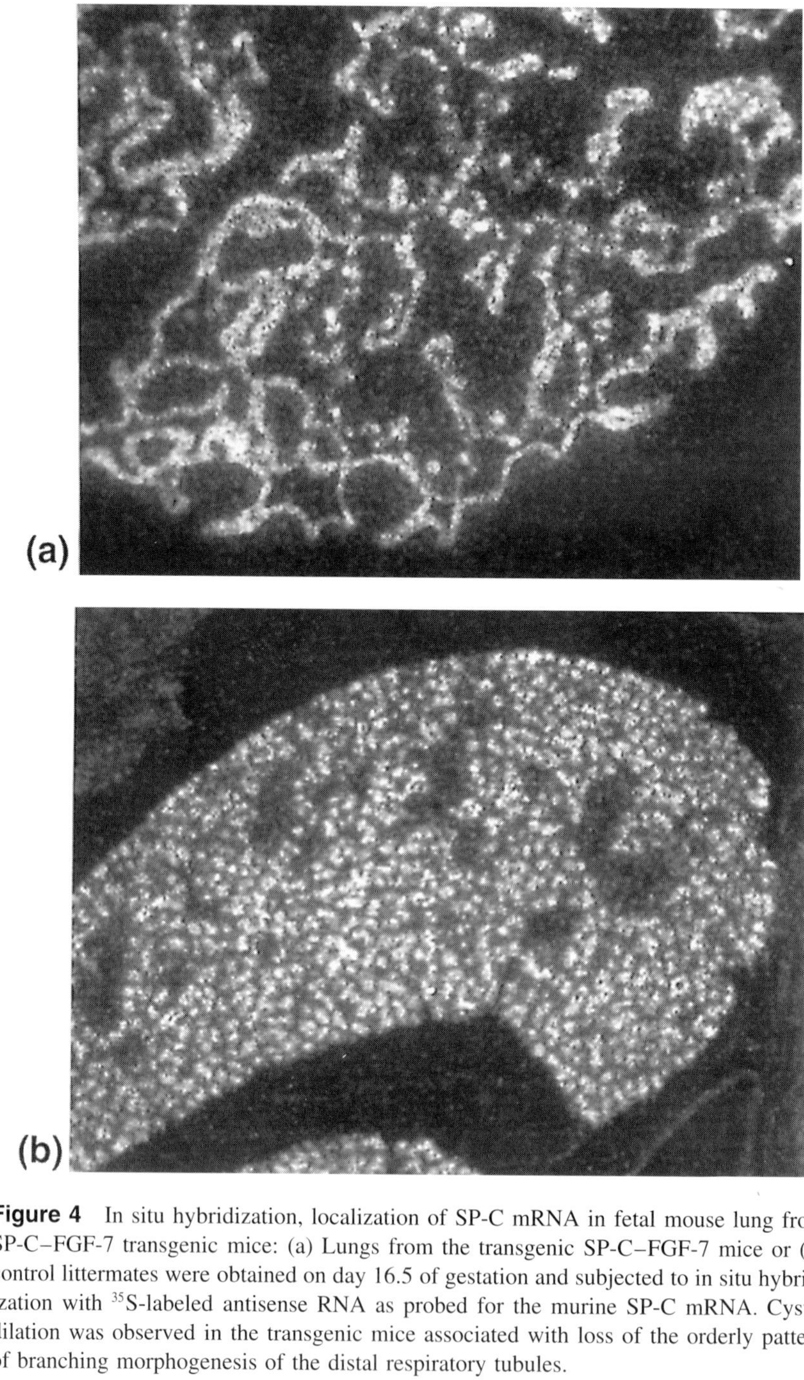

Figure 4 In situ hybridization, localization of SP-C mRNA in fetal mouse lung from SP-C–FGF-7 transgenic mice: (a) Lungs from the transgenic SP-C–FGF-7 mice or (b) control littermates were obtained on day 16.5 of gestation and subjected to in situ hybridization with ^{35}S-labeled antisense RNA as probed for the murine SP-C mRNA. Cystic dilation was observed in the transgenic mice associated with loss of the orderly pattern of branching morphogenesis of the distal respiratory tubules.

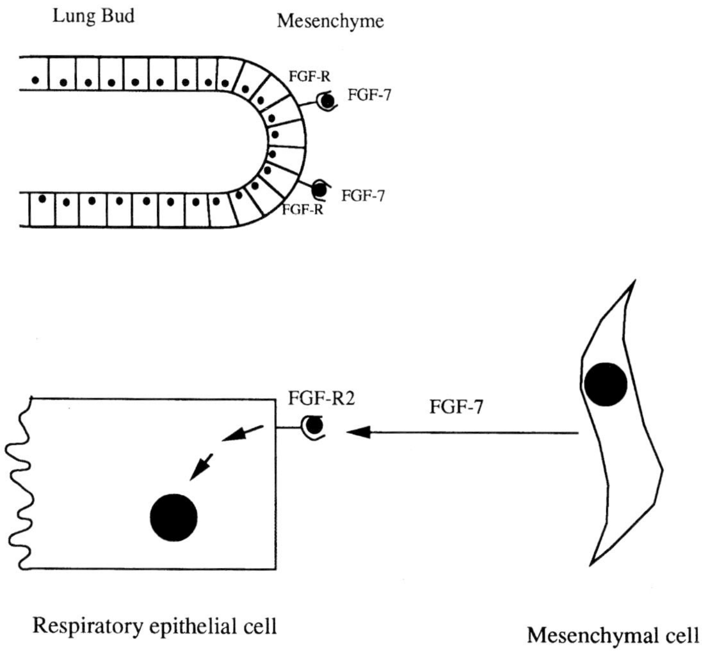

Figure 5 Proposed autocrine–paracrine signaling mediated by FGF-7 in branching morphogenesis of the lung: The precise temporal–spatial expression of FGF-7 by stromal cells leads to normal proliferation and branching morphogenesis of the respiratory epithelium, mediated by the interactions of FGF-7 with the FGF-R2 on respiratory epithelial progenitor cells.

DNA synthesis and changes in gene transcription. Both EGF receptors and EGF family members are expressed in developing and adult lung. EGF enhances type II cell proliferation and increases surfactant protein A synthesis (15,16). EGF, TGF-α, and other members of the EGF family are expressed by pulmonary epithelial cells following injury and have been postulated to play a role in lung fibrosis and repair (17,18).

Korfhagen et al. expressed human TGF-α under control of the SP-C promoter in alveolar cells of the developing respiratory epithelial cells of transgenic mice (20); (Fig. 6a). The SP-C–TGF-α transgenic mice developed marked pulmonary fibrosis. Peribronchial and pleural collagen deposition and alterations in elastin staining were noted in most animals. Alveolar airspaces were markedly enlarged. The effects of the TGF-α transgene were readily apparent within several weeks of age. The abnormalities of alveolar airspaces were observed at the time of birth, and the severity increased postnatally (Fig. 7). Pulmonary fibrosis ap-

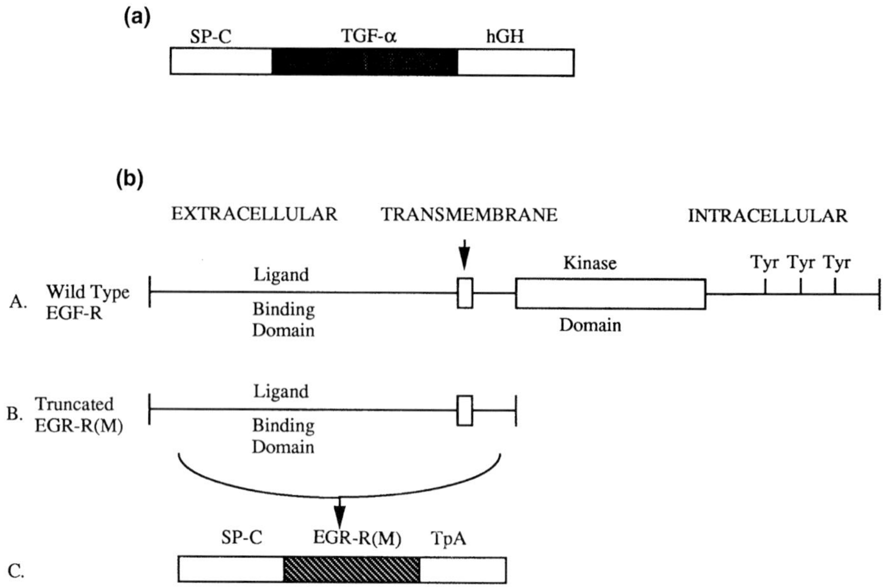

Figure 6 Transgenic constructs used to express TGF-α and the mutant EGF receptor. The SP-C promoter was used to drive expression of (a) the TGF-α cDNA construct, or (b) the dominant-negative EGF receptor generated by deletion of domains encoding the cytoplasmic kinase and phosphorylation sites (Tyr). Permanent transgenic lines were generated with each construct and were then crossed to generate bitransgenic mice expressing both TGF-α and the mutant EGF receptor in respiratory epithelial cells of mice.

peared later and was readily apparent by 3 or 4 weeks of age. The severity of pulmonary lesions correlated, in general, with the levels of TGF-α mRNA expression. Fibrotic lesions involve the airspaces, entrapping respiratory epithelial cells that express the TGF-α transgene. Although mRNA levels of TGF-β_1 were not altered in the TGF-α-expressing transgenic mice, the expression of EGF receptor mRNA was increased in the stromal cells of the fibrotic lesions. The finding that the EGF receptor was increased in the fibrotic lesions suggests that a local paracrine effect of TGF-α (produced by the epithelial cells under control of the SP-C promoter) increased EGF receptor expression on stromal cells. The mechanisms by which epithelial expression of TGF-α produces the pulmonary fibrosis and alveolar hypoplasia are still unclear, but do not appear to be related to inflammation. Pulmonary fibrosis and alveolar hypoplasia seen in the SP-C–TGF-α mice were associated with abnormalities in lung compliance.

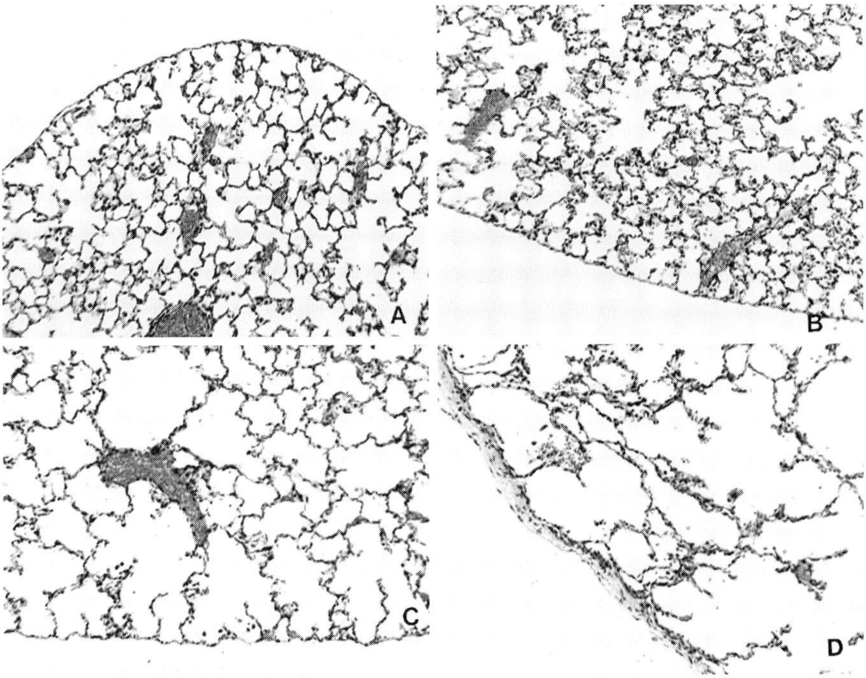

Figure 7 Lung histology of SP-C–TGF-α, SP-C–EGF-R/M, and bitransgenic mice: (A) Lung from an age-matched nontransgenic mouse; (B) lung tissue from an SP-C–EGF-R/M mouse, showing no histologically detectable lung abnormalities; (C) lung tissue from a bitransgenic SP-C–TGF-α × SP-C–EGF-R/M mouse showing correction of pleural fibrosis and airspace hypoplasia; (D) lung from an adult SP-C–TGF-α transgenic mouse showing pleural fibrosis and enlarged airspaces.

A. Role of Respiratory Epithelium in the Generation of Pulmonary Lesions in the TGF-α-Expressing Transgenic Mice

To assess whether autocrine or autocrine–paracrine mechanisms might contribute to the intracellular signaling involved in the TGF-α-induced lung lesions, transgenic mice were generated in which a mutated EGF receptor (EGF-R/M), lacking the cytoplasmic domain and tyrosine phosphorylation sites required for intracellular signaling of the EGF receptor, was expressed in the respiratory epithelium under control of the SP-C promoter in transgenic mice (see Fig. 6b). The EGF-R/M was designed to allow heterodimerization of the mutant receptor with the wild-type EGF receptors in respiratory epithelial cells. Such receptor heterodimers are capable of binding EGF-α, TGF-α, or other EGF family members; however, the intracellular signaling is inhibited owing to a dominant–negative effect of the mutant receptor on phosphorylation of the wild-type receptor. When expressed under control of the SP-C promoter; the transgene blocks receptor signaling only in the respiratory epithelium and is not expressed (see Fig. 6b). EGF dominant–negative receptors have been used previously in vitro, blocking EGF-mediated signal transduction and growth in several cell model systems (21–23). The SP-C promoter was used to express the mutant EGF-R in bronchiolar and alveolar epithelial cells of the developing and postnatal lungs of the transgenic mice. Several permanent lines of the SP-C–EGF-R/M transgenic mice were produced. The SP-C–EGF-R/M mice developed normally under routine laboratory conditions. No apparent abnormalities of lung morphology were observed in the SP-C–EGF-R transgenic mice, suggesting that the EGF receptors in the developing respiratory epithelium are not critical to lung development or function under normal conditions (see Fig. 7). These findings are supported by the findings of relatively normal branching morphogenesis and lung function noted in the lungs of wa-2/wa-2 mice, which are deficient in EGF-R signaling, and in EGF-R knockout mice (24,25).

B. Bitransgenic SP-C–EGF-R/M × SP-C–TGF-α Mice

Some SP-C–EGF-R mice were bred to the SP-C–TGF-α mice to assess whether inhibition of epithelial cell EGF-R signaling corrected the lung pathology characteristic of the SP-C–TGF-α mice. In breeding experiments with several distinct lines of SP-C–TGF-α and SP-C–EGF-R mutant mice, the TGF-α-induced lung disease was nearly completely ameliorated in the bitransgenic offspring (see Fig. 7). Both airspace remodeling and pulmonary fibrosis were nearly fully corrected in the bitransgenic mice. The levels of TGF-α mRNA in the lungs of the bitransgenic mice were not altered, suggesting that changes in TGF-α expression were not involved in the correction of the lesions. These findings strongly support the concept that TGF-α-induced pulmonary fibrosis and airspace remodeling, at least in part, involve an autocrine mechanism dependent on EGF receptors on the type II and distal bronchiolar epithelial cells expressing the transgene. TGF-α-induced pulmonary fibrosis and airspace remodeling was dependent on the function of EGF receptors in pulmonary epithelial cells. The stromal cell proliferation observed in the TGF-α transgenic mice is likely dependent on an autocrine signal (TGF-α) that enhances proliferative activity of stromal cells in a paracrine manner. Although TGF-α may exert a direct paracrine effect on stromal cells (as suggested by the increase in EGF receptors on stromal cells), paracrine signaling alone does not appear to be sufficient for the development of pulmonary lesions and requires the activity of EGF receptors on type II and bronchiolar epithelial cells.

These experiments support the presence of an autocrine–paracrine pathway by which epithelial cell TGF-α stimulates cell signaling pathways in the epithelium itself to signal, through paracrine mechanisms, stromal cell proliferation and pulmonary fibrosis, but they do not rule out a combined effect of a TGF-α-dependent paracrine loop that might also contribute to the pulmonary lesion seen in the SP-C–TGF-α mice. The SP-C–EGF-R/M mice provide a framework for future experimentation to assess the potential role of TGF-α and EGF receptors in the pathogenesis of pulmonary fibrosis in lung injury following a variety of injuries and diseases, including cystic fibrosis, idiopathic pulmonary fibrosis, bronchopulmonary dysplasia (BPD), and recovery from adult respiratory distress syndrome (ARDS). Expression of TGF-α and EGF has been demonstrated in the respiratory epithelium or alveolar macrophages after lung injury (26). The finding that the EGF receptor signaling is involved in pathogenesis of fibrosis in the TGF-α mice supports a framework for developing therapies to inhibit the autocrine–paracrine loop involved in EGF-dependent lung fibrosis and remodeling. Therapies designed to inhibit EGF receptor signaling, whether pharmacologic or genetic, may be of use for therapy of fibrotic lung disease in the future.

IV. Bronchopulmonary Dysplasia

Bronchopulmonary dysplasia (BPD) was first described by Northway et al. (26) in premature human infants treated for respiratory distress syndrome (RDS). Likewise, similar pulmonary lesions were observed in neonatal mice exposed to high concentrations of oxygen during the neonatal period (27). The pathogenesis of the fibrosis and parenchymal remodeling seen in the lungs of infants with BPD is complex and includes the influence of both oxygen injury, barotrauma, infection, and host responses. Ultimately, BPD is associated with decreased DNA content, alveolar airspace remodeling, pulmonary fibrosis, and emphysema. The repair of the lung in BPD is dependent on cell proliferation and remodeling of both epithelial and stromal compartments, ultimately leading to the reorganization of lung parenchyma that allows the close apposition of alveolar epithelial cells and capillary endothelial cells required for efficient gas exchange in the alveolus. Cell proliferation, remodeling, and differentiation of the cuboidal type II cells to form type I epithelial cells leads to restoration of epithelial–capillary surfaces in the alveoli. Recovery of the injured lung, therefore, is likely to depend on the restoration of interactions between stromal and epithelial cells that likely recapitulate many of the cellular interactions required for normal fetal and neonatal lung development. Although the precise molecules involved in the repair of the lung lesions in BPD are not fully established, several polypeptides, including TGF-α and FGF family members are expressed in both developing and injured lung and are likely to play critical roles in the pathogenesis and recovery from lung injury.

V. Summary

Transgenic mice have been used to explore potential roles of the FGF and EGF receptor systems in the fetal and postnatal lung. These studies demonstrate the usefulness of dominant–negative receptors and the expression of active polypeptides in the developing respiratory tract that have revealed unanticipated and profound roles of both FGF-7 and FGF-R2 in the morphogenesis of the lung. The finding that FGF-7 is a potent mitogen in the postnatal lung supports a potential role in repair following lung injury. Because FGF-7 is expressed in the developing mesenchyme of the lung, these findings support important paracrine regulation (mediated by FGF-7 binding to FGF receptors) as a requirement for the precise branching morphogenesis associated with lung development, a process that is likely recapitulated during recovery from lung injury. Disruption of the precise temporal–spatial expression of FGF-7 may also be a factor in abnormalities of fetal lung development. Although EGF receptors in the respiratory epithelium do not appear to be required for lung morphogenesis or function at birth, mice expressing TGF-α developed severe airspace remodeling and pulmonary fibrosis in the postnatal period. These transgenic mice have revealed a potential role of autocrine–paracrine signaling, dependent on the EGF receptor in the respiratory epithelium, in the pathogenesis of pulmonary fibrosis. Whether similar autocrine–paracrine interactions are involved in the pathogenesis of lung fibrosis in the developing and adult lung remains to be elucidated.

Cell-specific addition and deletion of the signaling molecules or their receptors in the lungs of transgenic mice provides a powerful bridge between in vitro and in vivo studies that are contributing to our understanding of the actions of polypeptide growth factors on cell proliferation and differentiation. Transgenic mice provide an unique in vivo model useful in the study of autocrine–paracrine-signaling pathways active during lung development. Such models may be useful in understanding the role of these signaling pathways in injury and repair of the developing and mature lung.

Acknowledgments

RDP Center for Cystic Fibrosis and Other Lung Diseases, Programs of Excellence in Molecular Biology (HL 51835), and Center for Gene Therapy (HL 38859).

References

1. Glasser SW, et al. Transgenic models for study of pulmonary development and disease. Am J Physiol 1994; 267:L489–L497.

2. Wessels NK. Mammalian lung development: interactions in formation and morphogenesis of tracheal buds. J Exp Zool 1979; 175:445–460.
3. Givol D, Yayon A. Complexity of FGF-receptors: genetic basis for structure diversity and functional specificity. FASEB J 1992; 6:3362–3369.
4. Gospodarowicz D. Fibroblast growth factor and its involvement in developmental processes. Curr Top Dev Biol 1990; 24:57–93.
5. Mason IJ, et al. FGF-7 (keratinocyte growth factor) expression during mouse development suggests roles in myogenesis, forebrain regionalization and epithelial–mesenchymal interactions. Mech Dev 1994; 45:15–30.
6. Peters KG, et al. Two FGF receptor genes are differentially expressed in epithelial and mesenchymal tissues during limb formation and organogenesis in the mouse. Development 1992; 114:233–243.
7. Panos RJ, et al. Keratinocyte growth factor and hepatocyte growth factor are heparin-binding growth factors for alveolar type II cells in fibroblast conditioned medium. J Clin Invest 1993; 92:969–977.
8. Deterding RR, Shannon JM. Proliferation and differentiation of total pulmonary epithelium in the absence of mesenchyme. J Clin Invest 1995; 95:2963–2972.
9. Nogawa H, Ito T. Branching morphogenesis of embryonic mouse lung epithelium in mesenchyme free culture. Development 1995; 121:1015–1022.
10. Ueno H, et al. Dominant–negative mutations of platelet-derived growth factor (PDGF) receptors. Inhibition of receptor function by ligand-dependent formation of heterodimers between PDGF α and β receptors. J Biol Chem 1993; 268:22814–22819.
11. Peters K, et al. Targeted expression of a dominant negative FGF receptor blocks branching morphogenesis and epithelial differentiation of the mouse lung. EMBO J 1994; 13:3296–3301.
12. Wert SE, et al. Transcriptional elements from the human SP-C gene direct expression in the primordial respiratory epithelium of transgenic mice. Dev Biol 1993; 156: 426–443.
13. Simonet WS, et al. Pulmonary malformation in transgenic mice expressing human keratinocyte growth factor in the lung. Proc Natl Acad Sci USA 1995; 92:12461–12465.
14. Ulich TR, et al. Keratinocyte growth factor is a growth factor for type II pneumocytes in vivo. J Clin Invest 1994; 93:1298–1306.
15. Ryan RM, et al. Growth factors alter neonatal type II cell alveolar epithelial cell proliferation. Am J Physiol 1994; 266:L17–L22.
16. Whitsett JA, et al. Differential effects of epidermal growth factor and transforming growth factor-β on synthesis of M_r = 35,000 surfactant-associated protein in fetal lung. J Biol Chem 1987; 262:7908–7913.
17. Stahlman MT, et al. Immunocytochemical localization of epidermal growth factor in the developing human respiratory system and in acute and chronic lung disease in the neonate. Lab Invest 1989; 60:539–547.
18. Madtes DK, et al. Expression of transforming growth factor-α and epidermal growth factor receptor is increased following bleomycin-induced lung injury in rats. Am J Respir Cell Mol Biol 1994; 11:540–551.
19. Vivekananda J, et al. Acute inflammatory injury in the lung precipitated by oxidant

stress induces fibroblasts to synthesize and release transforming growth factor-α. J Biol Chem 1994; 269:25057–25061.

20. Korfhagen TR, et al. Respiratory epithelial cell expression of human transforming growth factor-α induces lung fibrosis in transgenic mice. J Clin Invest 1994; 93: 1691–1699.
21. Kashles O, et al. A dominant negative mutation suppresses the function of normal epidermal growth factor receptors by heterodimerization. Mol Cell Biol 1991; 11: 1454–1463.
22. Honegger AM, et al. Evidence for epidermal growth factor (EGF)-induced intermolecular autophosphorylation of the EGF receptors in living cells. Mol Cell Biol 1990; 10:4035–4044.
23. Redemann N, et al. Anti-oncogenic activity of signalling-defective epidermal growth factor receptor mutants. Mol Cell Biol 1992; 12:491–498.
24. Threadgill DW, et al. Targeted disruption of mouse EGF receptor: effect of genetic background on mutant phenotype. Science 1995; 269:230–238.
25. Fowler KJ, et al. A mutation in the epidermal growth factor receptor in waved-2 mice has a profound effect on receptor biochemistry that results in impaired lactation. Proc Natl Acad Sci USA 1995; 92:1465–1469.
26. Northway WH, et al. Pulmonary disease following respirator therapy of hyaline membrane disease. N Engl J Med 1967; 276:357–358.
27. Northway WH, et al. Quantitative aspects of oxygen toxicity in the newborn: inhibition of lung DNA synthesis in the mouse. Pediatrics 1972; 50:67–72.
28. Madtes DK, et al. Induction of transforming growth factor-alpha in activated human alveolar macrophage. Cell 1988; 53:285–293.

38

Animal Models of Chronic Lung Injury

JACQUELINE J. COALSON and STEVEN R. SEIDNER

University of Texas Health Science Center
San Antonio, Texas

ROBERT A. De LEMOS*

University of Southern California,
Los Angeles, California

I. Introduction

The search for the appropriate experimental model for bronchopulmonary dysplasia (BPD) is ongoing owing to the complex multifactorial etiology and pathogenesis of the disease. In this era of prenatal glucocorticoid treatment and postnatal surfactant therapy, disruption of normal intrauterine lung growth yields an increasingly immature lung to which injury is augmented by exposure to oxygen levels above that of the uterine environment; tissue stress, induced by excessive pressure or stretch; and inflammation or infection. Clinicians readily recognize the difference in treating a 24-week–gestation human infant of borderline viability when compared with that of a 30-week–gestation infant. Considerable lung growth and differentiation normally occurs during this gestational period. At 24 weeks, lungs are still in a canalicular stage (1–3); for example, vascular development at the capillary level has been ongoing for only about 6 weeks (3), no alveolar macrophages are present (4), and surfactant secretion is negligible (5). Immaturity of nonpulmonary organ systems, such as the kidney, heart, and gastrointestinal tract, further complicate the pulmonary status of these immature infants. Finally, factors known to initiate preterm deliveries in the human, such as chorioamnionitis and premature rupture of membranes (6–8), probably influence the

*Deceased.

human disease, but are not likely to be modeled in another species. The advantages of an animal model remain that of the standardization of time, use of common etiologic initiators, availability and standardized sampling of tissues and body fluids, predictability of lung injury patterns, and a means by which interventional therapies can be used to study mechanisms of lung adaptation to extrauterine growth and differentiation.

II. What Is the Human Disease That Needs to Be Modeled?

A. BPD and Chronic Lung Disease of Infancy

In the past 15 years, there has been a dramatic change in the nature of chronic lung disease in surviving premature infants (9,10). In the classic description of BPD by Northway et al., all infants began with severe hyaline membrane disease (HMD), necessitating the use of high ventilator pressures and supplemental oxygen, and then evolved through the ''exudative'' phase to chronic lung illness (11). In 1977, over 40% of infants surviving until discharge ultimately died of the complications of cor pulmonale (12). Bonikos et al. more fully described the pathological features, which included squamous metaplasia, bronchiolar smooth-muscle hypertrophy, alternating areas of overinflation and atelectasis, fibroproliferative changes in the lung parenchyma, inflammation, and chronic vascular changes (13). Pulmonary immaturity, oxygen toxicity, pulmonary barotrauma, and infection were thought to be the major factors in pathogenesis.

The introduction of surfactant replacement therapy, use of antenatal glucocorticoids, and changes in ventilatory management have combined to change the incidence and nature of BPD (14–21). Ogawa reported that only 30% of infants with BPD followed the classic pattern, and another third had no clinically apparent lung disease at the time of birth (22). Recently, Rojas et al. noted that BPD developed most often in immature infants who initially had minimal pulmonary dysfunction (10). They determined that immaturity, persistence of a patent ductus arteriosus (PDA), and infection were major pathogenetic factors. The majority of this new generation of BPD infants are oxygen-independent and have normal chest radiographs by 2 months of age but, based on clinical and laboratory data, it is likely that all have significant and irreversible decreases in pulmonary reserve (23–26).

Both the classic and the milder patterns of BPD show clinical and radiographic evidence of pulmonary edema as a consistent feature of evolution into chronic lung disease. Although human pathological data in this window are not available, the clinical and laboratory findings are consistent with the diffuse alveolar damage (DAD) lesion described by Coalson et al. in the premature baboon with HMD–BPD (27). It is likely that the increase in alveolar–capillary permeability characteristic of this stage in the injury process is related to an active inflammatory response caused by oxygen toxicity, ventilator-related injury, infection, or some combination of these factors. The resultant changes in lung compliance, surface tension, and oxygenation increase the need for mechanical ventilation and supplemental oxygen, increasing the likelihood of additive injury. These factors can lead, singly or in combination, to the development of persistent lung injury, which then sets the stage for development of BPD.

B. Characteristics of Acute Versus Chronic Lung Injuries

A fairly consistent response of the lung to injury can be induced by several agents, and one pattern of an acute injury response is called diffuse alveolar damage (DAD; 28,29). This stereotypical pattern of lung injury and repair has an exudative phase, which includes congestion, edema, microatelectasis, and formation of hyaline membranes (29). During the 1960s, experimental studies of sepsis- and hemorrhage-induced shock elicited an exudative phase of DAD, but not the proliferative phase, during which changes of epithelial type 2 cell hyperplasia and interstitial fibroproliferation dominate (30,31). The proliferative phase of DAD is delayed (5–7 days following injury), and it has been difficult to "titrate" an experimental injury that will both induce exudative DAD lesions, and then persist into a proliferative phase without killing the animal.

However, the healing response in the immature infant may differ from that in the adult. Recent reports of lung pathology in humans and induced BPD in a baboon model show a relative lack of intramural organization (32,33), a specific type of healing response in which fibroblasts, myofibroblasts, and endothelial cells migrate into a fibrin-rich matrix in the alveolar space. This correlates with the work of Idell and Viscardi and their co-workers (34,35), who demonstrated increased fibrinolytic activity in human and baboon neonates with BPD, which likely enhanced the dissolution of the intra-alveolar proteinaceous exudate (hyaline membranes) that formed during the exudative phase of BPD.

Numerous agents have been used to induce experimental models of diffuse alveolar injury: *N*-nitroso-*N*-methylurethane (NNMU), oleic acid, bleomycin, paraquat, irradiation, and hyperoxia (reviewed in 36). Most of the studies using these agents have been performed in mature species, except for hyperoxia, which has been used in premature and newborn species (see later discussion). The response of the immature lung to acute alveolar injury has been examined in the rabbit, monkey, sheep, pig, and several rodents. In this review, models that include species of premature of neonatal age, chronicity of time, and mechanical ventilatory support for viability or maintenance will be emphasized.

III. Contributors to the Development of BPD

A. Immaturity

Special Features of Immaturity Affect Model Development

Bronchopulmonary dysplasia is the end result of lung injury in a developmentally unique host. Its uniqueness as a clinical and pathological entity is largely accounted for by several concurrent biological events: (1) the normal developmental profile of the fetal and newborn lung; (2) its perturbation by labor, delivery, and postnatal adaptation; and (3) the response of the immature lung to various insults. The challenge in developing an animal homologue of BPD is to bring these elements together in a model system that allows control of both the developmental variables and the injuries.

There are ample data to support the hypothesis that injury responses of the newborn lung are qualitatively or quantitatively different from those of adults. The coagulation–fibrinolytic responses differ (34). Newborn animals of most species are more resistant to pulmonary oxygen injury than adults (37). Although this may be partly related to the newborn's unique ability to undergo induction of antioxidant enzymes, recent data suggest that a less effective inflammatory response also may be contributory (38,39) (see Chap. 33). Regardless of the nature of the injury, alveolar capillary permeability is altered more in immature than mature animals (40,41). These observations, along with others, point to the need to have both species and developmental similarities between an animal model and the human disease.

Premature birth and survival alter the normal timetable of fetal development. Since the initial observation that administration of glucocorticoids to the fetal lamb accelerated lung maturation (42), much experimental data have documented the effects of several hormones on fetal lung development (43–47). Studies in preterm baboons demonstrated that birth and postnatal adaptation are associated with precocious maturation of multiple systems, presumably secondary to changes in gene expression. Following premature birth and survival, some genes upregulate in a "mature manner," and others either do not respond or are capable of only limited response (48). In one illustrative example, Minoo and co-workers demonstrated that the production of surfactant protein genes, SP-A, SP-B, and SP-C, all increase following preterm delivery, but that the abundance of mRNA for SP-A and levels of protein never reach that of a term infant (49–51). It is likely that this defect in expression of SP-A reflects injury to the premature lung.

More recently, Jones et al. (52) described decreased expression of the anti-inflammatory cytokine interleukin (IL)-10 in lung cells from premature human infants with HMD. This developmental delay in IL-10 had been observed earlier in neonatal blood monocytes and T cells (53). It is likely that additional aberrations in gene expression associated with premature birth will be discovered in the future, thus providing a molecular basis for the unique responses of the premature lung to injury. Once this molecular profile is fully defined, it may be possible to select models targeted to a homologous system of interest. Short of this futuristic goal, the only way to develop a homologue of the human disease is to mimic the human condition in which the injury responses are to be assessed.

B. Hyperoxia

In spite of considerable controversy surrounding the relative roles of ventilator-induced injury and oxygen toxicity in the pathogenesis of BPD in humans, there is no question that the triad of altered inflation pattern, airway lesions, and fibroproliferative change have been replicated in newborn and adult animals by prolonged exposure to various levels of hyperoxia (54–62). Likewise, a DAD lesion can be induced with acute or subacute exposure in most species (63). Thus, by using morphological endpoints as one way of defining BPD, it is possible to reproduce many of its pathological findings in hyperoxic, spontaneously breathing or mechanically ventilated animals.

Investigators have used preterm and term newborn rats, mice, rabbits, sheep, and piglets to study the mechanisms underlying developmental differences in injury response to hyperoxia. Several studies have shown that the newborn pig, rat, mouse, and rabbit are relatively oxygen-resistant (63,64). In 1966, Polger et al. exposed newborn mice to 100% oxygen for 8 days, following which the survivors showed no lung lesions, whereas adult mice comparably exposed died with exudative lung changes (65). Hellstrom and Nergardlt exposed mice to 100% oxygen for 5–25 days (54). The lack of an exudative response was noted, and in those animals exposed for the longer time periods, a mixed emphysema and patchy atelectasis pattern was described. Bonikos et al. reported ultrastructural changes of epithelial and endothelial cellular damage in newborn mice exposed to 100% oxygen for 7 days (66). In a longer 6-week exposure study, progressive pulmonary changes were demonstrated, with emphysema grossly apparent at 3 weeks. Forty weeks after removal from oxygen, airway lesions and alveolar septal fibrosis were present (58). The same investigators also looked at the effects of a 6-week exposure to an FIO_2 of 0.8 in newborn mice (60). Compared with their earlier 100% O_2-exposed group, there was less hyperplasia of type II and bronchiolar cells, with greater peribronchiolar and parenchymal fibrosis.

Newborn rats also have been used as models of hyperoxic lung injury. Because the newborn rat is incompletely alveolarized at birth, this has been a useful model with which to study postnatal influences on alveolarization. Exposure of 1-day-old rat pups to 46% oxygen resulted in decreased lung weight and volume, and decreased alveolar number and surface area (67). Prolonged higher levels of oxygen cause bronchiolar hyperplasia and metaplasia, bullae, and emphysema in 1-month-old rats (55). Randall et al. used newborn rats exposed for 1 week to an FIO_2 of 0.85. When examined at 40 days, these animals had abnormally large airspaces, suggesting perturbations of alveolar development (61). Tierney at al. studied adult rats exposed for 7 days to FIO_2 0.85 followed by FIO_2 1.0 for 6 weeks and found the survivors to have bullae, fibrosis, and emphysema (59). Roberts et al. (68) demonstrated decreased pulmonary capillaries after 6 days of exposure to FIO_2 of 1.0, but this lesion was reversible after 2 weeks of recovery. Chronic vascular changes of muscular extension into peripheral arteries, medial hypertrophy of muscular arteries, and loss of smaller arteries also have been produced in the newborn rat model by various investigators (69, reviewed in 70). The results of these and other studies demonstrate that hyperoxic lung injury mimics most of the pathological features of bronchopulmonary dysplasia in humans, and lends support to those who theorize that free radical injury plays a major role in pathogenesis of the human illness.

Susceptibility to pulmonary oxygen injury varies with development and among species (37,63,64). An understanding of the mechanisms underlying these developmental differences is useful, as it may give some insight into the specific vulnerabilities of the immature subject. Keeney et al. (71), in a preterm rat model, showed that antenatal dexamethasone induced antioxidant enzyme activity in the preterm rat, but that once induced, the responses were similar to the term animal. The same group has recently reported that resistance to oxygen injury in the term rat is related to decreased neonatal inflammatory responses, confirming the earlier observations of others who related various types of lung injury to inflammation in newborns (72). Frank et al. (73) demonstrated that tissue concentrations of the lung antioxidant enzyme activities in the rat fetus increased at approximately the same time as that of the surfactant system. In another study, Frank and his co-workers (74) showed that, unlike the term rabbit, preterm rabbits did not have an increase of antioxidant enzymes in the lungs when they were exposed to hyperoxia. If these data are applied to the human premature infant, they would imply extreme vulnerability to oxidant injury and the possibility that even exposure to ambient oxygen by the extremely immature infant might be injurious.

However, studies done with animals more immature than those used by Frank et al. (74) suggested that premature infants may be more resistant to hyperoxia than adults of the same species. Jenkinson and Idell and their co-workers (34,75) studied 140-day–premature baboons treated with positive-pressure ventilation and FIO_2 of 1.0 for periods from 6 to 10 days. The severity of lung injury, as measured by edema, inflammation, and changes in gas exchange, was much less severe in the premature animals than in comparably treated adult baboons. Antioxidant enzymes were increased by 6 days in hyperoxic premature baboons, compared with normoxic controls, and the relative resistance to hyperoxia in the immature animals was accompanied by considerably less inflammation (75). Idell and colleagues (34) demonstrated that fibrinolysis was enhanced in the bronchoalveolar lavage (BAL) samples from immature baboons treated with an FIO_2 of 1.0, whereas fibrinolysis was decreased in adult baboons treated comparably for the same time period (76).

Because it is likely that free radical injury plays a role in the final pathway of a number of injury mechanisms, models of oxygen injury can be used to study the efficacy and safety of therapies designed to modify or prevent such injury. Again, developmental issues play a critical role in determining the relevance of the model to the human premature infant. In some cases, biochemical pathways involved in injury of mature subjects may not be relevant or may play only a minimal role in immature subjects. For example, although iron-dependent lipid peroxidation plays a role in pulmonary oxygen injury in adult animals, neither Hansen et al. (77) nor deLemos et al. (78) could demonstrate its role in immature lambs or baboons, respectively. Drugs that are safe in adult subjects frequently have unforeseen toxicities in preterm or term newborns (79). A recent report showed that the iron-chelating agent deferoxamine, which has been used in the treatment of iron poisoning and hemosiderosis in children and adults, resulted in lethal cardiovascular complications in the premature baboon (78). As with models designed to study pathogenesis, drug toxicity studies must be conducted in a developmentally relevant animal model (80).

Although there is clearly value to the use of these models in understanding some developmental differences, most human disease occurs in infants who are physiologically more immature than the preterm rabbit or rat pup used by most investigators. As it is likely that the limitations of upregulation of gene expression associated with prematurity are developmentally related, selection of the developmental window is critical in selecting a model from which to extrapolate data to the human condition. Premature nonhuman primates serve as an ideal species for studying oxygen injury and its relevance to BPD because the investigator can control the developmental, adaptive, and injury variables and because the high degree of homology with humans allows use of most human reagents. However, these are expensive and scarce resources and, therefore, are not suitable for studies that need large numbers of animals.

C. Animal Models of Barotrauma

As ventilator-induced injury is thought to play a role in the pathogenesis of BPD, studies designed to examine its underlying mechanisms, even when performed in mature animals, should provide relevant information. However, the same issues discussed earlier prevail; namely, that the developmental status and species may affect the response to injury.

There are extensive data describing increased alveolar–capillary permeability, decreased compliance, decreased functional residual capacity, and increased intrapulmonary shunts in adult and newborn animals treated with conventional mechanical ventilation at high peak airway pressures (81,82). This effect can be modified, but not eliminated, by the use of continual distending pressure (83). Dreyfuss, in an adult rat model, showed that even short-term overdistension of the lung resulted in immediate and sustained changes in epithelial and endothelial permeability (84). The same group of investigators, in an elegant series of experiments, demonstrated that peak lung volume, rather than pressure, was the major determining factor (85).

Young animals manifest greater changes in alveolar–capillary permeability than do adults under similar experimental conditions (40,41,86). Because nonuniform distribution of intrapulmonary gas and an increased dead space/tidal volume ratio are characteristic of the ventilated immature lung, it is likely that focal acinar overdistension occurs in spontaneously breathing or mechanically ventilated preterm infants, and that the resulting excessive tissue stretch contributes to development of the exudative phase of BPD. In spite of major technical problems, some investigators have used preterm animals to determine the role of excessive pressure or volume in a developmentally relevant setting. Nilsson et al. (87) reported the development of epithelial necrosis shortly after the onset of tidal ventilation in surfactant-deficient premature rabbits. Meredith et al. (88) reported that the immediate institution of high-frequency oscillatory ventilation (HFOV) at a high mean airway pressure in the premature baboon prevented development of the pathological and physiological changes of HMD. They also noted an association between the presence of one inflammatory mediator, platelet-activating factor, and the development of lung injury. Several reports of the use of HFOV in adult experimental models also have demonstrated decreases in various mediators and cytokines when compared with conventional ventilation (89,90). Jackson et al. (91) demonstrated that the use of surfactant and HFOV together in the premature monkey was superior to either treatment alone. Davis et al. (92) used a neonatal piglet model and attempted to dissect the differential effects of oxygen and positive-pressure inflation, and concluded that hyperoxia caused more significant physiological, inflammatory, and histological changes than positive-pressure inflation alone. Although these studies and others suggest that the findings of Dreyfuss and others, who studied mature animals, have relevance to the pathogenesis of lung injury in immature subjects, the complex cardiopulmonary physiology of the premature animal makes it difficult to sort out any single factor in pathogenesis. What is left, therefore, is to try to define the underlying physiological and biochemical mechanisms of pressure-induced and stretch-induced injury in mature animal models, and then attempt to define them in the more complex setting of a developmentally relevant model.

D. Combination of Immaturity, Hyperoxia, and Barotrauma

Excellent homologues of HMD have been produced by premature delivery of surfactant-deficient rabbits, lambs, and nonhuman primates. With short-term ventilatory support, these animals manifest clinical, biochemical, physiological, and morphological features similar to HMD in human premature infants (reviewed in 93–96). The ability to maintain these animals for longer periods requires an intensive care environment, continuous nursing care, and the ability to deal with the diverse problems of prematurity. The size of the animal also influences the nature of the studies that can be performed. The value of these homologues lies in their similarities to the human condition. This is offset in part by many of the same problems that occur secondary to other manifestations of immaturity (e.g., cardiovascular instability, nosocomial infection, and such).

A well-characterized homologue of BPD is the premature baboon (27,97,98). When delivered at 140 days (term = 185 days gestation), premature baboons had HMD indistinguishable clinically, biochemically, and morphologically from that in humans, including the presence of a patent ductus arteriosus (PDA). If supported with positive-pressure ventilation (PPV) and intensive care techniques similar to those used in human premature infants, spontaneous pulmonary recovery begins at about 42 hr after birth and is associated with precocious maturation of multiple organ systems (95).

When treated with PPV and clinically appropriate oxygen (PRN), about 30% of the 140-day–delivered baboons die of airleak-associated complications, but the remainder recover without demonstrable clinical or morphological sequelae (96). The administration of surfactant or the use of high-frequency oscillatory ventilation, as in humans, reduces the incidence of airleak and improves survival (96). When treated with PPV and prolonged hyperoxia, this HMD homologue acquires clinical, radiographic, and morphological features consistent with severe lethal BPD of the classic type, in which death occurred within 2 weeks (27,98). The clinical course of these animals follows a biphasic pattern, with the animals initially manifesting severe HMD, followed by a blunted recovery, compared with PRN controls, and subsequent clinical deterioration after 6–8 days (95). The radiographic features of the second phase are consistent with the exudative phase of BPD as described by Northway (11).

A model of less severe BPD was created by treating 140-day–premature baboons with PPV and F_{IO_2} 1.0 for 7 days, followed by 14 days at 0.8 (33). Although, at 21 days, there were significant morphometric, physiological, and radiographic differences between the animals with the mild–moderate BPD lesion and PRN controls (33), most of these findings disappeared as the survivors matured. However, morphometric analysis of long-term survivors showed a significant decrease of alveolar number, suggesting that the early injuries had a long-term adverse effect on postnatal lung development (99).

Even though this is clearly an induced, rather than a natural, model of BPD because the levels of oxygen needed to produce the disease endpoint are in excess of those needed to maintain oxygenation, it has the distinct advantage of being developmentally relevant and having the ability to independently control the various injury variables in a way not possible in natural disease models. Various studies have examined the role of ventilator-induced injury, hyperoxia, and the PDA on the defined BPD endpoint in this model. One weakness of an animal model, which includes that delivery be cesarean section, is the lack of a predelivery stimulus to induce lung inflammation comparable with the usual scenario of preterm labor, sometimes with ruptured membranes or signs of infection, that often proceeds premature birth in humans. Data from various investigators suggest that maternal chorioamnionitis leads to an active inflammatory response that directly or indirectly triggers a response in the fetus (6–8).

Because of the high degree of homology between baboons and man, most probes directed against human protein, DNA, or RNA, will cross-react. This, coupled with the fact that the developing fetus is naive from point of view of environmentally stimulated gene expression, makes this an ideal model with which to sort the relative roles of development and injury in the pathogenesis of BPD. Construction of libraries and differential cloning, as well as other sophisticated molecular techniques, allow comparison of developmental and injury variables in a way not possible in newborn or adult animals of other species.

E. Combination of Immaturity, Normoxia, and Baro- or Volutrauma

The prolonged ventilated preterm lamb model, recently developed and described by a group of Utah researchers, should help further our understanding of certain aspects of the pathogenesis of BPD, especially those related to the pulmonary circulation (100), interstitial connective tissue elements (101,102), and lung fluid balance (see Chaps. 27 and 29). The normal lung maturation of fetal lambs results in a fully alveolarized lung, with a predominantly single capillary system at term, which differs from the human and baboon in which postnatal alveolization continues. Advantages of studying preterm lambs are that they are larger (2–3 kg), often with twins or triplets, thereby increasing tissue availability; and with permanently implanted vascular catheters, variables related to pulmonary hemodynamics and lung fluid balance can be monitored over time.

In this lung injury model, preterm lambs at 120 days gestational age (80% of 150-day–full-term gestation) are used. At this gestation in sheep, the stage of lung development is between saccular and alveolar. Lambs had their lungs instilled with calf lung surfactant immediately before birth, were stabilized, and then received mechanical ventilation for 3–4 weeks at a respirator rate of either 20 breaths per minute (tidal volume, 15 mL/kg) or 60 breaths per minute (tidal volume, 5 mL/kg). $Paco_2$ was maintained at 35–45 mmHg, with sufficient O_2 to keep Pao_2 at 60–90 mmHg (generally Fio_2 of 0.4–0.6). Their mean birth weight was 2.5 kg. Under anesthesia, the newborns underwent two thoracotomies in the first week for (1) surgical ligation of the ductus arteriosus, (2) placement of catheters in the pulmonary artery, left atrium, and main lung lymphatic, (3) placement of a thermistor wire in the pulmonary artery, and (4) placement of a silicone rubber balloon in the pleural space. After 4 weeks they were the same postconceptional age as a full-term lamb and their measurements were compared with those of five normal full-term lambs that received mechanical ventilation at 30 breaths per minute for 1 hr. Chronic lung injury with edema, decreased radial alveolar counts, and increased elastin deposition developed, irrespective of the ventilatory pattern (100). High pulmonary vascular resistance persisted throughout the 3- to 4-week studies. Mechanical ventilation of preterm animals at 20 breaths per minute and high tidal volumes resulted in higher peak and mean airway pressures, end-expiratory lung volumes, and lung lymph flow after 3–4 weeks than did the strategy of 60 breaths per minute and lower tidal volumes. Chest radiographs and lung histology demonstrated nonuniform inflation in the chronically ventilated preterm lambs compared with normal full-term controls (102). There was less atelectasis, but more overinflation in the preterm animals ventilated with the 20 breaths per minute strategy than in those given 60 breaths per minute at smaller tidal volumes. In addition to the decreased radial alveolar counts and reduced numbers of secondary crests, there were increased tropoelastin mRNA expression and increased elastin in the extended alveolar walls in animals ventilated at low frequency and high tidal volume.

F. Combination of Immaturity, Normoxia, and Low Tidal Volume Ventilation

As noted in Section II, the widespread availability and use of exogenous surfactant therapy has reduced the severity of RDS in many immature neonates, has led to increased survival rates in newborns who are born prematurely at less than 28 weeks gestation (during the canalicular stage of lung development; 103,104), and has increased the incidence of BPD (20). Recent autopsy series that include extremely premature human infants with BPD suggest that a ''new'' form of chronic lung disease is emerging, with histopathology that is dominated by arrested development of terminal respiratory units (32,105,106). The bronchial and bronchiolar components are less conspicuous than those described by Northway in the classic four stages of BPD (11), and there is more prominent, diffuse, uniform intersaccular fibroplasia, accompanied by significantly reduced radial alveolar counts (32,106).

When premature baboons that were delivered at 140 days gestational age (76% of 185-day–full-term gestation) were treated with clinically appropriate levels of oxygen and without postnatal surfactant administration, the 70% that survived their RDS had only minimal radiographic, morphological, and clinical sequelae after 10–21 days (27,33,75,98,99). Therefore, a new model of chronic lung injury was developed in baboons of borderline viability at 125 days gestational age (67% full-term) during the canalicular stage of lung development (107). In contrast to the 140-day–gestational age baboons, those delivered at 125 days gestational age required early exogenous surfactant instillation for survival (4/4 died of severe respiratory failure when surfactant was withheld for more than 4 hr). Therefore, these animals received surfactant (4 mL/kg of Survanta) at birth and again 6 hr later. They subsequently acquired clinical and radiographic features consistent with BPD, despite receiving only 25–40% O_2 during 14 days of mechanical ventilation (107). Most of these baboons had fused eyelids at birth, indicating that they were extremely premature. At birth, males weighed about 400 g and females about 350 g, and these animals had very immature skin, renal function, and capillary leak, with large fluid needs and massive edema during the first few days of life. Shunting across the PDA was variable, and closure of the PDA often was transient when it occurred. Chest radiographs typically progressed from diffuse granularity with air bronchograms (days 1–4) to diffuse haziness typical of injured, edematous lungs, and patchy infiltrates, presumably from segmental atelectasis or pneumonia. This radiographic progression was similar to the evolution of BPD in human infants.

In contrast to intrauterine development from 125 to 140 days gestational age, the 14-day–ventilated survivors showed no significant progression of secondary crest formation and alveolization. Enlarged simplified terminal airspaces and a lack of extensive airway epithelial hyperplasia and metaplasia were the remarkable histological features. The epithelial cells of baboons ventilated for 2 weeks had a wide spectrum of morphological configurations, ranging from undifferentiated cells, with no lamellar bodies and abundant glycogen, to type II cells with many and often atypical-appearing lamellar bodies. Thinning of the interstitium was less evident after 2 weeks of ventilation than it was after 2 weeks in utero and capillaries were situated variably, some central in the wall, others next to the epithelial basement membrane.

Recoveries of saturated phosphatidylcholine were surprisingly low from postmortem lung lavages of animals that were ventilated for 14 days. Despite instillation of surfactant containing about 120 μmol of Sat PC per kilogram body weight on the first day of life, only 3–7 μmol Sat PC per kilogram were recovered by lung lavage 2 weeks later. This compares with Sat PC pool sizes of 50–100 μmol/kg in untreated, spontaneously breathing full-term baboons, which is similar to values reported for full-term lambs (108) and rhesus monkeys (109). Whether the surfactant deficiency seen in these extremely premature animals is due to decreased recycling, increased clearance, decreased synthesis, or sequestration in unusable tissue compartments is under investigation. Treatment of this prolonged surfactant deficiency with exogenous surfactant may be complicated by the detrimental effects of instilling relatively large volumes into the very limited functional airspace of abnormal terminal respiratory units, although some human infants with chronic lung injury have benefited from late treatments (110).

The 14-day baboon model described earlier has been adapted to more closely approximate the disease seen in the extremely immature human infant with neonatal chronic lung disease (CLD; 111–113). Pregnant dams were treated with prenatal glucocorticoids, following which borderline viable fetuses were delivered at 125 days gestation. The infants received exogenous surfactant at birth, were maintained on appropriate oxygen and ventilatory support, and survived 1–2 months. The ventilatory strategy used small tidal volumes (4–6 mL/

kg) to maintain Pa_{CO_2} between 45 and 60 torr. Oxygenation strategy optimized lung volume with PEEP until the F_{IO_2} was decreased to 0.40, or lower. Parenteral nutrition with amino acids, electrolytes, multivitamins, and trace elements was initiated 24 hr after birth. A 20% lipid emulsion was initiated on day 7, and enteral nutrition with human breast milk also began on day 7. Chest radiographs showed resolution of early HMD, followed by progressive changes consistent with neonatal CLD over the first month.

All of the 125-day CLD animals showed a marked decrease in alveolization, whether they survived for 1 or 2 months (111). Only occasional secondary crests were identified, and mean linear intercepts and total internal surface area determinations showed that the CLD specimens had significantly decreased alveolization and decreased internal surface area measurements when compared with gestational and air-breathing controls. The saccular walls showed variable degrees of mild-to-moderate fibrosis (Fig. 1 and 2). Another developmental process that was interrupted in this CLD model was vasculogenesis. When compared with appropriate gestation age and air-breathing controls, the CLD specimens showed a dysmorphic pattern of vascular organization (112). Point-counting

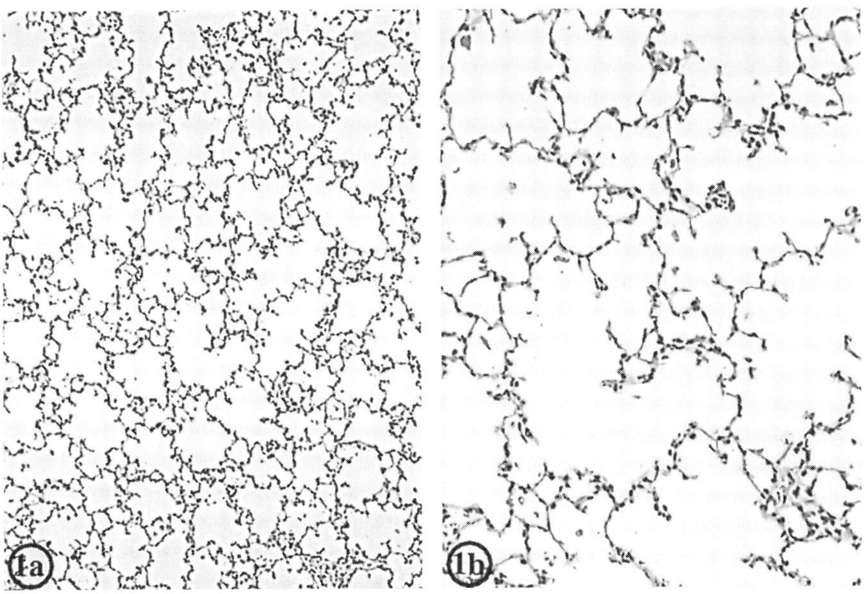

Figure 1 (a) The lung from a term + 2-month air-breathing control shows very thin saccular and alveolar walls, and abundant alveoli are evident. (b) The alveolar structures are better visualized (hematoxylin and eosin; original magnifications, 4 and 10×).

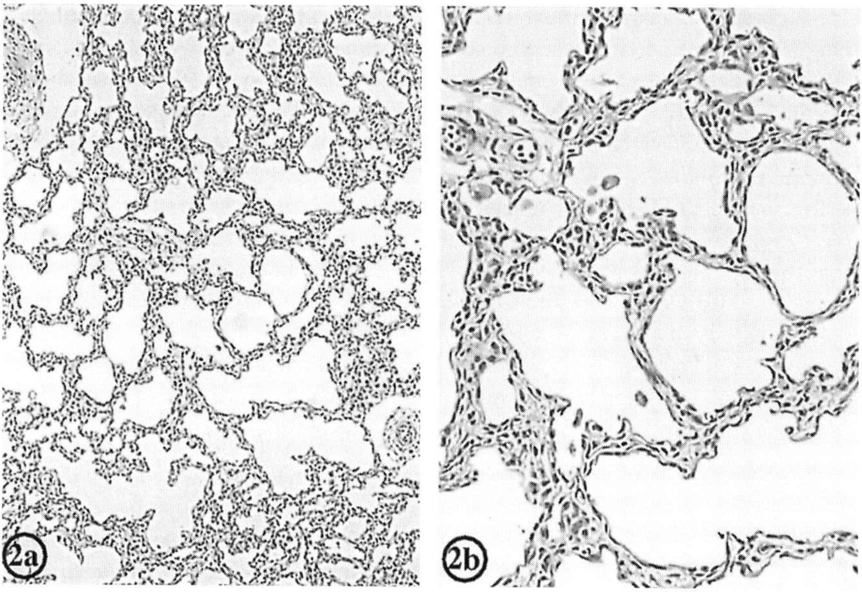

Figure 2 At the same magnifications shown in Figure 1 (a,b), a lung specimen from a CLD baboon that survived for 39 days is depicted. Enlarged air spaces, thickened saccular/alveolar walls, a few secondary crests, and no alveolar structures are the findings. Increased interstitial cells and connective tissue elements are evident in the thickened walls (hematoxylin and eosin; original magnifications, 4 and 10×).

quantitative data showed significantly decreased CD31 endothelial staining in the 125-day–gestation control and the CLD specimens when compared with term and term plus 2 month air-breathing controls. These data suggest that in spite of appropriate oxygenation (median F_{IO_2} at 28 days = 0.32, range = 0.21–0.50) and low tidal volume ventilation strategy, alveolar and capillary hypoplasia result in the extremely immature lung following premature delivery.

Studies with this model have suggested that an inflammatory autoinjury occurs early, and then persists over time, during development of CLD (113). Proinflammatory cytokines tumor necrosis factor (TNF)-α, IL-1β, IL-6, and IL-8, and the anti-inflammatory cytokine IL-10 were analyzed in tracheal aspirate specimens obtained sequentially from CLD baboons (113). The values were compared with values obtained from lung lavages of other normoxic baboons. The early appearance, marked elevation, and persistence of IL-6 and IL-8, plus the presence of other mediators, are probably indicative an ongoing inflammatory autoinjury and repair response in the neonatal lung.

Similar to previous studies in 140-day–gestational-age baboon homologues of BPD, experiments with the more immature baboons delivered at 125 days gestational age continue to have several major advantages over clinical studies in humans and other animal models: (1) gestations are timed with serial fetal ultrasound, facilitating delivery of normal fetuses at a single gestational age following normal intrauterine growth; (2) studies of pathophysiology are not complicated by numerous underlying causes of prematurity; (3) maturity of nonpulmonary organ systems are more homologous, compared with premature lambs and rabbits that have relatively delayed lung maturation and are typically studied at 80–90% of term gestation; (4) overall homology to humans and cross-reactivity to human probes facilitates evaluation of immunocytochemistry and in situ hybridization studies; and (5) histopathological findings are not skewed toward the most severe cases, nor is postmortem pathology influenced by prolonged periods of hypoxia and acidosis preceding death, as human autopsy data often are.

By overcoming the limitations of tissue availability in human trials and by allowing nontherapeutic interventions, animal models should help increase our knowledge of the molecular, biochemical, and cellular events that disrupt the normal program of growth and differentiation in the lungs following premature adaptation to the extrauterine environment. Their greatest strength is in providing the critical descriptive data to direct the more mechanistic studies in subsequent in vitro analyses and transgenic mouse studies.

IV. Potential Uses of Transgenic Models for Future Studies

The normal program of differentiation observed in utero is altered when a fetus is prematurely removed from the intrauterine environment. Air-breathing, surfactant instillation, positive–pressure-assisted ventilation, and varying degrees of subsequent injury, all may contribute to disease development. It is possible that recombinant DNA technology will provide important new insights into the pathophysiology of the dysregulated growth and development following these events. DNA constructs are now routinely integrated into "transgenic" offspring of mice that can be bred and used for studying the roles of both normal and mutated genes (114,115).

Overexpression of specific genes can be studied by injecting the DNA construct into the male pronucleus of a recently fertilized mouse oocyte. This "transgene" is then randomly integrated into the host genome, with inclusion of one to as many as 1000 copies at the site of integration. Altered oocytes are then injected into a surrogate mother, yielding offspring that are subsequently bred to homozygosity. With this technique, White et al. (116) showed improved resistance to hyperoxic damage following increased nonspecific transgene expression of copper–zinc superoxide dismutase (CuZn-SOD) in pulmonary and nonpulmonary tissues. Lung-specific promoters, such as the 5′-flanking sequence from surfactant protein C (SP-C), can be included in the transgene to direct the expression of the chimeric genes to specific lung cell types (117). Wispe et al. (118) showed increased protection from 95% O_2 following increased SP-C promoter-linked transgene expression of manganese superoxide dismutase (Mn-SOD) in respiratory epithelium.

Overexpression of various proteases, cytokines, and key synthetic enzymes of lipid mediators in transgenic mice may lead to sequelae that help explain the pathogenesis of histological abnormalities that develop in BPD. When transgenic mice were bred with increased expression of a human collagenase under the direction of a haptoglobin promoter, the affected offspring had histopathological changes that mimicked human emphysema, with disrupted alveolar walls and coalescence of alveolar spaces, but no evidence of fibrosis or inflammation (119). When transgenic mice were generated with overexpression of human transforming growth factor-α (TGF-α) in lung epithelial cells, increased collagen, and abnormal elastin were deposited in the interstitium and on the pleural surface (120). These SP-C promoter-linked TGF-α mice had fibrotic lesions of variable severity in their lungs that were dependent on the founder line and the magnitude of transgene expression, with increased epidermal growth factor (EGF) receptors also noted in the interstitial cells of the fibrotic lesions (121). In subsequent studies, fibrosis did not develop after TGF-α overexpression when bitransgenic mice were bred that overexpressed a mutant EGF receptor under the control of the SP-C promoter (122).

Immunoreactive EGF is also increased in the conducting airway epithelium of infants who have died with BPD in association with severe pulmonary fibrosis (123). Overexpression of porcine TGF-β_1, which does not bind to EGF receptors in lung epithelium, did not cause fibrosis, but led to arrested lung sacculation and epithelial cell differentiation despite normal lung and body weights (124). Recently, SP-C promoter-linked tumor necrosis factor-α (TNF-α) transgenic mice acquired lymphocytic and fibrosing alveolitis (125). In separate studies (126–128), IL-4 and IL-6 overexpression, directed by Clara cell CC10 promoters to airway epithelium, were accompanied by airway inflammation. However, no change in airway hyperreactivity to methacholine in the transgenic mice overexpressing IL-4 was seen, whereas decreased hyperreactivity to methacholine in the strain overexpressing IL-6 was noted. In addition, transgenic mice that overexpressed IL-4 in their B lymphocytes (128) had delayed viral clearance after infection with respiratory syncytial virus (RSV), a common pathogen in babies with BPD.

Once active genes and their products are identified by in situ hybridization and immunocytochemistry in clinically relevant human and modeled animal specimens, transcriptional regulation can be studied by linking promoters for these genes, to biologically inactive marker genes. Currently, the prokaryotic genes chloramphenicol acetyltransferase (*CAT*) and β-galactosidase (*lac Z*), and eukaryotic genes firefly luciferase and growth hormone have been the most widely employed because of their lack of toxicity in mammalian cells, their ease of detectability, and the specificity of their detection methods. By evaluating marker expression in lungs of mice containing transgenes with varying lengths of 5′-flanking sequences, the *cis*-acting elements controlling lung-specific and cell-specific transcription can be identified. In vitro transfections of lung explants or pulmonary and nonpulmonary cell lines can be used concurrently to identify regions of the 5′-flanking sequence that are critical for binding both ubiquitous and cell-selective *trans*-acting factors. Finally, the critical length of 5′-flanking sequence can be linked to a marker gene and used to generate transgenic mice that can be examined at various stages of fetal development to determine the normal program of differentiation for the gene being studied. Investigators already have used transgenic mouse models to make many of these determinations for surfactant protein C (129,130), Clara cell secretory protein (131), and α_1-collagen (132).

Once active genes and their products are identified in human and modeled animal specimens with BPD, their relevance can also be examined by altering or subtracting those genes through the use of embryonic stem (ES) cells (i.e., gene targeting or ''knockout'') or by generating mice with lung cell-specific, but randomly-integrated, ''dominant–negative'' receptor transgenes. Gene targeting in a locus-specific manner can be accomplished by linking a DNA construct with the desired deletion of the coding region or mutation to a piece of heterologous DNA that confers resistance to neomycin or another antibiotic. In addition, the construct also must contain DNA homologous to the targeted region to allow homologous recombination between large segments of the incoming transgene and cognate chromosomal DNA. The DNA construct is introduced into ES cells (pluripotent cell lines derived from mouse blastocysts) by electrophoration and then grown in media containing neomycin to select for cells that have integrated the targeting construct. Once clonally isolated, the correctly targeted ES cells are microinjected into blastocysts and transplanted into a pseudopregnant surrogate mother. The progeny mice are variably chimeric because the host blastocyst cells are also pluripotent, but can be sorted by coat color if one uses ES cells that carry a dominant coat-color gene that is absent from the host blastocyst. The site-specific mutation is passed through the germline to offspring, which can eventually be bred to homozygosity. This technique has already been used to produce murine models of cystic fibrosis (133–135), and targeted disruption of surfactant protein B causing respiratory failure in newborn mice (136).

Targeted disruption of granulocyte–macrophage colony-stimulating factor (GM-CSF) caused alveolar proteinosis in the affected progeny (137), with decreased catabolism and clearance of surfactant components, resulting in tenfold increases in alveolar and lung tissue pools of saturated phosphatidylcholine (138).

Surfactant proteins A and B were also increased severalfold in this knockout model, despite normal levels of mRNA for these proteins. These observations support the unexpected, but critical, role for GM-CSF in the normal catabolic pathways of surfactant components. Overexpression of GM-CSF in only respiratory epithelium of mice deficient in GM-CSF resulted in increased type II epithelial cell numbers, increased lung size, and normalization of alveolar saturated phosphatidylcholine pools. The increased incorporation of choline and palmitate was counterbalanced by decreased accumulation and increased reuptake of dipalmitoylphosphatidylcholine and SP-B, and demonstrated another unanticipated role for GM-CSF in the regulation of type 2 cell proliferation and differentiation (139,140).

Targeted disruption of surfactant proteins A and B in mice also has increased our knowledge of their roles in normal lung function, and SP-C–promoter-driven overexpression of various fragments has further elucidated the mechanisms involved. Targeted disruption of SP-B resulted in death from respiratory failure in homozygous newborn mice (136), whereas heterozygous mice survived, but had some air trapping and decreased lung compliance (141). When SP-B knockout mice were rescued with an SP-C–promoter-driven construct, encoding a truncated SP-B proprotein, they had a twofold increase in SP-B levels compared with wild-type littermates, and survived with normal lung function (142). However, saturated phosphatidylcholine pools and lamellar body size in the intracellular compartments of their lungs were increased, and the SP-C proprotein was processed abnormally, suggesting that the missing COOH-terminal propeptide of SP-B is not required for normal structure and function of extracellular surfactant, but may be an important determinant of intracellular surfactant pools.

Targeted disruption of SP-A was not lethal and had little effect on lung function and surfactant metabolism in full-term newborn mice (143,144). However, tubular myelin figures were abnormal and decreased in affected animals; at low concentrations of saturated phosphatidylcholine, in vitro surface tension lowering was also decreased. Therefore, the role of SP-A might become more significant in combination with surfactant deficiency or surfactant inhibition following preterm delivery or with lung injury. In another knockout model, bleomycin-induced fibrosis was lessened with targeted disruption of plasminogen activator inhibitor-1 and increased with its overexpression (145).

As an alternative approach to the ES cell-derived knockout, standard oocyte injections can be used to generate "dominant–negative" receptors into the lungs of transgenic mice by linking a lung cell-specific construct (such as the SP-C promoter) with a "dominant" defective receptor for the gene product of interest. Such a dominant–negative was generated by mutating a fibroblast growth factor (FGF) receptor, so that it dimerized with the normal wild-type FGF receptors in the plasma membrane, but failed to autophosphorylate its wild-type dimeric partner, thereby blocking the mitogenic effects of acidic fibroblast growth factor and keratinocyte growth factor, which usually bind to that particular FGF receptor (146). The resulting mice that expressed the transgene died at birth and had no lung components distal to the bronchi. Subsequently, transgenic mice that overexpressed keratinocyte growth factor had a pulmonary malformation resembling cystadenoma, with no normal distal lung epithelium (147). A dominant–negative strategy also was used in transgenic mice that overexpressed an SP-C–promoter-driven calmodulin inhibitor peptide that showed the critical role of calmodulin in branching morphogenesis, in that affected mice had underdeveloped lungs (146). Another critical factor in branching morphogenesis of the lung is N-*myc*, with hypoplastic lungs seen following its disruption in knockout mice (149–151). Future analysis of genes that must be present and those that must not be overexpressed for normal growth and differentiation may help elucidate some essential components contributing to arrested alveolar development during evolution of BPD.

Transgenic models are still somewhat limited by variable levels of transgene expression, by differences in human and murine physiology, and by possible effects that the site of integration may have on both the transgenes and the regulation of endogenous gene products at that locus. However, when premature animal models and human specimens lead to further understanding of the specific genes to target, transgenic models will become a much more powerful tool for dissecting the interrelation between molecular regulation and pathophysiology. Meanwhile, both expected and accidental findings in these models will lead us to important new areas of investigation.

V. Summary and Future Needs

The disease of BPD has changed dramatically over the years since its description in 1967. The original infants had severe HMD, received high inspired oxygen concentrations, and were mechanically ventilated with very high positive airway pressures. This severe form of BPD is now less common. Infants usually are not treated with high airway pressures or inspired oxygen concentrations in this era, and a much milder form of BPD, called by some workers neonatal chronic lung disease (CLD), is the common presentation. Despite advances in the prevention of RDS in infants, BPD, or CLD, remains a major complication in premature infants who require prolonged ventilatory support. Improvements in respiratory care and management and the introduction and use of exogenous surfactant has improved survival of very immature infants with BPD.

So what are the factors needed for a good experimental model of CLD/BPD in the 1990s and beyond? Fetal immaturity with borderline viability, use of maternal prenatal glucocorticoids and exogenous surfactant treatments postdelivery, appropriate oxygenation levels, ventilatory strategies to reduce volutrauma, and a prolonged study time to study the progression, especially the autoinflammatory component, of the disease, would be the desired elements. The immaturity factor has to be a requirement in any relevant model. Human infants born at 23–28 weeks of gestation are still in the canalicular stage of lung development, so vasculogenesis, especially the capillary vascular system, has been underway only a few weeks, and secondary crest formation commences only in the latter portion of this phase. However, relevance to the human disease is not the only reason the use of an extremely immature lung model is important in studying the pathogenesis of BPD. The fetal lung has some unique differences when compared with the adult lung. Newborn animals of most species are more resistant to pulmonary oxygen injury than adults, alveolar capillary permeability is more altered in the immature than mature animals, volu- or barotrauma induces unique lung injury features in neonates when compared with adults, and the inflammatory response in immature neonates is qualitatively and quantitatively blunted when compared with the adult. These observations, along with others, point to the need to have both species and developmental similarities between an animal model and the human disease.

Other models that exaggerate or focus on a particular etiologic factor generally believed to be relevant to the development of BPD or CLD (e.g., volutrauma, inflammation, or other) can dissect some of the cellular and molecular processes in lung injury. Ultimately though, it will be the elucidation of how several judiciously administered, but still injurious, insults of appropriate oxygenation and volume-sparing ventilatory strategies injure an extremely immature lung, that will determine the relevance of an appropriate model.

References

1. Langston C, Kida K, Reed M, Thurlbeck WM. Human lung growth in late gestation and in the neonate. Am Rev Respir Dis 1984; 129:607–613.
2. Langston C, Thurlbeck WM. Lung growth and development in late gestation and early postnatal life. Perspect Pediatr Pathol 1982; 7:203–235.
3. Roman J. Cell–cell and cell–matrix interactions in development of the lung vasculature. In: McDonald JA, ed. Lung Growth and Development. New York: Marcel Dekker, 1997:355–389.
4. Alenghat E, Esterly JR. Alveolar macrophages in perinatal infants. Pediatrics 1984; 74:221–223.
5. Avery ME, Mead J. Surface properties in relation to atelectasis and hyaline membrane disease. Am J Dis Child 1959; 97:517–523.
6. Gibbs RS, Romero R, Hillier SL, Eschenbach DA, Sweet RL. A review of premature birth and subclinical infection. Am J Obstet Gynecol 1992; 166:1515–1528.
7. Hillier SL, Witkin SS, Krohn MA, Watts DH, Kiviat NB, Eschenbach DA. The relationship of amniotic fluid cytokines and preterm delivery, amniotic fluid infec-

tion, histologic chorioamnionitis, and chorioamnion infection. Obstet Gynecol 1993; 81:941–948.
8. Watterberg KL, Demers LM, Scott SM, Murphy S. Chorioamnionitis and early lung inflammation in infants in whom bronchopulmonary dysplasia develops. Pediatrics 1996; 97:210–215.
9. Heneghan MA, Sosulski R, Baquero JM. Persistent pulmonary abnormalities in newborns: the changing picture of bronchopulmonary dysplasia. Pediatr Radiol 1986; 16:180–184.
10. Rojas MA, Gonzalez A, Bancalari E, Claure N, et al. Changing trends in the epidemiology and pathogenesis of neonatal chronic lung disease. J Pediatr 1995; 126: 605–610.
11. Northway WH Jr, Rosan RC, Porter DY. Pulmonary disease following respirator therapy of hyaline-membrane disease: bronchopulmonary dysplasia. N Engl J Med 1967; 276:357–368.
12. Edwards DK, Dyer WM, Northway WH Jr. Twelve years experience with BPD. Pediatrics 1977; 59:839–846.
13. Bonikos DS, Bensch KG, Northway WH Jr, Edwards DK. Bronchopulmonary dysplasia: the pulmonary pathologic sequel of necrotizing bronchiolitis and pulmonary fibrosis. Hum Pathol 1976; 7:643–666.
14. Avery ME, Tooley WH, Keller JB, Hurd SS, Bryan MH, Cotton RB, Epstein MF, Fitzhardinge PM, Hansen CB, Hansen TN, Hodson WA, James LS, Kitterman JA, Nielsen HC, Poirier TA, Truog WE, Wung J-T. Is chronic lung disease in low birth weight infants preventable? A survey of eight centers. Pediatrics 1987; 79:26–30.
15. Horbar JD, McAuliffe TL, Adler SM, Albersheim SA, Cassady G, Edwards W, Jones R, Kattwindel J, Kraybill EN, Krishnan V, Raschko P, Wilkinson AR. Variability in 28-day outcomes for very low birth weight infants: an analysis of 11 neonatal intensive care units. Pediatrics 1988; 82:554–559.
16. Horbar JD, Soll RF, Sutherland JM, Kotagal U, Philip AGS, Kessler DL, Little GA, Edwards WH, Vidyasagar D, Raju TNK, Jobe AH, Ikegami M, Mullett MD, Myerberg DZ, McAuliffe TL, Lucey JF. A multicenter randomized, placebo-controlled trial of surfactant therapy for respiratory distress syndrome. N Engl J Med 1989; 320:959–965.
17. Kraybill EN, Runyan DK, Bose CL, Khan JH. Risk factors for chronic lung disease in infants with birth weights of 751 to 1000 grams. J Pediatr 1989; 115:115–120.
18. Hack M, Horbar JD, Malloy MH, Tyson JE, Wright L. Very low birth weight outcome of National Institute of Child Health and Human Development Neonatal Network. Pediatrics 1991; 87:587–597.
19. Palta M, Gabbert D, Weinstein MR, Peters ME. Multivariate assessment of traditional risk factors for chronic lung disease in very low birth weight neonates. J Pediatr 1991; 119:285–292.
20. Parker RA, Lindstrom DP, Cotton RB. Improved survival accounts for most, but not all, of the increase in bronchopulmonary dysplasia. Pediatrics 1992; 90:663–668.
21. Van Marter LJ, Pagano M, Allred EN, Leviton A, Kuban KCK. Rate of bronchopulmonary dysplasia as a function of neonatal intensive care practices. J Pediatr 1992; 120:938–946.
22. Ogawa Y, Fujimura M, Goto A, Kawano T, Kondo T, Nakae N, Nishida A, Ohno

T, Takeuchi Y, Togari H, Maeta H, Oguchi K. Epidemiology of neonatal chronic lung diseases in Japan. Acta Paediatr Jpn 1992; 34:663–667.
23. Pelkonen AS, Hakulinen AL, Turpeinen M. Bronchial lability and responsiveness in school children born very preterm. Am J Respir Crit Care Med 1997; 156:1178–1184.
24. Gerhardt T, Hehre D, Feller R, Reifenberg L, Bancalari E. Serial determination of pulmonary function in infants with chronic lung disease. J Pediatr 1987; 110:448–456.
25. Mallory GB, Chaney H, Mutich RL, Motoyama EK. Longitudinal changes in lung function during the first three years of premature infants with moderate to severe bronchopulmonary dysplasia. Pediatr Pulmonol 1991; 11:8–14.
26. Jacob SV, Lands LC, Coates AL, Davis GM, MacNeish CF, Hornby L, Riley SP, Outerbridge EW. Exercise ability in survivors of severe bronchopulmonary dysplasia. Am J Respir Crit Care Med 1997; 155:1925–1929.
27. Coalson JJ, Kuehl TJ, Prihoda TJ, deLemos RA. Diffuse alveolar damage in the evolution of bronchopulmonary dysplasia in the baboon. Pediatr Res 1988; 24:357–366.
28. Katzenstein A-LA, Bloor CM, Liebow AA. Diffuse alveolar damage—the role of oxygen, shock, and related factors. Am J Pathol 1976; 85:219–228.
29. Katzenstein AA, Askin FB. Diffuse alveolar damage. In: Surgical Pathology of Non-neoplastic Lung Disease. Philadelphia: WB Saunders 1982:9–42.
30. Barkett VM, Coalson JJ, Greenfield LJ. Early effects of hemorrhagic shock on surface tension properties and ultrastructure of canine lungs. Johns Hopkins Med J 1969; 124:87–94.
31. Harrison LJ, Beller BA, Hinshaw LB, Coalson JJ, Greenfield LJ. Effects of endotoxin on capillary permeability, ultrastructure and surfactant. Surg Gynecol Obstet 1969; 269:723–733.
32. Chambers HM, Van Velzen D. Ventilator-related pathology in the extremely immature lung. Pathology 1989; 21:79–83.
33. Coalson JJ, Winter VT, Idell S, Gerstmann DR, King RJ, deLemos RA. Pathophysiologic, morphometric and biochemical studies in the premature baboon with bronchopulmonary dysplasia. Am Rev Respir Dis 1992; 145:872–881.
34. Idell S, Kumar A, Koenig KB, Coalson JJ. Pathways of fibrin turnover in lavage of premature baboons with hyperoxic lung injury. Am J Respir Crit Care Med 1994; 149:767–775.
35. Viscardi RM, Broderick K, Sun C-CJ, Yale-Loehr AJ, Hessamfar A, Taciak V, Burke KC, Doenig KB, Idell S. Disordered pathways of fibrin turnover in lung lavage of premature infants with respiratory distress syndrome. Am Rev Respir Dis 1992; 146:492–499.
36. Ryan SF. Acute alveolar injury: experimental models. In: Gil J, ed. Models of Lung Disease. Microscopy and Structural Methods. New York: Marcel Dekker, 1990: 641–733.
37. Frank L. Developmental aspects of experimental pulmonary oxygen toxicity. Free Radic Biol Med 1991; 11:463–494.
38. Wilson CB. Immunologic basis for increased susceptibility of the neonate to infection. J Pediatr 1986; 108:1–12.

39. Hill HR. Biochemical, structural, and functional abnormalities of polymorphonuclear leukocytes in the neonate. Pediatr Res 1987; 22:375–382.
40. Jobe A, Ikegami M, Jacobs H, Jones S. Permeability of premature lambs to protein and the effect of surfactant on that permeability. J Appl Physiol 1983; 55:169–176.
41. Jobe A, Jacobs H, Ikegami M, Berry D. Lung protein leaks in ventilated lambs: effects of gestational age. J Appl Physiol 1985; 58:1246–1251.
42. deLemos RA, Shermeta DW, Knelson JH, Kotas R, Avery ME. Acceleration of appearance of pulmonary surfactant in the fetal lamb by the administration of corticosteroids. Am Rev Respir Dis 1970; 102:459–461.
43. Schellenberg JC, Liggins GC, Manzai M, Kitterman JA, Lee CC. Synergistic hormonal effects on lung maturation in fetal sheep. J Appl Physiol 1988; 65:94–100.
44. Tabor BL, Ikegami M, Jobe AH, Yamada T, Oetomo SB. Dose response of thyrotropin-releasing hormone on pulmonary maturation in corticosteroid-treated preterm rabbits. Am J Obstet Gynecol 1990; 163:669–676.
45. Tabor BL, Rider ED, Ikegami M, Jobe AH, Lewis JF. Dose effects of antenatal corticosteroids for induction of lung maturation in preterm rabbits. Am J Obstet Gynecol 1991; 164:675–681.
46. Jobe AH, Polk D, Ikegami M, Newnham J, Sly P, Kohen R, Kelly R. Lung responses to ultrasound-guided fetal treatments with corticosteroids in preterm lambs. J Appl Physiol 1993; 75:2009–2105.
47. Polk DH, Ikegami M, Jobe AH, Newnham J, Sly P, Kohen R, Kelly R. Postnatal lung function in preterm lambs: effects of a single exposure to betamethasone and thyroid hormones. Am J Obstet Gynecol 1995; 172:872–881.
48. Hixson JE, Henkel RD, Britten ML, Vernier DR, deLemos RA, Vandeberg JL, Walsh RA. alpha-Myosin heavy chain cDNA structure and gene expression in adult, fetal, and premature baboon myocardium. J Mol Cell Cardiol 1989; 21:1073–1086.
49. Minoo P, Segura L, Coalson JJ, King R, deLemos RA. Alterations in surfactant protein gene expression associated with premature birth and exposure to hyperoxia. Am J Physiol 1991; 261:L386–L392.
50. King RJ, Coalson JJ, deLemos RA, Gerstmann DR, Seidner SR. SP-A deficiency in primate model of BPD. Biochemistry. Am J Respir Crit Care Med 1995; 151:1989–1997.
51. Coalson JJ, King RJ, Yang F, Winter V, Whitsett JA, deLemos RA, Seidner SR. SP-A deficiency in primate model of BPD and infection. In situ mRNA and immunostains. Am J Respir Crit Care Med 1995; 151:854–898.
52. Jones CA, Cayabyab RG, Kwong K, Stotts C, Wong B, Hamdan H, Minoo P, deLemos RA. Undetectable IL-10 and persistent IL-8 expression early in hyaline membrane disease: a possible developmental basis for the predisposition to chronic lung inflammation in preterm newborns. Pediatr Res 1996; 39:966–975.
53. Chheda S, Palkowetz KH, Garofalo R, Rassin DK, Goldman AS. Developmental delay in the production of IL-10 by human neonatal blood monocytes and T cells. Pediatr Res 1995; 37(suppl 2):285A.
54. Hellstrom B, Nergardlt A. The effect of high oxygen concentrations and hypothermia on the lung of the newborn mouse. Acta Paediatr Scand 1965; 54:457–466.
55. Brooksby GA, Dennis RL, Staley RW. Effects of continuous exposure of rats to

100 percent oxygen at 450 mmHg for 64 days. Aerospace Med 1966; 37:243–246.
56. Brooksby GA, Dennis RL, Datnow B, Clark D. Experimental emphysema: histologic changes and alterations in pulmonary circulation. Calif Med 1967; 107:391–395.
57. Ludwin SK, Northway WH Jr, Bensch KG. Oxygen toxicity in the newborn: necrotizing bronchiolitis in mice exposed to 100 percent oxygen. Lab Invest 1974; 31:425–435.
58. Bonikos DS, Bensch KG, Northway WH Jr. Oxygen toxicity in the newborn: the effect of chronic continuous 100 percent oxygen on the lungs of newborn mice. Am J Pathol 1976; 85:623–635.
59. Tierney DF, Ayers L, Kasuyama RS. Altered sensitivity to oxygen toxicity. Am Rev Respir Dis 1977; 115:59–65.
60. Pappas CTE, Obara H, Bensch KG, Northway WH Jr. Effect of prolonged exposure to 80% oxygen on the lung of the newborn mouse. Lab Invest 1983; 48:735–748.
61. Randell SH, Mercer RR, Young SL. Neonatal hyperoxia alters the pulmonary alveolar and capillary structure of 40-day-old rats. Am J Pathol 1990; 136:1259–1266.
62. Deneke SM, Fanburg BL. Normobaric oxygen toxicity of the lung. N Engl J Med 1980; 303:76–86.
63. Bucher FL Jr, Roberts RJ. Oxygen toxicity in neonatal and adult animals of various species. J Appl Physiol 1978; 45:669–704.
64. Frank L. Effects of oxygen on the newborn. Fed Proc 1985; 44:2328–2334.
65. Polgar G, Antagnoli W, Ferigan LW, Martin EA, Gregg WP. The effect of chronic exposure to 100% oxygen in newborn mice. Am J Med Sci 1966; 252:580–587.
66. Barlett D Jr. Postnatal growth of the mammalian lung: influence of low and high oxygen tensions. Respir Physiol 1970; 9:58–64.
67. Bonikos DS, Bensch KG, Ludwin SK, Northway. WH Jr. Oxygen toxicity in the newborn: the effect of prolonged 100 percent O_2 exposure on the lungs of newborn mice. Lab Invest 1975; 32:619–635.
68. Roberts RJ, Weesner K, Bucher JR. Oxygen-induced alterations in lung vascular development in the newborn rat. Pediatr Res 1983; 17:368–375.
69. Shaffer SG, O'Neill D, Bradt SK, Thibeault DW. Chronic vascular pulmonary dysplasia associated with neonatal hyperoxia-exposure in the rat. Pediatr Res 1987; 21:14–20.
70. Loppel R, Han RNN, Cox D, Tanswell AK, Rabinovitch M. α_1-Antitrypsin protects neonatal rats from pulmonary vascular and parenchymal effects of oxygen toxicity. Pediatr Res 1994; 36:763–770.
71. Keeney SE, Mathews MJ, Rassin DK. Antioxidant enzyme responses to hyperoxia in preterm and term rats after prenatal dexamethasone administration. Pediatr Res 1993; 33:177–180.
72. Keeney SE, Mathews MJ, Haque AK, Schmalstieg FC. Comparison of pulmonary neutrophils in the adult and neonatal rat after hyperoxia. Pediatr Res 1995; 38:857–863.
73. Frank L, Lewis PL, Sosenko IRS. Dexamethasone stimulation of fetal rat lung antioxidant enzyme activity in parallel with surfactant stimulation. Pediatrics 1985; 75:569–574.

74. Frank L, Sosenko IRS. Failure of premature rabbits to increase antioxidant enzymes during hyperoxic exposure: increased susceptibility to pulmonary oxygen toxicity compared to term rabbits. Pediatr Res 1991; 29:292–296.
75. Jenkinson SG, Roberts RJ, deLemos RA, Lawrence RA, Coalson JJ, King RJ, Null DM Jr, Gerstmann DR. Allopurinol-induced effects in premature baboons with respiratory distress syndrome. J Appl Physiol 1991; 70:1160–1167.
76. Idell S, Peters J, Gonzalez K, Fair D, Coalson J. Local abnormalities of coagulation and fibrinolytic pathways which promote alveolar fibrin deposition in the lungs of baboons with diffuse alveolar damage. J Clin Invest 1989; 84:181–193.
77. Hansen TN, Smith CV, Gest AL, Smith HW, Giesler M. Biochemical manifestations of oxygen toxicity in the newborn lamb. Pediatr Res 1990; 28:613–617.
78. deLemos RA, Roberts RJ, Coalson JJ, deLemos JA, Null DM Jr, Gerstmann DR. Toxic effects associated with the administration of deferoxamine in the premature baboon with hyaline membrane disease. Am J Dis Child 1990; 144:915–919.
79. Bove KE, Kosmetatos N, Wedig KE, Frank DJ, Whitlatch S, Saldivar V, Haas J, Bodenstein C, Balistreri WF. Vasculopathic hepatotoxicity associated with E-Ferol syndrome in low-birth-weight infants. JAMA 1985; 254:2422–2430.
80. deLemos RA, Kuehl TJ. Animal models for evaluation of drugs for use in the mature and immature newborn. Pediatrics 1987; 79:275–280.
81. Parker JC, Hernandez LA, Peevy KJ. Mechanisms of ventilator-induced lung injury. Crit Care Med 1993; 21:131–143.
82. Dreyfuss D, Saumon G. Ventilator-induced lung injury. Am J Respir Crit Care Med 1998; 157:294–323.
83. Dreyfuss D, Soler P, Basset G, Saumon G. High inflation pressure pulmonary edema. Respective effects of high airway pressure, high tidal volume and positive end expiratory pressure. Am Rev Respir Dis 1988; 137:1159–1164.
84. Dreyfuss D, Soler P, Saumon G. Spontaneous resolution of pulmonary edema caused by short periods of cyclic overinflation. J Appl Physiol 1992; 72:2081–2089.
85. Dreyfuss D, Saumon G. Role of tidal volume, FRC and end-inspiratory volume in the development of pulmonary edema following mechanical ventilation. Am Rev Respir Dis 1993; 148:1194–1203.
86. Carlton DP, Cummings JJ, Scheerer RS Poulain FR, Bland RD. Lung overexpansion increases pulmonary microvascular protein permeability in young lambs. J Appl Physiol 1990; 69:577–583.
87. Nilsson R, Grossmann G, Robertson B. Lung surfactant and the pathogenesis of neonatal bronchiolar lesions induced by artificial ventilation. Pediatr Res 1978; 12: 249–255.
88. Meredith KS, deLemos RA, Coalson JJ, King RJ, Gerstmann DR, Kumar R, Kuehl TJ, Winter DC, Taylor A, Clark RH, Null DM. Role of lung injury in the pathogenesis of hyaline membrane disease in premature baboons. J Appl Physiol 1989; 66: 2150–2158.
89. Imai Y, Kawano T, Miyasaka K, Takata M, Imai T, Okuyama K. Inflammatory chemical mediators during conventional ventilation and during high frequency oscillatory ventilation. Am J Respir Crit Care Med 1994; 150:1550–1554.
90. Takata M, Abe J, Tanaka H, Kitano Y, Doi S, Kohsaka T, Miyasaka K. Intraalveolar

expression of tumor necrosis factor-α gene during conventional and high-frequency ventilation. Am J Respir Crit Care Med 1997; 156:272–279.
91. Jackson JC, Truog W, Standaert TA, Murphy JH, Juul SE, Chi EY, Hildebrandt J, Hodson WA. Reduction in lung injury after combined surfactant and high-frequency ventilation Am J Respir Crit Care Med 1994; 150:534–539.
92. Davis JM, Dickerson B, Metlay L, Penney DP. Differential effects of oxygen and barotrauma on lung injury in the neonatal piglet. Pediatr Pulmonol 1991; 10:157–163.
93. Coalson JJ. Experimental models of acute lung injury. In: Bancalari E, Stocker JT, eds. Bronchopulmonary Dysplasia. Aspen Seminars in Pediatric Disease. Washington: Hemisphere Publishing, 1988:134–147.
94. Kessler DL, Truog WE, Murphy JH, Palmer S, Standaert TA, Woodrum DE, Hudson WA. Experimental hyaline membrane disease in the premature monkey: effects of antenatal dexamethasone. Am Rev Respir Dis 1982; 126:62–69.
95. deLemos RA, Coalson JJ, Gerstmann DR, Kuehl TJ, Null DM. Oxygen toxicity in the premature baboon with hyaline membrane disease. Am Rev Respir Dis 1987; 136:677–681.
96. Gerstmann DR, deLemos RA, Coalson JJ, Clark RH, Wiswell TE, Winter DC, Kuehl TJ, Meredith KS, Null DM. Influence of ventilatory technique on pulmonary baroinjury in baboons with HMD. Pediatr Pulmonol 1988; 5:82–91.
97. Escobedo MB, Hilliard JL, Smith F, Meredith K, Walsh W, Johnson D, Coalson JJ, Kuehl TJ, Null DM Jr, Robotham JL. A baboon model of bronchopulmonary dysplasia. Exp Mol Pathol 1982; 37:323–334.
98. Coalson JJ, Kuehl TJ, Escobedo MB, Hillard JL, Smith F, Meredith K, Null DM Jr, Walsh W, Johnson D, Robotham JL. A baboon model of bronchopulmonary dysplasia. II. Pathologic features. Exp Mol Pathol 1982; 37:335–350.
99. Coalson JJ, Winter V, deLemos RA. Decreased alveolarization in baboon survivors with BPD. Am J Respir Crit Care Med 1995; 152:640–646.
100. Bland RD, Kullama LK, Day RW, Carlton DP, MacRitchie AN, Albertine KH. Nitric oxide inhalation decreases pulmonary vascular resistance in preterm lambs with evolving chronic lung disease. Pediatr Res 1997; 41:247A.
101. Pierce RA, Albertine KH, Starcher BC, Bohnsack JF, Carlton DP, Bland RD. Chronic lung injury in preterm lambs: disordered pulmonary elastin deposition. Am J Physiol 1997; 272:L452–L460.
102. Albertine KH, Jones GP, Starcher BC, Bohnsack JF, Davis PL, Cho S-C. Carlton DP, Bland RD. Chronic lung injury in preterm lambs. Disordered respiratory tract development. Am J Respir Crit Care Med 1999; 159:945–958.
103. Hoekstra RE, Jackson JC, Myers TF, Frantz ID 3d, Stern ME, Powers WF, Maurer M, Raye JR, Carrier ST, Gunkel JH. Improved neonatal survival following multiple doses of bovine surfactant in very premature neonates at risk for respiratory distress syndrome. Pediatrics 1991; 88:10–18.
104. Liechty EA, Donovan E, Purohit D, Gilhooly J, Feldman B, Noguchi A, Denson SE, Sehgal SS, Gross I, Stevens D. Reduction of neonatal mortality after multiple doses of bovine surfactant in low birth weight neonates with respiratory distress syndrome. Pediatrics 1991; 88:19–28.
105. Van Lierde S, Cornelis A, Devlieger H, Moerman P, Lauweryns J, Eggermont E.

Different patterns of pulmonary sequelae after hyaline membrane disease: heterogeneity of bronchopulmonary dysplasia? Biol Neonate 1991; 60:152–162.
106. Margraf LR, Tomashefski JF, Bruce MC, Dahms BB. Morphometric analysis of the lung in bronchopulmonary dysplasia. Am Rev Respir Dis 1991; 143:391–400.
107. Seidner S, McCurnin D, Coalson J, Correll D, Castro R. A new model of chronic lung injury in surfactant-treated preterm baboons delivered at very early gestations. Pediatr Res 1993; 33:344A.
108. Glats T, Ikegami M, Jobe A. Metabolism of exogenously administered natural surfactant in the newborn lamb. Pediatr Res 1982; 16:711–715.
109. Jackson SC, Palmer S, Standaert TA. Developmental changes of surface active material in newborn nonhuman primates. Am Rev Respir Dis 1984; 129:A204.
110. Pandit PB, Dunn MS, Kelly EN, Perlman M. Surfactant replacement in neonates with early chronic lung disease. Pediatrics 1995; 95:851–854.
111. Coalson JJ, Winter V, Yoder B. Decreased alveoli and surface area in premature baboons with long term bronchopulmonary dysplasia (BPD). Am J Respir Crit Care Med 1998; 157:A373.
112. Coalson JJ, Winter V, Yodar B. Dysmorphic vascular development in premature baboons with bronchopulmonary dysplasia. Am J Respir Crit Care Med 1997; 155: A262.
113. Coalson JJ, Winter V, Siler-Khodr T, Yoder B. Cytokine profiles in tracheal aspirates of premature baboons with long term bronchopulmonary dysplasia (BPD). Am J Respir Crit Care Med 1998; 157:A373.
114. Glasser SW, Korfhagen TR, Wert SE, Whitsett JA. Transgenic models for study of pulmonary development and disease. Am J Physiol 1994; 267:L489–L497.
115. Ho YS. Transgenic models for the study of lung biology and disease. Am J Physiol 1994; 266:L319–L353.
116. White CW, Avraham KB, Shanley PF, Groner Y. Transgenic mice with expression of elevated levels of copper–zinc superoxide dismutase in the lungs are resistant to pulmonary oxygen toxicity. J Clin Invest 1991; 87:2162–2168.
117. Glasser SW, Korfhagen TR, Wert SE, Bruno MD, McWilliams KM, Vorbroker DK, Whitsett JA. Genetic element from human surfactant protein SP-C gene confers bronchiolar-alveolar cell specificity in transgenic mice. Am J Physiol 1991; 261:L349–L356.
118. Wispe JR, Warner BB, Clark JC, Dey CR, Neuman J, Glasser SW, Crapo TD, Chang LY, Whitsett JA. Human Mn-superoxide dismutase in pulmonary epithelial cells of transgenic mice confers protection from oxygen injury. J Biol Chem 1992; 267:23937–23941.
119. D'Armiento J, Dalal SS, Okada Y, Berg RA, Chada K. Collagenase expression in the lungs of transgenic mice causes pulmonary emphysema. Cell 1992; 71:955–961.
120. Korfhagen TR, Swantz RJ, Wert SE, McCarty JM, Kerlakian CB, Glasser SW, Whitsett JA. Respiratory epithelial cell expression of human transforming growth factor-alpha induces lung fibrosis in transgenic mice. J Clin Invest 1994; 93:1691–1699.
121. Hardie WD, Bruno MD, Huelsman KM, Iwamoto HS, Carrigan PE, Leikauf GD, Whitsett JA, Korfhagen TR. Postnatal lung function and morphology in transgenic

mice expressing transforming growth factor-alpha. Am J Pathol 1997; 151:1075–1083.

122. Hardie WD, Kerlakian CB, Bruno MD, Huelsman KM, Wert SE, Glasser SW, Whitsett JA, Korfhagen TR. Reversal of lung lesions in transgenic transforming growth factor-alpha mice by expression of mutant epidermal growth factor receptor. Am J Respir Cell Mol Biol 1996; 15:499–508.
123. Stahlman MT, Orth DN, Gray ME. Immunocytochemical localization of epidermal growth factor in the developing human respiratory system and in acute and chronic lung disease in the neonate. Lab Invest 1989; 60:539–547.
124. Zhou L, Dey CR, Wert SE, Whitsett JA. Arrested lung morphogenesis in transgenic mice bearing an SP-C-TGF-beta 1 chimeric gene. Dev Biol 1996; 175:227–238.
125. Miyazaki Y, Araki K, Vesin C, Garcia I, Kapanci Y, Whitsett JA, Piguet PF, Vassalli P. Expression of a tumor necrosis factor-alpha transgene in murine lung causes lymphocytic and fibrosing alveolitis. A mouse model of progressive pulmonary fibrosis. J Clin Invest 1995; 96:250–259.
126. DiCosmo BF, Geba GP, Picarella D, Elias JA, Rankin JA, Stripp BR, Whitsett JA, Flavell RA. Airway epithelial cell expression of interleukin-6 in transgenic mice. Uncoupling of airway inflammation and bronchial hyperreactivity. J Clin Invest 1994; 94:2028–2035.
127. Rankin JA, Picarella DE, Geba GP, Temann UA, Prasad B, DiCosmo B, Tarallo A, Stripp B, Whitsett J, Flavell RA. Phenotypic and physiologic characterization of transgenic mice expressing interleukin 4 in the lung: lymphocytic and eosinophilic inflammation without airway hyperreactivity. Proc Natl Acad Sci USA 1996; 93: 7821–7825.
128. Fischer JE, Johnson JE, Kuli-Zade RK, Johnson TR, Aung S, Parker RA, Graham BS. Overexpression of interleukin-4 delays virus clearance in mice infected with respiratory syncytial virus. J Virol 1997; 71:8672–8677.
129. Korfhagen TR, Glasser SW, Wert SE, Bruno MD, Daugherty CC, McNeish JD, Stock JL, Potter SS, Whitsett JA. *cis*-Acting sequences from a human surfactant protein gene confer pulmonary-specific gene expression in transgenic mice. Proc Natl Acad Sci USA 1990; 87:6122–6126.
130. Wert SE, Glasser SW, Korfhagen TR, Whitsett JA. Transcriptional elements from the human SP-C gene direct expression in the primordial respiratory epithelium of transgenic mice. Dev Biol 1993; 156:426–443.
131. Hackett BP, Gitlin JD. Cell-specific expression of a Clara cell secretory protein–human growth hormone gene in the bronchiolar epithelium of transgenic mice. Proc Natl Acad Sci USA 1992; 89:9079–9083.
132. Slack JL, Liska DJ, Bornstein P. An upstream regulatory region mediates high-level, tissue-specific expression of the human alpha 1(I) collagen gene in transgenic mice. Mol Cell Biol 1991; 11:2066–2074.
133. Clarke LL, Grubb BR, Gabriel SE, Smithies O, Koller BH, Boucher RC. Defective epithelial chloride transport in a gene-targeted mouse model of cystic fibrosis. Science 1992; 257:1125–1128.
134. Dorin JR, Dickinson P, Alton EW, Smith SN, Geddes DM, Stevenson BJ, Kimber WL, Fleming S, Clarke AR, Hooper ML. Cystic fibrosis in the mouse by targeted insertional mutagenesis. Nature 1992; 359:211–215.

135. Snouwaert JN, Brigman KK, Latour AM, Iraj E, Schwab U, Gilmour MI, Koller BH. A murine model of cystic fibrosis. Am J Respir Crit Care Med 1995; 151: S59–S64.
136. Clark JC, Wert SE, Bachurski CJ, Stahlman MT, Stripp BR, Weaver TE, Whitsett JA. Targeted disruption of the surfactant protein B gene disrupts surfactant homeostasis, causing respiratory failure in newborn mice. Proc Natl Acad Sci USA 1995; 92:7794–7798.
137. Huffman JA, Hull WM, Dranoff G, Mulligan RC, Whitsett JA. Pulmonary epithelial cell expression of GM-CSF corrects the alveolar proteinosis in GM-CSF–deficient mice. J Clin Invest 1996; 97:649–655.
138. Ikegami M, Ueda T, Hull W, Whitsett JA, Mulligan RC, Dranoff G, Jobe AH. Surfactant metabolism in transgenic mice after granulocyte macrophage–colony stimulating factor ablation. Am J Physiol 1996; 270:L650–L658.
139. Huffman Reed JA, Rice WR, Zsengeller ZK, Wert SE, Dranoff G, Whitsett JA. GM-CSF enhances lung growth and causes alveolar type II epithelial cell hyperplasia in transgenic mice. Am J Physiol 1997; 273:L715–L725.
140. Ikegami M, Jobe AH, Huffman Reed JA, Whitsett JA. Surfactant metabolic consequences of overexpression of GM-CSF in the epithelium of GM-CSF–deficient mice. Am J Physiol 1997; 273:L709–L714.
141. Clark JC, Weaver TE, Iwamoto HS, Ikegami M, Jobe AH, Hull WM, Whitsett JA. Decreased lung compliance and air trapping in heterozygous SP-B-deficient mice. Am J Respir Cell Mol Biol 1997; 16:46–52.
142. Akinbi HT, Breslin JS, Ikegami M, Iwamoto HS, Clark JC, Whitsett JA, Jobe AH, Weaver TE. Rescue of SP-B knockout mice with a truncated SP-B proprotein. Function of the C-terminal propeptide. J Biol Chem 1997; 272:9640–9647.
143. Korfhagen TR, Bruno MD, Ross GF, Huelsman KM, Ikegami M, Jobe AH, Wert SE, Stripp BR, Morris RE, Glasser SW, Bachurski CJ, Iwamoto HS, Whitsett JA. Altered surfactant function and structure in SP-A gene targeted mice. Proc Natl Acad Sci USA 1996; 93:9594–9599.
144. Ikegami M, Korfhagen TR, Bruno MD, Whitsett JA, Jobe AH. Surfactant metabolism in surfactant protein A-deficient mice. Am J Physiol 1997; 272:L479–L485.
145. Eitzman DT, McCoy RD, Zheng X, Fay WP, Shen T, Ginsburg D, Simon RH. Bleomycin-induced pulmonary fibrosis in transgenic mice that either lack or overexpress the murine plasminogen activator inhibitor-1 gene. J Clin Invest 1996; 97: 232–237.
146. Peters K, Werner S, Liao X, Wert S, Whitsett J, Williams L. Targeted expression of a dominant negative FGF receptor blocks branching morphogenesis and epithelial differentiation of the mouse lung. EMBO J 1994; 13:3296–3301.
147. Simonet WS, DeRose ML, Bucay N, Nguyen HQ, Wert SE, Zhou L, Ulich TR, Thomason A, Danilenko DM, Whitsett JA. Pulmonary malformation in transgenic mice expressing human keratinocyte growth factor in the lung. Proc Natl Acad Sci USA 1995; 92:12461–12465.
148. Wang J, Campos B, Kaetzel MA, Dedman JR. Expression of a calmodulin inhibitor peptide in progenitor alveolar type II cells disrupts lung development. Am J Physiol 1996; 271:L245–L250.
149. Moens CB, Auerbach AB, Conlon RA, Joyner AL, Rossant J. A targeted mutation

reveals a role for N-*myc* in branching morphogenesis in the embryonic mouse lung. Gene Dev 1992; 6:691–704.

150. Sawai S, Shimono A, Wakamatsu Y, Palmes C, Hanaoka K, Kondoh H. Defects of embryonic organogenesis resulting from targeted disruption of the N-*myc* gene in the mouse. Development 1993; 117: 1445–1455.

151. Stanton BR, Perkins AS, Tessarollo L, Sassoon DA, Parada LF. Loss of N-*myc* function results in embryonic lethality and failure of the epithelial component of the embryo to develop. Gene Dev 1992; 6:2235–2247.

AUTHOR INDEX

Italic numbers give the page on which the complete reference is listed.

A

B

C

D

F

G

H

I

J

K

L

M

N

O

P

S

W

X

Y

Z

SUBJECT INDEX

A

C

D

I

K

L

M

N

R

S

T

U

V

W